Surgery of the Liver and Biliary Tract

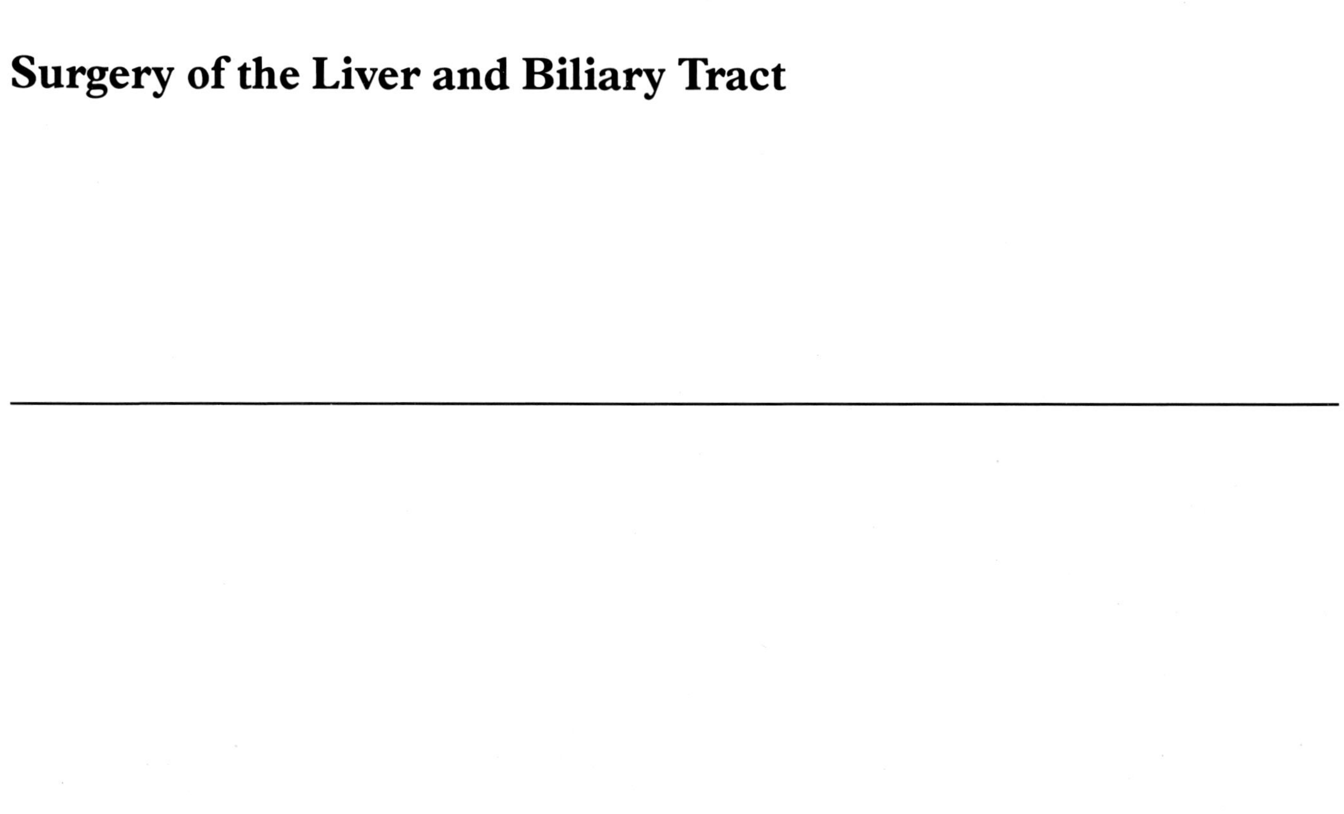

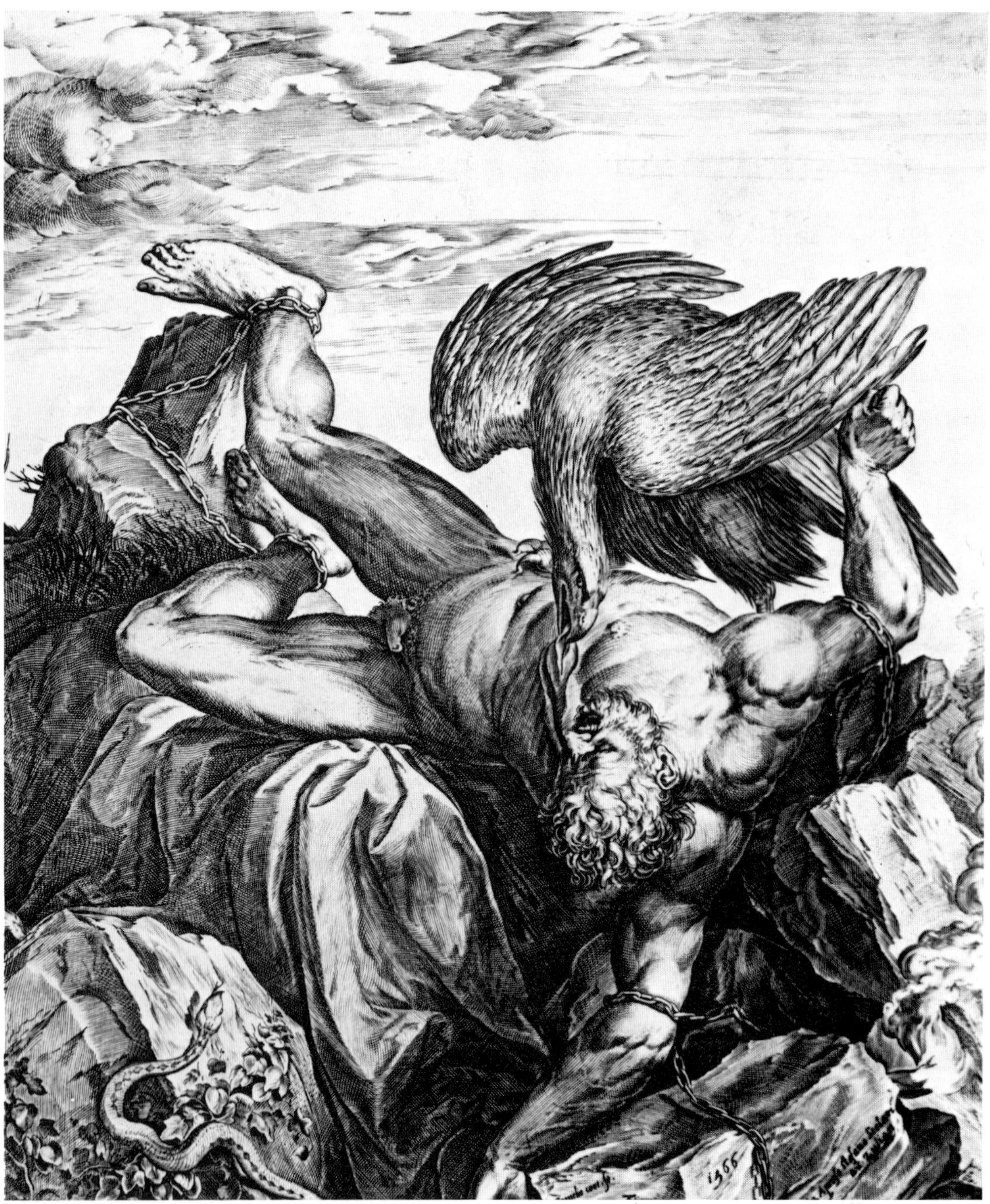

Prometheus, chained to the rocky Mount Caucasus, has his liver eaten by the vulture of Zeus. (Engraving, 1566, possibly after a work by Titian. Reproduced by permission of BBC Hulton Picture Library, London.)

Surgery of the Liver and Biliary Tract

EDITED BY

L. H. Blumgart BDS MD FRCS(Edin) FRCPS(Glas) FRCS(Eng)
Professor of Surgery
University of Bern;
Director, Clinic for Visceral and Transplantation Surgery
Inselspital
Bern
Switzerland

Illustrations by Doig Simmonds

VOLUME 1

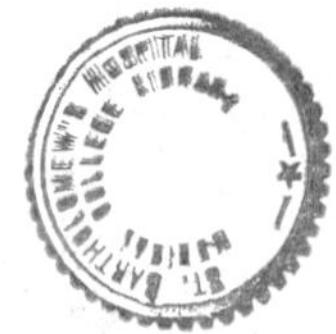

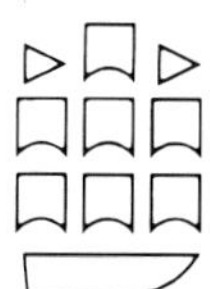

CHURCHILL LIVINGSTONE
EDINBURGH LONDON MELBOURNE AND NEW YORK 1988

CHURCHILL LIVINGSTONE
Medical Division of Longman Group UK Limited

Distributed in the United States of America by Churchill Livingstone Inc., 1560 Broadway, New York, N.Y. 10036, and by associated companies, branches and representatives throughout the world.

First published 1988

ISBN 0 443 031495 (2 volumes)

British Library Cataloguing in Publication Data
Surgery of the liver and biliary tract.
1. Biliary tract—Surgery
I. Blumgart, L.H.
617'.556059 RD546

Library of Congress Cataloging in Publication Data
Surgery of the liver and biliary tract.
Includes indexes.
1. Liver—Surgery. 2. Biliary tract—Surgery.
I. Blumgart, L. H. [DNLM: 1. Biliary Tract—surgery.
2. Liver—surgery. WI 770 S9605]
RD669.S87 1988 617'.556 87-21794
ISBN 0-443-03149-5

Printed and bound in Great Britain by
William Clowes Limited, Beccles and London

Preface

In the editing of this book I have attempted to cover comprehensively the surgical aspects of the management of liver and biliary tract disorders. The contributors were selected on the basis of a record of established and ongoing work in the field and they reflect a cross-section of those involved in the specialty management of liver and biliary tract disease. Thus the important, indeed essential, contributions of radiologists and endoscopists, the collaboration and assistance of hepatologists, of anaesthetists and of the pathologist were welcomed. All were asked to discuss their subject from the point of view of surgical management and to relate their views to the contributions of others. In many instances authors with conflicting opinions were chosen so as to allow the reader an opportunity to assess the views of enthusiasts for different approaches to the same problem. In some instances, for example in coverage of interventional radiological and endoscopic techniques and in drawing together a rational approach for the utilization of diagnostic imaging, balancing chapters were inserted in an attempt to draw together the extraordinary advances which have taken place in recent years. In many instances, for example in the management of injury to the liver and biliary tract, deliberate overlap between chapters has been encouraged, firstly to allow each contribution to be an encapsulated account which would stand on its own for the reader who wishes to consult the book as a reference, and secondly to allow display of different nuances of approach to particularly difficult problems.

There is an initial major section of the book devoted to applied anatomy of the liver and biliary tract, including its radiological demonstration. Throughout the book the anatomical contributions of Claude Couinaud are recognized, the liver anatomy and the nomenclature of various operative approaches being according to his descriptions. Normal function and pathophysiological aspects are covered with particular reference to measurement techniques, infections and to the response not only of the liver and biliary tract, but of the patient to disease. Preoperative and operative diagnostic approaches, including endoscopic techniques and intraoperative ultrasonography, are covered.

The recently introduced interventional endoscopic and radiological approaches to gallstones, biliary strictures and liver and biliary cancer are especially emphasized and are discussed in relation to surgical approaches. There is a full discussion and illustrated description of selected operative approaches to biliary disease with a special emphasis on the management of gallstones, biliary strictures and fistula, and of biliary, periampullary and pancreatic cancer. Liver and biliary infection due to pyogenic organisms, hydatid disease and tropical infestations are detailed. Liver and biliary cysts and their surgical management are fully described as are the management of injuries to the liver and associated biliary ducts, arteries and veins.

Primary and secondary liver tumours and the differences in approach in the Western World and in Asia are described. Surgical treatment and a variety of alternative approaches are covered in detail with a special emphasis on the techniques of liver resection and the newly introduced modality of intraoperative ultrasonically guided surgery in these conditions.

Cirrhosis of the liver and the management of portal hypertension, including operative descriptive techniques for the control of variceal haemorrhage, are illustrated. There is a discussion of metabolic disease affecting the liver from a surgical standpoint and a full discussion of the immunological, anaesthetic and technical aspects of liver transplantation and its results.

In short, I have attempted to include all aspects of the anatomy, pathology, diagnosis and surgically related therapeutic approaches to liver and biliary tract disorders and to provide a text which would be of value not only to the trainee surgeon and the established specialist, but also of interest to specialists in other disciplines concerned with management of diseases of the liver and its associated biliary system. I hope this book proves of value not only as a document of the current state of the art in surgical aspects of liver and biliary disease, but also acts as a stimulus to those interested in further study of the many unresolved problems which await investigation.

Bern, 1988 L.H.B.

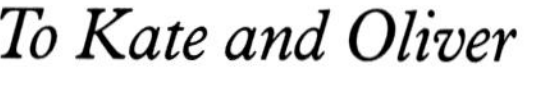

To Kate and Oliver

Acknowledgements

I am deeply grateful to all who have contributed to this publication. My colleagues in surgery, internal medicine, radiology, endoscopy, pathology and anaesthesia all responded enthusiastically and added the weight of their experience. I shall always be grateful to them for adding the spice of differing opinion and the aroma of international practice to the basic flavour of the work. Especial thanks are due to members of my own staff who have individually contributed or assisted me in a considerable number of the chapters and particularly to Mr I. S. Benjamin who undertook much of the proofreading.

In an attempt to render the illustrative work within the book of a uniform character nearly all the drawings were done by Mr Doig Simmonds, Medical Illustrator at the Royal Postgraduate Medical School, Hammersmith Hospital, London. He undertook the formidable task cheerfully and in discussion with the contributors and with me has produced a truly remarkable series of drawings.

Secretarial co-ordination for the book was done by Mrs Brigitte Studley. She typed, or re-typed, many of the manuscripts, organized the editor, jostled the contributors and collaborated with the publishers. I am very grateful to her for a major task so cheerfully undertaken.

Finally, my thanks and deep appreciation to my wife and family who have tolerated my preoccupation with this work during many evenings, over many a weekend and during our holidays.

Contributors

M A Adson MD
Department of Surgery,
Mayo Clinic,
Rochester,
Minnesota, USA

D J Allison BSc MD DMRD FRCR
Professor and Director,
Department of Diagnostic Radiology,
Royal Postgraduate Medical School and Hammersmith Hospital, London, UK

M E M Allison BSc MBChB MD FRCP(Edin) FRCP(Glas)
Senior Lecturer in Medicine and Honorary Consultant Physician,
Glasgow Royal Infirmary,
UK

R P Altman MD
Professor of Surgery,
Division of Pediatric Surgery,
The Babies Hospital,
New York,
USA

I B Angorn FRCS
Formerly, Professor of Surgery,
University of Natal,
Durban,
South Africa

M J P Arthur BM MRCP
Lecturer in Medicine,
Southampton General Hospital,
UK

N L Ascher MD
Director, Liver Transplant Program,
Department of Surgery,
Phillips-Wagensteen Building,
Minneapolis,
Minnesota, USA

L W Baker MD FRCS
Head of the Department of Surgery,
University of Natal,
Durban,
South Africa

D M Balfe MD
Assistant Professor in Radiology,
Mallinckrodt Institute of Radiology,
Washington University School of Medicine,
St Louis,
Missouri, USA

J R Batchelor MA MD MRCS LRCP
Head of Immunology,
Royal Postgraduate Medical School and Hammersmith Hospital,
London, UK

J N Baxter FRCS
Lecturer,
Department of Surgery,
University of Liverpool,
UK

R M Beazley MD
Louisiana State University Medical School,
Department of Surgery,
New Orleans,
Louisiana, USA

S Bengmark MD
Director and Professor of Surgery
University of Lund,
Sweden

J P Benhamou MD
Professor of Hepatology and Gastroenterology,
University of Paris;
Head, Department of Hepatology,
Hôpital Beaujon,
Clichy, France

I S Benjamin BSc FRCS
Senior Lecturer and Honorary Consultant in Surgery,
Royal Postgraduate Medical School and Hammersmith Hospital,
London, UK

G Berci MD FACS
Associate Director of Surgery,
Cedars-Sinai Medical Center,
Los Angeles,
CA, USA

T V Berne MD
Department of Surgery,
USC School of Medicine,
Los Angeles,
CA, USA

H Bismuth MD FACS
Professor of Hepatobiliary Surgery,
Hôpital Paul Brousse,
Villejuif,
France

J I Blenkharn MSc FIMLS
Senior Microbiologist,
Department of Surgery,
Royal Postgraduate Medical School and Hammersmith Hospital,
London, UK

S Bloom MA DSc MD FRCP
Professor of Endocrinology,
Royal Postgraduate Medical School and Hammersmith Hospital,
London, UK

L H Blumgart BDS MD FRCS(Edin) FRCPS(Glas) FRCS(Eng)
Professor of Surgery, University of Bern;
Director, Clinic for Visceral and Transplantation Surgery,
Inselspital,
Bern, Switzerland

I A D Bouchier MBChB MD FRCP(Eng) FRCP(Edin)
Professor of Medicine,
University of Edinburgh,
Royal Infirmary,
Edinburgh, UK

J W Braasch MD
Lahey Clinic Medical Center,
Burlington,
USA

T A Broughan MD
Department of General Surgery,
The Cleveland Clinic,
Cleveland,
Ohio, USA

H J Burhenne MD
Professor and Head,
Department of Radiology,
University of British Columbia,
Vancouver BC,
Canada

G M Bydder MRCP FRCR
Senior Lecturer,
Department of Diagnostic Radiology,
Royal Postgraduate Medical School and Hammersmith Hospital,
London, UK

Sir Roy Y Calne MA MS FRCS FRS
Professor of Surgery,
University of Cambridge;
Honorary Consultant Surgeon,
Addenbrooke's Hospital,
Cambridge, UK

J L Cameron MD
Professor and Chairman in Surgery,
Johns Hopkins Hospital,
Baltimore,
Maryland, USA

L C Carey MD
Chairman, Department of Surgery,
The Ohio State University,
Columbus,
USA

D L Carr-Locke MA MBBChir MRCP DObst RCOG
Consultant Physician in Gastroenterology,
Leicester Royal Infirmary,
UK

D Castaing MD
Department of Hepatobiliary Surgery,
Hôpital Paul Brousse,
Villejuif,
France

J L C Ch'ng MB BS MRCP
Formerly, Department of Endocrinology,
Royal Postgraduate Medical School and Hammersmith Hospital,
London, UK

T K Choi MD FACS
Reader in Surgery,
University of Hong Kong,
Queen Mary Hospital,
Hong Kong

M Classen
Direktor der Zweiten Medizinischen
Klinik Rechts der Isar,
Munich,
West Germany

N A Collier FRCS FRACS
The University of Melbourne,
Department of Surgery,
Royal Melbourne Hospital,
Victoria,
Australia

D O Cosgrove MA MSc MRCP
Consultant in Nuclear Medicine,
Royal Marsden Hospital,
Sutton,
Surrey, UK

P B Cotton MD FRCP
Consultant Physician,
Department of Gastroenterology,
The Middlesex Hospital,
London, UK

I R Crossley MD MRCP
Senior Registrar,
Liver Unit,
King's College Hospital,
London, UK

A Cuschieri MD ChM FRCS(Eng) FRCS(Edin)
Professor and Head,
Department of Surgery,
Ninewells Hospital and Medical School,
Dundee, UK

J Dawson MB BS MS FRCS
Consultant Surgeon,
King's College Hospital,
London, UK

S A Deane FRACS
Senior Lecturer,
Department of Surgery,
Westmead Centre,
Westmead, Australia

L Den Besten MD
Department of Surgery,
UCLA Medical Center,
Los Angeles,
CA, USA

A J Donovan MD
USC School of Medicine,
Department of Surgery,
Los Angeles,
CA, USA

J Edmond MD
Associate Professor,
Department of Hepatobiliary Surgery,
Hôpital Paul Brousse,
Villejuif,
France

H Ekberg MD
Department of Surgery,
University Hospital of Lund,
Sweden

E C Ellison MD
Department of Surgery,
The Ohio State University,
Columbus,
Ohio, USA

S Erlinger MD
Professor of Hepatology and Gastroenterology,
University of Paris;
Director of the Hepatic Physiopathology Research Unit,
Hôpital Beaujon,
Clichy,
France

O Farges MD
Resident Head,
Department of Hepatobiliary Surgery,
Hôpital Paul Brousse,
Villejuif,
France

J V Farman MB BS FSARCS
Consultant in Anaesthetics and Intensive Care,
Addenbrooke's Hospital,
Cambridge,
UK

G M Flannigan BSc MB ChB FRCS ChM
Urological Registrar,
Department of Urology,
The Middlesex Hospital,
London, UK

J H Foster MD
Professor and Chairman,
Department of Surgery,
University of Connecticut Health Center,
Farmington,
Connecticut, USA

R N Garrison MD
Department of Surgery,
University of Louisville,
Kentucky, USA

R N Gibson MB BS MD FRACR
Department of Diagnostic Radiology,
Royal Melbourne Hospital,
Parkville,
Victoria,
Australia

R M Girard MD
Hôpital Maisonneuve-Rosemont,
Montreal,
Canada

M L Gliedman MD
Professor and Chairman,
Department of Surgery,
Montefiore Hospital & Medical Center,
Bronx, NY
USA

P Grases MD
Gastrointestinal Pathology Unit,
The Pathology Institute,
Central University of Venezuela,
Caracas,
Venezuela

S Grundfest-Broniatowski MD
Department of General Surgery,
Cleveland Clinic,
Ohio, USA

J Gugenheim MD
Department of Hepatobiliary Surgery,
Hôpital Paul Brousse,
Villejuif,
France

P Gullstrand MD
Department of Surgery,
University of Lund,
Sweden

A A Gunn MB ChB FRCS(Edin) ChM(Edin)
Consultant Surgeon,
Bangour General Hospital,
Broxburn,
UK

N S Hadjis FRCS
Department of Surgery,
Royal Postgraduate Medical School and Hammersmith Hospital,
London, UK

A W Halliday MD FRCS
Research Fellow, Department of Surgery,
Royal Postgraduate Medical School and Hammersmith Hospital,
London, UK

J M Ham MD
Department of Surgery,
Prince of Wales Hospital,
Randwick,
NSW, Australia

H Hasegawa
5-1 Tsukiji, Chuo-Ku,
Tokyo National Cancer Center,
Tokyo,
Japan

A P Hemingway MRCP DMRD FRCR
Consultant Radiologist,
Department of Diagnostic Radiology,
Royal Postgraduate Medical School and Hammersmith Hospital,
London, UK

R E Hermann MD
Chairman, Department of General Surgery,
Cleveland Clinic,
Ohio, USA

K E F Hobbs ChM FRCS
Professor of Surgery,
Academic Department of Surgery,
Royal Free Hospital,
London, UK

H J F Hodgson MA BM BCh FRCP
Consultant Physician,
Department of Gastroenterology,
Royal Postgraduate Medical School and Hammersmith Hospital,
London, UK

D Houssin MD
Department of Hepatobiliary Surgery,
Hôpital Paul Brousse,
Villejuif,
France

E R Howard, MB BS MS FRCS
Consultant Surgeon,
King's College Hospital,
London, UK

K Huibregtse
Division of Gastroenterology,
Academisch Ziekenhuis,
University of Amsterdam,
The Netherlands

C W Imrie BSc MBChB FRCS
Consultant Surgeon,
Department of Surgery,
Glasgow Royal Infirmary,
UK

S Iwatsuki MD
Department of Surgery,
University of Pittsburgh,
School of Medicine,
Pittsburgh, PA,
USA

J J Jakimowicz MD PhD
Department of Surgery,
Catharina Hospital,
Eindhoven,
The Netherlands

B Jeppsson MD
Department of Surgery,
University Hospital of Lund,
Sweden

P J Johnson MB ChB MRCP
Consultant Physician and Honorary Senior Lecturer,
Liver Unit,
King's College Hospital,
London, UK

G W Johnston MB BCh MCh FRCSI FRCS DObst RCOG DCH
Consultant Surgeon,
Royal Victoria Hospital,
Belfast, UK

R M Katon
Academisch Ziekenhuis,
University of Amsterdam,
The Netherlands

M R B Keighley MS FRCS(Eng) FRCS(Edin)
Professor of Surgery,
The General Hospital,
Birmingham,
UK

R K Kerlan MD
Assistant Professor in Radiology,
University of California School of Medicine,
San Francisco,
CA, USA

J Korula MD FRCPC
Assistant Professor of Clinical Medicine,
University of Southern California School of Medicine,
Los Angeles,
CA, USA

G A Kune FRACS
Professor of Surgery,
Repatriation General Hospital,
Heidelberg,
Victoria,
Australia

M Lavelle-Jones FRCS
Fellow in Surgery,
University of California, San Diego Medical Center,
San Diego,
CA, USA

J P Lavender MRCP(Lond) DMRD FRCR FRCP
Honorary Professor of Diagnostic Radiology,
Royal Postgraduate Medical School and Hammersmith Hospital,
London, UK

J K Lee MD
Associate Professor in Radiology,
Mallinckrodt Institute of Radiology,
St Louis,
Missouri, USA

G Legros MD FRCS
Chief, General Surgery,
Associate Professor of Surgery,
Maisonneuve-Rosemont Hospital,
Montreal,
Canada

P Lief MD
Department of Medicine,
Albert Einstein College of Medicine,
Bronx, NY,
USA

J R Lilly MD
Chief, Pediatric Surgery,
University of Colorado School of Medicine,
Denver,
Colorado, USA

J M Little MD
Professor and Chairman of Surgery,
Westmead Centre,
Westmead,
NSW, Australia

D A Lloyd MD
Associate Professor, Department of Pediatric Surgery,
Children's Hospital,
Pittsburgh, PA,
USA

M S Losowsky MD FRCP MB ChB
Professor of Medicine and Honorary Consultant Physician,
Department of Medicine,
St James's Hospital,
Leeds, UK

A Lunderquist MD
Head and Professor of Gastrointestinal and Interventional Radiology,
University Hospital of Lund,
Sweden

F M Luvuno FRCS
Lecturer, Department of Surgery,
University of Natal,
Durban,
South Africa

E Mack MD
Associate Professor of Surgery,
University of Wisconsin School of Medicine,
Clinical Sciences Center,
Madison, Wisconsin,
USA

M Makuuchi
Tokyo National Cancer Center,
Tokyo,
Japan

R T Mathie BSc PhD
Lecturer in Physiology,
Experimental Surgery Unit,
Royal Postgraduate Medical School and Hammersmith Hospital,
London, UK

R F McCloy BSc MD FRCS
Senior Lecturer and Honorary Consultant,
University Department of Surgery,
Manchester Royal Infirmary,
UK

J O'D McGee MD PhD FRCPath MA
Professor and Head,
Nuffield Department of Pathology,
John Radcliffe Hospital,
Oxford, UK

N McIntyre MD FRCP
Professor of Medicine,
Academic Department of Medicine,
Royal Free Hospital,
London, UK

G A D McPherson MCh MD FRCS
Senior Registrar in Surgery,
Royal Postgraduate Medical School and Hammersmith Hospital,
London, UK

C K McSherry MD
Director of Surgery,
Beth Israel Medical Center,
New York,
USA

Y Menu MD
Consultant, Department of Radiology,
Hôpital Beaujon,
Clichy,
France

A R Moossa MD FRCS(Eng) FRCS(Edin) FACS
Professor and Chairman, Department of Surgery,
Surgeon-in-Chief,
University of California at San Diego Medical Center,
California, USA

M Morgan MB BS FFARCS
Reader in Anaesthetics,
Royal Postgraduate Medical School and Hammersmith Hospital,
London, UK

K P Morrissey MD
Associate Professor of Clinical Surgery,
Cornell University Medical College,
New York, NY,
USA

D M Nagorney MD
Department of Surgery,
Mayo Clinic,
Rochester,
Minnesota,
USA

J S Najarian MD
Department of Surgery,
University of Minnesota,
Minneapolis,
Minnesota,
USA

F Nakayama
Professor and Chairman,
Department of Surgery,
Kyushu University Faculty of Medicine,
Fukuoka,
Japan

A Nobin MD
Department of Surgery,
University Hospital of Lund,
Sweden

D J Nolan MD MRCP FRCR
Consultant Radiologist,
Department of Radiology,
John Radcliffe Hospital,
Oxford, UK

M J Orloff MD
Professor of Surgery,
University of California Medical Center,
San Diego, CA,
USA

L R Pennington MD
Assistant Professor,
Department of Surgery,
Johns Hopkins Hospital,
Baltimore,
Maryland, USA

J Perissat MD
Chirurgien des Hôpitaux,
Bordeaux,
France

J Phillip
Zweite Medizinische Klinik Rechts der Isar,
Munich,
West Germany

J Polak MD DSc
Consultant Histopathologist and Professor of
Endocrine Pathology,
Royal Postgraduate Medical School and Hammersmith Hospital,
London, UK

H C Polk Jr MD
Professor and Chairman,
Department of Surgery,
University of Louisville,
Kentucky, USA

M C Posner MD
Department of Surgery,
University of Colorado Health Sciences Center,
Denver, Colorado,
USA

F Procacciante MD
Policlinico Umberto I,
11 Clinica Chirurgica,
Roma,
Italy

T B Reynolds MD
Professor of Medicine,
University of Southern California,
Los Angeles, CA,
USA

G Ribotta MD
Policlinico Umberto 1,
11 Clinica Chirurgica,
Roma,
Italy

E J Ring MD
Professor and Chief of Radiology,
University of California,
San Francisco,
USA

B Rotoli MD
Sezione Autonoma di Ematologia Clinica,
Clinica Medica,
Nuovo Policlinica,
Naples,
Italy

P R Salmon MB BSc FRCP FRCP(Edin)
Consultant Physician and Gastroenterologist,
The Middlesex Hospital,
London, UK

Ph Sandblom
Lausanne,
Switzerland

J P Schuppisser MD
Associate Professor of Surgery,
Department of Surgery,
St Claraspital,
Basel,
Switzerland

S I Schwartz MD
Professor of Surgery,
University of Rochester,
New York,
USA

R Scott Jones MD
Professor and Chairman,
Department of Surgery,
University of Virginia,
Charlottesville, Virginia,
USA

C E M Sharrock BSc PhD
Special Training Fellow in Recombinant DNA Technology,
Lymphocyte Molecular Biology Laboratory,
Imperial Cancer Research Fund,
St Bartholomew's Hospital,
London, UK

B W Shaw Jr MD
Department of Surgery,
University of Pittsburgh Health Center,
Pennsylvania,
USA

R Shields MB ChB MD FRCS(Eng) FRCS(Edin)
Professor of Surgery,
University of Liverpool,
UK

C Smadja MD
Service de Chirurgie Digestive,
Hôpital Bicêtre,
Le Kremlin Bicêtre,
France

O Søreide
Department of Surgery,
Haukeland University Hospital,
Bergen,
Norway

T E Starzl MD PhD
Professor of Surgery,
University of Pittsburgh School of Medicine,
Pennsylvania,
USA

H Harlan Stone MD
Professor and Chief,
Division of General Surgery,
University of Maryland,
Baltimore,
USA

J A Summerfield MB BS MD MRCP(UK)
Consultant Physician,
Royal Free Hospital,
London, UK

I Taylor MD ChM FRCS
Professor of Surgery and Honorary Consultant Surgeon,
University Surgery Unit,
Southampton General Hospital,
UK

J Terblanche ChM FCS(SA) FRCS(Eng) FRCPS(Glas)
Head of Department and Professor of Surgery,
University of Cape Town Medical School,
Observatory, Cape Town
South Africa

J N Thompson MA FRCS
Senior Registrar,
Department of Surgery,
St Mary's Hospital,
London, UK

P Tondelli MD
Leiter der Chirurgischen Klinik,
St Claraspital,
Basel,
Switzerland

J Toouli MD FRACS
Senior Lecturer in Surgery,
Flinders Medical Centre, Bedford Park,
SA, Australia

K G Tranberg MD
Department of Surgery,
University Hospital of Lund,
Sweden

D E F Tweedle MB ChB ChM FRCS
Consultant Surgeon,
Withington Hospital,
Manchester,
UK

G N Tytgat
Professor, Division of Gastroenterology,
Academic Medical Centre,
Amsterdam,
The Netherlands

S Wapnick MD
Clinical Associate Professor,
Department of Surgery,
Albert Einstein College of Medicine,
Bronx, NY,
USA

J McK Watts MD FRCS
Professor of Surgery,
Flinders Medical Centre, Bedford Park,
SA, Australia

K Weinbren MD
Professor, Department of Surgical Pathology,
Royal Postgraduate Medical School and Hammersmith Hospital,
London, UK

M J Whiting
Department of Clinical Biochemistry,
Flinders Medical Centre, Bedford Park,
SA, Australia

J G Whitwam MB ChB PhD FRCP FFARCS
Director, Department of Anaesthetics,
Royal Postgraduate Medical School and Hammersmith Hospital,
London, UK

R Williams MD FRCP
Director and Consultant Physician,
Liver Research Unit,
King's College Hospital,
London, UK

J Wong PhD FRACS FRCS(Edin) FACS
Professor, University of Hong Kong,
Department of Surgery,
Queen Mary Hospital,
Hong Kong

R Wright MB ChB MD FRCP
Professor of Medicine,
University of Southampton,
Southampton General Hospital,
UK

S Yamazaki
Tokyo National Cancer Center,
Tokyo,
Japan

R Zeppa MD
Professor of Surgery,
University of Miami/Jackson Memorial Medical Center,
Miami,
Florida,
USA

Contents

SECTION 1

Anatomy and pathophysiology

Surgical anatomy and anatomical surgery of the liver

A good knowledge of the anatomy of the liver is a prerequisite for modern surgery of the liver (Bismuth 1982).

ANATOMY OF THE LIVER

Liver anatomy can be described according to different aspects: morphological anatomy and functional anatomy and, now that ultrasound allows precise intraoperative display in individual cases, the real anatomy.

Morphological anatomy

The liver, as it appears at laparotomy, is divided by the umbilical fissure and by the falciform ligament into two lobes: the right lobe, which is the larger, and the left lobe (Fig. 1.1). At the inferior surface of the right lobe is the transverse hilar fissure which constitutes the posterior limit of this lobe. The portion of the right lobe located anteriorly to this fissure is called the quadrate lobe, limited on the left by the umbilical fissure and on the right by the gallbladder fossa. Posterior to the hilar transverse fissure is a fourth lobe, the Spigel lobe.

Thus, the liver is comprised of two main lobes and two accessory lobes which are individualised by visible well defined fissures. This corresponds to the true definition of a lobe: 'part of parenchyma limited by fissures or grooves' (Stedman's medical dictionary).

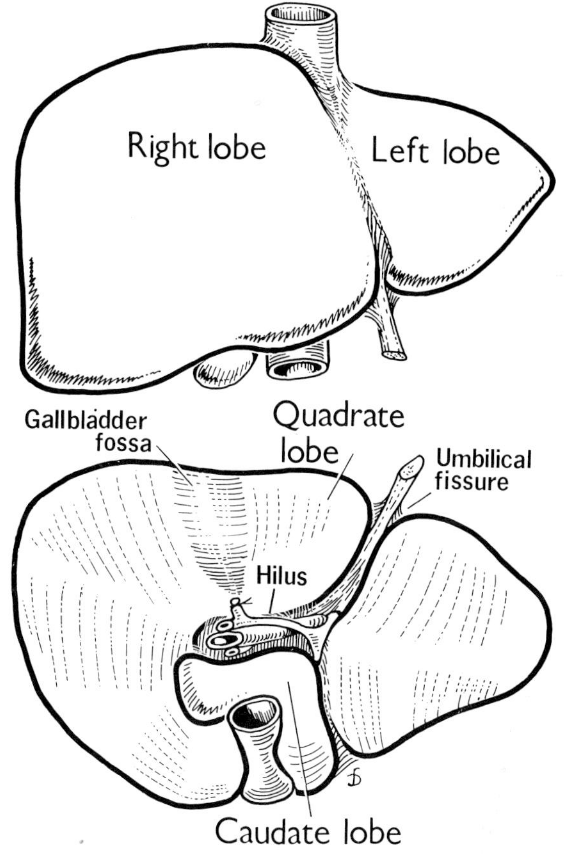

Fig. 1.1 Morphological aspect of the liver. Note that the liver is divided into a right and left lobe as seen from the anterior aspect. From the inferior aspect the right lobe is bounded posteriorly by the transverse fissure, a portion of the right lobe lying anterior to this being the quadrate lobe limited on the left by the umbilical fissure and on the right by the gallbladder fossa. Posteriorly to the hilar fissure is a fourth lobe, the caudate (Spigelian) lobe

Functional anatomy

Besides this classical description of the anatomy of the liver, there is now a second more recent mode of description which can be called the functional anatomy of the liver. This description, initiated by Cantlie in 1898 was followed by the works of McIndoe & Counseller (1927), Ton That Tung (1939), Hjörstjö (1931), Couinaud (1957), and Goldsmith & Woodburne (1957). Although somewhat complex, the description by Couinaud is the most complete and its exactitude and usefulness for the surgeon have been proven by a large experience (Ch. 97). It is that description which is used in this chapter and throughout this book.

The study of the functional anatomy of the liver permits the description of hepatic segmentation based upon the distribution of the portal pedicles and the location of the hepatic veins (Fig. 1.2). The three main hepatic veins divide the liver into four sectors, each of which receives a portal pedicle, with an alternation between hepatic veins and portal pedicles. The four sectors individualised by the three hepatic veins are called portal sectors, for these portions of parenchyma are supplied by independent portal pedicles. For the same reason, the scissurae containing the hepatic veins are called *portal scissurae*, while the scissurae containing portal pedicles are called *hepatic scissurae*: the umbilical fissure corresponds to an hepatic scissura. According to this functional anatomy, the liver appears to be separated into two livers (or hemilivers), the right and left livers, by the main portal scissura, also called Cantlie's line (Fig. 1.3). It is better to call them right and left livers rather than right and left lobes, for this last nomenclature causes some confusion with the anatomical lobes and is erroneous since, as mentioned, there is no visible mark that permits individualization of a true lobe. The main portal scissura goes from the middle of the gallbladder bed anteriorly to the left side of the vena cava posteriorly. This scissura describes an angle of 75° with the horizontal plane opened to the left. The right and left livers individualised by the main portal scissura are independent as regards the portal and arterial vascularization and the biliary drainage. The middle hepatic vein follows this main portal scissura.

These right and left livers are themselves divided into two parts by two other portal scissurae. These four subdivisions are usually called *segments* in the Anglo-Saxon nomenclature (Goldsmith & Woodburne 1957). According to Couinaud's nomenclature (1957), which we are using here, they are called *sectors*.

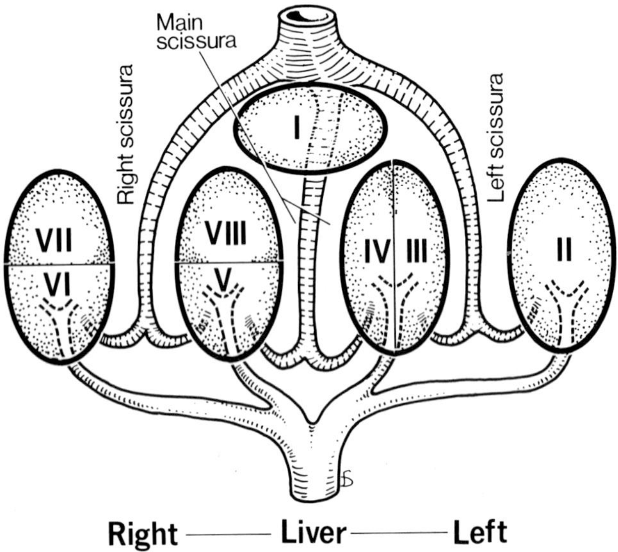

Fig. 1.2 Schematic representation of the functional anatomy of the liver. There are three main hepatic veins lying within the liver scissurae and dividing the liver into four sectors each receiving a portal pedicle. The hepatic veins and portal pedicles are intertwined as are the fingers of the two hands

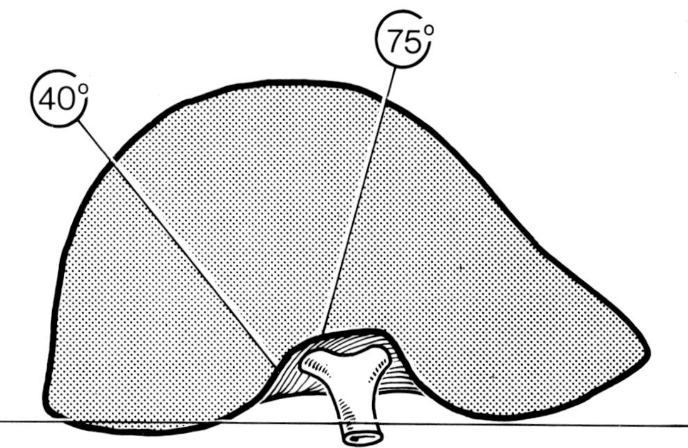

Fig. 1.3 The obliquity of the middle and right portal scissurae

The right portal scissura divides the right liver into two sectors: anteromedial or anterior and posterolateral or posterior. Along the right portal scissura runs the right hepatic vein. The right portal scissura is inclined 40° to the right (Fig. 1.3). With the liver in its normal place in the abdominal cavity, the posterolateral sector is behind the anteromedial sector and the scissura is almost in a frontal plane: in the patient, it is better to speak of anterior and posterior sectors for in all the morphological examinations of the liver (ultra-sound, CT scan, arteriography, etc.) the posterolateral sector projects exactly behind the anteromedial sector (Fig. 1.4a). By contrast, medial and lateral are better denominations when the liver is removed at autopsy for pathology or anatomical study and put flat on a table (Fig. 1.4b). The exact location of the right portal scissura is not well defined because it has no external landmark. According to Couinaud (1957), it extends, at the anterior surface of the liver, from the anterior border of the liver at the middle of the distance between the right angle of the liver and the right side of the gallbladder bed, to the confluence between the inferior vena cava and the right hepatic vein posteriorly. According to Ton That Tung (1939), this scissura follows a line parallel to the right lateral edge of the liver, three fingers' breadth more anteriorly.

The left portal scissura divides the left liver into two sectors: superior and posterior. This left portal scissura is not the umbilical fissure, since this fissure is not a portal scissura; in a portal scissura, there is an hepatic vein whereas in the umbilical fissure there is a portal pedicle. The left portal scissura is, in fact, located posteriorly to the teres ligamentum and is found inside the left lobe of the liver where the left hepatic vein runs. Thus, the anterior sector of the left liver is composed of the part of the right lobe which is to the left of the main portal scissura and of the anterior part of the left lobe.

In conclusion, the liver appears to be divided into two livers by the main hepatic scissura within which the middle hepatic vein runs (Fig. 1.4).

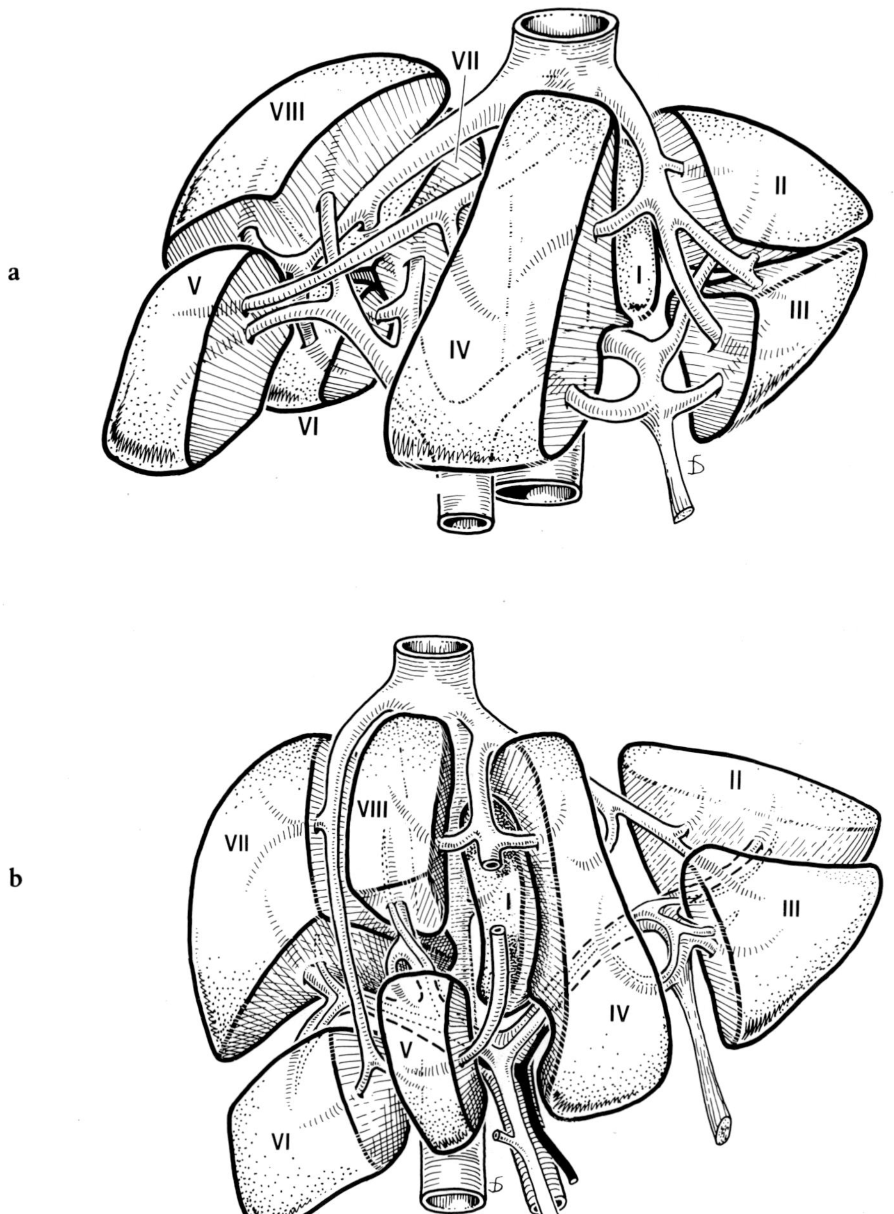

Fig. 1.4 The functional division of the liver and of the liver segments according to Couinaud's nomenclature: a. as seen in the patient; b. in the ex-vivo position (see text)

1. The right liver is divided into two sectors by the right portal scissura within which runs the right hepatic vein. Each of these two sectors is divided into two segments: anterior sector — segment V inferiorly and segment VIII superiorly; and the posterior sector — segment VI inferiorly and segment VII superiorly.

2. The left liver is also divided into 2 sectors by the left portal scissura where the left hepatic vein runs. The anterior sector is divided by the umbilical fissure into two segments: medially segment IV, the anterior part of which is the quadrate lobe, and laterally segment III, which is the anterior part of the left lobe. The posterior sector is comprised of only one segment, segment II which is the posterior part of the left lobe. This is an exception to the nomenclature where each sector is divided in two segments (see Fig. 1.2): as a result the two hemilivers, each of them divided into two sectors, comprises seven segments (segment II to VIII).

3. The Spigel lobe (or segment I) must be considered from the functional point of view as an autonomous segment, for its vascularization is independent of the portal division and of the three main hepatic veins. It receives its vessels from the left but also from the right branches of the portal vein and hepatic artery: its hepatic veins are

independent and drain directly into the inferior vena cava. The anatomy of this third liver is revealed in some pathological circumstances, e.g. in Budd-Chiari disease: due to the obstruction of the three main hepatic veins, the hepatic blood outflow is ensured through the Spigel lobe which hypertrophies.

In most countries, the segments and their numbers have become very popular among surgeons. This definition of the segments according to Couinaud's nomenclature (1957) is different from that of Goldsmith & Woodburne (1957): for these last authors Couinaud's sector is called a segment and a segment according to Couinaud is called a subsegment. This is a cause of confusion in the world literature as the Goldsmith & Woodburne nomenclature is usually used in Anglo-Saxon literature.

The real anatomy

Progress has recently been made which allows the surgeon to know the precise anatomy of the liver he is operating on with the use of *operative ultrasound* (Castaing et al 1985). By this investigation, during the operation, the surgeon is able to see the exact anatomy of the liver he has in his hands (Ch. 96).

Recognition of the vascular distribution inside the liver is the first step in liver resection. With precise location of the three main hepatic veins, the portal scissurae are identified and their projections on the anterior surface of the liver are marked by small incisions on Glisson's capsula. Operative ultrasound is even more useful for segmental resection as division inside the liver of the main portal branches can be located easily. More precise definition of segments can be done by injection of dye under ultrasound guidance into the segmental portal branch or by balloon catheter occlusion (Ch. 96, 97).

CLASSIFICATION OF HEPATECTOMIES (see also Ch. 97)

Classification according to the anatomy

Liver resections can be separated into two groups:

1. *Typical* hepatectomies also called hepatectomies 'réglées', which are defined by the resection of a portion of liver parenchyma following one or several anatomical scissurae. These resections are called hepatectomies (left or right), sectoriectomies, and segmentectomies.

2. *Atypical* hepatectomies which consist of the resection of a portion of parenchyma not limited by anatomical scissurae.

The most common typical hepatectomies can be separated into two groups (Fig. 1.5). Firstly, there are right and left hepatectomies in which the line of transection is the main portal scissura separating the right and the left livers. Secondly, there are right and left lobectomies in which the line of transection is the umbilical fissure. In the classification of Couinaud, right lobectomy corresponds to a right hepatectomy extended to segment IV. The terms left or right lobectomy are frequently used in the Anglo-Saxon literature to define what is, in fact, a left or right hepatectomy. It is preferable, in our opinion, to avoid referring to as 'lobectomy' the resection of a part of the liver that does not fit with the anatomical definition of the lobe. In order to avoid confusion the author has recently proposed the omission of the words 'right lobectomy' for any kind of *right* liver resection and to use the word right

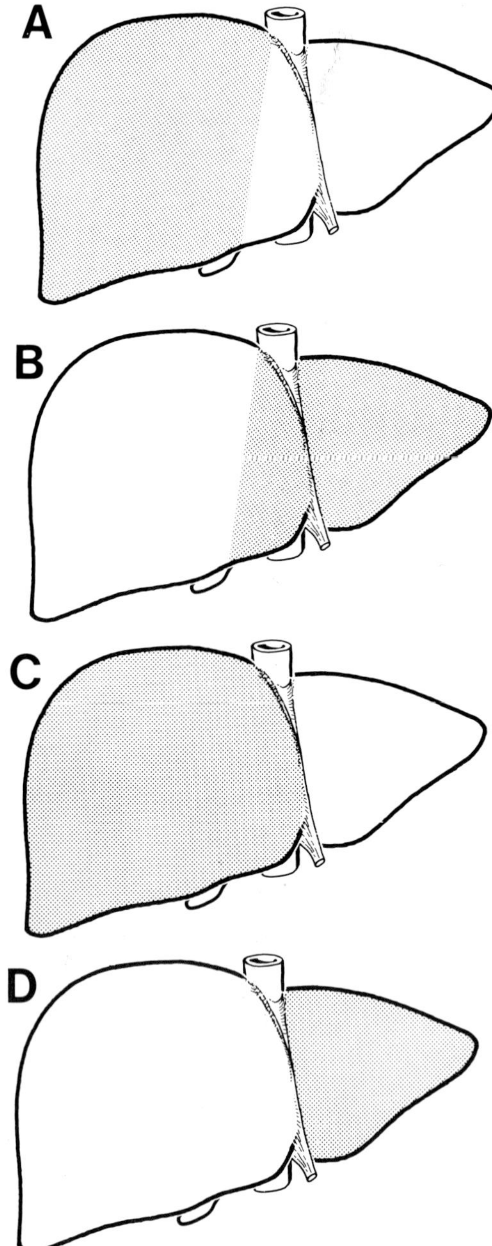

Fig. 1.5 The four common hepatectomies: A and B right and left hepatectomy as defined by the main portal scissura; C and D right and left lobectomy as defined by the umbilical fissure (see also Ch. 97)

hepatectomy extended to the segment IV (equivalent of right lobectomy or right trisegmentectomy of Starzl et al 1975) or right hepatectomy extended to the segments IV and I when the Spigel lobe (segment I) is also removed. On the left, for the resection of the classical left lobe (segment II and III), its seems difficult to avoid speaking of left lobectomy: left lateral segmentectomy is anatomically wrong for the true left lateral segment (or sector) is only segment II. Fig. 1.6 illustrates the differences in definition of hepatectomies.

The other liver resections are numerous. Indeed, according to the anatomical segmentation of the liver, all the individual or associated segmentectomies can be described (Bismuth, Houssin & Castaing 1982).

Classification according to surgical technique

Two opposing technical conceptions of typical hepatectomies can be described (Fig. 1.7) (Ch. 97).

Hepatectomy with preliminary vascular control

This technique was first described by Lortat-Jacob, Robert & Henry (1952) at the time of the first right typical hepatectomy. This technique consists in ligating and dividing the portal pedicle and the hepatic vein prior to transecting the parenchyma. Using this technique, a right

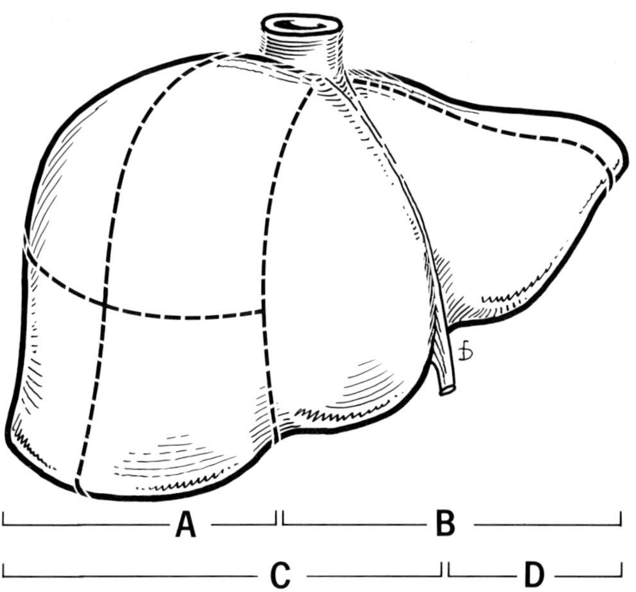

Fig. 1.6 Differences in definition of hepatectomies.

	Couinaud 1957	*Goldsmith & Woodburne 1957*
A	right hepatectomy	right hepatic lobectomy
B	left hepatectomy	left hepatic lobectomy
C	right lobectomy	right extended lobectomy*
D	left lobectomy	left lateral segmentectomy

*Also called trisegmentectomy (Starzl et al 1975). The horizontal line within the right lobe and the vertical line marking the right scissura show demarcation of segmentectomies and postero-lateral sectoriectomy (see above Ch. 97)

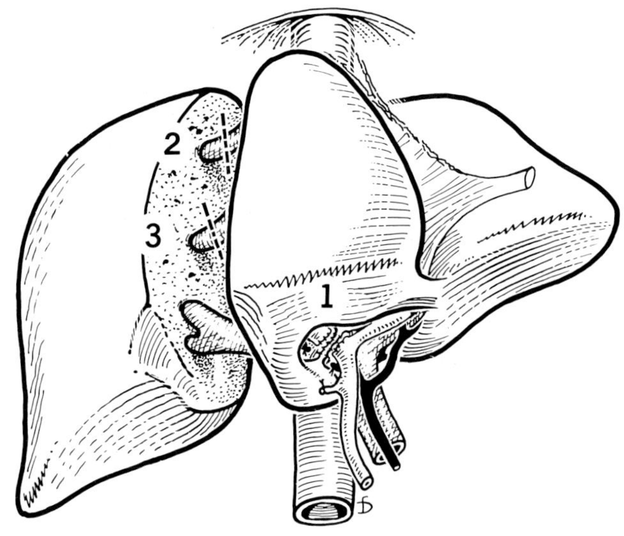

a

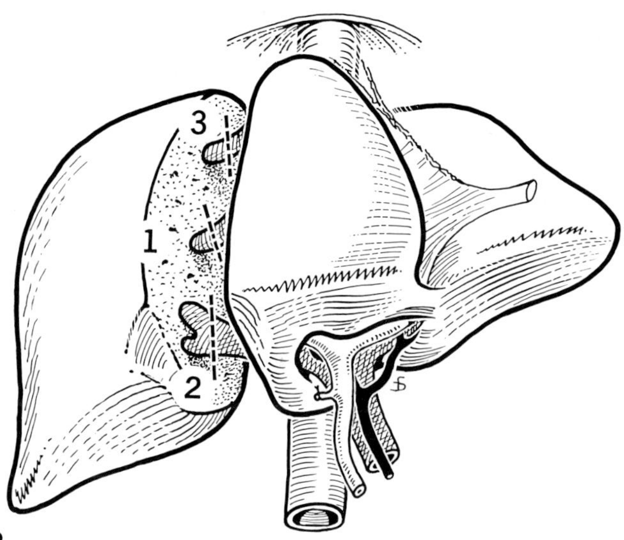

b

Fig. 1.7 The two basic procedures of right hepatectomy. a. Primary division of the vessels (Lortat-Jacob's technique) (1) followed by transection of the liver substance with subsequent control of the hepatic vein (2) and then parenchymatous transection (3). b. Primary parenchymatous transection (Ton That Tung's technique) (1) followed by intraparenchymal control of the portal pedicles (2) and hepatic veins (3)

hepatectomy starts with the ligation and section of the right portal pedicle at the hilus, continues with the ligation and section of the right hepatic vein, and ends with the transection of the parenchyma. The dissection of the hepatic vein is dangerous in that there is a major risk of tearing or penetrating this large vein or the vena cava itself, leading to massive bleeding which is difficult to control, and to the danger of air embolism. For this reason, in the initial technique of Lortat-Jacob, it was suggested that the dissection of the right hepatic vein be preceded by the control of the inferior vena cava above and below the liver. This technique has two advantages: the primary vascular control permits visualization of the borderline between the two livers by the darkening of the right liver: and good vascular control results in a decrease in intraoperative bleeding. However, the technique has two disadvantages: on one hand, the risk of causing an injury to the hepatic vein; and on the other, the risk of devitalizing the remaining liver by an erroneous ligation of an element of the porta hepatis, a risk which is increased by the frequency of anatomical abnormalities.

Hepatectomy by primary parenchymatous transection

The principle of this technique, described by Ton That Tung (1979), is to begin with the opening of the parenchyma along the line of the scissura. The hilar elements are approached and ligated within the liver. Section of the hepatic vein is performed in the same fashion at the end of the procedure inside the liver. This technique has two advantages: it excises the amount of liver parenchyma 'à la demande' according to the nature and the location of the lesion; and ligation of the vessels is not hampered by anatomical abnormalities, since the vessels are approached above the hilus inside the liver. There are two disadvantages: intraoperative bleeding can be considerable owing to the lack of preliminary vascular control and thus quick performance is mandatory; clamping of the porta hepatis may be necessary, either during the whole procedure or intermittently.

From the combination of these two basic procedures are derived the other techniques of hepatectomy. The author's technique of liver resection illustrates this association of the two methods: it combines the advantages of both procedures, while seeking to avoid their disadvantages (Fig. 1.7). Its principle is to begin with a hilar dissection in order to control the arterial and portal elements of the right pedicle (in the case of a right hepatectomy) and *to clamp these elements without ligating them*. The right flank of the retrohepatic inferior vena cava is freed without attempting systematically to dissect the right hepatic vein. Then the liver is opened along the main scissural line and, as in Ton That Tung's technique, the portal elements are located by a superior approach inside the parenchyma: thus ligation of these vessels is performed distally to the clamps (Fig. 1.8). At the end of the liver transection, the hepatic vein is ligated inside the liver. This technique has the advantage of proceeding with control of the vessels before the liver transection, as in Lortat-Jacob's technique; and of dividing the vessels inside the parenchyma, as in Ton That Tung's technique.

There are two other techniques of liver resection, less frequently used. Their indications are limited to some specific cases.

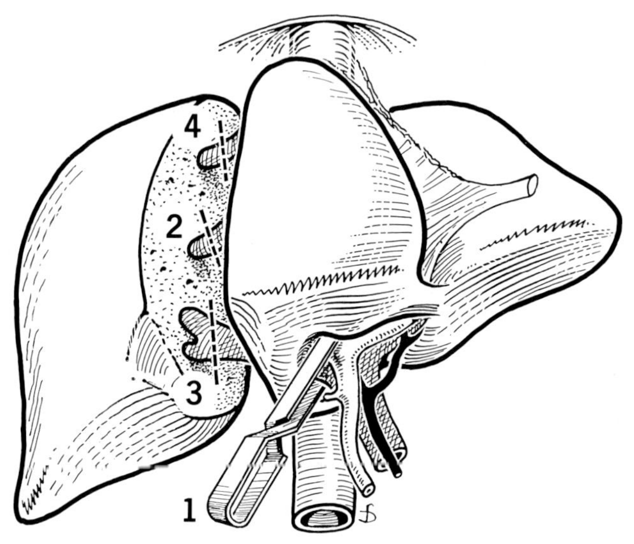

Fig. 1.8 The author's procedure for right hepatectomy which combines the two techniques with temporary clamping of the main portal pedicle (1) followed by parenchymatous transection (2) with control of the portal pedicles (3) and hepatic veins (4)

1. In huge tumours, when a right extended hepatectomy is indicated, complete vascular exclusion of the liver can be beneficial. This procedure, described by Heaney & Jacobson (1975), is achieved by simultaneous clamping of the hepatic pedicle and of the vena cava below and above the liver. It has been shown that clamping the aorta is not necessary (Huguet et al 1976).

2. For the small or atypical liver resections, the control of bleeding at the level of the parenchymatous transection by a clamp placed across the liver substance can be useful (Lin 1974).

The finger-fracture is often thought of as a type of liver resection. Actually, it is only a means of cutting the liver much as a knife or scissors is used; in fact, we formerly used a Kelly clamp which, used with small bites, progressively divides the parenchyma, exposing the small vessels (we call this method of section 'Kellyclasy' by analogy with 'digitoclasy').

In conclusion, there are now many types of liver resections according to the amount of liver to be excised and the surgical technique selected. The surgeon must choose between them in order to elect the best management for every case of hepatic lesion in which hepatic resection is indicated. Always bearing in mind the principle of an anatomical operation, the surgeon can choose between a major and a minor hepatectomy and between resection with primary ligation of the vessels or with primary parenchymatous transection.

REFERENCES

Bismuth H 1982 Surgical anatomy and anatomical surgery of the liver. World Journal of Surgery 6: 3–9

Bismuth H, Houssin D, Castaing D 1982 Major and minor segmentectomies-'règlées' in liver surgery. World Journal of Surgery 6: 10–24

Castaing D, Kunstlinger F, Habib N, Bismuth H 1985 Intra-operative ultrasound study of the liver: Methodology and anatomical results. American Journal of Surgery 149: 676–682

Couinaud C 1957 Le foie. Etudes anatomiques et chirurgicales. Masson, Paris

Goldsmith N A, Woodburne R T 1957 Surgical anatomy pertaining to liver resection. Surgery, Gynecology and Obstetrics 195: 310–318

Heaney J P, Jacobson A 1975 Simplified control of upper abdominal haemorrhage from the vena cava. Surgery 78: 138–141

Hjôrstjô C H 1931 The topography of the intrahepatic duct systems. Acta Anatomica 11:599

Huguet C, Gallot D, Offenstadt G, Coloigner M 1976 Exclusion vasculaire totale du foie dans la chirurgie d'exérèse hépatique large. Nouvelle Presse Médecine 5: 1189–1192

Lin T Y 1974 A simplified technique for hepatic resection. Annals of Surgery 180: 285–290

Lortat-Jacob J L, Robert H G, Henry C 1952 Un cas d'hépatectomie droite réglée. Memoires del'Academie de Chirurgie 78: 244–251

McIndoe A H, Counseller V X 1927 A report on the bilaterality of the liver. Archives of Surgery 15:589

Starzl T E, Bell R H, Beart R W, Putman C W 1975 Hepatic trisegmentectomy and other liver resections. Surgery, Gynecology and Obstetrics 141: 429–437

Ton That Tung 1939 La vascularisation veineuse du foie et ses applications aux résections hépatiques. Thèse Hanoi

Ton That Tung 1979 Les résections majeures et mineures du foie. Masson, Paris

2

C. Smadja, L. H. Blumgart

The biliary tract and the anatomy of biliary exposure

INTRODUCTION

Biliary exposure is the most important step in any biliary operative procedure. A thorough knowledge of the anatomy of the biliary tract is essential if dissection is to be precise and error avoided. Thus, bile duct injury during cholecystectomy is generally due to inadequate bile duct exposure or failure to recognize variations in anatomy. Moreover, cholangitis following high biliary ductal repair is not infrequently due to incomplete biliary drainage as a result of erroneous interpretation of the hepatic cholangiogram. Indeed some operative approaches, e.g. the mucosal graft procedure for biliary repair, have been developed because of a failure to appreciate biliary ductal anatomy at the hilus and within the umbilical fissure and of the possibilities of surgical access (Ch. 58, 70).

Several authors have thoroughly described the anatomy of the biliary tract (Couinaud 1957, Healey & Schroy 1953, Hjortsjö 1951) but the surgical implications have been incompletely described and understood.

In this chapter the anatomy of the biliary tract will be detailed after the descriptions of Couinaud (1957) and of Healey & Schroy (1953). This description will be followed by an analysis of the surgical implications and of surgical exposure.

INTRAHEPATIC BILE DUCT ANATOMY

The liver is divided into two major portions and a dorsal lobe (Fig. 2.1, Fig. 2.2). The right liver and the left liver are respectively drained by the right and the left hepatic

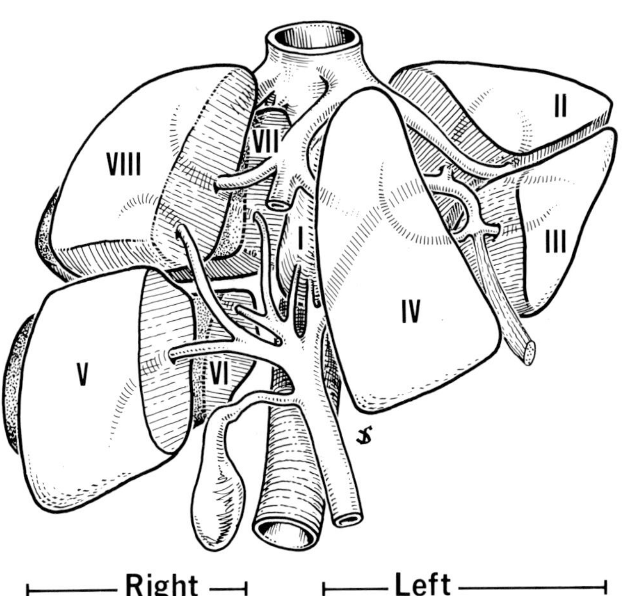

Fig. 2.1 Diagram showing the biliary drainage of the two functional hemilivers. Note the position of the right anterior and right posterior sectors (see also Ch. 1). The caudate lobe drains into the right and left ductal system

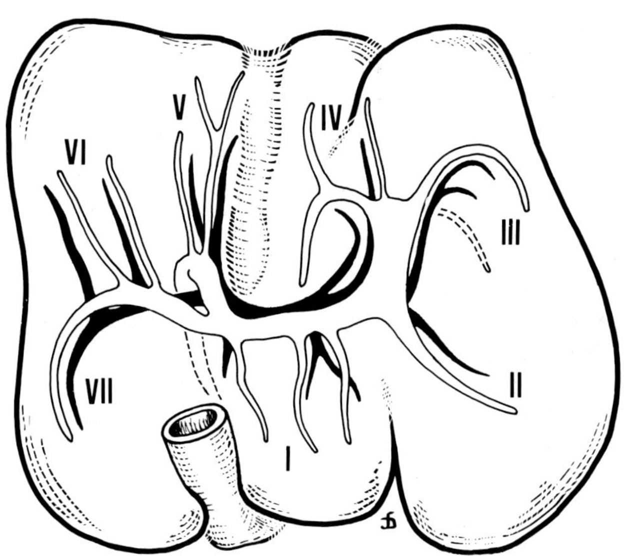

Fig. 2.2 Diagram showing the inferior aspect of the liver. The biliary tract is represented in black and the portal branches in white. Note the biliary drainage of segment IV. Segment VIII is not represented because of its anterior location

ducts whereas the dorsal lobe (caudate lobe) is drained by one or several ducts joining both the right and left hepatic ducts (Healey & Schroy 1953). The intrahepatic ducts are tributaries of the corresponding hepatic ducts which form part of the major portal tracts and which penetrate the liver invaginating Glisson's capsule at the hilus. Of the different biliary and vascular elements of the major portal triads, the hepatic arterial branches, portal veins and biliary tract, the least liable to variation are the portal venous components. In particular, the left branch of the portal vein tends to be consistent in location (Couinaud 1957). Bile ducts are usually located above the corresponding portal branches whereas hepatic arterial branches are situated inferior to the veins. Each branch of the intrahepatic portal veins corresponds to one or two bile ducts which form outside the liver, the right and left hepatic ductal systems converging at the liver hilus to constitute the common hepatic duct. The umbilical fissure divides the left liver passing between segment III and segment IV where it may be bridged at its base by a tongue of liver tissue. The ligamentum teres passes through the umbilical fissure to join the left branch of the portal vein within the recessus of Rex (Fig. 2.1), (Fig. 2.18a see below). All these biliary and vascular elements are liable to anatomical variation.

The left hepatic duct drains the three segments (II, III & IV) which constitute the left liver (Fig. 2.1, Fig. 2.2). The duct draining segment III is located slightly behind the left horn of the umbilical recessus, running backwards (Ch. 58, 70) to join the duct of segment II to the left of the main portal branch to segment II at the point where the left branch of the portal vein turns forward and caudally at the recessus of Rex (Couinaud 1957), (Fig. 2.3). The left hepatic duct traverses beneath the left liver at the base of segment IV, just above and behind the left branch of the portal vein (Ch. 70), crosses the anterior edge of that vein and joins the right hepatic duct to constitute the hepatic ductal confluence. In its transverse portion it receives one to three small branches from segment IV (Couinaud 1957).

The right hepatic duct drains segments V, VI, VII, & VIII (Fig. 2.1 & 2.2) and arises from the junction of two main sectoral ductal tributaries: the posterior or lateral duct and the anterior or medial duct, each a satellite of its corresponding vein. The right posterior sectoral duct has an almost *horizontal* course (Ton That Tung 1979) (Fig. 2.4) and is constituted by the confluence of the ducts of segments VI & VII. The duct then runs to join the right anterior sectoral duct as it descends in a *vertical* manner (Ton That Tung 1979). The right anterior sectoral duct is formed by the confluence of the ducts draining segment V and segment VIII. Its main trunk is located to the left of the right anterior sectoral branch of the portal vein which pursues an ascending course. The junction of these two main right biliary channels usually takes place above the right branch of the portal vein (Couinaud 1957).

The right hepatic duct is short and joins the left hepatic duct to constitute the confluence lying in front of the right portal vein and forming the common hepatic duct.

The dorsal (caudate) lobe (segment I) has its own biliary drainage. According to Healey & Schroy (1953) the dorsal lobe comprises two portions, a caudate lobe proper located at the posterior aspect of the liver and a caudate process passing behind the portal structures to join the right liver (Fig. 2.5). The caudate lobe proper is divided into right and left portions. In 44% three separate ducts drain these

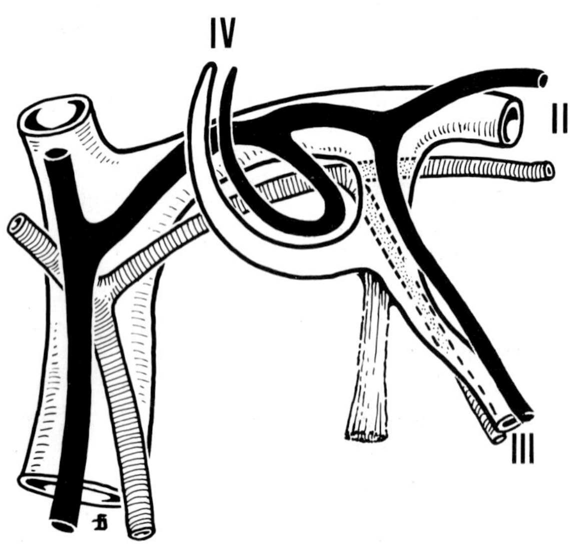

Fig. 2.3 Biliary and vascular anatomy of the left liver. Note the location of the segment III duct above the corresponding vein and its relationship to the recessus of Rex. The anterior branch of the segment IV duct is not represented

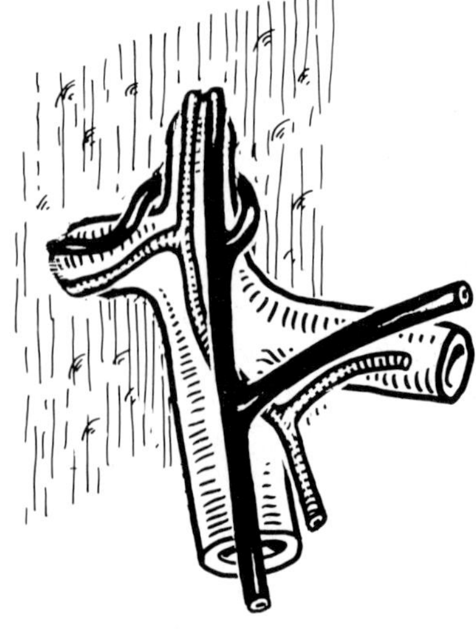

Fig. 2.4 Biliary vascular anatomy of the right liver. Note the horizontal course of the posterior sectoral duct and the vertical course of the anterior sectoral duct

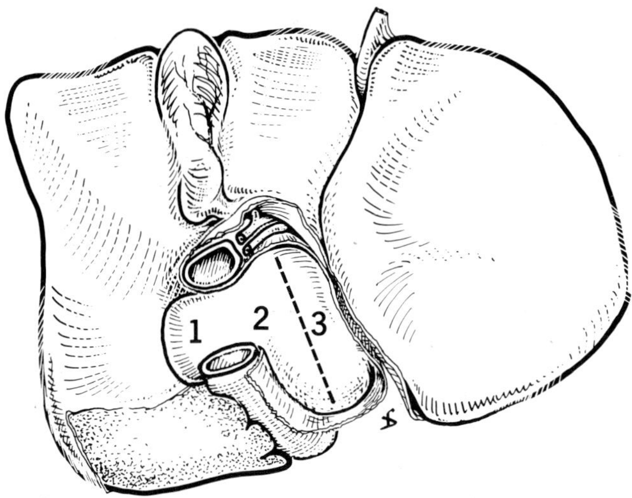

Fig. 2.5 Diagram showing the anatomy of the caudate lobe which is divided into a caudate process (1) and a caudate lobe proper which is itself sub-divided into a right (2) and left (3) portion. Note the relationship of the caudate process to the inferior vena cava and the portal triad

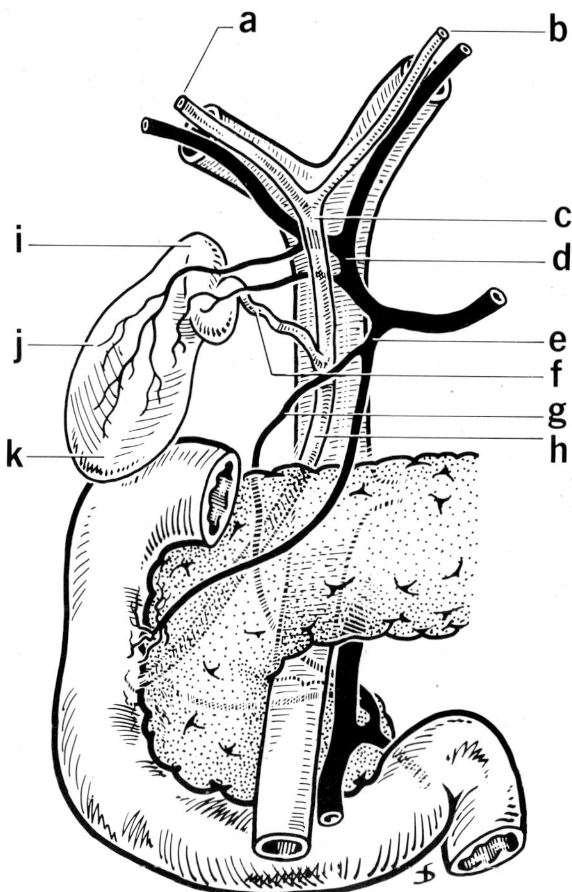

Fig. 2.6 Anterior aspect of the biliary anatomy: (a) right hepatic duct, (b) left hepatic duct, (c) common hepatic duct, (d) hepatic artery, (e) gastroduodenal artery, (f) cystic duct, (g) retroduodenal artery, (h) common bile duct, (i) neck of the gallbladder, (j) body of the gallbladder, (k) fundus of the gallbladder.

Note particularly the situation of the hepatic bile duct confluence anterior to the right branch of the portal vein, the posterior course of the cystic artery behind the common hepatic duct and the relationship of the neck of the gallbladder to the right branch of the hepatic artery

three parts of the lobe, while in 26% there is a common duct between the right portion of the caudate lobe proper and the caudate process and an independent duct draining the left part of the caudate lobe. The site of drainage of these ducts is variable. In 78% of cases, drainage of the caudate lobe is into both right and left hepatic ducts but in 15% drainage is by the left hepatic ductal system only. In about 7% the drainage is into the right hepatic system.

Surgical resection of hilar cholangiocarcinoma (Ch. 65, 97) necessitates thorough knowledge of hilar anatomy and of the caudate lobe since following resection there must be complete reconstruction and biliary-enteric drainage of all intrahepatic ducts. Incomplete drainage leads either to biliary fistula or cholangitis. The techniques of biliary-enteric bypass have been described in detail (Voyles & Blumgart 1982, Blumgart & Kelley 1984) (Ch. 70). Moreover Hasegawa (1984) has recently proposed removal of the caudate lobe if performing resection of hilar cholangiocarcinoma since its close and variable connections with the biliary ductal confluence render tumour clearance and avoidance of subsequent biliary leakage difficult. On the other hand, Blumgart and his co-workers (1984) have resected cholangiocarcinoma at the confluence of the bile ducts without undertaking removal of the caudate lobe as a routine and with good results (Ch. 97).

EXTRAHEPATIC BILIARY ANATOMY

The extrahepatic bile ducts are represented by the extrahepatic segments of the right and left hepatic ducts joining to form the biliary confluence and the main biliary channel draining to the duodenum. The accessory biliary apparatus, which constitutes a reservoir, comprises the gallbladder and cystic duct (Fig. 2.6).

The confluence of the right and left hepatic ducts takes place at the right of the hilus of the liver anterior to the portal venous bifurcation and overlying the origin of the right branch of the portal vein (Fig. 2.6). The extrahepatic segment of the right duct is short but the left duct has *a much longer extrahepatic course* (Ch. 70). The biliary confluence is separated from the posterior aspect of the quadrate lobe (segment IV) of the liver by the hilar plate, which is the fusion of connective tissue enclosing the biliary and vascular elements with Glisson's capsule (Fig. 2.7). Because of the absence of any vascular interposition it is possible to open the connective tissue constituting the hilar plate at the inferior border of the quadrate lobe (segment IV) and by elevating it to display the biliary convergence and left hepatic duct (Fig. 2.8) (Hepp & Couinaud 1956) (Ch. 70).

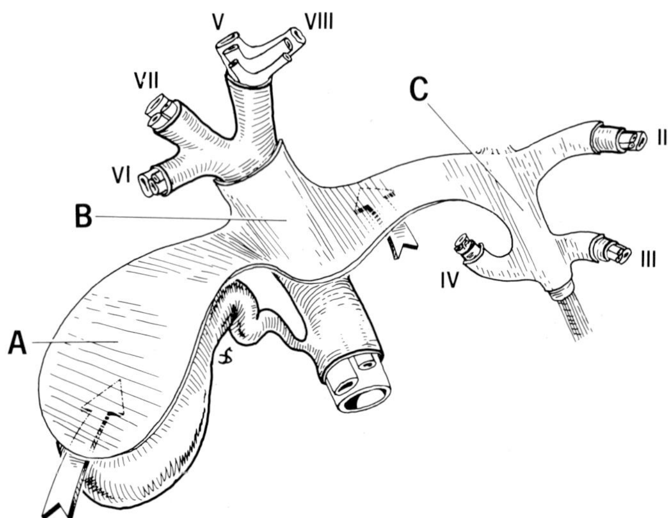

Fig. 2.7 Sketch of the anatomy of the plate system. Note the cystic plate (A) above the gallbladder, the hilar plate (B) above the biliary confluence and at the base of the quadrate lobe and the umbilical plate (C) above the umbilical portion of the portal vein. Large curving arrows indicate the plane of dissection of the cystic plate during cholecystectomy and of the hilar plate and approaches to the left hepatic duct

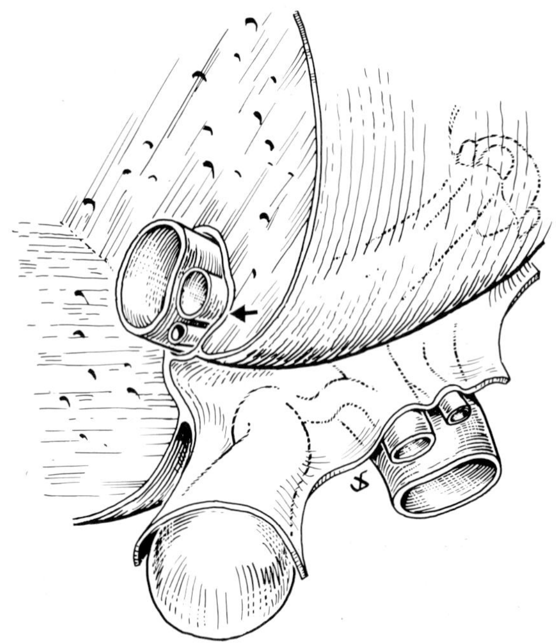

a

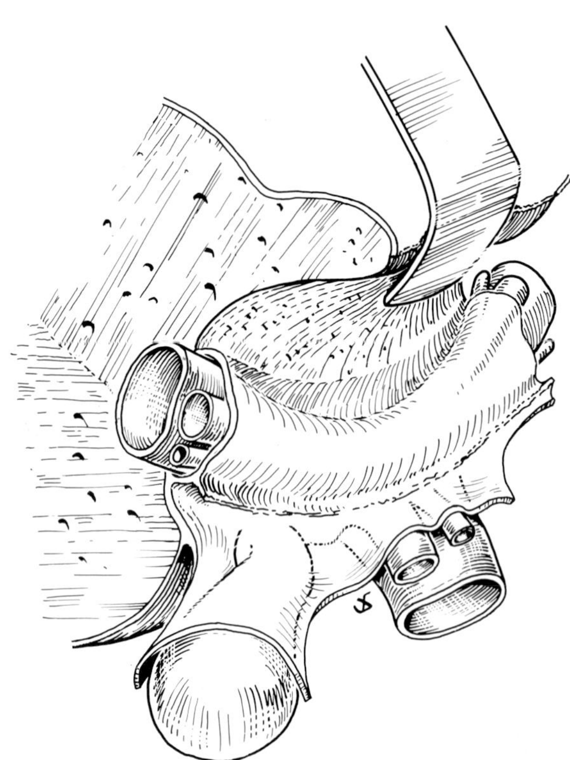

b

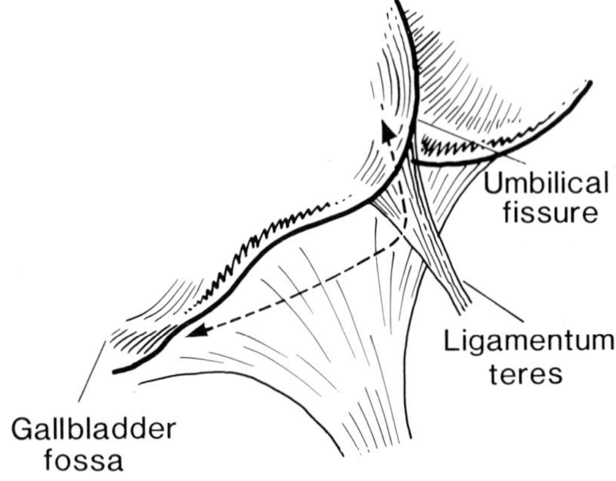

c(1)

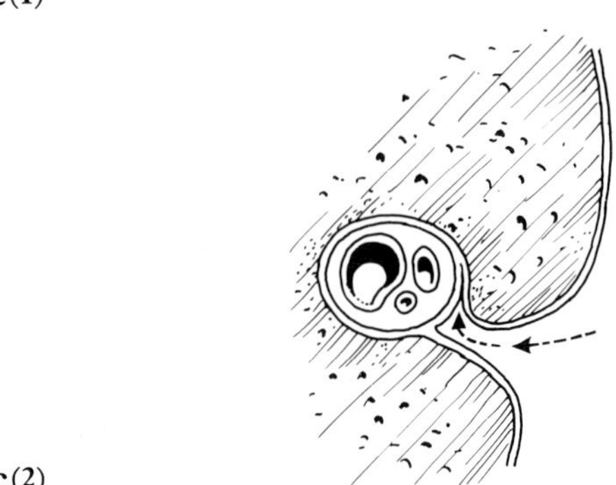

c(2)

Fig. 2.8 a. Diagram showing the relationship between the posterior aspect of the quadrate lobe and the biliary confluence. The hilar plate (arrow) is formed by the fusion of the connective tissue enclosing the biliary and vascular elements with Glisson's capsule. b. Diagram showing the biliary confluence and left hepatic duct exposed by lifting the quadrate lobe upwards after incision of Glisson's capsule at its base. This technique (lowering of the hilar plate) (Hepp & Couinaud 1956) is generally used to display dilated bile ducts above an iatrogenic stricture or hilar cholangiocarcinoma. c. (1) Sketch showing the line of incision to allow extensive mobilization of the quadrate lobe. This manoeuvre is of particular value for high bile duct stricture and in the presence of liver atrophy/hypertrophy. The procedure consists of lifting the quadrate lobe upwards (see a & b above) and then opening not only the umbilical fissure but incising the deepest portion of the gallbladder fossa. (2) Diagram showing incision of Glisson's capsule in order to gain access to the biliary system (arrow)

The main bile duct and the sphincter of Oddi

The main bile duct (Fig. 2.6), the mean diameter of which is about 6 mm, is divided into two segments: the upper segment is called the common hepatic duct and is situated above the cystic duct, which joins it to form the common bile duct. The common duct courses downwards anterior to the portal vein in the free edge of the lesser omentum and is closely applied to the hepatic artery which runs upwards on its left, giving rise to the right branch of the hepatic artery which crosses the main bile duct usually posteriorly, though sometimes anteriorly. The cystic artery, arising from the right branch of the hepatic artery, may cross the common hepatic duct posteriorly or anteriorly. The common hepatic duct constitutes the left border of the triangle of Calot, the other borders of which were originally described as the cystic duct below and the cystic artery above (Rocko, Swan & Di Gioia 1981). However, the commonly accepted working definition of Calot's triangle recognizes the inferior surface of the right lobe of the liver as the upper border and the cystic duct as the lower (Wood 1979). Dissection of Calot's triangle is of key significance during cholecystectomy (Ch. 44) since in this triangle runs the cystic artery, often the right branch of the hepatic artery and occasionally a bile duct which should be displayed prior to cholecystectomy. In the event of an anomalous hepatic artery arising from the superior mesenteric trunk (Ch. 3), this vessel usually courses upwards in the groove posterolateral to the common biliary channel, appearing in the medial side of Calot's triangle and usually running just behind the cystic duct where it is vulnerable during cholecystectomy or portacaval shunt. The union between the cystic duct and the common hepatic duct may be located at various levels. At its lower extrahepatic portion the common bile duct crosses the pyloric vessels and the retroduodenal artery (Fig. 2.9) and then traverses the posterior aspect of the pancreas running in a groove or tunnel. The retropancreatic portion of the common bile duct approaches the second portion of the duodenum obliquely accompanied by the terminal part of the duct of Wirsung. This duct courses from left to right within the pancreas, curves downwards approaching the common bile duct, and runs parallel with but separated from it by the transampullary septum to enter the duodenum at the papilla of Vater after traversing the sphincter of Oddi.

The sphincter of Oddi has been thoroughly studied (Ch. 9) (Boyden 1957, Delmont 1979) and consists of a unique cluster of smooth muscle fibres (Fig. 2.10) distinguishable from the adjacent smooth muscle of the duodenal wall. The papilla of Vater at the termination of the common bile duct is a small nipple-like structure protruding into the duodenal lumen and marked by a longitudinal fold of duodenal mucosa. The duct of Wirsung as it runs down parallel with the common bile

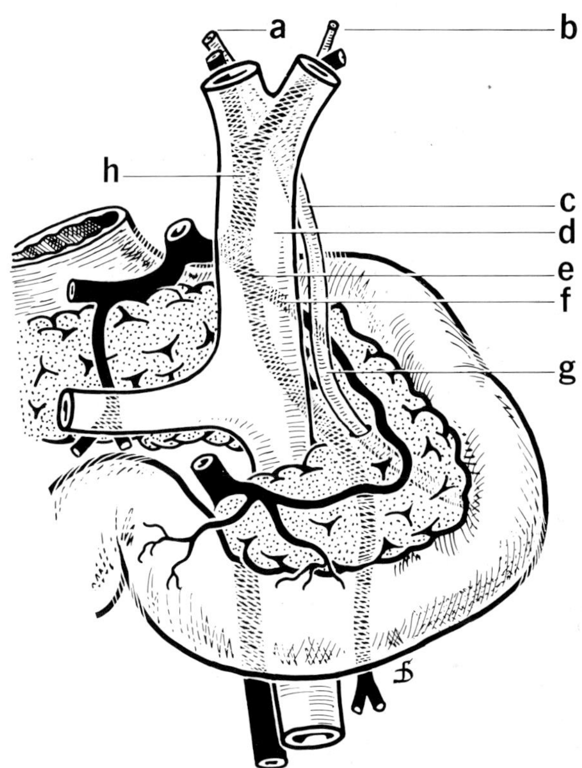

Fig. 2.9 Posterior aspect of the biliary tree: (a) left hepatic duct, (b) right hepatic duct, (c) common hepatic duct, (d) portal vein, (e) gastroduodenal artery, (f) retroduodenal artery, (g) common bile duct, (h) hepatic artery

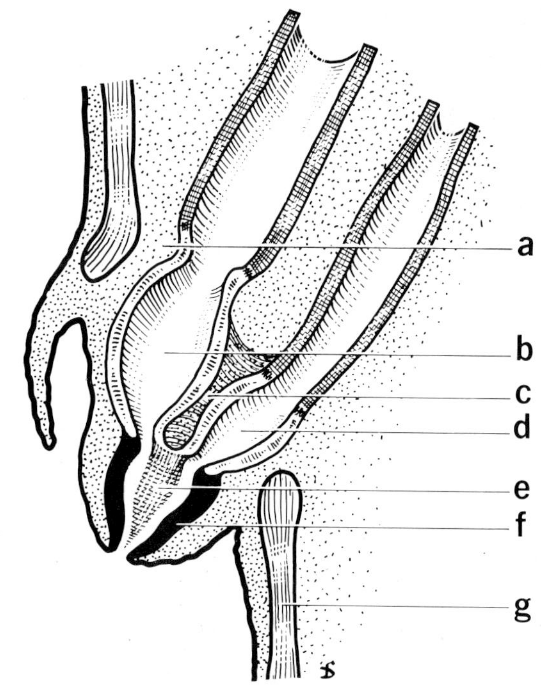

Fig. 2.10 Schematic representation of the sphincter of Oddi: (a) notch, (b) biliary sphincter, (c) transampullary septum, (d) pancreatic sphincter, (c) membranous septum of Boyden, (f) common sphincter, (g) smooth muscle of duodenal wall.

duct for some 2 cm joins it within the sphincteric segment in some 70–85% of cases (Anacker, Weiss & Kamann 1977), enters the duodenum independently in 10–13% of patients and in only 2% is replaced by the duct of Santorini (Phillip, Koch & Classen 1974). Further details of the anatomy and function of the sphincter of Oddi are found in Chapters 9, 28, 53 and 56.

Gallbladder and cystic duct

The gallbladder is a reservoir located on the undersurface of the right lobe of the liver within the cystic fossa and separated from the hepatic parenchyma by the cystic plate, which is constituted of connective tissue closely applied to Glisson's capsule and prolonging the hilar plate (see Fig. 2.7). Sometimes the gallbladder is deeply embedded in the liver but occasionally presents on a mesenteric attachment and may then be liable to volvulus. The gallbladder varies in size and consists of a fundus, a body and a neck. The tip of the fundus usually, but not always, reaches the free edge of the liver and is closely applied to the cystic plate. The cystic fossa is a precise anterior guide mark to the main liver scissura (Ch. 1). This is of major importance in the performance of right and left liver resection (Ch. 1, 97). The neck of the gallbladder makes an angle with the fundus. A large gallstone lodged in this part of the neck of the gallbladder creates a Hartmann's pouch (Wood 1979), which may obscure the common hepatic duct and constitute a real danger point during cholecystectomy (Ch. 58). Indeed erroneous common hepatic duct resection has been recorded during this step of the operation (Bismuth & Lazorthes 1981). Sometimes, freeing of the neck of the gallbladder during cholecystectomy may threaten the right branch of the hepatic artery (or an aberrant right hepatic artery) and rarely the right hepatic duct.

The cystic duct arises from the neck or infundibulum of the gallbladder and extends to join the common hepatic duct. Its lumen is usually some 1 to 3 mm. Its length is variable depending upon the type of union with the common hepatic duct (see below). The mucosa of the cystic duct is arranged in spiral folds known as the valves of Heister (Wood 1979). Its wall is surrounded by a sphincteric structure called the sphincter of Lutkens. While the cystic duct joins the common hepatic duct in its supraduodenal segment in 80% of cases (Moosman 1970), it may extend downwards to the retroduodenal or even retroprancreatic area. Occasionally the cystic duct may join the right hepatic duct or a right hepatic sectoral duct (see below) (Ch. 58).

The blood supply of the gallbladder is by the cystic artery, which has multiple variations (Fig. 2.11). Ignorance of these may provoke unexpected haemorrhage during cholecystectomy and may result in bile duct injury during efforts to secure haemostasis (Ch. 44, 58).

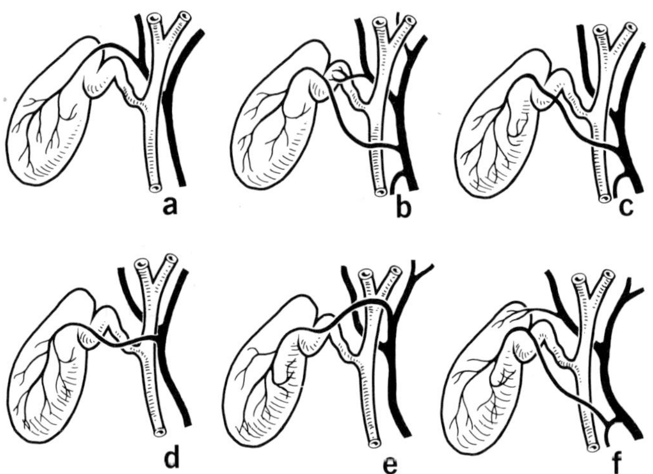

Fig. 2.11 Sketch showing the main variations of the cystic artery: (a) typical course, (b) double cystic artery, (c) cystic artery crossing anterior to main bile duct, (d) cystic artery originating from the right branch of the hepatic artery and crossing the common hepatic duct anteriorly, (e) cystic artery originating from the left branch of the hepatic artery, (f) cystic artery originating from the gastroduodenal artery

BILIARY DUCTAL ANOMALIES

Full knowledge of the frequent variations from the described normal biliary anatomy is required while performing any hepatobiliary procedure.

The constitution of a normal biliary confluence by union of the right and left hepatic ducts as described above is reported in only 57% (Couinaud 1957) to 72% (Healey & Schroy 1953) of cases. This difference in figures is probably due to the fact that the study of Healey & Schroy did not recognize a triple confluence of the right posterior sectoral duct, the right anterior sectoral duct and the left hepatic duct, recorded in 12% of instances by Couinaud (1957) (Fig. 2.12). In addition Couinaud records a right sectoral duct joining the main bile duct directly in 20% of individuals (Couinaud 1957). In 16% the right anterior sectoral duct and in 4% the right posterior sectoral duct may approach the main bile duct in this fashion. Furthermore, in 6% a right sectoral duct may join the left hepatic duct (the posterior duct in 5% and the anterior duct in 1%). In 3% there is an absence of the hepatic duct confluence and in 2% the right posterior sectoral duct may join the neck of the gallbladder or may be entered by the cystic duct (Couinaud 1957) (Fig. 2.12). Similarly, Healey & Schroy (1953) describe an ectopic drainage of the anterior sectoral duct in 22% and of the right posterior sectoral duct in 6% of cases. In any event these multiple biliary ductal variations at the hilus are important to recognize, both in resective and reconstructive surgery of the biliary tree at the hilus and also during partial hepatectomy (Ch. 97).

Intrahepatic bile duct variations are also common.

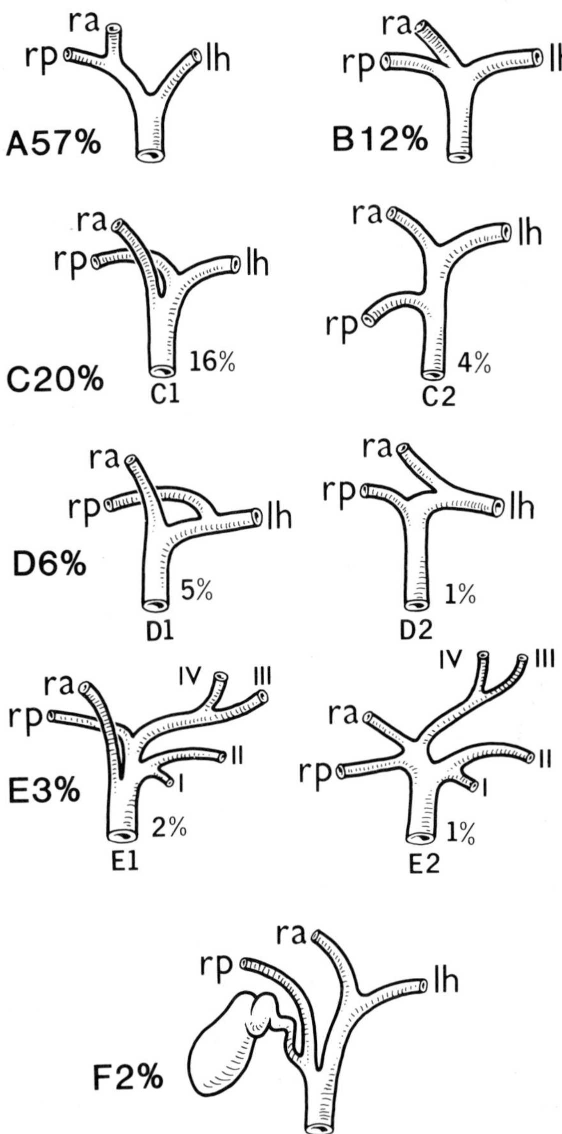

Fig. 2.12 Main variations of the hepatic duct confluence (Couinaud 1957): (A) typical anatomy of the confluence, (B) triple confluence, (C) ectopic drainage of a right sectoral duct into the common hepatic duct, (C 1) right anterior duct draining into the common hepatic duct, (C 2) right posterior ducts draining into the common hepatic duct, (D) ectopic drainage of a right sectoral duct into the left hepatic ductal system, (D 1) right posterior sectoral duct draining into the left hepatic ductal system, (D 2) right anterior sectoral duct draining into the left hepatic ductal system, (E) absence of the hepatic duct confluence, (F) absence of right hepatic duct and ectopic drainage of the right posterior duct into the cystic duct

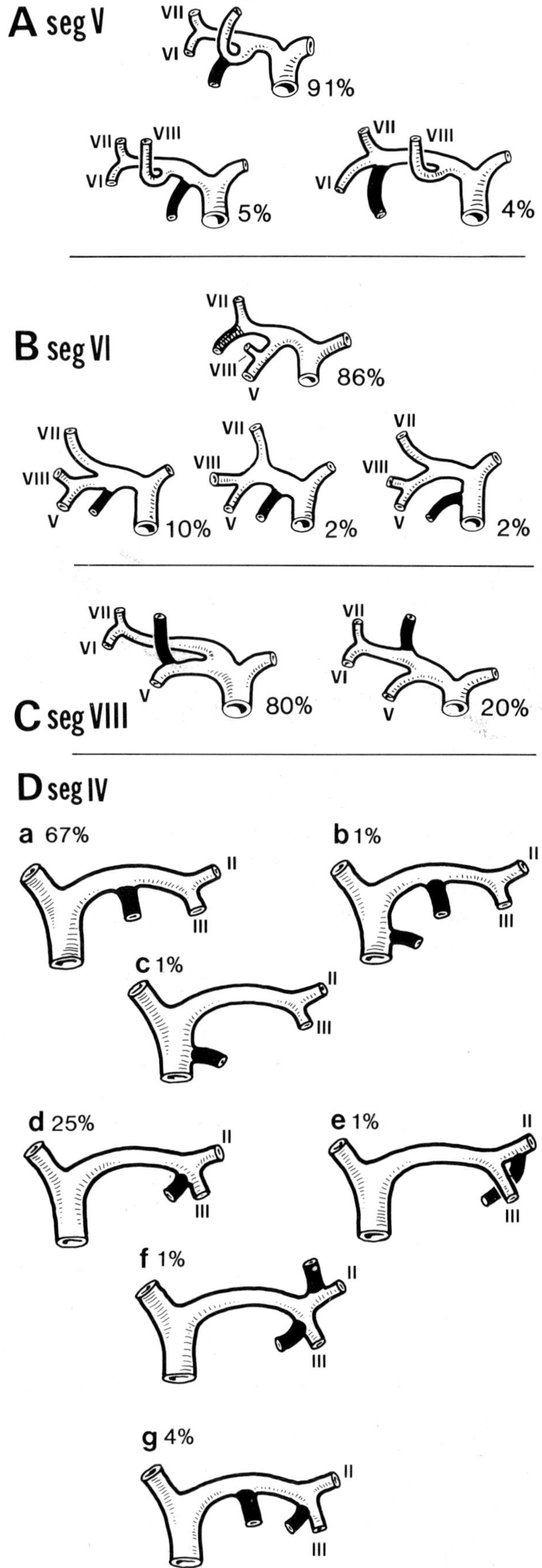

Fig. 2.13 A sketch to show the main variations of the intrahepatic ductal system (Healey & Schroy 1953): (A) variations of segment V, (B) variations of segment VI, (C) variations of segment VIII, (D) variations of segment IV. Note that there is no variation of drainage of segments II, III and VII

According to Healey & Schroy (1953) (Fig. 2.13), the main right intrahepatic duct variations are represented by an ectopic drainage of segment V in 9%, of segment VI in 14%, and of segment VIII in 20%. According to these authors there is no variation of the duct of segment VII. In addition, a subvesical duct has been described in 20% to 50% of cases (Healey & Schroy 1953, Champetier et al 1982). This duct, sometimes deeply embedded in the cystic plate, joins either the common hepatic duct or the right hepatic duct (Ch. 44). This duct does not drain any specific liver territory, never communicates with the gallbladder, and is not a satellite of an intrahepatic branch of the portal vein or hepatic artery. Although not of major anatomical significance, injury may occur during cholecystectomy if the cystic plate (see below) is not preserved and this may lead to a postoperative biliary leak (Ch. 60). Sometimes there is also injury to a branch of the portal vein.

According to Healey & Schroy (1953) (Fig. 2.13) there is in 67% of instances a classical distribution of the main left intrahepatic biliary ductal system. The main variation in this region is represented by a common union between the ducts of segment III and IV in 25%. In only 2% does the duct of segment IV join the common hepatic duct independently (Fig. 2.13).

Several anomalies of drainage of the intrahepatic ducts into the neck of gallbladder or cystic duct have been reported (Fig. 2.14) (Albaret et al 1981, Couinaud 1957) and these must be kept in mind during cholecystectomy.

Although the surgical importance of all these variations has already been emphasized, it should be mentioned that a precise knowledge is mandatory during bile duct repair following iatrogenic injury, resection of hilar cancer or the surgical treatment of intrahepatic stone disease. Analysis of hepatic cholangiography will avoid incomplete drainage of intrahepatic ducts, or residual intrahepatic stones leading to persistent postoperative cholangitis.

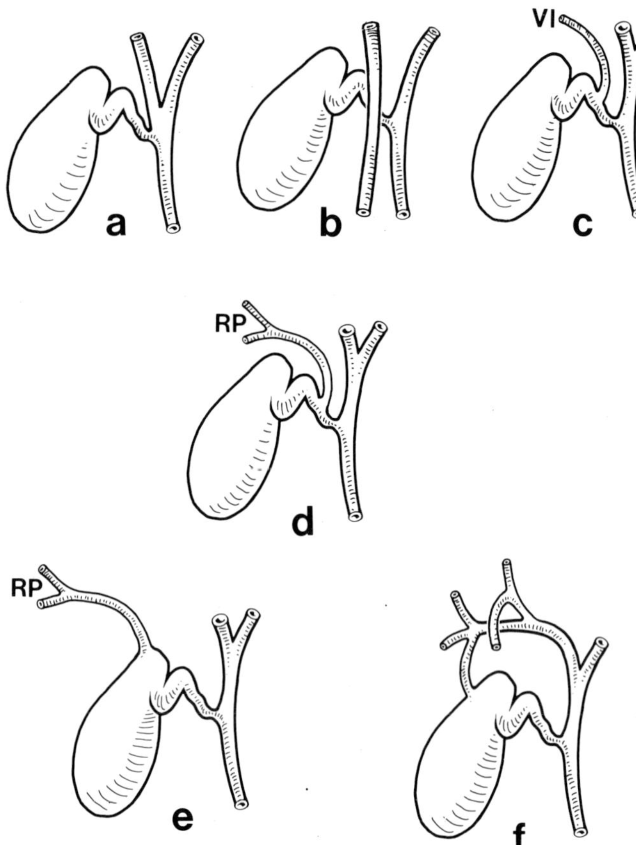

Fig. 2.14 The main variations of ectopic drainage of the intrahepatic ducts into the gallbladder and cystic duct: (a) drainage of the cystic duct into the biliary confluence, (b) drainage of cystic duct into the left hepatic duct associated with no biliary confluence, (c) drainage of segment VI duct into the cystic duct, (d) drainage of the right posterior sectoral duct into the cystic duct, (e) drainage of the distal part of the right posterior sectoral duct into the neck of the gallbladder, (f) drainage of the proximal part of the right posterior sectoral duct into the body of the gallbladder

ANOMALIES OF THE ACCESSORY BILIARY APPARATUS

A number of anomalies have been described by Gross (1936) (Fig. 2.15).

While rare, agenesis of the gallbladder (Boyden 1926, Rogers, Crews & Kalser 1975), bilobar gallbladders with a single cystic duct but two fundi (Hobby 1970) and duplication of the gallbladder with two cystic ducts (Rachad-Mohassel et al 1973) have all been described. Finally a double cystic duct may drain a unilocular gallbladder as described by Perelman (1961). Congenital diverticulum of the gallbladder with a muscular wall is also to be found (Eelkema, Staar & Good 1958).

More frequently reported are anomalies of position of the gallbladder, which may lie either in an intrahepatic position completely surrounded by normal liver tissue or may be found on the left of the liver (Newcombe & Henley 1964). This may give rise to diagnostic and technical problems (Weill et al 1983).

The mode of union of the cystic duct with the common hepatic duct may be angular, parallel or spiral (Fig. 2.16). An angular union is the most frequent and is found in 75% of patients (Kune 1970). The cystic duct may run a parallel course to the common hepatic duct in 20% with connective tissue ensheathing both ducts. Finally, the cystic duct may approach the common bile duct in a spiral fashion curving about it usually from the posterior aspect. All these anatomical variations may lead to biliary ductal injury during cholecystectomy especially if persistent attempts are made to display the union between cystic duct and the common biliary channel — a practice to be discouraged (Ch. 44, 58). The absence of a cystic duct is probably an acquired anomaly representing a choledocho-cholecystic fistula (Ch. 61, 58).

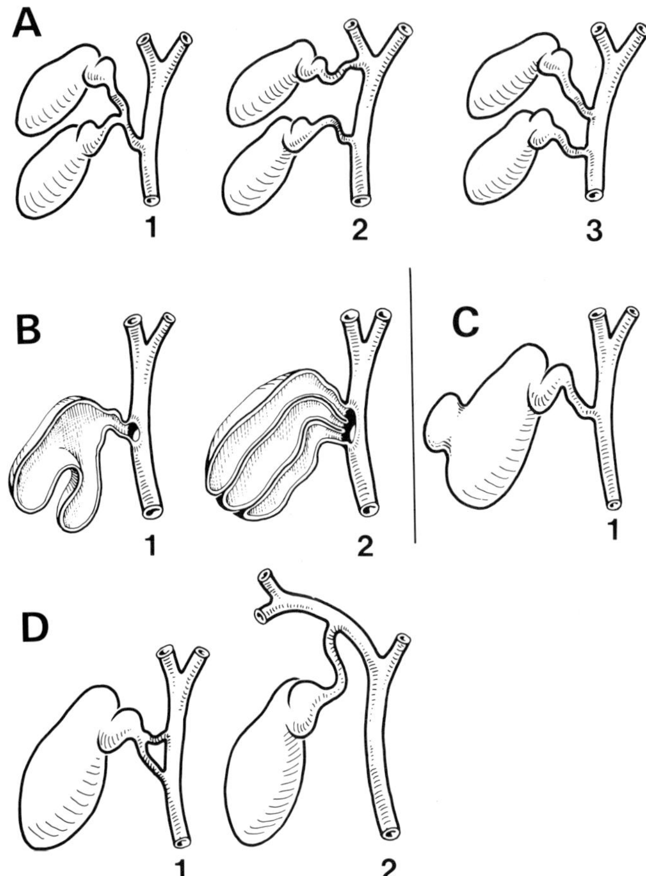

Fig. 2.15 Main variations in gallbladder and cystic duct anatomy: (A) bi-lobed gallbladder, (B) septum of the gallbladder, (C) diverticulum of the gallbladder, (D) variations in cystic ductal anatomy

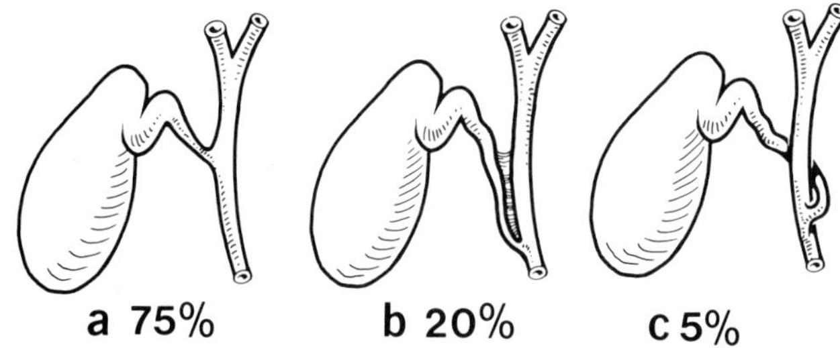

Fig. 2.16 Different types of union of the cystic duct and common hepatic duct: (a) angular union (b) parallel union (c) spiral union

BILE DUCT BLOOD SUPPLY

The blood supply of the bile duct has recently received attention (Northover & Terblanche 1979). Indeed, despite the presence of a rich biliary ductal vasculature, it is proposed that arterial damage during cholecystectomy may cause ischaemia and result in postoperative bile duct stricture (Northover & Terblanche 1982) and possibly be related to the biliary complications encountered after transplantation (Calne 1972).

It seems unlikely that ischaemia alone is a major mechanism in the causation of bile duct stricture but may be contributory especially in the retraction of the common hepatic duct seen after injury. (Ch. 58).

According to Northover & Terblanche (1979) the bile duct may be divided into three segments: hilar, supraduodenal and retropancreatic (lower common bile duct). The blood supply of the supraduodenal duct is essentially axial (Fig. 2.17): most vessels to the supraduodenal duct arise from the retroduodenal artery, the right branch of the hepatic artery, the cystic artery, the gastroduodenal artery and the retroportal artery. On average, eight small arteries measuring each about 0.3 mm diameter supply the supraduodenal duct. The most important of these vessels run along the lateral borders of the duct and have been called the 3 o'clock and 9 o'clock arteries (Fig. 2.17). 60% of the blood vessels vascularizing the supraduodenal duct run upwards from the major inferior vessels and only 38% of arteries run downwards, originating from the right branch of the hepatic artery and other vessels. Only 2% of the arterial supply is non-axial, arising directly from the main trunk of the hepatic artery as it courses up parallel to the main biliary channel. The hilar ducts receive a copious supply of arterial blood from surrounding vessels

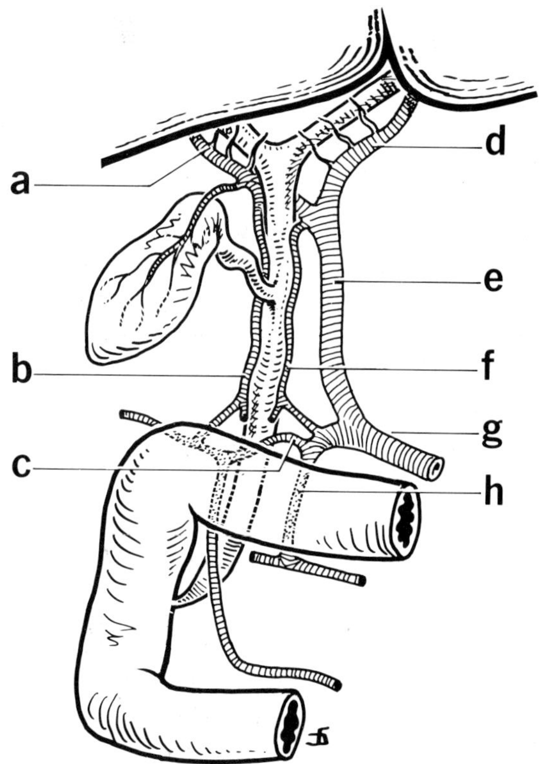

Fig. 2.17 The bile duct blood supply (Northover & Terblanche 1979). Note the axial arrangement of the vasculature of the supraduodenal portion of the main bile duct and the rich network enclosing the right and left hepatic ducts: (a) right branch of the hepatic artery, (b) 9 o'clock artery, (c) retroduodenal artery, (d) left branch of the hepatic artery, (e) hepatic artery, (f) 3 o'clock artery, (g) common hepatic artery, (h) gastroduodenal artery

forming a rich network on the surface of the ducts in continuity with the plexus around the supraduodenal duct. The source of the blood supply of the retropancreatic common bile duct is from the retroduodenal artery, which provides multiple small vessels running around the duct to form a mural plexus.

The veins draining the bile ducts are satellite to the corresponding described arteries, draining into 3 o'clock and 9 o'clock veins along the borders of the common biliary channel. Veins draining the gallbladder empty into this venous system and not directly into the portal vein. The biliary tree seems to have its own portal venous pathway to the liver (Northover & Terblanche 1982).

THE ANATOMY OF BILIARY EXPOSURE

Surgical exposure of the bile ducts, and especially the approach to the biliary ductal confluence, the left hepatic duct at the hilus and the segment III duct, are based on precise anatomical landmarks. Recently, ultrasonography (Okuda & Tsuchiya 1983), has allowed improvement in methods for the location of intrahepatic biliary radicles. Biliary-enteric bypass necessitates precise bile duct exposure in order to allow the construction of a mucosa-to-mucosa anastomosis (Bismuth et al 1978, Bismuth & Lazorthes 1981, Voyles & Blumgart 1982, Blumgart & Kelley 1984). This section deals with procedures that do not require hepatic resection and should be read in conjunction with Ch. 70.

Biliary-vascular sheaths and exposure of the hepatic bile duct confluence

The fusion of Glisson's capsule with the connective tissue sheaths surrounding the biliary and vascular elements at the inferior aspect of the liver constitute the plate system (Fig. 2.7) which includes the hilar plate above the biliary confluence, the cystic plate related to the gallbladder, and the umbilical plate situated above the umbilical portion of the left portal vein (Couinaud 1957).

Hepp & Couinaud (1956) described a technique where, by lifting the quadrate lobe upwards and incising the Glisson's capsule at its base, a good exposure of the hepatic hilar structures could be obtained (Fig. 2.8a, 2.8b). This technique was referred to as lowering of the hilar plate. It can be carried out with safety since there is only exceptionally (in 1% of cases) any vascular interposition between the hilar plate and the inferior aspect of the liver (Couinaud 1957). This manoeuvre is of particular value in exposing the extrahepatic segment of the left hepatic duct since it has a long course beneath the quadrate lobe. It is not as effective in exposing the extrahepatic right duct or its secondary branches, which are short. The technique is of major importance for the identification of proximal biliary mucosa during bile duct repair following injury (Bismuth & Lazorthes 1981, Blumgart & Kelley 1984). Basically, an incision is required at the posterior edge of the quadrate lobe where Glisson's capsule is attached to the hilar plate (Fig. 2.8c) (Ch. 70). The upper surface of the hilar plate can then be separated from the hepatic parenchyma and by lifting the quadrate lobe upwards display of the hepatic duct convergence, which is *always* extrahepatic, is effected. Bile duct incision then allows performance of a mucosa-to-mucosa anastomosis (Bismuth et al 1978, Voyles & Blumgart 1982, Blumgart & Kelley 1984). In some rare instances it may be hazardous to approach the biliary confluence in this manner especially when anatomical deformity has been created by atrophy/hypertrophy of liver lobes (Ch. 6) and in patients where there appears to be a very deep hilus which is displaced upwards and rotated laterally (Bismuth & Lazorthes 1981). Frequently by a simultaneous opening of the deepest portion of the gallbladder fossa and the umbilical fissure (Fig. 2.8c), a good exposure of the biliary duct confluence and especially the right hepatic duct can be obtained without the necessity for full hepatotomy.

The umbilical fissure and the segment III (ligamentum teres) approach

The round ligament, which is the remnant of the obliterated umbilical vein, runs through the umbilical fissure to connect with the left branch of the portal vein within the recessus of Rex (Fig. 2.18a). The termination of the round ligament is sometimes deeply embedded in the umbilical fissure. At its termination the round ligament spreads somewhat in the manner of a goose's foot, the prolongations containing small channels which are elements of the left portal system. The bile ducts of the left lobe of the liver (Fig. 2.3, Fig. 2.18a) are located above the left branch of the portal vein and lying behind these prolongations, whereas the corresponding artery is situated below the vein. Dissection of the round ligament on its *left* side with division of one or two fibrous and usually vascular prolongations allows display of the pedicle or anterior branch of the duct of segment III (Fig. 2.18b). (Soupault & Couinaud 1957) (Ch. 70).

The procedure is carried out by mobilizing the round ligament and pulling it downwards, freeing it from the depths of the umbilical fissure (Fig. 2.18b). The umbilical fissure is opened and this often requires preliminary division of a bridge of liver tissue which usually runs between segments IV and III. This manoeuvre with downward traction of the ligamentum teres allows exposure on its left side of an anterior branch of the segment III duct (Fig. 2.18b). However, it may be necessary to perform a superficial left liver split in order to gain access to the duct. In the event of biliary obstruction with intrahepatic biliary ductal dilatation, the segment III duct is generally easily

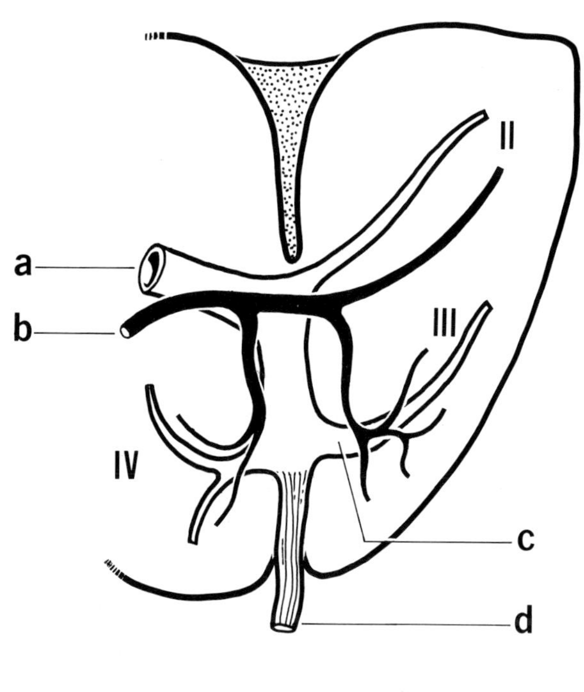

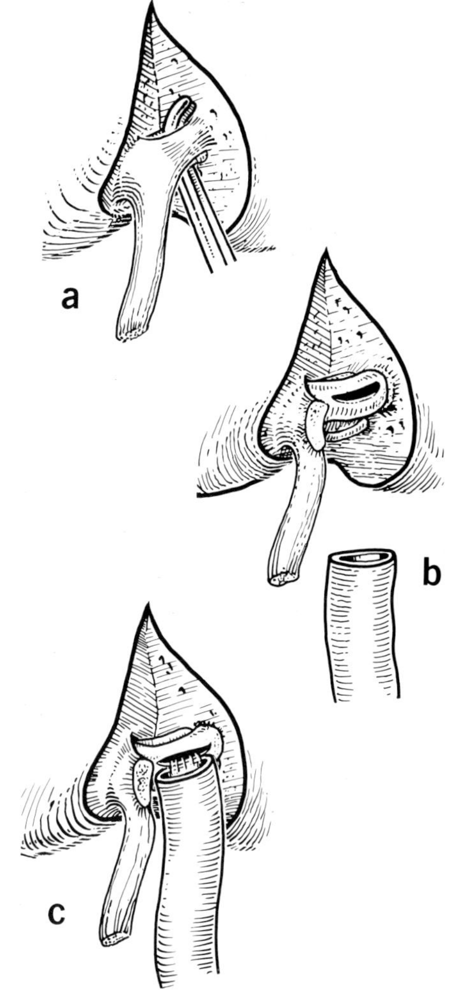

Fig. 2.18 A. The biliary and vascular anatomy of the left liver. Note the relationship of the left horn of the umbilical recess with the segment III ductal system: (a) left portal vein, (b) left hepatic duct, (c) segment III system, note the duct (black) lies adjacent to the portal venous branch indicated (d) ligamentum teres. **B.** Segment III ductal approach: (a) exposure of the left horn of the umbilical recess, (b) division of the left horn of the umbilical recess. Exposure and opening of segment III duct: (c) hepaticojejunostomy using the segment III ductal system

located above the left branch of the portal vein. Sometimes, however, in the case of left liver hypertrophy, it may be necessary to split the normal liver tissue more extensively just to the left of the umbilical fissure in order to widen the fissure further and allow access to the ductal system.

Surgical approaches to the right hepatic biliary ductal system

Because of the lack of precise anatomical guide marks, exposure of the right intrahepatic ductal system is much more hazardous and imprecise than the left. Recently, however, peroperative ultrasonography has afforded improvement in the localization of dilated intrahepatic ductal radicles. Bleeding which may be difficult to control and the poor bile duct exposure obtained through this approach has led many to abandon the technique but some surgeons (Smith & Sherlock 1964, Nagasue et al 1983) have renewed interest in this approach.

The gallbladder is separated from the liver and the cystic plate incised. In order to detect the right intrahepatic duct, needle puncture is first carried out. Once this is localized, a longitudinal incision is made through the liver substance down to the duct and bypass performed (Nagasue et al 1983) (Fig. 2.19).

Exposure of the bile ducts by liver resection

This chapter does not detail exposure of the bile ducts by resection of liver substance, details of which are to be found in Chapter 70. However, in essence a segment of the left lobe may be amputated to expose the segments II or III ducts (Longmire & Sandford 1949) or a similar procedure carried out after removal of the inferior tip of the right lobe. Finally, in some instances removal of the quadrate lobe (Blumgart, Drury & Wood 1979) may be carried out to effect exposure of the biliary confluence. This procedure really represents a simple extension of the mobilization of the quadrate lobe after opening of the principal scissura and the umbilical fissure as described above (Ch. 70).

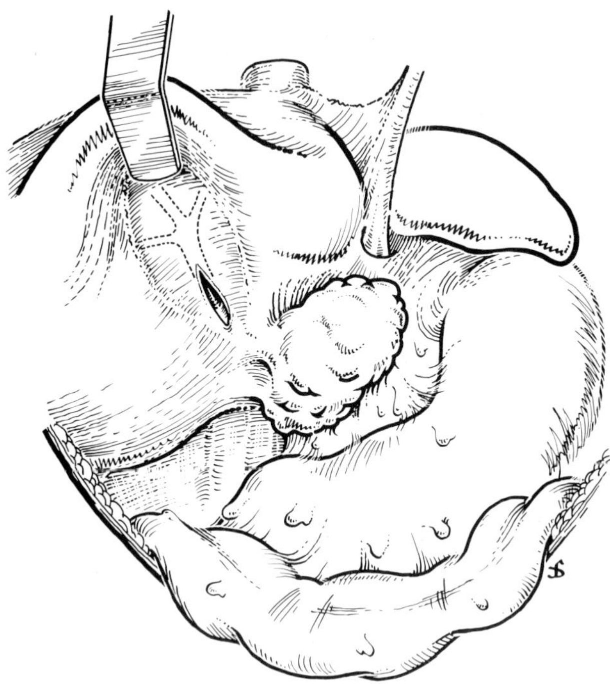

Fig. 2.19 Illustration of the right intrahepatic ductal approach through the gallbladder bed (Nagasue et al 1983)

REFERENCES

Albaret P, Chevalier J M, Cronier P, Enon B, Moreau O, Pillet J 1981 A propos des canaux hépatiques directement abouchés dans la voie biliaire accessoire. Annales de Chirurgie 35: 88–92

Anacker H, Weiss H D, Kamann B 1977 Endoscopic retrograde pancreatico-cholangiography (ERCP). Springer, Berlin

Bismuth H, Franco D, Corlette N B, Hepp J 1978 Long term results of Roux-en-Y hepaticojejunostomy. Surgery, Gynecology and Obstetrics 146: 161–167

Bismuth H, Lazorthes F 1981 Les traumatismes opératoires de la voie biliaire principale. Vol 1. Masson, Paris

Blumgart L H, Drury J K, Wood C B 1979 Hepatic resection for trauma, tumour and biliary obstruction. British Journal of Surgery 66: 762–769

Blumgart L H, Kelley C J 1984 Hepaticojejunostomy in benign and malignant high bile duct stricture: approaches to the left hepatic ducts. British Journal of Surgery 71: 257–261

Blumgart L H, Hadjis N S, Benjamin I S, Beazley R 1984 Surgical approaches to cholangiocarcinoma at confluence of hepatic ducts. Lancet 1: 66–70

Boyden E A 1926 The accessory gallbladder. An embryological and comparative study of aberrant biliary vesicles occurring in man and the domestic mammals. American Journal of Anatomy 38: 177–231

Boyden E A 1957 The anatomy of the choledochoduodenal junction in man. Surgery, Gynecology and Obstetrics 104: 641–652

Calne R Y 1972 Observations on experimental and clinical liver transplantation. Transplantation Proceedings 4: 773–779

Champetier J, Davin J L, Yver R, Vigneau B, Letoublon C 1982 Aberrant biliary ducts (vasa aberrantia): Surgical implications. Anatomica Clinica 4: 137–145

Couinaud C 1957 Le foie. Etudes anatomiques et chirurgicales. Vol 1. Masson, Paris

Delmont J 1979 Le sphincter d'Oddi: Anatomie traditionelle et fonctionnelle. Gastroéntrologie Clinique et Biologique 3: 157–165

Eelkema H H, Staar G F, Good C A 1958 Partial duplication of the gallbladder, diverticulum type. Report of a case. Radiology 70: 410–412

Gross R E 1936 Congenital anomalies of the gallbladder. A review of a hundred and forty-eight cases with report of a double gallbladder. Archives of Surgery 32: 131–162

Hasegawa H 1984 Personal communication.

Healey J E, Schroy P C 1953 Anatomy of the biliary ducts within the human liver. Analysis of the prevailing pattern of branchings and the major variations of the biliary ducts. American Medical Association Archives of Surgery 66: 599–616

Hepp J, Couinaud C 1956 L'abord et l'utilisation du canal hépatique gauche dans les réparations de la voie biliaire principale. Presse Médicale 64: 947–948

Hjortsjö C H 1951 The topography of the intrahepatic duct systems. Acta Anatomica 11: 599–615

Hobby J A E 1979 Bilobed gallbladder. British Journal of Surgery 57: 870–872

Kune G A 1970 The influence of structure and function in the surgery of the biliary tract. Annals of the Royal College of Surgeons of England 47: 78–91

Longmire W P Jr. Sandford M C 1949 Intrahepatic cholangiojejunostomy for biliary obstruction — further studies: Report of 4 cases. Annals of Surgery 130: 455–460

Moosman D A 1970 The surgical significance of six anomalies of the biliary duct system. Surgery, Gynecology and Obstetrics 131: 665–660

Nagasue N, Hirose S, Yukaya H 1983 Right hepatic duct-duodenostomy in the treatment of non resectable carcinoma of the hepatic hilus. Chirurgia Epato Biliare 2: 36–67

Newcombe J F, Henley F A 1964 Left-sided gallbladder. A review of the literature and a report of a case associated with hepatic duct carcinoma. Archives of Surgery 88: 494–497

Northover J M A, Terblanche J 1979 A new look at the arterial blood supply of the bile duct in man and its surgical implications. British Journal of Surgery 66: 379–384

Northover J M A, Terblanche J 1982 Applied surgical anatomy of the biliary tree. In: Blumgart L H (ed) Biliary tract, Vol 5. Churchill Livingstone, Edinburgh

Okuda K, Tsuchiya Y 1983 Ultrasonic anatomy of the biliary system. Clinics in Gastroenterology 12: 49–63

Perelman H 1961 Cystic duct reduplication. Journal of the American Medical Association 175: 710–711

Phillip J, Koch H, Classen M 1974 Variations and anomalies of the papilla of vater, the pancreas and the biliary duct system. Endoscopy 6: 70–77

Rachad-Mohassel M A, Baghieri F, Maghsoudi H, Nik Akhtar B 1973 Duplication de la vésicule biliaire. Archives Françaises des Maladies de l'Appareil Digestif 62: 679–683

Rocko J M, Swan K G, Di Gioia J M 1981 Calot's triangle revisited. Surgery, Gynecology and Obstetrics 153: 410–414

Rogers H I, Crews R D, Kalser M H 1975 Congenital absence of the gallbladder with choledocholithiasis. Literature review and discussion of mechanisms. Gastroenterology 48: 524–529

Smith R, Sherlock S 1964 Surgery of the gallbladder and bile ducts. Butterworth, London

Soupault R, Couinaud C 1957 Sur un procédé nouveau de dérivation bilaire intra-hépatique. Les cholangio-jéjunostomies gauches sans sacrifice hépatique. Presse Médicale 65: 1157–1159

Ton That Tung 1979 Les résections majeures et mineures du foie, Vol 1. Masson, Paris

Voyles C R, Blumgart L H 1982 A technique for construction of high biliary-enteric anastomoses. Surgery, Gynecology and Obstetrics 154: 885–887

Weill G, Quilichini F, Comiti J, Arnaud A, Vinson M F 1983 Cholécystites aigues lithiasiques intra-hépatiques. A propos d'un cas. Journal de Chirurgie 20: 111–113

Wood D 1979 Eponyms in biliary tract surgery. American Journal of Surgery 138: 746–754

3

A. P. Hemingway, R. N. Gibson

Radiological anatomy of the liver and biliary tract

INTRODUCTION

This chapter will outline the anatomy of the liver and biliary system as demonstrated by a variety of radiological imaging techniques. Although individual techniques are discussed in detail elsewhere, this section is intended to indicate the areas in which each respective modality is of greatest benefit in demonstrating anatomical detail.

PLAIN RADIOGRAPHY

The radiographic identification of any structure depends on the differential attenuation of the X-ray beam by that structure and the surrounding tissues. The 'true' borders of the normal liver can only be identified if outlined against fat or fat-containing tissue, such as the extraperitoneal, retroperitoneal, properitoneal and intraperitoneal fat (Gelfand 1983). The true lateral margin of the right lobe of the liver is usually delineated by properitoneal fat as far as its inferior angle. The visceral surface of the liver faces downwards, posteriorly and to the left; the inclination of this surface determines how well this inferior surface is seen on a plain radiograph (Fig. 3.1). The inferior margin of the left lobe of the liver is only rarely seen on the plain radiograph (Bowley & Malmud 1986).

In the absence of supradiaphragmatic or subdiaphragmatic disease the position of the superior surface of the right lobe of the liver can be inferred from the position of the gas/tissue interface between the lungs and the diaphragm.

A common, normal variant of liver structure, a Reidel's lobe, is also frequently visible on the plain radiograph. Other structures are not normally identified unless calcified, abnormal or diseased. The plain abdominal radiograph will of course reveal the site of the gallbladder when cholelithiasis is present (Fig. 3.2a), when the bile is radio-opaque ('limey bile'), or when its wall is calcified (porcelain gallbladder) (Fig. 3.2b). Hepatomegaly can be inferred from the plain film because of its effects on other structures, such as diaphragmatic elevation, or colonic and renal displacement. Similarly disease in the surrounding organs may temporarily displace or distort the normal contours of the liver.

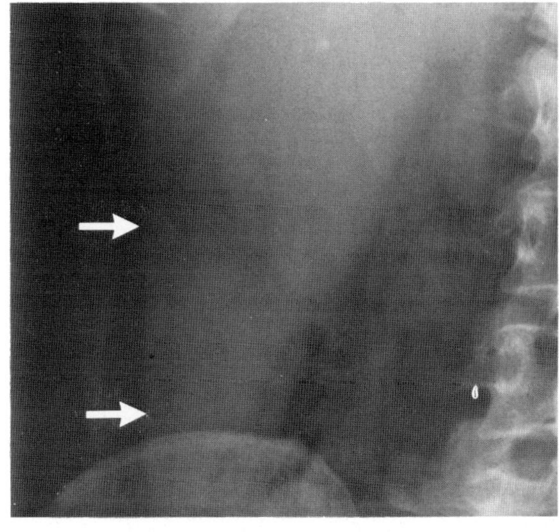

Fig. 3.1 Plain abdominal radiograph showing the liver outline delineated by fat (arrows). This patient has a Reidel's lobe

The plain radiograph may also provide clues to disease relevant to the patient's presenting condition, e.g. splenomegaly or pancreatic calcification may provide valuable information in patients with portal hypertension. Gas within the biliary tree (Fig. 3.3) may indicate the presence of disease or previous surgery.

ULTRASOUND

Ultrasound of the liver and biliary tract is discussed in great detail in Chapter 14. The advantage of this modality is that it is non-invasive and does not employ ionizing radiation. A knowledge of cross-sectional anatomy is essential for both the radiologist performing and interpreting

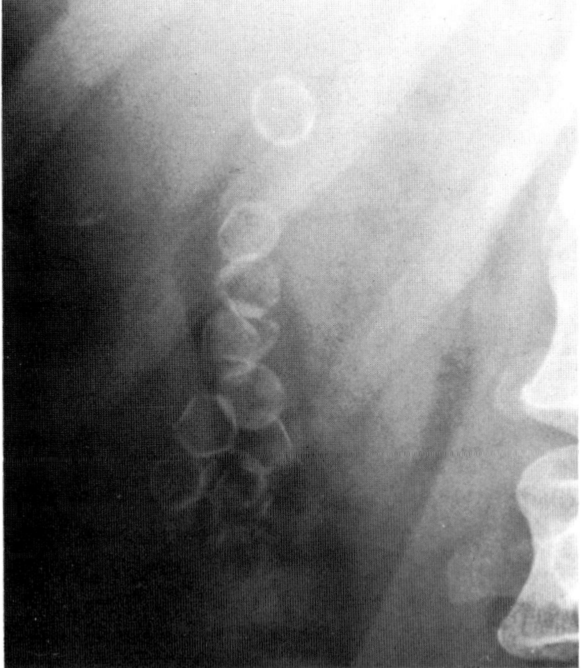

a

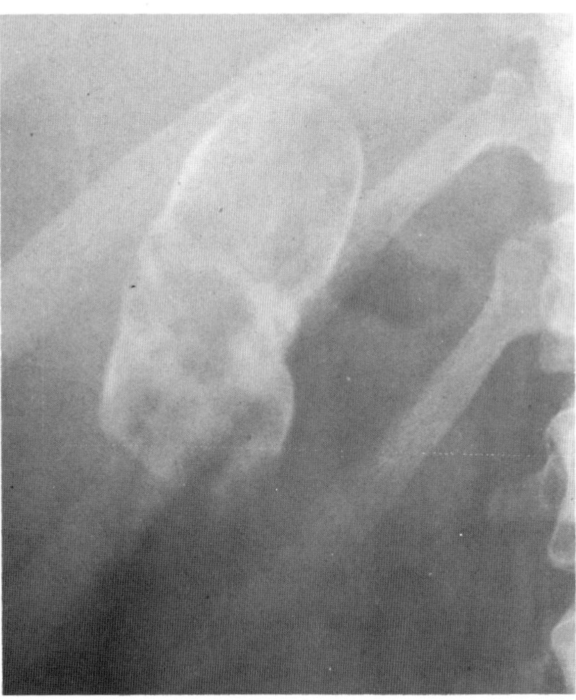

b

Fig. 3.2 a. Plain abdominal film showing faceted, opaque gallstones in the right hypochondrium; b. plain film showing calcification in the wall of the gallbladder (porcelain gallbladder)

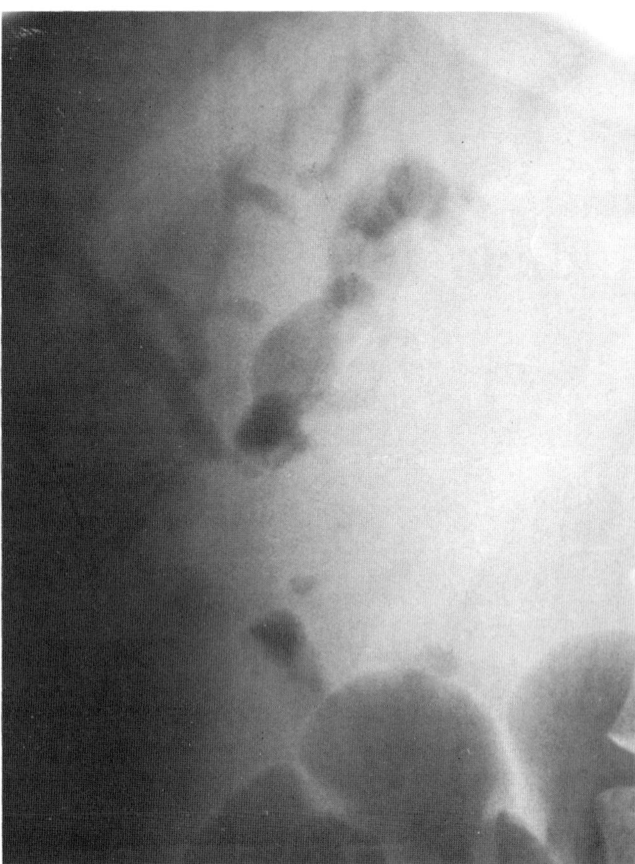

Fig. 3.3 Gas within the biliary tree from a choledochoduodenal fistula; some of the ducts are dilated

the scan and the clinician viewing the images. A detailed knowledge of biliary anatomy and vascular anatomy is also necessary when interpreting ultrasound examinations if the maximum possible information is to be obtained from the scan. The segmental anatomy of the liver and biliary tree has been discussed in detail in Chapters 1 & 2 and the same nomenclature (Couinaud 1957) will be employed throughout this chapter when referring to liver segments and bile ducts. Arterial and venous anatomy is discussed below. It is essential that the scan plane is indicated on the image produced or in the report as scans may be obtained in the longitudinal, transverse or oblique planes. Ultrasound is able to demonstrate vascular and biliary structures, as well as parenchymal detail.

The gallbladder and bile ducts

The normal gallbladder is demonstrated on ultrasound as a thin-walled echolucent structure lying infero-medially to the right lobe of the liver. Folds within the gallbladder wall may sometimes be detected and should not be mistaken for pathology (Fig. 3.4). A number of anomalies of gallbladder development exist, some of which may be detectable or at least suspected on ultrasound examination. *Agenesis* is very rare occurring in about 0.03 to 0.07% of the population; it is associated with other congenital defects such as imperforate anus, rectovaginal fistula and absence of one or more bones (Bowley et al 1986). *Double gallbladder* is rare occurring in 1 in 4000 cases; the organs

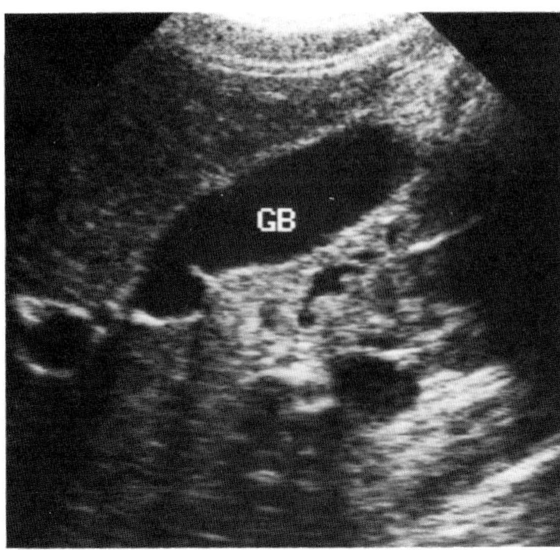

Fig. 3.4 Oblique ultrasound scan through the right hypochondrium showing a normal gallbladder (GB) lying infero-medially to the right lobe of the liver

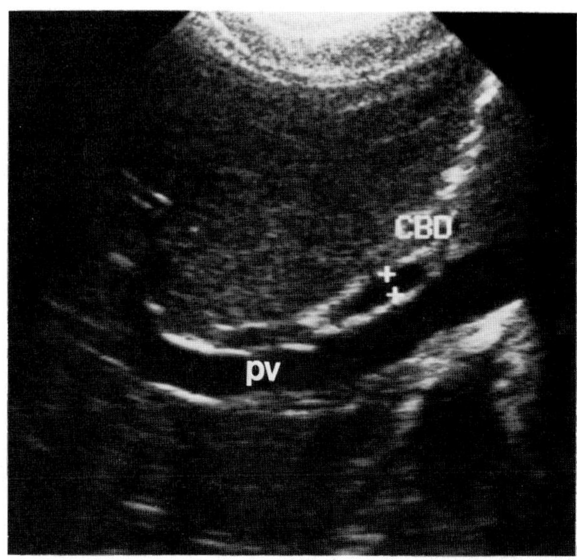

Fig. 3.5 Oblique ultrasound scan obtained with the patient in the right anterior oblique projection. The common bile duct (CBD) is visualized anterior to the portal vein (PV). The CBD measures 4 mm in diameter

may have separate cystic ducts or more commonly share a duct. *Anomalous intrahepatic ducts* may drain into the gallbladder, and are of significance at cholecystectomy. Hayes et al (1985) detected such ducts in 7–14% of biliary operations. *Diverticula* of the gallbladder may occur in the fundus, body and neck of the gallbladder and must be differentiated from Rokitansky-Aschoff sinuses which are usually multiple. The gallbladder is *intrahepatic* up to the second month of intra-uterine life. When this position persists into adult life the gallbladder is frequently diseased. The detection of this anomaly is important in any patient who is to undergo percutaneous biliary puncture or drainage. Occasionally, the gallbladder may be in a retrohepatic or suprahepatic position or may even be left-sided.

The cystic duct is not usually seen in the non-dilated state but the knowledge that it may have an anomalous communication with the common duct must be borne in mind when examining patients prior to intervention or surgery in this area. The cystic duct is usually short but in a proportion of patients may be as long as 25 mm. The cystic duct may also enter the right or left hepatic ducts which may then be damaged at surgery if this anomaly is not recognized.

The confluence of left and right hepatic ducts and the common ducts should be demonstrable on ultrasound examination in the normal non-dilated state. The extra-hepatic ducts are most reliably identified in the right anterior oblique projection (Behan 1978). In this projection the common duct (it is not usually possible to distinguish between common hepatic and common bile ducts) lies ventral to the portal vein, and allows both to be identified on the same image (Fig. 3.5). The diameter of the normal common duct, as shown on ultrasound, has been the subject of some debate with reports ranging from 1–4 mm (Cooperberg 1978) to 8 mm (Koeningsberg 1979). It would seem that ducts measuring between 6 and 8 mm fall into a grey area between the upper limit of normal and marginal dilatation. The right and left intrahepatic ducts are identified ventral to the branches of the portal venous system. Calibres of between 1 and 3 mm for the main ducts are within normal limits.

Vascular structures

Ultrasound plays an important role in the identification of vascular structures. It is possible to identify the coeliac axis as it arises from the aorta (Fig. 3.6) and its division into splenic and hepatic arteries. It is important to be aware of and look for normal anatomical variants. By far the most important common arterial anomaly is that the right hepatic artery arises from the superior mesenteric artery and this variant is detectable on ultrasound. Prior knowledge of this anomaly is important in biliary or hepatic surgery.

Details of portal anatomy can be readily demonstrated on ultrasound. The main portal vein is seen on transverse section anterior to the aorta and inferior vena cava (IVC), and posterior to the hepatic artery and common bile duct (Fig. 3.7). In an oblique plane the division of the right vein into anterior and posterior trunks is also visualized (Fig. 3.8). It is possible to identify intrahepatic portal branches. The main branches follow the same segmental pattern as the bile ducts and can be numbered in the same way (Fig. 3.9).

The systemic veins can also be visualized. On a high

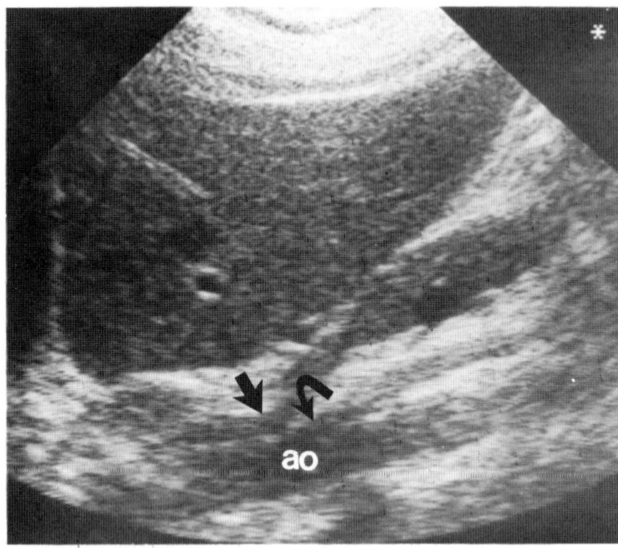

Fig. 3.6 Longitudinal ultrasound scan showing the coeliac axis (arrow) and superior mesenteric artery (curved arrow) arising from the aorta (ao)

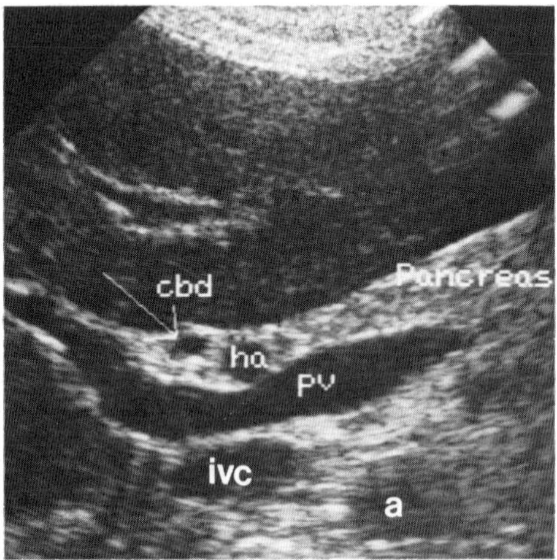

Fig. 3.7 Oblique transverse section of the upper abdomen shows the relationship of the portal vein (pv), to the hepatic artery (ha), common bile duct (cbd), inferior vena cava (ivc) and aorta (a)

transverse section the confluence of the three main hepatic veins with the IVC can be demonstrated (Fig. 3.10). In longitudinal section it is possible to demonstrate the 'normal' narrowing of the IVC as it passes behind the caudate lobe (Fig. 3.11).

A normal appearance on ultrasound which must not be interpreted as representing pathology is the well-defined area of bright echoes caused by the ligamentum teres (Fig. 3.12).

COMPUTERIZED TOMOGRAPHY (CT)

This subject is covered in detail in Chapter 16. Computerized tomography has the advantage over many other imaging modalities in that it is able to demonstrate all

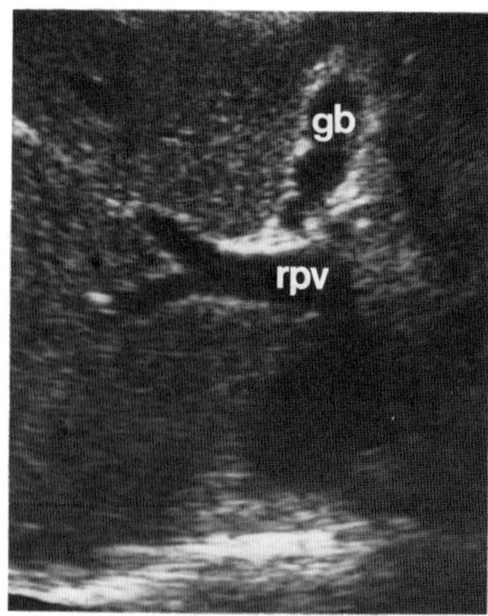

Fig. 3.8 An oblique ultrasound scan through the liver shows the division of the main right portal vein (rpv) into anterior and posterior sectoral trunks. The neck of the gallbladder (gb) is seen anteriorly

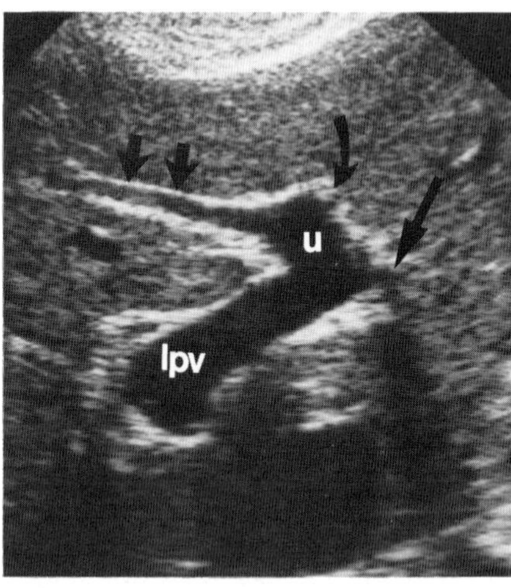

Fig. 3.9 Ultrasound scan. Transverse section through the left portal vein showing its branching pattern which follows the same segmental distribution as the bile ducts. lpv = left portal vein; u = umbilical portion of left portal vein. Segment II duct (long arrow), segment III duct (curved arrow), segment IV duct (double arrow)

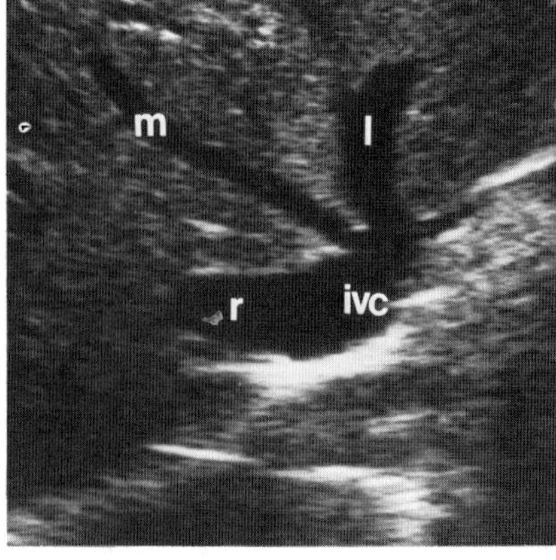

Fig. 3.10 Ultrasound scan. High transverse section through the liver shows the confluence of the right (r), middle (m) and left (l) hepatic veins with the inferior vena cava (ivc)

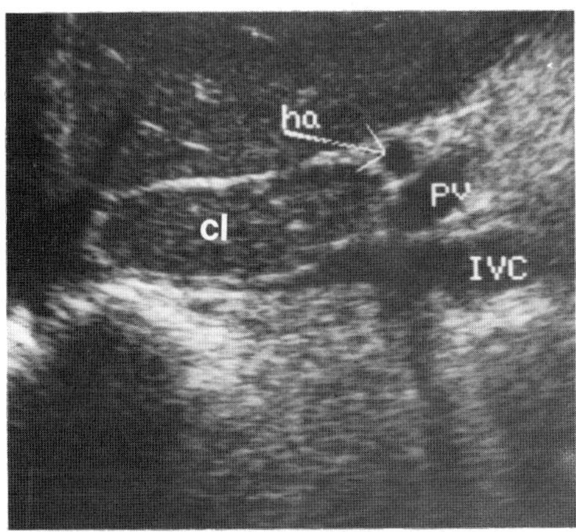

Fig. 3.11 Ultrasound scan. Longitudinal section just to the right of the midline shows the inferior vena cava (ivc) passing behind the caudate lobe (cl). The portal vein (pv) and hepatic artery (ha) are also seen. The bright echoes immediately anterior to the caudate lobe and dividing it from the rest of the liver substance represent the fissure for the ligamentum venosum

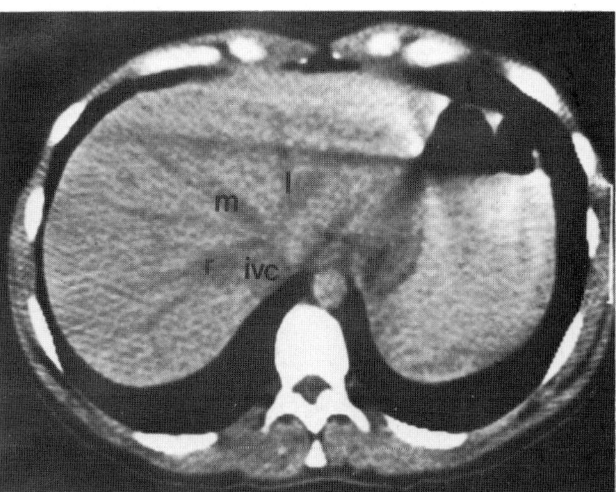

Fig. 3.13 CT scan through the upper abdomen shows the liver surrounded by lung. The confluence of the right (r), middle (m) and left (l) hepatic veins with the inferior vena cava (ivc) is seen.

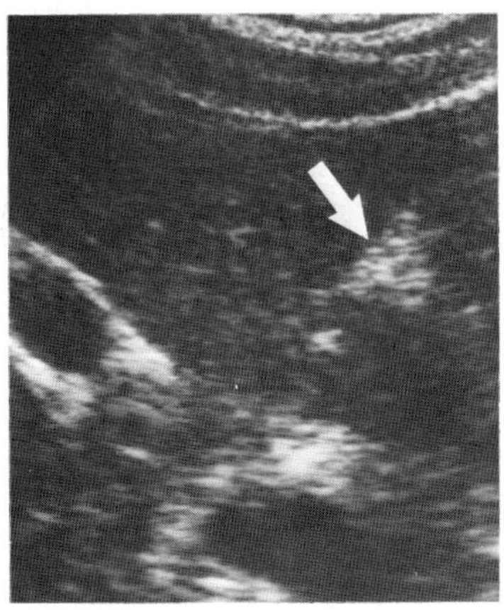

Fig. 3.12 Ultrasound scan. Transverse section through the liver showing the bright echoes caused by the ligamentum teres (arrow)

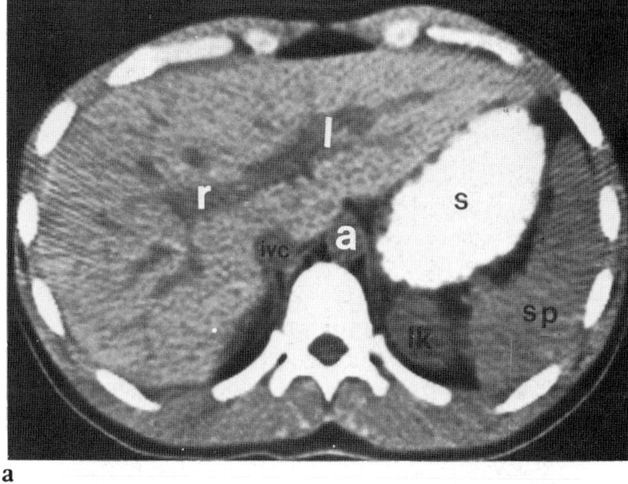

a

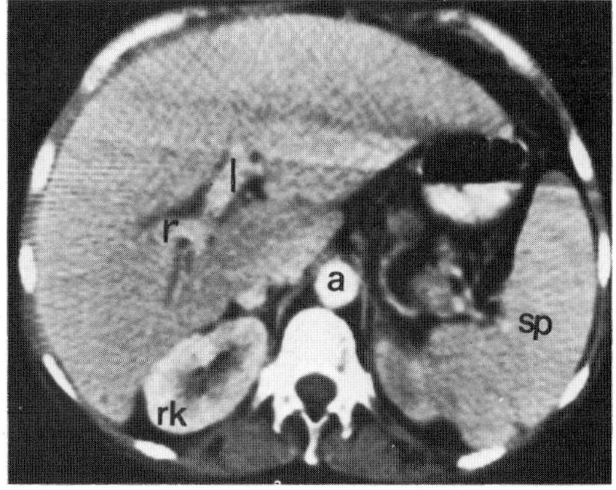

b

Fig. 3.14 a. Unenhanced CT scan through the main body of the liver shows the left (l) and right (r) portal veins as dark (low attenuation) structures in a lighter (high attenuation) background. The relationship of the liver to the inferior vena cava (ivc), the aorta (a), stomach (s), spleen (sp) and left kidney (lk) is clearly shown b. CT scan through the liver following enhancement with intravenous contrast medium. The portal veins now appear as high attenuation (light) structures

structures (bone, soft tissues and fluid) at the level being imaged and demonstrates very clearly the relations of the liver to the surrounding organs. Intravenous contrast medium can be employed to aid in the visualization of vascular structures. Normally the entire liver is examined in contiguous slices (8–10 mm). As with ultrasound, a detailed knowledge of cross-sectional anatomy is required. A high cut through the liver shows the dome of the right lobe surrounded by lung. The confluence of the hepatic veins as they enter the IVC is visualized (Fig. 3.13). A cut through the main body of the liver will usually demonstrate the main portal venous radicles, these appear as low attenuation (dark) structures in a high attenuation (light) background (Fig. 3.14a); following the administration of intravenous contrast medium this contrast difference is reversed (Fig. 3.14b). The main left portal vein frequently appears to pass directly forward from the bifurcation (Fig. 3.14b) and indeed its umbilical portion runs ventrally

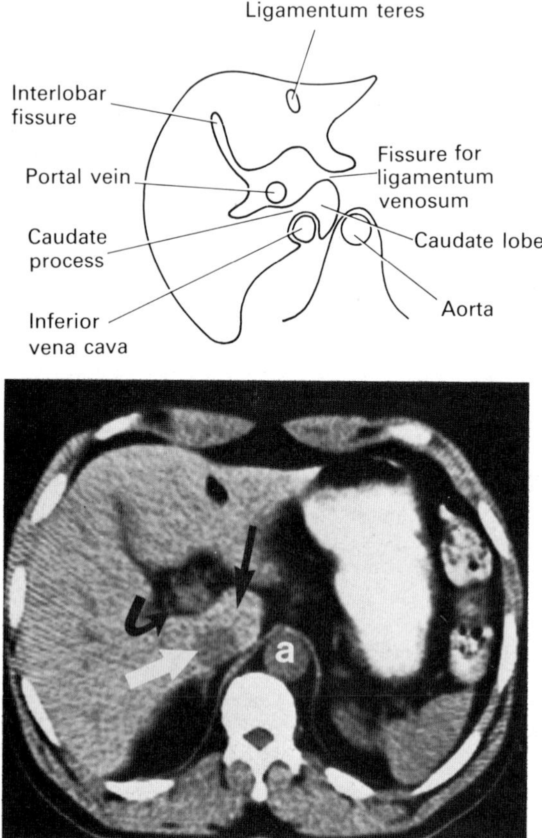

Fig. 3.15 Unenhanced CT scan through the liver which demonstrates very clearly the intimate relationship between the caudate lobe (black arrow), inferior vena cava (white arrow) and portal vein (curved arrow)

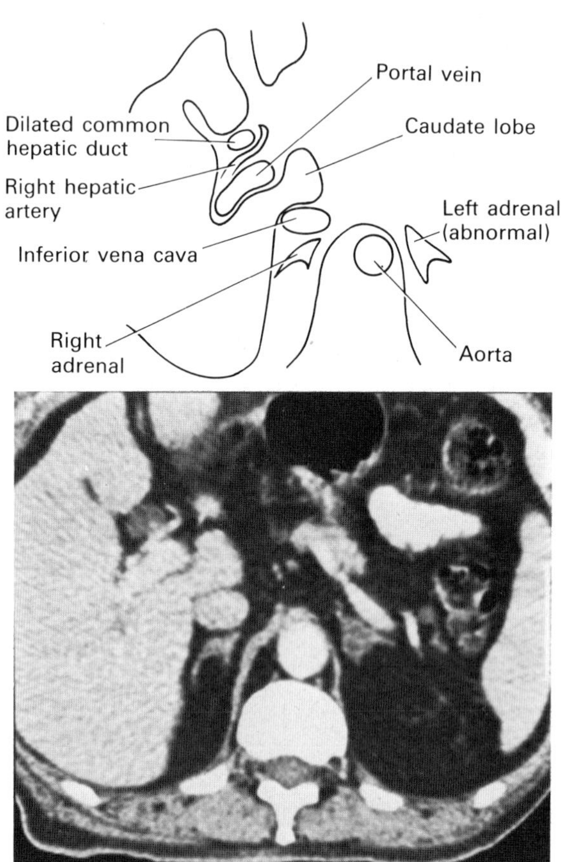

Fig. 3.16 Enhanced CT scan through the liver showing the relationship of the common hepatic duct, right hepatic artery and portal vein to each other and to the caudate lobe and inferior vena cava

and caudally. This may produce a very confusing appearance on portal venography (See below).

Slightly lower cuts demonstrate the relationships of the liver to the IVC, portal vein, right hepatic artery, common bile duct and adrenal glands (Figs. 3.15 & 3.16). A 'slice' through the gallbladder delineates the division between the right and left liver (Fig. 3.17). Low cuts through the uncinate process of the pancreas (Fig. 3.18) show the relationship of the common bile duct to the pancreatic duct.

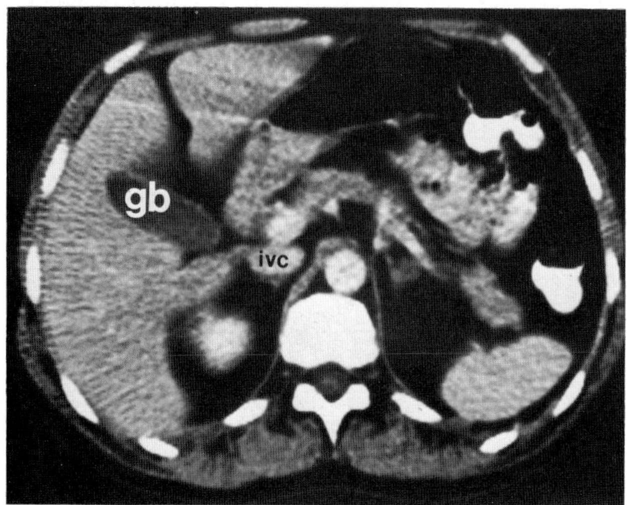

Fig. 3.17 Enhanced CT scan through the liver showing the gallbladder (gb). A line drawn through the gallbladder and the inferior vena cava (ivc) delineates the boundary between the right and left liver

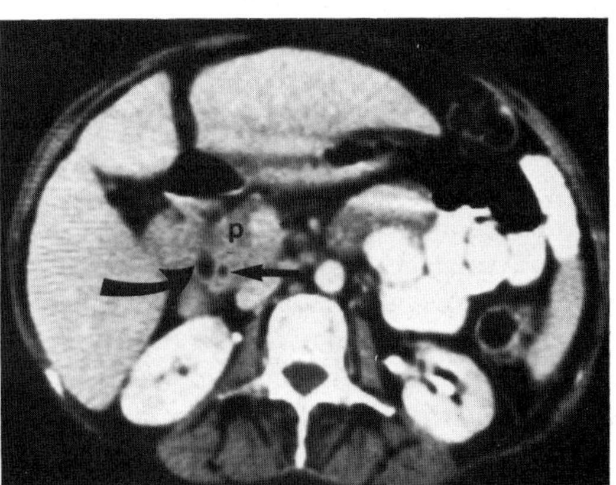

Fig. 3.18 Enhanced CT scan shows the common bile duct (curved arrow) and pancreatic duct (straight arrow) in the head of the pancreas (p)

MAGNETIC RESONANCE IMAGING (MRI) (See Chapter 17)

Because the principals of image formation in MRI are completely different from those of CT, the appearances of the many structures related to the liver are different; their anatomy and relationships are, however, unchanged and the accurate interpretation of the images again depends on a knowledge of cross-sectional anatomy.

SCINTIGRAPHY (See Chapter 15)

Only gross anatomical detail can be demonstrated on a sulphur colloid isotope liver scan. In the anterior view the liver is seen to occupy most of the space between the diaphragm and the costal margin. The falciform ligament may be identified as an area of decreased isotope uptake and the gallbladder fossa appears as an indentation on the inferior surface of the liver (Fig. 3.19) (Herlinger et al 1986). Gross intrahepatic and extrahepatic biliary anatomy may be demonstrated by ^{99m}Tc-HIDA studies, but this is predominantly a functional rather than an anatomical investigation.

CHOLANGIOGRAPHY (Lunderquist 1983)

As with any radiological examination the aim of the study is usually to demonstrate the presence or absence of pathology. When performing a cholangiogram it is essential therefore to have a knowledge of ductal anatomy and to attempt to delineate *all* the major branches. Failure to do so can lead to a missed or mis-diagnosis. A knowledge of this anatomy also enables one to detect anatomical variants which may have very important surgical implications. The detailed anatomy of the biliary tract is discussed in chapters 1 and 2. The common hepatic duct is formed by the junction of the right and left hepatic ducts (Fig. 3.20) in approximately 57% of patients (Couinaud 1957). In a further 13% of cases the right hepatic duct is absent and the common duct is formed by the junction of the right anterior and posterior sectoral ducts with the left hepatic duct (Heloury et al 1985). In a further 22% of patients the right posterior sectoral duct drains into the left hepatic duct (Fig. 3.21) and in 6% the right anterior sectoral duct drains into the left hepatic duct (Healey & Schroy 1953). There are of course many more anomalies that have been recognized and described (Couinaud 1957, Heloury et al 1985), e.g., a low insertion of a right sectoral duct into the common hepatic duct (Hand 1973) which may have very serious implications for the surgeon (Fig. 3.22).

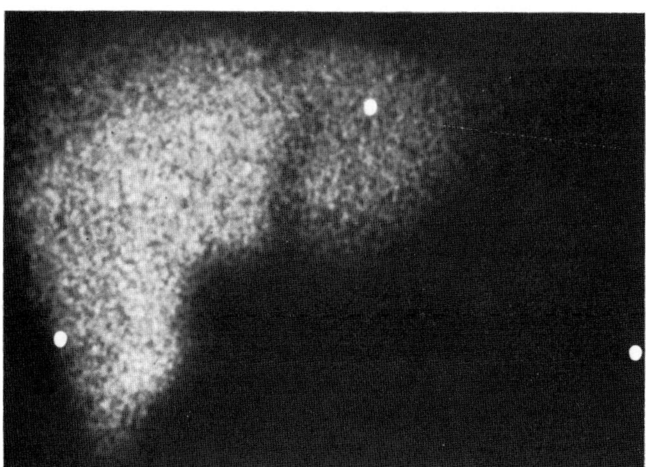

Fig. 3.19 Sulphur colloid isotope liver scan. The white markers indicate the costal margins and the xyphisternum. Note the linear defect in the scan due to the falciform ligament and the indentation on the inferior surface for the gallbladder

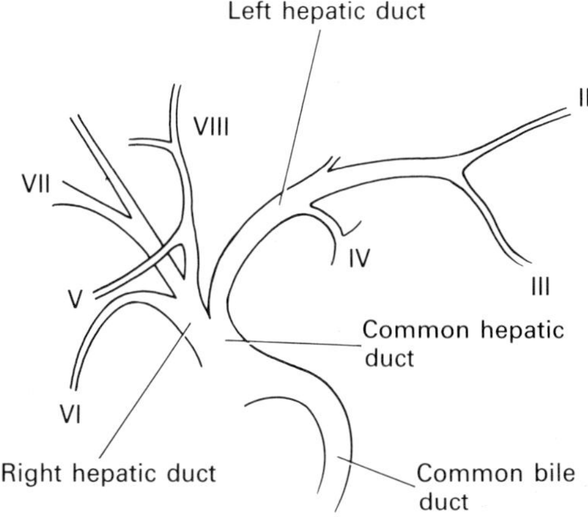

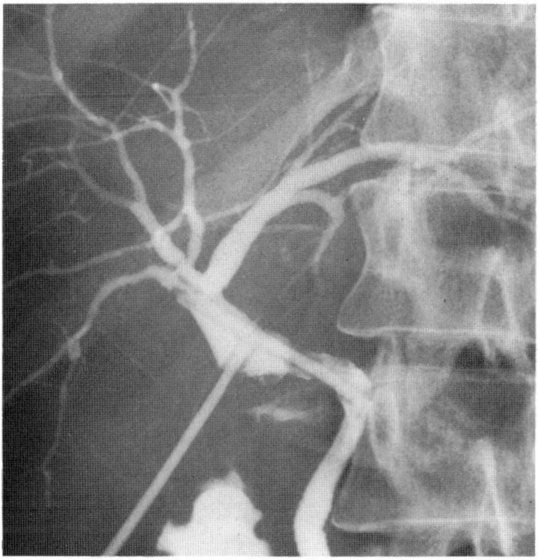

Fig. 3.20 T-tube cholangiogram showing the commonest arrangement of hepatic ducts

Oral cholangiography

The advent of ultrasound has, in many centres, rendered

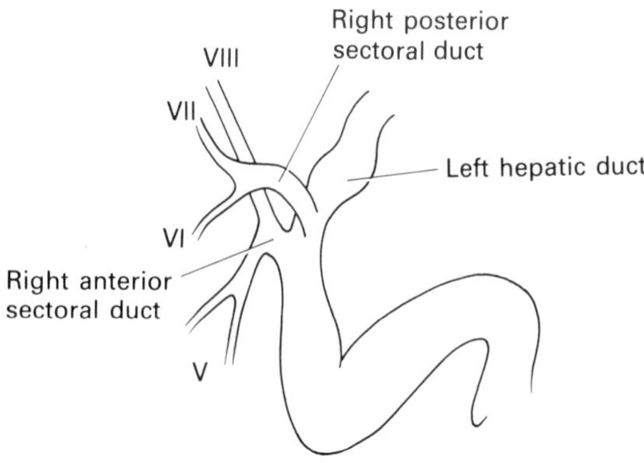

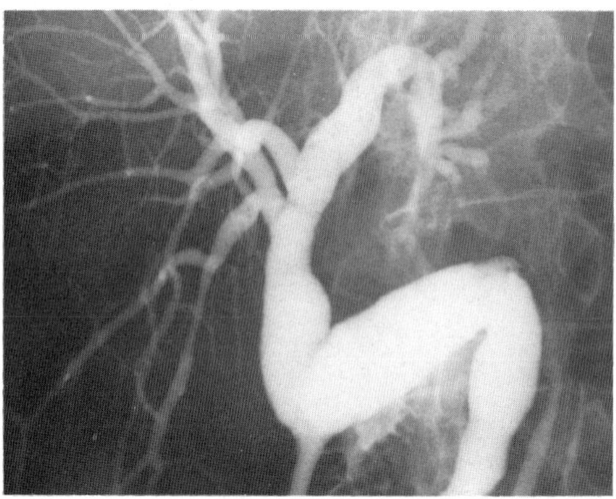

Fig. 3.21 Transtubal cholangiography showing a common normal variant where the right posterior sectoral duct drains into the left hepatic duct

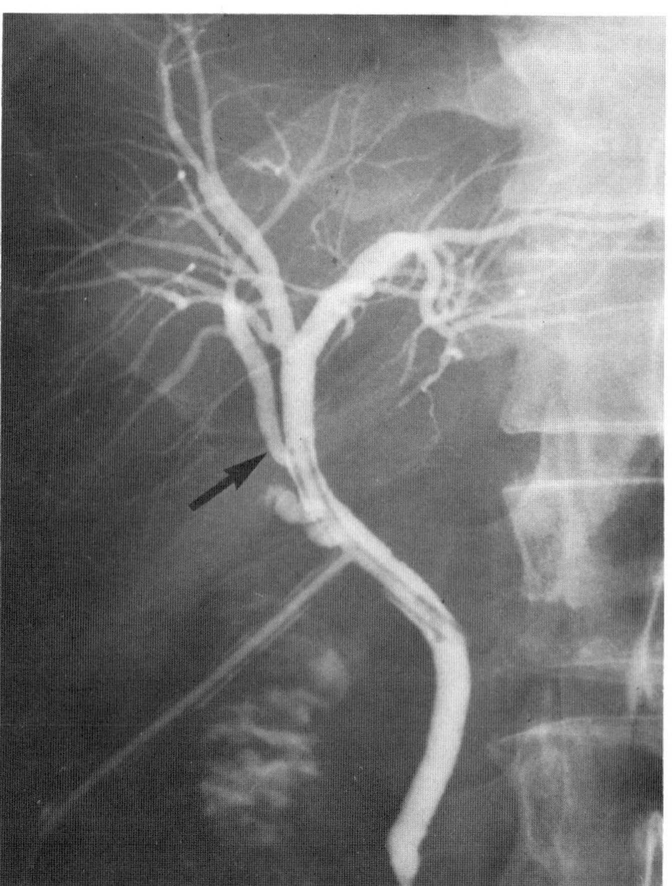

Fig. 3.22 T-tube cholangiogram showing a very low insertion of a right sectoral duct into the common hepatic duct (arrow)

this examination obsolete. On those occasions when it is still performed it is essential to obtain a plain abdominal radiograph, prior to the administration of contrast medium, to exclude the presence of radio-opaque calculi. The gallbladder is then examined following the ingestion of oral contrast agents. In the ideal situation the gallbladder, cystic duct, common hepatic and common bile ducts are visualized (Fig. 3.23a & b). Details of intrahepatic biliary anatomy cannot be determined by this method.

Intravenous cholangiography

The advent of the techniques of ultrasound, PTC and ERCP have rendered this investigation virtually obsolete.

Trans-tubal cholangiography

Following definitive or palliative intervention in the liver and biliary tract a temporary or permanent drainage tube may be left within the biliary tree. Contrast medium may be injected into these tubes to check that they are in a satisfactory position and that drainage is adequate. Knowledge of any surgery that has been performed is essential for the correct interpretation of such images.

Endoscopic retrograde choledochopancreatography (ERCP)

This subject is covered in detail in Chapter 20. There are many clinical reasons in addition to the avoidance of a direct hepatic puncture, why ERCP may be chosen to examine the biliary tree rather than PTC, e.g. it is possible to inspect the stomach and duodenum during the same examination. It is also possible to completely outline not just the biliary tract but also the pancreatic duct system (Fig. 3.24).

Percutaneous transhepatic cholangiography (PTC)

The details of this technique are discussed in chapter 19.

It is worth reiterating at this point the necessity of attempting to delineate the entire biliary tree when performing a cholangiogram. The value of both patient rotation and gravity in helping to delineate ducts (Fig. 3.25) should not be forgotten and it may be necessary to puncture the right and left duct systems separately to obtain a satisfactory study.

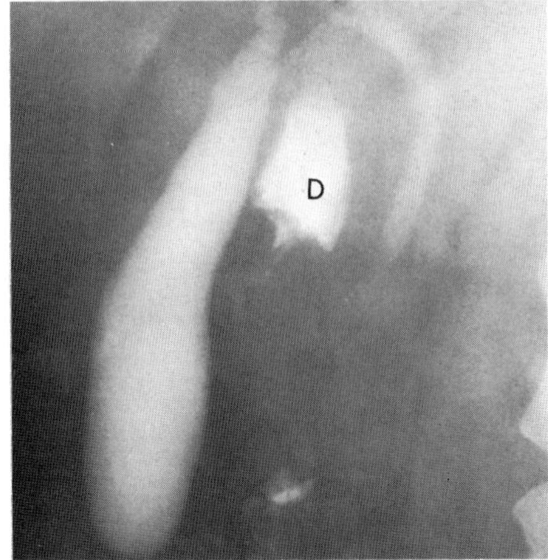

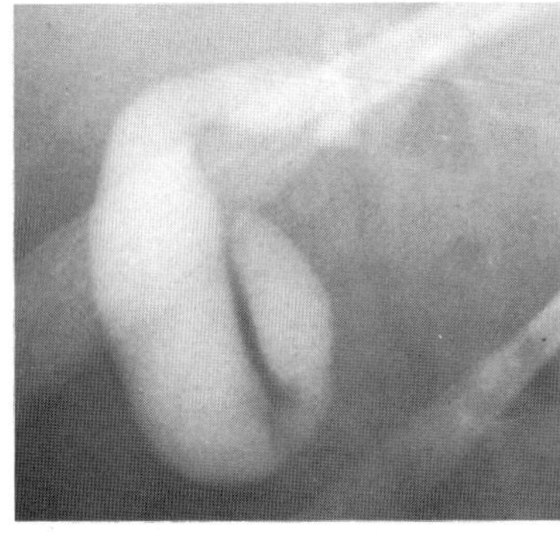

Fig. 3.23 a. Oral cholangiogram showing a normal gallbladder, cystic duct and common duct. Some contrast medium (calcium ipodate) still remains in the duodenal cap (D). b. Oral cholecystogram showing a Phrygian cap deformity

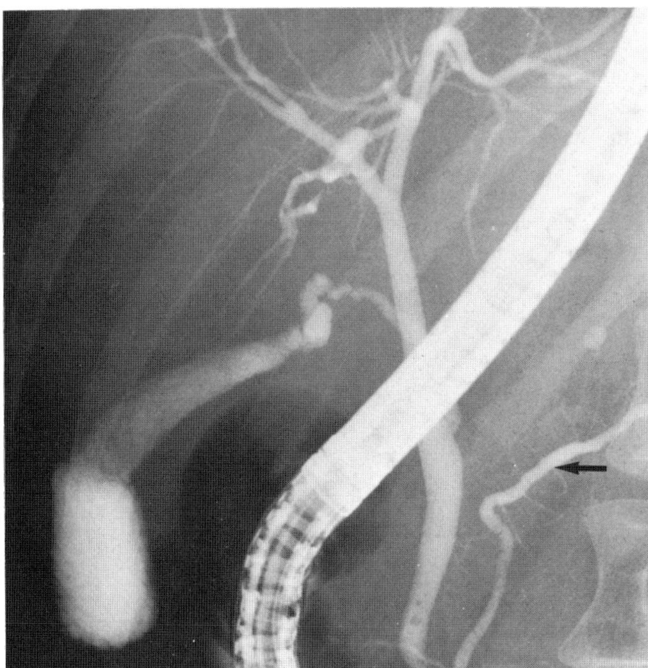

Fig. 3.24 ERCP showing the pancreatic duct (arrow), gallbladder and biliary tree

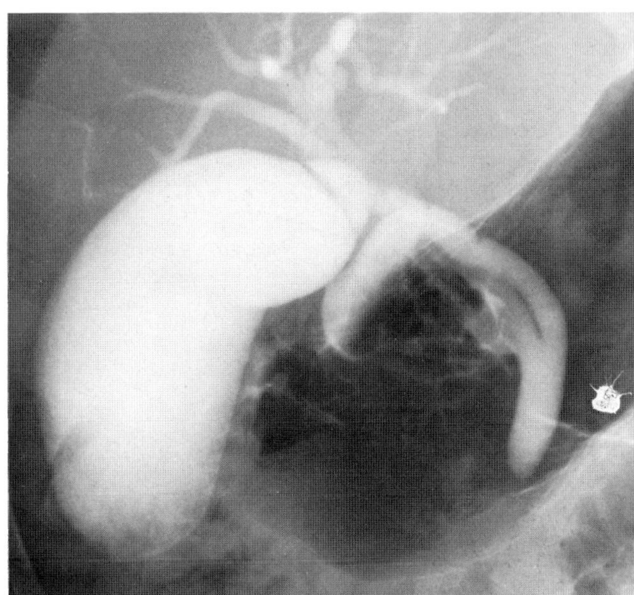

Fig. 3.25 PTC (needle removed). The patient has been turned into a shallow right anterior oblique projection. This clearly shows that the cystic duct is inserted low into the antero-medial aspect of the common hepatic duct. This feature could not be delineated with the patient supine

ANGIOGRAPHY (Abrams 1983, Allison 1986)

Arteriography (Lunderquist 1967, Nebesar et al 1969)

Arteriographic technique is discussed in Chapter 21.

There is considerable variation in the arterial supply to the liver owing to the complex embryological development of the coeliac axis and superior mesenteric artery. It is important for both the angiographer and surgeon to be aware of the possible anomalies that exist and a complete vascular study must be obtained when arteriography is performed. Failure to demonstrate all the arteries feeding the liver may not only result in errors of diagnosis (e.g. missed pathology) but may also seriously mislead the surgeon or the interventional radiologist.

The coeliac axis (Allison 1986a & b, Ring 1983, Nebesar et al 1969)

The coeliac axis is the artery that supplies those structures derived from the primitive foregut, and supplies, through its three branches (common hepatic, left gastric and splenic) the liver, gallbladder, pancreas, stomach and spleen.

The normal coeliac axis arises from the front of the aorta just below the aortic opening of the diaphragm. The main trunk, about 1.25 cm long, passes forwards above the pancreas and splenic vein and divides immediately into its true terminal branches (Fig. 3.26a & b). Occasionally one or both phrenic arteries may also arise from the coeliac axis instead of the aorta.

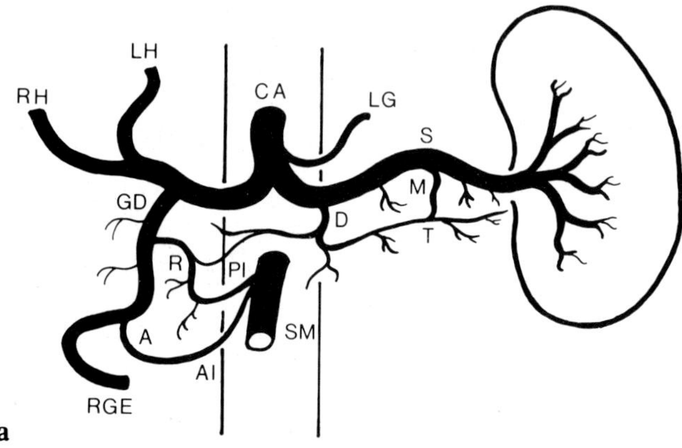

a

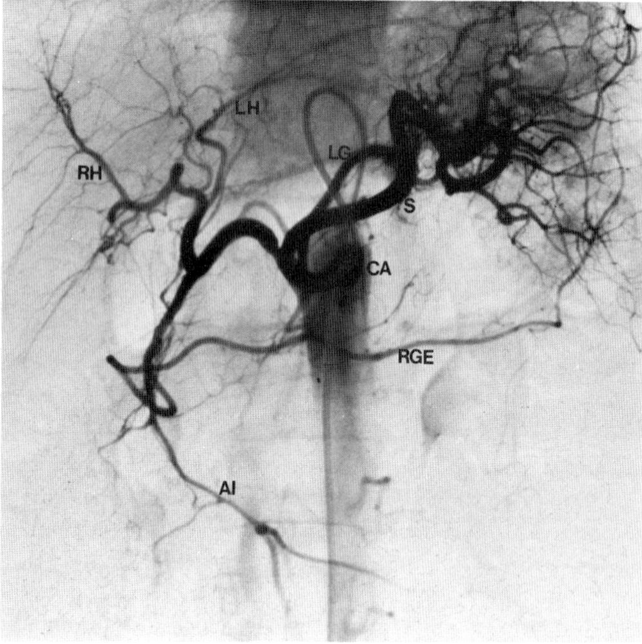

b

Fig. 3.26 a. Diagram to show the branches of the coeliac axis. CA = coeliac axis; LG = left gastric artery; S = splenic artery; M = arteria pancreatica magna; D = dorsal pancreatic artery; SM = superior mesenteric artery; T = transverse pancreatic artery; PI = posterior inferior pancreatico-duodenal artery; AI = anterior inferior pancreatico-duodenal artery; A = anterior superior pancreatico-duodenal artery; R = retroduodenal artery; GD = gastroduodenal artery; RH = right hepatic artery; LH = left hepatic artery; RGE = right gastroepiploic artery b. Normal coeliac axis angiogram (see above for key to abbreviation). Arterial spasm is noted at the origin of the hepatic artery; this is secondary to catheterisation of the vessel

The *left gastric artery*, the smallest of the three coeliac branches, passes upwards and to the left behind the lesser sac to the cardia of the stomach. There it gives off branches to the oesophagus and then turns downwards and forwards to run along and supply the lesser curve of the stomach.

The *common hepatic artery* (Nebesar et al 1969, Herlinger et al 1983) passes forwards and then to the right below the medial end of the opening of the lesser sac. It crosses in front of the portal vein and ascends between the two layers of lesser omentum to the porta hepatis where it divides into right and left branches, supplying the corresponding lobes of the liver (Fig. 3.27). The common hepatic artery gives off the right gastric artery (Fig. 3.28) (often not identi-

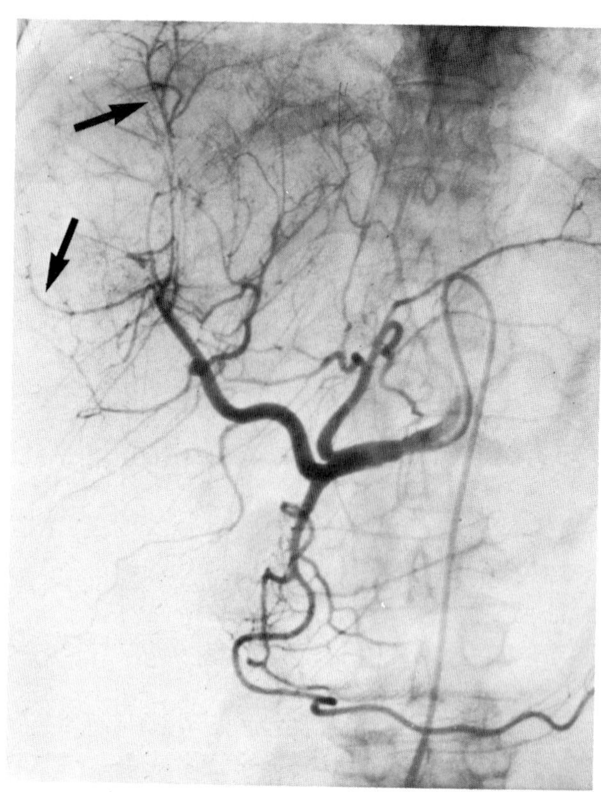

Fig. 3.27 Normal hepatic arterial anatomy. An avascular tumour is displacing some branches of the right hepatic artery (arrowed)

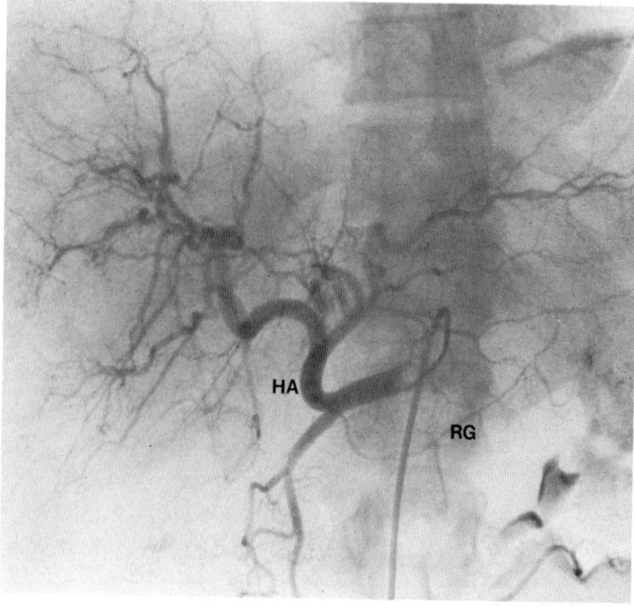

Fig. 3.28 Right gastric artery (RG) arising from the proper hepatic artery (HA)

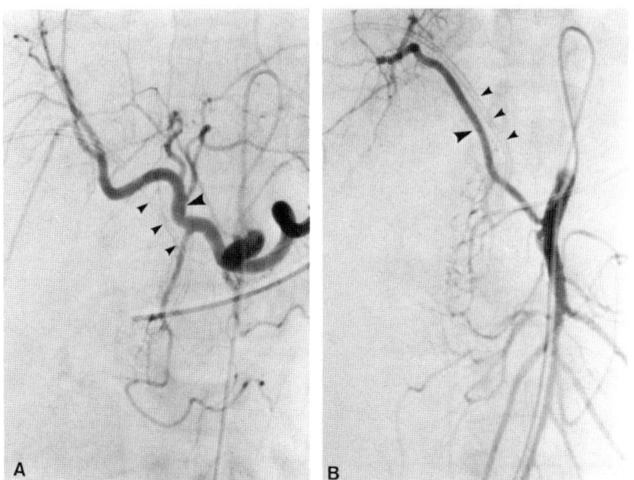

Fig. 3.29 Angiogram. (A) The hepatic artery (large arrow) arises from the coeliac axis. The small arrows indicate a drainage catheter in the bile duct. (B) The same patient. An accessory right hepatic artery (large arrow) is arising from the superior mesenteric artery and lies lateral to the catheter (small arrows) in the common bile duct

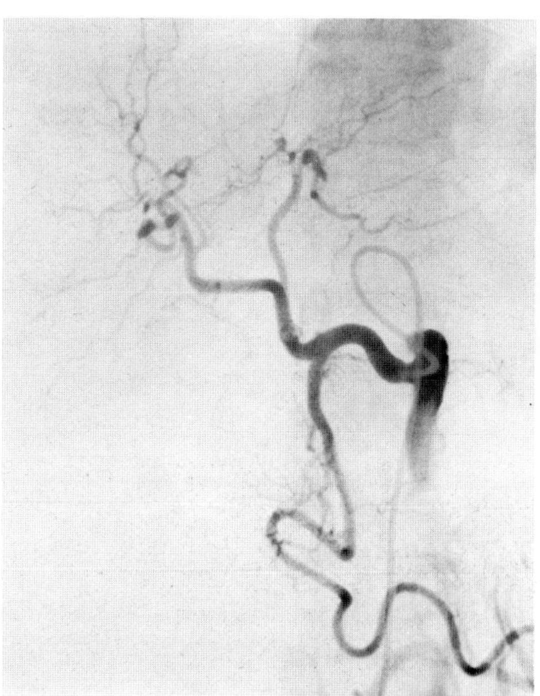

Fig. 3.30 Replaced common hepatic artery. The common hepatic vessel is shown arising from the superior mesenteric artery instead of from the coeliac axis

fied angiographically), the gastroduodenal artery and the cystic artery after which it is referred to as the proper hepatic artery (Lunderquist 1983). In the majority of people the proper hepatic artery divides into right and left hepatic branches. In approximately 18% of arteriographic examinations a middle hepatic artery arises from the proper hepatic artery and supplies part of the left liver. In approximately 18% of individuals the right hepatic artery arises partially (8%) or completely (10%) from the superior mesenteric artery (SMA) (Fig. 3.29) and in a similar proportion the left hepatic artery may be partially or completely replaced by a branch of the left gastric artery.

An artery which exists in addition to the normal artery is referred to as an *accessory* artery; an artery which takes the place of the normal artery is called a *replaced* artery. In 2.5% of patients the entire common hepatic artery arises from the superior mesenteric artery (Fig. 3.30) and very rarely (0.2%) from the left gastric artery.

An hepatic artery which arises from the SMA passes lateral to the portal vein and frequently lies posterior and lateral to the common bile duct (Fig. 3.29b) in the hepatoduodenal ligament where it may be susceptible to operative injury if not recognized (Bowley & Benjamin 1982).

Other variations include the separate origin of the common hepatic artery from the aorta (Fig. 3.31) and the persistence of primitive embryological links between the coeliac and superior mesenteric systems (Fig. 3.32). The anatomy of the coeliac and superior mesenteric arteries is reviewed by Nebesar et al (1969).

The normal cystic artery is not often identified at arteriography but in most patients a characteristic blush may be identified in the wall of the gallbladder (Fig. 3.33).

The rich pancreatic anastomoses between the coeliac axis and superior mesenteric artery are shown diagramatically in Fig. 3.26a, and are particularly well demonstrated on selective gastroduodenal and dorsal pancreatic arteriography (Fig. 3.34 & 3.35).

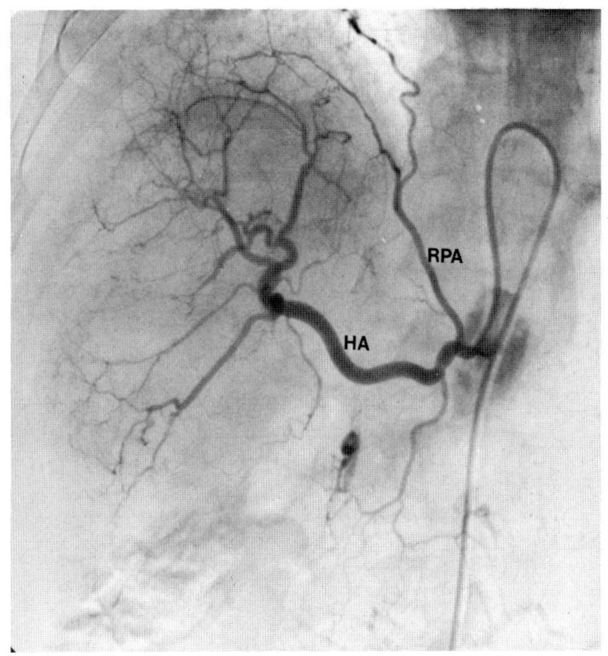

Fig. 3.31 Hepatic artery (HA) and right phrenic artery (RPA) arising directly from the aorta. Note reflux into the aorta and adjacent splenic artery

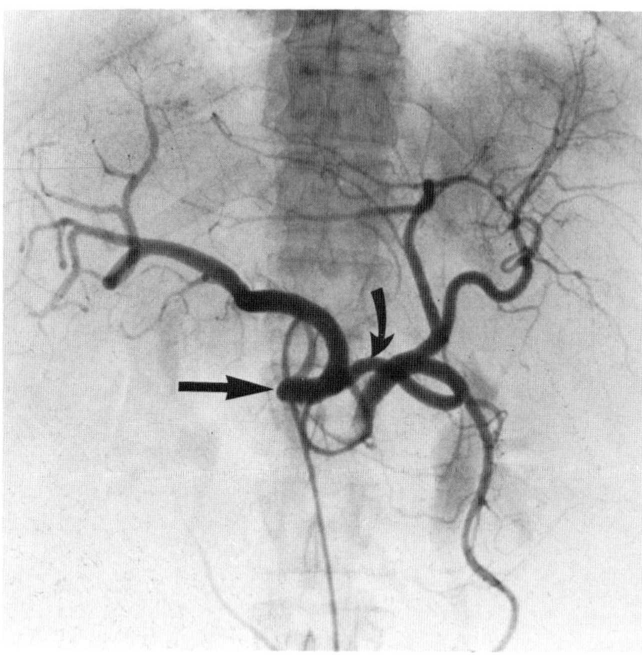

Fig. 3.32 Arc of Buhler: the patient has a combined hepato-mesenteric trunk and an arc of Buhler. The catheter lies in the superior mesenteric artery and is opacifying a common hepatic artery (straight arrow) arising from the SMA (hepatomesenteric trunk). In addition a link vessel (curved arrow), which represents a persistent ventral longitudinal anastomosis connects the hepato-mesenteric trunk to the coeliac axis which is also opacified

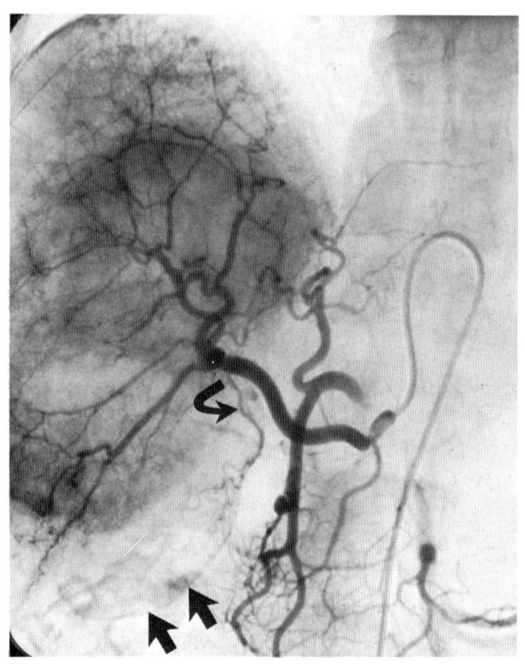

Fig. 3.33 Selective hepatic arteriography shows the outline of the normal gallbladder and a blush in the gallbladder wall (arrows). A cystic artery could be identified in this patient (curved arrow). The liver parenchyma is abnormal

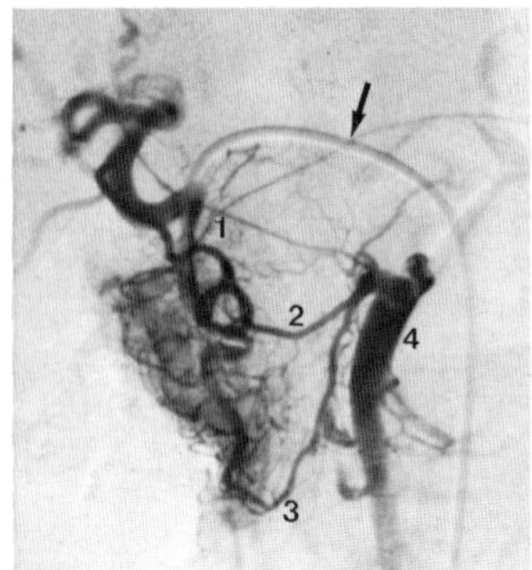

Fig. 3.34 A catheter (arrow) is selectively placed in the gastroduodenal artery (1) The posterior (2) and anterior (3) pancreatico-duodenal arcades are demonstrated and there is filling of the superior mesenteric artery (4)

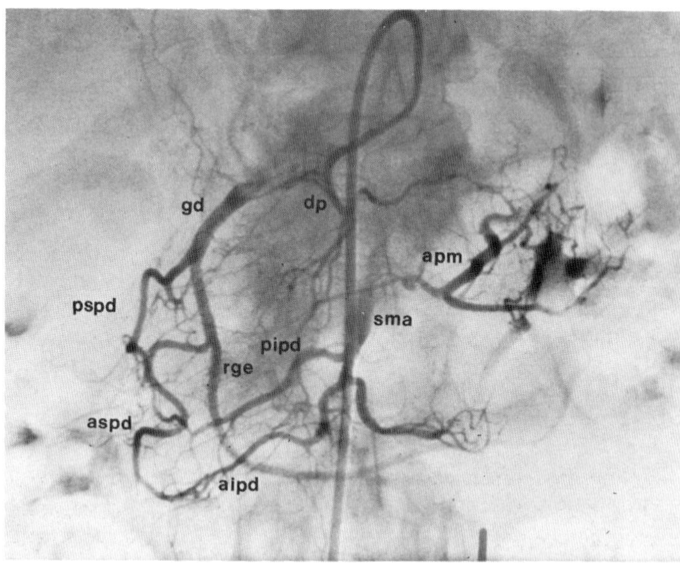

Fig. 3.35 Selective dorsal pancreatic arteriogram. gd = gastroduodenal artery; dp = dorsal pancreatic; apm = arteria pancreatica magna; sma = superior mesenteric artery; rge = right gastroepiploic artery; pspd, aspd, pipd, aipd = posterior superior, anterior superior, posterior inferior, anterior inferior pancreatico-duodenal arteries

The *gastroduodenal artery* descends between the first part of the duodenum and the neck of the pancreas and gives off the posterior superior pancreatico-duodenal artery at the upper border of the first part of the duodenum. At the lower border of the duodenum it divides into its two terminal branches, the right gastro-epiploic artery and the anterior superior pancreatico-duodenal artery. Rarely the pancreatic vessels may link with the inferior mesenteric artery, an important fact to detect especially if embolisation is being considered. Selective injection of the gastroduodenal artery may give rise to a dense vascular blush in the duodenal mucosa and pancreatic head which should not be mistaken for a pathological change (Fig. 3.36).

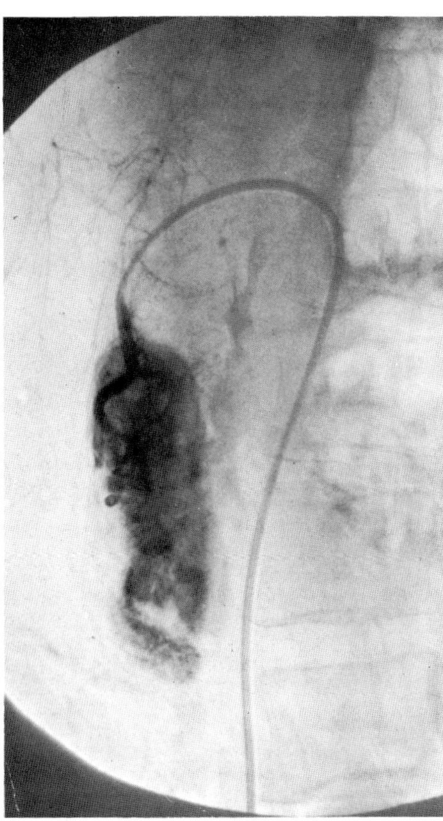

Fig. 3.36 Capillary phase of a selective gastroduodenal arteriogram. There is a dense blush in the wall of the duodenum; this is a normal appearance and should not be confused with pathology

The *splenic artery* is the largest branch of the coelic axis (Fig. 3.26b). It passes horizontally to the left behind the stomach and lesser sac and along the upper border of the pancreas adjacent to the splenic vein. It crosses in front of the left adrenal gland and upper pole of the left kidney and, entering the lieno-renal ligament, terminates at the hilum of the spleen by dividing into five or six splenic branches. During its course it gives off several pancreatic branches. At or near its termination it gives rise to the left gastro-epiploic artery and several short gastric arteries.

The superior mesenteric artery (Nebesar et al 1969)

The superior mesenteric artery supplies that part of the gastrointestinal tract derived from the primitive mid-gut, i.e. from the Ampulla of Vater to the splenic flexure of the colon. It arises from the front of the aorta 1 cm below the coeliac axis and is crossed at its origin by the splenic vein and the body of the pancreas. Just beyond its origin the left renal vein separates it from the aorta. It passes downwards and forwards anterior to the uncinate process of the pancreas and the third part of the duodenum and descends to the right iliac fossa (Fig. 3.37). The artery is accompanied by the superior mesenteric vein which lies on

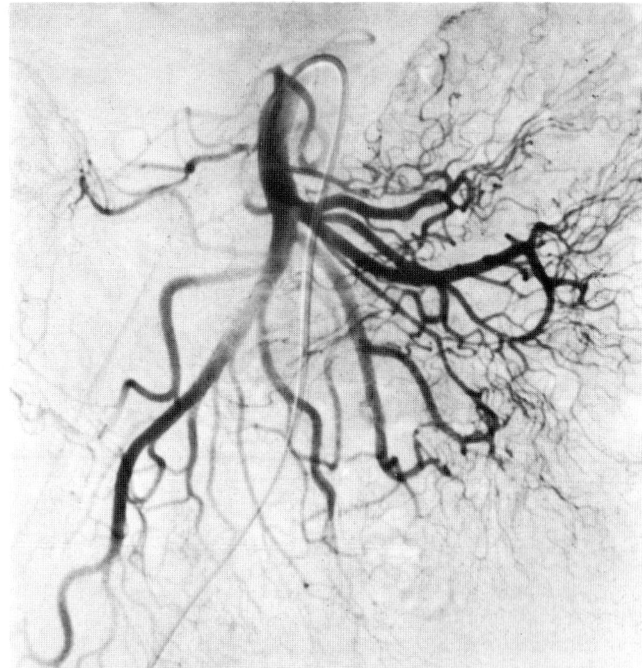

Fig. 3.37 Normal superior mesenteric arteriogram

its right side. The inferior pancreatico-duodenal artery arises either as a common stem (82%) or as separate anterior and posterior branches from the SMA or its first jejunal branch.

Venography

System and portal venography is discussed in detail in Chapter 21.

Systemic veins (Lunderquist 1983)

The hepatic veins (right, middle and left) drain into the inferior vena cava just below the diaphragm and some 3 cm before the junction of the IVC with the right atrium. The middle and left veins frequently unite before draining into the cava. The normal radiological appearance of the veins is shown in Fig. 3.38. It is not always possible to demonstrate all three veins angiographically, but the right vein, unless diseased, should be readily demonstrated (Hemingway 1986).

Portal veins

The main portal vein is formed by the junction of the splenic vein and the superior mesenteric vein. The splenic vein is formed from the anastomosis of smaller intrasplenic radicles. It passes towards the midline along the pancreas adjacent to the splenic artery. The inferior mesenteric vein and left gastric veins drain into the splenic vein. The

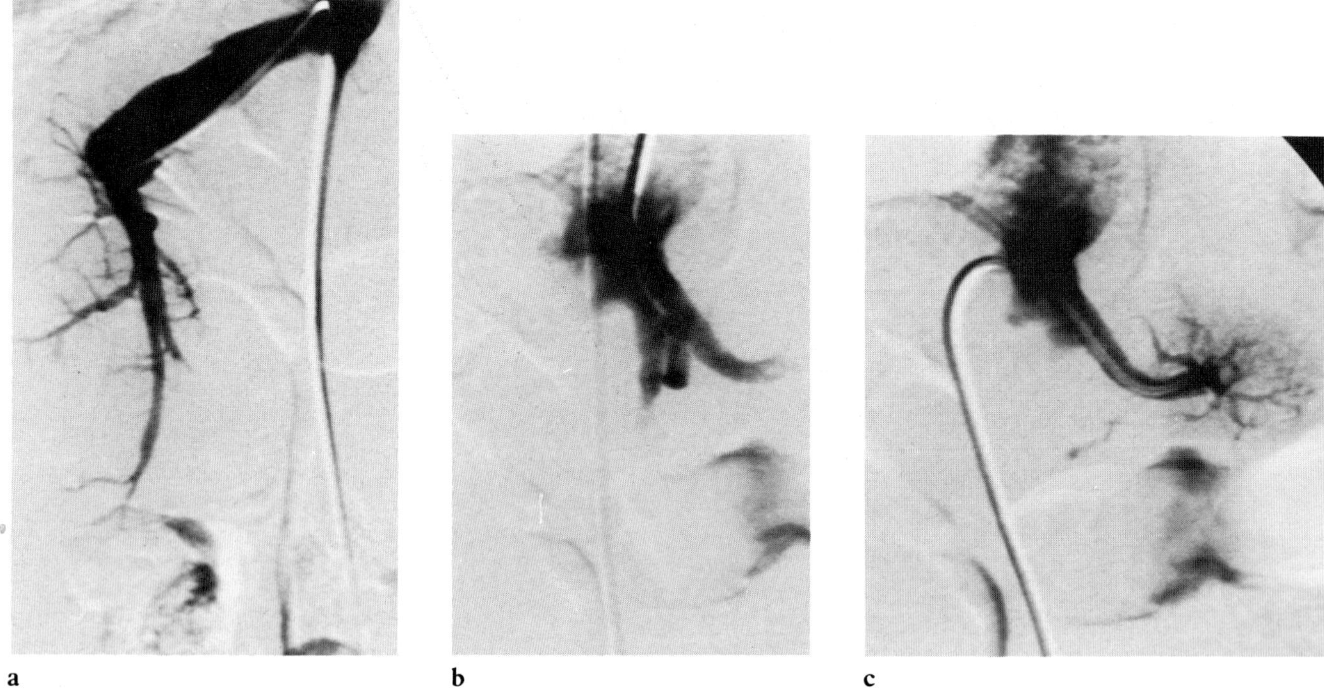

a b c

Fig. 3.38 Normal hepatic veins: (a) right, (b) middle and (c) left hepatic veins

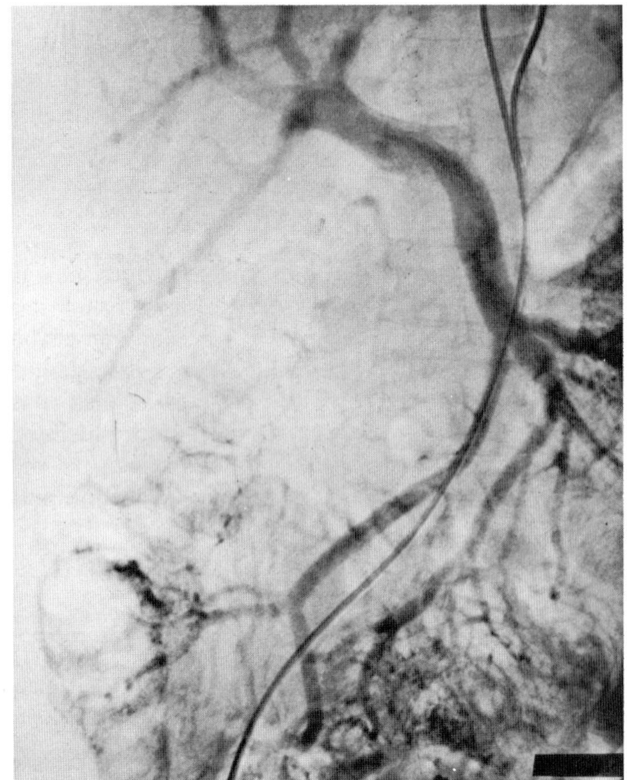

Fig. 3.39 Normal superior mesenteric vein

splenic vein then unites with the superior mesenteric vein (Fig. 3.39) to form the portal vein. The portal vein ascends behind the neck of the pancreas, the first part of the duodenum and the gastroduodenal artery. It then enters the lesser omentum where the bile duct and hepatic artery lie anterior to it. Behind the portal vein lies the inferior vena cava. Having reached the porta hepatis the vein then divides into left and right branches (Hjortsjo 1956) and then into sectoral and segmental branches within a sheath containing branches of the hepatic artery and bile ducts (Fig. 3.40).

The left portal vein passes obliquely to the left, its

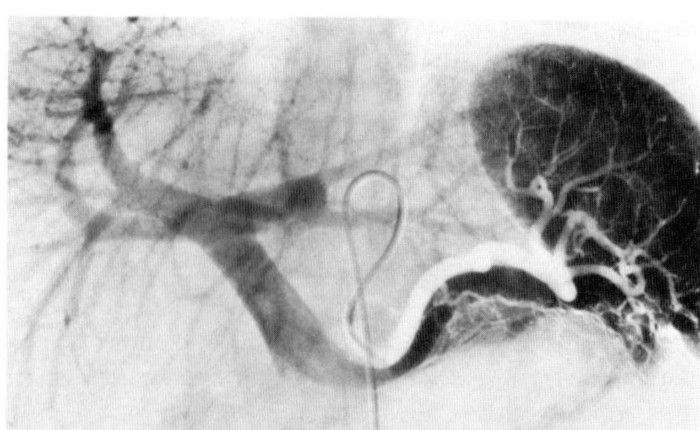

Fig. 3.40 Normal indirect splenoportogram, subtracted study. The splenic artery is seen in white, the adjacent splenic vein is black. Note the branching pattern of the intrahepatic portal radicles

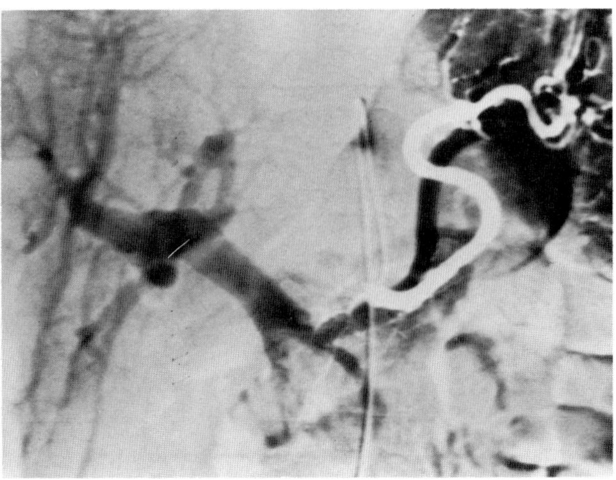

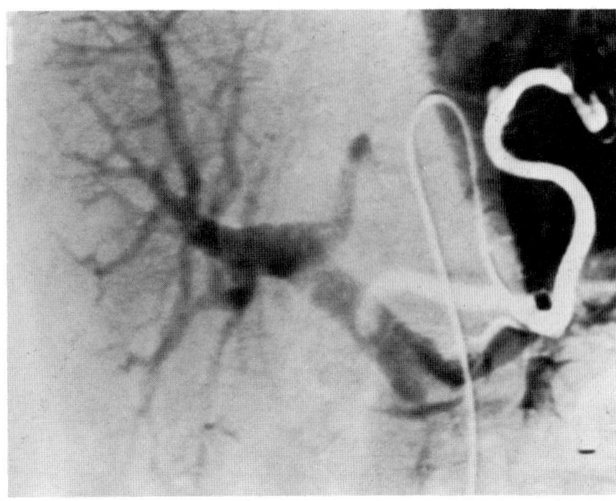

Fig. 3.41 The left portal vein is foreshortened in the AP projection (A). A right anterior oblique projection shows the main trunk more clearly (B)

umbilical portion running ventrally (see Fig. 3.14b), and it may be necessary to perform portal venography in the right anterior oblique projection in order to see the origin of the left vein clearly (Fig. 3.41).

The advent of digital subtraction angiography (see Ch. 21) allows both the arterial and venous systems to be demonstrated on the same image, a useful feature when assessing vessel involvement by tumour.

REFERENCES

Abrams H L 1983 Angiography, 3rd ed. Little, Brown, Boston

Allison D J 1986a Arteriography. In: Grainger R G, Allison D J (eds) Diagnostic radiology: An Anglo-American textbook of imaging. Churchill Livingstone, Edinburgh, ch 94, p 1987–2059

Allison D J 1986b Arteriography. In: Grainger R G, Allison D J (eds) Diagnostic radiology: An Anglo-American textbook of imaging. Churchill Livingstone, Edinburgh, ch 94, p 1987–2059

Behan M, Kazam 1978 Sonography of the common bile duct: value of the right anterior oblique view. American Journal of Roentgenology 130: 701–709

Bowley N B, Benjamin I S 1982 Diagnostic approaches in the biliary tract In: Blumgart L H (ed) The biliary tract. Churchill Livingstone, Edinburgh

Bowley N B, Malmud L S 1986 The biliary tract. In: Grainger R G, Allison D J (eds) Diagnostic radiology: An Anglo-American textbook of imaging. Churchill Livingstone, Edinburgh, ch 51, p 955–987

Cooperberg P L 1978 High-resolution real-time ultrasound in the evaluation of the normal and obstructed biliary tract. Radiology 129: 477–480

Couinaud C 1957 Le Foie. Etudes anatomiques et chirurgicales. Masson, Paris

Gelfand D W, 1983 Plain film radiographic anatomy of the liver. In: Herlinger H, Lunderquist A, Wallace S (eds) Clinical Radiology of the Liver. Marcel Dekker, New York

Hand B H 1973 Anatomy and function of the extrahepatic biliary system. Clinics in Gastroenterology 2: 3–29

Hayes M A, Goldenberg I S, Bishop C C 1985 The developmental basis for bile duct anomalies. Surgery, Gynecology and Obstetrics 107: 447–456

Healey J E, Shroy P C 1953 Anatomy of the bilary ducts within the human liver. AMA Archives of Surgery 66: 599–616

Hemingway A P 1986 Venography. In: Grainger R G, Allison D J (eds) Diagnosis radiology: An Anglo-American textbook of imaging. Churchill Livingstone, Edinburgh

Heloury Y, Leborgne J, Roges J M, Robert R, Lehur P A, Parmer M, Borbin J Y 1985 Radiological anatomy of the bile ducts based on intra-operative investigation in 250 cases. Anatomica Clinica 7: 93–102

Herlinger L, Lunderquist A, Wallace S (eds) 1983 Clinical radiology of the liver. Marcel Dekker, New York

Herlinger H 1986 The Liver. In: Grainger R G, Allison D J (eds) Diagnostic radiology: An Anglo-American textbook of imaging. Churchill Livingstone, Edinburgh, ch 50, p 925–953

Hjortsjo C H 1956 The intrahepatic ramification of the portal vein. *Fysiogr. Sallsk. Handl*: 67 No 20

Koeningsberg M, Wiener S W, Walzer A 1979 The accuracy of sonography in the differential diagnosis of obstructive jaundice: a comparison with cholangiography. Radiology 133: 157–165

Lunderquist A 1967 Arterial segmental supply of the liver. An angiographic study. Acta Radiologica (suppl): 272

Lunderquist A 1983 Vascular anatomy of the liver. In: Herlinger H, Lunderquist A, Wallace S (eds) Clinical radiology of the liver. Marcel Dekker, New York

Nebesar R A, Kornblith P L, Pollard J J, Michels M A, 1969a Coeliac and superior mesenteric arteries. J & A Churchill, London

Ring E J 1983 Vascular disease of the liver. In: Herlinger H, Lunderquist A, Wallace S (eds) Clinical radiology of the liver. Marcel Dekker, New York, ch 29, p 953–974

4

N. McIntyre

Liver function

The liver serves many important functions: it secretes bile into the intestine, adds substances to the blood and removes others, stores many compounds and conducts a large number of important metabolic reactions. This chapter gives a brief and highly selected account of the functions of the liver and may be read in conjunction with the account of liver failure (Ch. 102).

The liver has a special blood supply; it is fed directly by the hepatic artery but in addition receives venous blood from the gut, pancreas and spleen via the portal vein. Many nutrients and drugs absorbed from the intestine, and substances added to blood by the gut and pancreas, are thus presented to the liver in relatively high concentration and may be largely removed during the 'first pass' of portal venous blood through the liver. Small arteries and portal vein tributaries open into one end of the hepatic sinusoids; these communicate with central veins which drain via the hepatic veins into the inferior vena cava. The epithelial wall of the sinusoids is separated from hepatocytes by the space of Disse and it is penetrated by many fenestrations (*c* 100 nm) which allow transit of large molecules and particles into and out of the blood (Motta 1982).

Hepatocytes close to the portal tract remove some substances from the blood and add others to it; thus the concentrations of substances to which they are exposed (including oxygen) are different from the concentrations experienced by hepatocytes close to the central veins; there is other evidence for functional differentiation of hepatocytes depending on their position along the sinusoid (Gumucio & Miller 1982).

CARBOHYDRATE METABOLISM (Alberti, Johnston and Taylor 1985, Katz & McGarry 1984)

The liver helps to control the blood glucose concentration. During a meal it removes glucose; in the fasting state it releases glucose to supply tissues like the brain and erythrocytes which are glucose dependent. Released glucose comes from the breakdown of stored glycogen (a glucose polymer) or from gluconeogenesis (glucose production from glucogenic amino-acids, particularly alanine, and from metabolic intermediates such as lactate, pyruvate and glycerol). During a short fast about 60–75% of the glucose leaving the liver (approximately 7.5 g/h), comes from glycogenolysis, the rest from gluconeogenesis. As the normal adult liver contains only about 5–7 g of glycogen per 100 g wet weight after a meal, this reserve would be depleted within a day. With prolonged fasting a greater proportion of glucose comes from gluconeogenesis and the kidneys also begin to contribute significantly to the blood glucose pool. The body adapts and its obligatory requirement for glucose falls by 50–70%; the brain, for example, supplements its energy supply by using ketone bodies which are produced in the liver from acetyl CoA.

One might expect fasting hypoglycaemia with liver disease but it is rare except in patients with acute hepatic failure due to viruses and toxins; then, prevention of hypoglycaemia is an important aspect of management. Impaired hepatic glycogenolysis (due to low glycogen stores or impaired response to glucagon) is probably a major factor in this hypoglycaemia, but reduced gluconeogenesis may play a part, and increased peripheral glucose utilization may also be important as very large amounts of intravenous glucose are sometimes required to correct the hypoglycaemia.

Following the ingestion of glucose or glucose-containing compounds such as sucrose, starch and glycogen, there is an increased concentration of glucose in portal venous blood. Most of it passes through the liver and the arterial blood glucose rises. Glucose uptake is increased in peripheral tissues where it is metabolized or stored (as glycogen in muscles, or triglyceride in adipose tissue). The increase in peripheral glucose uptake and a reduction in hepatic gluconeogenesis are triggered by the rise in plasma insulin which accompanies an increased blood glucose; this rise in insulin is greater if the glucose is absorbed from the intestine. Glycogen storage and fat synthesis after glucose ingestion appears to arise, not from hepatic glucose uptake, but from the uptake of three-carbon fragments (e.g. lactate) produced in the gut, muscle and erythrocytes.

Many patients with liver disease have an exaggerated plasma glucose response to oral glucose and it has been assumed that the damaged liver fails to take up portal glucose during its first passage through the liver. However, a portacaval shunt has relatively little effect on oral glucose tolerance. The main reason for the glucose intolerance of liver disease seems to be a peripheral insensitivity to insulin which has been demonstrated by many workers. The mechanism is unknown.

The intracellular hepatic concentration of glucose is relatively high and it diffuses out of the liver even in the face of relatively high glucose levels in fasting blood. The two other major monosaccharides, fructose and galactose, are present in liver cytoplasm at very low concentrations. When the portal venous concentration of fructose and galactose rises after a meal there is rapid transfer into the liver which explains the marked first pass uptake of these sugars, and the striking 'intolerance' to oral fructose and galactose which occurs following a portacaval shunt. Both sugars are phosphorylated rapidly prior to their subsequent metabolism. Lack of the enzymes which deal with fructose-l-phosphate and galactose-l-phosphate cause the diseases hereditary fructose intolerance and galactosaemia.

In the past intravenous fructose has been used as an energy source in place of intravenous glucose. This is dangerous in patients with liver disease. It does not prevent or help in the management of hypoglycaemia and it may cause or contribute to the development of lactic acidosis (Tygstrup 1983).

Galactose is of value as a quantitative test of one particular aspect of hepatic function. If sufficient galactose is injected intravenously its rate of removal from the blood stream can be used to measure the hepatic maximum transport capacity (Vmax) for the sugar (Tygstrup 1983).

LACTATE AND PYRUVATE METABOLISM (Cohen & Woods 1976)

Glucose, fructose and galactose are converted after phosphorylation to fructose 1-6 diphosphate; this is cleaved to triose phosphates which in turn are converted to pyruvic acid (Fig. 4.1). In the presence of NAD^+ and coenzyme A, pyruvate is converted to acetyl CoA which enters the citric acid cycle (Krebs cycle) for complete oxidation to carbon dioxide and water. When there is a shortage of oxygen, NADH rather than NAD^+ accumulates and pyruvate is reduced to lactate. These reactions occur in most tissues; peripheral tissues such as muscle and erythrocytes add a large amount of lactate to the blood each day. This lactate is removed by the liver where it is oxidized or converted back to glucose. This process is physiologically very important. The production of lactate ions from glucose is accompanied by the release of H^+ ions; hepatic utilization of lactate removes these H^+ ions. If the liver's ability to remove lactate is impaired, e.g. with hypoxia or severe hepatocellular necrosis, lactate and H^+ ions may accumulate in the blood causing lactic acidosis, particularly if peripheral tissues produce more lactate than usual because of hypoxaemia or poor perfusion. Lactate is quantitatively the most important source of newly synthesized glucose but as the lactate is derived mainly from glucose (by anaerobic glycolysis) it serves mainly as a method of conserving glucose during fasting; unlike amino acids, it is not an important source of new glucose molecules.

Fat metabolism

Bile secretion and fat absorption (Gray 1983, Hoffman 1983)

Hepatic bile is secreted into canaliculi and modified during passage through the bile ducts and gallbladder before entering the duodenum through the ampulla of Vater (Ch. 8). Bile contains bile salts, phospholipid and cholesterol in micellar solution (as well as bilirubin, copper and other substances). In the small intestine bile salts cause 'emulsification' of dietary fat, i.e. its breakdown into much smaller particles. This increases the surface area of the fat and so facilitates the hydrolysis of triglyceride by pancreatic lipase, a process aided by colipase, another pancreatic protein. The fatty acids and monoglyceride released by lipase combine with bile salts to form small particles called micelles which have a polar surface and a hydrophobic core. Cholesterol and fat-soluble vitamins are incorporated into the hydrophobic core. The micelles are taken up by the mucosal brush border and most of the constituents are absorbed. The bile acids return to the lumen to participate again in the process of micelle formation; a large proportion are actively absorbed in the distal ileum, transported to the liver in the portal blood and re-excreted in bile.

The monoglycerides and fatty acids are reconverted into triglycerides by the mucosal cells and packaged into chylomicrons which have a hydrophobic core, e.g. triglyceride and cholesteryl ester, and a polar surface made up of free cholesterol, phospholipid and apoproteins (B and C). The chylomicrons enter the blood via the intestinal lymphatics and the thoracic duct. Their triglyceride is hydrolyzed in the tissues where fatty acids are taken up, and the chylomicron remnants, the surface of which is enriched with apoprotein E within the circulation, are taken up by the liver together with their cholesteryl esters and other hydrophobic substances such as Vitamin A esters: chylomicron remnants are removed via receptors for apoprotein E.

Cholesterol and bile acid metabolism (Hoffman 1983, Norum et al 1983)

Cholesterol and phospholipids are the main structural components of the lipid bilayer of plasma membranes and intracellular membranes. Cholesterol is absorbed from the intestine. It can be synthesized by all tissues and many tissues, including the liver, can minimize synthetic requirements by using plasma cholesterol acquired by the uptake of cholesterol rich lipoproteins. Cholesterol is removed from the body in bile and in cells shed from skin and mucosal surfaces. A small amount is converted to steroid hormones; the liver converts a larger amount to bile acids which are eventually lost in the faeces. The liver is the major organ for cholesterol removal from the body. It removes absorbed cholesterol via chylomicron remnants, and tissue cholesterol by uptake of other cholesterol rich lipoproteins (see later).

The liver makes two main bile acids, cholic acid and chenodeoxycholic acids (primary bile acids). These are conjugated with taurine and glycine before secretion into bile. In the intestine these conjugated bile acids play their role in fat absorption and are then re-absorbed passively in the jejunum and by an efficient active transport process in the ileum. They return to the liver via the portal vein, are rapidly removed and resecreted in the bile (an entero-hepatic circulation). A small proportion escapes ileal absorption and enters the colon where bacteria deconjugate the bile acids, and also remove the 7α-hydroxyl group thus converting cholic and chenodeoxycholic acids to deoxy-cholic and lithocholic acids (secondary bile acids). These are absorbed into portal blood and on return to the liver the deoxycholate is conjugated and secreted in bile, joining the conjugated forms of cholic and chenodeoxycholic acids in their enterohepatic recirculation. Lithocholic acid is sulphated by the liver before biliary secretion and this sulphation prevents intestinal reabsorption.

Where there is bacterial contamination of the small intestine deconjugation of bile acids may occur and, as the deconjugated bile acids are less effective micelle formers than the conjugated forms, there may be impaired absorption of fat and fat-soluble vitamins.

Synthesis: metabolism of lipoproteins (Glickman & Sabesin 1982, Eisenberg 1984)

The liver synthesizes lipids, including fatty acids and cholesterol, and takes up free fatty acids and lipoproteins from plasma. Where there is an excess of fatty acids they are converted to triglyceride which is packaged in large particles (but smaller than chylomicrons) called very low density lipoproteins (VLDL) which are secreted into the blood. Their surface is made up of cholesterol, phospholipid and apoprotein B and C. Their triglyceride, like that of chylomicrons, is hydrolysed by lipoprotein lipase in the periphery, where fatty acids are utilized or stored. In the process VLDL are converted to low density lipoprotein particles (LDL) which retain the apo B of the VLDL and the particles are enriched with cholesteryl ester. Many tissues, including the liver, have cell surface receptors which recognize apo B (and apo E), so they are called apo B, E receptors. The LDL are taken up by these tissues and their cholesteryl ester is hydrolysed, releasing cholesterol which can be used by the cells.

The liver is a major site of cholesterol catabolism via conversion into bile acids. When intestinal bile acid reabsorption is impaired (with ileal resection or bypass, or by the use of resins such as cholestyramine) bile acid synthesis in the liver is increased, and there is an increased demand for cholesterol. This is met by increased synthesis and by increased removal of cholesteryl ester rich LDL which occurs because of an increase in apo B, E receptors on the surface of the hepatocytes (Brown & Goldstein 1984).

The liver secretes high density lipoproteins (HDL) into plasma, and also an enzyme called lecithin cholesterol acyl transferase (LCAT). LCAT catalyzes the transfer of a fatty acid from the beta position of lecithin to the hydroxyl group of cholesterol with the production of cholesteryl ester and lysolecithin. This reaction occurs on the surface of HDL. The cholesteryl ester is transferred from HDL to VLDL and LDL.

Patients with liver disease may show reduced secretion of VLDL, HDL and LCAT, the extent of abnormality depending on the severity of hepatocellular dysfunction. Low LCAT activity is associated with accumulation of cholesterol and lecithin in plasma, in the membranes of erythrocytes and platelets and in tissues. There is an increase in the cholesterol : phospholipid ratio of cell membranes and this results in a change in the fluidity of cell membranes. This may have important effects on cell function (Owen et al 1984).

Fatty acids

Fatty acids have varying chain lengths and most fatty acids in foods and in tissues are long chain acids with 16 or more carbon atoms in their backbone. Palmitic (C16) and stearic (C18) acids have fully saturated hydrocarbon chains. Some fatty acids have a single double bond in the carbon chain (e.g. oleic — C18△9 where the △ signifies the position of the double bond). These three fatty acids (and others) can be synthesized by the mammalian body. Some fatty acids have more than one double bond. The body can and does insert new double bonds into fatty acids and it can elongate the carbon chain; the liver plays a major role in these processes. But it cannot insert double bonds into the end of the fatty acid molecule furthest from the carboxyl group. Fatty acids containing such bonds are needed by the body and are thus 'essential' fatty acids (Sinclair 1984). The main ones in the diet are linoleic (C18, △9, 12) and

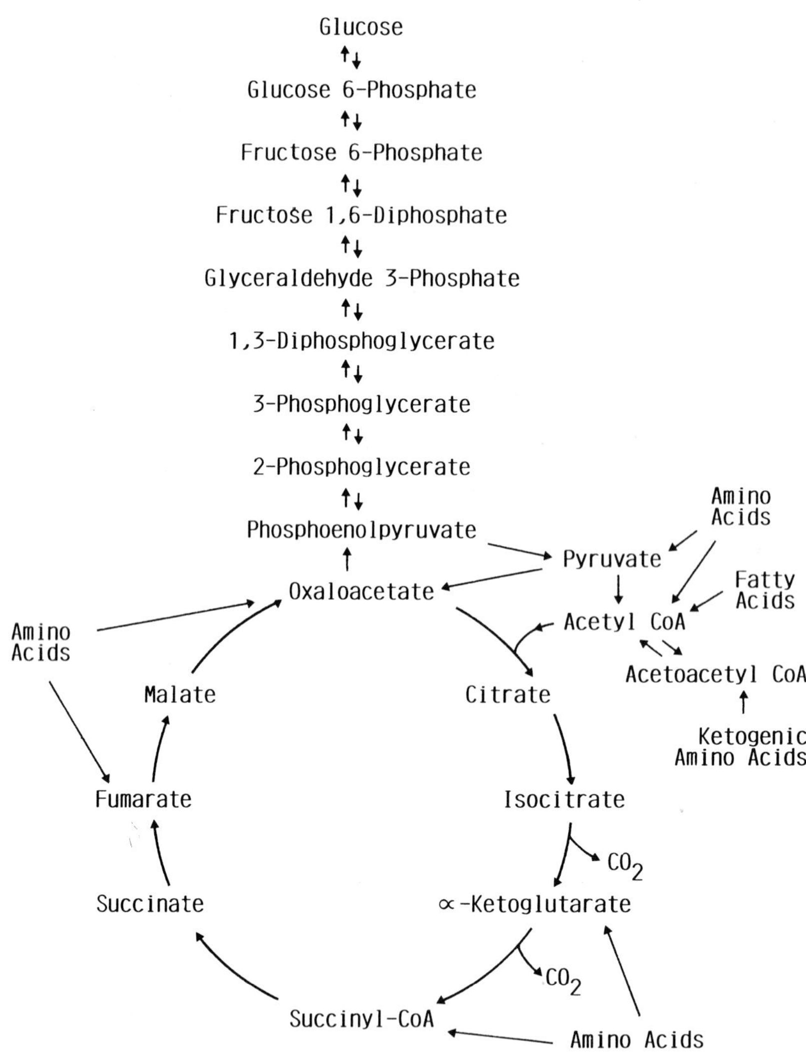

Fig. 4.1 A simplified summary of some aspects of intermediary metabolism within hepatocytes

linolenic acids (C18, △9, 12, 15). One important fate of linoleic acid is its conversion to arachidonic acid (C20, △5, 8, 11, 14) which is the precursor of the 2-series prostaglandins (PGE_2, PGl_2 etc). Essential fatty acids and their derivatives are also important constituents of the structural phospholipids of cellular membranes and seem to be important in the regulation of many enzymatic reactions. Essential fatty acid deficiency is common in liver disease; the pathogenesis and consequences are poorly understood, but impairment of renal prostaglandin production (secondary to arachidonic acid deficiency) may play an important role in the pathogenesis of renal failure (Ch. 31), a common and serious complication of liver disease.

Fatty acids are a major energy source in the body's intermediary metabolism. Esterified fatty acids are transported in blood as triglycerides (in which fatty acids are esterified with the three hydroxyl groups of glycerol), as phospholipids and in cholesteryl ester. These substances are components of lipoprotein particles. Adipose tissue is a major store of fatty acid, in the form of triglyceride. During fasting the triglyceride of adipose tissue is hydrolyzed, releasing free fatty acids into the blood, where they are bound to albumin which has specific sites for fatty acid binding. Plasma free fatty acids are present in very small amounts but have a very rapid turnover as they are taken up by peripheral tissues and used to provide energy. Their uptake by the liver appears to be facilitated by binding of the albumin-free fatty acid complex (Weisiger et al 1982).

Liver and peripheral tissues break down fatty acids by beta-oxidation in which successive 2-carbon fragments are released from the carboxyl end of the fatty acid in the form of acetyl CoA. This is cleaved by the citric acid cycle to yield CO_2, and H_2O and energy which is stored as ATP (Fig. 4.1). Fatty acids cannot be converted to sugar in animal cells. When there is active gluconeogenesis, oxaloacetate tends to be converted to phosphoenolpyruvate which undergoes further conversion to glucose. Increased utilization of oxaloacetate depletes Krebs cycle intermediates and if beta-oxidation is active at the same time, as in insulin-deficient diabetes or in starvation, the acetyl CoA produced cannot all be converted to CO_2. Instead, large amounts of acetyl-CoA are converted to ketone bodies, aceto-acetic acid, beta-hydroxybutyrate and acetone; the relative proportion of these substances depends on the redox state of the liver cell (Foster 1984). The production of ketone bodies occurs exclusively in the liver; they are an important source of energy for peripheral tissues.

Excess fatty acids taken up by the liver may be reconverted into triglyceride (their major storage form in the periphery) for incorporation into VLDL and secretion into the plasma. Excess carbohydrate (e.g. glucose, fructose) may also be converted to fatty acids for incorporation into triglyceride and VLDL. In the periphery the VLDL triglyceride is hydrolyzed and the fatty acids are utilized or re-stored in adipose tissue triglyceride. Some subjects accumulate triglyceride in liver cells with the production of fatty liver, of which there is more than one type. The pathogenesis of fatty liver is poorly understood and may involve excess synthesis of triglyceride and/or impaired release of VLDL.

AMINO ACID AND PROTEIN METABOLISM
(Albers et al 1983, Tavill 1979.)

The common amino acids have a carboxylic acid group and an amino group joined to the same carbon atom. Hydrogen occupies the third carbon bond, and either a hydrogen atom (in glycine) or a more complex side chain completes the fourth bond. The side chains vary in composition and thus in size, chemical properties and charge. (Lysine, arginine and histidine have basic side chains, aspartic acid and glutamic acids have acidic side chains. Glycine, asparagine, glutamine, cysteine, serine, threonine and tyrosine have uncharged but polar side chains; the other eight common amino acids have non-polar side chains). Proteins and polypeptides are linear polymers of amino acids which are joined by peptide bonds between the carboxyl group of one amino acid and the amino group of the next. Only 20 amino acids are used in protein synthesis. The polypeptide chain formed by translation of the messenger RNA which codes for protein synthesis may be modified in various ways following translation. The liver is a very active site of protein and polypeptide synthesis. Some are local proteins for incorporation within liver cells. The liver also makes secretory proteins which are transported into plasma: they may remain there or they may be taken up by peripheral tissues (see later).

In the liver (and in other tissues) amino acids are involved in many chemical reactions not directly related to protein synthesis. They cannot be stored as such (except in peptides and proteins) and surplus amino acids are used to provide energy or for conversion to other compounds. They are first deaminated and the remaining carbon skeletons are converted to a variety of intermediary metabolites, namely pyruvate, acetyl CoA, acetoacetyl CoA, alpha-ketoglutarate, succinyl CoA, fumarate and oxaloacetate. The last four of these are intermediates in the citric acid cycle (Fig. 4.1). The amino group may be transferred to an alpha-ketoacid to form a different amino acid. (This transamination is an important function of the liver.) Amino acids which can be formed by such interconversions are not essential components of the diet. However, threonine, methionine, lysine, valine, isoleucine, histidine, phenylalanine and tryptophan cannot be synthesized in the body; these are essential amino acids and must be supplied in the diet.

The liver can handle all amino acids but the processes and interactions are complex. Individual amino acids are handled quite differently; some are removed by the liver, others are released into the blood stream. Alanine, which is released by muscles, is avidly taken up by hepatocytes and deaminated to pyruvate which is then converted to glucose. The liver takes up most amino-acids from portal blood but the branched chain amino acids, leucine, isoleucine and valine, are not extracted to any great extent and they are taken up by peripheral tissues. Glutamine is also released from muscles in relatively large amounts and removed in the intestine and kidney. The liver can use glutamine for urea synthesis (in periportal cells) but it also synthesizes glutamine (from NH_4^+ ions and glutamate in perivenular cells) and there is little net hepatic uptake (Haussinger et al 1984).

Most of the nitrogen of ingested protein is excreted as urea and urea is synthesized only in the liver. Urea production occurs through a complex series of reactions which take place in hepatic mitochondria and in the cytosol (Fig. 4.2). Nitrogen atoms enter urea from two sources. Mitochondrial deamination of glutamate (by glutamate dehydrogenase) provides NH_4^+ ions which interact with ATP to produce carbamoyl phosphate. This combines with ornithine to produce citrulline which transfers to the cytosol; there it combines with aspartate (the source of the second nitrogen atom) to give argininosuccinate. This is cleaved to give arginine which in turn is hydrolyzed by arginase to produce urea and ornithine (which returns to the mitochondria to complete the 'urea cycle'). Glutamate plays a key role in urea synthesis as it is produced within the cytoplasm by transfer of an amino group (from many amino-acids) to alpha-ketoglutarate. It is not only the source of intramitochondrial NH_4^+ but it is also a precursor of the aspartate which combines with

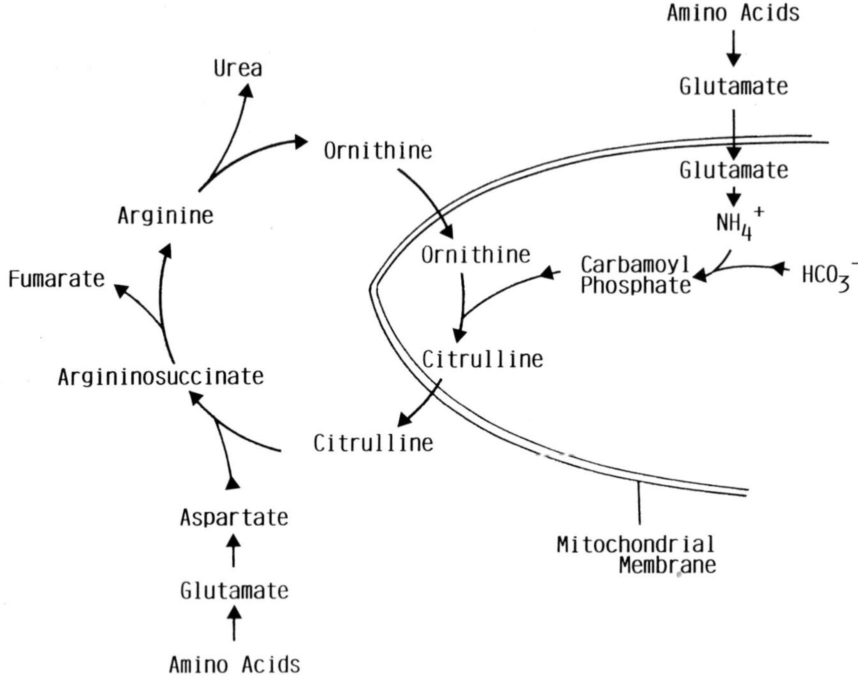

Fig. 4.2 The urea cycle

citrulline (via a transamination catalyzed by aspartate aminotransferase, i.e. AST or SGOT).

Urea production is normally considered to be a mechanism for the excretion of nitrogen. Recently there has been a re-evaluation of the metabolic role of urea production with an emphasis on its role in the regulation of acid-base balance (Atkinson & Camien 1982). It has been assumed that protein catabolism results in the production of H^+ ions which must be removed either by renal excretion of H^+ (titratable urinary acidity) or by removal of NH_4^+ ions (which have been assumed to represent H^+ ion excretion in association with NH_3). The sum of H^+ and NH_4^+ has been called total urinary acidity. In the metabolism of the zwitterionic amino acids the COO^- and NH_3^+ groups are converted to HCO_3^- and NH_4^+ ions (about 1000 mmol of each per day). The NH_4^+ ions have little effect on pH; HCO_3^+ ions, however, are part of the major buffer sytem of plasma and would have a profound effect on pH if they were to accumulate in plasma. The formation of urea by the liver (summarized as $2HCO_3^- + 2NH_4^+ \rightarrow H_2N{-}CO{-}NH_2 + CO_2 + 3H_2O$) is seen as a method of neutralizing the large amounts of HCO_3^- produced from proteins. Impairment of urea production would explain the metabolic alkalosis seen in patients with acute and chronic hepatocellular failure, as well as the accumulation of NH_4^+ which occurs. This concept also has important implications for our understanding of the kidney's role in H^+ ion excretion. It suggests that renal NH_4^+ excretion is not a means of excreting H^+ ions but rather that it is a way of excreting NH_4^+ ions produced in the tissues.

COAGULATION FACTORS AND VITAMIN K
(Liebman et al 1982, Austen 1983)

The processes of blood clotting and of lysis of clots are very complicated. The liver plays a key role (Ch. 12) because it synthesizes many of the proteins involved in coagulation including fibrinogen and factors II (prothrombin), V, VII, IX and X. The synthetic process within the liver is complex. The polypeptide chains are synthesized from messenger RNA (translation) but may undergo a variety of post-translational modifications prior to secretion into the blood. Carbohydrate chains are added. Fibrinogen is secreted as a complex of polypeptide chains.

The polypeptide chains of newly synthesized factors II, VII, IX and X contain a number of glutamic acid residues near the N-terminal end which are carboxylated by a Vitamin K dependent mechanism and thus converted into a new amino acid, gammacarboxyglutamic acid; this has an extra negative charge which enhances bonding to calcium and to platelets and is essential for coagulant activity. Vitamin K is oxidized during the process of carboxylation but is regenerated by processes which are inhibited by anticoagulants such as warfarin (Roka et al 1983).

Vitamin K occurs naturally as K1 (in vegetables) and K2 (synthesized by intestinal bacteria). It is fat-soluble and depends on micellar solubilization for absorption. With biliary obstruction Vitamin K deficiency occurs quickly. Synthesis of the polypeptide chains of factors II, VII, IX and X continues and with immunological methods they can be detected in plasma; however, their function is impaired as reflected in the prothrombin time and partial thromboplastin time. If Vitamin K is given there is rapid improvement in function. Damage of hepatocytes may impair the synthesis or release of the polypeptide chain; this type of abnormality is not corrected by administration of Vitamin K.

METABOLISM OF OTHER VITAMINS

Fat-soluble vitamins (Goodman 1982, Smith 1982, Bieri et al 1983)

Vitamins A, D and E, like Vitamin K, depend for their absorption on micellar solubilization and their absorption is impaired when bile flow is impaired, particularly with bile duct obstruction. There are usually large stores of these vitamins and clinical evidence of deficiency occurs only with long-standing impairment of absorption.

Vitamin A activity is present in the diet as retinyl esters and as beta carotene; both are hydrolyzed in the small intestine to retinol which is esterified before transfer to the liver via chylomicrons. Retinyl ester is stored in the liver. Before release from the liver it is hydrolyzed to retinol which is bound to retinol binding protein (RBP) in plasma. This in turn is complexed with the larger pre-albumin molecule which serves to minimize urinary losses of RBP. In the tissues retinol is oxidized to its native form retinal by retinol dehydrogenase, a zinc-dependent enzyme; this has great affinity for ethanol which therefore acts as a competitive inhibitor of the enzyme.

Retinal is important for the function of rods in the retina, in spermatogenesis, epithelial growth and the glycosylation of protein. In biliary obstruction evidence of Vitamin A deficiency is usually found only with prolonged biliary obstruction; overt night blindness is rare but impaired dark adaptation may be found by special testing.

Vitamin D is transported from the gut in chylomicrons and is stored unchanged in liver, muscle and adipose tissue. In the liver Vitamin D is hydroxylated to 25-OH cholecalciferol. This is the major circulating form of Vitamin D and is bound to a vitamin D binding protein. Renal hydroxylation leads to the production of 1-25 dihydroxycholecalciferol, a highly active metabolite. Vitamin D promotes intestinal calcium and phosphorus absorption, mobilizes them from bone and increases renal calcium reabsorption. Patients with long-lasting biliary absorption may develop osteomalacia, responsive to Vitamin D, but this is not a major cause of bone disease in chronic obstructive jaundice; its pathogenesis is poorly understood.

Vitamin E activity is found in naturally occurring tocopherols. Free tocopherols are incorporated in chylomicrons and then into other lipoproteins and stored in liver, fat and muscle. Vitamin E inhibits oxidation of unsaturated fatty acids and other oxygen sensitive compounds and has free radicle scavenging properties. It is clearly important but the clinical consequences of Vitamin E deficiency in adults are not obvious, though low plasma levels are found with chronic biliary obstruction. Children with chronic cholestasis develop a neurological syndrome involving peripheral neuropathy and cerebellar signs which appear to respond, in part, to treatment with Vitamin E.

Water soluble vitamins (Morgan & McIntyre 1965)

The metabolism of water soluble vitamins appears to be less affected by liver disease than that of the fat soluble vitamins, although the liver is involved in many important reactions involving these vitamins. It phosphorylates thiamine, riboflavin and the pyridoxine compounds of the vitamin B_6 group. Folate is stored in the liver. The liver is the main store of Vitamin B_{12}. Vitamin B_{12} levels in plasma rise with various forms of liver disease, due presumably to release from damaged cells. Overt evidence of deficiency of water soluble vitamins is rare in liver disease, unless there are other factors, such as alcoholism or poor nutrition. But biochemical evidence of disturbance of the metabolism of water soluble vitamins is relatively common. Although the consequences of this are unknown, it seems sensible to give supplements of water soluble vitamins to patients with liver disease.

Iron, transferrin and ferritin (Aisen 1984, Bacon & Tavill 1984)

Within the normal liver iron is stored either as ferritin (in the cytosol and lysosomes) or haemosiderin (in lysosomes), and is present in haem (in haem-containing proteins), in iron-containing enzymes, and in an 'intracellular transit pool.' Iron in plasma is carried mainly on transferrin, an iron-binding protein synthesized mainly in the liver. The liver, and other tissues such as red cell precursors and placenta, bear receptors with a high affinity for ferric-transferrin. The transferrin-receptor complex enters the liver by invagination of clathrin-coated pits on the cell surface, a mechanism which is important in the uptake of many other circulating proteins. The resulting vesicles lose their clathrin coat; hydrogen ions are pumped into the vesicle and iron, released from the ferric transferrin, enters the iron pool within the hepatocyte. The residual apotransferrin returns to the cell surface to re-enter the plasma.

When there is an excess of iron the synthesis of ferritin proteins is increased and iron is stored in the core of spherical particles which have ferritin protein molecules on the surface. With further excess of iron haemosiderin particles are formed.

Hepatic iron contributes only a few per cent of the normal daily turnover of plasma iron but hepatic iron can be released if there is a requirement for iron in other tissues (e.g. liver iron is removed when haemochromatosis is treated by venesection). The mechanism of this removal is not understood but it is assumed that transferrin may be involved and that it can take iron out of the hepatocyte as well as bring it in. In iron deficiency transferrin levels in the blood are elevated but its saturation with iron is decreased; the opposite holds in states of iron overloading. By contrast serum ferritin is increased with iron loading and decreased with iron deficiency. The high serum ferritin in iron overload has a low iron content and may represent an 'overflow' of new ferritin molecules into plasma because of the high ferritin synthesis in the tissues.

Copper (Epstein 1983)

Copper is an important mineral. It is present in a number of enzymes such as caeruloplasmin and superoxide dismutase (both antioxidants) and in a number of other oxidases. Body stores are regulated by controlling intestinal absorption and by excretion of copper in bile in which it is complexed with ligands and is not available for reabsorption. In the liver copper is incorporated into enzymes; caeruloplasmin is released into plasma where it accounts for 90% of circulating copper. With biliary obstruction there is marked accumulation of copper in the liver, where it is found in lysosomes, but it seems to be non-toxic. There is a hereditary disorder of copper metabolism, Wilson's disease, in which copper also accumulates in the liver; for reasons which are not clear the copper appears to be toxic in this condition, leading to the development of chronic active hepatitis and cirrhosis (Ch. 100, 101).

Zinc (Burch et al 1978)

Zinc is an important nutrient; it is a component of many enzymes, is involved in microtubular and microfilament production, and helps to stabilize microsomal and lysosomal membranes. It plays a role in the storage and secretion of insulin, and in the metabolism of Vitamin A. Only about 3% of the body's zinc is found in the liver where it is associated with zinc-binding metalliothioneins. Following intestinal absorption zinc is transported in the portal blood bound to albumin. There may normally be a rapid hepatic uptake of absorbed zinc; chronic liver disease is associated with high urinary zinc levels and low hepatic zinc concentrations. There is dispute over the whole body zinc status in liver disease; the levels in liver, plasma and leucocytes may be low and urinary excretion high, but radioactive zinc studies suggest increased retention in the rest of the body. The consequence of impaired zinc metabolism in chronic liver disease, e.g. for normal healing, remain to be established.

BILIRUBIN METABOLISM (Billing 1983, Hauser & Gollan 1984)

Bilirubin is produced in the reticuloendothelial system from the haem of haemoglobin, and a smaller amount is produced, mainly in the liver, from turnover of hepatic haem and haemoproteins such as the cytochromes P-450. Unconjugated bilirubin is carried in the blood tightly bound to albumin, transported across the hepatocyte membrane, and enters the cytoplasm where it is bound to proteins such as ligandin. In the endoplasmic reticulum it is conjugated with one or two molecules of glucuronic acid prior to excretion in the bile as either bilirubin monoglucuronide or the major form, bilirubin diglucuronide.

When there is excessive red cell breakdown there is an increase in the bilirubin concentration of blood but, as this is largely due to insoluble unconjugated bilirubin which is bound to albumin, there is no bilirubinuria (i.e. there is acholuric jaundice). However, the commonest cause of unconjugated hyperbilirubinaemia is not haemolysis but a benign condition, Gilbert's syndrome, in which there is impairment both of hepatic uptake of bilirubin and of its conjugation with glucuronic acid.

With hepatocellular damage (as in hepatitis or cirrhosis) most steps in hepatic bilirubin metabolism remain intact but, as in obstructive jaundice, there is an impairment of biliary excretion and regurgitation of conjugated bilirubin into the blood. When the conjugated bilirubin accumulates in liver cells a small amount is deconjugated; thus unconjugated as well as conjugated bilirubin accumulates in the plasma. Conjugated bilirubins are water soluble and when they increase in blood they are excreted in the urine giving it its characteristic dark colour in many jaundiced patients. While the presence of bilirubinuria implies a conjugated hyperbilirubinaemia its absence does not rule out the possibility of parenchymal disease or biliary obstruction in jaundiced patients. When conjugated bilirubin levels rise there is a covalent linkage of bilirubin to albumin (bili-ALB); the proportion of bili-ALB increases with time while conjugated bilirubin levels may fall. Bill-ALB is not excreted in the urine (Weiss et al 1983).

The bilirubin excreted in bile is converted in the intestine to urobilinogen which may be absorbed, transported to the liver in portal blood and resecreted. If hepatocellular function is impaired urobilinogen appears in the urine where it may be detected. Although it is absent with complete biliary obstruction the measurement of urinary urobilinogen is now of little clinical value.

THE METABOLISM OF EXOGENOUS COMPOUNDS

One important function of the liver is the metabolism of exogenous compounds. It can usually be considered as a beneficial function leading to removal of the foreign substance but occasionally the biochemical reactions carried out by the liver lead to the production of more toxic intermediates.

Ethanol (Zakim et al 1982)

Ethanol is usually metabolized by the hepatic cytosolic enzyme alcohol dehydrogenase; this oxidizes ethanol to acetaldehyde which is further oxidized by acetaldehyde dehydrogenase. Both of these oxidations involve the production of NADH from NAD^+; many sequelae of ethanol ingestion are thought to be due to the increase in the $NADH/NAD^+$ ratio. Ethanol can also be converted to acetaldehyde by a microsomal ethanol oxidizing system which uses NADPH and molecular oxygen, and by catalase which uses hydrogen peroxide. Blood acetaldehyde increases during ethanol metabolism and it is thought that acetaldehyde is a toxic substance. Its role in ethanol toxicity is uncertain, and there is as yet no good explanation for the long-term liver damage produced by excessive ethanol ingestion.

Drugs (Bentley & Oesch 1982)

Drugs and other foreign compounds are handled mainly by the liver and kidneys, the role of the kidneys being the excretion of water soluble drugs or metabolites. Many compounds are relatively lipophilic and need to be converted into more hydrophilic substances prior to renal or biliary excretion. This is a major function of the liver. Four main types of process are involved: oxidation, reduction, hydrolysis and conjugation.

There are two groups of oxygenases involved in drug metabolism:

1. Mixed function amine oxidase which catalyzes the oxidation of nitrogen and sulphur atoms;
2. The more important cytochrome P-450 dependent mono-oxygenases which have very broad substrate specificity and which consist of NADPH-cytochrome P-450 (cytochrome C) reductase together with a variety of terminal oxygenases, the cytochromes P-450.

These proteins are present in the endoplasmic reticulum and tranfer reducing equivalents from NADPH to the P-450 so that eventually an oxygen molecule is split; one atom of oxygen is reduced to water, the other added to the drug or other substance metabolized. Drugs which are metabolized by this system can increase the amount of cytochromes P-450 or change their relative proportions, a phenomenon known as enzyme induction. It is important because administration of one drug may lead to increased metabolism of others and this has important therapeutic implications, e.g. barbiturates, phenytoin and rifampicin are inducing agents which diminish the effects of warfarin by increasing its metabolism; larger doses are given for anticoagulant effect and these may prove toxic when the inducing agent is withdrawn. Some reductions are also mediated through P-450 enzymes, and a number of compounds are handled by hydrolytic reactions.

Finally, many compounds are made more water soluble by conjugation with an amino acid, glucuronic acid, sulphate or glutathione. Drugs can also be acetylated or methylated. Conjugation with glutathione is the most versatile form of conjugation and it is particularly important for the handling of reactive intermediates; there are a number of proteins with glutathione S-transferase activity and they have different substrate specificities. Glutathione has a number of other important functions particularly in the protection of cells against oxidative stress (Meister & Anderson 1983).

When drugs have been altered by the liver they may be suitable for renal excretion. Alternatively, they may be excreted in bile and some drugs can be re-absorbed from the intestine, returning to the liver via the portal vein. This enterohepatic recirculation of drugs is occasionally of clinical importance as the effect of the drug is minimized if the enterohepatic circulation is broken, e.g. by biliary drainage.

The hepatic metabolism of drugs is not always beneficial, particularly if the drug is taken in excess. The predictable hepatotoxic effects of paracetamol and carbon tetrachloride are thought to result from the formation of reactive intermediates. Therapeutic doses of paracetamol are thought to be handled mainly by conjugation with glucuronide or sulphate. Large doses exceed the capacity of these systems and oxidation via the cytochrome P-450 (P-448) pathway plays an increasing role in the metabolism of the drug. The toxic intermediate, thought to be N acetyl-imidoquinone, is conjugated with glutathione, but if glutathione reserves are also exhausted then the toxic compound is free to damage the hepatocyte. Support for this theory comes from experimental observations showing that enzyme induction with phenobarbitone reduces the dose required to give paracetamol toxicity while inhibitors of cytochrome P-450, such as cimetidine, protect against injury. Clinical treatments designed to replenish the glutathione supply, or to provide other substrates for conjugation of the toxic metabolite, such as N-acetyl cysteine or methionine, are also effective in preventing liver damage (Black 1983).

REFERENCES

Aisen P 1984 Transferrin metabolism and the liver. Seminars in Liver Disease 4: 193–206

Albers B, Bray D, Lewis J, Raff M, Roberts K, Watson J D 1983 Molecular biology of the cell. Garland, New York

Alberti K G, Johnston D G, Taylor R 1985 Carbohydrate metabolism in liver disease. In: Wright R, Alberti K G, Karran S, Millward-Sadler G H (eds) Liver and biliary disease, 2nd edn. W B Saunders, London, Ch. 3

Atkinson D E, Camien M N 1982 The role of urea synthesis in the removal of metabolic bicarbonate and the regulation of blood pH. Current Topics in Cellular Regulation 21:261

Austen D E G 1983 The clinical biochemistry of blood coagulation. In: Williams D L, Marks V (eds) Biochemistry in clinical practice. Heinemann, London, p 251–268

Bacon B R, Tavill A S 1984 Role of the liver in normal iron metabolism. Seminars in Liver Disease 4: 181–192

Bentley P, Oesch F 1982 Foreign compound metabolism in the liver. In: Popper H, Schaffner F (eds) Progress in liver diseases, Vol 7. Grune and Stratton, New York, p 157–178

Bieri J G, Corash L, Husband V S 1983 Medical use of vitamin E. New England Journal of Medicine 308: 1063–1071

Billing B H 1983 Assessment of the value of bile pigment determinations in the diagnosis of jaundice. Postgraduate Medical Journal 59: (suppl. 4) 19–25

Black M 1983 Drug induced liver damage. Postgraduate Medical Journal 59: 116–122

Brown M S, Goldstein J L 1984 How LDL receptors influence cholesterol and atherosclerosis. Scientific American 251: 52–60

Burch R E, Hahn H K J, Sullivan, J F 1978 Other metals and the liver, with particular reference to zinc. In: Powell L (ed) Metals and the liver. Decker, New York, p 333–361

Cohen R D, Woods H F 1976 Clinical and biochemical aspects of lactic acidosis. Blackwell, Oxford

Eisenberg S 1984 High density lipoprotein metabolism. Journal of Lipid Research 25: 1017–1058

Epstein O 1983 Liver copper in health and disease. Postgraduate Medical Journal 59: (suppl. 4) 88–94

Foster D W 1984 From glycogen to ketones — and back. Diabetes 33: 1188–1199

Glickman R M, Sabesin S M 1982 Lipoprotein metabolism. In: Arias I M, Popper H, Schachter D, Shafritz D (eds) The liver: biology and pathobiology. Raven Press, New York, 123–142

Goodman D S 1982 Vitamin A metabolism. In: Arias I M, Popper H, Schachter D, Shafritz D (eds) In: The liver: biology and pathobiology. Raven Press, New York, p 347–352

Gray G M 1983 Mechanisms of digestion and absorption of food. In: Sleisinger M H, Fordtran J S (eds) Gastrointestinal disease: pathophysiology, diagnosis, management. W B Saunders, Philadelphia, p 844–858

Gumucio J J, Miller D L 1982 Liver cell heterogeneity. In: Arias I A, Popper H, Schachter D, Shafritz D (eds) The liver: biology and pathobiology. Raven Press, New York, p 647–661

Hauser S, Gollan J 1984 Recent developments in hyperbilirubinaemia and bilirubin metabolism. In: Gitnick G Current hepatology Vol 4. J Wiley, New York

Haussinger D, Gerok W, Sies H 1984 Hepatic role in pH regulation: role of the intracellular glutamine cycle. Trends in Biochemical Sciences 9: 300–302

Hoffman A F 1983 The enterohepatic circulation of bile acids in health and disease. In: Sleisenger M H, Fordtran J S (eds) Gastrointestinal disease: pathophysiology, diagnosis, management. W B Saunders, Philadelphia, p 115–134

Katz J, McGarry J D 1984 The glucose paradox; is glucose a substrate for liver metabolism? Journal of Clinical Investigation 74: 1901–1909

Liebman H A, Furie B C, Furie B 1982 Hepatic vitamin K-dependent carboxylation of blood clotting proteins. Hepatology 2: 488–494

Meister A, Anderson M E 1983 Glutathione. Annual Review of Biochemistry 52: 711–760

Morgan M Y, McIntyre N 1985 Nutritional aspects of liver disease. In: Wright R, Alberti K G, Karran S, Millward-Sadler G H (eds) Liver and biliary disease, 2nd edn. W B Saunders, London, p

Motta P M 1982 Scanning electron microscopy of the liver. In: Popper H, Schaffner F (eds) Progress in liver diseases Vol 7. Grune and Stratton, New York, p 1

Norum K R, Bert T, Helgerud P, Drevon C A 1983 Transport of cholesterol. Physiological Reviews 63: 1343–1419

Owen J S, McIntyre N, Gillet M P T 1984 Lipoproteins, cell membranes and cellular functions. Trends in Biochemical Sciences 9: 238–242

Roka L, Dehler G, Stibora M, Bleyl H 1983 Vitamin K in liver disease. In: Bianchi L, Gerok W, Landmann L, Sickinger K, Stalder G A (eds) Liver in metabolic diseases. MTP Press, Boston, p 429

Sinclair H M 1984 Essential fatty acids in perspective. Human Nutrition: Clinical Nutrition 38c: (4) 245–260

Smith J E 1982 Vitamin D metabolism. In: Arias A, Popper H, Schachter D, Shafritz D (eds) The liver: biology and pathobiology. Raven Press, New York, p 353–357

Tavill A S 1979 Protein metabolism and the liver. In: Wright R, Alberti K G, Karran S, Millward-Sadler G H (eds) Liver and biliary disease 2nd edn. W B Saunders, London, p 83–107

Tygstrup N 1983 Galactose and fructose metabolism in liver disease. In: Bianchi L, Gerok W, Landmann L, Sickinger K, Stalder G A (eds) Liver in metabolic diseases. MTP Press, Boston, p 255

Weisiger R A, Gollan J L, Ockner R K 1982 The role of albumin in hepatic uptake processes. In: Popper H, Schaffner F (eds) Progress in liver diseases. Grune and Stratton, New York, p 71

Weiss J S, Gautam A, Lauff J J, Sundberg M W, Jatlow P, Boyer J L, Seligson D 1983 The clinical importance of a protein bound fraction of serum bilirubin in patients with hyperbilirubinaemia. New England Journal of Medicine 309: 147–150

Zakim D, Boyer T D, Montgomery C, Kanas N 1982 Alcoholic liver disease. In: Zakim D, Boyer T D (eds) Hepatology. W B Saunders, Philadelphia, p 739–789

5

K. Weinbren, N. S. Hadjis

Compensatory hyperplasia of the liver

INTRODUCTION

Compensatory enlargement of liver tissue after damage to, or loss of a part, is a major hepatic reaction on which much of modern surgical therapy relies. The phenomenon of growth of the remnant after partial resection has been described in most species in which the necessary manipulations have been undertaken (Fishback 1929, Higgins & Anderson 1931, Higgins et al 1932, Grindlay & Bollman 1952, Yokoyama et al 1953, Pack et al 1962) and, as far as can be assessed from published works (Bucher 1963), there is no known species or strain in which uncomplicated surgical reduction of a substantial part of the liver is not attended by enlargement of the remnant. The nature of the phenomenon, first described almost a century ago (Ponfick 1889, Von Meister 1894) is comparable in different species and in different circumstances and there is now little conflict about the morphological (Harkness 1952, Grisham 1962, Brues & Marble 1937) and biochemical changes which have been found (Baserga 1974, Lewan et al 1977, McGowan & Fausto 1978, MacManus et al 1973). The mechanisms underlying the development of the changes are not understood and there remains a considerable diversity of opinion about the key enzymatic and humoral factors which may be responsible. Nor is it clear why there is so little concordance of views after so much intensive investigation of a reproducible biological phenomenon. It is proposed therefore in this chapter to identify what facts may be relevant to the process and to attempt an analysis of the postulates proposed and the experimental phenomena on which these are based.

PROLIFERATION OF HEPATOCYTES

The increase in mass of the remnant after partial hepatectomy is repeatedly confirmed and in general, increases in DNA content (Bucher et al 1964, Grisham 1962) and in numbers of liver cells are regarded as the basic changes. The response is therefore referred to as a compensatory hyperplasia, the latter term justified by the measurable increase in genetic units or DNA (Schulte-Hermann 1974) which may be expressed as absolute values or as a ratio to body weight (Bucher & Malt 1971), organ weight or protein content (Rabes & Brändle 1969). The rate of incorporation of precursors into DNA (Weinbren & Woodward 1964) and the incidence of hepatocyte mitoses (Weinbren & Tarsh 1964) are also used as indices of the response. There are sometimes microscopic rearrangements of hepatocytes in a liver which has undergone hyperplastic changes (Morgan & Hartroft 1961, Weinbren & Mutum 1984) and these may provide a means of recognizing the process in tissue sections; some changes which simulate those found in neoplastic conditions have been observed in experiments associated with continued compensatory proliferation of cells (Weinbren 1982). On a macroscopic level, in certain circumstances changes may be observed in hepatic contours on an image generated by one of the clinical imaging procedures (Aronsen et al 1970).

While it is possible to detect cellular proliferation after evident damage to liver tissue, it has to be remarked that proliferation of liver cells may also be observed in other conditions. The process of somatic growth, easily recognizable in terms of bodily stature alterations, includes, according to well-defined and allometric formulae, a predictable enlargement of the liver with age and with increases in bodily length, surface area and weight (Deland & North 1968, Kennedy & Pearle 1958, Donaldson 1924). Increases in liver mass are noted also, even when liver tissue is not surgically removed or damaged (Barka & Popper 1967). Proliferation of liver cells may thus occur in different circumstances and, among the difficulties encountered in defining the structural, metabolic and mechanical phenomena of compensatory hyperplasia, is that of distinguishing these from the effects of other forms of adaptive liver growth and also from somatic growth (Echave Llanos et al 1971, Rabes & Brandle 1969). These processes are similar in some but not all respects.

Somatic growth, that which is genetically programmed, is detectable in the post-organogenesis embryonic period and proceeds throughout life in some species, e.g. the male rat (McKellar 1949), and only for a restricted time, until epiphyseal fusion, in other species, such as man. If adaptive growth is initiated, this takes place at a different rate and often assumes a different form from somatic growth but these processes may possibly be confused. Chemically induced adaptive growth may also show differences from compensatory enlargement after surgical resection and damage by disease or toxins and mechanistic views derived from the study of one of these reactions may not be applicable to the other (Schulte-Hermann 1974). Neoplastic growth also involves proliferation of hepatocytes and this process, too, must be distinguished from compensatory hyperplasia (Cayama et al 1978).

The superimposition of compensatory hyperplasia on one or other of the afore-mentioned proliferative processes is an obvious possibility since it is conceivable that an acute injury or disease may affect a young growing individual or acute toxic damage may develop in an organism in which adaptive proliferation of liver cells is already in progress in association with enzyme induction. The characteristics therefore of somatic liver growth require some attention in this regard, because of the possible concurrence of the two processes. The changes observed in the otherwise normal growing liver have been outlined (Doljanski 1960) and some of the regulating factors are agreed (Walter & Addis 1939). Liver mass bears a predictable relationship with body weight in man and in several other species, a sex difference being observed after puberty (Boyd 1933). The main component in the proliferative process is an increase in cell number, but not in average amount of structural protein per hepatocyte (Bucher 1963). A significant conformational change occurs in the organization of the hepatocytes as the liver grows and it has become important in recent years to note this arrangement both in healthy and in diseased tissue or in hyperplastic liver. In essence, liver tissue in embryos of most vertebrates is made up of two-cell thick plates of liver cells separated by vascular channels or sinusoids and this pattern is retained during maturity and even in ageing in birds, fish and reptiles but not in non-aquatic mammals (Elias & Sherrick 1969). In these last, the double plates are transformed into plates of only one-cell thickness during early development in different species, this change occurring, e.g. at about five years in man (Morgan & Hartroft 1961). Part of normal somatic growth therefore is cellular proliferation and part involves remodelling of the liver structure. The mechanism by means of which this transformation is effected is still unknown and so far no evidence has been presented which indicates an enzymic or any other form of cytolysis which is operative at the appropriate times. In addition, there appears to be no reference to any reaction consequent on cellular necrosis at the relevant times when two-cell thick (embryonic or juvenile) plates are converted to single-cell thick adult type plates. The mechanisms involved in this remodelling process are not known, but the questions posed by the transformation are of interest not only to those whose interest lies in pathogenesis; it seems possible that a failure in this aspect of development may allow survival of thick plates, the presence of which may complicate interpretation of the microscopic changes in abnormalities of the liver. Nonetheless it has become customary to consider the development of hepatocyte plates which are more than one-cell thick in a human adult as representing the effects of hyperplasia (Weinbren 1978), and in most instances a reflection of compensatory hyperplasia. Such a conformational change is found in many forms of chronic liver disease and may be identified purely on structural grounds and it is reasonable to refer to the thickened hepatocyte plates in positional terms, such as 'periportal hepatocyte hyperplasia' or 'diffuse hepatocyte hyperplasia'. The prognostic importance of the integrity of vascular supply and drainage in chronic liver disease is generally agreed (Weinbren 1978) and a further categorization of the hyperplastic changes therefore depends on the identification of a normal spatial relationship between portal tracts and efferent veins (Weinbren et al 1985). Thus, diffuse thickening of 'hyperplastic' plates associated with normal vascular relations is referred to as 'lobular hyperplasia' and that in which a normal vascular relationship is lost, as 'nodular hyperplasia', the latter term including a range from large nodules, as seen in some forms of cirrhosis, to very small, sublobular nodules, usually noted in diffuse nodular hyperplasia (Weinbren & Mutum 1984). The types of chronic hepatic disease associated with thickening of liver plates, usually considered to represent compensatory hyperplasia, include almost any condition in which substantial cellular damage or destruction is known to have taken place, such as direct toxic action of chemicals like paracetamol (Black 1980), accidental trauma or surgical resection (Blumgart et al 1971), replacement of tissue by tumour, inflammatory destruction of liver cells in duct obstruction (Weinbren et al 1985) and also conditions in which loss of liver cells is presumed to have taken place, such as cirrhosis (Popper 1954), and even in circumstances in which evidence of previous cellular necrosis is not persuasive or completely lacking, such as focal nodular hyperplasia (Knowles & Wolff 1976). The term 'hyperplasia' may not be applicable in this last condition as the possibility of a hamartomatous change is strongly supported (Stocker & Ishak 1981). The same may be considered for both diffuse nodular hyperplasia and for partial nodular transformation (Sherlock et al 1966) but structural evidence supporting a hamartomatous origin is not as compelling in these circumstances. Changes in the liver which are considered to represent compensatory hyperplasia therefore are frequently observed in a variety of chronic liver diseases and also as an immediate response to removal of or damage to part of the liver.

INVESTIGATIONS INTO PROLIFERATIVE RESPONSES

Investigations into the mechanisms which regulate the phenomena involved in compensatory hyperplasia have been presented for many years and have in general involved four lines of study:

1. Observations made on in vivo changes in subjects undergoing the hyperplastic response.
2. Attempts made to modify the response by in vivo manipulation.
3. In vitro studies to identify growth factors for the hepatocyte.
4. Attempted correlations between in vitro and in vivo phenomena.

1. Observations on hepatic and other changes in subjects in whom compensatory hyperplasia was known to be taking place

Such studies have been in progress for almost a century. They have generated a large body of data about some of which there is now agreement, it being conceded that many of the observations which were not readily confirmed usually reflected experimental weaknesses or represented forms of proliferation other than compensatory hyperplasia. In general terms, the involvement of the whole remnant (Fishback 1929), the timing and magnitude of the DNA synthetic response (Weinbren & Woodward 1964) and the spatial distribution of the hepatocytes exhibiting mitoses (Harkness 1952), the proportion of cells taking part in the acute proliferative response after two-thirds partial hepatectomy at different ages (Bucher et al 1964) and a wide variety of biochemical changes are generally not disputed (Francavilla et al 1978). The biochemical and physical changes in the intact organism have stimulated much speculation about the proliferative mechanisms, membrane and sublemmal activity (Deliconstantinos & Ramantanis 1983), ornithine decarboxylase (ODC) (McGowan & Fausto 1978), non-histone nucleoproteins (Baserga 1974, Martinez-Sales & Baguena 1981), alpha-fetoprotein (Watanabe et al 1976, Sell et al 1974), surface charge activity (Eisenberg et al 1962, Wondergem & Harder 1980) and changes in gap junction formation (Yee & Revel 1978, Meyer et al 1981) are of particular interest in this regard. Other variables, such as water and fat content (Simek et al 1968), cyclic AMP (Short et al 1975, Friedman 1976), although not so frequently featuring in postulates about growth mechanisms, are becoming more relevant to the identification of proliferating tissue particularly in view of the detection capacity of the newer imaging procedures using electromagnetic field changes (de Certaines et al 1982) and the part assigned to phosphorylated compounds in experimental in vitro studies (Koch et al 1976). While the many excellent biochemical studies on the liver remnant after partial hepatectomy have helped to elucidate several of the key reactions involved in the cellular proliferation, none, so far as we can tell, has convincingly led to the identification of the initiator of the process. Postulated flow-charts (Leffert et al 1982) have indeed indicated the order of biochemical reactions and the most likely enzymatic activities, and have suggested possible mechanisms for the regulation of reactions at particular post-initiation times, but the essential primary stimulus is so far elusive. This is perhaps not surprising for the tissue remnant activity must perforce reflect the reaction to a deprivation mechanism, the removal of normal tissue somehow initiating the process and at the same time depriving the organism of a host of unidentified factors.

Changes in other tissues and in the serum have also been observed after partial hepatectomy. These include alterations in levels of insulin (Bucher & Weir 1976), glucagon (Leffert et al 1975), VLDL (Leffert & Weinstein 1976), as well as structural changes in the pituitary of some species (Echave Llanos et al 1971) and changes apparently in the biological activity of the serum (Moolten & Bucher 1967). The main finding here is the reproducible stimulatory effect on hepatocyte proliferation of serum taken from rats which have undergone partial hepatectomy (Michalopoulos et al 1984, Nakamura 1984).

2. Attempts made to modify the proliferative response by in vivo manipulation

Many experiments have been carried out in which the environment of the hepatocyte has been modified by endocrine ablation or hormone administration (Starzl et al 1978, Starzl et al 1975, Rixon & Whitfield 1976), vascular or ductal occlusion (Mizumoto et al 1970, Weinbren 1953), or interference with nervous activity (Weinbren et al 1967), by the administration of enzyme inhibitors (Weinbren & Fitschen 1959), the use of radiation (Weinbren et al 1960) infusion of serum from other animals (Adibi et al 1959, Nadal 1975) or administration of putative stimulating or inhibiting agents (Terblanche et al 1980). The considerable experimental activity in this field has not yet yielded a consensus view about the main in vivo growth mechanism. What seems to have emerged is that several hormones are capable of modulating the proliferative response to partial hepatectomy in the experimental animal, but so far no individual compound, including those which may show conspicuous biological activity in other respects, such as insulin (Starzl et al 1973), glucagon (Starzl et al 1973), heparin (Zimmerman & Celozzi 1961, Short et al 1972), epidermal growth factor (St. Hilaire & Jones 1982), nerve growth factor (Yanker & Shooter 1982), appears to be the certain initiator of compensatory hyperplasia as tested in vivo.

3. In vitro studies to identify growth factors for the hepatocyte

The conditions governing the growth of hepatocytes in vitro usually require precise control and changes are effected by chemical and physical variations even without addition of putative stimulating or inhibitory factors (Leffert & Koch 1979). There are several attributes of monolayer cultures, apparently closely related to cellular proliferation, which are completely understood and which complicate the interpretation of changes which may be observed with the addition of compounds under test. One such phenomenon is known as contact inhibition (Holley & Kiernan 1968) and is reflected in the progressive decrease in synthesis of macromolecules as cellular monolayers fill an area (Hasegawa et al 1982) and which is reversed by experimentally creating a separation between the cells (James & Bradshaw 1984). This latter procedure may be effected by subdividing or wounding the culture so that cells are freed from tight contact with their neighbours. The mechanism on which this reaction is based is not understood, but several plausible views have been adduced which so far have not been seriously challenged. One such theory implicates changes in the rate of diffusion of molecules between cells because of variations in intrinsic cellular oscillations of asynchronous cells during different parts of the cell cycle, which depend on confluency, and another suggests reduced pinocytosis and uptake of mitogenic serum molecules in contacting neighbour cells (James & Bradshaw 1984). While it is an important aspect of in vitro cellular activity, and its effects have necessarily to be controlled if possible in experiments on growth factors, the phenomenon of contact inhibition has so far not provided an understanding of the initiation of the compensatory hyperplastic response. This however does not deny that basic observations in this field which relate to the free passage of a current of ions between normal and growing but not malignant cells and may be of relevance to the initiation mechanism (Loewenstein & Kanno 1967).

A second and probably connected phenomenon relates to the dependency of the culture on the addition of fresh medium (Rozengurt & Collins 1983). A change of medium is often associated with a wave of division in cultures and has been considered to be due to a serum factor which reduces contact inhibition, or by a change in pH or by an alteration in the availability of surface receptors possibly due to proteolytic activity of fresh medium (Holley & Kiernan 1968). This phenomenon has attracted much investigation, has led to the singularly important suggestion that tumour cells probably release 'autocrine' or self growth-promoting factors, whereas non-neoplastic cells do not (Sporn & Roberts 1985) and may introduce a confounding factor in experiments on in vitro hepatocyte growth, but so far has not provided the key to the initiation of compensatory hyperplasia.

Reports of studies in this field have indicated that a number of factors are effective in stimulating DNA synthesis in density-inhibited cultures of several different cell types and the questions about the underlying mechanisms require elucidation. Several groups of chemicals have been tested for activity in culture systems and these have formed the basis for several hypotheses about sequences of activity, receptor sites and devices for translating plasmalemmal changes into mitogenic stimuli (Rozengurt & Collins 1983). Some of the postulated factors are known hormones already familiar because of other more clearly defined in vivo activity; some, although transported by the blood stream and probably effective in stimulating cells which are different from the tissues or cells from which they were released, are considered separately from conventional hormones and several are derived from a variety of tissues in different circumstances and have been tested on several culture systems (Leffert et al 1982). The test systems used have included hepatocytes and although specificity has not been a primary consideration, a body of evidence has been acquired which supports a link between these compounds and cellular proliferation. The established hormones with mitogenic effects on cultured cells include insulin (Leffert 1974, Leffert et al 1979) glucagon, growth hormone, thyroxine and cortisol (Leffert 1974), all of which stimulate adult or neonatal rat hepatocyte DNA synthesis or 3HdT incorporation into DNA (Leffert et al 1979).

A second class of proliferogenic compounds which are not conventional hormones have been grouped together on the basis of their property of stimulating DNA synthesis in cultured hepatocytes (Leffert et al 1982). These are generally peptides and several aspects of their activity have been defined and suggestions have been made about their possible interdependence and sequential activity (Antoniades & Owen 1982). There is some overlap with the group of known hormones as glucagon and insulin are generally included with this group, but the main growth factors which reproducibly stimulate DNA synthesis in hepatocytes are epidermal growth factor (EGF) (St Hilaire & Jones 1982), Insulin-like growth factor (IGF) previously referred to as Non-suppressible insulin-like action (NSILA) (Zapf et al 1978) and Somatomedin C (Daughaday 1977, Rechler & Nissley 1977). These factors possess a number of common properties, besides the capacity to stimulate rat hepatocyte DNA synthesis in vitro, which include a single chain polypeptide structure of about MW of 7500 daltons, insulin-like activity on adipocytes, and anabolic processes in cartilage in vitro; all react strongly with IGF receptors and weakly with insulin receptors (Daughaday 1977, Rechler & Nissley 1977). They generally cross-react extensively, apart from IGF II (Daughaday 1977). The relationship to insulin is further underlined by the strong homology of amino acid sequences between human pro-insulin and IGF II, and striking similarities between IGF I and Somatomedin C in radioreceptor assays and in chemical structure (Rinderknecht & Humbel 1978, Svoboda et al 1980, Van Wyk et al 1980). All these factors are very weak mitogens alone, even in vitro, but they are now regarded as possible supporters of proliferation once cells are committed and, without them, some cultured cells may not progress through their cycle (Stiles et al 1979). They cannot therefore be regarded as inducers of proliferation either in cultures or in vivo.

Epidermal growth factor (EGF) peptide, first extracted from salivary glands, is a proliferogenic factor whose effect is reproducibly demonstrable in culture system. Many studies of this peptide have now been made, and it is reported that it has a MW of 6100 daltons, appears to be active early in the cell-cycle and shows conspicuous biological synergism with glucagon and IGF I and II (McGowan et al 1981). The substance is probably identical with urogastrone (Hollenberg & Gregory 1976) and there appears to be a wide distribution of receptors for EGF, which can be distinguished from those for other hormones (Carpenter & Cohen 1979). These factors, which have formed the basis for many speculations about mechanisms underlying compensatory hyperplasia in the intact organism, show activity on cell lines other than hepatocytes and there is some difficulty therefore in reconciling this observation with the organ-specific reaction in vivo.

Several mechanisms have been considered as the possible basis for the proliferogenic effects of these factors (Leffert et al 1982) but these are so far not fully supported by the data available and are unable to encompass all the observations made. Ligand receptor complexes are thought to be endocytosed and degraded by lysosomes (Pastan & Willingham 1981) and changes are observed in the phosphorylation of membranes (King & Cuatrecasas 1981), with changes in Na^+, K^+ and ATPase levels (Koch & Leffert 1979). Other membrane-associated changes include reorganization of actin microfilaments (Schlessinger & Geiger 1981) and increased activity of ornithine decarboxylase (Tomita et al 1981). Thus it seems that there are membrane-associated changes (Leffert & Koch 1980) and there is clear mitogenic activity when an appropriate factor is added to a culture system. It is not clear however how these two phenomena are related. The recognition of cell-membrane associated receptors has been the principal impetus for the refinement of views about the action of growth factors (Brown & Goldstein 1979, Bradshaw & Rubin 1980) and the properties of receptors form an agreed basis for attempted analyses of the process. The properties so far generally accepted are the ability to recognize specific chemical structures (Lauffenburger & DeLisi 1983), to control cellular responsiveness and to generate intracellular signals which include the stimulus to DNA synthesis.

The first step in the process is a reversible binding to the ligand which however is saturable and generally specific, although able to be blocked by related molecules which may have occupied relevant receptor sites. Such occupancy has been referred to as 'down-regulation' and as such may have profound effects on anticipated cellular activity (Earp & O'Keefe 1981). Receptor-ligand complexes appear to require functioning microtubules as tubule damaging agents may reduce ligand activity (Brown et al 1980). It is postulated also that the post-ligand receptor binding steps involve endocytosis of the complex and degradation by lysosomes (Goldstein et al 1979). The mitogenic ligands are thus supposed to enter the cytoplasm but the possibility of desensitization of such factors at this stage is not excluded and has been considered a possibly added regulatory mechanism for the proliferative response. The actual intracellular changes which may play a part in the translation of the ligand-receptor complex or cell-surface activity include increases in ion fluxes (Rozengurt & Mendoza 1980) and in cAMP levels, changes more easily observed in Swiss 3T3 cells, but probably also relevant to liver cells (Lopes Rivas et al 1982). The cAMP levels are thought to relate to an increase in protein kinase activity, an activity which parallels ligand complexing in several in vitro culture systems. The ligands remarked as stimulating this activity are varied, and there may be a synergism between ion fluxes and cAMP (Rozengurt & Mendoza 1980, Whitfield et al 1980). Nor is it clear what part may be played by the possible increased passage of nutrients from the medium into the cell as a result of altered membrane activity (Leffert et al 1978).

A third rather less compact group of proliferogenic factors has been described as showing effects on cell culture systems, but not all appear to have been tested or are found to be active in hepatocyte systems. Nonetheless the activities described seem to be relevant to the problem of ligand-receptor complexing and mitosis-stimulation, and tentative conclusions drawn have been derived from data generated by several different cell types. Platelet derived growth factor (PDGF) (Kaplan et al 1979) is contained in the alpha granules of platelets, has a MW of 30 000 daltons (larger than IGF), is able to induce proliferation in a variety of cells, and thought to render cells competent to the action of later proliferogenic factors. Fibroblast growth factor (FGF) (Gospodarowicz & Mescher 1980) (MW 13 400 daltons) derived either from pituitary or brain is similar in some respects to PDGF (Gospodarowicz et al 1978). FGF is also active in blastemal cells of frogs in vivo, but its activity is inhibited by proteolytic digestion (Westall et al 1978). It is effective in low densities of cells, may enhance clonogenic activity and stimulates cell migration.

Extracellular factors (referred to as extracellular matrix-ECM) also play some part (Kleinman et al 1981). It is not clear exactly how extracellular factors, including collagens, proteoglycans, basement membrane collagen and glycoprotein, affect the sensitivity of cultured cells but there are differences between cells on plastic or glass and cells on collagen (Yamada 1983). The molecules of the substrate responsible for the modification of the response are not defined.

A variety of other facts play some part in the cellular proliferation induced in density-inhibited or serum-depleted culture systems, some of which are physical (temperature dependency), others are chemical and derived from intact organisms (proteolytic agents) in serum which may render membranes more permeable or expose more receptors (Ham 1981); but although advantages are claimed for the use of cell cultures in terms of the absence of the 'complexities' of in vivo work, it has to be acknowledged that any synthesis of mechanisms derived from cell culture data is not confirmed in whole animal experiments (Leffert et al 1976). Even the most enthusiastic proponents of the view that the hormones or other known growth factors which act sequentially to such striking effect in vitro, may also be relevant to the biological phenomenon of compensatory hyperplasia, acknowledge the irritating 'paradoxes' (Leffert et al 1976).

4. Attempted correlations between in vitro and in vivo observations

Alterations in the liver tissue undergoing hepatocyte hyperplasia are similar in several respects to those noted in culture systems, notably increased activity in the ornithine decarboxylase-putrescine system (Russel & Snyder 1968, Demetriou et al 1983), lipid (Harkness 1957), alpha-fetoprotein (Madsen et al 1980), actin filaments (Schlessinger & Geiger 1981) and electrical charge; and the changes in the serum which correlate include VLDL depression (Leffert et al 1976), AFP increase and proliferogenic activity in recipients of supernatant (LaBrecque & Pesch 1975, LaBrecque 1982). Of these changes, it seems reasonable to regard most as reflecting the proliferating process in which the cells are involved, either in the organ in situ, or in a monolayer system, and it is not likely that any of these changes represents the factor which initiates the replicating process with such reproducibility and precision. In this regard, studies on rats with congenitally high levels of VLDL do not in fact show a substantial change in their reaction to partial resection (Leffert & Weinstein 1976); and raised levels of AFP in both in vivo and in vitro conditions are recognized as indicating an early post-mitotic cellular marker (Sell et al 1974, Madsen et al 1980). Delayed responses have been noted in instances of deprivation in vivo of hormones which show activity in culture system but these are invariably temporary and may be matched by metabolic changes such as variations in blood glucose levels (Leffert et al 1976).

There is, however, some supportive evidence of a type of correlation between the two main experimental activities, as the administration of a mixture of amino acids, heparin, thyroxine and glucagon was reported to stimulate hepatocyte proliferation in intact livers (Short et al 1972) but the exact interpretation of the proliferogenic effect of this bizarre mixture is not certain.

Irreversible inhibition of ODC by the administration of difluoro-methylornithine (DFMO) was found to block DNA synthesis in vivo (Pösö & Jänne 1976) which was restored in regenerating liver by the addition of putrescine (Pösö & Pegg 1982). Comparable decrease in the rate of DNA synthesis has been observed by inhibition of the polyamine synthetic pathway by diaminopropane and DL-hydrazine-amino-valeric acid (DL-AVA) (Pegg et al 1978), but this cannot be regarded as evidence in favour of the regulating molecule being a substance involved in the ODC-polyamine pathway, as polyamines, spermine and putrescine do not appear to initiate cellular proliferation when administered in vivo.

In a comparable way, insulin has been administered to intact animals without the desired effect of initiating a wave of hepatocyte proliferation (Bucher et al 1978), but an interesting anomaly has been observed in relation to the administration of insulin to rats previously rendered diabetic by the administration of alloxan (Younger et al 1966). In such circumstances, after 30 days of diabetes, administration of insulin was associated with the initiation of DNA synthesis of the hepatocytes, by a mechanism which is so far not clear.

The administration of various amines, either in combination with other factors or in the form of isoproterenol, has also been attended by a proliferative response in hepatocytes (Pipkin et al 1982). The substance is strikingly associated with an increase in cell size and also in DNA synthesis in the salivary gland as well as in the liver (Baserga 1970). Mediation by the autonomic nervous system has been excluded (Morley & Royse 1981) and the phenomenon suggests a parallel to that noted after exposure to phenobarbital or other enzyme inducers (Kenda & Lambotte 1981). In such circumstances proliferation of endoplasmic reticulum sometimes in the perivenous (Staubli et al 1969) regions and sometimes in other regions (Willson et al 1984) accompanies DNA synthesis and mitoses in the same regions of the lobule. None of these findings, however, sheds light on the mechanism underlying the initiation of DNA synthesis after liver cells have been damaged or destroyed. They do indicate that the process of cellular proliferation, once initiated, may be influenced by a variety of factors and that several different circumstances may lead to hepatocyte DNA synthesis when liver tissue has not been destroyed or damaged.

THICK HEPATIC PLATES IN THE HUMAN

The question of the morphological expression of cells which have proliferated in the human liver has already been raised, but it perhaps ought to be remarked that since the general acceptance of the view that plates consisting of two thicknesses of hepatocytes might represent the effects of cellular division in the adult, this feature has been increasingly referred to in disease states (Weinbren et al 1985). The finding then of thick plates, involving the whole liver, albeit affecting specific spatial regions within the lobules, indicates hyperplasia, apart from the unusual conditions already referred to in which thick hepatocyte plates may reasonably be considered to represent the outcome of a process other than hyperplasia, and associated changes may be better interpreted.

Hyperplastic liver plates, by this definition, are observed in the human in a wide variety of pathological conditions and very often impart characteristic macroscopic appearances which may be encountered during surgical procedures or in biopsy specimens. The characteristic first noticed about hyperplastic liver was the pallor, as compared with normal liver tissue, and next was the proliferative phenomenon which imparts a convexity to the part of the lobe or the surviving liver which is thus affected. These two attributes are found in many liver diseases and an appreciation of their significance may help to assess the underlying condition.

Neoplastic tissue may sometimes resemble hyperplasia but tumours do not generally possess a regular and patterned arrangement of cells and are more frequently affected by larger or smaller foci of necrosis. The two processes, even in cirrhosis, are usually distinguishable although difficulties are occasionally encountered.

The conditions with which hyperplasia is associated include changes in the liver in which cellular damage or loss plays some part, but this feature is sometimes difficult to identify amidst the other processes, such as inflammation and repair, macrophage activity, necrosis or atrophy. However, the presence of structural reorganization which is interpreted as hyperplasia is an important observation in the analysis of the pathological entity and may represent a reaction to a variety of different types of damage to liver cells. The lesions to which compensatory hyperplasia may be consequential include cellular necrosis either of the coagulative or cytolytic types (Majno et al 1960), these in turn being caused by vascular insufficiency, toxins, viral infection or tumour replacement (Bianchi et al 1979, Black 1980). In all these circumstances hyperplastic tissue may be found as diffuse or zonal changes usually depending on the degree of severity and survival of hepatocytes in different regions of the liver.

Obstruction to tributaries or ostia of hepatic veins results in severe changes in cells and sinusoids surrounding hepatic venous radicles with periportal hepatocyte survival and hyperplasia, as well as hyperplasia of liver cells in regions with intact hepatic venous drainage systems. These last regions may undergo striking cellular hyperplasia sometimes seriously distorting liver contour and substance (Rensing et al 1984). Caudate lobes are frequently reported as undergoing much enlargement, in some cases of ostial occlusion, because of the separate venous drainage of the caudate lobe directly into the inferior vena cava (Tavill et al 1975).

It is generally agreed that branch portal venous occlusion, if involving large enough regions, is associated with hyperplasia of liver tissue in which portal blood flow is maintained in both experimental animals and man (Rous & Larimore 1920, Gautier-Benoit & Houcke 1973), but there is some disagreement about the nature of the changes which develop after deprival of portal blood flow to part or all of the liver. Most reports stress the atrophy of the parenchyma without particular development of cellular necrosis (Weinbren 1955, Dubuisson et al 1982) but there is one view which suggests that the main change is a form of 'shrinkage necrosis', by means of which separate hepatocytes become necrotic without a general reaction and with only a minor component of atrophy (Kerr 1971). This disagreement may reflect a profound difference in the direction of research into the mechanism involved in the initiation of the compensatory hyperplastic response. For if the striking cellular proliferation so reproducibly observed after portal venous obstruction is a consequence of multiple necroses, then the sequence is probably little different from that which occurs after a large part of the liver is infarcted by interruption of its arterial blood supply and subsequent loss by necrosis of all cellular elements. But if atrophy is the major effect of portal venous occlusion, then the hyperplastic reaction takes place in response to changes in cytoplasmic but not nuclear elements within hepatocytes. The ultimate elucidation of the mechanism will therefore take account of the generation of the proliferation signal in altered hepatocyte cytoplasmic organelles, membranes or cytosol and not one arising from nuclear changes (Starzl et al 1975). The available evidence points to cytoplasmic changes as more likely to be the source than nuclear loss (Weinbren 1982).

It therefore appears that, in these circumstances, a negative net protein accretion rate may be the primary initiating phenomenon in the sequence of changes culminating in compensatory hyperplasia (Weinbren et al 1972). Deprivation of portal blood may exert its effect by decreased protein synthesis or by increased lysosomal-autophagosomal activity (Pfeifer 1978) since both probably occur with reproducible regularity and qualitative analytical procedures have been devised for quantifying the autophagosomes (Pfeiffer 1978). Difficulty in adopting this line of reasoning lies in the observation that atrophy as a consequence of fasting or hypophysectomy does not appear to stimulate a hyperplastic response, although portacaval anastomosis in rats (Weinbren & Washington 1976) and dogs (Starzl et al 1976) and diversion of portal flow in man (Klemperer 1928) apparently do have a proliferogenic effect. Hepatocyte atrophy perhaps is associated with a compensatory hyperplastic response when the liver is inappropriately reduced in size by a local effect but not when the whole organism undergoes an atrophic process such as fasting, in which case the hepatic atrophy is appropriate to the generalized changes.

The incidence of hyperplastic changes is therefore moderately frequent, being noted in many chronic liver diseases and clearly anticipated after major injury or surgical resection, or other forms of hepatocyte trauma. The recognition of these hyperplastic changes in terms of structural alteration is made only when the hyperplastic process has been of sufficient intensity to result in the formation of thick hepatocyte plates, many minor hepatocyte losses clearly being repaired and cells being replenished without diffuse conformational changes. When these features are recognized possible further developments may be considered. With regard to immediate effects of hyperplastic plates, there is as yet no evidence which incriminates such plate changes as a cause for portal hypertension, unless there are other accompanying structural changes, such as distortion of the vascular relations, as in cirrhosis (Kelty et al 1950) or Diffuse Nodular Hyperplasia (Weinbren & Mutum 1984), or with severe fibrosis, as occurs in chronic obstructive bile duct disease (Weinbren et al 1985) (Ch. 10, 58). It is probable that plates will remodel to one-cell thickness if the stimulus abates but this is not proven in man; it seems unlikely however that recovery and restitution to single-cell thick hepatocyte plates will occur if cirrhosis is present. It may be that the vascular distortion found in cirrhosis maintains a stimulus to hyperplasia because of the constant hypoperfusion but this is not certain (Kelty et al 1950).

The question of progression of hyperplastic plates was raised nearly 80 years ago (Turnbull & Worthington 1908), but there is as yet no acceptable evidence that the hyperplastic process may be converted into a neoplastic lesion *sui generis*. In instances of apparent conversion of hyperplastic nodules into neoplasms in general, another factor such as a virus or a toxin operates, or at least such intervention is not excluded (Farber 1980; Ogawa et al 1979).

There are several practical issues which relate to the reproducible and predictable process of compensatory hyperplasia and these may be of some consequence in clinical diagnosis and therapy. First, it is inevitable that a liver harbouring or invaded by a large primary or secondary tumour, will itself undergo an enlargement based on cellular proliferation. The response will usually be proportional to the quantity of liver tissue destroyed by the expanding or invading tumour mass, but will often also reflect the effects of the tumour on adjacent vessels with consequent hepatocyte atrophy or necrosis. It becomes difficult in such circumstances to construct a therapeutic staging system within the liver based on the proportion of liver involved.

A severe distortion may be a further reflection of compensatory hyperplasia of part of the liver and anatomical landmarks and visceral relations may be difficult to assess during imaging or other investigative or therapeutic procedures. This is not a new observation and, for well over a century, compression atrophy of part of the liver has resulted in a compensatory elongation of the right lobe of the liver (Rolleston & McNee 1929), a phenomenon not known to be associated with clinical symptoms.

The recognition of hyperplastic plates does not indicate the basis of the process or even the diagnosis. It does however imply that hepatocytes have been stimulated to proliferate. The thick plates are probably a more accurate indication of hyperplasia even than the presence of mitoses within liver cells. The main reason for this preference is that it is often impossible to exclude the phenomenon of 'mitotic arrest' as a result of toxins or metabolites and the changes may be spurious (Clarke 1971). The preferred site of the hyperplastic plate-change is generally the periportal region and in more severe instances this phenomenon may be diffuse, involving also perivenous hepatocytes, irrespective of the cause. Only occasionally are perivenous regions preferentially involved and the diagnosis of enzyme induction is possible, although the selective effect on cellular populations in different lobular sites has been challenged (Burger & Herdson 1966, Willson et al 1984).

REFERENCES

Adibi S, Paschkis K E, Cantarow A 1959 Stimulation of liver mitosis by blood serum from hepatectomized rats. Experimental Cell Research 18: 396–398

Antoniades H N, Owen A J 1982 Growth factors and regulation of cell growth. Annual Review of Medicine 33: 445–463

Aronsen K F, Ericsson B, Nosslin B, Nylander G, Pihl B, Waldeskog B 1970 Evaluation of hepatic regeneration by scintillation scanning, cholangiography and angiography in man. Annals of Surgery 171: 567–574

Barka T, Popper H 1967 Liver enlargement and drug toxicity. Medicine 46: 103–117

Baserga R 1970 Induction of DNA synthesis by a purified chemical compound. Federation Proceedings 29: 1443–1446

Baserga R 1974 Non-histone chromosomal proteins in normal and abnormal growth. Life Sciences 15: 1057–1071

Bianchi L, Zimmerli-Ning M, Gudat F 1979 Viral hepatitis. In: MacSween R N M, Anthony P P, Scheuer P J (eds) Pathology of the liver, Churchill Livingstone, London, p 164–191

Black M 1980 Acetaminophen hepatotoxicity. Gastroenterology 78: 382–392

Blumgart L H, Leach K G, Karran S J 1971 Observations on liver regeneration after right hepatic lobectomy. Gut 12: 922–928

Boyd E 1933 Normal variability in weight of the adult human liver and spleen. Archives of Pathology 16: 350–372

Bradshaw R A, Rubin J S 1980 Polypeptide growth factors: some structural and mechanistic considerations. Journal of Supramolecular Structure 14: 183–199

Brown K D, Friedkin M, Rozengurt E 1980 Colchicine inhibits epidermal growth factor degradation in 3T3 cells. Proceedings of the National Academy of Sciences of the United States of America 77: 480–484

Brown M S, Goldstein J L 1979 Receptor-mediated endocytosis:

insights from the lipoprotein receptor system. Proceedings of the National Academy of Sciences of the United States of America 76: 3330–3337

Brues A M, Marble B B 1937 An analysis of mitosis in liver restoration. Journal of Experimental Medicine 65: 15–27

Bucher N L R 1963 Regeneration of mammalian liver. International Review of Cytology 15: 245–300

Bucher N L R, Swaffield M N, Di Troia J F 1964 Influence of age upon incorporation of thymidine-2-C^{14} into DNA of regenerating rat liver. Cancer Research 24: 509–512

Bucher N L R, Malt R A 1971 Regeneration of liver and kidney. Little, Brown, Boston, p 55–77

Bucher N L R, Weir G C 1976 Insulin, glucagon, liver regeneration and DNA synthesis. Metabolism 25: 1423–1425

Bucher N L R, Patel V, Cohen St 1978 Hormonal factors concerned with liver regeneration. In: Ciba Foundation Symposium 55. Elsevier, Amsterdam, p 95–110

Burger P C, Herdson P B 1966 Phenobarbital-induced fine structural changes in rat liver. American Journal of Pathology 48: 793–803

Carpenter G, Cohen S 1979 Epidermal growth factor. Annual Review of Biochemistry 48: 193–216

Cayama E, Tsuda H, Sarma D S R, Farber E 1978 Initiation of chemical carcinogenesis requires cell proliferation. Nature 275: 60–62

Clarke R M 1971 A comparison of metaphase arresting agents and tritiated thymidine in measurement of the rate of entry into mitosis in the crypts of Lieberkuhn of the rat. Cell Tissue Kinetics 4: 263–272

Daughaday W H 1977 Hormonal regulation of growth by somatomedin and other tissue growth factors. Clinics in Endocrinology and Metabolism 6: 117–135

de Certaines J D, Moulinoux J P, Benoist L, Bernard A M, Rivet P 1982 Proton nuclear magnetic resonance of regenerating rat liver after partial hepatectomy. Life Sciences 31: 505–508

Deland F H, North W A 1968 Relationship between liver size and body size. Radiology 91: 1195–1198

Deliconstantinos G, Ramantanis G 1983 Alterations in the activities of hepatic plasma-membrane and microsomal enzymes during liver regeneration. Biochemical Journal 212: 445–452

Demetriou A A, Seifter E, Levenson S M 1983 Ornithine decarboxylase as an early indicator of in vitro hepatocyte DNA synthesis. Journal of Surgical Research 35: 163–167

Doljanski F 1960 The growth of the liver with special reference to mammals. International Review of Cytology 10: 217–241

Donaldson H H 1924 The rat. Data and reference tables. Wistar Institute of Anatomy and Biology, Philadelphia

Dubuisson L, Bioulac P, Saric J, Balabaud C 1982 Hepatocyte ultrastructure in rats with portacaval shunt. Digestive Diseases and Sciences 27: 1003–1010

Earp H S, O'Keefe E J 1981 Epidermal growth factor receptor number decreases during rat liver regeneration. Journal of Clinical Investigation 67: 1580–1583

Echave Llanos J M, Gomez-Dumm C L, Surur J M 1971 Growth hormone release after hepatectomy. Experientia 27: 574–575

Eisenberg S, Ben-Or S, Doljanski F 1962 The electrophoretic behaviour of liver cells during regeneration and post-natal growth. Experimental Cell Research 26: 451–461

Elias H, Sherrick J C 1969 Morphology of the liver. Academic Press, New York

Farber E 1980 The sequential analysis of liver cancer induction. Biochimica et Biophysica Acta 605: 149–166

Fishback F C 1929 A morphologic study of regeneration of the liver after partial removal. Archives of Pathology 7: 955–977

Francavilla A, Porter K A, Benichou J, Jones A F, Starzl T E 1978 Liver regeneration in dogs: morphologic and chemical changes. Journal of Surgical Research 25: 409–419

Friedman D L 1976 Role of cyclic nucleotides in cell growth and differentiation. Physiological Reviews 56: 652–708

Gautier-Benoit C, Houcke M 1973 Atrophie du lobe gauche du foie par thrombose de la branche gauche de la veine porte. Medecine et Chirurgie Digestives 2: 157–160

Goldstein J L, Anderson R G W, Brown M S 1979 Coated pits, coated vesicles and receptor mediated endocytosis. Nature 279: 679–685

Gospodarowicz D, Bialecki H, Greenburg G 1978 Purification of the fibroblast growth factor activity from bovine brain. Journal of Biological Chemistry 253: 3736–3743

Gospodarowicz D, Mescher A L 1980 Fibroblast growth factor and the control of vertebrate regeneration and repair. Annals of the New York Academy of Sciences 399: 151–174

Grindlay J H, Bollman J L 1952 Regeneration of the liver in the dog after partial hepatectomy. Surgery, Gynecology and Obstetrics 94: 491–496

Grisham J W 1962 Morphologic study of deoxyribonucleic acid synthesis and cell proliferation in regenerating rat liver: Autoradiography with thymidine-H^3. Cancer Research 22: 842–849

Ham R G 1981 Survival and growth requirements of nontransformed cells. Handbook of Experimental Pharmacology 57: 13–88

Harkness R D 1952 The spatial distribution of dividing cells in the liver of the rat after partial hepatectomy. Journal of Physiology 116: 373–379

Harkness R D 1957 Regeneration of liver. British Medical Bulletin 13: 87–93

Hasegawa K, Watanabe K, Koga M 1982 Induction of mitosis in primary cultures of adult rat hepatocytes under serum free conditions. Biochemical and Biophysical Research Communications 104: 259–265

Higgins G M, Anderson R M 1931 Experimental pathology of liver. I. Restoration of liver of white rat following partial surgical removal. Archives of Pathology 12: 186–202

Higgins G M, Mann F C, Priestley J T 1932 Restoration of the liver of the domestic fowl. Archives of Pathology 14: 491–497

Hollenberg M D, Gregory H 1976 Human urogastrone and mouse epidermal growth factor share a common receptor site in cultured human fibroblasts. Life Sciences 20: 267–274

Holley R W, Kiernan J A 1968 "Contact inhibition" of cell division in 3T3 cells. Proceedings of the National Academy of Sciences of the United States of America 60: 300–304

James R, Bradshaw R A 1984 Polypeptide growth factors. Annual Review of Biochemistry 53: 259–292

Kaplan D R, Chao F C, Stiles C D, Antoniades H N, Scher C D 1979 Platelet a-granules contain a growth factor for fibroblasts. Blood 53: 1043–1052

Kelty R H, Baggenstoss A H, Butt H R 1950 The relation of the regenerated liver nodule to the vascular bed in cirrhosis. Gastroenterology 15: 285–295

Kenda J F, Lambotte L 1981 Oxidative phosphorylation, enzyme induction and rat liver regeneration: effect of phenobarbital. European Surgical Research 13: 169–173

Kennedy G C, Pearce W M 1958 The relation between liver growth and somatic growth in the rat. Journal of Endocrinology 17: 149–157

Kerr J F R 1971 "Shrinkage necrosis": a distinct mode of cellular death. Journal of Pathology 105: 13–20

King A C, Cuatrecasas P 1981 Peptide hormone induced receptor mobility, aggregation, and internalisation. New England Journal of medicine 305: 77–88

Kleinman H K, Klebe R J, Martin G R 1981 Role of collagenous matrices in the adhesion and growth of cells. Journal of Cell Biology 88: 473–485

Klemperer P 1928 Cavernomatous transformation of the portal vein: its relation to Banti's disease. Archives of Pathology 6: 353–377

Knowles D M, Wolff M 1976 Focal nodular hyperplasia of the liver. Human Pathology 7: 535–545

Koch K S, Leffert H L, Moran T 1976 Hepatic proliferation control by purines, hormones, and nutrients. In: Fishman W H, Sell S (eds) Oncodevelopmental gene expression. Academic Press, New York, p 21–33

Koch K S, Leffert H L 1979 Increased sodium ion influx is necessary to initiate rat hepatocyte proliferation. Cell 18: 153–163

LaBrecque D R 1982 In vitro stimulation of cell growth by hepatic stimulator substance. American Journal of Physiology 242: G289–295

LaBrecque D R, Pesch L A 1975 Preparation and partial characterization of hepatic regenerative stimulator substance (ss) from rat liver. Journal of Physiology 248: 273–284

Lauffenburger D, DeLisi C 1983 Cell surface receptors: physical chemistry and cellular regulation. International Review of Cytology 84: 269–302

Leffert H L 1974 Hormonal control of DNA synthesis and its possible significance to the problem of liver regeneration. Journal of Cell Biology 62: 792–801

Leffert H L, Alexander N M, Faloona G, Rubalcava B, Unger R 1975 Specific endocrine and hormonal receptor changes associated with liver regeneration in adult rats. Proceedings of the National Academy of Sciences of the United States of America 72: 4033–4036

Leffert H L, Weinstein D B 1976 Growth control of differentiated fetal rat hepatocytes in primary monolayer culture. IX. Specific inhibition of DNA synthesis initiation by very low density lipoprotein and possible significance to the problem of liver regeneration. Journal of Cell Biology 70: 20–32

Leffert H L, Koch K S, Rubalcava B 1976 Present paradoxes in the environmental control of hepatic regeneration. Cancer Research 36: 4250–4255

Leffert H L, Koch K S, Rubalcava B, Sell S, Moran T, Boorstein R 1978 Hepatocyte growth control: in vitro approach to problems of liver regeneration and function. National Cancer Institute, Monographs 48: 87–101

Leffert H L, Koch K S 1979 Regulation of growth of hepatocytes. In: Popper H, Schaffner F (eds) Progress in liver diseases. Grune and Stratton, New York, p 123–134

Leffert H L, Koch K S, Moran T, Rubalcava B 1979 Hormonal control of rat liver regeneration. Gastroenterology 76: 1470–1482

Leffert H L, Koch K S 1980 Ionic events at the membrane initiated rat liver regeneration. Annals of the New York Academy of Sciences 339: 201–215

Leffert H L, Koch K S, Lad P J, Skelly H, de Hemptinne B 1982 Hepatocyte regeneration, replication, and differentiation. In: Arias I, Popper H, Schachter D, Shafritz D A (eds) The Liver: Biology and pathobiology. Raven Press, New York, p 601–614

Lewan L, Yngner T, Engelbrecht C 1977 The biochemistry of the regenerating liver. International Journal of Biochemistry 8: 477–487

Loewenstein W R, Kanno Y 1967 Intercellular communication and tissue growth. I Cancerous growth. Journal of Cell Biology 33: 225–234

Lopez-Rivas A, Adelberg E A, Rozengurt E 1982 Intracellular K^+ and the mitogenic response of 3T3 cells to peptide factors. Proceedings of the National Academy of Sciences of the United States of America 79: 6275–6279

McGowan J, Fausto N 1978 Ornithine decarboxylase activity and the onset of deoxyribonucleic acid synthesis in regenerating liver. Biochemical Journal 170: 123–127

McGowan J A, Strain A J, Bucher N L R 1981 DNA synthesis in primary cultures of adult rat hepatocytes in a defined medium: effects of epidermal growth factor, insulin, glucagon and cyclic-AMP. Journal of Cellular Physiology 108: 353–363

McKellar M 1949 The postnatal growth and mitotic activity of the liver of the albino rat. American Journal of Anatomy 85: 263–307

MacManus J P, Braceland B M, Youdale T, Whitfield J F 1973 Adrenergic antagonists and a possible link between the increase in cyclic adenosine 3′:5′ monophosphate and DNA synthesis during liver regeneration. Journal of Cellular Physiology 82: 157–164

Madsen A C, Rikkers L F, Moody F G, Wu J T 1980 Alpha-fetoprotein as a marker for hepatic regeneration in the dog. Journal of Surgical Research 28: 71–76

Majno G, La Gattuta M, Thompson T E 1960 Cellular death and necrosis: chemical, physical and morphologic changes in rat liver. Virchows Archiv A 333: 421–465

Martinez-Sales V, Baguena J 1981 Changes in non-histone proteins during mouse liver regeneration. Cellular and Molecular Biology 27: 223–229

Meyer D J, Yancey S B, Revel J-P 1981 Intercellular communication in normal and regenerating rat liver: a quantitative analysis. Journal of Cell Biology 91: 505–523

Michalopoulos G, Houck K A, Dolan M L, Luetteke N C 1984 Control of hepatocyte replication by two serum factors. Cancer Research 44: 4414–4419

Mizumoto R, Wexler M, Slapak M, Kojima Y, McDermott W V 1970 The effect of hepatic artery inflow on regeneration, hypertrophy, and portal pressure of the liver following 50 per cent hepatectomy in the dog. British Journal of Surgery 57: 513–517

Moolten F L, Bucher N L R 1967 Regeneration of rat liver: transfer of humoral agent by cross-circulation. Science 158: 272–273

Morgan J D, Hartroft W S 1961 Juvenile liver. Archives of Pathology 71: 86–88

Morley C G D, Royse V L 1981 Adrenergic agents as possible regulators of liver regeneration. International Journal of Biochemistry 13: 969–973

Nadal C 1975 Inhibition of rat hepatocyte multiplication by serum factors. Physiological significance. Virchows Archiv B 18: 273–280

Nakamura T, Nawa K, Ichihara A 1984 Partial purification and characterization of hepatocyte growth factor from serum of hepatectomized rats. Biochemical and Biophysical Research Communications 122: 1450–1459

Ogawa K, Medline A, Farber E 1979 Sequential analysis of hepatic carcinogenesis: the comparative architecture of preneoplastic, malignant, prenatal, postnatal and regenerating liver. British Journal of Cancer 40: 782–790

Pack G T, Islami A H, Hubbard J C, Brasfield R D 1962 Regeneration of human liver after major hepatectomy. Surgery 52: 617–623

Pastan I, Willingham M C 1981 Receptor mediated endocytosis of hormones. Annual Review of Physiology 43: 239–250

Pegg A E, Conover C, Wrona A 1978 Effects of aliphatic diamines on rat liver ornithine decarboxylase activity. Biochemical Journal 170: 651–660

Pfeifer U 1978 Inhibition by insulin of the formation of autophagic vacuoles in rat liver. A morphometric approach to the kinetics of intracellular degradation by autophagy. Journal of Cell Biology 78: 152–167

Pipkin J L, Hinson W G, Anson J F, Hudson J L 1982 Isoproterenol modulation of nuclear protein synthesis during rat liver regeneration. Cell Biology International Reports 6: 205–214

Ponfick E 1889 Experimentelle Beiträge zur Pathologie der Leber. Virchows Archiv fur Pathologische Anatomie 188: 209–249

Popper H 1954 Liver disease — morphologic considerations. American Journal of Medicine 16: 98–117

Pösö H, Jänne J 1976 Inhibition of polyamine accumulation and deoxyribonucleic acid synthesis in regenerating rat liver. Biochemical Journal 158: 485–488

Pösö H, Pegg A E 1982 Effect of alpha-difluoromethylornithine on polyamine and DNA synthesis in regenerating rat liver: reversal of inhibition of DNA synthesis by putrescine. Biochimica et Biophysica Acta 696: 179–186

Rabes H, Brändle H 1969 Synthesis of RNA, protein, and DNA in the liver of normal and hypophysectomized rats after partial hepatectomy. Cancer Research 29: 817–822

Rechler M M, Nissley S P 1977 Somatomedins and related growth factors. Nature 270: 665–666

Rensing V, Wimmer B, Lesch R, Wenz W 1984 Budd-Chiari-Stuart Bras syndrome. Hepato-gastroenterology 31: 218–226

Rinderknecht E, Humbel R E 1978 The amino acid sequence of human insulin-like growth factor I and its structural homology with proinsulin. Journal of Biological Chemistry 253: 2769–2776

Rixon R H, Whitfield J F 1976 The control of liver regeneration by para-thyroid hormone and calcium. Journal of Cellular Physiology 87: 147–155

Rolleston H, McNee J W 1929 Diseases of the liver, gall-bladder and bile-ducts, 3rd edn. Macmillan, London

Rous P, Larimore L D 1920 Relation of the portal blood to liver maintenance. Journal of Experimental Medicine 31: 609–632

Rozengurt E, Mendoza S 1980 Monovalent ion fluxes and the control of cell proliferation in cultured fibroblasts. Annals of the New York Academy of Sciences 339: 175–190

Rozengurt E, Collins M 1983 Molecular aspects of growth factor action: receptors and intracellular signals. Journal of Pathology 141: 309–331

Russell D H, Snyder S H 1968 Amine synthesis in rapidly growing tissues: Ornithine decarboxylase activity in regenerating rat liver, chick embryo and various tumors. Proceedings of the National Academy of Sciences of the United States of America 60: 1420–1427

St. Hilaire R J, Jones A L 1982 Epidermal growth factor: its biologic and metabolic effects with emphasis on the hepatocyte. Hepatology 2: 601–613

Schlessinger J, Geiger B 1981 Epidermal growth factor induces redistribution of actin and alpha-actinin in human epidermal carcinoma cells. Experimental Cell Research 134: 273–279

Schulte Hermann R 1974 Induction of liver growth by xenobiotic compounds and other stimuli. Critical Reviews in Toxicology 3: 97–158

Sell S, Nichols M, Becker F F, Leffert H L 1974 Hepatocyte proliferation and alpha$_1$-fetoprotein in pregnant, neonatal and partially hepatectomized rats. Cancer Research 34: 865–871

Sherlock S, Feldman C A, Moran B, Scheuer P J 1966 Partial nodular transformation of the liver with portal hypertension. American Journal of Medicine 40: 195–203

Short J, Brown R F, Husakova A, Gilbertson J R, Zemel R, Lieberman I 1972 Induction of deoxyribonucleic acid synthesis in the liver of the intact animal. Journal of Biological Chemistry 247: 1757–1766

Short J, Tsukada K, Rudert W A, Lieberman I 1975 Cyclic adenosine 3′–5′ monophosphate and the induction of deoxyribonucleic acid synthesis in liver. Journal of Biological Chemistry 250: 3602–3606

Simek J F, Rubin F, Lieberman I 1968 Synthesis of DNA after partial hepatectomy without changes in the lipid and glycogen contents of the liver. Biochemical and Biophysical Research Communications 30: 571–575

Sporn M B, Roberts A B 1985 Autocrine growth factors and cancer. Nature 313: 745–747

Starzl T E, Francavilla A, Halgrimson C G et al 1973 The origin, hormonal nature, and action of hepatotrophic substances in portal venous blood. Surgery, Gynecology and Obstetrics 137: 179–199

Starzl T E, Porter K A, Putnam C W 1975 Intraportal insulin protects from the liver injury of partacaval shunt in dogs. Lancet ii: 1241–1242

Starzl T E, Watanabe K, Porter K A, Putnam C W 1976 Effects of insulin, glucagon, and insulin glucagon infusions on liver morphology and cell division after complete portacaval shunt in dogs. Lancet i: 821–825

Starzl T E, Francavilla A, Porter K A, Benichou J, Jones A F 1978 The effect of splanchnic viscera removal upon canine liver regeneration. Surgery, Gynecology and Obstetrics 147: 193–207

Staubli W, Hess R, Weibel E R 1969 Effects of phenobarbital on rat hepatocytes. Journal of Cell Biology 42: 92–112

Stiles C D, Capone G T, Scher C D, Antoniades H N, Van Wyk J J, Pledger W J 1979 Dual control of cell growth by somatomedins and "competence factors". Proceedings of the National Academy of Sciences of the United States of America 76: 1279–1283

Stocker J T, Ishak K G 1981 Focal nodular hyperplasia of the liver: a study of 21 pediatric cases. Cancer 48: 336–345

Svoboda M E, Van Wyk J J, Klapper D G, Fellows R E, Grisson F E, Schlueter R J 1980 Purification of somatomedin-C from human plasma: chemical and biological properties, partial sequence analysis, and relationship to other somatomedins. Biochemistry 19: 790–797

Tannock I F 1967 A comparison of the relative efficiencies of various metaphase arrest agents. Experimental Cell Research 47: 345–356

Tavill A S, Wood E J, Kreal L, Jones E A, Gregory M, Sherlock S 1975 The Budd-Chiari syndrome: correlation between hepatic scintigraphy and the clinical, radiological, and pathological findings in nineteen cases of hepatic venous outflow obstruction. Gastroenterology 68: 509–518

Terblanche J, Porter K A, Starzl T E, Moore J, Patzelt L, Hayashida N 1980 Stimulation of hepatic regeneration after partial hepatectomy by infusion of a cytosol extract from regenerating dog liver. Surgery, Gynecology and Obstetrics 151: 538–544

Tomita Y, Nakamura T, Ichihara A 1981 Control of DNA synthesis and ornithine decarboxylase activity by hormones and amino acids in primary cultures of adult rat hepatocytes. Experimental Cell Research 135: 363–371

Turnbull H M, Worthington R 1908 Three cases illustrating the transition from regeneration to carcinoma in cirrhosis of the liver. Archives of the Pathological Institute of the London Hospital 2: 59–74

Van Wyk J J, Svoboda M E, Underwood L E 1980 Evidence from radioligand assays that somatomedin-C and insulin-like growth factor I are similar to each other and different from other somatomedins. Journal of Clinical Endocrinology and Metabolism 50: 206–208

Von Meister V 1894 Recreation des Lebergewebes nach Abtragung ganzer Leberlappen. Beitrage zur Pathologischen Anatomie and zur Allgemeinen Pathologie 15: 1

Walter F, Addis T 1939 Organ work and organ weight. Journal of Experimental Medicine 69: 467–483

Watanabe A, Miyazaki M, Taketa K 1976 Differential mechanisms of increased alpha$_1$-fetoprotein production in rats following carbon tetra chloride injury and partial hepatectomy. Cancer Research 36: 2171–2175

Weinbren K 1953 The effect of bile duct obstruction on regeneration of the rat's liver. British Journal of Experimental Pathology 34: 280–289

Weinbren K 1955 The portal blood supply and regeneration of the rat liver. British Journal of Experimental Pathology 36: 583–591

Weinbren K 1978 The liver. In: Symmers W St C (ed) Systemic pathology, 2nd edn. Churchill Livingstone, London, Vol 3, p 1207

Weinbren K 1982 Experimental diffuse nodular hepatic hyperplasia. Toxicologic Pathology 10: 81–92

Weinbren K, Fitschen W 1959 The influence of sodium fluoroacetate on regeneration of the rat's liver. British Journal of Experimental Pathology 40: 107–112

Weinbren K, Fitschen W, Cohen M 1960 The unmasking by regeneration of latent irradiation effects in the rat liver. British Journal of Radiology 33: 419–425

Weinbren K, Tarsh E 1964 Mitotic response in rat liver after different regenerative stimuli. British Journal of Experimental Pathology 45: 475–480

Weinbren K, Woodward E 1964 Delayed incorporation of ^{32}P from orthophosphate into deoxyribonucleic acid of rat liver after subtotal hepatectomy. British Journal of Experimental Pathology 45: 442–449

Weinbren K, Bezmalinovic Z, Daniller A I 1967 The effect of catecholamines on the delay of the restorative response after subtotal hepatectomy. British Journal of Experimental Pathology 48: 305–308

Weinbren K, Stirling G A, Washington S L A 1972 The development of a proliferative response in liver parenchyma deprived of portal blood flow. British Journal of Experimental Pathology 53: 54–58

Weinbren K, Washington S L A 1976 Hyperplastic nodules after protacaval anastomosis in rats. Nature 264: 440–442

Weinbren K, Mutum S S 1984 Pathological aspects of diffuse nodular hyperplasia of the liver. Journal of Pathology 143: 81–92

Weinbren K, Hadjis N S, Blumgart L H 1985 Structural aspects of the liver in patients with biliary disease and portal hypertension. Journal of Clinical Pathology 38: 1013–1020

Westall F C, Lennon V A, Gospodarowicz D 1978 Brain-derived fibroblast growth factor: identity with a fragment of the basic protein of myelin. Proceedings of the National Academy of Sciences of the United States of America 75: 4675–4678

Whitfield J F, Boynton A L, MacManus J P et al 1980 The roles of calcium and cyclic AMP in cell proliferation. Annals of the New York Academy of Sciences 339: 216–240

Willson R A, Wormsley S B, Muller-Eberhard V 1984 A comparison of hepatocyte size distribution in untreated and phenobarbital-treated rats as assessed by flow cytometry. Digestive Diseases and Sciences 29: 753–757

Wondergem R, Harder D R 1980 Membrane potential measurements during rat liver regeneration. Journal of Cellular Physiology 102; 193–197

Yamada K M 1983 Cell surface interactions with extracellular materials. Annual Review of Biochemistry 52: 761–799

Yanker B A, Shooter E M 1982 The biology and mechanism of action of nerve growth factor. Annual Review of Biochemistry 51: 845–868

Yee A G, Revel J-P 1978 Loss and reappearance of gap junctions in regenerating liver. Journal of Cell Biology 78: 554–564

Yokoyama H O, Wilson M E, Tsuboi K K, Stowell R E 1953 Regeneration of mouse liver after partial hepatectomy. Cancer Research 13: 80–85

Younger L R, King J, Steiner D F 1966 Hepatic proliferative response to insulin in severe alloxan diabetes. Cancer Research 26: 1408–1413

Zapf J, Rinderknecht E, Humbel R E, Froesch E R 1978 Nonsuppressible insulin-like activity (NSILA) from human serum: recent accomplishments and their physiologic implications. Metabolism 27: 1803–1828

Zimmerman M, Celozzi E 1961 Stimulation by heparin of parenchymal liver cell proliferation in normal adult rats. Nature 191: 1014–1015

6

N. S. Hadjis L. H. Blumgart

Liver hyperplasia, hypertrophy and atrophy; clinical relevance

INTRODUCTION

Although the terms hypertrophy and atrophy have been used to identify conditions in a static sense, the fundamental processes underlying hypertrophy and atrophy are also important and, in the following, use of these terms implies their static and dynamic meaning. The question arises as to how the quality of the state of normotrophy, i.e. the starting point of hypertrophy and atrophy (Pfeifer 1982), can be described. Under normotrophic conditions the liver cell is in a steady state resulting from the continuous addition of cytoplasmic constituents and a simultaneous withdrawal of constituents destined for degradation. In this steady state accretion or loss of cytoplasm can occur consequent on metabolic changes in the cells associated with shifts in enzymatic activities; the critical point is the balance. A shift in balance will result in cellular atrophy or hypertrophy. Two metabolic processes are involved in maintaining the balance: anabolism and catabolism. Hypertrophy is induced either when anabolic processes are enhanced or when anabolism remains constant but catabolism is reduced; atrophy, or a negative protein balance, on the other hand, can result from increased catabolism or a reduction of anabolic processes if catabolism continues at a constant rate (Pfeifer 1982).

Virchow's concept of hypertrophy distinguished between the increase in mass of an organ by increase in cell size and by increase in cell number. Since then, the term hypertrophy has come to imply increase in mass due to increase in cell size without an increase in genetic substance. By contrast, the term hyperplasia indicates an increase in mass due to cell division and increase in cell numbers. Atrophy, being the reverse of hypertrophy, may also be defined in terms of cell size or cytoplasmic protein content. Indeed, hepatocyte atrophy and hypertrophy may be regarded as aspects of the same process, differing in degree. In this context, the term atrophy signifies loss of cytoplasm but not loss of liver cells. The implication is that reduction of size of an organ consequent on ischaemic cell necrosis followed by organization and the development of fibrosis is not considered to represent atrophy. Hyperplasia, however, is a separable process and it can be associated with either atrophy or hypertrophy (Weinbren 1955, Sigel et al 1967, Weinbren et al 1972, Starzl et al 1976).

Following acute loss of liver substance through injury or surgical resection, the restoration of liver mass to its former size involves a combination of hyperplasia and hypertrophy (Ch. 5). However, adaptive hepatic growth is basically a hyperplastic process, although in the following the term hypertrophy will be retained for descriptive purposes.

This chapter concerns itself primarily with clinical aspects of lobar or segmental liver atrophy and concomitant hypertrophy (hyperplasia) of the unaffected parenchyma. It is this 'atrophy/hypertrophy complex' that gives rise to particular diagnostic problems and accounts for the management difficulties associated with the condition.

DEFINITIONS

For the purpose of this chapter, atrophy is defined in terms of reduction in mass of a recognized lobe or segment of the liver by at least an estimated 50%, irrespective of the histological features. However, the microscopic picture is important and of clinical significance and will be discussed according to the underlying cause of atrophy. Manifest enlargement of a lobe is considered to represent hypertrophy.

AETIOLOGY

Many cases of lobar or segmental liver atrophy have been reported in association with primary hepatocellular disease, predominantly cirrhosis (Ham 1979), affecting the entire liver and therefore of little surgical significance since the disease process is by definition irreversible. Furthermore, the atrophy/hypertrophy complex is usually absent in these cases.

The common causes of the atrophy/hypertrophy complex encountered in surgical practice are bile duct obstruction or portal venous occlusion, or both, to the atrophied area (Braasch et al 1972, Longmire & Tompkins 1975, Bismuth & Malt 1979). Less common causes include occlusion of the hepatic veins and space occupying hepatic lesions, compressing or invading vascular channels from without (Meyer 1950, Hueston 1953, Galloway et al 1973). Of 48 cases of liver atrophy seen in the Hepatobiliary Unit at the Hammersmith Hospital over a period of five years, 44 had bile duct obstruction secondary to benign or malignant bile duct strictures. Indeed, the incidence of atrophy in hilar cholangiocarcinoma is around 20% (Carr et al 1985), with about half of the patients having concomitant ipsilateral portal venous occlusion. Postcholecystectomy bile duct strictures head the list of benign causes, with an incidence of atrophy of around 10% (Fig. 6.1). Similar figures have been reported from France (Bismuth 1982).

a

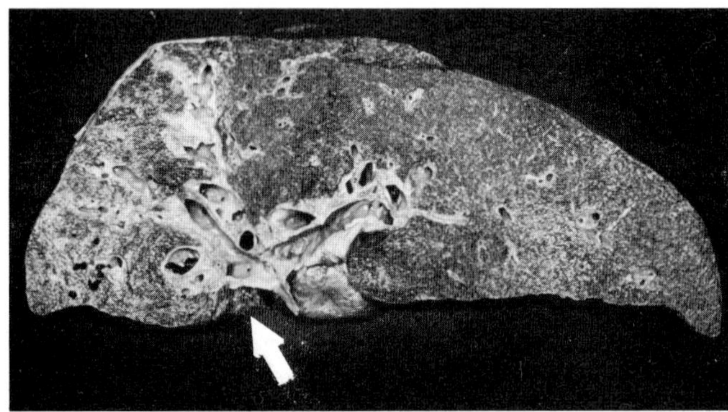

b

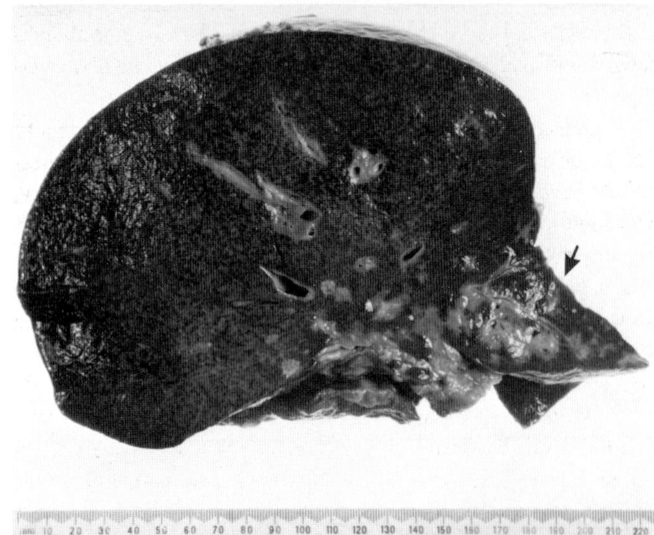

Fig. 6.1 a. Coronal-section of liver specimen from a patient with benign bile duct stricture who died of liver failure. Gross atrophy of right liver (arrow), with evident fibrosis. Marked left liver hypertrophy. b. Coronal-section of liver specimen from a patient with hilar cholangiocarcinoma, showing pronounced left lobe atrophy (arrow) and compensatory enlargement of right lobe

PATHOGENESIS

With regard to atrophy consequent on diversion of portal flow, the consensus view is that portal blood controls hepatocyte size and the lack of it results in loss of hepatocyte cytoplasmic mass (Rous & Larimore 1920a, Weinbren 1955, Weinbren & Tarsh 1964, Starzl et al 1976, Dubuisson et al 1982a) through mechanisms as yet not fully defined (Cole et al 1971, Pfeifer 1978, 1982). However, some investigators have shown ligation of the portal vein to be associated with hepatocyte necrosis (Steiner & Batiz 1961, Kerr 1971, Rozga et al 1985). Although the idea that obliteration of individual branches of the portal vein induces atrophy of the corresponding parts of the hepatic parenchyma was discussed as early as 1858 (Frerichs 1861), the matter remained in dispute until the classical experimental work of Rous & Larimore (1920a). Others, subsequently, have confirmed the invariable liver atrophy associated with deprivation of portal blood flow in many species (Schalm et al 1956, Steiner & Batiz 1961, Starzl et al 1975, Putnam et al 1976).

Liver atrophy secondary to bile duct obstruction was first studied experimentally by Nasse (1894) and later by Harley & Barratt (1901), Rous & Larimore (1920b), and McMaster & Rous (1921). In contrast to portal occlusion, the response to bile duct ligation differs substantially among species (Harley & Barratt 1901, McMaster & Rous 1921, Stewart et al 1937, Steiner & Batiz 1961, Braasch et al 1972), and this has been attributed to the variation in the amount of bile produced (Rous & Larimore 1920b). The pathogenesis of the development of atrophy is poorly understood. Experimental data suggest a reduction in the number of hepatocytes and atrophy of the hepatic lobules (Harley & Barratt 1901, Swanson et al 1967, Johnstone & Lee 1976), but a decrease in hepatocyte size, although described in animals (Rous & Larimore 1920b), is less well established in man. Preliminary results obtained in our laboratory from an animal model of induced liver atrophy indicate that ligation of a bile duct draining part of the liver is associated with considerable reduction in perfusion of the relevant liver tissue by portal blood, as was initially suggested by Rous & Larimore (1920b). Benz et al (1952) reported seven cases of left lobe atrophy secondary to bile duct obstruction and considered, on the limited available anatomical evidence, that this was effected by compression of the long slender left branch of the portal vein by the dilated left hepatic duct. They reasoned that this accounted for the more common affliction of the left lobe, at least in cases of biliary atrophy. However, in the Hammersmith Hospital series, right and left lobe atrophy occurs with equal frequency; furthermore, in 15 cases of left lobe atrophy for whom there was angiographic information available, no vascular compression was observed that could not be accounted for by previous surgical injury or invasion by tumour.

PATHOLOGICAL ASPECTS OF THE ATROPHY/HYPERTROPHY COMPLEX

Although deviation of portal blood may be a common pathophysiological mechanism in the development of atrophy secondary to portal venous or bile duct obstruction, the parenchymal and connective tissue reaction is entirely different in the two situations. Portal vein occlusion results in atrophy of the affected hepatocytes and striking hyperplasia of cells enjoying an intact portal flow. It is perhaps worth noting that the compensatory cellular proliferation initiated by atrophied hepatocytes is reproducible and comparable in time and intensity to the adaptive DNA synthetic response observed after liver resection (Weinbren & Tarsh 1964). Although striking ultrastructural changes have been described in hepatocytes deprived of portal blood, among them depletion of the rough endoplasmic reticulum and reduction in the membrane-bound polyribosomes (Putnam et al 1976, Starzl et al 1976), the mechanism by which atrophy initiates hepatic DNA synthesis is unclear. Since there is no significant reduction in total DNA in the lobes deprived of portal flow, it has been postulated that the generation of the mitotic stimulus does not depend on reduced nuclear material but that it is likely that a cytoplasmic component, within the atrophying hepatocyte, is involved in the production of the initiating signal which results in DNA synthesis (Weinbren & Tarsh 1964). Unlike the hepatocytes, the Kupffer cells appear not to be affected by portoprivation either in terms of number or function (Dubuisson et al 1982b, Edgcomb et al 1982).

The response to inhibition of bile flow depends on the level of bile duct obstruction. Obstruction below the confluence of the hepatic ducts results in enlargement of the entire liver. By contrast, lobar or segmental duct obstruction leads, like portal venous occlusion, to atrophy of the affected liver and compensatory hyperplasia of the parenchyma with unimpaired bile drainage (Rous & Larimore 1920b, Ogawa et al 1960, Braasch et al 1972, Longmire & Tompkins 1975). However, cellular loss rather than hepatocyte atrophy is likely to be the primary initiating phenomenon in the sequence of events culminating in cellular proliferation. The microscopic picture of biliary atrophy, unlike portal atrophy, includes bile duct proliferation and periportal fibrosis with expansion of the portal tracts and destruction of adjacent liver cells (Rous & Larimore 1920b). The remaining hepatocytes may show variable degrees of atrophy but in general the size of the hepatocytes does not correlate with the degree of lobar atrophy (Benz et al 1952).

The clinical situation however is often more complex. Lobar biliary atrophy can be asymptomatic until such time as the other hepatic duct also becomes obstructed. With the two lobes sequentially obstructed and 'disadvantaged' (Schalm et al 1956), the loss of hepatocytes consequent on the expanding portal tracts generates the stimulus for compensatory hyperplasia affecting the hepatocytes of both lobes. The result is interesting in the sense that, given time, the hepatocytes of the atrophied lobe as well as those of the contralateral lobe become hyperplastic, even if the former cells were previously atrophied (Weinbren et al 1985). This microscopic picture confirms experimental data that bile duct obstruction does not inhibit hepatocyte proliferation (Weinbren 1953, Swanson et al 1967), and supports existing experimental evidence that hepatocyte protein synthesis controlling atrophy or hypertrophy and DNA synthesis leading to hyperplasia are independent processes, i.e. atrophic hepatocytes can also be hyperplastic (Fisher et al 1962, Sigel et al 1967, Weinbren et al 1972, Starzl et al 1976, Weinbren 1982).

CLINICAL ASPECTS

The clinical presentation depends on the underlying cause of atrophy. Most patients with lobar atrophy secondary to bile duct obstruction present with jaundice. The shortest interval that we have encountered between the time a bile duct injury was recorded and the subsequent diagnosis of atrophy is one year. However, this is likely to be an overestimation of the time required for atrophy to develop since prompt diagnosis of atrophy is an unusual event. Our experience indicates that, unless one is aware of its existence, atrophy may be missed even at surgery. Of the laboratory tests the serum alkaline phosphatase is of interest. Although the enzyme is invariably raised in the presence of jaundice, anicteric patients with unilateral hepatic duct obstruction show an early rise (an important diagnostic feature), but as atrophy is gradually established serum enzyme levels return to normal. We have observed this pattern in four patients with benign stricture.

In malignant obstruction, lobar atrophy is commonly associated with a neoplasm arising in one hepatic duct (Ch. 65). This results in atrophy of the affected liver, although the patient may remain asymptomatic or with non-specific constitutional complaints. In time, the tumour grows into the contralateral duct leading to the development of jaundice (Marshall 1932). Although the incidence of lobar atrophy (indicating initial unilateral hepatic duct obstruction) in hilar cholangiocarcinoma is about 20% (Carr et al 1985), only two out of 116 patients admitted to the Hammersmith Hospital with this disease were diagnosed during the anicteric phase when the tumour was limited to one hepatic duct, and in both cases the lesions were successfully resected. It is therefore possible that an awareness of lobar atrophy as a feature of hilar biliary obstruction might result in earlier diagnosis and a higher resectability rate of malignant lesions.

Inadvertent damage to a bile duct, be it sectoral or lobar, during biliary surgery is the commonest cause of atrophy in patients with benign biliary disease (Ch. 58). However, in countries where recurrent pyogenic cholangitis is prevalent, intrahepatic stones are just as important a cause (Chen et al 1984) (Ch. 77). Reconstructive surgery at the hilum may be followed by atrophy if anastomotic repair is complicated by recurrent fibrous stenosis of one or other hepatic duct. Atrophy may also complicate a particular surgical procedure. Six out of 22 patients with postcholecystectomy bile duct stricture, reoperated on at the Hammersmith Hospital following a previous mucosal graft procedure, were found to have gross lobar atrophy. On the other hand, of 48 patients with a stricture of the same cause who had not been treated by this procedure, only five were found to have atrophy. The number of previous explorations was similar in the two groups. It is possible that the pulling-up of the jejunal loop into the liver obstructs side ducts leading to atrophy (Ch. 58). Lobar atrophy consequent on portal venous occlusion may be asymptomatic, e.g. after injury to the portal vein during cholecystectomy (Blumgart et al 1984), or the patient may complain of symptoms associated with a space occupying hepatic lesion which is obstructing a branch of the portal vein causing atrophy.

Liver atrophy as part of the atrophy/hypertrophy complex is associated with particular diagnostic problems which may be clinical or radiological. Of 48 cases with the atrophy/hypertrophy complex, 10 presented with a palpable abdominal mass; seven in the epigastrium, the result of right lobe atrophy with compensatory enlargement of the left lobe producing a 'mass' effect, and three below the lateral half of the right hypochondrium indicating the obverse. Three of the 'masses' were thought on referral to be neoplastic. It is important that patients with a history of jaundice and previous biliary surgery presenting with an epigastric or right subcostal mass are investigated with the possibility in mind that this may be due to lobar hypertrophy. This mass effect is not unique to biliary atrophy; portal venous obstruction, hepatic venous occlusion, and ischaemic liver necrosis may cause and present as an undiagnosed abdominal mass (Tsuzuki et al 1973). In most cases of Budd-Chiari syndrome both lobes are affected, with the exception of the caudate lobe which drains directly into the inferior vena cava (Tavill et al 1975). Compensatory enlargement of the caudate lobe (Rensing et al 1984) can be mistaken for a liver tumour (Wilkinson & Sherlock 1984) (Fig. 6.2). Occasionally, one of the main hepatic veins remains patent, in which case disparity in size develops between the right and the left liver (Meyer 1950, Galloway et al 1973). It is perhaps worthy of note that the palpable mass in liver atrophy represents the functionally competent or least impaired hepatic parenchyma.

Further diagnostic confusion can result from gross hypertrophy of the left liver misinterpreted as splenomegaly and from the appearance of a radio-isotope liver scan obtained to investigate suspected hepatobiliary disease or an abdominal mass. Depending on the degree to which hepatocytes and Kupffer cells have been replaced by periportal fibrosis, the atrophied lobe or segment may imitate a 'cold' area on the scan and be erroneously interpreted as a space occupying lesion with metastases (mass) (Ham 1979, Makler et al 1980, Hadjis et al 1986b).

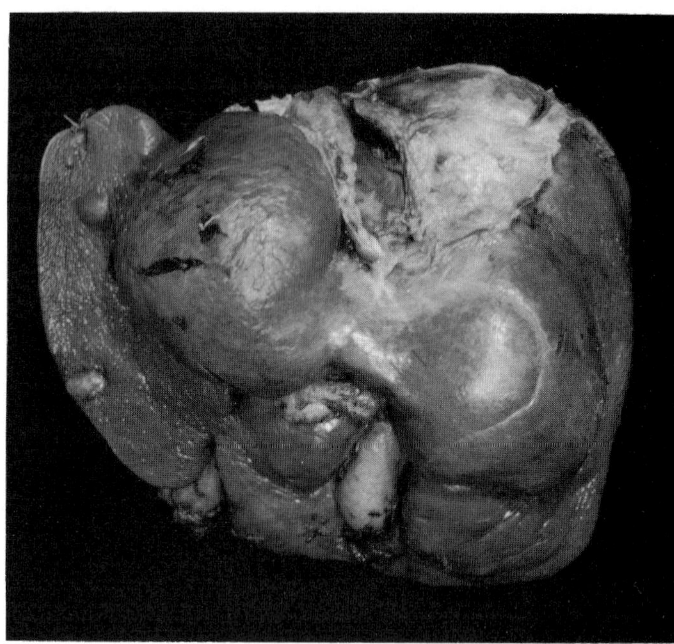

Fig. 6.2 Gross liver specimen of a patient with Budd-Chiari syndrome. The right and left lobes are small, while the caudate lobe is grossly hypertrophied

RADIOLOGICAL DIAGNOSIS

The diagnosis of liver atrophy can be made preoperatively by several radiological modalities, a reduction in lobe size being the common finding. CT scanning is probably the best single non-invasive investigation in revealing atrophy, particularly left liver atrophy (Carr et al 1985) (Fig. 6.3a, b, c). It is less accurate in the diagnosis of right liver atrophy but this should always be suspected whenever there is marked left sided hypertrophy shown on CT. Furthermore, since the imaginary line between the gallbladder fossa and the inferior vena cava demarcates the left from the right liver, atrophy of the right liver is likely to be missed in rare cases where the gallbladder is attached to the left liver (Fig. 6.3d). Segmental atrophy is usually indicated by a concave change in the outline of the liver over the affected segment. Changes in the anatomical relations of the hilar structures consequent on the development of the atrophy/hypertrophy complex can also be demonstrated by CT.

Percutaneous cholangiography (PTC) is complementary

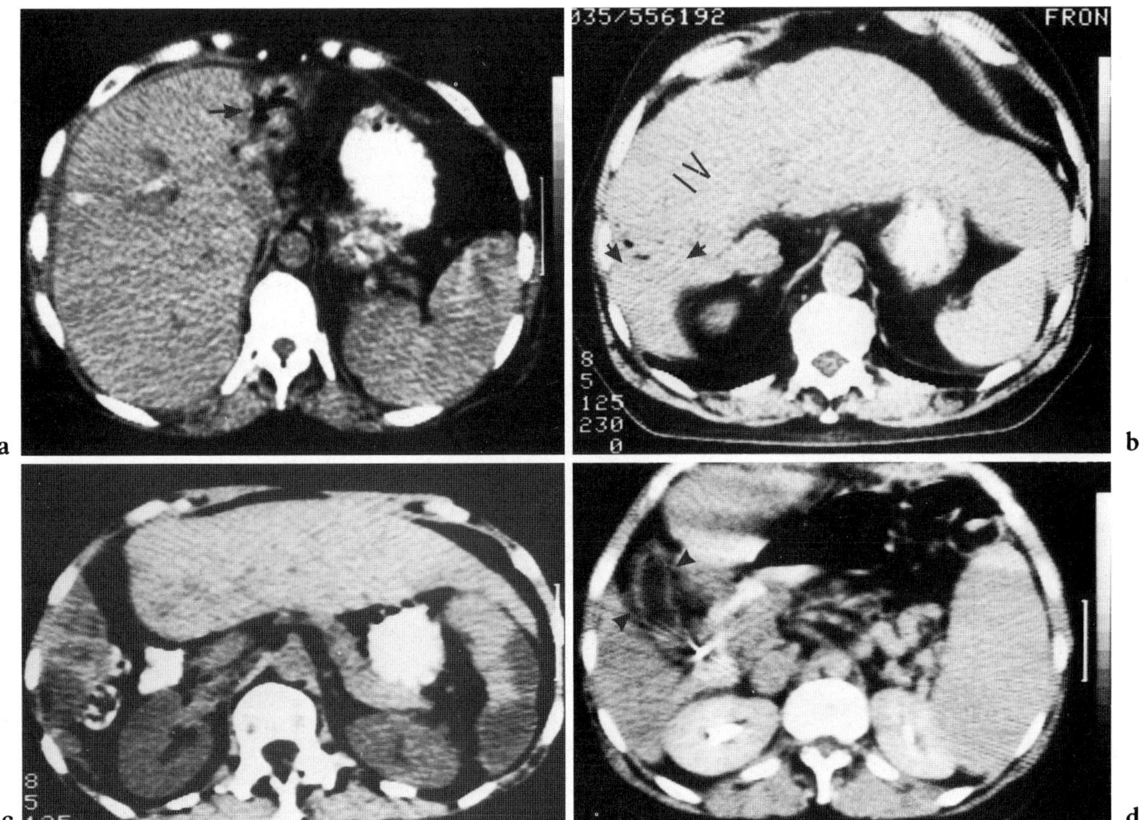

Fig. 6.3 a. CT scan illustrating a very small left lobe with dilated ducts (arrow), in a patient with postcholecystectomy bile duct stricture. b. CT scan showing marked right liver atrophy and considerable hypertrophy of segment IV and the left lobe, in a patient with benign stricture of the right hepatic duct. c. Gross hypertrophy of the left lobe in a patient with right liver atrophy secondary to occlusion of the right branch of the portal vein by an hepatocellular carcinoma. d. CT scan of a patient with a left-sided gallbladder and a very small right liver. The quadrate lobe (segment IV) and the left lobe, on either side of the gallbladder (arrowed), were misinterpreted to be the right and left liver

to CT scanning. The intrahepatic ducts of the affected lobe appear crowded together and may or may not be dilated even in the presence of obstruction (Ham 1979, Myracle et al 1981) (Fig. 6.4a). PTC is more sensitive than CT in showing segmental and right liver atrophy provided that all ducts have been demonstrated (Fig. 6.4b, c). The hypertrophied lobe extends across the midline, and the relevant hepatic duct may or may not be obstructed. Angiography demonstrates tortuous vessels packed together and provides information on the underlying cause of the atrophy (Ham 1979) (Fig. 6.5). Ultrasonography does have the potential of accurately diagnosing lobar atrophy and it can point to the cause.

Liver scintigraphy (Ch. 15) can contribute significantly to the diagnosis and differential diagnosis of liver atrophy. The uptake curve of a HIDA scan gives an indication of parenchymal dysfunction. On the basis of experimental evidence that portoprivation is compatible with normal uptake of HIDA and colloid preparations by hepatocytes and Kupffer cells respectively, and given the striking destruction of hepatocytes and Kupffer cells common to atrophy consequent on biliary obstruction but absent in atrophy associated with portoprivation, we have used a combination of HIDA and colloid scans to differentiate the two conditions (Hadjis et al 1986b). As would have been predicted, a small lobe with normal uptake of both radionuclides is indicative of portal atrophy (Fig. 6.6). By contrast, the scintigraphic picture of biliary atrophy reflects the variable degree of hepatocyte and Kupffer cell replacement by proliferating bile duct cells and fibrosis; reduced, patchy uptake of both HIDA and colloid characterizes cases of moderate severity (Fig. 6.7), but with marked fibrosis there may be no uptake at all (Ham 1979, Makler et al 1980, Hadjis et al 1986b) (Fig. 6.8, 6.9). In cases with ipsilateral occlusion of the bile duct and portal vein, the scintigraphic findings are those of biliary atrophy.

SURGICAL MANAGEMENT

The management of patients with liver lobe disparity consequent on atrophy, as exemplified by the atrophy/hypertrophy complex, calls for an understanding of the anatomical and functional changes associated with this condition. An appreciation of these changes is particu-

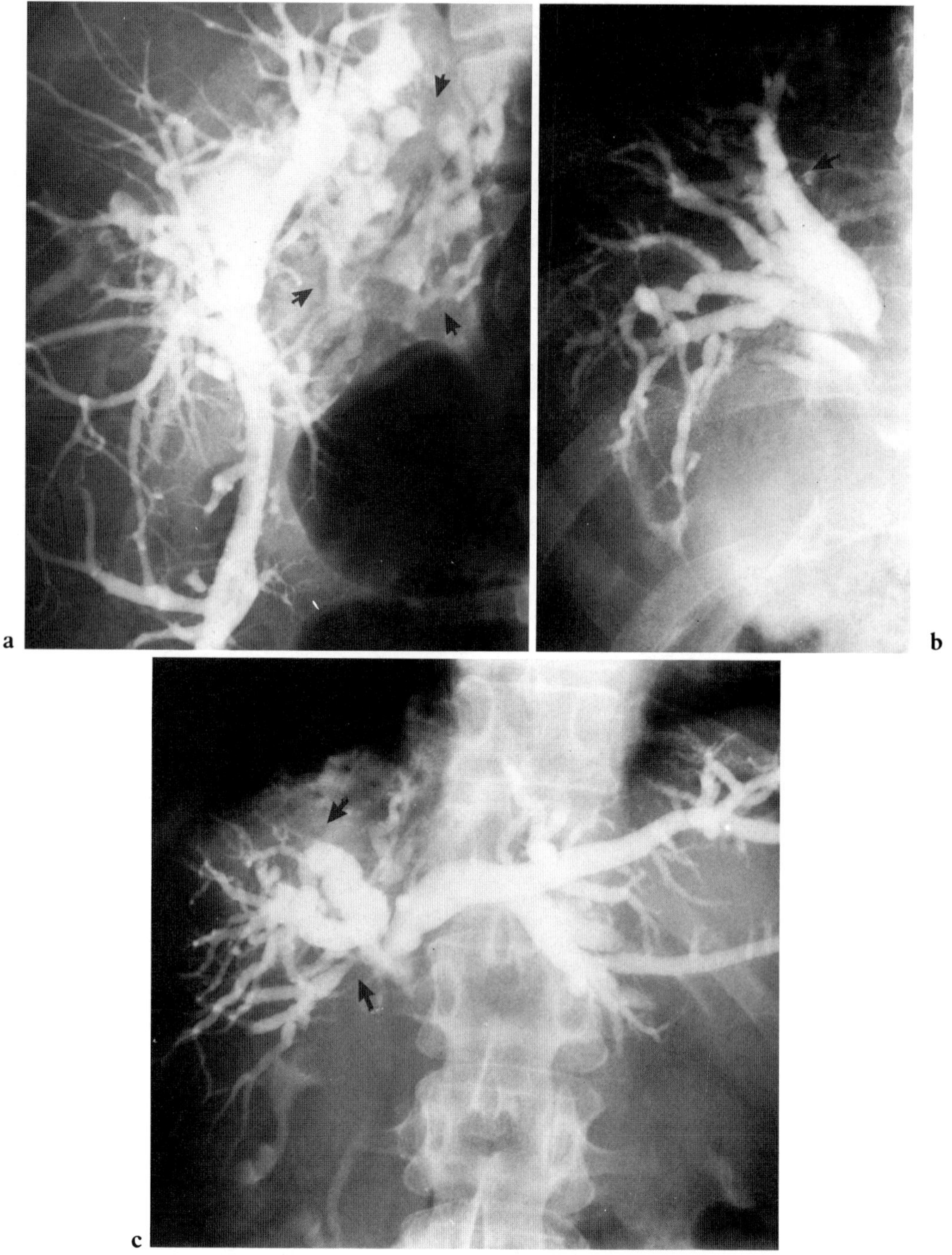

Fig. 6.4 a. Percutaneous cholangiogram of a patient with hilar cholangiocarcinoma showing crowding of the intrahepatic ducts in the left lobe indicative of atrophy (arrowed). The right lobe is enlarged. b. Percutaneous cholangiogram of the right hepatic ductal system. The superior ducts are crowded together (arrows) consistent with segmental atrophy, which was confirmed at surgery. c. Percutaneous cholangiogram of a patient with hilar cholangiocarcinoma. Gross atrophy of the right liver is indicated by the crowding of the intrahepatic ducts (arrows). There is hypertrophy of the left liver

larly important whenever surgery is required to relieve symptoms usually related to bile duct disease.

The surgical problems can be conveniently divided into operative difficulty, arising from poor access to the ducts, and those related to the functional reserve of the atrophied liver. Although 30% of normal parenchyma is adequate to maintain a normal serum bilirubin (Bismuth & Malt 1979), the functional capacity of the atrophied lobe to relieve jaundice after drainage is questionable. In the same context, the presence of lobar atrophy precludes resection of an otherwise resectable lesion sited in the contralateral lobe and requiring lobectomy. The authors have studied the effect of biliary decompression on the atrophied liver in terms of function by performing HIDA and colloid

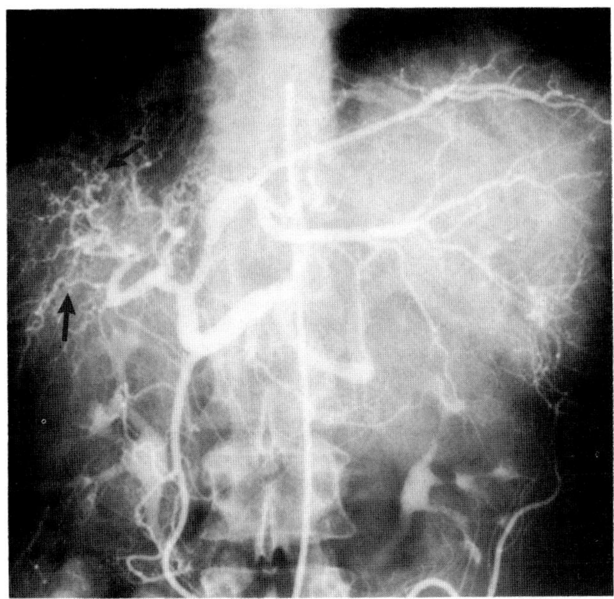

Fig. 6.5 Typical angiographic appearance of atrophy of the right liver (case as in 6.4c). Note crowded, tortuous arteries (arrows), and hypertrophy of the left liver with enlarged arteries

scans before and after surgery (Hadjis et al 1986b). The results can be summarized as follows:

1. Drainage of an atrophied lobe secondary to unilateral hepatic duct obstruction is unlikely to improve its function (Fig. 6.10).
2. Drainage of an atrophied lobe associated with ipsilateral portal venous occlusion and obstruction below the confluence of the hepatic ducts may increase its functional capacity (Fig. 6.6).
3. Drainage of an atrophied lobe associated with ipsilateral occlusion of the hepatic duct and portal vein is unlikely to result in any functional improvement.

Operative difficulties emanate from the distorted configuration of the liver and the tendency of the lobe undergoing hypertrophy to rotate and extend across the midline, particularly in right liver atrophy. Vessels and ducts conform to this spatial lobar re-arrangement with the following consequences: firstly, the portal vein lies more superficially and is therefore at risk of being injured; and secondly the portal venous branches develop an anterior relation to the bile ducts making access to these ducts exceedingly difficult. In effect, the hilar structures come to course obliquely upwards, the hepatic artery and portal vein anteriorly and the bile duct posteriorly (Fig. 6.11). Furthermore, the atrophied right liver tends to be hidden high under the costal margin making mobilization a tedious undertaking, while the convex edge of the hypertrophied left liver extends forwards and downwards in an overhanging fashion with the hilar structures obscured beneath it. Similar anatomical changes in the vascular and ductal channels take place after partial hepatectomy and any future approach, e.g. to correct a post-traumatic bile duct stricture, will be hampered by the same problems of access.

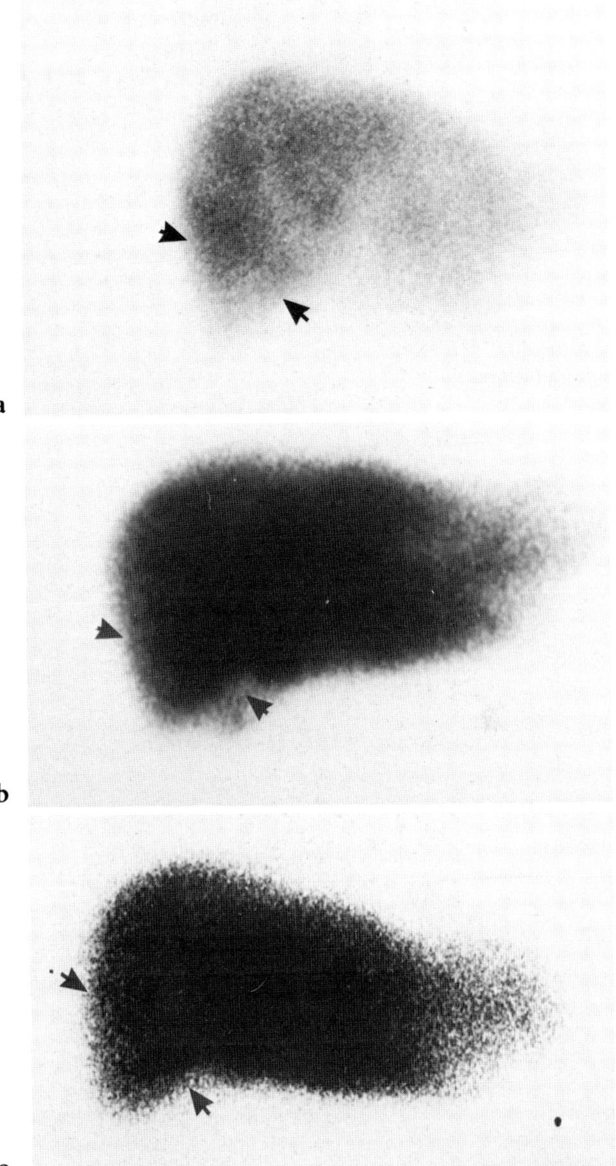

Fig. 6.6 Patient with postcholecystectomy stricture of the common hepatic duct and occlusion of the right branch of the portal vein, demonstrated angiographically. a. HIDA scan prior to repair of the stricture. There is reduced uptake of the radionuclide by the whole liver. The right liver appears to be small (arrows). b. HIDA scan six months after repair of the stricture. Normal uptake by the right liver which remains small (arrows). Hypertrophy of the left liver. c. Sulphur colloid scan confirming normal function of an atrophied right liver (arrows)

In general, the primary pathology whether benign or malignant, the site of atrophy and the nature and severity of symptoms are the main factors determining the options of treatment. It is important to note that demonstration of

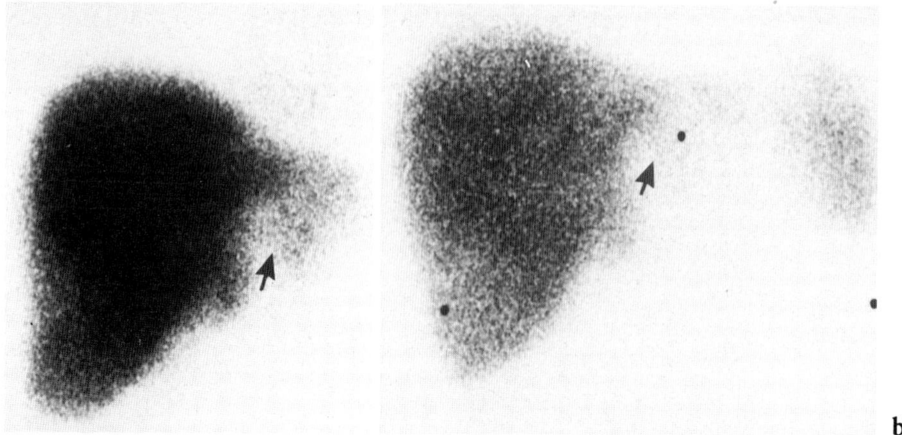

Fig. 6.7 Patient with hilar cholangiocarcinoma and left lobe atrophy. Note reduced uptake of the tracer in (a) HIDA scan (arrow) and (b) colloid scan (arrow)

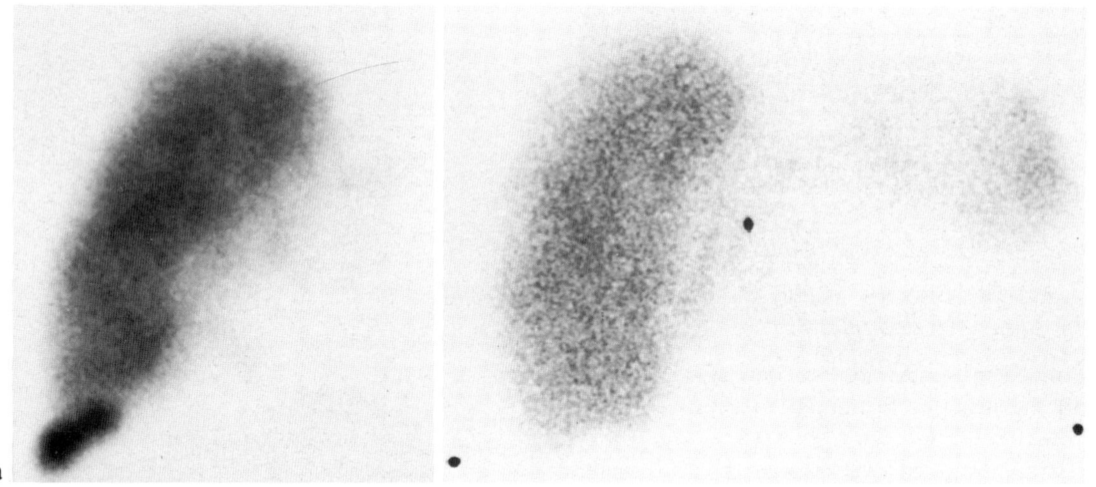

Fig. 6.8 Patient with hilar cholangiocarcinoma and left lobe atrophy. No radionuclide uptake by the atrophied lobe in either (a) HIDA or (b) colloid scan

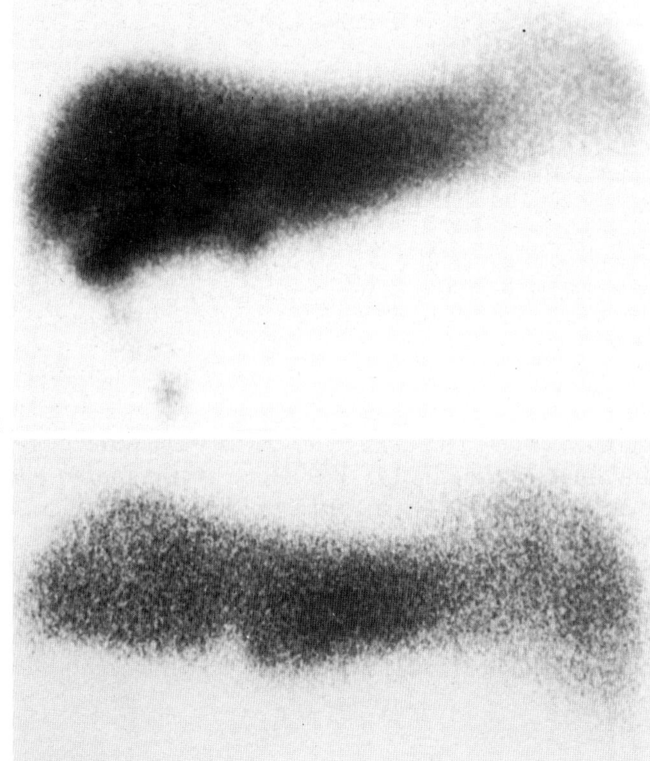

atrophy does not imply irresectability of a neoplastic lesion provided there is no vascular or second order duct involvement in the contralateral lobe. The options of palliation available with malignant obstruction and left liver hypertrophy include percutaneous, endoscopic or surgical intubation and formal anastomosis to the left ducts either by the round ligament approach or by a left intrahepatic hepaticojejunostomy (Ch. 70). Access to the right hepatic ductal system is normally poor because of the short extrahepatic course of the right hepatic duct and anatomical inaccessibility of the segmental ducts; hypertrophy of the right lobe accentuates these problems. Intubation or intrahepatic hepaticojejunostomy to the right liver may be considered. However, the latter procedure may not completely relieve symptoms where second order ducts are involved or a substantial part of the parenchyma drains

Fig. 6.9 Patient with right liver atrophy secondary to benign stricture of the right hepatic duct. There is no uptake of (a) HIDA, or (b) colloid by the atrophied liver. Segment IV and the left lobe are markedly hypertrophic

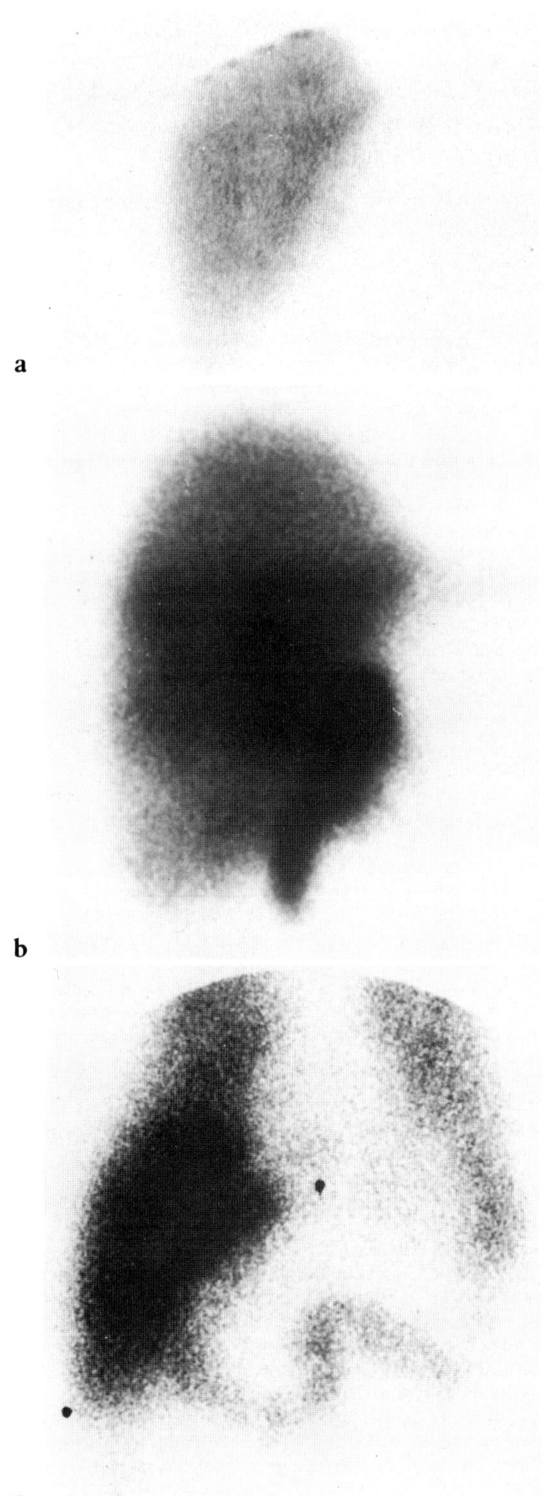

Fig. 6.10 Patient with postcholecystectomy high bile duct stricture and left lobe atrophy. a. HIDA scan before repair of the stricture. Note reduced uptake by the right lobe. There is no function in the left lobe. b. HIDA scan 18 months after repair of the stricture. (The patency of the anastomosis was confirmed on cholangiography.) The function of the right lobe has returned to normal, but the left lobe remains 'silent'. c. Colloid scan confirming the findings on HIDA (HIDA tracer is present in the bowel)

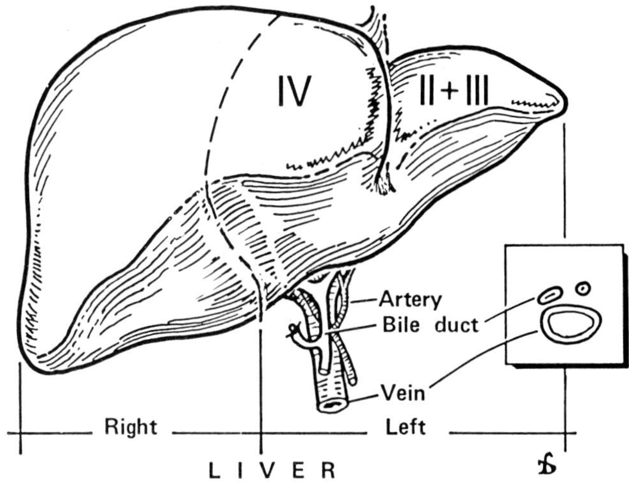

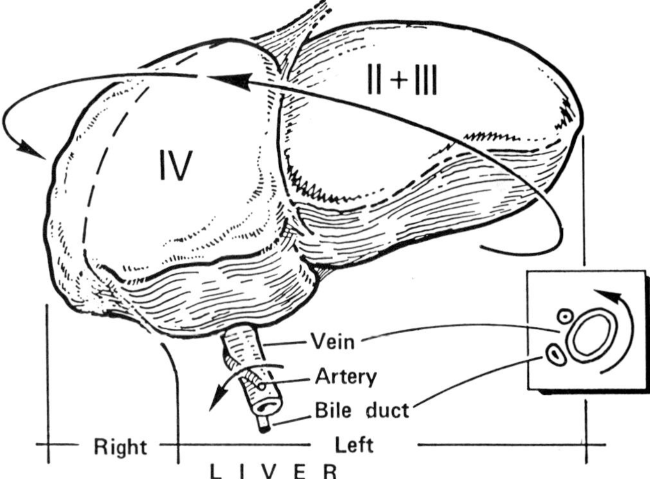

Fig. 6.11 (top) Normal size of the right and left liver and anatomical relation of vascular and ductal structures. Note the common bile duct anterior to the portal vein. (bottom) Schematic representation of the altered relation of vessels and duct as seen with right liver atrophy/left hypertrophy. Note rotation of hilar structures so that the portal vein comes to lie somewhat ventral to the duct

into the left duct; such variations of drainage occur in about 30% of cases (Healey & Schroy 1953).

In benign disease every effort should be made to construct a hilar mucosa-to-mucosa anastomosis since intrahepatic biliary-enteric anastomoses away from the hilum tend to have a higher rate of stricture recurrence. Interventional radiology has a place in the treatment of these patients, especially when combined with initial surgical repair (Czerniak et al 1986). Where atrophy is secondary to unilateral hepatic duct obstruction and provided that the contralateral lobe functions normally, expectant therapy may be warranted (Hadjis et al 1986a). Episodes of cholangitis and pain should be treated with antibiotics and analgesics. Details of management are to be found in Ch. 70.

Finally, liver lobe disparity secondary to biliary disease nearly always indicates hilar pathology. Preoperative diagnosis is important and should be precise in every case so that operative difficulties are anticipated and a clear plan of action is formulated. However, it is perhaps worth noting that liver atrophy secondary to bile duct obstruction is usually indicative of advanced disease, diagnostic delay or therapeutic mismanagement. Therapy, whether curative or palliative, is usually complicated and good results are correspondingly difficult to obtain.

REFERENCES

Benz E J, Baggenstoss A H, Wollaeger E E 1952 Atrophy of the left lobe of the liver. Archives of Pathology 53: 315–330

Bismuth H, Malt R A 1979 Carcinoma of the biliary tract. New England Journal of Medicine 301: 704–706

Bismuth H 1982 Postoperative strictures of the bile duct. In: Blumgart L H (ed) The biliary tract. Clinical Surgery International, Vol 5, Churchill Livingstone, Edinburgh, p 209–218

Blumgart L H, Kelley C J, Benjamin I S 1984 Benign bile duct stricture following cholecystectomy: critical factors in management. British Journal of Surgery 71: 836–843

Braasch J W, Whitcomb F F, Watkins E, Maguire R R, Khazei A M 1972 Segmental obstruction of the bile duct. Surgery, Gynecology and Obstetrics 134: 915–920

Carr D, Hadjis N S, Banks L, Hemingway A, Blumgart L H 1985 Computed tomography of hilar cholangiocarcinoma. American Journal of Roentgenology 145: 53–56

Chen H H, Zhang W H, Wang S S 1984 Twenty-two year experience with the diagnosis and treatment of intrahepatic calculi. Surgery, Gynecology and Obstetrics 159: 519–524

Cole S, Matter A, Karnovsky M J 1971 Autophagic vacuoles in experimental atrophy. Experimental and Molecular Pathology 14: 158–175

Czerniak A, Soreide O, Gibson R, Hadjis N S et al 1986 Liver atrophy complicating benign bile duct strictures. Surgical and interventional radiological approaches. American Journal of Surgery 152: 294–300

Dubuisson L, Bioulac P, Saric J, Balabaud C 1982a Hepatocyte ultrastructure in rats with portacaval shunt. Digestive Diseases and Sciences 27: 1003–1010

Dubuisson L, Bioulac-Sage P, Hemet J, Dubois J P, Balabaud C 1982b Ultrastructure of sinusoidal cells in rats with long term portacaval shunt. In: Knook D L, Wisse E (eds) Sinusoidal liver cells, Elsevier, Amsterdam, p 109–116

Edgcomb L P, Knol J A, Strodel W E, Eckhauser F E 1982 Differential effects of portal diversion on hepatoctle function (HF) and hepatic reticuloendothelial cell (HRES) activity in the dog. Journal of Surgical Research 33: 233–244

Fisher B, Lee S H, Fisher E R, Saffer E 1962 Liver regeneration following portacaval shunt. Surgery 52: 88–102

Frerichs F T 1861 Diseases of the Liver, Vol II, The Sydenham Society, London, p 396

Galloway S, Casarella W J, Price J B 1973 Unilobar veno-occlusive disease of the liver. American Journal of Roentgenology 119: 89–94

Hadjis N S, Carr D, Banks L M, Gibson R, Blumgart L H 1986a Expectant management of patients with unilateral hepatic duct obstruction and liver atrophy. Gut 27: 1223–1227

Hadjis N S, Fitzpatrick M, Henderson B, Lavender J P, Blumgart L H 1986b Scintigraphic, pathological and radiological aspects of liver atrophy. (submitted for publication)

Ham J M 1979 Partial and complete atrophy affecting hepatic segments and lobes. British Journal of Surgery 66: 333–337

Harley V, Barratt W 1901 The experimental production of hepatic cirrhosis. Journal of Pathology and Bacteriology 7: 203–213

Healey J E, Schroy P 1953 The anatomy of the bile ducts within the human liver; an analysis of the prevailing patterns of branching and their major variants. Archives of Surgery 66: 599–616

Hueston J T 1953 The production of liver lobe atrophy by hydatid cysts. British Journal of Surgery 41: 427–430

Johnstone J M S, Lee E G 1976 A quantitative assessment of the structural changes in the rat's liver following obstruction of the common bile duct. British Journal of Experimental Pathology 57: 85–94

Kerr J F R 1971 'Shrinkage necrosis': a distinct mode of cellular death. Journal of Pathology 105: 13–20

Longmire W P, Tompkins R K 1975 Lesions of the segmental and lobar hepatic ducts. Annals of Surgery 182: 478–495

McMaster P D, Rous P 1921 The biliary obstruction required to produce jaundice. Journal of Experimental Medicine 33: 731–750

Makler P T, Lewis E, Cantor R, Charkes N D, Malmud L S 1980 Nonvisualization of the left lobe of the liver due to atrophy or aplasia. Clinical Nuclear Medicine 5: 63–65

Marshall J M 1932 Tumors of the bile ducts. Surgery, Gynecology and Obstetrics 54: 6–12

Meyer W W 1950 Unilaterale leberschwunde oder lappenhypoplasien der leber? Virchows Archiv 319: 127–230

Myracle M R, Stadalnik R C, Blaisdell F W, Farkas J P, Matin P 1981 Segmental biliary obstruction: diagnostic significance of bile duct crowding. American Journal of Roentgenology 137: 169–171

Nasse 1894 Ueber experimente an der leber und den gallenwegen. Archiv fur Klinische Chirurgie 48: 885–893

Ogawa T, Jefferson N C, Necheles H 1960 Comparative study of bile drainage in dogs and man. American Journal of Surgery 99: 57–62

Pfeifer U 1978 Inhibition by insulin of the formation of autophagic vacuoles in rat liver. A morphometric approach to the kinetics of intracellular degradation by autophagy. Journal of Cell Biology 78: 152–167

Pfeifer U 1982 Kinetic and subcellular aspects of hypertrophy and atrophy. International Review of Experimental Pathology 23: 1–45

Putnam C W, Porter K A, Starzl T E 1976 Hepatic encephalopathy and light and electron micrographic changes of the baboon liver after portal diversion. Annals of Surgery 184: 155–161

Rensing U, Wimmer B, Lesch R, Wenz W 1984 Budd-Chiari-Stuart-Bras syndrome: clinical, sonographic, radiological reexaminations in occlusive diseases of hepatic veins. Hepato-gastroenterology 31: 218–226

Rous P, Larimore L D 1920a Relation of the portal blood to liver maintenance. Journal of Experimental Medicine 31: 609–632

Rous P, Larimore L D 1920b The biliary factor in liver lesions. Journal of Experimental Medicine 32: 249–272

Rozga J, Jeppsson B, Bengmark S 1985 Hepatotrophic factors in liver growth and atrophy. British Journal of Experimental Pathology 66: 669–678

Schalm L, Bax H R, Mansens B J 1956 Atrophy of the liver after occlusion of the bile ducts or portal vein and compensatory hypertrophy of the unoccluded portion and its clinical importance. Gastroenterology 31: 131–155

Sigel B, Baldia L B, Menduke H, Feigl P 1967 Independence of hyperplastic and hypertrophic responses in liver regeneration. Surgery, Gynecology and Obstetrics 125: 95–100

Starzl T E, Porter K A, Kashiwagi N, Putnam C W 1975 Portal hepatotrophic factors, diabetes mellitus and acute liver atrophy, hypertrophy and regeneration. Surgery, Gynecology and Obstetrics 141: 843–858

Starzl T E, Watanabe K, Porter K A, Putnam C W 1976 Effects of insulin, glucagon, and insulin/glucagon infusions in liver morphology and cell division after complete portacaval shunt in dogs. Lancet i: 821–825

Steiner P E, Martinez Batiz J 1961 Effects on the rat liver of bile duct, portal vein and hepatic artery ligations. American Journal of Pathology 39: 257–289

Stewart H L, Cantarow A, Morgan D R 1937 Changes in the liver of the cat following ligation of single hepatic ducts. Archives of Pathology 23: 641–652

Swanson E A, Millians W S, Sotus P C, Skandalakis J E 1967 Liver cell regeneration and degeneration after lobar biliary obstruction in dogs. American Journal of Gastroenterology 47: 280–286
Tavill A S, Wood E J, Kreal L, Jones E A, Gregory M, Sherlock S 1975 The Budd-Chiari syndrome: correlation between hepatic scintigraphy and the clinical radiological and pathological findings in nineteen cases of hepatic venous outflow obstruction. Gastroenterology 68: 509–518
Tsuzuki T, Hoshino Y, Uchiyama T, Kitazima M, Mikata A, Matsuki S 1973 Compensatory hypertrophy of the lateral quadrant of the left hepatic lobe due to atrophy of the rest of the liver, appearing as a mass in the left upper quadrant of the abdomen: report of a case. Annals of Surgery 177: 406–410
Weinbren K 1953 The effect of bile duct obstruction on regeneration of the rat's liver. British Journal of Experimental Pathology 34: 280–289
Weinbren K 1955 The portal blood supply and regeneration of the rat's liver. British Journal of Experimental Pathology 36: 583–591
Weinbren K, Tarsh E 1964 The mitotic response in the rat liver after different regenerative stimuli. British Journal of Experimental Pathology 45: 475–480
Weinbren K, Stirling G A, Washington S L A 1972 The development of a proliferative response in liver parenchyma deprived of portal blood flow. British Journal of Experimental Pathology 53: 54–58
Weinbren K 1982 Experimental diffuse nodular hepatic hyperplasia. Toxicologic Pathology 10: 81–92
Weinbren K, Hadjis N S, Blumgart L H 1985 Structural aspects of the liver in patients with biliary disease and portal hypertension. Journal of Clinical Pathology 38: 1013–1020
Wilkinson M, Sherlock S 1984 A case of ascites. Hospital Update 10: 712–726

7

R. T. Mathie, D. M. Nagorney, L. H. Blumgart

Liver blood flow: physiology, measurement and clinical relevance

The hepatic circulation is both large and complex. This chapter describes the nature and physiological control of the liver's blood supply, outlines the techniques used for its measurement in experimental animals and in man, and explores its importance in a variety of clinical situations.

PHYSIOLOGY

LIVER BLOOD SUPPLY

The liver normally receives about one quarter of the total cardiac output, and obtains its supply from two main sources, the hepatic artery and the portal vein. Mixing of arterial and portal blood takes place in the sinusoids which are drained by the hepatic venous system into the inferior vena cava. In addition, a large number of smaller arteries provide a small blood supply to the liver, but, in the event of hepatic arterial occlusion, are a potent source for the formation of a collateral circulation.

Hepatic artery

The hepatic arterioles empty directly or via the peribiliary plexus into the sinusoids and terminal portal venules. Direct artery to hepatic vein connections do not usually exist, but may arise in some liver diseases such as cirrhosis. Reduction of pressure in the arterial system towards that existing in the portal circulation is probably achieved mainly by: 1. the pre-sinusoidal arteriolar resistance (especially that provided by the peribiliary plexus), and 2. the intermittent closure of the arterioles, which effectively shields the portal bloodstream from the arterial pressure (Rappaport 1973).

The hepatic artery normally supplies about 30 ml/min per 100 g liver tissue, approximately 25% of the total blood flow to the liver. However, it may provide up to 30–40% of the liver's normal oxygen requirement, largely because the arterial blood has a greater oxygen content than portal blood (see below).

Portal vein

The tributaries of the portal vein collect the venous outflow from the entire intestinal tract from the lower oesophagus to the rectum, as well as from the pancreas and spleen. Until recently it had been the widespread belief that blood from the splenic vein supplies mainly the left lobe of the liver while blood from the superior mesenteric vein passes mainly to the right lobe. It is now believed, however, that any constant streamlining is most unlikely, but that a partial streamline may occur in certain circumstances, for example by changing the patient's posture. It is thus improbable that the pattern of hepatic distribution of portal inflow can explain the localization of blood-borne hepatic lesions seen in some patients (Groszmann et al 1971).

The portal vein normally carries about 75% of the total blood flow to the liver, or 90 ml/min per 100 g liver weight. Normal portal pressure is in the region of 5–10 mmHg. Portal blood is post-capillary and therefore partly deoxygenated but, because of its large volume flow rate, may supply 60–70% of the liver's normal oxygen requirement. Hepatic oxygen supply may be at risk if portal blood flow is significantly reduced, but the effect is minimized by an increase in oxygen extraction from the hepatic arterial blood and/or by an increase in the arterial blood flow rate to the liver (see below).

Hepatic veins

The hepatic venous system is the final common pathway of hepatic arterial and portal venous blood after sinusoidal mixing in the normal liver. It is therefore the drainage tract of the entire splanchnic vascular bed, and carries in the region of 1.5 l/min. The free pressure in an hepatic vein is 1–2 mmHg. Wedged hepatic venous pressure is a useful method of estimating sinusoidal pressure, and may also indicate portal venous pressure (Boyer et al 1977).

Hepatic venous blood is normally about two-thirds saturated with oxygen; this may be markedly reduced during periods of low delivery of oxygen to the liver, when an increased proportion of the available supply is extracted by the liver cells. Under normal conditions, the liver accounts for some 20% of the total oxygen consumption of the body.

CONTROL OF LIVER BLOOD FLOW

The majority of investigations responsible for the information outlined in this section have been carried out in experimental animals rather than in man, since human studies have largely concentrated on the changes in the hepatic circulation in disease.

The control of liver blood flow takes place in three distinct areas: the hepatic arterioles, the portal venules, and the mesenteric arterioles. The arterial blood supply of the liver is subject to active control by the normal array of factors influencing the peripheral vasculature; the portal venous blood supply normally encounters minimal resistance in the portal venules and is therefore effectively controlled outside the liver by the action of the arterial resistance vessels within the organs of the digestive tract and spleen.

Reciprocal relationship between hepatic artery and portal vein blood flow

Studies of the individual control mechanisms of the hepatic arterial and portal venous circulations are frequently complicated by the complex haemodynamic interaction between the two bloodstreams occurring within the organ (usually known as the 'reciprocal' relationship). Many workers have observed an increase in arterial blood flow after portal flow reduction (e.g. Schenk et al 1962, Kock et al 1972, Mathie et al 1980a); the converse response (i.e. an increase in portal flow after arterial flow reduction) has only rarely been found, and it is now proposed that the relationship be referred to as the 'hepatic arterial buffer response' (Lautt 1981). Hepatic arterial blood flow hyperaemia following serious loss of portal inflow is unable to provide complete haemodynamic compensation (Mathie & Blumgart 1983a), but may be of vital importance in conditions such as portal hypertension (see below). However, the certainty that such a hyperaemic arterial response occurs is unfortunately not matched by a clear view of the mechanism controlling the reaction, and hypotheses remain 'at best speculative and at worst completely obscure' (Lautt 1977).

Metabolism

The presumption that hepatic arterial blood flow is linked to liver metabolism has recently been challenged (Lautt 1983, Mathie & Blumgart 1983a). It has been shown, for example, that neither altered oxygen supply nor bile secretion causes a dependent change in arterial flow (Lautt 1983), and it has been concluded that the hepatic artery acts as a 'buffer' to prevent significant changes in total liver blood flow, thereby tending to maintain a constant level of hepatic clearance of blood-borne drugs and hormones. Thus the hepatic artery may uniquely be regarded as subservient to the metabolic requirements of the entire organism rather than to those of the perfused tissue. As stated previously, however, the hepatic artery is still highly important for the supply of oxygen to the liver, and uptake may increase according to local requirements, particularly in situations of low portal blood flow; by contrast, its blood flow *control* appears to be independent of the oxygen demands of the liver.

Blood gas tensions

Recent experimental studies in dogs have clarified the influence of arterial blood gas tensions and pH on the hepatic circulation. Hypercarbia ($PaCO_2>70$ mmHg) increases portal venous flow and decreases hepatic arterial flow (Hughes et al 1979a), while hypocarbia ($PaCO_2<30$ mmHg) decreases both (Hughes et al 1979b). Systemic hypoxia ($PaO_2<70$ mmHg) causes a fall in arterial flow but no change in the portal venous contribution (Hughes et al 1979c). The hepatic haemodynamic reaction to metabolic acidosis is similar to that induced by hypercarbia, while metabolic alkalosis has little biologically significant effect (Hughes et al 1980b). The mechanisms for these responses are not totally understood, though it is evident that the sympathetic nervous system is responsible for the hepatic arterial vasoconstriction observed in both hypercarbia and hypoxia (Mathie & Blumgart 1983b).

Neural control and catecholamines

Hepatic sympathetic nervous stimulation causes hepatic arterial vasoconstriction and reduced blood flow, but this is not maintained and 'autoregulatory escape' occurs (Greenway & Stark 1971). Portal pressure rises due to an increase in portal venous resistance but portal flow does not decrease unless there is a decrease in intestinal or splenic blood flow caused by simultaneous sympathetic stimulation of these vascular beds.

Both alpha- and beta-adrenergic receptors exist in the hepatic artery; the portal venous system is thought to contain only alpha-receptors (Richardson & Withrington 1981). The haemodynamic response to noradrenaline is very similar to that produced by nerve stimulation. The effect of adrenaline is complicated by the dose-dependency of its action on alpha- and beta-receptors: at low doses, hepatic and mesenteric arterial vasodilatation predominate, whereas at high doses vasoconstriction occurs in both the hepatic arterial and portal venous vascular beds as well as in the mesenteric circulation (Greenway & Stark 1971, Richardson & Withrington 1981).

Hormones and drugs

Hepatic blood flow is profoundly increased by glucagon; the flow increase is a consequence of its strong vasodilatory action on the mesenteric vasculature and a lesser vasodilatory influence on the hepatic arterial system. Insulin has little haemodynamic effect on the hepatic circulation. Histamine causes hepatic arterial dilatation, and, in the dog only, hepatic venous constriction or outflow block. Bradykinin is a potent hepatic arterial vasodilator but has little effect on the portal venous system. The hepatic arterial vascular bed is dilated by the majority of prostaglandins. Angiotensin decreases both hepatic arterial and portal blood flows, and indeed is one of the few substances to produce a significant vasoconstrictor effect on the hepatic artery. Vasopressin decreases portal flow and pressure mainly by mesenteric arterial vasoconstriction but the pressure reduction is also the result of direct portal venous vasodilatation; it has variable effects on the hepatic artery (Richardson & Withrington 1981).

Anaesthetic agents

Most investigations of the effects of general anaesthetic agents on liver blood flow have concentrated attention on halothane, though the newer products have been the subject of some recent study. Both hepatic arterial and portal venous blood flow decrease passively in parallel with cardiac output during halothane inhalation, with little change in vascular resistance (Thulin et al 1975, Hughes et al 1980a). Hepatic oxygen consumption is not diminished by halothane, but at the cost of a marked increase in the oxygen extraction rate from the reduced blood supply (Andreen et al 1975). The more recent agent enflurane has been found to have somewhat similar effects to those of halothane, though there is a decrease in hepatic arterial vascular resistance as part of a generalized decrease in peripheral vascular resistance (Hughes et al 1980a). Both cyclopropane and methoxyflurane reduce liver blood flow, mainly by increasing the mesenteric vascular resistance (Batchelder & Cooperman 1975). Nitrous oxide in concentrations of 30–70% reduces both hepatic artery and portal vein flow, possibly as a result of a generalized stimulatory action on alpha-adrenergic receptors (Thomson et al 1982).

MEASUREMENT OF LIVER BLOOD FLOW

Many different techniques have been employed in attempts to measure the hepatic blood flow in experimental animals and in man. The earliest workers approached the problem using direct techniques which had no application in clinical investigations. Subsequent developments allowed an indirect determination of blood flow by the use of a variety of indicator clearance techniques which could also be applied to the clinical situation, but with diminished accuracy in the presence of liver disease. More sophisticated technology now enables liver blood flow or tissue perfusion to be determined either directly or indirectly in animals or in man with greater accuracy and fewer difficulties than before. Continuing efforts are being made to improve methodology still further. Methods are listed in Table 7.1 and will be discussed under two broad headings: total flow measurement (ml/min) and tissue perfusion measurement (ml/min per gram of liver tissue).

Total flow measurement

Early methods

Burton-Opitz (1910, 1911) directly measured blood flow rate in the portal vein and the hepatic artery using the intravascular stromuhr. Other early workers adopted a venous outflow collection method to assess total hepatic blood flow (MacLeod & Pearce 1914). Both methods give quantitative data about total flow but involve extensive

Table 7.1 Methods used for measuring liver blood flow

TOTAL FLOW MEASUREMENT
Early methods
Intravascular stromuhr
Venous outflow
Transillumination
Clearance techniques
Hepatocyte excretory clearance
Bromsulphthalein
Rose Bengal (^{131}I)
Indocyanine green
Reticulo-endothelial particle clearance
Colloidal gold (^{198}Au)
Heat-denatured serum albumin (^{131}I)
Sulphur colloid (^{99m}Tc)
Hepatic drug extraction
Lignocaine
Propranolol
Indicator dilution
Red blood cells (^{51}Cr)
Serum albumin (^{131}I)
Indicator fractionation
Potassium (^{42}K)
Rubidium (^{86}Rb)
Microspheres (various labels)
Electromagnetic flowmeter
Ultrasound (Doppler)
TISSUE PERFUSION MEASUREMENT
Inert gas clearance
Krypton (^{85}Kr)
Xenon (^{133}Xe)

operative procedures which prevent their application in man. Transillumination is another direct method, in which an edge of the liver is illuminated from below by a quartz rod and the intrahepatic vessels examined by microscopy (Wakim & Mann 1942).

Clearance techniques

Hepatic blood flow was estimated in man for the first time using an indirect method based on the Fick principle (Bradley et al 1945). The Fick principle allows an assessment of organ blood flow by dividing the rate of removal of a substance by its arterio-venous concentration difference across the organ. The measurement obtained by Bradley's group depended on the fact that intravenously injected bromsulphthalein (BSP) is removed from the bloodstream entirely by the hepatocytes into the bile. They derived a value for the rate of hepatic BSP removal indirectly by determining the rate of intravenous infusion of dye that maintained the peripheral arterial concentration at a constant level, and by also measuring the arterio-venous concentration difference of BSP they were thus able to calculate hepatic blood flow. The mean value obtained in a group of 23 normal subjects was 1.5 l/min, a figure still considered to be the 'normal' total liver blood flow in healthy men of average weight. Since 1945, this technique has been used extensively for hepatic blood flow measurements, sometimes substituting BSP with other substances dependent on hepatocyte extraction into bile such as ^{131}I-labelled Rose Bengal (Combes 1960) and indocyanine green (Caesar et al 1961). None of these substances actually enjoys complete hepatic removal and so hepatic venous cannulation is necessary to allow calculation of true extraction efficiency. Two other hepatic clearance techniques have therefore been employed: colloidal clearance by the hepatic reticulo-endothelial (Kupffer) cells (Dobson & Jones 1952), and hepatocyte removal of highly extracted drugs (George 1979). The more complete hepatic extraction of these materials overcomes the need to cannulate an hepatic vein in patients with normal liver function.

Though these methods may be accurate in normal subjects, problems arise in patients with liver disease, when there may be reduced cellular uptake of the marker and a variable degree of extrahepatic removal of dyes and colloids. There may also be vascular shunts within or around the liver, allowing bypass of the liver cells. In these circumstances, the clearance methods become increasingly useful as tests of hepatic *function* rather than blood flow.

Recent experimental adaptations of the colloid uptake method may in future offer the possibility of measuring two very important aspects of the hepatic circulation in the clinical context: the arterial and portal components of total liver blood flow (Karran et al 1982); and the quantitation of portal-systemic shunting of splanchnic venous blood (Rikkers 1981).

Indicator dilution

Reichman et al (1958) were the first to apply an indicator dilution technique to the measurement of total liver blood flow in man. The method involves the portal venous or hepatic arterial injection of a labelled substance that is not removed by the liver (red blood cells or serum albumin), and either measuring the changes in hepatic vein concentration by blood sampling, or monitoring the hepatic isotope activity with an external detector. Portal venous blood flow may be determined separately using a modification of the original technique, by sampling portal venous blood after splenic vein or superior mesenteric artery injection (Chiandussi et al 1968, Huet et al 1973); hepatic arterial flow may then be calculated as the difference between total and portal flows. In addition, a modification of the thermal dilution technique has recently been used to measure portal blood flow in man (Biber et al 1983). Indicator dilution methods are not affected by hepatocellular function, but may be rendered inaccurate in the presence of portal-systemic collateral channels.

Indicator fractionation

Sapirstein (1956) was responsible for developing a method for the measurement of the distribution of cardiac output using the principle of indicator fractionation. Substances used have been ^{42}K and ^{86}Rb, but more recently radioactive microspheres have enjoyed widespread application for experimental investigations of the peripheral circulation in animals. The hepatic arterial blood flow is easily determined by this method, but the portal flow contribution can only be found by addition of the flow values obtained in all the other splanchnic organs (Gurll et al 1980). Examination of the intrahepatic distribution of microspheres also provides a means of assessing the pattern of blood flow in different regions of the liver (Greenway & Oshiro 1972).

Electromagnetic flowmeter

The direct and continuous measurement of both hepatic arterial and portal venous blood flows with electromagnetic flow probes is probably the most valuable means of assessing liver blood flow currently available. The technique has found widespread application in experiments using large animals, but its employment in clinical situations has been prevented both by the relatively extensive vascular dissection required for placement of the flow probes and by the overestimation of sinusoidal flow in the presence of portal-systemic shunts. Using the method, Schenk and colleagues (1962) found normal hepatic flow in man to be about 1 l/min, of which approximately 25% was supplied by the hepatic artery. All subsequent clinical studies have concentrated on haemodynamic investigations of liver diseases such as cirrhosis. A typical experimental

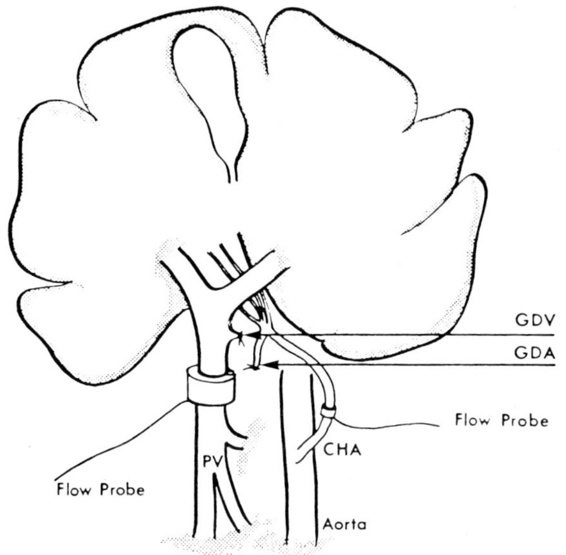

Fig. 7.1 Experimental arrangement for measuring liver blood flow in the dog with electromagnetic flow probes. Probes are shown on the portal vein (PV) and common hepatic artery (CHA). The gastroduodenal vein (GDV) and gastroduodenal artery (GDA) are ligated as illustrated, to ensure that the flows measured by the probes are those which actually perfuse the liver

preparation utilizing the electromagnetic flowmeter is illustrated in Figure 7.1.

Ultrasound

There have been few attempts as yet to measure liver blood flow using Doppler ultrasound. Successful animal studies have been reported however (Loisance et al 1973), and recent investigations have achieved Doppler measurements of portal and arterial blood flow in conscious dogs on multiple occasions over periods of up to eight months (Anderson 1981). Advances in Doppler technology may eventually allow the accurate and non-invasive clinical measurement of blood flow in the major hepatic vessels as well as in extrahepatic portal-systemic shunt channels.

Tissue perfusion measurement

Inert gas clearance

The last decade has seen the successful application of the inert gas clearance technique to the measurement of hepatic tissue perfusion in animals and man. The method, employing either Krypton (^{85}Kr) or Xenon (^{133}Xe), requires only the measurement of the rate of clearance of gas after its injection into the hepatic blood supply. After injection, the gas diffuses rapidly throughout the liver and reaches equilibrium between the tissue and blood. The gas then 'clears' from the tissue into the blood, and is almost completely eliminated from the body after a single passage through the lungs. The clearance rate is proportional to the hepatic tissue perfusion rate (derived from both hepatic artery and portal vein), and the clearance is monitored using an appropriate detector placed over the liver: a Geiger-Müller tube for detecting the beta emissions of ^{85}Kr, or a scintillation crystal or gamma camera for detecting the gamma emissions of ^{133}Xe. Hepatic tissue perfusion (expressed in ml/min per gram of liver tissue) is calculated from a standard formula after determining the clearance half-time ($T\frac{1}{2}$) from the logarithmic replot of the exponential clearance:

$$\text{Tissue perfusion (ml/min per gram)} = \frac{\lambda . \log_e 2}{T\frac{1}{2}},$$

where $T\frac{1}{2}$ is expressed in minutes, and λ (the liver : blood partition coefficient of the gas) is generally taken as 0.91 for ^{85}Kr (Leiberman et al 1978a) and 0.74 for ^{133}Xe (Conn 1961). Figure 7.2 illustrates the ^{85}Kr clearance curve that is typically obtained in clinical or experimental studies.

Inert gas clearance methods involve minimal trauma to the subject being investigated, are not affected by the presence of hepatic cellular disease or shunts, and provide a quantitative assessment of actual tissue perfusion derived from the combined hepatic arterial and portal venous blood supply (Leiberman et al 1978b). The first workers to use the method for liver blood flow measurement in man were Aronsen et al (1966), who recorded the gamma emissions of ^{133}Xe after the injection of a saline solution of the isotope into the portal vein. Other routes of administration may be employed, including hepatic artery, liver parenchyma, splenic pulp, or gas inhalation; however, each of these routes tends to lead to erroneous perfusion values, and direct portal vein injection is recommended as the preferred and accurate method. Because of the lipophilic nature of inert gases, it is also important to take account of the changes in hepatic fat content known to occur in certain clinical conditions (Mathie et al 1977).

Individual assessment of the hepatic arterial and portal venous components of hepatic tissue perfusion may be achieved only by briefly occluding one vessel and observing the clearance rate due to the perfusion from the other supply. With this approach, it must be accepted that the residual hepatic blood flow after occlusion of one vessel may be significantly different from basal flow in the remaining vessel with an entirely intact system. This particularly applies in the case of portal vein occlusion since this causes a significant hyperaemic response of the hepatic artery (see above).

CLINICAL RELEVANCE

HAEMORRHAGIC SHOCK

Much has been written about the effect of haemorrhage and shock on the hepatic circulation, particularly in exper-

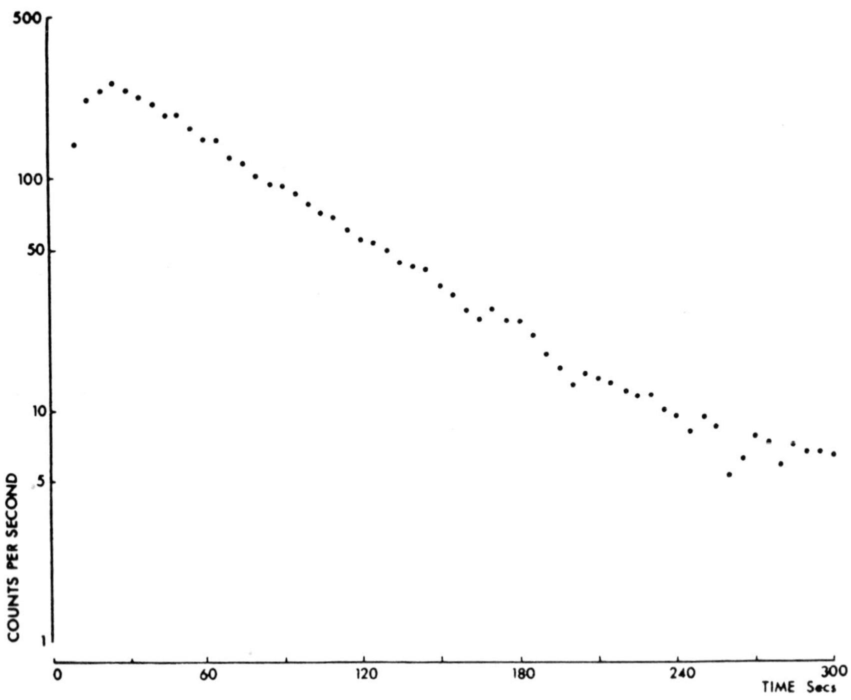

Fig. 7.2 Typical ^{85}Kr clearance curve obtained after portal venous injection of the isotope in the anaesthetized dog. The mono-exponential clearance generally obtained with this technique allows the clearance half-time ($T\frac{1}{2}$) to be readily obtained. $T\frac{1}{2}$ is the time required for activity to decrease to one-half any given value on the straight part of the curve, and in this case is 0.74 min, enabling hepatic tissue perfusion to be calculated as 0.85 ml/min per gram liver (85 ml/min per 100 gram). Reproduced with permission from Academic Press (Leiberman et al 1978a)

imental animals (Greenway & Stark 1971), and only a brief account is given here. Total liver blood flow decreases approximately in relation to the severity of the haemorrhagic hypotension. Portal venous blood flow decreases in parallel to the cardiac output, but, in common with the coronary, pulmonary and cerebral circulations, hepatic arterial flow does not fall until quite severely low blood pressures are reached. As a result the hepatic oxygen supply tends to be maintained, though oxygen extraction greatly increases in order to preserve normal total oxygen consumption (Smith et al 1979). Hepatic outflow block has been reported to occur with retransfusion of the shed blood after haemorrhagic hypotension, but this phenomenon appears to be a feature specific to the hepatic venous anatomy of the dog, and is therefore a complication unlikely to arise in the clinical situation.

Clinically, ischaemic hepatitis or shock liver is generally recognized following cardiogenic or haemorrhagic shock (Birgens et al 1978, Bynum et al 1979). Hepatic dysfunction caused by hepatic hypoperfusion is characterized morphologically by centrilobular necrosis and clinically with abdominal pain, cholestatic jaundice, and marked elevation of serum transaminases. These findings typically resolve within seven to 10 days of injury. Recently, Gottlieb et al (1983) showed that hepatic dysfunction in man following trauma was inversely related to the hepatic blood flow rate. They found that hepatic blood flow was markedly reduced after injury and that, although oxygen delivery was decreased, splanchnic oxygen consumption remained normal due to increased extraction by the liver.

LIVER ATROPHY

Alterations in liver blood flow which significantly reduce either the volume flow or the composition or concentration of hepatotrophic substances result in liver atrophy (Ch. 6). The degree of atrophy is dependent upon the degree of blood flow deprivation. Atrophy of the liver resulting from reduced blood flow may either be segmental, lobar or diffuse and results from a sustained reduction in either portal venous or hepatic artery blood flow, or both.

Atrophy and fatty degeneration of the canine liver after total portal diversion through an Eck fistula was initially reported almost a century ago (Hahn et al 1893). Numerous experimental studies in a variety of species have confirmed that both partial and complete diversion of portal vein blood flow from the liver results in atrophy. Complete portal venous flow diversion with interruption of all portal venous collaterals results in more profound liver atrophy than the partial deviation of portal venous flow resulting from side-to-side portacaval anastomoses (Bollman 1961). An accurate quantitative relationship for the degree of liver atrophy relative to the reduction of portal venous blood flow remains to be determined primarily because changes in both volume flow and composition of portal blood are involved, but also because of attendant changes in hepatic arterial flow.

Nevertheless, there is accumulating evidence that liver atrophy following portal diversion is not the result of a decrease in absolute volume flow but the consequence of the effective loss of hepatotrophic constituents in the portal blood. Rats subjected to portal flow diversion with portacaval transposition underwent a decrease in relative liver weight (Guest et al 1977), despite the effective preservation of portal perfusion from the inferior vena cava (Ryan et al 1978). Dogs with 'partial portacaval transposition' (Marchioro et al 1967) or 'splanchnic flow division' (Starzl et al 1973, 1975) revealed atrophy in those liver lobes deprived of pancreatic venous drainage, despite subsequent demonstration of normal tissue perfusion in all regions of the liver (Mathie et al 1979). Thus liver size depends critically on its portal circulation, but this is due predominantly to the quality of the blood it supplies to the liver rather than the quantity of flow it provides.

Regardless of degree, the effect of portal blood flow deprivation occurs rapidly. Atrophy is essentially complete within four days of total diversion of portal venous flow (Starzl et al 1983). Although hepatocyte size decreases rapidly, other histological abnormalities are uncommon (Lee et al 1974, Weinbren & Washington 1976). However, depletion and disruption of the rough endoplasmic reticulum and reduction of membrane-bound polyribosomes have been demonstrated ultrastructurally in atrophic hepatocytes (Starzl et al 1983).

The fate of the liver after ligation of the hepatic artery depends largely upon the extent of a functional collateral arterial circulation (Rappaport & Schneiderman 1976). If collaterals are few, liver infarction and necrosis may occur after hepatic artery ligation and may result in death. However, with an adequate collateral supply, hepatic artery ligation results only in transient ischaemic changes in the periphery of the hepatic acinus (zone 3). Atrophy after hepatic artery ligation occurs grossly in liver segments which have sufficient collateral supply to prevent complete necrosis but insufficient collaterals to compensate completely for arterial ligation. The effects of hepatic artery interruption are compounded by low portal venous blood flow and oxygen saturation, superimposed infection, and complicated by species-specific differences (Rappaport & Schneiderman 1976). Histologically, arterial obstruction rapidly causes ischaemic changes with mitochondrial swelling, cell membrane disruption, platelet aggregation, and widening of the spaces of Disse (Mallet-Guy et al 1972).

The collateral arterial supply of the liver has been studied extensively in both animals and man by means of angiography and corrosion casts. In a detailed autopsy study, Michels (1955) has demonstrated 26 distinct collateral pathways in man. Following hepatic arterial ligation, the major potential arterial collaterals arise from the inferior phrenic arteries, which can develop connections with hepatic arteries within the liver, and from the gastroduodenal arteries, which derive blood flow from the superior mesenteric artery and supply the liver via the peribiliary arterial plexus around the intrahepatic bile ducts (Rappaport & Schneiderman 1976). The site of flow interruption has traditionally been thought to influence the effect of arterial ligation on the liver. Certainly, the precise nature of the functional collateral supply after hepatic arterial ligation is dependent on the site of occlusion: if the common hepatic artery is interrupted, revascularisation occurs through both major routes indicated above; if only the right or left hepatic artery is interrupted however, intrahepatic translobar anastomoses re-establish arterial flow in the ligated system (Mays & Wheeler 1974). Ligation of the proper hepatic arteries leads to revascularisation solely via an hypertrophied inferior phrenic circulation (Jefferson et al 1956). Clearly therefore, complete dearterialisation of the liver by any form of arterial vascular occlusion is extremely unlikely, and it is probable that the effect of arterial ligation on the liver is in fact independent of the actual site of flow interruption (Mays 1974).

Clinically, ligation of either the portal vein or hepatic artery is tolerated as an isolated injury. Survival has been documented following portal vein ligation carried out to control haemorrhage after traumatic injury (Pachter et al 1979) or during difficult biliary tract surgery. Similarly, survival after hepatic artery ligation for either trauma, aneurysm, haemobilia, or neoplasms has been confirmed (Rappaport & Schneiderman 1976). However, the outcome after ligation of either the portal vein or the hepatic artery in the face of shock, infection or concomitant organ failure is much less certain.

LIVER RESECTION AND REGENERATION

A number of studies in man have confirmed that hepatic regeneration of the normal in situ liver remnant proceeds rapidly following partial hepatic resection (Blumgart et al 1971, Aronsen et al 1970). Histologically, the regenerated liver is normal, though morphologically it is globular in shape. Importantly, however, Lin & Chen (1965) have suggested that neither significant regeneration, hypertrophy, nor improved function occurs in the cirrhotic liver after major resection.

Partial liver resection without devascularisation would normally be expected to produce little change in total liver blood flow. This occurs because the major contributor to total flow, the portal vein, is affected less by events taking place within the liver than by control mechanisms in the arterial resistance vessels of the pre-hepatic splanchnic bed. Because essentially the same total blood flow is therefore redistributed to a smaller mass of liver tissue, a

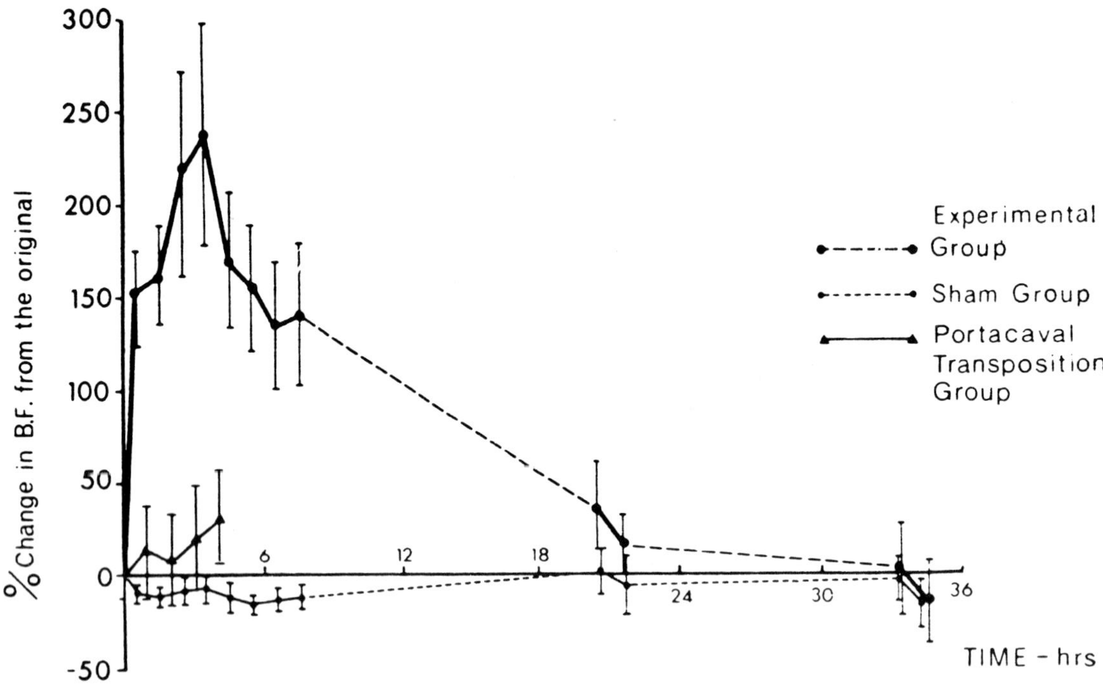

Fig. 7.3 Changes in hepatic tissue perfusion (ml/min per gram liver) in three groups of rats following two-thirds hepatectomy. Normal rats ('Experimental Group') showed a striking increase in perfusion during the first eight hours, whereas animals subjected to a prior portacaval transposition demonstrated no significant change. Perfusion in rats which had sham partial hepatectomy did not alter throughout the period of measurement. Error bars indicate ± 1 S.D. Reproduced with permission from Elsevier Scientific Publishers (Blumgart 1978)

corresponding increase in tissue perfusion (ml/min per unit tissue weight) would be anticipated in the non-resected remnant. Experimental studies support these expectations: using the ^{85}Kr clearance technique, an increase in hepatic tissue perfusion of 150–250% was observed in rats immediately following two-thirds hepatectomy (Rice et al 1977) (Fig. 7.3). Moreover, similar studies in three patients during right hepatic lobectomy or right hepatectomy demonstrated an increase in tissue perfusion of approximately 120% in the remnant (Mathie & Blumgart 1982) (Table 7.2). The latter investigation also showed that four patients with compromised portal flow to the subsequently

Table 7.2 Hepatic tissue perfusion in seven patients before and after partial hepatectomy (^{85}Kr clearance measurements)

Group	Case	Age	Condition	Operation	Hepatic tissue perfusion (ml/min/100 g liver) Before	After	Change	Mean change
	1	59	Cholangiocarcinoma	Right hepatic lobectomy	130	291	+124%	
Normal portal vein	2	53	Secondary – right lobe	Right hepatectomy	176	378	+115%	+118%
	3	42	Secondary – right lobe	Right hepatectomy	205	445	+117%	
	4	59	Hepatocellular carcinoma – right lobe	Right hepatectomy	176	237	+35%	
	5	16	Hepatocellular carcinoma – left lobe	Left hepatectomy	261	223	−15%	+10%
Obstructed portal vein	6	50	Cholangiocarcinoma	Right hepatic lobectomy	148	194	+31%	
	7	33	Cholangiocarcinoma	Right hepatic lobectomy	158	140	−11%	

Adapted from Mathie & Blumgart (1982)

resected lobes exhibited little change in tissue perfusion after resection (Table 7.2), indicating the presence of maximal perfusion in the non-resected lobes of these patients even before partial hepatectomy was carried out.

The significance of blood flow in relation to liver regeneration has frequently been debated during the 40 years since Mann (1944) suggested that regenerative hyperplasia of the liver after partial resection was a function of portal blood flow and that the process could be prevented by portal flow diversion. As discussed elsewhere (Ch. 5, 6), however, it is now believed that regenerative hyperplasia is not dependent on either the increase in tissue perfusion normally seen after partial hepatectomy, or, in contrast to the requirements for the prevention of liver atrophy, the direct supply of portal venous blood to the liver cells (Blumgart 1978). The most important evidence to uphold this hypothesis arises from studies of hepatic haemodynamics and metabolic activity in rats (Guest et al 1977, Ryan et al 1978): regenerative hyperplasia takes place normally following partial liver resection in portacavally transposed animals, despite the absence of a direct supply of portal blood or the usual post-hepatectomy rise in hepatic tissue perfusion (Fig. 7.3).

Some of these recent concepts have been confirmed in the clinical situation, where segmental portal obstruction leads to hypoperfusion and atrophy in the corresponding liver segment, accompanied by a regenerative hyperplastic response in the contralateral segment of liver tissue. In such patients there has been a long-standing stimulus to regenerative hyperplasia, probably in the absence of increased tissue perfusion (see Table 7.2). Personal clinical observations (e.g. the excellent postoperative response which occurred in Case 6, Table 7.2) also suggest that this long standing situation may be associated with a better liver reserve after resection, there being no lag period to accommodate the metabolic changes associated with regeneration (Vajrabukka et al 1975).

PORTAL HYPERTENSION

Portal hypertension is a state of sustained increase in the intraluminal pressure of the portal vein and its collaterals. Haemodynamic factors which influence portal hypertension are best understood by application of the pressure-flow-resistance relationship to the portal venous system. Portal pressure depends upon two basic components: portal blood flow, and hepatic portal vascular resistance. Thus, portal hypertension may result from a significant and sustained increase in either portal flow or hepatic vascular resistance, or both. Although simple in concept, multiple factors may influence both components of the system and thus the pathophysiology of portal hypertension (Blendis 1981). Discussion here will therefore be limited to the known general features of hepatic haemodynamics during elevated portal pressure caused by increased resistance to portal blood flow, without attempting to specify the particular form or site of the anatomical lesion.

Major disturbances of liver blood flow in patients with portal hypertension and cirrhosis have been postulated on the basis of increased portal pressure and resistance, anatomical and functional shunting, and hepatic artery flow compensation. Indeed, reduction of total liver blood flow, if the hepatic arterial compensation response is incomplete, would be anticipated following a decrease in portal flow. However, accurate clinical measurements of liver blood flow or its components are lacking in patients with portal hypertension of any aetiology.

Most preoperative studies on portal haemodynamics have been restricted to measurements of portal and hepatic vein pressures and angiographic estimates of portal blood flow. Alternatively, hepatic blood flow has been measured by clearance techniques based on the Fick principle. As discussed above, however, the accuracy of these methods is dependent upon complete extraction of the marker compound by the liver, which is generally affected by hepatic function. Reported decreases in liver blood flow utilizing these methods are therefore difficult to interpret in patients with portal hypertension and abnormal liver function.

Intraoperative measurements of hepatic artery and portal vein flow with electromagnetic flowmeters have also been employed. Such studies have shown that portal flow in cirrhosis is usually substantially reduced (often by more than 50%) and that the hepatic artery provides a greater relative contribution to the total blood flow supplying the liver (Moreno et al 1967). However a review of the data from 54 patients with portal hypertension reported in the literature illustrated that absolute hepatic arterial flow varied widely (91–1100 ml/min), and that the calculated mean flow (414 ml/min) was in fact similar to that in patients without liver disease (Reynolds 1982). Nevertheless, as discussed previously, there are limitations to the electromagnetic flowmeter technique, since blood flow is inclusive of intrahepatic shunted flow and therefore probably overestimates true blood flow to the hepatocyte in patients of this type.

Recent investigations have succeeded in quantifying the magnitude of intra- and extrahepatic shunt flow in small groups of patients with cirrhosis. Data from 15 patients revealed that nearly 80% of portal blood flow bypassed the sinusoidal bed within the liver, while evidence from eight patients indicated that up to 50% of the portal flow circulated through extrahepatic shunt pathways (Okuda et al 1977). Other workers have demonstrated that 10–30% of the hepatic arterial blood in five subjects flowed through intrahepatic shunt channels to the systemic venous circulation (Groszmann et al 1977).

Thus, few estimates of total liver blood flow obtained

in patients with portal hypertension and cirrhosis reflect actual hepatocyte or 'sinusoidal' flow. Only the inert gas clearance method, described earlier, has been used to measure true hepatic tissue perfusion in cirrhosis (Leiberman et al 1978c), but information is as yet limited to just a few patients. A relationship between hepatic dysfunction and decreased liver blood flow in portal hypertension therefore remains speculative.

The direction of portal blood flow has been postulated as both a consequence of and contributor to the pathophysiology of portal hypertension. Normally, portal blood flows towards the liver (prograde or hepatopetal flow). With progression of intrahepatic disease and increasing sinusoidal pressure, Warren & Muller (1959) postulated the potential for reverse portal blood flow (retrograde or hepatofugal portal flow). Thus, portal blood flow could be diverted away from the liver as a result of cirrhosis and could accelerate the disease by depriving the liver of nutrient flow. Although portal vein blood flow probably does decrease with progressive portal hypertension, measurements indicate that spontaneous reversal of portal vein flow does not in fact occur to any significant degree. Using a variety of non-quantitative radiographic techniques, hepatofugal flow has actually been demonstrated in only two cirrhotic patients, while measurement of portal flow magnitude and direction in 273 such patients collected in the literature revealed no case of spontaneous flow reversal (Moreno et al 1975).

Surgical relief of portal hypertension is achieved by carrying out of one of many portal-systemic shunt procedures (Ch. 108, 112, 113, 114). First performed experimentally by Eck in 1897 (Child 1953), the initial clinical application of the portacaval shunt was reported nearly 50 years later (Whipple 1945). The haemodynamic consequences of shunt surgery are complex, and depend on the particular shunt performed, the nature and severity of the disease, and the pre-existing haemodynamic conditions in the individual patient. In general, liver blood flow falls after portacaval shunt. End-to-side shunt diverts all portal blood flow away from the liver, while less severe procedures reduce portal blood flow in proportion to the degree to which the shunt reduces portal pressure (Reynolds 1982). The hepatic artery flow may increase by 20–105% (Reynolds 1982), but this can only partly compensate for loss of portal flow (Mathie & Blumgart 1983a); hepatic oxygen consumption tends to be maintained however (Redeker et al 1958), though at the expense of increased oxygen extraction from the available arterial supply.

Total portacaval shunt is clearly effective in reducing portal pressure, and indeed is the most effective treatment for the prevention of bleeding from oesophageal varices. However, as this form of shunt deprives the liver entirely of inflow from the portal venous system and allows splanchnic venous blood to reach the systemic circulation, liver failure and encephalopathy are common complications of the operation (Ch. 108). Such problems led to the search for alternative operations which would not compromise the liver in this manner.

Side-to-side shunt, mesocaval shunt, and proximal or distal splenorenal shunts have all enjoyed varying degrees of clinical popularity. The side-to-side shunt has frequently been associated with reversed portal flow (Moreno et al 1967, Reynolds 1970). Direction of portal vein flow has been used clinically as an indirect indicator of hepatic perfusion and has been related to liver dysfunction. Clinically, hepatic encephalopathy has most often been related to direction of hepatic flow. Both Moreno et al (1967) and Reynolds (1970) have shown that nearly two-thirds of patients with side-to-side portacaval shunts have hepatofugal flow and 30% of survivors develop severe encephalopathy. Chandler & Fechner (1983) recently described complete resolution of encephalopathy following restoration of hepatopetal flow after take-down of side-to-side portacaval shunt and construction of distal splenorenal shunts in two patients. Although the above findings suggest that the direction of portal blood flow, documented angiographically, corresponds roughly to volume of liver blood flow, and thus may be correlated with hepatic dysfunction, it is important to be aware that angiographic findings may be misleading (Fulenwider et al 1979, Koolpe et al 1981). Nevertheless, recent quantitative haemodynamic studies in dogs with side-to-side shunt demonstrate that portally drained blood following the operation traverses metabolically inefficient hepatic pathways, suggesting a long-term detrimental influence on liver function (Mathie & Blumgart 1986).

Distal splenorenal shunt (Ch. 113) selectively decompresses the oesophageal varices via the splenic circulation and allows venous blood from the intestine to continue to perfuse the liver (Warren et al 1967). The incidence of postoperative hepatic failure and encephalopathy has been reported to be lower than for the more complete portacaval shunt procedures (Galambos et al 1976). Maintenance of hepatic tissue perfusion immediately after the Warren shunt has been demonstrated quantitatively (Reichle & Owen 1979, Mathie et al 1980b, Rikkers et al 1981) (Table 7.3), though other studies have suggested that a gradual reduction of liver blood flow occurs over a period of several months following the operation (Maillard et al 1979).

Many authors have attempted to utilize preoperative or intraoperative haemodynamic parameters to predict morbidity and mortality in patients undergoing portal-systemic shunts for portal hypertension. In general, static portal pressures, corrected portal or hepatic vein wedge pressures (Reynolds 1970, Price et al 1967) and portal and hepatic arterial blood flows before shunting (Burchell et al 1974, Moreno et al 1967, Price et al 1967) have not been predictive of survival (Ch. 108). However, more recent blood flow studies suggest that certain haemodynamic data

Table 7.3 Hepatic tissue perfusion in six patients before and after distal splenorenal shunt (^{85}Kr clearance measurements)

Case	Age	Condition	Hepatic tissue perfusion (ml/min/100 g liver) Before	After	Change
1	55	Alcoholic cirrhosis	53	53	0
2	59	Chronic active hepatitis	135	93	−42
3	20	Wilson's disease	161	158	− 3
4	58	Primary biliary cirrhosis	115	130	+15
5	45	Cryptogenic cirrhosis	184	194	+10
6	32	Portal vein thrombosis	194	161	−33
Mean	45		140.3	131.5	−8.8

The data from patients 1–4 were previously reported by Mathie et al (1980b)

may in fact have prognostic value for survival and encephalopathy. Burchell et al (1976) retrospectively correlated immediate intraoperative changes in hepatic artery blood flow with early postoperative deaths and encephalopathy in patients with portacaval shunts. They found that over 90% of patients who had less than a 100 ml/min increase in hepatic arterial flow immediately after portacaval shunting subsequently died or developed encephalopathy.

Although Burchell's group showed that morbidity, mortality, and long-term survival were directly related to the magnitude of the post-shunt increment in hepatic artery flow, recognition of some form of predictive haemodynamic response preoperatively rather than intraoperatively after portacaval shunting would be of more clinical value. Zimmon & Kessler (1980) reported just such a predictive response by studying the effect on intrahepatic pressure of acute changes in portal venous blood flow achieved through a temporary extracorporeal umbilical vein to saphenous vein portal-systemic shunt. They divided patients into two groups based on their response to diversion of blood flow from the portal to systemic circulations. Compensating patients (type A) were able to maintain a relatively constant intrahepatic pressure with acute increase or decrease in portal vein flow. In contrast, noncompensating patients (type B) exhibited a sharp increase in intrahepatic pressure when portal flow was increased and a decrease in pressure when portal flow was decreased. In a subsequent review of 40 patients with portacaval shunts, they found longer survival and less encephalopathy in patients who had maintained a high intrahepatic pressure than in patients in whom intrahepatic pressure had decreased; moreover they considered that maintenance of intrahepatic pressure was achieved by means of a compensatory increase in hepatic arterial blood flow after loss of portal flow.

Intraoperative data have been utilized by other workers to predict hepatic haemodynamics after portacaval shunt, and have been shown to provide some practical benefit: Leiberman et al (1979c) and Mathie et al (1980b) have employed the inert gas clearance method and temporary portal vein occlusion before undertaking portal-systemic shunt to allow a prediction of the hepatic tissue perfusion (by the hepatic artery) immediately after a total portacaval shunt and to provide a rough estimate of the relative arterial and portal contributions to basal total hepatic blood flow. This information may be derived from a single isotope injection into the portal vein if the portal occlusion procedure is carried out during the course of the gas clearance recording (Fig. 7.4). In accordance with the principle of maintaining total liver blood flow, patients showing a substantial decrease in tissue perfusion did not receive a total portacaval shunt, but side-to-side or distal splenorenal shunt instead. No direct correlations with patient prognosis were carried out however.

BILE DUCT OBSTRUCTION

Bile duct obstruction can significantly affect hepatic haemodynamics. In general, liver blood flow is reduced in the presence of chronic biliary obstruction. Indeed, reduction of liver blood flow in this setting may contribute to hepatic dysfunction. Conversely, *acute* increases in bile duct pressure following obstruction result in a reactive increase in liver blood flow which may represent an attempt by the liver to maintain adequate function against an increase in the pressure gradient opposing secretion and excretion of bile. Most evidence suggests that the haemodynamic response of the liver to biliary obstruction is related, directly or indirectly, to changes in bile duct pressure.

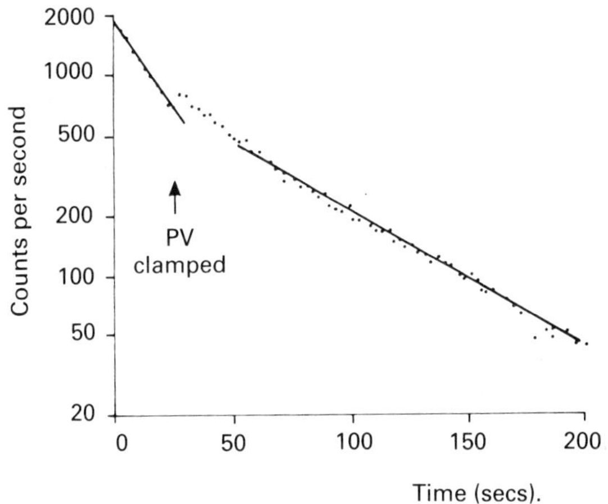

Fig. 7.4 ^{85}Kr clearance curve obtained in patient with cryptogenic cirrhosis after single portal vein (PV) injection of isotope, showing immediate effect of PV occlusion on the rate of gas clearance. The clearance half-time ($T\frac{1}{2}$) changed from 20.5 to 37.0 sec, implying a decrease in hepatic tissue perfusion from 184 to 102 ml/min per 100 g. Reproduced with permission from Castle House Publications (Mathie 1982)

Hepatic haemodynamics after complete bile duct obstruction are unaffected acutely (< four hours) unless bile duct pressure is increased abruptly. Nagorney et al (1982) showed that acute increases in bile duct pressure in dogs with complete bile duct obstruction could significantly increase hepatic arterial blood flow but did not affect portal venous blood flow. They found that a sigmoid relationship between hepatic arterial blood flow and bile duct pressure existed and that a 250% increase in hepatic artery blood flow was obtainable with serial increases in bile duct pressure.

Chronic bile duct obstruction is associated with a decrease in total liver blood flow. Aronsen et al (1969), using a ^{198}Au clearance technique, first showed a decrease in the total effective hepatic blood flow. In addition, Ohlsson et al (1970) demonstrated dilatation of the sinusoids and elevation of portal pressure in dogs after four weeks of complete bile duct obstruction. Relief of long-term obstruction is not associated with a return of normal haemodynamics, suggesting irreversible intrahepatic vascular damage (Aronsen et al 1969). Indeed, Aronsen (1968) further showed that a 23% reduction in effective liver blood flow persisted for one to five years after operative decompression in patients with choledocholithiasis and jaundice if cholestasis was evident more than two weeks preoperatively. Hunt (1979) serially measured liver blood flow daily for one week following bile duct ligation in rats, using the ^{133}Xe clearance technique to document the early haemodynamic response. Total liver blood flow decreased steadily after the first postoperative day to a plateau level of approximately 50% of the preoperative value five days after operation. Recently, Mathie et al (1986) confirmed the decrease in total liver blood flow following bile duct ligation and extended Hunt's findings by measuring the individual portal venous and hepatic arterial components of liver blood flow. Using electromagnetic flow meters in dogs with complete bile duct ligation, hepatic arterial and portal venous blood flow were observed to decrease by 36% and 44%, respectively. Moreover, they showed a 200% increase in intrahepatic portal vein resistance without similar increases in hepatic arterial resistance. Similarly, Bosch et al (1983) have also demonstrated that dogs with chronic bile duct ligation had decreased portal venous flow, and had developed sinusoidal portal hypertension and extensive portal-systemic shunting.

The mechanism for reduction in liver blood flow following chronic bile duct obstruction is unknown. Reuter & Chuang (1976) have shown a disproportionate increase in corrected portal vein pressure (CPVP) over corrected wedge hepatic vein pressure (CWHVP) (37% versus 117% increase, respectively) 28 days after biliary obstruction, suggesting that the primary site of resistance to the portal vein blood flow is pre-sinusoidal. Portal venograms, which revealed narrowing of the portal vein radicles and delayed emptying of portal vein contrast after obstruction, supported their hypothesis that compression of the terminal portal vein radicles by distended bile ducts is the pre-sinusoidal site of portal venous flow resistance.

In contrast, Tamakuma et al (1975) postulated that post-obstructive increases in bile duct pressure, leading to bile duct dilatation, affected the hepatic haemodynamics by a post-sinusoidal route. They showed that both CWHVP and CPVP were directly related to biliary pressure, implicating an interaction of biliary pressure and the intrahepatic vasculature. Similarly, Bosch et al (1983) showed comparable elevations in both CPVP and CWHVP after eight weeks of bile duct ligation in dogs, supporting a sinusoidal block. Their histological findings also supported a sinusoidal block. They found fibrosis in both the portal and central areas of the liver lobule, ranging from broadening of the portal zones to frank bridging fibrosis with nodular regeneration. Moderate congestion and dilatation of the sinusoids were also present. In addition, capillary proliferation of the sinusoids was also evident with marked peri-sinusoidal collagen deposition. Finally, Bosch et al (1983) also showed the development of significant portal-systemic shunting with an inverse correlation between shunting and portal venous blood flow, suggesting that the reduced portal flow was related to a large fraction of the portal inflow being diverted through portal-systemic collaterals. Both Bosch (1983) and Ohlsson (1972) have confirmed that the site of shunting is predominantly extrahepatic.

Clinically, haemodynamic abnormalities associated with chronic biliary obstruction are encountered in two situations: portal hypertension associated with secondary biliary fibrosis; and shock following biliary tract decompression. Approximately 20% of patients with prolonged biliary obstruction develop clinically significant portal hypertension (Sedgwick et al 1966, Adson & Wychulis 1968, Blumgart et al 1984). The operative risk of biliary decompression in these patients is significant (Ch. 58). Technical difficulties of stricture repair (dense fibrous adhesions, hilar ductal involvement, infection) are compounded with the risk of haemorrhage from sub-hepatic and periductal varices and the potential of post-operative liver failure. These complex problems warrant a careful and thorough preoperative evaluation. Decisions on surgical decompression of either the biliary or the portal system must be based on the exclusion of hepatic failure from other causes. Portal-systemic shunts are advocated prior to biliary decompression in patients with bleeding oesophageal varices or previous intraoperative haemorrhage which precluded successful stricture repair (Sedgwick et al 1966, Adson & Wychulis 1968). Generally, splenorenal shunts are preferred technically. Non-operative tubal decompression and dilatation of the obstructed biliary tract now allows another option. Operation can thus be carried out electively and after an initial improvement in general status has been allowed (Ch. 58).

In addition to the haemodynamic consequences of chronic bile duct obstruction, sudden decompression of the obstructed biliary tree may also have profound haemodynamic effects. Tamakuma et al (1975) have studied the significance of clinical shock following biliary decompression. They noted that hypotension and shock could develop in the immediate postoperative period following biliary decompression, even though no apparent cause of shock, such as haemorrhage, infection or cardiac failure, was evident. They hypothesized that factors associated with sudden release of biliary obstruction and establishment of biliary drainage might affect both hepatic and systemic haemodynamics. They showed that biliary decompression resulted in an abrupt decrease in wedged hepatic vein pressure, portal vein pressure, and arterial pressure within 30 minutes of decompression. Similarly, Steer et al (1968) reported that rapid needle decompression of an obstructed biliary tree in jaundiced dogs induced a decreased arterial pressure, central venous pressure, and portal venous pressure within one hour, and concluded that sudden decompression of chronic biliary obstruction permitted sequestration of fluid within the liver, leading to a decrease in the effective circulating plasma volume, resulting in hypotension. Clinically, the potential for haemodynamic changes and sequestration of large volumes of fluid into the perivascular spaces within the liver and the portal system following decompression of an obstructed bile duct should be anticipated and compensated perioperatively by adequate hydration.

REFERENCES

Adson M A, Wychulis A R 1968 Portal hypertension in secondary biliary cirrhosis. Archives of Surgery 96: 604–612

Anderson M F 1981 Pulsed Doppler ultrasonic flowmeter: Application to the study of hepatic blood flow. In: Granger D N, Bulkley G B (eds) Measurement of blood flow. Applications to the splanchnic circulation. Williams & Wilkins, Baltimore p 395–398

Andreen M, Irestedt L, Thulin L 1975 The effect of controlled halothane anaesthesia on splanchnic oxygen consumption in the dog. Acta Anaesthesiologica Scandinavica 19: 238–244

Aronsen K F 1968 Late effects of biliary stasis on the effective liver blood flow. Acta Chirurgica Scandinavica 134: 278–281

Aronsen K F, Ericsson B, Fajgelj A, Lindell S E 1966 The clearance of ^{133}Xenon from the liver after intraportal injection in man. Nuclear Medicine 5: 241–245

Aronsen K F, Ericsson B, Nosslin B, Nylander G, Phil B, Waldeskog B 1970 Evaluation of hepatic regeneration by scintillation scanning, cholangiography and angiography in man. Annals of Surgery 171: 567–574

Aronsen K F, Nylander G, Ohlsson E G 1969 Liver blood flow studies during and after various periods of total biliary obstruction in the dog. Acta Chirurgica Scandinavica 135: 55–59

Batchelder B M, Cooperman L H 1975 Effects of anesthetics on splanchnic circulation and metabolism. Surgical Clinics of North America 55: 787–794

Biber B, Holm C, Winsö O, Gustavsson B 1983 Portal blood flow in man during surgery, measured by a modification of the continuous thermodilution method. Scandinavian Journal of Gastroenterology 18: 233–239

Birgens H S, Henriksen J, Matzen P, Poulsen H 1978 The shock liver. Acta Medica Scandinavica 204: 417–421

Blendis L M 1981 Portal hypertension. In: Lautt W W (ed) Hepatic circulation in health and disease. Raven Press, New York, p 329–350

Blumgart L H 1978 Liver atrophy, hypertrophy and regenerative hyperplasia in the rat: the relevance of blood flow. In: Ciba Foundation Symposium 55 (new series): Hepatotrophic factors. Elsevier Excerpta Medica, North-Holland and Elsevier, North Holland, p 181–215

Blumgart L H, Leach K G, Karran S J 1971 Observations on liver regeneration after right hepatic lobectomy Gut 12: 922–928

Blumgart L H, Kelley C J, Benjamin I S 1984 Benign bile duct stricture following cholecystectomy: Critical factors in management. British Journal of Surgery 71: 836–843

Bollman J L 1961 The animal with an Eck fistula. Physiological Reviews 41: 607–621

Bosch J, Enriquez R, Groszmann R J, Storer E H 1983 Chronic bile duct ligation in the dog: Hemodynamic characterization of a portal hypertensive model. Hepatology 3: 1002–1007

Boyer T D, Triger D R, Horisawa M, Redeker A G, Reynolds T B 1977 Direct transhepatic measurement of portal vein pressure using a thin needle. Comparison with wedged hepatic vein pressure. Gastroenterology 72: 584–589

Bradley S E, Ingelfinger F J, Bradley G P, Curry J J 1945 The estimation of hepatic blood flow in man. Journal of Clinical Investigation 24: 890–897

Burchell A R, Moreno A H, Panke W F, Nealon T F 1974 Hemodynamic variables and prognosis following portacaval shunts. Surgery, Gynecology and Obstetrics 138: 359–369

Burchell A R, Moreno A H, Panke W F, Nealon T F 1976 Hepatic artery flow improvement after portacaval shunt: A single hemodynamic clinical correlate. Annals of Surgery 184: 289–302

Burton-Opitz R 1910 The vascularity of the liver. I. The flow of blood in the hepatic artery. Quarterly Journal of Experimental Physiology 3: 297–313

Burton-Opitz R 1911 The vascularity of the liver. IV. The magnitude of the portal inflow. Quarterly Journal of Experimental Physiology 4: 113–125

Bynum T E, Boitnott J K, Maddrey W C 1979 Ischaemic hepatitis. Digestive Diseases and Sciences 24: 129–135

Caesar J, Shaldon S, Chiandussi L, Guevara L, Sherlock S 1961 The use of indocyanine green in the measurement of hepatic blood flow and as a test of hepatic function. Clinical Science 21: 43–57

Chandler J G, Fechner R E 1983 Hepatopetal flow restoration in patients intolerant of total portal diversion. Annals of Surgery 197: 574–583

Chiandussi L, Greco F, Sardi G, Vaccarino A, Ferraris C M, Curti B 1968 Estimation of hepatic arterial and portal venous blood flow by direct catheterisation of the vena porta through the umbilical cord in man. Acta Hepatosplenologica 15: 166–171

Child C G 1953 Eck's fistula. Surgery, Gynecology and Obstetrics 96: 375–376

Combes B 1960 Estimation of hepatic blood flow in man and in dogs by I^{131}-labelled rose bengal. Journal of Laboratory and Clinical Medicine 56: 537–543

Conn H L Jr 1961 Equilibrium distribution of radioxenon in tissue: xenon-hemoglobin association curve. Journal of Applied Physiology 16: 1065–1070

Dobson E L, Jones H B 1952 The behaviour of intravenously injected particulate material. Its rate of disappearance from the blood stream as a measure of liver blood flow. Acta Medica Scandinavica (Supplementum) 273: 1–71

Fulenwider J T, Nordlinger B M, Millikan W J, Sones P J, Warren W D 1979 Portal pseudoperfusion. An angiographic illusion. Annals of Surgery 189: 257–268

Galambos J T, Warren W D, Rudman D, Smith R B, Salam A A 1976 Selective and total shunts in the treatment of bleeding varices. A randomized controlled trial. New England Journal of Medicine 295: 1089–1095

George C F 1979 Drug kinetics and hepatic blood flow. Clinical Pharmacokinetics 4: 433–448

Gottlieb M E, Sarfeh I J, Stratton H, Goldman M L, Newell J C, Shah D M 1983 Hepatic perfusion and splanchnic oxygen consumption on patients postinjury. The Journal of Trauma 23: 836–843

Greenway C V, Stark R D 1971 Hepatic vascular bed. Physiological Reviews 51: 23–65

Greenway C V, Oshiro G 1972 Intrahepatic distribution of portal and hepatic arterial blood flows in anaesthetized cats and dogs and the effects of portal occlusion, raised venous pressure and histamine. Journal of Physiology (London) 227: 473–485

Groszmann R J, Kotelanski B, Cohn J N 1971 Hepatic lobar distribution of splenic and mesenteric blood flow in man. Gastroenterology 60: 1047–1052

Groszmann R J, Kravetz D, Paryson O 1977 Intrahepatic arteriovenous shunting in cirrhosis of the liver. Gastroenterology 73: 201–204

Guest J, Ryan C J, Benjamin I S, Blumgart L H 1977 Portacaval transposition and subsequent partial hepatectomy in the rat: effects on liver atrophy, hypertrophy and regenerative hyperplasia. British Journal of Experimental Pathology 58: 140–146

Gurll N J, Reynolds D G, Coon D, Shirazi S S 1980 Acute and chronic splanchnic blood flow responses to portacaval shunt in the normal dog. Gastroenterology 78: 1432–1436

Hahn M, Massen O, Nencki M, Pawlow J 1893 Die Eck'sche Fistel zwischen der unteren Hohlvene und der Pfortader und ihre Folgen für den Organismus. Archiv für Experimentelle Pathologie und Pharmakologie 32: 161–210

Huet P M, Lavoie P, Viallet A 1973 Simultaneous estimation of hepatic and portal blood flows by an indicator dilution technique. Journal of Laboratory and Clinical Medicine 82: 836–846

Hughes R L, Mathie R T, Campbell D, Fitch W 1979a The effect of hypercarbia on hepatic blood flow and oxygen consumption in the greyhound. British Journal of Anaesthesia 51: 289–296

Hughes R L, Mathie R T, Fitch W, Campbell D 1979b Liver blood flow and oxygen consumption during hypocapnia and IPPV in the greyhound. Journal of Applied Physiology 47: 290–295

Hughes R L, Mathie R T, Campbell D, Fitch W 1979c Systemic hypoxia and hyperoxia, and liver blood flow and oxygen consumption in the greyhound. Pflügers Archiv. 381: 151–157

Hughes R L, Campbell D, Fitch W 1980a Effects of enflurane and halothane on liver blood flow and oxygen consumption in the greyhound. British Journal of Anaesthesia 52: 1079–1086

Hughes R L, Mathie R T, Fitch W, Campbell D 1980b Liver blood flow and oxygen consumption during metabolic acidosis and alkalosis in the greyhound. Clinical Science 60: 355–361

Hunt D R 1979 Changes in liver blood flow with development of biliary obstruction in the rat. Australian and New Zealand Journal of Surgery 49: 733–737

Jefferson N C, Hassan M I, Popper H L, Necheles H 1956 Formation of effective collateral circulation following excision of hepatic artery. American Journal of Physiology 184: 589–592

Karran S J, Fleming J S, Humphries N L M 1982 Non-invasive assessment of hepatic perfusion and of the relative arterial and portal components. In: Mathie R T (ed) Blood flow measurement in man. Castle House Publications, Tunbridge Wells, p 155–167

Kock N G, Hahnloser P, Roding B, Schenk W G Jr 1972 Interaction between portal venous and hepatic arterial blood flow: an experimental study in the dog. Surgery 72: 414–419

Koolpe H A, Embil W, Koolpe L, Russell E, Williams C O 1981 Hemodynamic guidelines for surgical therapy of portal hypertension. Annals of Surgery 194: 553–561

Lautt W W 1977 The hepatic artery: subservient to hepatic metabolism or guardian of normal hepatic clearance rates of humoral substances. General Pharmacology 8: 73–78

Lautt W W 1981 Role and control of the hepatic artery. In: Lautt W W (ed) Hepatic circulation in health and disease. Raven Press, New York, p 203–226

Lautt W W 1983 Relationship between hepatic blood flow and overall metabolism: the hepatic arterial buffer response. Federation Proceedings 42: 1662–1666

Lee S, Chandler J M, Broelsch C E, Flamant Y M, Orloff M J 1974 Portal-systemic anastomosis in the rat. Journal of Surgical Research 17: 53–73

Leiberman D P, Mathie R T, Harper A M, Blumgart L H 1978a Measurement of liver blood flow in the dog using krypton-85 clearance: A comparison with electromagnetic flowmeter measurements. Journal of Surgical Research 25: 147–153

Leiberman D P, Mathie R T, Harper A M, Blumgart L H 1978b The hepatic arterial and portal venous circulations of the liver studied with a krypton-85 clearance technique. Journal of Surgical Research 25: 154–162

Leiberman D P, Mathie R T, Harper A M, Blumgart L H 1978c An isotope clearance method for measurement of liver blood flow during portasystemic shunt in man. British Journal of Surgery 65: 578–580

Lin T-Y, Chen C-C 1965 Metabolic function and regeneration of cirrhotic and non-cirrhotic livers after hepatic lobectomy in man. Annals of Surgery 162: 959–972

Loisance D Y, Peronneau P A, Pellet M M, Lenriot J P 1973 Hepatic circulation after side-to-side portacaval shunt in dogs: Velocity pattern and flow rate changes studied by an ultrasonic velocimeter. Surgery 73: 43–52

MacLeod J J R, Pearce R G 1914 The outflow of blood from the liver as affected by variations in the condition of the portal vein and hepatic artery. American Journal of Physiology 35: 87–105

Maillard J N, Flamant Y M, Hay J M, Chandler J G 1979 Selectivity of the distal splenorenal shunt. Surgery 86: 663–671

Mallet-Guy Y, Paillot J M, Switalska C, Mallet-Guy P 1972 Note sur les lésions ultrastructurales immédiates du foie après clampage expérimentale de l'artère hépatique. Lyon Chirurgical 68: 170–175

Mann F C 1944 The William Henry Welch Lectures: II. Restoration and pathologic reactions of the liver. Journal of Mount Sinai Hospital 11: 65–74

Marchioro T L, Porter K A, Brown B I, Otte J-B, Starzl T E 1967 The effect of partial portacaval transposition on the canine liver. Surgery 61: 723–732

Mathie R T 1982 Measurement of liver blood flow in man. In: Mathie R T (ed) Blood flow measurement in man. Castle House Publications, Tunbridge Wells, p 139–149

Mathie R T, Blumgart L H 1982 Hepatic tissue perfusion studies during partial hepatectomy in man. Surgical Gastroenterology 1: 297–302

Mathie R T, Blumgart L H 1983a The hepatic haemodynamic response to acute portal venous blood flow reductions in the dog. Pflügers Archiv 399: 223–227

Mathie R T, Blumgart L H 1983b Effect of denervation on the hepatic haemodynamic response to hypercapnia and hypoxia in the dog. Pflügers Archiv 397: 152–157

Mathie R T, Blumgart L H 1986 Haemodynamic and metabolic consequences of reversed portal venous blood flow after side-to-side portacaval shunt in the dog: A comparison with end-to-side shunt. (in press)

Mathie R T, Leiberman D P, Harper A M, Blumgart L H 1977 The solubility of ^{85}Krypton in the regenerating liver of the rat. British Journal of Experimental Pathology 58: 231–235

Mathie R T, Leiberman D P, Harper A M, Blumgart L H 1979 The role of blood flow in the control of liver size. Journal of Surgical Research 27: 139–144

Mathie R T, Lam P H M, Harper A M, Blumgart L H 1980a The hepatic arterial blood flow response to portal vein occlusion in the dog: The effect of hepatic denervation. Pflügers Archiv 386: 77–83

Mathie R T, Toouli J, Smith A, Harper A M, Blumgart L H 1980b Hepatic tissue perfusion studies during distal splenorenal shunt. American Journal of Surgery 140: 384–386

Mathie R T, Nagorney D M, Lewis M H, Blumgart L H 1986 Hepatic haemodynamics after chronic biliary obstruction in the dog. (in press)

Mays E T 1974 The hepatic artery. Surgery, Gynecology and Obstetrics 139: 595–596

Mays E T, Wheeler C S 1974 Demonstration of collateral arterial flow after interruption of hepatic arteries in man. New England Journal of Medicine 290: 993–996

Michels N A 1955 Blood supply and anatomy of the upper abdominal organs: With a descriptive atlas. J B Lippincott Philadelphia

Moreno A H, Burchell A R, Rousselot L M, Panke W F, Slafsky S F, Burke J H 1967 Portal blood flow in cirrhosis of the liver. Journal of Clinical Investigation 46: 436–445

Moreno A H, Burchell A R, Reddy R V, Steen J A, Panke W F, Nealon T F Jr 1975 Spontaneous reversal of portal blood flow: The call for and against its occurrence in patients with cirrhosis of the liver. Annals of Surgery 181: 346–358

Nagorney D M, Mathie R T, Lygidakis N J, Blumgart L H 1982 Bile duct pressure as a modulator of liver blood flow after common bile duct obstruction. Surgical Forum 33: 206–208

Ohlsson E G 1972 The arterial circulation in the liver after total biliary obstruction in dogs. Acta Chirurgica Scandinavica 138: 51–58

Ohlsson E G, Rutherford R B, Boitnott J K, Haalebos M M P, Zuidema G D 1970 Changes in portal circulation after biliary obstruction in dogs. American Journal of Surgery 120: 16–22

Okuda K, Suzuki K, Musha H, Arimizu N 1977 Percutaneous transhepatic catheterization of the portal vein for the study of portal haemodynamics and shunts. A preliminary report. Gastroenterology 73: 279–284

Pachter H L, Drager S, Godfrey N, LeFleur R 1979 Traumatic injuries of the portal vein: The role of acute ligation. Annals of Surgery 189: 383–385

Price J B, Voorhees A B, Britton R C 1967 Operative hemodynamic studies in portal hypertension. Significance and limitations. Archives of Surgery 95: 843–852

Rappaport A M 1973 The microcirculatory hepatic unit. Microvascular Research 6: 212–228

Rappaport A M, Schneiderman J H 1976 The function of the hepatic artery. Reviews of Physiology, Biochemistry and Pharmacology 76: 129–175

Redeker A G, Geller H M, Reynolds T B 1958 Hepatic wedge pressure, blood flow, vascular resistance and oxygen consumption in cirrhosis before and after end-to-side portacaval shunt. Journal of Clinical Investigation 37: 606–618

Reichle F A, Owen O E 1979 Hemodynamic patterns in human hepatic cirrhosis. A prospective randomized study of the hemodynamic sequelae of distal splenorenal (Warren) and mesocaval shunts. Annals of Surgery 190: 523–534

Reichman S, Davis W D, Storaasli J P, Gorlin R 1958 Measurement of hepatic blood flow by indicator dilution techniques. Journal of Clinical Investigation 37: 1848–1856

Reuter S R, Chuang V P 1976 The location of increased resistance to portal blood flow in obstructive jaundice. Investigative Radiology 11: 54–59

Reynolds T B 1970 Hepatic circulatory changes after shunt surgery. Annals of the New York Academy of Sciences 170: 379–391

Reynolds T B 1982 Portal hypertension. In: Schiff L, Schiff E R (eds) Diseases of the liver, 5th edn. J B Lippincott, Philadelphia, p 393–431

Rice G C, Leiberman D P, Mathie R T, Ryan C J, Harper A M, Blumgart L H 1977 Liver tissue blood flow measured by ^{85}Kr clearance in the anaesthetized rat before and after partial hepatectomy. British Journal of Experimental Pathology 58: 243–250

Richardson P D I, Withrington P G 1981 Liver blood flow. II. Effects of drugs and hormones on liver blood flow. Gastroenterology 81: 356–375

Rikkers L F, Miller F J, Christian P 1981 Effect of portasystemic shunt operations on hepatic portal perfusion. American Journal of Surgery 141: 169–174

Ryan C J, Guest J, Harper A M, Blumgart L H 1978 Liver blood flow measurement in the portacavally transposed rat before and after partial hepatectomy. British Journal of Experimental Pathology 59: 111–115

Sapirstein L A 1956 Fractionation of the cardiac output of rats with isotopic potassium. Circulation Research 4: 689–692

Schenk W G Jr, McDonald J C, McDonald K, Drapanas T 1962 Direct measurement of hepatic blood flow in surgical patients: with related observations on hepatic flow dynamics in experimental animals. Annals of Surgery 156: 463–469

Sedgwick C E, Poulantzas J K, Kune G A 1966 Management of portal hypertension secondary to bile duct strictures: Review of 18 cases with splenorenal shunt. Annals of Surgery 163: 949–953

Smith A, Mathie R T, Hughes R L, Harper A M, Blumgart L H 1979 Effect of haemorrhagic hypotension on liver blood flow and oxygen consumption in the dog. Gut 20: A454

Starzl T E, Francavilla A, Halgrimson C G, Francavilla F R, Porter K A, Brown T H et al 1973 The origin, hormonal nature and action of hepatotrophic substances in portal venous blood. Surgery, Gynecology and Obstetrics 137: 179–199

Starzl T E, Porter K A, Kashiwagi N, Lee I Y, Russell W J I, Putnam C W 1975 The effect of diabetes mellitus on portal blood hepatotrophic factors in dogs. Surgery, Gynecology and Obstetrics 140: 549–562

Starzl T E, Porter K A, Francavilla A 1983 The Eck fistula in animals and humans. Current Problems in Surgery 20: 687–752

Steer M L, Thomas A N, Rosson C T, Ketchum S A, Hall A D 1968 Chronic biliary obstruction: Hemodynamic effects of decompression. Surgical Forum 19: 342–344

Tamakuma S, Wada N, Ishiyama M, Suzuki H, Kanayama T, Okinaga K et al 1975 Relationship between hepatic hemodynamics and biliary pressure in dogs: Its significance in clinical shock following biliary decompression. Japanese Journal of Surgery 5: 255–268

Thomson I A, Hughes R L, Fitch W, Campbell D 1982 Effects of nitrous oxide on liver haemodynamics and oxygen consumption in the greyhound. Anaesthesia 37: 548–553

Thulin L, Andreen M, Irestedt L 1975 Effect of controlled halothane anaesthesia on splanchnic blood flow and cardiac output in the dog. Acta Anaesthesiologica Scandinavica 19: 146–153

Vajrabukka T, Bloom A L, Sussman M, Wood C B, Blumgart L H 1975 Postoperative problems and management after hepatic resection for blunt injury to the liver. British Journal of Surgery 62: 189–200

Wakim K G, Mann F C 1942 The intrahepatic circulation of blood. Anatomical Record 82: 233–253

Warren W D, Muller W H 1959 A classification of some hemodynamic changes in cirrhosis and their surgical significance. Annals of Surgery 150: 413–427

Warren W D, Zeppa R, Fomon J J 1967 Selective trans-splenic decompression of gastroesophageal varices by distal splenorenal shunt. Annals of Surgery 166: 437–455

Weinbren K, Washington S L A 1976 Hyperplastic nodules after portacaval anastomosis in rats. Nature 264: 440–442

Whipple A O 1945 The problem of portal hypertension in relation to the hepatosplenopathies. Annals of Surgery 122: 449–475

Zimmon D S, Kessler R E 1980 Effect of portal venous blood flow diversion on portal pressure. Journal of Clinical Investigation 65: 1388–1397

Bile secretion

INTRODUCTION

Bile secretion is one of the major functions of the liver. Bile is an aqueous solution of organic and inorganic compounds. Bile acids, bile pigments, cholesterol and phospholipids are the chief organic compounds. Bile also contains small amounts of protein. Because of the peculiar aggregation properties of the bile acids, which readily form micelles at physiological concentrations, bile is more complex than most other secretions, especially with regard to the osmotic properties of its constituents. Bile formed by the hepatocytes is secreted into the bile canaliculi. It is then modified during its passage in the bile ductules and ducts, and in the gallbladder, where water and inorganic electrolytes are reabsorbed, with, as a result, concentration of the organic constituents. Most conclusions regarding canalicular bile formation are derived from indirect evidence and are hypothetical. In this chapter, the available experimental data are summarized and the current theories of hepatic bile formation discussed. More detailed references may be found in several recent reviews (Blitzer & Boyer 1982, Erlinger 1982a, 1982b, Scharschmidt & Van Dyke 1983).

BILE COMPOSITION

In general, inorganic electrolytes are present in common duct bile at concentrations closely reflecting those in plasma (Table 8.1). Bile concentrations of sodium, potassium, calcium, and bicarbonate may, however, be appreciably higher than in plasma, while the chloride level may be lower.

In spite of these variations, bile osmolality, as measured by freezing point depression, is usually approximately 300 mosmol/kg and it varies in parallel with plasma osmolality. The total osmotic activity is accounted for only by the inorganic electrolytes because it is generally assumed that bile acids, which are in micellar form, have little or no osmotic activity.

The concentration of bicarbonate in bile is often higher than that in plasma. This may be due to bicarbonate transport mechanisms, which have been postulated in the hepatocytes and in the bile ductules and ducts, in response to secretin (see below).

The major organic constituents of bile are the conjugated bile acids, the bile pigments, cholesterol and phospholipids. The concentration and physicochemical properties of these compounds, which are important for the understanding of cholesterol and pigment gallstone formation, will be discussed in Chapter 38.

STRUCTURE–FUNCTION RELATIONSHIPS IN THE BILIARY SYSTEM

Bile is secreted primarily by the hepatocytes into bile canaliculi which are formed by a groove of the lateral

Table 8.1 Flow and electrolyte concentrations of hepatic bile

Species	Flow (μl.min^{-1} kg^{-1})	Concentrations (mmol/l)						
		Na^+	K^+	Ca^{2+}	Mg^{2+}	Cl^-	HCO^-_3	Bile acids
Man	1.5–15.4	132–165	4.2–5.6	0.6–2.4	0.7–1.5	96–126	17–55	3–45
Dog	10	141–230	4.5–11.9	1.5–6.9	1.1–2.7	31–107	14–61	16–187
Sheep	9.4	159.6	5.3	—	—	95	21.2	42.5
Rabbit	90	148–156	3.6–6.7	1.3–3.3	0.15–0.35	77–99	40–63	6–24
Rat	30–150	157–166	5.8–6.4	—	—	94–98	22–26	8–25
Guinea pig	115.9	175	6.3	—	—	69	49–65	—

Numbers indicate range or means of published values.

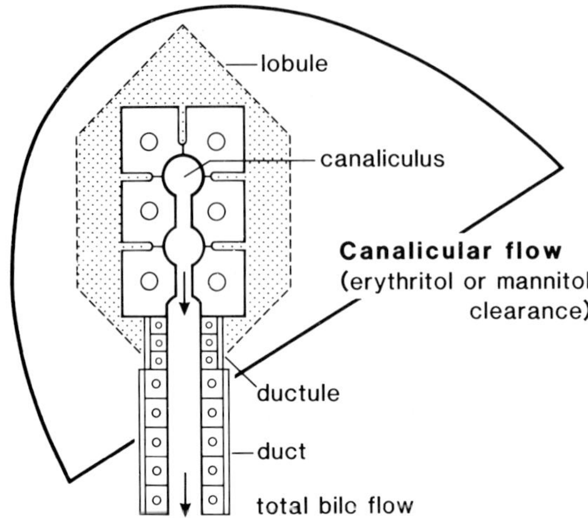

Fig. 8.1 Schematic diagram of the biliary system

plasma membrane between two hepatocytes and are about 1 μm in diameter. The membrane forms numerous microvilli which increase the surface area. The bile canalicular membrane represents about 13% of the hepatocyte plasma membrane. The bile canaliculi connect to bile ducts, lined by biliary epithelial cells. The smallest bile duct, the ductule, connects the canaliculus with the portal (interlobular) bile ducts. The interlobular bile ducts drain into larger bile ducts which form the intra- and extrahepatic biliary tree (Fig. 8.1). With respect to bile secretion, the liver may be regarded as an epithelium transporting a variety of substrates from blood to bile. This vectorial transport is made possible by the high degree of polarization of the hepatocyte plasma membrane. As in other transporting epithelia, the canalicular lumen is sealed by intercellular junctions.

The polarization of the hepatocyte plasma membrane

Three domains of the hepatocyte plasma membrane may be recognized: sinusoidal (facing the blood sinusoids), lateral (or intercellular) and canalicular. They demonstrate important morphological, biochemical and enzymatic differences. Especially important for transepithelial transport is the localization of the Na^+,K^+-activated adenosine triphosphatase (Na^+,K^+-ATPase) which is mainly in the sinusoidal and intercellular membrane, with little or no activity in the canalicular membrane (Blitzer & Boyer 1978, Latham & Kashgarian 1979, Meier et al 1984). A wide range of epithelia, including iso-osmotic and hyperosmotic absorbers and secretors, have (with the exception of the choroid plexus) the Na^+ pump (the Na^+,K^+-ATPase) preferentially on the basolateral surface of the epithelial cells. In the hepatocyte, the sinusoidal and intercellular membrane is the equivalent of the basolateral membrane of other epithelial cells: the liver is therefore no exception among transporting epithelia regarding the localization of the enzyme. Alkaline phosphatase, whose role in transport and in bile secretion is unknown, is, in contrast, preferentially located on the canalicular membrane (Blitzer & Boyer 1978).

The tight junction and the paracellular pathway

A substrate in plasma can enter canalicular bile in one of two ways: by the transcellular pathway (entering the hepatocyte through the sinusoidal membrane, crossing the hepatocyte and entering the canaliculus through the canalicular membrane) or by the paracellular pathway. In the latter case, the solute crosses the intercellular junction. The junction includes the tight junction, which is a sealing structure between the lumen of the bile canaliculus and the intercellular space and, hence, the sinusoidal blood. Tight junctions differ among epithelia. In impermeable epithelia (such as the toad bladder), the tight junction provides a high transepithelial resistance to the movement of water and ions (and, hence, to electrical current) whereas in relatively permeable epithelia (such as the gallbladder, intestine or proximal kidney tubule), the tight junction is 'leaky' permitting some passage of water and ions with, as a result, a low electrical resistance. The liver is of an intermediate type and there is evidence for a paracellular ion and fluid flux into bile which could play an important role in choleresis and possibly cholestasis.

The hepatocyte cytoskeleton

The canaliculus is surrounded by a narrow zone of organelle-poor cytoplasm, known as a pericanalicular ectoplasm, where actin microfilaments, 7 nm in diameter, are particularly present. They form a pericanalicular network, insert in the intercellular junction and extend into the microvilli where they appear to insert on the inner part of the membrane. They may have a key role in maintaining the shape of the cell, particularly its microvilli. Agents that interfere with the structure and function of microfilaments affect bile flow, which suggests a role for these organelles in secretion.

Microtubules, which are 24 nm in diameter, are more randomly distributed within the liver cell cytoplasm than are microfilaments. They play a role in the intracellular transport and secretion by the liver cell of proteins and lipoproteins. Antimicrotubular agents may also affect bile formation (see below).

CANALICULAR BILE FLOW

The maximal bile secretory pressure (about 25–30 cm H_2O) exceeds the sinusoidal perfusion pressure (about 5–10 cm H_2O), which excludes hydrostatic filtration as an important mechanism of canalicular bile secretion. Canalicular bile flow is regarded mainly as an osmotic water flow in response to active solute transport. Bile acids, which are potent choleretics, are most probably one of these solutes but the active transport of inorganic ions also plays a role.

Estimation of canalicular bile flow

Canalicular bile flow may be estimated by measuring the biliary clearance of non-metabolized solutes that enter canalicular bile by passive processes and are neither secreted nor reabsorbed by the biliary epithelium (Forker 1967, Wheeler et al 1968). The most widely used of such solutes are erythritol and mannitol (labelled with ^{14}C). In brief, when injected into the systemic circulation, the biliary secretion rate of such a solute during a steady state should depend on the permeability of the canaliculus and on canalicular bile flow. The biliary clearance (C) is calculated as $C = F \times (B)/(P)$ where F is bile flow, (B) and (P) the biliary and plasma concentrations respectively. The technique implies that the selected solute: (1.) is unable to cross the biliary epithelium; (2.) has a permeability in the canaliculi high enough to achieve diffusion equilibrium at the highest rates of canalicular flow. Neither of these assumptions is presently accessible to direct experimental testing. However, an operational test of adequate canalicular permeability is the finding that increments in bile flow induced by bile acids are accompanied by parallel increases in solute clearance. Depending on the species, erythritol (MW 122) and mannitol (MW 182) meet these requirements.

The original assumption that erythritol and mannitol do not cross the biliary epithelium was based on the observation that their clearance was not modified by secretin (Forker 1967, Wheeler et al 1968) which acts presumably on the ductules or ducts. However, small increases in erythritol and mannitol biliary clearance in response to secretin have been observed in dogs because either canalicular bile flow is stimulated by this hormone, or there is some permeability of the bile ductules or ducts to erythritol and mannitol.

The observation that the biliary clearance of polyethylene glycol 900 (a solute much larger than erythritol and mannitol) is greater than that of erythritol and mannitol suggests that reabsorption of water may occur either in the canaliculus itself or distally (Javitt & Wachtel 1981).

Bile acids and bile flow

Bile acid transport by the liver

The liver has an extraction efficiency for bile acids of approximately 90%. The uptake of bile acids by the hepatocyte is a saturable, carrier-mediated process (Glasinovic et al 1975, Reichen & Paumgartner 1975) exhibiting (especially for conjugated bile acids) a strong sodium dependence (Ruifrok & Meijer 1982). Such Na^+ dependence is highly suggestive of a sodium-coupled transport (or symport) process which is energized by the Na^+ gradient maintained by the Na^+ pump (or Na^+,K^+-ATPase). It allows accumulation of bile acids within the hepatocyte against their electrochemical gradient: it is therefore referred to as *active*. (Because it is not directly linked to the energy source — ATP — but rather to an ion gradient, it is called *secondary* active).

Once concentrated into the cell, the bile acid anion will tend to move out of the cell into the canalicular lumen along its electrochemical gradient, a movement favoured by the negative membrane potential which will drive anions out of the cell. Because canalicular secretion is limited by a maximal secretory capacity it is assumed that the process is carrier-mediated. It is not known whether the putative carrier, possibly the bile acid binding protein identified by Accatino & Simon (1976), uses an additional source of energy or is a passive carrier-mediated transport, for example facilitated diffusion. The very high biliary bile acid concentration (up to the 100 mmol/l range) is probably related to the formation of micelles.

Effect of bile acid secretion on canalicular flow

An apparently linear relationship between bile acid secretion rate and bile flow has been demonstrated in many animal species, including the dog (Preisig et al 1962) and man (Prandi et al 1975) (Fig. 8.2). Bile acid-induced choleresis is presumably of canalicular origin; it is accompanied by a parallel increase in erythritol clearance and a linear relationship is also found between erythritol clearance and bile acid secretion.

The hypothesis that bile acids increase bile flow by providing an osmotic driving force for water and electrolytes was proposed by Sperber (1959), but because bile acids are in the micellar form most of the osmotic activity

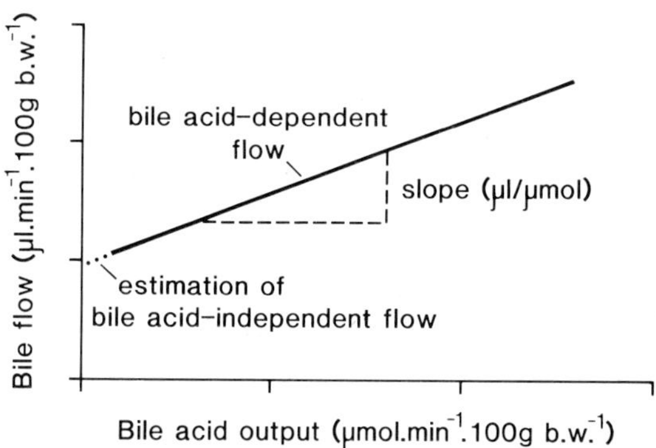

Fig. 8.2 Relationship between bile flow and bile acid output in bile. Note the linear relationship between bile flow and bile acid output (bile acid-dependent flow) and the positive intercept, which is a rough estimation of the bile acid-independent bile flow

must be accounted for by their counter-ions (cations accompanying the bile acid anions to maintain electroneutrality). Alternatively their choleretic effect could be due, at least in part, to their regulating the activity of other solute pumps. Experimental studies of selective biliary obstruction demonstrated an increased bile acid flux through the non-obstructed liver and a disproportionate increase in bile flow, together with an increase in Na^+,K^+-ATPase activity of liver cell plasma membranes. In other experiments ursodeoxycholic acid (and 7-ketolithocholic acid) was hyper-choleretic (more choleretic than physiological bile acids) and, simultaneously, stimulated biliary bicarbonate secretion (Dumont et al 1981), an apparently important flow-generating system (see below).

Pathway of fluid movement

Because bile acids are transported through the canalicular membrane of the hepatocyte, it is often thought that the associated osmotic water flow also occurs through the canalicular membrane. However, the ionic composition of bile closely resembles that of the extracellular fluid; so it is necessary to postulate either an equilibration downstream along the biliary channels, or a paracellular water and ionic pathway from the intercellular space into the bile canaliculi. The first possibility seems unlikely but as discussed earlier, the tight junction between liver cells is probably relatively 'leaky'. The bile-to-plasma concentration ratio of large solutes stabilized well before the liver-to-plasma ratio (Forker 1970), suggesting either a restricted (e.g., vesicular) pathway within the hepatocytes, or, alternatively, a direct passage through the paracellular pathway. Polyethylene glycol 4000 appears very rapidly in bile even though its size precludes a rapid entry into the hepatocytes. Experiments with the potent choleretics, dehydrocholate and taurodehydrocholate, have demonstrated a progressive increase in the bile-to-plasma concentration ratio of sucrose, penetration of ionic lanthanum from plasma into the tight junctions and increase in the number of intercellular 'blisters'. These observations suggest that the paracellular pathway may be an important site for bile acid-induced water and ion movement into bile (Layden et al 1978).

Other mechanisms in canalicular bile flow (canalicular bile acid–independent flow)

Although there is a good correlation between bile flow and bile acid secretion under physiological circumstances, studies at low bile acid secretion rates have shown an increase in slope of the bile flow–bile acid secretion relationship, possibly due to a fall in the concentration of bile acids below the critical micellar concentration and, hence, an increase in their osmotic activity. Because of endogenous bile acid synthesis, it is practically impossible to obtain bile without bile acids. Therefore, one can postulate either a fall of bile flow to zero, or a positive extrapolation of the bile flow–bile acid secretion relationship for a zero bile acid secretion (Fig. 8.2).

In the former case, bile acids would be the only active flow-generating solute ('one component theory'). In the latter case, flow could be generated without bile acids by one (or even several) other mechanisms ('two component theory'). The best piece of evidence in favour of the second view is the possibility of an increase in canalicular bile flow without any increase in bile acid secretion, e.g. with phenobarbital (Berthelot et al 1970) and a variety of other agents. The term canalicular bile acid–independent flow is generally used to describe this fraction of bile flow but this may not be adequate because interrelationships between the two fractions have been observed. Better terms must await the identification of the cellular mechanisms involved.

Role of Na^+,K^+-ATPase

The question of the role of Na^+,K^+-ATPase in canalicular transport processes other than bile acid transport remains controversial. Evidence for a role for this enzyme was originally derived from studies of the effect of inhibitors of Na^+ transport on bile flow. However, interpretation of the effect of drugs such as ouabain, ethacrynic acid or amiloride in vivo is complex, the overall effect being the result of both a choleretic and an inhibitory effect.

More direct evidence for a role of Na^+,K^+-ATPase has been sought by studying the relationship between bile flow and Na^+,K^+-ATPase in liver cell plasma membranes and a good correlation has been found between bile flow and Na^+,K^+-ATPase activity (Layden & Boyer 1976, Reichen & Paumgartner 1977, Simon et al 1977). It is difficult to understand the mode of coupling between enzyme activity and secretion because the bulk of Na^+,K^+-ATPase activity is located not on the canalicular membrane, but on the sinusoidal and intercellular membrane opposite to the net direction of Na^+ transport. Two ways of coupling between enzyme activity and transport are proposed (Erlinger 1981): firstly active transport of Na^+ into the intercellular space followed by passive movement into the canalicular lumen; secondly the transport of an anion, such as Cl^- or $HCO^-{}_3$ (or some other), using the Na^+ gradient. Sodium-driven Cl^- transport is widespread among epithelia. However, studies on cultured hepatocytes do not support the latter mechanism. Bicarbonate transport is also conceivable.

Role of bicarbonate transport

A bicarbonate transport mechanism may have a role in the elaboration of canalicular bile (Dumont et al 1981, Scharschmidt & Van Dyke 1983). The cellular mechanism is not known. Attempts to demonstrate a bicarbonate-sensitive ATPase in liver cell plasma membranes have failed but other mechanisms (such as the Na^+/H^+ antiport of the kidney tubule) are possible.

ROLE OF DUCTULES AND DUCTS

Secretion (ductular/ductal bile acid-independent flow)

Secretion occurs in the ductules and ducts in many species including man, mostly in response to secretin administration (Preisig et al 1962). Secretin choleresis is generally accompanied by changes in bile composition, chiefly a rise in bicarbonate and pH, and a fall in bile acids (Hardison & Norman 1968). The intraduodenal infusion of HCl in dogs induces the same response as endogenous secretin. The evidence for a ductular/ductal site of action of secretin is:

1. secretin choleresis does not enhance the maximal biliary secretory capacity of BSP whereas bile acids, which act on the bile canaliculi, do;
2. the biliary 'wash-out' volume during constant rate BSP infusions is less with secretin choleresis than bile acid choleresis suggesting that secretin acts distal to the canaliculi;
3. biliary clearances of erythritol and mannitol are increased during bile acid choleresis and not during secretin choleresis.

The secretory activity of the bile ductules and ducts explains the choleresis that occurs in certain diseases. Elevated bile flows have been recorded in patients with cirrhosis, other chronic liver diseases associated with ductular proliferation, and in congenital dilatation of the intrahepatic biliary tree. An augmented surface of the biliary epithelium is common to these conditions.

Reabsorption

The bile ductules or ducts may also have a reabsorptive function. Thus in cholecystectomized dogs, the composition of bile stored in the common bile duct was similar to typical gallbladder bile. Bile-to-plasma concentration ratios above unity in the steady state have been found for mannitol and erythritol in various species which suggest there is water reabsorption distal to the canaliculi because neither solute is thought to be transported by concentrative processes. This could be important in man after cholecystectomy.

MECHANISMS OF CHOLESTASIS

Cholestasis is defined as a diminution (or cessation) of bile flow and is subdivided as extrahepatic and intrahepatic. *Extrahepatic cholestasis* is the result of mechanical obstruction of the extrahepatic bile ducts usually by a gallstone or a tumour. *Intrahepatic cholestasis* may be the result of two different mechanisms: 1. mechanical obstruction of intrahepatic bile ducts, e.g. by a primary or secondary liver tumour, granulomas, infiltration by lymphoma or any other space-occupying lesion; 2. disturbance of canalicular bile flow, e.g. during viral or drug-induced hepatitis, or drug-induced cholestasis. Cholestasis must be distinguished from necrosis during liver parenchymal disease: both can occur separately or together. For instance, during viral hepatitis, necrosis can occur alone (anicteric hepatitis), or in association with cholestasis (common acute hepatitis with jaundice), while cholestasis can occur alone or predominantly (cholestatic hepatitis).

The cellular mechanisms of intrahepatic cholestasis due to disturbance of canalicular bile flow are not well understood (Erlinger 1985) and it is possible that there are several. Experimentally, three main mechanisms have been implicated.

1. A decrease in Na^+,K^+-ATPase

In this case, cholestasis could result from decreased bile acid secretion due to a decreased Na^+ gradient, or from decreased Na^+,K^+-ATPase mediated transport. Drugs which affect the Na^+,K^+-ATPase activity to produce cholestasis include oestrogens, chlorpromazine, and 17α-alkylated steroids. Interference with hepatocyte membrane transport processes is a common mechanism of cholestasis.

2. An alteration of the cytoskeleton

Interference with microfilament structure and function by cytochalasin B or phalloidin (Dubin et al 1978) causes a decrease or even a complete cessation of bile flow, and provides circumstantial evidence that microfilament dysfunction leads to cholestasis and that microfilaments may have a role in secretion. This could be by a. altering the structural organization necessary for normal secretion, particularly microvilli; b. interfering with a contractile function; c. modifying the permeability of the paracellular pathway that may be regulated by microfilaments.

The role of microtubules has been studied with colchicine and vinblastine. No effect on basal (spontaneous) bile flow was observed but colchicine markedly decreased bile flow and bile acid secretion induced by a bile acid load.

3. An increase in the permeability of the paracellular pathway

This was first postulated to explain oestrogen-induced cholestasis (Forker 1969). Any increased permeability may allow regurgitation of bile constituents (such as bile acids or bilirubin, and water) from the canalicular lumen into the circulation. Structural evidence that absorption (regurgitation) can also take place in human bile ductules has been obtained in cholestasis from various causes.

CHOLERETICS: MECHANISMS OF ACTION

A choleretic drug might act by one of several possible mechanisms:
1. concentrative (usually active) secretion into bile canaliculi followed by osmotic filtration of water and electrolytes. This process may be conveniently called 'bile acid-like choleresis' and operates for most commercial choleretics. However, this type of choleresis is not accompanied by an increase in biliary lipid secretion, in contrast to the choleresis induced by physiological bile acids.
2. Stimulation of 'bile acid-independent mechanisms' as with phenobarbital and other drugs (spironolactone or clofibrate in the rat) that are microsomal enzyme inducers.
3. Stimulation of secretion by the ductules or ducts, e.g. with secretin.

There is no evidence that any of these choleretics are of therapeutic value in patients with cholestasis, with the possible exception of phenobarbitone (phenobarbital) in children with intrahepatic cholestasis.

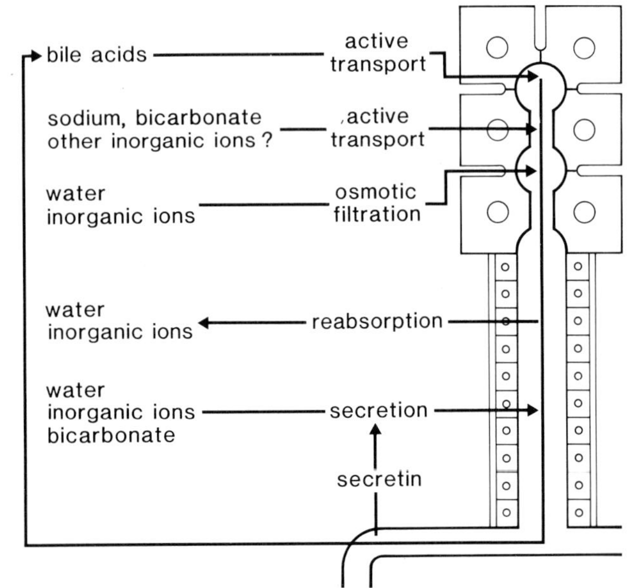

Fig. 8.4 Schematic representation of the main processes responsible for bile flow

BILIARY SECRETION IN MAN

Although the existence of most of the processes described previously has been inferred from animal studies, similar processes may well operate in man (Fig. 8.3). Patients with T-tubes in the common bile duct show a linear relationship between bile flow (and erythritol or mannitol clearance) and bile acid secretion rate, with a mean of 11 μl of canalicular bile secreted per μmol of bile acids. When the enterohepatic circulation is intact, a mean of approximately 15 μmol of bile acids is secreted per min, which gives a mean flow associated with bile acids of 0.15–0.16 ml/min. The estimated canalicular bile acid-independent flow is 0.16–0.17 ml/min, and the estimated ductular/ductal secretion is about 0.11 ml/min. The daily hepatic bile production under these circumstances (i.e. after cholecystectomy) is therefore approximately 600 ml.

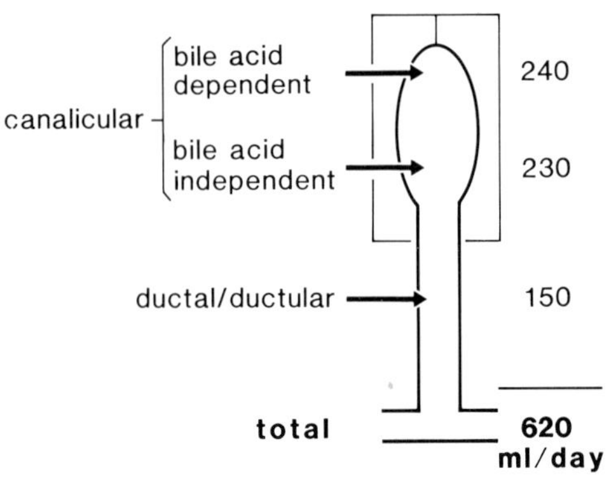

Fig. 8.3 The three major components of hepatic bile flow in man

SUMMARY

Bile is an isotonic aqueous solution of bile acids, cholesterol, phospholipids, bile pigments and inorganic electrolytes. It is secreted by the hepatocytes into the bile canaliculi and modified in the bile ductules or ducts. The three main processes identified in the generation of bile flow are schematized in Fig. 8.4. They are defined as follows:
1. Active transport (concentrative) of bile acids from blood into bile canaliculi. This is responsible for the bile acid-dependent canalicular bile flow. Coupling between water flow and bile acid secretion is probably effected mainly through an osmotic mechanism. There is evidence that water flows (at least in part) through the interhepatocytic junctions. The bile acid-dependent flow accounts for 30 to 60% of spontaneous basal bile flow.
2. A canalicular, bile acid-independent secretion, probably due to active electrolyte transport. The ions responsible (possibly bicarbonate and sodium) are not fully identified. This fraction of bile flow is stimulated by phenobarbital. It represents 30 to 60% of basal bile flow. Normal canalicular bile flow also depends on the integrity of intracellular cytoskeletal organelles, mostly microfilaments.
3. Reabsorption and secretion of fluid and inorganic electrolytes by the ductules and ducts. Secretion chiefly occurs in response to secretin and represents 30% of basal bile flow.

Cholestasis may be extrahepatic or intrahepatic. Extrahepatic cholestasis results from mechanical obstruction of extrahepatic bile ducts, usually by a stone or a tumour.

Intrahepatic cholestasis may be the result of:
1. mechanical obstruction of intrahepatic bile ducts;
2. alteration of the flow-generating systems by the hepatocytes (due, for instance, to a virus or a drug). The basis of this alteration is not well understood and might be an interference with the sodium pump (Na^+,K^+-ATPase) in hepatocytes, an alteration of the permeability of the biliary system (possibly of the paracellular pathway) or a lesion of the cytoskeleton.

REFERENCES

Accatino L, Simon F R 1976 Identification and characterization of a bile acid receptor in isolated liver surface membranes. Journal of Clinical Investigation 56: 496–508

Berthelot P, Erlinger S, Dhumeaux D, Préaux A M 1970 Mechanism of phenobarbital-induced hypercholeresis in the rat. American Journal of Physiology 219: 809–813

Blitzer B L, Boyer J L 1978 Cytochemical localization of Na^+,K^+-ATPase in the rat hepatocyte. Journal of Clinical Investigation 62: 1104–1108

Blitzer B L, Boyer J L 1982 Cellular mechanisms of bile formation. Gastroenterology 82: 346–357

Dubin M, Maurice M, Feldmann G, Erlinger S 1978 Phalloidin-induced cholestasis in the rat: relation to changes of microfilaments. Gastroenterology 75: 450–455

Dumont M, Uchman S, Erlinger S 1981 Hypercholeresis induced by ursodeoxycholic acid and 7-ketolithocholic acid in the rat. Possible role of bicarbonate transport. Gastroenterology 79: 82–89

Erlinger S 1981 Hepatocyte bile secretion: current views and controversies. Hepatology 1: 352–359

Erlinger S 1982a Bile flow. In: Arias I, Popper H, Schachter D, Shafritz D A (eds) The Liver: biology and pathobiology. Raven Press, New York, p 407–427

Erlinger S 1982b Secretion of bile. In: Schiff L, Schiff E (eds) Diseases of the liver, 5th edn. Lippincott, Philadelphia, p 93–119

Erlinger S 1985 What is cholestasis in 1985? Journal of Hepatology 1: 687–693

Forker E L 1967 Two sites of bile formation as determined by mannitol and erythritol clearance in the guinea pig. Journal of Clinical Investigation 46: 1189–1195

Forker E L 1969 The effect of estrogen on bile formation in the rat. Journal of Clinical Investigation 48: 654–663

Forker E L 1970 Hepatocellular uptake of insulin, sucrose and mannitol in rats. American Journal of Physiology 219: 1568–1573

Glasinović J C, Dumont M, Duval M, Erlinger S 1975 Hepatocellular uptake of taurocholate in the dog. Journal of Clinical Investigation 55: 419–426

Hardison W G M, Norman J C 1968 Electrolyte composition of the secretin fraction of bile from the perfused pig liver. American Journal of Physiology 214: 758–763

Javitt N B, Wachtel N 1981 Hepatic bile formation: quantitative estimates of canalicular water flow. In: The Liver: Dynamics of structure and function: Abstracts of the Fourth International Gstaad Symposium, Gstaad, p 23

Latham P S, Kashgarian M 1979 The ultrastructural localization of transport ATPase in the rat liver at non-bile canalicular plasma membranes. Gastroenterology 76: 988–996

Layden T J, Boyer J L 1976 The effect of thyroid hormone on bile salt-independent bile flow and Na^+,K^+-ATPase activity in liver plasma membranes enriched in bile canaliculi. Journal of Clinical Investigation 57: 1009–1018

Layden T J, Elias E, Boyer J L 1978 Bile formation in the rat. The role of the paracellular shunt pathway. Journal of Clinical Investigation 62: 1375–1385

Meier P J, Sztul E S, Reuben A, Boyer J L 1984 Structural and functional polarity of canalicular and basolateral plasma membrane vesicles isolated in high yield from rat liver. Journal of Cell Biology 98: 991–1000

Prandi D, Erlinger S, Glasinović J C, Dumont M 1975 Canalicular bile production in man. European Journal of Clinical Investigation 5: 1–6

Preisig R, Cooper H L, Wheeler H O 1962 The relationship between taurocholate secretion rate and bile production in the unanesthetized dog during cholinergic blockade and during secretin administration. Journal of Clinical Investigation 41: 1152–1162

Reichen J, Paumgartner G 1975 Kinetics of taurocholate uptake by the perfused rat liver. Gastroenterology 68: 132–136

Ruifrok P G, Meijer D K 1982 Sodium ion-coupled uptake of taurocholate by rat-liver plasma membrane vesicles. Liver 2: 28–34

Scharschmidt B F, Van Dyke R W 1983 Mechanism of hepatic electrolyte transport. Gastroenterology 85: 1199–1214

Simon F R, Sutherland E, Accatino L 1977 Stimulation of hepatic sodium and potassium-activated adenosine triphosphatase activity by phenobarbital. Its possible role in regulation of bile flow. Journal of Clinical Investigation 50: 849–861

Sperber I 1959 Secretion of organic anions in the formation of urine and bile. Pharmacological Reviews 11: 109–134

Wheeler H O, Ross E D, Bradley S E 1968 Canalicular bile production in dogs. American Journal of Physiology 214: 866–874

J. Toouli

The function of the biliary tract and factors in the production of biliary pain

INTRODUCTION

The liver and the biliary tract are mentioned in the earliest recorded observations of man (Glenn & Grafe 1966). The Babylonians (2000 BC) described the gallbladder, cystic, hepatic and common bile ducts but their role in digestion was not appreciated. In 1543 Vesalius reported the presence of a membrane near the distal end of the common bile duct thought to impede reflux of duodenal contents into the bile duct, and in 1879 this structure was described as a sphincter and named after Rugero Oddi who in 1887 published a detailed description of its anatomy (Oddi 1887). In 1928 Ivy and Oldberg reported the successful extraction from hog duodenal mucosa of the hormone cholecystokinin which was shown to contract the gallbladder and reduce sphincter of Oddi resistance. These and subsequent studies firmly established that an intimate relationship existed between gallbladder contraction, sphincter of Oddi function and the flow of bile into the duodenum.

ANATOMY

Embryology

Embryological studies have demonstrated that the gallbladder and bile ducts arise from the caudal portion of a diverticular anlage that originates from the ventral floor of the foregut. The pancreas develops from two foregut buds in the region of the future duodenum. In 1957 Boyden confirmed that the distal muscularis propria of the bile duct and pancreatic duct are independent from duodenal musculature. In studies of the human fetus he showed that the sphincter of Oddi musculature arises de novo from mesenchyme, appearing approximately five weeks after the intestinal musculature.

Morphology

Bile from the hepatocytes is secreted into canaliculi which communicate with numerous interlobular ducts, which in turn drain into two main hepatic ducts. The main right and left hepatic ducts fuse at the porta hepatis into the common hepatic duct and the cystic duct joins the common hepatic duct at a variable distance caudal to the porta hepatis to form the common bile duct.

The human gallbladder is a pear-shaped sac nestled along a fossa on the right inferior surface of the liver. The gallbladder is divided anatomically into the blunt ended fundus, the body and the neck, which leads to the cystic duct. A sacculation at the neck of the gallbladder is known as Hartman's pouch. The cystic duct is of variable length, usually joining the common hepatic duct at an acute angle to form the common bile duct.

The common bile duct (Ch. 2) passes dorsal to the first part of the duodenum lying in a groove either within or posterior to the head of the pancreas and enters the second part of the duodenum through the major duodenal papilla in association with the pancreatic duct of Wirsung. The junction of the terminal common bile duct, pancreatic duct and duodenum at the papilla assumes one of three configurations that may be likened to a Y, V, or U (Ch. 2). In approximately 70% of subjects the ducts open into a common channel and thus have a Y configuration. This common channel drains into the duodenum through a single orifice on the duodenal papilla of Vater. In approximately 20% of subjects the common channel is almost non-existent and the two ducts have a common V shape opening on the papilla. In 10% of subjects the common bile duct and pancreatic duct have separate openings on the tip of the papilla; these openings lie adjacent to each other and give a U-shaped configuration. The terminal parts of the common bile duct and pancreatic duct, the common channel and major duodenal papilla of Vater are invested by varying thickness of smooth muscle and together form the sphincter of Oddi segment.

The major part of the human sphincter of Oddi lies within the duodenal wall, and anatomically has been shown to be distinctly separate from it. Boyden (1937), in a series of publications on the anatomy of the sphincter of

Oddi, described distinct sphincters at the terminal end of the common bile duct (sphincter choledochus), the terminal end of the pancreatic duct (sphincter pancreaticus) and the common channel (sphincter ampullae). However more recently Hand (1963), using a combination of radiological, duct cast techniques and histological sectioning methods, did not distinguish separate sphincters. Hand concluded from his human autopsy studies that the common bile duct and pancreatic duct become fused in a common connective tissue sheath outside the duodenal wall and pass together through a slit in the duodenal muscle known as the 'choledochal window'. The lumina, however, do not join at this level but are separated by a thick muscular septum. In most subjects fusion of the two lumina occurs in the submucosal layer of the duodenum to form a common channel varying in length between 2 and 17 mm. Before entering the duodenum each duct becomes completely surrounded by circular muscle, some of which forms a figure of eight pattern around the two ducts. The point at which the smooth muscle starts on each duct is readily identified radiologically as a notch (Fig. 9.1). Distal to the notch each lumen becomes narrow as it traverses the duodenal wall, this narrowing being associated with a thickening of the duct wall due to smooth muscle, connective tissue and mucous glands. As the ducts pass through the duodenal wall longitudinal muscle fibres inter-digitate between the circular ductular muscle fibres and the duodenal muscle. The ducts emerge from the duodenal muscle layers to have a course of variable length through the duodenal submucosa before opening on to the papilla of Vater; throughout this submucosal course the ducts are ensheathed by circularly orientated smooth muscle (Fig. 9.2). Recent manometric studies in man support Hand's description of the sphincter of Oddi in that separate sphincteric zones have not been identified (Toouli et al 1982a).

The mucosa of the human sphincter of Oddi segment is lined by columnar epithelium and contains numerous mucus-secreting glands. The mucosa is thrown into longitudinal folds likened to mucosal valvules (Tansy et al 1975). These folds are least marked proximally and increase distally becoming maximal in the common

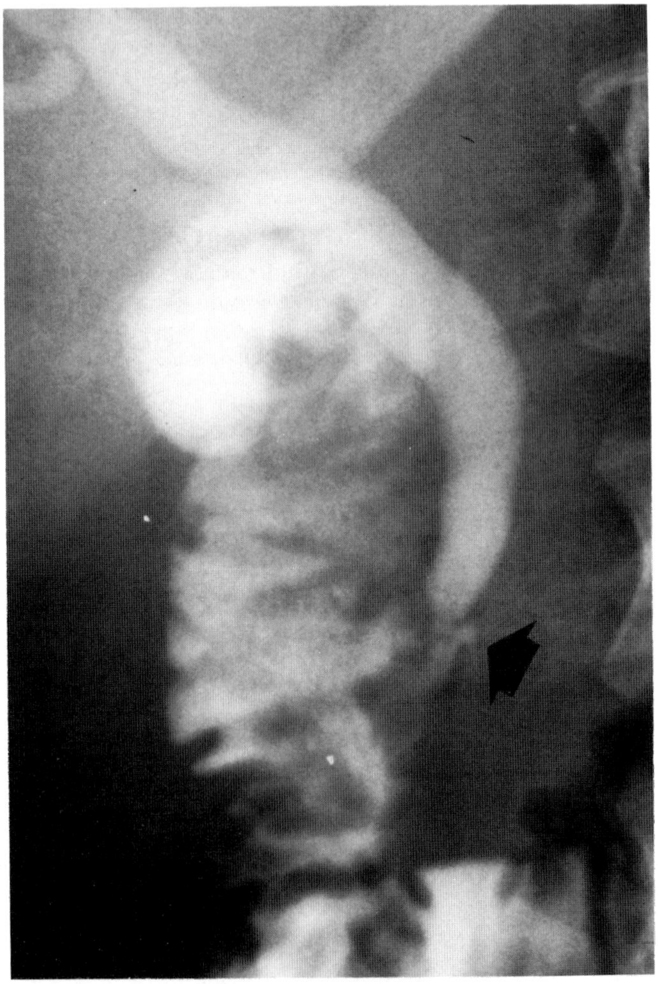

Fig. 9.1 Choledochogram demonstrating the notch at the terminal end of the bile duct. This notch identifies the uppermost margin of the sphincter of Oddi. Reproduced with permission from the publishers, Butterworth. London, and The British Journal of Surgery 71: 251–256

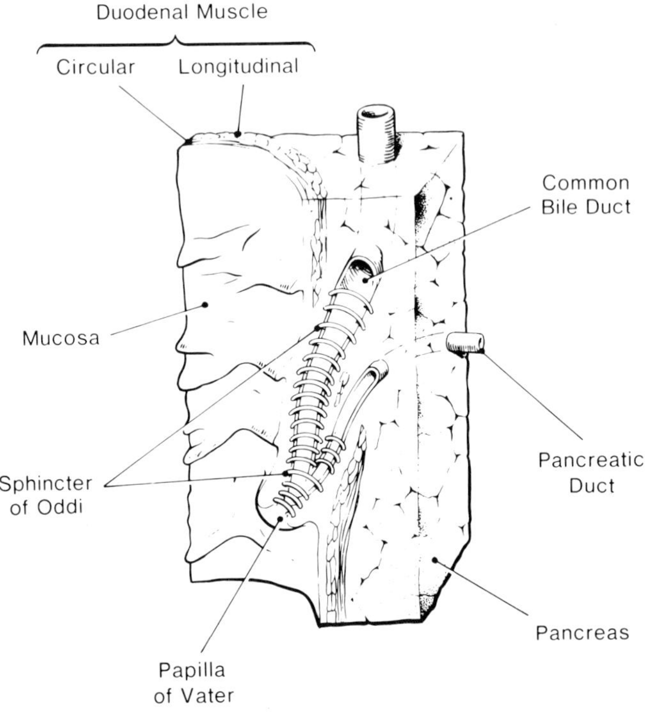

Fig. 9.2 Diagram of the human sphincter of Oddi demonstrating the circular smooth muscle which surrounds the terminal common bile duct and pancreatic duct. The length of the sphincter along the pancreatic duct is shorter than the length investing the terminal common bile duct. The major part of the sphincter lies within the duodenal wall and enters the duodenum through a slit in the duodenal muscle

channel. The mucosal folds may occasionally be seen projecting through the orifice of the duodenal papilla.

Innervation

The gallbladder and extrahepatic bile ducts are supplied by both extrinsic sympathetic and parasympathetic nerves. The coeliac ganglia contribute both motor and sensory nerves made up of sympathetic fibres which originate in the T7 to T10 spinal segments. Nerve fibres from both vagal nerves merge to form the hepatic plexus which supplies parasympathetic motor nerves to the extrahepatic biliary system (Burnett et al 1964).

Intrinsic nerve plexuses are found throughout the extrahepatic biliary system. These plexuses contain cells with histological features consistent with ganglia and are believed to be analogous to the submucosal and muscular plexuses of the gut. Histochemical labelling has shown that the gallbladder is richly supplied with both adrenergic and cholinergic ganglia. In addition, recent studies (Sundler et al 1977, Wen-Qin & Gabella 1983) have shown the presence of immunoreactive peptidergic nerves which label with vasoactive intestinal polypeptide (VIP). The sphincter of Oddi has a rich ganglionic plexus which appears to have a predominance of cholinergic ganglia and a smaller number of adrenergic ganglia. Future histochemical studies for peptidergic nerves should demonstrate their presence in the sphincter region as pharmacological evidence has suggested.

METHODS OF STUDY

A number of different techniques have been used in the study of biliary physiology and pathophysiology, and the following is an overview of some of the most useful methods.

Radiography

Cholecystography has been used extensively for the study of gallbladder motility. Estimations of gallbladder volume are made and the effects of ingested food substances, intravenous injection of gastrointestinal hormones, and parasympathetic and sympathetic nerve stimulation recorded. The kinetics of common bile duct and sphincter of Oddi motility are studied by infusing the contrast medium into the biliary system via a tube inserted in the common bile duct, and making a continuous record by cineradiography (Ch. 28) (Caroli et al 1960).

Manometry

Measurement of pressure changes from within the extrahepatic biliary system has been the basic investigation for understanding biliary dynamics. Intraluminal gallbladder pressures have been recorded with the cystic duct either patent or occluded in both anaesthetized and awake animals. Recently intraluminal gallbladder pressures have also been recorded in anaesthetized humans undergoing surgery for gallbladder disease, and the effect of intravenously administered drugs on the gallbladder pressures determined (Csendes & Sepulveda 1980).

Pressure measurements from the bile ducts have been obtained in animals and man anaesthetized or awake by inserting a tube into the bile duct. Pressures have been read visually from fluid-filled manometers or recorded by a transducer linked to a polygraph (Hess 1979). Investigators have determined the opening, passage and closing pressures of the sphincter of Oddi by either increasing or decreasing the height of the fluid reservoir connected in series with the tube inside the bile duct. From measurements of common bile duct pressure inferences were drawn about sphincter of Oddi function (Ch. 28) (Cushieri et al 1972).

Accurate direct pressure measurements from the sphincter of Oddi became possible by miniaturization of manometry catheters and the development of manometric systems of low compliance. A triple lumen constantly perfused catheter is inserted into the sphincter of Oddi segment and intraluminal pressure changes reflecting the activity of the sphincter recorded (Geenen et al 1980). These pressure measurements are made in awake humans under mild sedation by introducing the catheter into the papilla of Vater via an endoscope (Fig. 9.3). In addition intraoperative studies are possible by passage of the catheter through the cystic duct and positioning it in the sphincter of Oddi segment. Similarly in animals manometry catheters are positioned within the sphincter of Oddi segment either through the bile duct or from the duodenum.

Electromyography

Extracellular bipolar or monopolar electrodes sutured to the outside surface of the biliary tract have been used to record contractile activity from both animals and man (Sarles et al 1975). Studies have shown that the biliary tree, like the rest of the gastrointestinal tract, is characterized by two basic types of myoelectrical activity, i.e. slow regular changes in membrane potential known as 'slow waves', and rapid depolarization spikes called 'spike bursts' (Honda et al 1982). In general, spike bursts are virtually always associated with a phasic smooth muscle contraction and as such reflect intraluminal pressure changes.

Radioisotope imaging

A variety of Technetium^{99m} IDA (iminodiacetic acid) compounds are cleared through the liver into bile after intravenous administration (Ch. 15). Technetium^{99m} gives off 140 Kev gamma photons that are ideally suited for

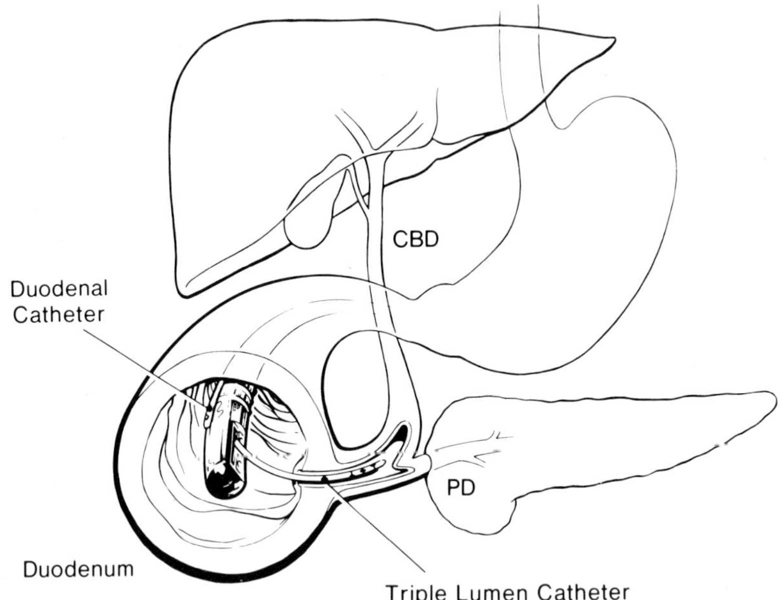

Fig. 9.3 Diagram illustrating endoscopic sphincter of Oddi manometry. A triple lumen catheter is inserted into either the common bile duct or the pancreatic duct and withdrawn so that all three lumens are stationed within the sphincter. A separate single lumen catheter records duodenal pressures. Reproduced with permission from the publishers, Butterworth, London, and The British Journal of Surgery 71: 251–256

imaging and counting by a gamma camera. These properties of the T^{99m}IDA compounds have been used to image the gallbladder and by producing temporal profiles monitoring of gallbladder filling and emptying can be studied (Shaffer et al 1980). Adaptation of these techniques to the study of bile flow through the bile duct in post-cholecystectomy subjects also has been possible. A major advantage of the isotope method is its non-invasive nature, which makes it suitable for use in humans.

Ultrasonography

The major use of ultrasonography in the study of biliary dynamics has been in the determination of gallbladder volume. In order to calculate gallbladder volume at a point in time, the maximal length and corresponding transverse diameter of the gallbladder are determined. Volume then is calculated from the ultrasound images as the sum of a series of cylinders (Everson et al 1980). Repeated measurements of gallbladder volume determine changes with various stimuli. Application of this technique to estimation of bile duct calibre has not been in common use, but may provide a non-invasive method for studying the biliary ducts.

PHYSIOLOGY

Gallbladder

Fluid transport and its regulation

Studies in animals and man have demonstrated that the gallbladder concentrates hepatic bile by selective reabsorption of bile constituents. However, in addition, recent studies have shown that both under physiological and pathological conditions reversal of fluid transport across the gallbladder mucosa occurs and net secretion into the gallbladder lumen results.

Sodium and chloride ions are absorbed from the gallbladder lumen by both active and passive transport mechanisms. Water absorption is thought to be passive and secondary to active solute movement resulting from osmotic equilibration of transported solute within the epithelium. The secretion of water and electrolytes by the gallbladder mucosa is an active process which can take place against hydrostatic and osmotic gradients (Wood & Svanvik 1983).

Animal in vitro and in vivo studies have demonstrated that a number of gastrointestinal peptides affect gallbladder fluid transport. Cyclic AMP has been proposed as a second messenger for the effects of several mediators and has been implicated in sodium and chloride transport in rabbit and necturus gallbladder. Vasoactive inhibitory polypeptide (VIP) and secretin have been shown to modify gallbladder fluid transport at concentrations which suggest a physiological role. However, other peptides such as glucagon, cholecystokinin, neurotensin, bombesin, motilin and somatostatin, which have been shown to enhance absorption in vitro, may act to potentiate or inhibit the effects of the major peptides (Wood et al 1982).

Application of prostaglandins of the E and F series to in vitro animal gallbladder preparations have demonstrated inhibition of fluid absorption and enhanced secretion from the gallbladder mucosa. Prostaglandins have been isolated from gallbladder mucosa, and indomethacin, a prostaglandin synthatase inhibitor, antagonizes inhibition of gallbladder fluid absorption by arachidonic acid (Thornell et al 1979). In animal studies bile salts, female sex hormones and autonomic nerve stimulation also have been shown to influence fluid transport.

Accumulating evidence suggests that normally during fasting the gallbladder absorbs fluid at a rate corresponding to one third of the fasting gallbladder volume. After feeding there is reversal of the direction of gallbladder transport from a net absorption to a net secretion into the gallbladder lumen. The net water transport across the gallbladder wall may be influenced by both humoral factors and autonomic nerves. During inflammation of the gallbladder, often associated with cystic duct obstruction, the absorptive capacity of the gallbladder mucosa is lost and net secretion into the lumen results, producing a hydrops. This pathological effect appears to be mediated by prostaglandin release possibly due to formation of lysolecithin by hydrolysis of phospholipid in the gallbladder. Recent evidence suggests that this process can be reversed by indomethacin, supporting the belief that at least part of the change in fluid transport may result from endogenous prostaglandin formation.

Gallbladder motility

Estimations of human fasting gallbladder volume by ultrasound techniques have shown a mean volume of approximately 17 ml in normal subjects. Until recently it was thought that the gallbladder volume gradually increased during fasting until the mean maximal volume was reached and only emptied after a food stimulus. However, recent studies in dogs (Takahashi et al 1982b) and opossums have shown that the gallbladder contracts up to 40% of maximal contractile capacity during the interdigestive period, and that these gallbladder contractions occur during phase II of the migrating motor complex (MMC). The periodic gallbladder contractions during fasting empty concentrated viscous bile and enable gallbladder refilling with dilute hepatic bile. Preliminary studies in man using ultrasound estimation of gallbladder volume confirm that a similar cyclical pattern of gallbladder volume changes occurs in man, in association with phase II of the MMC. The controlling mechanism which produces gallbladder volume changes during fasting is unknown. A potential candidate is motilin, a hormone produced by the mucosa of proximal small intestine. Serum motilin levels show cyclic changes during MMC cycles with the peak values preceeding phase III MMC activity. In animal studies motilin has been shown to produce gallbladder contraction (Takahashi et al 1982b).

The flow of bile into the gallbladder is modulated by hepatic secretory pressure, sphincter of Oddi tone, and cystic duct resistance. Only 50% of secreted hepatic bile enters the gallbladder during fasting, the remaining bile passing into the duodenum without concentration by the gallbladder. Gallbladder emptying produced by a meal or exogenous cholecystokinin occurs as a slow steady contraction which delivers bile into the duodenum for 20 minutes or longer while generating an intraluminal gallbladder pressure that is generally only a few cm H_2O above that in the common bile duct. The slow emptying of the gallbladder is typical of a graded tonic smooth-muscle contraction, such as that which occurs in the fundus of the stomach during gastric emptying of liquids.

The ability of a fatty meal to elicit gallbladder contraction has been well documented in man and a number of animal species. Recent evidence has shown that proteins entering the duodenum also produce gallbladder contraction but carbohydrates have only a minimal effect. Endogenous cholecystokinin is released from the mucosa of proximal small intestine and studies which measure serum CCK levels by radio-immunoassay have shown that gallbladder contraction induced by intraduodenal infusion of fat correlates directly with the level of circulating CCK (Weiner et al 1981).

The role of autonomic nerves in regulating gallbladder volume is not clear. In one study increased fasting volume of the human gallbladder was demonstrated after vagotomy (Johnson & Boyden 1952). A number of studies have investigated the effect of vagal stimulation and vagotomy on gallbladder contractility (Benevantano & Rosen 1969), but the results generally have been inconclusive. Similarly, studies of sympathetic innervation have produced inconstant and variable findings, and the role of the sympathetic autonomic nervous system in gallbladder motility requires further study (Persson 1972).

Cystic duct

Accumulating evidence suggests that the cystic duct is not merely a passive conduit between the gallbladder and the common bile duct, but may play an active role in the flow of bile into and out of the gallbladder. Histologically an anatomically prominent sphincter, as described by Lutken, does not appear to be present; however, a thin layer of smooth muscle is evident in the wall of the duct, and, along with the prominent mucosal folds which make up the valves of Heister, the cystic duct may act as a variable resistor to flow.

Flow studies in dogs have demonstrated resistance to flow across the cystic duct, the resistance being equal whether perfusion was carried either into or out of the gallbladder (Scott & Otto 1979). Significant reductions in flow were induced following systemic intravenous or local intra-arterial injection of morphine, adrenalin or cholecystokinin, suggesting that the cystic duct performs like a sphincter in modulating flow through its lumen. Studies in the prairie dog gallstone model have shown that cystic duct resistance to flow increases prior to gallstone formation in these animals (Pitt et al 1981a). These studies suggest that abnormalities in cystic duct function may be implicated in the pathophysiology of gallstone formation.

Common bile duct

The role of the common bile duct in the control of bile flow remains unclear. As in the cystic duct, histological studies in man have demonstrated only thin longitudinally orientated layers of smooth muscle within the wall of the common bile duct (Toouli & Watts 1971). The major tissue component appears to be elastic fibres. However, species differences exist, and the sheep common bile duct is invested with circularly orientated smooth muscle which exhibits peristaltic activity.

The weight of experimental evidence suggests that the human common bile duct does not have a primary propulsile function. However, the elastic fibres and the longitudinally orientated smooth muscle probably provide a tonic pressure that may help overcome the tonic resistance of the sphincter of Oddi.

The diameter of the human common bile duct before and after cholecystectomy has been the subject of controversy. Part of the controversy has been due to methodology used in determining duct size. It has become quite obvious that duct size as determined by ultrasonography cannot be equated to duct size determined by endoscopic retrograde cholangiography or intraoperative extraluminal measurements. In general the normal diameter of the common bile duct as determined by ultrasound is less than 6 mm, by retrograde cholangiography less than 10 mm, and by intraoperative extraluminal measurements less than 12 mm. What has become clear from recent studies, however, is that the common bile duct does not increase in diameter significantly following cholecystectomy (Le Quesne et al 1959). The major cause of dilated common bile duct is increased intraluminal pressure, which generally is produced by obstruction at the sphincter of Oddi.

Sphincter of Oddi

The mechanism by which the sphincter of Oddi controls the flow of the bile and pancreatic secretion has been uncertain. Studies which recorded sphincter of Oddi function by indirect means, such as observing the rate of inflow of fluid into the common bile duct, concluded that the sphincter of Oddi remains closed during fasting, thus diverting bile flow into the gallbladder. After a meal the sphincter relaxed and bile flowed from the common bile duct into the duodenum propelled by pressure generated by the gallbladder. This description of sphincter of Oddi function, however, does not take into account the observation that only 50% of hepatic bile is stored in the gallbladder during fasting, and hence the remainder must pass through the sphincter into the duodenum. Furthermore, the description does not explain what happens to sphincter of Oddi function following cholecystectomy when the storage capacity of the gallbladder has been lost. Recent methodological advances in manometric techniques have allowed direct study of sphincter of Oddi motility in both animals and man and clearer understanding of sphincter of Oddi physiology has emerged.

Sphincter of Oddi motility studies in animals

In vivo studies in dogs, cats, rabbits, monkeys and opossums have demonstrated that the sphincter of Oddi exhibits muscle contractions which are independent of duodenal activity. The results from the dog studies suggested that the sphincter of Oddi has a milking effect on bile, thus propelling small volumes of fluid from the common bile duct into the duodenum (Watts & Dunphy 1966). Manometric and electromyographic studies of the opossum sphincter of Oddi demonstrated phasic contractions which propagate along the entire length from the cephalic to the caudal end (Toouli et al 1983a). The common bile duct and pancreatic duct proximal to the sphincter do not demonstrate spontaneous motor activity.

Analysis of simultaneous cineradiography, transsphincteric flow and electromyographic recordings from the opossum sphincter of Oddi has demonstrated the effect of the phasic contractions on flow of bile into the duodenum (Fig. 9.4). The predominant mechanism of common bile duct emptying in the opossum is the antegrade sphincter of Oddi phasic contraction. A wave of contraction begins at the junction of the common bile duct and sphincter of Oddi stripping the contents of the sphincter of Oddi segment into the duodenum. During the period of sphincter of Oddi contraction, flow into the common bile duct ceases and there is no flow from the common bile duct into the sphincter of Oddi segment. Next, the sphincter of Oddi relaxes and passive flow of bile occurs from the common bile duct into the sphincter of Oddi segment. After filling of the sphincter of Oddi segment, a wave of contraction again begins at the junction of the common bile duct and sphincter segment, and the cycle repeats itself. The overall effect of the phasic contractions is to promote flow from the common bile duct into the duodenum. During sphincter contraction, or systole, flow from the common bile duct into the sphincter of Oddi segment stops and flow into the sphincter segment occurs only during sphincter relaxation or diastole. Increasing the frequency of sphincter contractions by administering the sphincter agonists phenylephrine (50 μg/kg IV) and bethanechol (30 μg/kg IV) decreased the diastolic interval between contractions and decreased the time available for passive flow of fluid from the common bile duct into the sphincter segment. Initially, an increase in the frequency of sphincter phasic contractions produced an increase in flow across the sphincter. However, as the frequency of

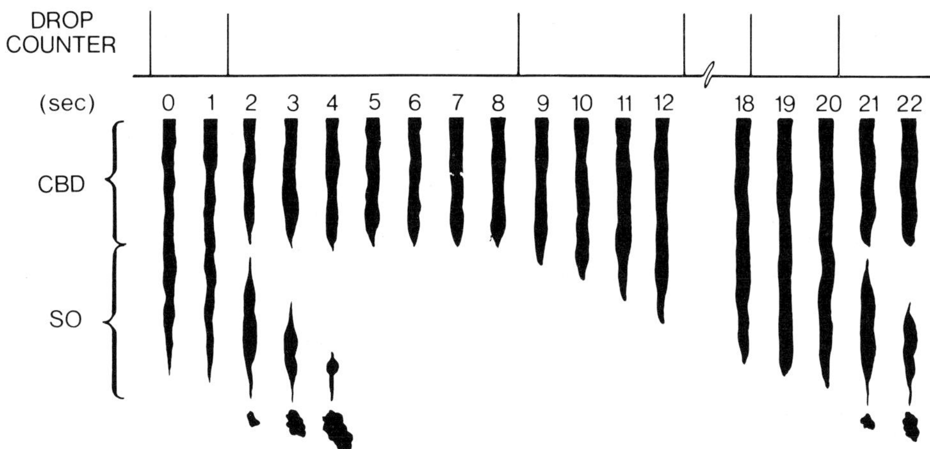

Fig. 9.4 Schematic representation of images from a cineradiographic recording illustrating flow through the sphincter of Oddi (SO). Contrast flowed into the common bile duct (CBD) at a rate of approx 6 drops/min (0.1 ml/min) from a reservoir and each drop is indicated by a vertical line. In this example contrast flows into the CBD and fills the SO segment. A phasic contraction begins at the junction of the CBD and SO, expelling contrast into the duodenum. Simultaneously flow from the CBD is interrupted and there is no flow from the reservoir into the CBD. On completion of the SO phasic contraction the SO segment relaxes and fluid passes from the CBD into the SO. The cycle then repeats itself. J. C. I. 1987 71: 208–220

contractions increases further, flow decreases due to the decrease in the diastolic interval. When the frequency of contractions exceeds eight per minute, the diastolic interval is abolished and there is no flow across the sphincter of Oddi segment of the opossum.

Following the ingestion of a meal, neuronal and hormonal stimuli influence the motor activity of the sphincter of Oddi and the hormone cholecystokinin plays a major role in the control of this activity. Its mechanism of action on the sphincter of Oddi has been studied in the cat (Behar & Biancani 1980). In this animal, an intravenous bolus of cholecystokinin inhibited the phasic contractions and produced a fall in sphincter tone. Following administration of the neurotoxin tetrodotoxin, cholecystokinin administration no longer produced inhibition, but instead caused contraction in the sphincter of Oddi. The investigators concluded that cholecystokinin produces its effect by stimulation of non-adrenergic non-cholinergic inhibitory neurones, this effect overriding a lesser, direct smooth muscle stimulatory action of the hormone.

Neurohistochemical studies have demonstrated both adrenergic and cholinergic neurones within the sphincter of Oddi and experiments in animals have determined the pharmacological effects of histamine, cholinergic and adrenergic stimulation on the sphincter muscle (Toouli et al 1983a). However, the physiological significance of these drug actions on the sphincter of Oddi requires further investigation.

The function of the vagus nerve in sphincter of Oddi physiology remains obscure. Studies in dogs suggested that following vagal transection the resistance to flow across the sphincter of Oddi is decreased (Pitt et al, 1981b). However, recent studies in the prairie dog have demonstrated increased resistance to flow through the sphincter of Oddi after truncal vagotomy. Results from vagal stimulation studies have failed to define clearly the role of the vagus in biliary dynamics.

Studies carried out in opossums with chronically implanted electrodes positioned on the sphincter of Oddi and the small intestine have demonstrated that the phasic activity of the sphincter of Oddi is omnipresent (Honda et al 1982). However, the frequency of the phasic contractions varies periodically during fasting. Four phases which are analagous to the phases of the intestinal interdigestive migrating motor complexes have been described for the sphincter of Oddi. Food ingestion and the intravenous infusion of cholecystokinin and pentagastrin abolish the periodic nature of the interdigestive sphincter of Oddi contractions. The physiological function of the periodic sphincter of Oddi contractions might be similar to that proposed for intestinal migrating motor complexes and that is to act as a housekeeper to eliminate any debris which may accumulate at the lower end of the bile duct. In addition, this activity of the sphincter may modulate the volume of bile passing into either the duodenum or gallbladder during fasting.

Sphincter of Oddi motility in man

Cineradiographic studies of the human sphincter of Oddi exhibit rhythmic contractions which propel contrast into the duodenum (Hess 1979). Sphincter of Oddi pressure studies conducted at the time of biliary tract surgery demonstrated variations in pressure thought to be the manometric equivalent of the cineradiographic contractions (Ch. 28) (Cushieri et al 1972). Resistance to outflow of fluid from the common bile duct into the duodenum also was demonstrated by the intraoperative studies. This resistance was reduced after administration of cholecystokinin octapeptide or smooth muscle relaxants such as amylnitrite (Butsch et al 1936).

Manometric recordings from within the sphincter of Oddi segment (Geenen et al 1980) have demonstrated that the human sphincter of Oddi is characterized by prominent phasic contractions superimposed on a basal sphincter of Oddi pressure 3 mmHg above the pressure in the common bile duct and pancreatic duct (Fig. 9.5). The amplitude of the phasic contractions is approximately 130 mmHg and the mean frequency is four per minute. Analysis of the direction of propagation of the phasic contractions during a continuous three-minute period demonstrated that the majority of contractions (60%) are orientated in an antegrade direction from the common bile duct towards the duodenum. A smaller number of contractions occurred either simultaneously (25%) or had a retrograde orientation (15%). Intravenous bolus injection of cholecystokinin octapeptide (20 ng/kg) normally produces inhibition of the phasic contractions and a fall in the basal sphincter of Oddi pressure (Fig. 9.6). Preliminary studies from patients with T-tubes inserted in the common bile duct following bile duct exploration have shown that the frequency of sphincter of Oddi phasic contractions during fasting may exhibit a periodicity in relation to duodenal migrating motor complexes, similar to that demonstrated in the opossum.

These studies in man suggest that the peristaltic type of sphincter of Oddi phasic contractions propel bile into the duodenum and possibly act to prevent reflux of duodenal contents into the bile and pancreatic ducts. Similar to findings in the opossum, bile flows passively into the sphincter segment during sphincter diastole and is expelled into the duodenum by the sphincter systolic contractions. Cholecystokinin inhibits the phasic contractions and produces a fall in basal pressure, which allows passive movement of bile across the sphincter segment into the duodenum. The effect of cholecystokinin on the human sphincter of Oddi is probably mediated via non-adrenergic non-cholinergic inhibitory neurones.

Overview of biliary tract physiology

During fasting approximately 50% of secreted hepatic bile is stored in the gallbladder whilst the remaining bile passes into the duodenum. The contractile activity of the sphincter of Oddi appears to modulate bile flow and either diverts small volumes into the gallbladder or expels it into the duodenum. This function of the sphincter of Oddi is probably produced by the prominent phasic contractions

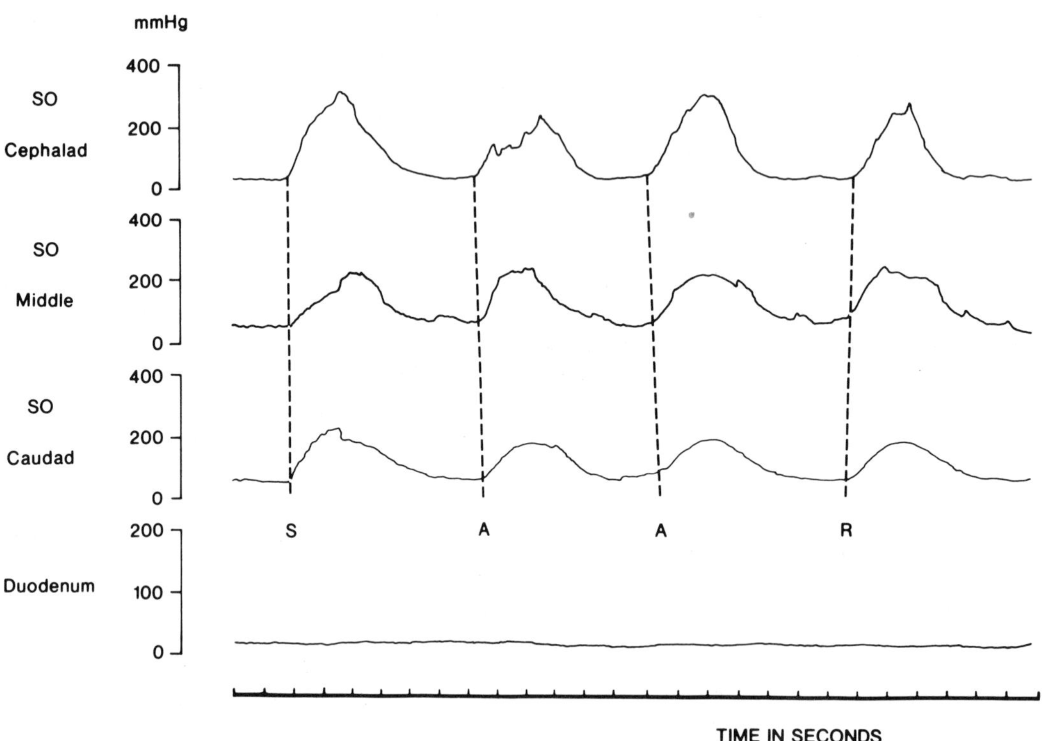

Fig. 9.5 Manometric recording of sphincter of Oddi (SO) and duodenal pressure changes in man. The top three recordings are from a triple lumen catheter stationed in the SO. The SO recording sites are spaced 2 mm apart. A line is drawn at the commencement of each phasic wave starting from the cephalic recording site to the caudal recording site. The phasic contractions show simultaneous (S), antegrade (A) and retrograde (R) orientations and are independent of duodenal pressure changes

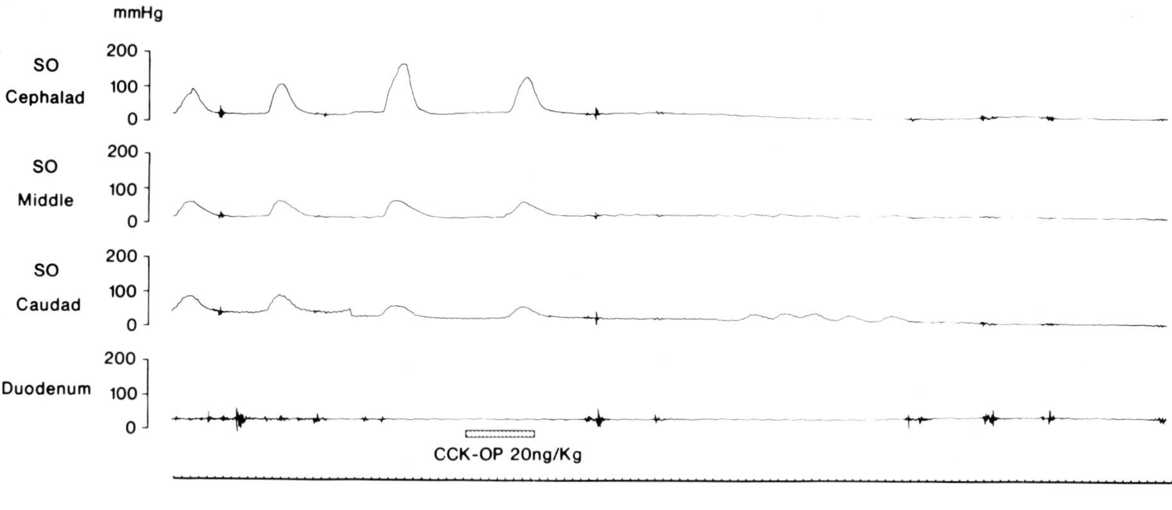

Fig. 9.6 Manometric recording showing the effect of a bolus IV injection of cholecystokinin-octapeptide (CCK-OP) on sphincter of Oddi (SO) phasic contractions. CCK-OP caused inhibition of the SO phasic contractions and no change in duodenal pressure. Reproduced with permission from the publishers, Butterworth, London, and The British Journal of Surgery 71; 251–256

which may be antegrade in direction and thus propel fluid into the duodenum, or retrograde and simultaneous which inhibit flow. The cystic duct generates a small resistance which can readily be overcome either by the strong sphincter of Oddi contractions or in reverse by the tonic contractions of the gallbladder. Bile stored in the gallbladder is concentrated by absorption of water and electrolytes. Both the gallbladder and sphincter of Oddi demonstrate a periodicity respectively with regard to volume changes and frequency of phasic contractions. This periodicity is related to the duodenal migrating motor complexes and its role might be as a housekeeper in eliminating small microcrystals which may develop in supersaturated fasting bile.

Following a meal, neuronal and hormonal stimuli produce slow gallbladder contraction and inhibition of the sphincter of Oddi contractions. This response allows flow of bile into the duodenum actively propelled by pressure generated from the gallbladder and hepatic secretion of bile.

PATHOPHYSIOLOGY — PRODUCTION OF BILIARY PAIN

Biliary pain characteristically is felt in the epigastrium and radiates to the right hypochondrium and to the right subscapular region (Doran 1967). The pain is erroneously labelled as a colic, although it is most commonly constant in nature with only minor fluctuations in intensity. Occasionally the site of the pain may differ from its classical position and be felt in the chest, left hypochondrium or lower abdomen. Pain originates from inflammation of the gallbladder and cystic duct, from distension of the gallbladder or bile duct and from direct irritation of the sphincter of Oddi.

The commonest and most readily understood cause of biliary pain is that which occurs in association with gallstones. Gallbladder stones impact in Hartman's pouch to produce obstruction of the cystic duct, thereby causing stasis of gallbladder bile. This initiating factor sets into motion a train of events in which prostaglandins appear to have an important role. Transport of fluid across the gallbladder mucosa is reversed, distension of the gallbladder and inflammation occurs and biliary pain of a visceral nature is felt. In most people the pain resolves spontaneously within hours, and this is due to relief of the cystic duct obstruction. Administration of a prostaglandin synthetase inhibitor, such as indomethacin, appears to promote early resolution of the symptoms (Thornell et al 1979). If the cystic duct obstruction is not relieved, the inflammatory process continues leading to acute cholecystitis with involvement of the parietal peritoneum in the right hypochondrium and pain of somatic origin is experienced.

When a stone migrates into or originates in the bile duct, obstruction of bile outflow may result if the stone impacts at the lower end of the common bile duct. Acute obstruction of the bile duct causes bile duct distension which gives rise to biliary pain. Similar pain may be produced inadvertently in patients with a T-tube in the common bile duct following bile duct exploration, if fluid is rapidly infused through the T-tube into the bile duct to produce acute distension.

The pathophysiology of non-calculous biliary pain is not as readily understood and the mechanisms by which such pain may originate remain the subject of investigation and controversy. A major problem in understanding non-calculous biliary pain has been the lack of objective evidence to incriminate biliary pathology as the cause.

Gallbladder dyskinesia

Abnormalities of gallbladder contraction are postulated to comprise either decreased contraction (hypokinesia) or excessive contraction (hyperkinesia) with or without production of biliary pain. Diagnosis of gallbladder dyskinesia has centred upon the visualization of the gallbladder either by contrast or isotope, followed by the administration of a standard stimulus such as cholecystokinin. A record is made of pain reproduction and the extent of gallbladder contractility in relation to time. In one study (Valberg et al 1971), 13 women who presented with biliary-type symptoms had their pain reproduced by administration of cholecystokinin. Cholecystokinin infusion given to 20 age-matched normal controls and 10 patients with anxiety neurosis and established functional disorder of the alimentary tract did not produce pain. Changes in gallbladder configuration were not taken into account in this study. Twelve of the 13 women who had a positive response to cholecystokinin administration underwent cholecystectomy and a median follow-up of 23 months (range 3–44 months) demonstrated resolution of the symptoms. There were no abnormalities of the gallbladder or cystic duct noted either at operation or on pathological examination. Goldstein & co-workers (1974) diagnosed gallbladder dyskinesia if pain was reproduced by cholecystokinin and the gallbladder emptied less than 50%. Cholecystectomy was performed in 25 of 28 patients studied with relief of symptoms in all but three patients. Histology revealed varying degrees of chronic cholecystitis with kinks or narrowing of the cystic duct in 10 of the 25 patients. In 17 controls the gallbladder contracted 50% or more and none of the patients reported upper abdominal pain.

Despite these favourable reports, others (Dunn et al 1974) have emphasized that in none of these studies were the results interpreted without knowledge of the patient's clinical condition. In a prospective study of 44 controls and 74 patients both the clinicians who administered the CCK and the radiologists who assessed the gallbladder contractions were blinded as to the patient's diagnosis. Twenty-nine patients had cholecystectomy for pain and the decision to operate was not based on the results of the CCK cholecystogram. After reviewing the results of the CCK cholecystography in relation to improvement of symptoms, there was no statistical difference in those patients who improved after cholecystectomy between patients having a positive or a negative test.

Therefore, at present the specificity of the cholecystokinin provocation test is questionable in that most studies that have used it to diagnose gallbladder dyskinesia comprised small groups of selected patients who were followed up only for short periods of time after cholecystectomy. Prospective randomized studies with appropriate follow-up of patients are required in order to better define its role in the diagnosis of gallbladder dyskinesia.

Cystic duct stump syndrome

Episodes of recurrent biliary pain occurring after cholecystectomy have been attributed in a small number of patients to continuing or recurrent disease in the cystic duct stump. A long cystic duct stump per se does not appear to be the cause of pain. However, stump neuromas, persistent chronic inflammation, retained stone in the stump, or inflammation around a non-absorbable suture have all been shown to be associated with recurrent post-cholecystectomy biliary pain. To date there are no investigations which allow diagnosis of this entity prior to surgery; thus laparotomy and excision of the stump is performed usually on clinical suspicion.

Sphincter of Oddi dysfunction

Dysfunction of sphincter of Oddi motility may be responsible for the production of biliary pain in patients who have previously had cholecystectomy performed for calculous or non-calculous biliary disease. In addition, sphincter of Oddi dysfunction may contribute to non-calculous gallbladder disease and the formation of primary common bile duct stones. Diagnosis of sphincter of Oddi dysfunction has lacked objectivity and pain provocative tests such as the Morphine-neostigmine test have not lived up to early expectations. Endoscopic sphincter of Oddi manometry recently has provided an objective method for evaluating sphincter of Oddi activity (Toouli 1984). However, its role in selecting patients with abnormalities for treatment remains under scrutiny. Based on the endoscopic manometric data, sphincter of Oddi disorders are categorized into two major groups:

1. Structural stenosis of the sphincter of Oddi

Manometrically this group of patients is characterized by an abnormally elevated sphincter of Oddi basal pressure suggestive of stenosis (Fig. 9.7). The sphincter stenosis may produce increased resistance to flow through the spincter giving rise to bile stasis. Although correlative pathological evidence is lacking, it is postulated that the sphincter of Oddi of these patients may be narrowed by a fibrotic stenosis, smooth muscle hypertrophy or mucosal hyperplasia.

2. Sphincter of Oddi dyskinesia

An abnormally functioning sphincter of Oddi is character-

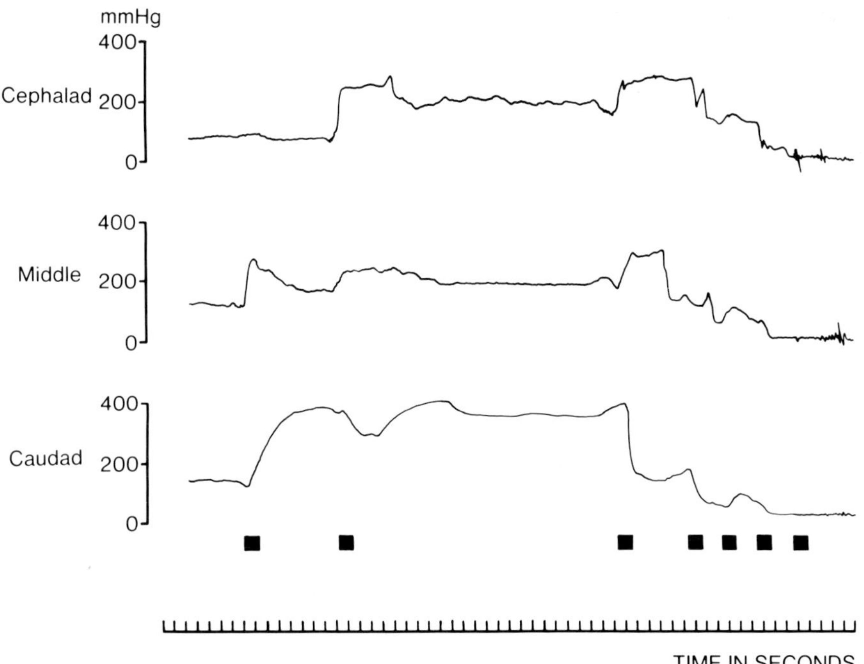

Fig. 9.7 Manometric recording showing a station pull through from the CBD through the SO to the duodenum using a triple lumen catheter. The square marks indicate withdrawal of the triple lumen catheter by 2 mm steps. A high basal pressure is demonstrated in all three lumens as the catheter is being withdrawn through a high pressure zone

ized manometrically by one or more of the following findings:

a. *Excessive retrograde contractions*

In control subjects the majority of the sphincter of Oddi phasic waves have an antegrade orientation towards the duodenum. When the percentage of retrograde contractions exceeds 50%, flow through the sphincter of Oddi may be impeded, giving rise to a relative obstruction to outflow that may produce bile duct distension and pain (Toouli et al 1982a).

b. *Rapid phasic contraction frequency*

Spontaneously occurring bursts of rapid phasic contractions or spasm may also produce acute obstruction to outflow resulting in bile duct distension and pain (Toouli et al 1983b). The obstruction results from a decrease in the diastolic interval between rapidly contracting phasic waves.

c. *Paradoxical response to cholecystokinin*

Cholecystokinin normally produces inhibition of the sphincter of Oddi phasic contractions with decrease in resistance to flow from the bile duct into the duodenum. In a group of patients with suspected sphincter of Oddi dyskinetic disorders and not those patients with a structural stenosis. However, the symptoms experienced by the patients with sphincter of Oddi dyskinesia tend to be episodic with variable intervals of time between attacks of pain. Therefore, an effective medication would need to be rapidly absorbed and effective in aborting an episode of pain.

Treatment of patients with suspected sphincter of Oddi dysfunction

Smooth muscle relaxants have been used without success in the treatment of patients with suspected sphincter of Oddi dysfunction. If medical therapy were to have a place in the management of these patients then it is expected that it might be most effective in the patients with the dyskinetic disorders and not those patients with a structural stenosis. However, the symptoms experienced by the patients with sphincter of Oddi dyskinesia tend to be episodic with variable intervals of time between attacks of pain. Therefore, an effective medication would need to be rapidly absorbed and effective in aborting an episode of pain.

A structural stenosis of the sphincter of Oddi might best be treated by division of the sphincter either endoscopically or by transduodenal operation. In a prospective randomized study, the effect of endoscopic sphincterotomy in the treatment of patients with suspected sphincter of Oddi dysfunction was evaluated (Geenen et al 1984). Post-cholecystectomy patients were selected for the study on the basis of clinical symptoms suggestive of biliary disease plus one or both objective signs of common bile duct dilatation and/or liver function test abnormality with episodes of pain. All patients underwent endoscopic manometry as part of their diagnostic work-up; however, the manometric findings were not used to determine treatment. 22 patients were randomized to endoscopic sphincterotomy and 23 patients served as controls. Neither group of patients were told whether a sphincterotomy was performed as the endoscope and papillotome were introduced into all patients whilst under sedation. Follow-up of symptoms was carried out prospectively for a period of 12 months. The results revealed that 10 out of 11 patients with an abnormally elevated sphincter of Oddi basal pressure became totally asymptomatic, whilst only three of the 12 controls with this manometric abnormality responded. Eleven patients with manometric findings suggestive of sphincter of Oddi dyskinesia did not improve significantly when compared to 11 controls with this disorder.

Long term results from two surgical studies (Moody et al 1983, Nardi et al 1983) in which patients underwent transduodenal sphincteroplasty and transampullary septectomy for treatment of chronic incapacitating upper abdominal pain also suggest that division of the sphincter of Oddi may alleviate pain in patients having a stenosis of the sphincter of Oddi. These results support the hypothesis that dysfunction of the sphincter of Oddi produces recurrent episodes of biliary pain, and it appears that endoscopic manometric assessment of sphincter of Oddi activity offers an objective method for selecting patients for treatment by either endoscopic or transduodenal division of the sphincter of Oddi.

SUMMARY

The biliary tract is a complex system made up of well orchestrated components which act in concert to control flow of bile from the ducts into the duodenum. Extrinsic and intrinsic nerves and circulating hormones modulate its activity; however, their precise and individual roles are still to be defined. The most common pathological conditions giving rise to pain from the biliary tract are associated with inflammation secondary to stone formation. However, motility disorders of the gallbladder and sphincter of Oddi may explain the aetiology of non-calculous biliary symptoms. Future prospective studies should define with greater precision the prevalence of these disorders and their role in the production of biliary pain.

REFERENCES

Behar J, Biancani P 1980 Effect of cholecystokinin and the octapeptide of cholecystokinin on the feline sphincter of Oddi and gallbladder. Mechanisms of action. Journal of Clinical Investigation 66: 1231–9

Benevantano T C, Rosen R G 1969 The physiological effect of acute vagal section on canine biliary dynamics. Journal of Surgical Research 9: 331–4

Boyden E A 1937 The sphincter of Oddi in man and certain representative mammals. Surgery 1: 25–37

Boyden E A 1957 The anatomy of the choledochoduodenal junction in man. Surgery, Gynecology and Obstetrics 104: 641–652

Burnett W, Gairns F W, Bacsich 1964 Some observations on the innervation of the extrahepatic biliary system in man. Annals of Surgery 159: 8–26

Butsch W L, McGowan J M, Walters W 1936 Clinical studies on the influence of certain drugs in relation to biliary pain and to the variations in intrabiliary pressure. Surgery, Gynaecology and Obstetrics 63: 451–6

Caroli J, Porcher P, Pequignot G, Delattre M 1960 Contribution of cineradiography to study of the function of the human biliary tract. American Journal of Digestive Diseases 5: 677–696

Csendes A, Sepulveda A 1980 Intraluminal gallbladder pressure measurements in patients with chronic or acute cholecystitis. American Journal of Surgery 139: 383–384

Cuschieri A, Hughes J H, Cohen M 1972 Biliary pressure studies during cholecystectomy. British Journal of Surgery 59: 267–73

Doran F S 1967 The sites to which pain is referred from the common bile duct in man and its implication for the theory of referred pain. British Journal of Surgery 54: 599–606

Dunn F H, Christensen E C, Reynolds J et al 1974 Cholecystokinin cholecystography. Journal of the American Medical Association 228: 997–999

Everson G T, Braverman D Z, Johnson M L, Kern F Jnr 1980 A critical evaluation of real-time ultrasonography for the study of gallbladder volume and contraction. Gastroenterology 79: 40–46

Geenen J E, Hogan W J, Dodds W J, Steward E T, Arndorver R C 1980 Intraluminal pressure recording from the human sphincter of Oddi. Gastroenterology 78: 317–324

Geenen J E, Hogan W J, Toouli J, Dodds W J, Venu R 1984 A prospective randomized study of the efficacy of endoscopic sphincterotomy for patients with presumptive sphincter of Oddi dysfunction. Gastroenterology 86: 1086

Glenn F, Grafe W R Jr 1966 Historical events in biliary tract surgery. Archives of Surgery 93: 848–852

Goldstein F, Grunt R, Margulies M 1974 Cholecystokinin Cholecystography in the differential diagnosis of acalculous gallbladder disease. American Journal of Digestive Diseases 19: 835–839

Hand B H 1963 An anatomical study of the choledochoduodenal area. British Journal of Surgery 50: 486–494

Hess W 1979 Physiology of the sphincter of Oddi. In: Classen M, Geenen J, Kawai K (eds) The papilla Vateri and its diseases. Proceedings of the International Workshop of the World Congress of Gastroenterology held in Madrid 1978. Verlag Gerhard Witzshock, Kohn: 14–21

Honda R, Toouli J, Dodds W J, Sarna S, Hogan W J, Itoh Z 1982 Relationship of sphincter of Oddi spike bursts to gastro-intestinal myoelectric activity in conscious opossums. Journal of Clinical Investigation 69: 770–778

Ivy A C, Oldberg E 1928 A hormone mechanism for gallbladder contraction and evacuation. American Journal of Physiology 86: 599–613

Johnson F E, Boyden E A 1952 The effect of double vagotomy on the motor activity of the human gallbladder. Surgery 32: 591–601

Le Quesne L P, Whiteside C G, Hand B T 1959 The common bile duct after cholecystectomy. British Medical Journal 1: 329–332

Moody F G, Becker J M, Potts J R 1983 Transduodenal sphincteroplasty and transampullary septectomy for post-cholecystectomy pain. Annals of Surgery 197: 627–36

Nardi G L, Michelassi F, Zannini P 1983 Transduodenal sphincteroplasty 5–25 year follow-up of 89 patients. Annals of Surgery 198: 453–461

Oddi R 1887 D'une disposition a sphincter speciale de l'ouverture du canal cholidoque. Archives of Italian Biology 8: 317–322

Persson C G A 1972 Adreno receptors in the gallbladder. Acta Pharmacologia 32: 177–185

Pitt H A, Roslyn J J, Kuchenbecker S L, Doty J E, DenBesten L 1981a The role of cystic duct resistance in the pathogenesis of cholesterol gallstones. Journal of Surgical Research 30: 508–514

Pitt H A, Doty J E, Roslyn J J, DenBesten L 1981b The role of altered extrahepatic biliary function in the pathogenesis of gallstones after vagotomy. Surgery 90: 418–425

Sarles J C, Midejean A, Devaux M A 1975 Electromyography of the sphincter of Oddi. American Journal of Gastroenterology 63: 221–231

Scott G W, Otto W J 1979 Resistance and sphincter-like properties of the cystic duct. Surgery, Gynecology and Obstetrics 149: 177–182

Shaffer E A, McOrmond P, Duggan H 1980 Quantitative cholescintigraphy: assessment of gallbladder filling and emptying and duodenogastric reflux. Gastroenterology 79: 899–906

Sundler F, Alumets J, Hakanson R, Ingemansson S, Fahrenkrug J, Schaffalitzky O B 1977 VIP innervation of the gallbladder. Gastroenterology 72: 1375–1377

Takahashi I, Nakaya M, Suzuki T, Itoh Z 1982a Postprandial changes in contractile activity and bile concentration in gallbladder of the dog. American Journal of Physiology 6: G365–G371

Takahashi I, Suzuki T, Aizawa I, Itoh Z 1982b Comparison of gallbladder contractions induced by motilin and cholecystokinin in dogs. Gastroenterology 82: 419–424

Tansy M F, Salkin L, Innes D L, Martin J S, Kendall F M, Litwack D 1975 The mucosal lining of the intramural common bile duct as a determinant of ductal opening pressure. American Journal of Digestive Disease 20: 613–625

Thornell E, Jansson R, Kral J G, Svanvik J 1979 Inhibition of prostaglandin synthesis as a treatment of biliary pain. Lancet i: 584

Toouli J 1984 Sphincter of Oddi motility. British Journal of Surgery 71: 251–256

Toouli J, Watts J Mck, 1971 In vitro motility studies on the canine and human extrahepatic biliary tracts. Australian and New Zealand Journal of Surgery 40: 380–387

Toouli J, Dodds W J, Honda R, Hogan W J 1981 Effect of histamine on motor function of opossum sphincter of Oddi. American Journal of Physiology 241: G122–8

Toouli J, Geenen J E, Hogan W J, Dodds W J, Arndorfer R C 1982a Sphincter of Oddi motor activity: A comparison between patients with common bile duct stones and controls. Gastroenterology 82: 111–117

Toouli J, Hogan W J, Geenen J E, Dodds W J, Arndorfer R C 1982b Action of cholecystokinin octapeptide on sphincter of Oddi basal pressure and phasic wave activity in humans. Surgery 92: 497–503

Toouli J, Dodds W J, Honda R, Sarna S, Jogan W J, Komorowski R A, Linehan J H, Arndorfer R C 1983a Motor function of the opossum sphincter of Oddi. Journal of Clinical Investigation 71: 208–220

Toouli J, Roberts-Thomson I, Dent J, Watts J 1983b Endoscopic biliary manometry in patients with suspected sphincter of Oddi dysfunction. Gastroenterology 84: 1335

Valberg L S, Jabbari M, Kerr J W, Curtis A C, Ramchard S, Prentice R S A 1971 Biliary pain in the absence of gallstones. Gastroenterology 60: 1020–1026

Watts J McK, Dunphy J E 1966 The role of the common bile duct in biliary dynamics. Surgery, Gynecology and Obstetrics 122: 1207–81

Weiner I, Kazutomo I, Fagan C J, Lilja P, Watson L C, Thompson J C 1981 Release of cholecystokinin in man, correlation of blood levels with gallbladder contraction. Annals of Surgery 194: 321–327

Wen-Qin Cai, Gabella G 1983 Innervation of the gallbladder and biliary pathways in the guinea pig. Journal of Anatomy 136: 97–109

Wood J R, Brennan L J, Hormbrey J M, McLoughlin T A 1982 Effects of regulatory peptides on gallbladder function. Scandinavian Journal of Gastroenterology 17: (suppl) 78–528

Wood J R, Svanvik J 1983 Gallbladder water and electrolyte transport and its regulation. Gut 24: 579–593

10

I. S. Benjamin

Biliary tract obstruction — pathophysiology

DEFINITION

Obstruction of the biliary tract in one of its many forms is a problem frequently encountered by the general surgeon. While clearly the most obvious presentation of biliary tract obstruction is that of the patient with obstructive jaundice due to tumour or to choledocholithiasis, there has been increasing recognition of the more subtle forms of this entity. Clear recognition and understanding of the problem demands adoption of a broader view of biliary tract obstruction than that presented by the jaundiced patient. The author has previously proposed (Benjamin 1983) a classification which has proved useful in practice, and which recognizes four categories of biliary obstruction:

Type I *Complete obstruction*, producing jaundice

Type II *Intermittent obstruction*, which produces symptoms and typical biochemical changes, but may or may not be associated with attacks of clinical jaundice.

Type III *Chronic incomplete obstruction*, with or without classic symptoms or the observation of biochemical changes, which will eventually produce pathological changes in the bile ducts or the liver.

Type IV *Segmental obstruction*, in which one or more anatomical segments of the intrahepatic biliary tree are obstructed. In its turn, this segmental obstruction may take the form of (a) complete, (b) intermittent, or (c) chronic incomplete obstruction, as defined above.

Advances in biliary tract imaging have allowed increasing recognition of these categories of biliary tract obstruction, and these are further discussed in Ch. 25. It is inappropriate to attempt comprehensive listing of the specific causes of these types of obstruction, but it may be helpful in forming a concept of these categories to refer to the examples of lesions commonly associated with them shown in Table 10.1.

The aim of this chapter is to review some of the pathophysiological effects of biliary tract obstruction, and to discuss their relevance to the clinical situation and to the therapeutic options available to the surgeon.

Table 10.1 Lesions commonly associated with biliary tract obstruction

Type	Lesions
Type I	Complete obstruction
	Tumours, especially of the pancreatic head
	Ligation of the common bile duct
	Cholangiocarcinoma
	Parenchymal liver tumours, primary or secondary
Type II	Intermittent obstruction
	Choledocholithiasis
	Periampullary tumours
	Duodenal diverticula
	Papillomas of the bile duct
	Choledochus cyst
	Polycystic liver disease
	Intrabiliary parasites
	Haemobilia
Type III	Chronic incomplete obstruction
	Strictures of the common bile duct
	Congenital
	Traumatic (iatrogenic)
	Sclerosing cholangitis
	Post-radiotherapy
	Stenosed biliary-enteric anastomoses
	Stenosis of the sphincter of Oddi
	Chronic pancreatitis
	Cystic fibrosis
	? Dyskinesia
Type IV	Segmental obstruction
	Traumatic (including iatrogenic)
	Hepatodocholithiasis
	Sclerosing cholangitis
	Cholangiocarcinoma

PHYSICAL EFFECTS

Increased pressure

The normal secretory pressure of bile is 120–250 mm of water (Papageorgiou & Lynn 1985). Following total bile duct obstruction bile secretion will continue until the common bile duct pressure rises to 170–220 mm of water, at which time inhibition of the various elements of bile production commences. Cholesterol and phospholipid secretion are more readily reduced by high pressure than bile salt secretion, so that the composition of hepatic bile is altered and becomes less lithogenic (Strasberg et al 1971). The reduction in bile salt dependent canalicular bile flow under high pressure conditions results in inhibition of bile salt synthesis. Following relief of obstruction and return to normal pressure, the recovery of secretion rate for cholesterol and phospholipid is more rapid than that for bile salts so that bile becomes more lithogenic during this period. Some of these observations may be relevant to the clinical situations in which intermittent or incomplete obstruction occur. Manometric studies in man show that common bile duct pressures may intermittently rise above the maximal secretory pressure for bile, resulting in fluctuations in lithogenecity of the bile so produced (Ch. 8, 9).

Complete obstruction of the main extrahepatic bile ducts or of a major segmental duct will normally lead to proximal dilatation of the bile duct or of intrahepatic biliary radicles. However, this is not invariably the case, and the degree of dilatation will depend on the extent and the duration of obstruction, and also on the capacity of the bile ducts and surrounding hepatic parenchyma to expand. The lack of intrahepatic ductal dilatation constitutes a pitfall in the radiological diagnosis of biliary obstruction, and in particular in the use of ultrasound to distinguish between intrahepatic and extrahepatic cholestasis (Ch. 25). In a series of 100 cases of proven biliary obstruction studied at Mount Sinai Hospital in New York, 16 showed no evidence of ductal dilatation (Beinart et al 1981). Such findings should alert the clinician to the possibility of either secondary hepatic fibrosis or cirrhosis, or to co-existing unrelated hepatic parenchymal disease (such as alcoholic or post-hepatitic cirrhosis). Chronic obstruction which has undergone a slow evolution may fail to produce significant proximal dilatation, particularly when associated with marked chronic cholangitis and ductal fibrosis.

Hepatic blood flow

Argument from first principles would suggest that total hepatic tissue perfusion might be reduced in the face of increasing hydrostatic pressure within the liver in association with increased intra-ductal pressure and ductal dilatation. However, actual clinical evidence in this regard is negligible, and experimental studies are conflicting. Following bile duct ligation in the rat, one group has shown decreased liver blood flow (Hunt 1979), while other workers have shown no such change in the dog (Hall et al 1977). Interesting work in our own laboratory has shown that in the dog increases in bile duct pressure below 25 mmHg have no perceptible effect, while increases between 25 and 45 mmHg result in a linear increase of hepatic arterial flow, reaching a maximum of 3.5 times the resting value (Nagorney et al 1982). The mechanism of these changes has not been determined.

Alterations in hepatic tissue perfusion may be of some importance in relation to liver resection. Liver resection in the presence of obstructive jaundice carries a higher risk than in the anicteric patient, and it may be that some of this risk relates to secondary hepatocellular dysfunction which may be compounded by reduced hepatic tissue perfusion. Unfortunately, clinical studies are difficult to undertake in this area, although such studies are in progress in this department.

Pain

'Painless' progressive jaundice is the clinical hallmark of malignant biliary tract obstruction. However, it is by no means uncommon to elicit a history of abdominal pain in this group of patients. Pain was a feature in 27 of 94 patients with hilar cholangiocarcinoma studied in the Hepatobiliary Surgical Unit at Hammersmith Hospital (Blumgart et al 1984b). Similarly, 11 out of 19 patients with carcinoma of the gallbladder had pain as a presenting feature, and in six this was typical of biliary 'colic'. The origin of pain in biliary obstruction may be distension of the gallbladder or bile duct or may be associated with stretching of the liver capsule in cases of rapidly progressive obstruction. Nevertheless, severe pain of a spasmodic nature is more characteristic of calculous obstruction than of malignancy. This subject, and the more difficult subject of pain due to biliary dyskinesia, is covered in more detail in Ch. 9.

PATHOLOGICAL EFFECTS

Bile ducts and canaliculi

The ravages brought about by unrelieved biliary tract obstruction on the entire liver and biliary system begin at the level of the bile duct canaliculi. The canaliculus is formed by a groove in the lateral plasma membranes of two adjacent hepatocytes and is a tubular structure about one micron in diameter penetrating the hepatocyte plate, whose plasma membrane contains numerous microvilli projecting into the lumen. This membrane is a highly active structure involved in complex mechanisms for production of both bile salt dependent and bile independent bile flow (Ch. 8). There is some evidence that in both biliary obstruction (extrahepatic cholestasis) and intrahepatic cholestasis the initial pathological changes at the level of the canalicular microvilli are essentially the same (Schaffner & Popper 1985). The bile canaliculi become dilated and the microvilli distorted and swollen. Bile pigment 'thrombi' may be seen in the canaliculi and in the adjacent hepatocytes. If cholestasis is prolonged, there is an apparent proliferation of the canaliculi, with an increase in length and tortuosity. It is interesting that all of these changes can be induced not only by ligation of the bile duct in experimental animals but also by injection or feeding of lithocholic acid (Schaffner & Javitt 1966). In both cases it appears that the pathological effects may be initiated by high local concentrations of bile salts at the canalicular membrane (Schaffner et al 1971). Thus, many of the morphological and biochemical findings are similar in cholestasis of both extrahepatic and intrahepatic origin, and it may be difficult in some cases for the histopathologist to distinguish between these two in a biopsy specimen.

Reabsorption of bile constituents from the ductules leads to a marked inflammatory reaction in the portal tracts, with a polymorphonuclear leucocyte infiltrate. This 'acute cholangiolitis' does not necessarily imply ascending bacterial cholangitis, but is a tissue reaction to an irritant chemical stimulus. These cholangiolitic changes are followed by increased fibrogenesis with deposition of reticulin fibres and eventually of collagen bundles.

In the hepatocytes of the peri-portal zones both bilirubin and bile acid retention occur, and both exert toxic effects within the hepatocyte. Bile salts in particular cause both inhibition of cytochrome P450 and transformation into the inactive cytochrome P420 (Schaffner & Popper 1985). Both smooth and rough endoplasmic reticulum are disrupted and canalicular membrane components become solubilized, which explains in part the increased release of canalicular alkaline phosphatase into the bloodstream. Cytoplasmic hyaline deposits are seen, and feathery degeneration may eventually proceed to destruction of the hepatocytes around the portal tracts associated with leucocyte infiltration, the so-called 'biliary piecemeal necrosis'. Experimental observations have shown that if obstruction is relieved within two weeks these morphological changes are readily reversible, and that the appearance of the mitochondrial cristae may be useful in assessing this reversibility (Yokoi 1983).

Fibrotic changes

If obstruction continues, the reticulin laid down in the peri-portal areas matures to hard type I collagen, causing scarring fibrosis around the bile ducts, which may further aggravate the cholestasis. The extrahepatic ducts are also subject to these changes, and mucosal atrophy and squamous metaplasia followed by inflammatory infiltration and fibrosis in the sub-epithelial layers of the ducts may supervene, particularly in the presence of superadded infection.

When the intrahepatic fibrotic changes have progressed beyond this point, mechanical obstruction to sinusoidal flow may result in secondary portal hypertension. Fibrous septa may ultimately produce a severe peri-lobular fibrosis, but the lobular architecture of the liver is usually well preserved and only infrequently proceeds to a true pattern of secondary biliary cirrhosis. Because of this, we believe that many of the fibrotic changes are at least potentially reversible, and have observed a return to near normality of liver architecture on biopsy following relief of biliary obstruction (Blumgart 1978). Since it takes weeks to months of biliary obstruction to produce this degree of fibrotic change, this extreme situation is more likely to arise with chronic incomplete obstruction which does not produce a clamant clinical picture of obstructive jaundice. It is thus important that the clinician should not lightly accept continuing incomplete obstruction, since cholangitic and fibrotic changes may be progressing relentlessly with little biochemical or clinical evidence, but may yet be arrested or reversed by complete and adequate biliary drainage.

In this context it is relevant to note that benign iatrogenic biliary strictures, which are often chronic and incomplete, have a high association with portal hypertension. In a report from the Lahey Clinic, 19% of patients with biliary strictures had some degree of portal hypertension (Sedgwick et al 1966). At Hammersmith Hospital (Ch. 58) 14% of patients with iatrogenic biliary strictures had portal hypertension on referral, as evidenced by endoscopic, radiological or operative findings (Blumgart et al 1984a). Some authors have reported such changes as early as two years from the onset of obstruction (Kune 1972), but in our experience portal hypertension has been related to the length of history. The median duration of obstruction in 11 patients with portal hypertension was 48 months, significantly higher than that in 67 patients from our series without portal hypertension (15.5 months). Moreover, all the patients with portal hypertension gave a history of frequent and severe episodes of cholangitis, while only 16 of 67 patients without portal hypertension gave this history. These findings appeared also to be significantly related to the number of previous operations, which in turn influenced the occurrence of major infective episodes by the time of presentation (Blumgart et al 1984a).

It is important to note in passing that iatrogenic bile duct strictures may also be associated with direct operative damage to the hepatic arteries or portal veins (Ch. 58), and such damage to the portal vein may result in portal hypertension. Since the management of this type of portal hypertension may be different from that caused by hepatic fibrosis, it is important to consider this variant during the investigation of these patients.

Cholangitis

Although the neutrophil infiltrate associated with cholangiolitis is a chemical reaction associated with biliary obstruction, and does not imply bacterial inflammation, in the presence of biliary stasis secondary bacterial colonization may produce the additional element of infective cholangitis. Although classically referred to as 'ascending' cholangitis, the actual mechanism for entry of bacteria into the unoperated biliary tract may not always be clear (Ch. 11). Organisms are found in the bile in approximately one-third of patients with malignant biliary tract obstruction (McPherson et al 1982b). In the presence of previous biliary surgery, instrumentation, intubation or biliary-enteric anastomosis, this rate may be much higher. The highest rate of bile colonization is found in patients with choledocholithiasis or with benign bile duct strictures, where as many as 80% of patients may have positive cultures (Jackaman et al 1980). Following biliary intubation our own early data showed colonization of transhepatic biliary tubes in every case, with polymicrobial growth in 79% (McPherson et al 1982b). This type of contamination may go on to produce serious invasive sepsis, and this subject is covered in more detail in Ch. 37.

In the presence of acute cholangitis, there is marked portal oedema and neutrophil leucocyte infiltration not only around the ductules but also between the epithelial cells. In severe infection micro-abscesses may form leading to progressive duct destruction. The perilobular fibrotic changes already described become more marked in the presence of superadded infection.

The combination of biliary bacterial colonization and bile stasis may also be important in the pathogenesis of choledocholithiasis. *Escherichia coli* (the commonest species found in the biliary tree) is a producer of beta-glucuronidase which may lead to deconjugation of bilirubin in bile. This may lead to the formation of primary common bile duct stones with a high bile pigment content, and indeed the formation of such stones has been shown to correlate highly with the presence of *E. coli* in the bile duct (Saharia et al 1977). Once again the most potent clinical situation for the production of such stones is that of chronic obstruction due to an incomplete stricture and more particularly to partial stenosis of a biliary-enteric stoma such as a hepaticojejunostomy or choledochoduodenostomy. In contrast, an adequately draining stoma rarely if ever produces cholangitis and primary duct stones, even in the presence of free reflux of intestinal content in and out of the bile duct.

Atrophy

Although the early stages of unilateral hepatic duct obstruction may produce enlargement of the obstructed lobe, the characteristic effect is atrophy of the obstructed liver parenchyma with compensatory hyperplasia of the unaffected segments of the liver (Ch. 6). Indeed, a grossly hypertrophied left lobe palpable in the epigastrium in association with unilateral obstruction and right lobe atrophy may be interpreted as a hepatic tumour. Such unilateral or segmental ductal obstruction may fail to produce clinically significant hyperbilirubinaemia in the presence of the normal contralateral lobe. Thus four cases in a series of 116 patients with hilar cholangiocarcinoma were anicteric at presentation, because of asymmetrical ductal obstruction (Hadjis et al 1986): three of these patients were not jaundiced on admission despite obstruction of more than 70% of the liver. Such lobar or segmental atrophy can be demonstrated radiologically in some 20% of patients with hilar cholangiocarcinoma (Carr et al 1985). These findings have considerable surgical importance, and this is considered elsewhere (Ch. 6, 65).

The mechanism of the atrophy-hypertrophy complex remains somewhat obscure. The secondary effects of obstruction of the bile duct on hepatocytes have already been considered, and certainly the hepatocyte necrosis produced by local bile salt effects may be sufficient to trigger the well-recognized though incompletely explained compensatory hyperplastic response in the unobstructed liver segments. Secondary effects on portal blood flow may also be important, since portal factors are at least permissive and possibly regulatory in the control of hepatocyte growth (Bucher & McGowan 1985).

The practical importance of lobar atrophy in a surgical context lies in the fact that an atrophic liver lobe may be inadequate to support life following resection of normal or hyperplastic liver tissue, and moreover biliary drainage of such an obstructed lobe may also fail to produce resolution of jaundice.

BIOCHEMICAL EFFECTS

Bilirubin

Conjugated hyperbilirubinaemia is the classic biochemical feature of obstructive jaundice. However, in complex cases with prolonged partial obstruction of the biliary tract, functional effects on the hepatocytes may produce a mixed biochemical picture, with elevation of circulating unconjugated bilirubin. This diagnostic conundrum stems from the fact already noted that the basic lesion of cholestasis at the subcellular level is similar irrespective of the mechanical or metabolic nature of the agent producing cholestasis (Schaffner & Popper 1985). Cholestasis is defined as 'bile secretory failure of the liver cell with concomitant accumulation of bile constituents in the blood' (Desmet 1979). There must therefore exist a pathway for regurgitation of accumulated bile constituents from the biliary compartment to the bloodstream. The mechanism whereby this occurs is complex: it is probable that the early stages of obstruction produce biliary-lymphatic regurgitation, and that, as the pressure rises, biliary-venous regurgitation supervenes, but much of this pathway remains speculative. In addition to this intercellular escape, transhepatocytic regurgitation by means of reversal of the secretory polarity of the hepatocyte has been proposed (Desmet 1979). Finally, as a late event dilated canaliculi and inspissated bile thrombi may rupture into the sinusoids by necrosis of surrounding liver cells.

Even the actual mechanisms of transport of conjugated bilirubin within the hepatocyte and its secretion into the canaliculus are incompletely understood. Although the secretory mechanisms for bile acids and for bilurubin and a variety of exogenous organic anions (such as BSP and some dyes used in cholecystography) are functionally distinct, they are not entirely independent. This is considered further below.

It must be stated again that segmental or lobar obstruction even to a very major degree may fail to produce jaundice in the presence of one or more functioning and possibly hyperplastic liver segments. Nonetheless, a completely normal plasma bilirubin is the exception in any case of extrahepatic biliary obstruction.

Alkaline phosphatase

When the obvious pitfalls of sources of alkaline phosphatase apart from the liver and biliary tract are excluded, elevation of this enzyme is the most widely used and probably the most sensitive indicator of biliary tract obstruction. Certainly high levels of alkaline phosphatase are found in patients with complete obstruction and elevation of this enzyme may be the only biochemical indicator of incomplete or segmental obstruction. However, the true situation is more complex than this. Elevation of serum alkaline phosphatase is not entirely due to true regurgitation from the biliary compartment. Acute obstruction of the bile duct causes a prompt increase in hepatic synthesis of alkaline phosphatase (Kaplan et al 1983), and the sinusoidal cell membranes become histochemically strongly positive for the enzyme. There is a large and complex literature on the isoenzymes of alkaline phosphatase in patients with liver disease. However, it appears certain that there are two principal fractions of alkaline phosphatase found in bile: one fraction is derived from the liver cell, and the other only appears when there is obstruction to the flow of bile (Price & Sammons 1974). It has been suggested that this second component of alkaline phosphatase may allow better differentiation of patients with extrahepatic obstruction from those with intrahepatic cholestasis than total levels of the enzyme. Moreover, there is now considerable evidence that the large molecular size isoenzyme which appears in cholestasis is actually alkaline phostphatase of hepatocyte origin which is attached to circulating membrane fragments which also contain a number of other enzymes, including 5′-nucleotidase, gammaglutamyl transpeptidase and lipoprotein X (Desmet 1979, Price & Alberti 1985). These large enzyme-containing membrane fragments are probably released from the liver cell as one of the local effects of the detergent action of bile salts already discussed above.

While elevation of alkaline phosphatase is a sensitive marker of biliary obstruction, its return to normal following relief of obstruction is extremely variable. Long after the hyperbilirubinaemia has subsided levels of alkaline phosphatase may remain two or more times higher than normal despite an apparently successful clinical result (Smith 1978, Way et al 1981). The reason for this persistence is not always clear, but in using HIDA scanning to assess the long-term patency of biliary-enteric anastomosis in the follow-up of patients who have had repair of bile duct strictures, the author has found a number of patients in whom elevated alkaline phosphatase is associated with minor segmental obstruction or established lobar atrophy, in the presence of adequately functioning biliary-enteric drainage. Thus while alkaline phosphatase is a useful and sensitive test in the follow-up of such patients, it is not always necessary to proceed to invasive investigation on the basis of continued elevation.

Protein synthesis

The liver occupies a central role in protein synthesis, and albumin is quantitatively the most important plasma protein synthesized by the liver. However, because of the long half-life of albumin in the circulation (20 days) only minimal changes may occur secondary to the hepatocyte damage produced by biliary tract obstruction. Nonetheless, since biliary obstruction is frequently associated with other factors, such as malignancy and inadequate nutrition, hypoalbuminaemia remains an important feature of the patient with biliary obstruction. Moreover, several studies have now shown that low serum albumin levels represent a significant risk factor in the patient undergoing major biliary surgery (Dixon et al 1983, Blamey et al 1983).

As an acute marker of hepatic protein synthetic levels, serum prealbumin is more valuable since the half-life of this protein in the circulation is 1.9 days. This factor and others have been shown to be important prognostic factors in obstructive jaundice: this is considered in more detail in the chapter on nutrition (Ch. 32).

A most important aspect of protein synthesis relates to the role of the liver in the maintenance of the normal blood coagulation process (Ch. 12). Thus fibrinogen, prothrombin and Factor VII may all be affected in severe and prolonged obstructive jaundice. Of course, the major deficit in most cases of biliary obstruction relates to failure of vitamin K absorption due to absence of bile salts from the intestine. In cases of long-standing biliary obstruction with severe secondary hepatocyte malfunction, coagulopathy may fail to be corrected by parenteral administration of vitamin K. This should alert the clinician to the possibility of severe secondary changes or pre-existing alcoholic or other parenchymal liver disease.

Lipids

Cholesterol levels may be elevated in long-standing biliary obstruction. A number of alterations in low density lipoproteins have been observed, but these appear to be neither of great specific diagnostic value nor of major functional importance. The abnormal low density lipoprotein X has already been referred to above in relation to the membrane fragments associated with high molecular weight alkaline phosphatase. While this has been suggested as a valuable test in differentiating between intrahepatic and extrahepatic cholestasis, not all workers have found this to be so (Harry et al 1985).

Carbohydrate metabolism

Abnormal glucose tolerance may be seen in patients with impaired liver function, and impaired gluconeogenesis has been found after bile duct ligation in the rat (Lee et al 1972). This has been confirmed in patients with biliary tract obstruction due to malignancy, but it is suggested that the malignant disease might be the primary mechanism and that biliary tract obstruction causes no further deterioration in glucose tolerance in these patients (Flannigan 1986).

Bile salt circulation

The enterohepatic circulation of bile salts is completely interrupted by total biliary tract obstruction, and this may lead to gross elevation of serum bile acid levels, up to 60 times normal (Neale et al 1971). This is associated with a decrease in hepatic synthesis of bile acids, increased urinary excretion and the formation of abnormal bile acids by the liver (including ursodeoxycholate), which are more easily excreted in the urine than the normal bile acids. The role of the bile acids in producing hepatocellular damage at the canalicular level has already been noted.

There are two important consequences of these liver/bile salt relationships. Firstly, the absence of bile salts from the intestine is associated with altered small bowel microflora and increased absorption of endotoxin. Secondly, following external biliary drainage the secretion of bile is under an altered physiological drive, which may be modified by administration of oral bile salts. These aspects are considered below.

OTHER FUNCTIONAL EFFECTS

Hepatocyte function

It has already been noted that severe and prolonged biliary tract obstruction has effects on hepatocytes which may be reflected in gross biochemical abnormalities such as hypoalbuminaemia and unconjugated hyperbilirubinaemia. However, these are relatively non-specific and insensitive tests of 'liver function' and apart from their relationships with malnourishment and malignancy do not appear to have specific prognostic value. More recently the value of drugs as indicators of hepatic function has been recognized (Branch 1982) and the long-term objective must be to produce for hepatology the equivalent of the nephrologist's ability to measure renal blood flow, glomerular filtration rate and tubular function. Various approaches have been adopted. Elimination of aminopyrine by N-demethylation is a measure of hepatic microsomal function, and is a sensitive and quantitative indicator of liver dysfunction: its elimination may be estimated by breath analysis after oral administration of ^{14}C-aminopyrine, the aminopyrine breath test. Gill and his colleagues (1983) demonstrated that the aminopyrine breath test could predict the surgical risk in patients with known liver disease undergoing major surgery. Monroe and his colleagues (1982) also showed that the aminopyrine breath test reflects histological severity in patients with chronic hepatitis. Antipyrine (phenazone) is a minor analgesic which is eliminated by oxidation within the hepatocytes, and its clearance has been shown to correlate well with cytochrome P450 levels in the liver (McPherson et al 1982a). Because of the known effects on cytochrome P450 of obstructive jaundice, antipyrine elimination is a particularly appropriate means of assessing hepatic function in the jaundiced patient. Our studies show that antipyrine clearance was significantly impaired in patients with obstructive jaundice, and moreover that antipyrine clearance was better correlated with the subsequent rate of fall of plasma bilirubin following relief of obstruction than were standard liver function tests. Moreover, the degree of impairment of antipyrine clearance was significantly related to the risk of surgical mortality in a series of patients with obstructive jaundice (McPherson et al 1985).

Endotoxaemia and reticulo-endothelial function

Endotoxin is a lipopolysaccharide derived from the cell walls of gram negative bacteria present in the gut. Normally only minute amounts of endotoxin enter the portal circulation and these traces are cleared by the hepatic reticulo-endothelial system. In obstructive jaundice endotoxin has been found in the peripheral circulation in up to 50% of patients (Bailey 1976). Experimental evidence has shown that endotoxaemia is due to two principal factors: firstly, the absence of bile salts from the small intestine encourages endotoxin formation both by loss of a specific binding function of bile salts, and by alteration of the small bowel microflora; and secondly, to depressed reticulo-endothelial cell function within the liver, resulting in decreased clearance of absorbed endotoxin from the portal circulation. The first of these factors is further compounded by an actual increase in the rate of absorption from the intestine which can be demonstrated following administration of labelled endotoxin, probably due to increased vascular permeability (Ingoldby 1980). Circulating endotoxin has widespread pathological effects within the systemic circulation, which are reviewed elsewhere (Ch. 12, 31): these include renal vasoconstriction, redistribution of intra-renal blood flow away from the cortex and activation of complement, leucocytes, macrophages and platelets resulting in a tendency to disseminated intravascular coagulation.

External biliary drainage (Ch. 37) has not been shown to reduce the mortality from acute renal failure following surgery for obstructive jaundice, and this may be partly because it fails to correct the lack of bile salts in the small intestine. Administration of bile salts in rats (Bailey 1976) and in man (Cahill 1983) significantly reduced the incidence of endotoxaemia. However, the use of preoperative bowel preparation or of the anti-toxin polymixin B had no significant effect on endotoxaemia, although some changes in renal function were observed in each case (Hunt & Blumgart 1982, Ingoldby 1980). Gouma and his colleagues (1985) showed that endotoxaemia in rats with biliary obstruction was significantly reduced after *internal* biliary drainage, while both portal and systemic endotoxaemia persisted after external drainage. There is thus an increasing body of evidence to suggest the prime importance of bile salts in the gut in the management of patients with biliary obstruction. However, a controlled study from the Department of Surgery at Hammersmith Hospital of preoperative ursodeoxycholic acid administration in jaundiced patients showed a reduction in portal (but not systemic) endotoxaemia, but no significant effect on renal function or serum FDP levels, nor on the outcome of surgery. However, preoperative elevated FDP levels were associated with postoperative mortality (Thompson et al 1986). This subject is covered in greater depth in Ch. 12.

CHANGES AFTER RELIEF OF OBSTRUCTION

Following relief of biliary tract obstruction, whether surgical or by means of interventional radiological or endoscopic techniques, a return to normal biliary secretion, liver structure and function might be anticipated. However, these events do not occur at a predictable or constant rate, and the important features of each will be considered below.

Bile secretion

Bile secretion following relief of obstruction is best observed after insertion of an external percutaneous transhepatic biliary drain. There is frequently a prompt and major choleresis, and bile volumes may exceed four litres per day. Failure to replace the large fluid and electrolyte losses at this time may result in dehydration and electrolyte depletion with a metabolic acidosis. While sometimes this may necessitate intravenous fluid replacement, it may be sufficient to administer an oral electrolyte solution. The replacement of bile salts, if desired, may also be undertaken in the form of commercially available capsule preparations. While all of these results may also be achieved by encouraging patients to consume their own bile, the flavour being masked with stout or lager, we have found the majority of patients resistant to this method. Even nasogastric tube administration may result in biliary gastritis or oesophagitis.

During the first few days of biliary drainage the bile produced is of low bilirubin and bile salt concentration, although the total bilirubin and bile salt output may be high because of the large volume. This may partly be due to a slow return of the impaired liver to normal function, but also relates to loss of the enterohepatic circulation of bile salts. In experimental animals it has been shown that external diversion of biliary flow produces a decrease in the bile salt dependent canalicular flow within 30 minutes. This is promptly restored to normal by intravenous infusion of low concentrations of bile acids, which are taken up very rapidly from the plasma, 60–90% being cleared at the first passage through the liver (Heaton 1985). While it is known that bile salts thus stimulate the bile salt dependent component of canalicular flow, it is less widely appreciated that bile salts also stimulate more rapid excretion of bilirubin (Goresky et al 1974). We have examined this phenomenon in jaundiced patients following external tubal biliary drainage: oral administration of ursodeoxycholic acid in a dose of 300 mg four times daily gave rise not only to increased total bile flow but also to a reproducible increase in excretion of bilirubin and more rapid bilirubin clearance during the period of administration (Lewis et al 1986). This additional useful effect of oral bile salt administration may provide a further rationale for administration of bile salts in patients in whom external biliary decompression is necessary, and who have no endogenous intestinal bile salts.

Recovery of function

In the majority of cases, plasma bilirubin begins to fall promptly after insertion of a drainage catheter or an internal biliary bypass procedure and this is accompanied by clinical improvement. However, return of hepatocyte function to normal is not instantaneous. We examined plasma antipyrine clearance serially after surgical relief of obstructive jaundice in a group of patients in whom the clinical postoperative course was uncomplicated. The return of antipyrine clearance to normal was not seen until six weeks after relief of obstruction and the time taken to recover did not correlate well with other standard preoperative liver function tests nor with postoperative changes in these tests. Koyama et al (1981) have also suggested that preoperative biliary decompression may have to be continued for at least six weeks to allow recovery of hepatocellular function. Furthermore, excretion of antibiotics in the bile, severely impaired or even absent in the presence of total biliary obstruction, was still greatly reduced up to three weeks after external tubal drainage (Blenkharn et al 1985). Thus if the beneficial effects of preoperative biliary drainage in reducing the morbidity of subsequent surgery rely upon a return to normal hepatocyte function, a period of drainage of up to six weeks may be required to achieve this effect. There is no information on the equivalent time taken for return of reticulo-endothelial function.

These results apply to uncomplicated biliary obstruction, but other factors may have a further adverse influence on recovery. In dogs, infection of the obstructed biliary tract results in impaired biliary mannitol clearance and bilirubin UDP-glucuronyl transferase activity of the liver after relief of biliary obstruction (Higashino & Nagakawa 1985), so that pre-existing cholangitis may be a significant complicating factor. Moreover, in patients with severely impaired hepatic function following long-standing biliary obstruction, one should anticipate slow bilirubin clearance as well as impairment of the more subtle forms of hepatocyte function for many weeks after biliary decompression. This may be particularly important when relief of obstruction is accompanied by resection of liver tissue as in patients with obstructive jaundice due to hilar cholangiocarcinoma.

Structural changes

There has been little study of the physiology of the intra- and extrahepatic bile ducts after decompression. One study has demonstrated return to near normal bile duct diameter 24 hours after decompression by a variety of methods (Scudamore et al 1985). Certainly recent ultrasonographic experience suggests that the extrahepatic bile ducts may display rapid fluctuations in size with intermittent obstruction. However, it has not been our experience in patients with long-standing biliary obstruction to see a rapid return to normal diameter of the intrahepatic bile ducts. These bile ducts, which have been subject to oedema, inflammatory infiltration, cholangitis and fibrotic change, are likely to retain some rigidity for a considerable time after decompression. Indeed, there is evidence of continued poor emptying and intrahepatic ductal abnormalities on barium studies even several months after choledochoduodenostomy for long-standing biliary obstruction (Lygidakis 1981). In this study some patients had barium retained in the biliary tree up to one month after ingestion.

As regards reversal of intrahepatic fibrotic changes following drainage, it is difficult to obtain clear clinical evidence since this would rely upon serial liver biopsies in asymptomatic patients. Nevertheless, we have seen at least one patient with biliary obstruction and associated fibrosis in whom the fibrotic changes had resolved to normality on a subsequent biopsy. If such fibrotic changes, so long as they remain short of true secondary biliary cirrhosis, remain reversible by adequate drainage, then it is also possible that portal hypertension secondary to such fibrosis may be improved with adequate drainage and obviate the need for definitive treatment by portal-systemic shunting. Thus a reasonable approach in such difficult cases with long-standing obstruction and portal hypertension may be to ensure complete biliary decompression by the safest means and if necessary to treat associated varices by sclerotherapy, and to pursue an expectant policy in anticipation of a progressive fall in portal pressure as the liver changes resolve. Nonetheless, these patients with chronic biliary obstruction and supervening portal hypertension remain the highest risk group of patients with biliary obstruction, and pose both the most complex operative technical problems and the most difficult clinical decisions (Blumgart et al 1984).

REFERENCES

Bailey M E 1976 Endotoxin, bile salts, and renal function in obstructive jaundice. British Journal of Surgery 63: 774–778

Beinart C, Efremedis S, Cohen B, Mitty H A 1981 Obstruction without dilation. Importance in evaluating jaundice. Journal of the American Medical Association 245: 353–356

Benjamin I S 1983 Biliary tract obstruction. Surgical Gastroenterology 2: 105–120

Blamey S L, Feavon K C N, Gilmour W H, Osborne D H, Carter D C 1983 Prediction of risk in biliary surgery. British Journal of Surgery 70: 535–538

Blenkharn J I, Habib N, Mok D, John L, McPherson G A D, Gibson R, Blumgart L H, Benjamin I S 1985 Decreased biliary excretion of piperacillin following percutaneous relief of extrahepatic obstructive jaundice. Antimicrobial Agents and Chemotherapy 28: 778–780

Blumgart L H 1978 Biliary tract obstruction — new approaches to old problems. American Journal of Surgery 135: 19–31

Blumgart L H, Kelley C J, Benjamin I S 1984a Benign bile duct stricture following cholecystectomy: critical factors in management. British Journal of Surgery 71: 836–843

Blumgart L H, Benjamin I S, Hadjis N S, Beazley R M 1984b Surgical approaches to cholangiocarcinoma at the confluence of hepatic ducts. Lancet i: 66–70

Branch R A 1982 Drugs as indicators of hepatic function. Hepatology 2: 97–105

Bucher N L R, McGowan J A 1985 Regulatory mechanisms in hepatic regeneration. In: Wright R, Alberti K G M M, Karran S, Millward-Sadler G D T, (eds) Liver and biliary disease: Pathophysiology, diagnosis, management, 2nd edn. Saunders, London, Ch 11, p 251–265

Cahill C J 1983 Prevention of postoperative renal failure in patients with obstructive jaundice — the role of bile salts. British Journal of Surgery 70: 590–595

Carr D, Hadjis N S, Banks L, Hemingway A, Blumgart L H 1985 Computed tomography of hilar cholangiocarcinoma. American Journal of Radiology 145: 53–56

Desmet V J 1979 Cholestasis: extrahepatic obstruction and secondary biliary cirrhosis. In: MacSween R N M, Anthony P P, Scheuer P J (eds) Pathology of the liver. Churchill Livingstone, London, Ch 13, p 272–305

Dixon J M, Armstrong C P, Duffy S W, Davies G C 1983 Factors affecting morbidity and mortality after surgery for obstructive jaundice: a review of 373 patients. Gut 24: 845–852

Flannigan M 1986 Glucose metabolism in obstructive jaundice. (Data in preparation)

Gill R A, Goodman M W, Golfus G R, Onstad G R, Bubrick M P 1983 Aminopyrine breath test predicts surgical risk for patients with liver disease. Annals of Surgery 198: 701–704
Goresky C A, Haddad H H, Kluger W S, Nadleau B E, Bach G G 1974 The enhancement of maximal bilirubin excretion with taurocholate-induced increments in bile flow. Canadian Journal of Physiological Pharmacology 52: 389–403
Gouma D J, Goelho J C U, Fisher J D, Schlegel J F, Li Y F, Moody F G 1985 Endotoxaemia after relief of biliary obstruction by internal-external drainage in rats. Italian Journal of Surgical Science 15: 111
Hadjis N S, Benjamin I S, Blenkharn J I, Blumgart L H 1986 Anicteric presentation of hilar cholangiocarcinoma: anatomical and pathological observations. Digestive Surgery (in press)
Hall L, Bergen A, Henriken J E 1977 Blood flow in normal and cholestatic dogs as measured by intraparenchymal injection of Xenon-133. European Surgical Research 9: 357–363
Harry D S, Owen J S, McIntyre N 1985 Plasma lipoproteins and the liver. In: Wright R, Alberti K G M M, Karran S, Millward-Sadler G D T (eds) Liver and biliary disease: Pathophysiology, diagnosis, management, 2nd edn. Saunders, London, Ch 4, p 65–85
Heaton K W 1985 Bile salts. In: Wright R, Alberti K G M M, Karran S, Millward-Sadler G D T (eds) Liver and biliary disease: Pathophysiology, diagnosis, management, 2nd edn. Saunders, London, Chapter 13, p 277–299
Higashino Y, Nagakawa N 1985 Influence of biliary tract infection on bile secretion in dogs after relief from obstructive jaundice. Italian Journal of Surgical Science 15:111
Hunt D R 1979 Changes in liver blood flow with development of biliary obstruction in the rat. Australian and New Zealand Journal of Surgery 49: 733–737
Hunt D R, Blumgart L H 1982 Sodium homeostasis with obstructive jaundice: a randomized trial or preoperative bowel preparation. Chirurgia Epatobiliare 1: 99–102
Ingoldby C J H 1980 The value of polymyxin B in endotoxaemia due to experimental obstructive jaundice and mesenteric ischaemia. British Journal of Surgery 67: 565–567
Ingoldby C J H, McPherson G A D, Blumgart L H 1984 Endotoxaemia in human obstructive jaundice: effect of Polymixin B. American Journal of Surgery 144: 766–771
Jackaman F R, Hilson G R F, Lord Smith of Marlow 1980 Bile bacteria in patients with benign bile duct stricture. British Journal of Surgery 67: 329–332
Kaplan M M, Ohkubo A, Quaroni E G, Szetu D 1983 Increased synthesis of rat liver alkaline phosphatase by bile duct ligation. Hepatology 3: 368–376
Koyama K, Takagi Y, Ito K, Sato T 1981 Experimental and clinical studies on the effect of biliary drainage in obstructive jaundice. American Journal of Surgery 142: 293–299
Kune G A (ed) 1972 Current practice of biliary surgery. Little Brown, Boston
Lee E, Ross B D, Haines J R 1972 The effect of experimental bile-duct obstruction on critical biosynthetic function of the liver. British Journal of Surgery 59: 564–568
Lewis M H 1986 (Data in preparation)
Lygidakis N J 1981 Histological changes and intrahepatic biliary abnormalities in extrahepatic biliary tract obstruction. Surgery, Gynecology and Obstetrics 153: 532–536
McPherson G A D, Benjamin I S, Boobis A R, Brodie M J, Hampden C, Blumgart L H 1982a Antipyrine elimination as a dynamic test of hepatic functional integrity in obstructive jaundice. Gut 23: 737–738
McPherson G A D, Blenkharn J I, Nathanson B, Bowley N B, Benjamin I S, Blumgart L H 1982b Significance of bacteria in external biliary drainage systems: a possible role for antisepsis. Journal of Clinical Surgery 1: 22–26
McPherson G A D, Benjamin I S, Boobis A R, Blumgart L H 1985 Antipyrine elimination in patients with obstructive jaundice: a predictor of outcome. American Journal of Surgery 149: 140–143
Mathie R T, Blumgart L H 1972 Hepatic tissue perfusion studies during partial hepatectomy in man. Surgical Gastroenterology 1: 297–302
Monroe P S, Baker A L, Schneider J F, Krager P S, Klein P D, Schoeller D 1982 The aminopyrine breath test and serum bile acids reflect histologic severity in chronic hepatitis. Hepatology 2: 317–322
Nagorney D M, Mathie R T, Lygidakis N J, Blumgart L H 1982 Bile duct pressure as a modulator of liver blood flow after common bile duct obstruction. Surgical Forum 33: 206–208
Neale G, Lewis B, Weaver V, Panvelliwalla D 1971 Serum bile acids in liver disease. Gut 12: 145–152
Papageorgiou G, Lynn J A 1985 Physiology of the extrahepatic biliary tree. In: Wright R, Alberti K G M M, Karran S, Millward-Sadler G D T (eds) Liver and biliary disease: Pathophysiology, diagnosis, management, 2nd edn. Saunders, London, Ch 11, p 267–276
Price C P, Sammons H G 1974 The nature of the serum alkaline phosphatases in liver disease. Journal of Clinical Pathology 27: 392–398
Price C P, Alberti K G M M 1985 Biochemical assessment of liver function. In: Wright R, Alberti K G M M, Karran S, Millward-Sadler G D T (eds) Liver and biliary disease: Pathophysiology, diagnosis, management, 2nd edn. Saunders, London, Ch 18, p 455–493
Saharia P C, Zuidema G D, Cameron J L 1977 Primary common duct stones. Annals of Surgery 185: 598–604
Schaffner F, Javitt N B 1966 Morphologic changes in hamster livers during intrahepatic cholestasis induced by taurolithocholate. Laboratory Investigations 15: 1783–1966
Schaffner F, Bacchin P G, Hutterer F, Scharnbeck H H, Sarkozi L L, Denk H, Popper H 1971 Mechanism of cholestasis: 4. Structural and biochemical changes in the liver and serum in rats after bile duct ligation. Gastroenterology 60: 888–897
Schaffner F, Popper H 1985 Classification and mechanism of cholestasis. In Wright R, Alberti K G M M, Karran S, Millward-Sadler G D T (eds) Liver and biliary disease: Pathophysiology, diagnosis, management, 2nd edn. Saunders, London, Ch 15, p 359–386
Scudamore C H, Azad A, Cooperberg P 1985 The changes of the intra and extrahepatic bile duct diameter after decompression. Italian Journal of Surgical Science 15: 110
Sedgwick C E, Poulantzas J K, Kune G A 1966 Management of portal hypertension secondary to bile duct stenosis: review of 18 cases with splenorenal shunt. Annals of Surgery 163: 949–953
Smith, Lord 1978 Injuries of the liver, biliary tree and pancreas. British Journal of Surgery 65: 673–677
Strasburg S M, Dorne B C, Redinger R N, Small D N, Egdall R H 1971 Effect of alteration of biliary pressure on bile composition — a method for study: primate biliary physiology. V. Gastroenterology 61: 357–362
Thompson J N, Cohen J, Blenkharn J I, McConnell J S, Matkin J, Blumgart L H 1986 A randomized clinical trial of preoperative oral ursodeoxycholic acid in obstructive jaundice. British Journal of Surgery 73: 634–636
Way L W, Bernhoft R A, Thomas J M 1981 Biliary stricture. Surgical Clinics of North America 61: 963–972
Yokoi H 1983 Morphological changes of the liver in obstructive jaundice and its reversibility — with special reference to morphometric analysis of ultrastructure of the liver in dogs. Acta Hepatologica 24: 1381–1391

11

M. R. B. Keighley, J. I. Blenkharn

Infection and the biliary tree

Infection is still one of the most serious complications of operations on the biliary tract. Some infections, confined to a drain site or wound, may seem trivial. However, the serious complications of infection include septicaemia, liver abscess, hepatic and renal failure, endotoxaemia and disseminated intravascular coagulation and it is these which threaten the life of patients having surgical treatment for biliary disease.

The presence of bacteria in bile at the time of surgery or invasive diagnostic radiological procedures predisposes to septic complications. The judicious use of prophylactic antibiotics will significantly reduce morbidity and mortality due to infection. Prolonged antibiotic administration, e.g. throughout a period of external biliary decompression, can rarely be shown to sterilize heavily colonized bile and is of no proven value in the prevention of infection.

Septic complications are less frequently reported following invasive radiological procedures than following biliary surgery. However, fatal septicaemia has been recorded after percutaneous transhepatic cholangiography (PTC) and after endoscopic retrograde cholangiography. In both, the pathogenesis of septicaemia appears to be due to the introduction of contrast material under pressure into a heavily infected biliary tract. Intraperitoneal bile leakage following the percutaneous insertion of external biliary drainage catheters and endoprostheses occurs in up to 10% of patients. This may remain clinically silent but if bacteria are present in the bile this is a serious complication often requiring urgent surgical intervention and appropriate antibiotic therapy.

Patients with biliary disease may present for the first time with clinical signs of active infection. Local pain, fever and rigors are common presenting symptoms of acute cholecystitis, cholangitis and pyogenic abscess and these patients will benefit from full therapeutic courses of an appropriate antibiotic whether or not early surgical intervention is indicated. The selection of antibiotics for the treatment of active infection and for the prophylaxis of post-surgical sepsis is dependent upon the nature and sensitivity of the pathogens involved. In the vast majority of cases infection is due to bacteria originating from the biliary tract. The incidence and type of bacteria involved and their susceptibility to antibiotics can be accurately predicted and a suitable antibiotic regimen selected. Consideration should be given to the spectrum of activity, dosage and pharmacokinetics of the drug to be used. The route and timing of administration of antibiotics should also be considered, especially when these drugs are given for the prevention of post-surgical sepsis.

THE BACTERIOLOGY OF THE BILIARY TREE

Incidence of bacteria in the biliary tract

The reported incidence of bacteria in the bile is extremely variable ranging from 8–42% (Elkeles & Mirrizi 1942, Anderson & Priestley 1951, Flemma et al 1967, Watson 1969, Engstrom et al 1971, Maddocks et al 1973, Elliott 1980). The reasons for this enormous variation include the types of patients being studied and the use of antibiotics preoperatively. It is now well established that bacteria are more common in bile if the patient is jaundiced particularly if biliary obstruction is due to stones or a benign bile duct stricture. Infection is also more common in elderly patients and if there has been a recent acute attack of cholecystitis (Table 11.1). Bacteria are invariably present if there is an anastomosis between the bile ducts and the bowel. We have performed a comprehensive microbiological survey on the incidence of bacteria in the bile (Table 11.2). The greatest incidence of bacterial proliferation in the biliary tract occurred in patients with resolving acute cholecystitis, choledocholithiasis or stricture and in patients with a previous choledochoduodenostomy, with significantly lower numbers of bacteria in the bile of patients with malignant obstruction.

The incidence of bacteria throughout the biliary tree has been assessed at the General Hospital, Birmingham, by sampling material for microbiological study from the bile ducts, liver biopsies, gallbladder wall and cystic lymph

Table 11.1 Incidence of bacteria in bile according to biliary disease and age

Biliary pathology	% Positive bile cultures by age in decades <20yrs	20–30	30–40	40–50	50–60	60–70	70–80	>80yrs
Uncomplicated gallstones (n=412)	18	10	0	7	14	17	33	50
Acute cholecystitis (n=55)	0	0	—	23	36	70	33	100
Common duct stones, no jaundice (n=36)	—	66	66	25	80	55	0	66
Common duct stones, with jaundice (n=29)	—	0	0	20	50	—	100	100

Table 11.2 The incidence of bacteria in bile

	n	% positive bile culture
Acute cholecystitis (emergency operation)	29	82
Resolving acute cholecystitis	41	48
Mucocele of the gallbladder	17	29
Empyema of the gallbladder	14	34
Normal gallbladder with stones		
Age <50 yrs	42	11
50–70 yrs	37	13
>70 yrs	42	17
Choledocholithiasis	70	84
Benign bile duct stricture	86	90
Tumour of the distal common bile duct	45	29
High bile duct obstruction from malignancy	57	32
Previous choledochoduodenostomy	4	75
Previous hepaticojejunostomy Roux-en-Y	47	73

node, and from needle aspirates of duodenal contents (Fig. 11.1). When the lumen of the gallbladder was infected the bile ducts were invariably colonized by the same bacteria. In patients with bacteria in the gallbladder, organisms were also recovered from 80% of liver biopsy specimens, from 80% of duodenal aspirates, from the wall of the gallbladder in 88% of cases and from the cystic lymph node in 60%. Conversely, when the gallbladder bile was sterile so were all other sites in the biliary tract with the exception of the duodenum and the gallbladder wall (colonized by bacteria in 55% and 30% respectively).

Number and types of bacteria in infected bile

Most accounts of the bacterial isolates from patients with infected bile concur with one another (Edlund et al 1959, Mason 1968, Keighley 1977). The predominant organisms in bile are *Escherichia coli*, *Klebsiella* species and *Streptococcus faecalis* (Table 11.3). There is, however, some discrepancy in the literature on the isolation rate of anaerobic bacteria from bile. These differences can be partly explained by the techniques used to culture strict anaerobes and also by the selection of patients studied. Obligate anaerobes, particularly *Bacteroides fragilis*, *Bifidobacterium* species and *Fusobacterium* species appear to be extremely uncommon in Europe and in North America in patients with gallstones. On the other hand *B. fragilis* is commonly recovered after a previous biliary-enteric anastomosis particularly in the presence of a recurrent stricture (Elliott 1980).

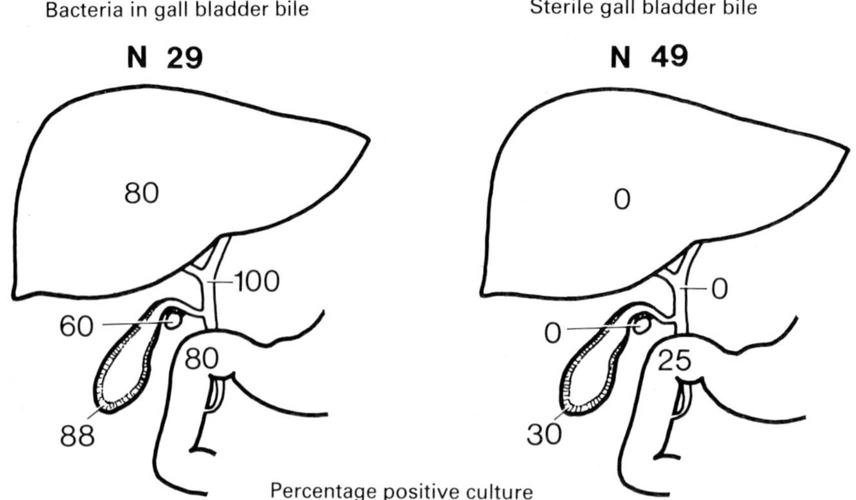

Fig. 11.1 The incidence of bacteria throughout the biliary tract in relation to the presence of infected gallbladder bile

Table 11.3 The frequency and type of bacteria in bile

	Malignant obstruction	Cholelithiasis	Benign Stricture	Previous bypass operation
Aerobic:				
Gram positive:				
Streptococcus faecalis	9 (9%)	51 (15%)	14 (13%)	6 (7%)
Viridans streptococci	4	12	3	4
Staphylococcus aureus	4	3	0	2
Staphylococcus epidermidis	2	5	1	7
Gram negative:				
Escherichia coli	28 (28%)	127 (37%)	31 (29%)	19 (21%)
Klebsiella aerogenes	15 (15%)	36 (10%)	15 (14%)	18 (20%)
Enterobacter species	4	10	4	5
Proteus species	5	19	8	2
Pseudomonas aeruginosa	6	5	5	9
others	7	14	7	6
Anaerobic:				
Gram positive:				
Clostridium perfringens	6 (6%)	29 (8%)	4 (4%)	5 (5%)
Clostridium species	2	4	1	0
Anaerobic cocci	3	19	1	2
Gram negative:				
Bacteroides fragilis	3 (3%)	6 (2%)	11 (10%)	7 (8%)
Bacteroides species	1	1	1	0
Fusobacterium species	1	4	1	0
TOTAL	100	245	107	92

Anaerobic bacteria can be recovered from bile following choledochoduodenostomy and Roux-en-Y hepaticojejunostomy in up to 30% of cases. Anaerobes are also common in the bile of patients with Asiatic cholangio-hepatitis and from liver abscesses is of biliary origin. Anaerobic cocci such as *Peptococcus* and *Peptostreptococcus* species are more common and *Clostridium* species, especially *Clostridium perfringens*, is well recognized as a frequent pathogen in acute acalculous cholecystitis and in chronic cholecystitis.

Bile is usually colonized by more than one organism and in our experience a single bacterial species was isolated in only 38% of patients with a positive bile culture. Two species were identified together in 29%, three species in 20%, four species occurred together in 12% and in a small proportion (1%) more than four different isolates were recovered from the bile.

The counts of bacteria in bile vary up to approximately 10^9 organisms per ml. The highest counts are usually found in the common bile duct but similar numbers of bacteria are also recovered from gallbladder bile and from infected T-tube bile (Fig. 11.2). It has been noted at the Surgical Hepatobiliary Unit, Hammersmith Hospital, that patients presenting with complete extrahepatic biliary obstruction, whether malignant or benign in nature, occasionally have extremely low counts of bacteria ($<10^2$ organisms per ml) in bile collected at the time of initial percutaneous transhepatic cholangiography. When obstruction is relieved either by insertion of a transhepatic drainage catheter or by definitive surgery, counts of bacteria in bile increase within a few days up to 10^8 to 10^9 organisms per ml. If results of the culture of bile collected at the time of PTC are to be used as a guide to antibiotic prophylaxis for subsequent surgical procedures (Peska 1980) laboratory techniques must be suitable for the recovery of these low numbers of organisms.

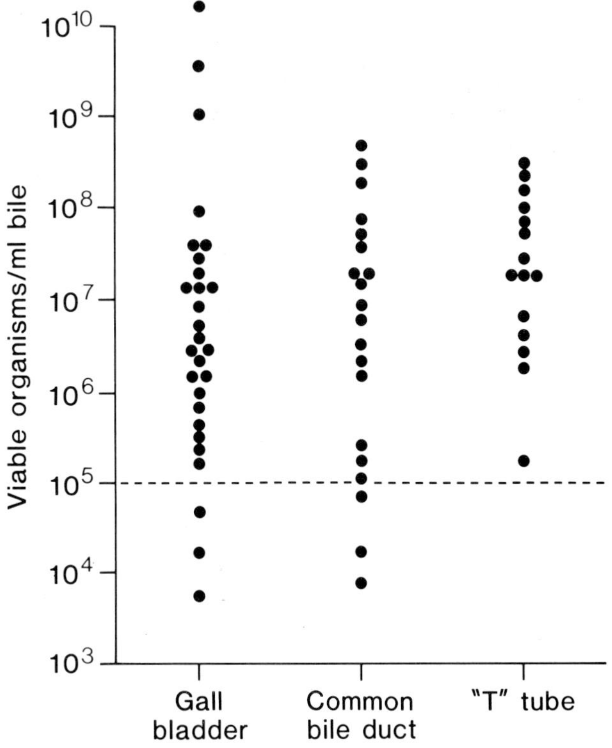

Fig. 11.2 Counts of bacteria from gallbladder, common bile duct and T-tube bile

Infected bile and post-operative sepsis

The close association between the presence of organisms in bile and infection following biliary surgery has been observed by many groups (Mason 1968, Edlund et al 1959) who have investigated the pathogenesis of post-surgical sepsis. The close correlation between positive bile cultures and the morphology of organisms recovered from infected wounds and positive blood cultures was demonstrated conclusively at the General Hospital, Birmingham, before prophylactic antibiotics were routinely used in biliary surgery (Fig. 11.3). 64% of wound infections and 90% of the episodes of bacteraemia occurring after biliary surgery were caused by an organism previously identified in the bile. When organisms were found in the bile at operation the incidence of wound sepsis (39%) and bacteraemia (20%) was significantly greater than in patients with sterile bile (11% and 3% respectively). The majority of wound infections in patients in whom the bile was sterile were staphylococcal and therefore presumably exogenous in origin. Episodes of bacteraemia in patients with sterile bile were either anaerobic and associated with coincidental appendicectomy or they occurred later in the postoperative period as a complication of T-tube drainage.

Incidence of postoperative sepsis

The principal postoperative infections associated with biliary surgery are wound sepsis, abscess and septicaemia. Respiratory infection is common but cannot be regarded as a specific complication of biliary surgery. The overall incidence of wound sepsis amongst patients undergoing biliary surgery in the General Hospital, Birmingham, between the years 1970–1973 when no antibiotic prophylaxis was used was 20% and there was a significantly higher incidence after emergency surgery (41%) than after elective operation (18%). In elective operations the incidence of wound sepsis was three times greater when choledochotomy was performed (31%) than after cholecystectomy alone (10%). Similarly the 12% incidence of bacteraemia during elective operations was significantly higher after exploration of the common bile duct than after cholecystectomy alone (1%). Bacteraemia was recorded before or after biliary surgery in 27 (6.2%) of 436 patients who were not receiving antibiotic cover. Five of these patients developed septicaemia within six hours of transhepatic cholangiography and in two patients septicaemia followed endoscopic retrograde cholangiography. Septicaemia was also recorded in two patients after choledochoscopy and in two others in whom an operative cholangiogram had demonstrated an impacted calculus in the distal common bile duct. There were also seven episodes of rigors and cholangitis after T-tube cholangiography. Of the 27 patients with bacteraemia nine developed endotoxic shock, complicated by acute renal failure in six, and five died. This represents an overall mortality from septicaemia in patients undergoing biliary surgery of 1.5%. The bacteria responsible for septicaemia are listed in Table 11.4 and are generally indistinguishable from those isolated concomitantly from bile.

Sepsis of biliary origin

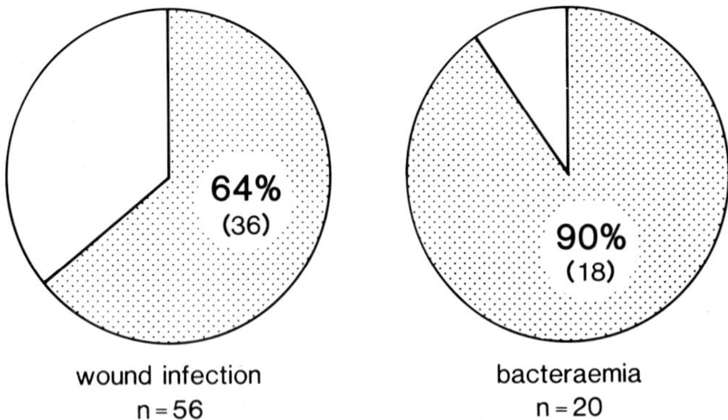

Fig. 11.3 The correlation of wound sepsis and bacteraemia in patients undergoing biliary surgery without antibiotics with the presence of bacteria in bile

Table 11.4 Aetiology of septicaemia

	Organisms isolated from blood culture	Same organism in the bile
Escherichia coli	28	26 (93%)
Klebsiella species	7	7 (100%)
Streptococcus faecalis	3	3 (100%)
Pseudomonas aeruginosa	1	1 (100%)
Serratia species	2	2 (100%)
Clostridium perfringens	2	2 (100%)
Bacteroides fragilis*	3	1 (33%)
TOTAL	46	42 (93%)

* Two patients had appendicectomy

Abscess occurred in only five of 181 patients (2%) who received no antibiotic cover; two cases occurred after emergency cholecystectomy for empyema of the gallbladder, one after a routine elective cholecystectomy and the remaining two after choledochotomy for stones.

BACTERIA IN BILE AFTER EXTERNAL BILIARY DRAINAGE

There has been recent interest in the role of external biliary drainage for patients with obstructive jaundice since it has been claimed that preoperative drainage may reduce the operative mortality in patients with profound jaundice. Postoperative decompression with T-tubes is widely used after exploration of the common bile duct. However, both of these procedures involve creating an external biliary fistula with a foreign body in the bile ducts. Some years ago it was shown that postoperative sepsis was more common following T-tube drainage and that many of these infections may have originated from bacteria in the external drainage system (Keighley & Graham 1971). Furthermore, septicaemia is still an occasional complication of T-tube cholangiography particularly if contrast material is introduced into the biliary tract under high pressure. For these reasons it is appropriate to consider the problems of bacteria in bile after external biliary drainage.

T-tube bile

The microflora of T-tube bile after choledochotomy was studied in 50 patients. Although the bile was infected in only 24 cases (48%) at the time of the operation, by the fifth postoperative day organisms were recovered from T-tube bile in 40 cases (80%). The bacteria recovered from T-tube bile frequently differed from those found in bile at the time of operation. 'New' organisms were recovered from the T-tube in 25 patients (50%) and in only 15 cases (30%) did the T-tube contain the same organisms as those previously isolated at operation. The 'new' bacteria found in the T-tube were intestinal organisms and not surface pathogens and it is probable that these new organisms were introduced through the drainage system. T-tube bile remained sterile in only 10 out of 50 patients (20%). Once bacteria colonized the T-tube they remained in the bile even though appropriate antibiotics were given (Keighley & Graham 1971). Hence once an external biliary drainage system becomes infected, these organisms are likely to persist despite antibiotic administration until the drainage tube is removed.

Preoperative percutaneous transhepatic drainage in malignant bile duct obstruction

At least two-thirds of patients with bile duct obstruction due to malignancy have a sterile biliary tract. Nevertheless, transhepatic biliary drainage catheters frequently become infected (Ch. 36, 37). Colonization of the biliary tract is a serious complication further predisposing to postoperative infective complications since the bacteria recovered from transhepatic drains are often of environmental origin and frequently resistant to many antibiotics.

In a consecutive study of 49 patients with obstructive jaundice undergoing preoperative percutaneous transhepatic biliary drainage the incidence of bacteria in bile at the time of insertion of the drainage catheter was 29% (Blenkharn et al 1984). At this time *E. coli* and *S. faecalis* were the most frequent isolates. Fifteen patients managed with a conventional open drainage system showed an increase to 100% positive bile cultures after 20 days' drainage (Table 11.5). In these cases, and in 16 patients managed with an open drainage system but incorporating a povidone-iodine antiseptic barrier to the collecting bag

Table 11.5 The influence of the type of drainage system on sepsis rates in patients with malignant obstructive jaundice undergoing preoperative percutaneous transhepatic drainage

	Type of drainage system		
	Open	Open plus antiseptic	Closed
Positive bile culture			
at initial PTC	6/15 (40%)	4/16 (25%)	4/18 (22%)
after 20 days drainage	14/14 (100%)	6/12 (50%)	5/18 (28%)
at operation	11/13 (85%)	7/11 (64%)	5/14 (36%)
Positive blood culture			
preoperative	7/15 (47%)	3/12 (25%)	1/18 (6%)
postoperative	9/13 (69%)	3/11 (27%)	1/14 (7%)
Positive wound culture	11/13 (85%)	9/11 (82%)	3/14 (21%)

there was a two-fold decrease in positive bile cultures (McPherson et al 1982), the additional organisms being of proven environmental origin. Towards the end of the drainage period the isolation rates of *Klebsiella aerogenes* and *Pseudomonas aeruginosa* had increased whilst that for *E. coli* and *S. faecalis* remained unchanged. There was unequivocal evidence of exogenous colonization of these systems with *K. aerogenes* and *P. aeruginosa* first appearing in the contents of the collecting bag and later being recovered from the proximal connecting tube also. This high incidence of positive bile cultures after a period of external decompression was associated with increased rates of bacteraemia both pre- and postoperatively and of wound sepsis. The subsequent development and introduction of an entirely closed biliary drainage system (Blenkharn et al 1981) enabled 18 patients to be drained for up to 36 days preoperatively with the acquisition of 'new' organisms in the bile of only one patient (Table 11.5). The use of this new closed drainage system (Fig. 11.4) in the management of patients undergoing preoperative percutaneous transhepatic biliary drainage was associated with a significant reduction in the incidence of bacteraemia pre- and post-

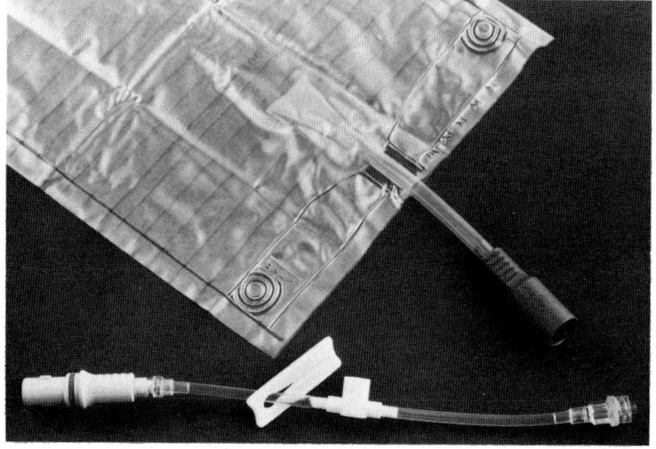

operatively and in the rate of wound infection. Furthermore, selection of prophylactic antibiotics for subsequent surgical procedures was not complicated by the acquisition of antibiotic resistant 'hospital strains' of aerobic gram negative bacteria.

The Hammersmith closed biliary drainage system is flexible and can be successfully employed with a wide variety of external drainage tubes including T-tubes and transanastomotic stents. Single-use, odour-proof collecting bags enable easy and safe disposal of potentially infected bile. Attachment to the drainage tube is via a unique twist-action, bayonet-fitting slit valve (Fig. 11.5) which seals automatically on removal of the bag. A multiple-use injection port has been incorporated in the upper part of the drainage tube to enable the introduction of X-ray contrast medium and saline flushing solutions should this be necessary without prejudice to the integrity of the closed system. Patient acceptance has been good and many patients adequately manage their own drainage system with some returning home during the period of preoperative decompression. Subsequent studies of this new closed biliary drainage system in the Hammersmith Hospital Surgical Hepatobiliary Unit confirm the value of closed drainage in the prevention of septic complications associated with external biliary drainage in over 100 high risk patients.

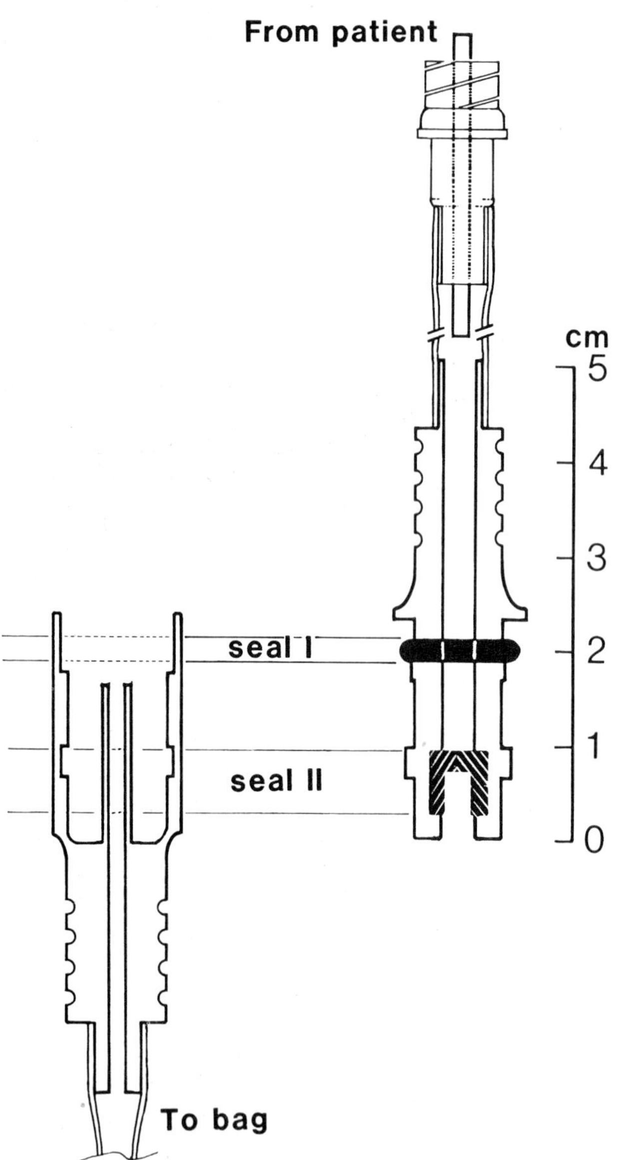

Fig. 11.5 Twist-action, bayonet-fitting slit valve incorporated in the Hammersmith closed drainage system (see also Fig. 11.4)

ANTIBOTICS IN BILIARY SURGERY

Principles of antibiotic therapy

It is important to differentiate antibiotic therapy from antibiotic prophylaxis. The term prophylaxis is quite inappropriate if there is established infection, for instance in patients requiring operations for acute cholecystitis, cholangitis and subhepatic or intrahepatic abscess associated with biliary disease. By contrast, patients having operations where bacteria may be disseminated from the biliary tract deserve to be protected from the postoperative infections which may occur as a consequence of endogenous intraoperative bacterial contamination. The dose, timing and duration of antibiotic administration for prophylaxis differs from their use in the therapy of established infection and for this reason they will be considered separately.

Therapy

For therapeutic purposes, an antibiotic must penetrate inflamed tissues and there should be a normally functioning immune mechanism. A therapeutic antibiotic should be bactericidal and preferably excreted in bile as well as providing adequate plasma and tissue concentrations. It is an advantage if the agent is weakly bound to protein since penetration of abscesses is facilitated if the antibiotic is freely diffusible (Wise 1981). It is also desirable to use an antibiotic with a narrow spectrum of activity provided the pathogen is known or can be accurately predicted.

It is necessary to prescribe a therapeutic antibiotic for a number of days (usually at least five) so that there is complete penetration of the infective process allowing repair to occur without further bacterial invasion. The duration of antibiotic administration will need to be longer if host defences are impaired as for distance in neutropenic patients, patients with poor hepatic or renal function, in immunosuppressed patients and in those with severe nutritional depletion. Prolonged antibiotic therapy may also be necessary in rare cases if the infective process is walled off and where prompt surgical drainage is contra-indicated.

The therapeutic agent should be non-toxic and have minimal side effects. It is particularly important to avoid agents such as the first generation cephalosporins which may give rise to renal failure when used with a diuretic, since jaundiced patients are at increased risk from developing renal damage. By the same token, the indiscriminate use of aminoglycosides is to be avoided, not only because of the risks of toxicity to the kidney and VIIIth cranial nerve but also because they may interfere with non-depolarizing muscle relaxants. Chloramphenicol would not be advised for general usage because of the risk of bone marrow depression. Similarly, newer broad spectrum agents such as cefoxitin would not be advised because of the risk of antibiotic-associated pseudomembranous colitis.

Finally it is desirable to choose an antibiotic which may be prescribed by the systemic as well as the oral route since parenteral therapy may not be necessary for more than a few days, whereas the antibiotic may need to be continued for longer.

Prophylaxis

The term prophylaxis is applicable only if there is no active preoperative infection by micro-organisms in tissues. For this reason only a single dose of antibiotic is generally necessary since the aim of prophylaxis is to provide high plasma and tissue levels of antibiotic at the time of risk of endogenous bacterial contamination from the bile (Keighley & Burdon 1979). Since only one or two doses of antibiotic are necessary it is possible to prescribe very high doses of an agent without the fear of toxicity.

The purpose of antibiotic prophylaxis is to prevent infection with bacteria liberated into the circulation from the operation site and it is mandatory that blood and tissue antibiotic levels are adequate when the operation is being performed. Furthermore as septicaemia is the complication which is most feared by biliary surgeons operating on the jaundiced patient it is crucial that the plasma antibiotic concentration should be at least five times greater than the minimum inhibitory concentrations for most biliary pathogens.

Routes of administration

There is a variety of routes for antibiotic administration. Oral antibiotics such as neomycin and metronidazole may be given for two or three days before operation in an attempt to suppress faecal flora (Arabi et al 1978). Such a regimen is popular in colorectal surgery and it has a theoretical application in operations for obstructive jaundice. It has been suggested that the endotoxaemia common in obstructive jaundice and associated with renal failure may be due to abnormal absorption of endotoxin from the colon due to the absence of intraluminal bile salts (Bailey 1976). Attempts to suppress the faecal flora might therefore reduce the risk of endotoxin release in jaundiced patients. This practice has not been widely accepted and it may be of dubious clinical benefit. Studies in animals (Ingoldby 1980) highlight the role of polymyxin B in the protection against endotoxaemia. Oral administration of polymyxin B was shown to afford greater protection than parenteral administration possibly due to intraluminal binding of endotoxin prior to absorption from the gut. An alternative and possibly more attractive approach is to administer oral bile salts preoperatively. This has been shown to prevent endotoxin absorption and to improve renal function (Evans et al 1982). However, the role of oral polymyxin B and bile salt administration in the protection against the clinical manifestations of endotoxaemia remains unproven and warrants further study. Certainly, with the possible exception of polymyxin B, the oral administration of antibiotics is not advised for prophylaxis against infection since the aim is to provide high blood levels at the time of surgery.

The intravenous route is to be preferred to intramuscular injection since this achieves much higher and predictable blood levels. It is also an advantage to use an antibiotic with long half-life since the use of an antibiotic rapidly excreted by the kidneys will be associated with insufficient plasma levels after three to four hours. These considerations are particularly important for patients requiring prolonged operations and it is generally advised that, if the procedure extends beyond four hours or if an excessive blood loss occurs, a second dose of antibiotic should be used. There are some who still consider that topical antibiotics have a place in biliary surgery. Topical agents may be used in the peritoneal cavity or in the incision. Antibiotic irrigation of the peritoneal cavity may be dangerous since some agents are rapidly absorbed and can reach toxic levels in the plasma (Ericsson et al 1978). Intra-incisional antibiotics are certainly extremely effective at reducing wound sepsis (Finch et al 1979). However since the antimicrobial is administered too late they do not therefore protect against septicaemia and intra-abdominal abscess (Hares et al, 1981). Moreover, topical antimicrobials may encourage the development of bacterial resistance. There have, however, been some interesting recent developments regarding the use of topical antibiotics, principally by the technique of pre-incisional infiltration of the wound before operation. Two recent trials report very low rates of wound sepsis when this technique has been used (Armstrong et al 1982, Taylor et al 1982).

The following policy of antibiotic prophylaxis is advised:

Choose a safe intravenous antibiotic with low protein binding and with a long half-life.

Give the antibiotic intravenously in the anaesthetic room just before the operation and repeat the antibiotic dose if the operation takes more than four hours.

No further antibiotics are recommended, since single

dose prophylaxis has been shown to be as good as (if not a little better than) five-day cover (Strachan et al 1977).

Use a big dose of antibiotic.

If someone has forgotten to give the antibiotic it is pointless giving antibiotics postoperatively since their use will not protect patients from postoperative sepsis (Stone et al 1976).

Antibiotics cannot be expected to provide a bad surgeon with good results. Every effort must therefore be made to prevent spillage of infected bile, the operative field should be packed away from the rest of the abdomen, there must be efficient haemostasis to avoid haematoma, tissues should be handled gently, non-absorbable suture materials should be avoided whenever possible and if gross contamination occurs it may be advisable to leave the skin and subcutaneous tissues open.

Antibiotic sensitivities

In patients undergoing elective surgery who have never had a previous biliary operation the principal pathogens which are likely to be encountered are *E. coli*, *Klebsiella* species, *S. faecalis* and staphylococci. Many clinicians do not consider that *S. faecalis* is a pathogen since it is infrequently isolated from blood culture and is rarely associated with monomicrobial postoperative sepsis (Watson 1969). Staphylococci certainly play an important role in the pathogenesis of wound sepsis amongst diabetic patients. If on the other hand the patient requires an emergency operation for acute cholecystitis, cholangitis or an abscess or if there is a history of previous biliary surgery (particularly with an anastomosis between the bile ducts and the small bowel), then other important pathogens are likely to be encountered. These include *Proteus* species, *Peptostreptococcus* species, *C. perfringens* and occasionally *B. fragilis*.

Four groups of antimicrobials are potentially useful in biliary surgery: penicillins, cephalosporins, aminoglycosides and the sulphonamides. Most early penicillins had a narrow spectrum of activity and, with the exception of flucloxacillin, were unstable to beta-lactamases. The newer agents such as a mecillinam, mezlocillin, piperacillin and ticarcillin are active against most of the aerobic gram negative organisms likely to be encountered in bile but they are generally not suitable for coagulase positive staphylococci. The ureido-penicillins have been particularly effective in biliary surgery and seem to be free from serious side effects. The earlier cephalosporins such as cephaloridine or cephazolin have a wide range of activity and most aerobic biliary pathogens including staphylococci are sensitive. The newer third generation cephalosporins such as cefotaxime, moxalactam, ceftriaxone, and cefotetan are very active against gram negative aerobes but are less active against staphylococci. In addition some of these agents are effective against the anaerobes likely to be isolated from infected bile. Hence these are valuable agents for the management of the high risk biliary patients already referred to. It is a universal feature of cephalosporin antibiotics that none has significant in vivo activity against *S. faecalis*. Whilst this may have little significance in the management of patients undergoing elective cholecystectomy, serious sepsis due to *S. faecalis* may occur in other groups of patients. Over a three-year period 64 episodes of bacteraemia were recorded in patients undergoing treatment for obstructive jaundice (Blenkharn & Blumgart 1984). Fifteen (23%) of these episodes were due to *S. faecalis* and in all cases the biliary tract was the source of bacteraemia. Septic episodes followed PTC in two patients and the percutaneous insertion of an endoprosthesis across a malignant bile duct stricture in a further two, despite antibiotic prophylaxis with cephalosporin plus aminoglycoside antibiotics. Six patients had bacteraemia in the immediate postoperative period and in five bacteraemia followed tube cholangiography. Other organisms, such as *E. coli*, *K. aerogenes* and *P. aeruginosa*, were isolated from the bile of all but one of these patients concomitantly with *S. faecalis*, although none other than *S. faecalis* was isolated from blood cultures. This represents therefore a significant gap in the spectrum of activity of both cephalosporin and aminoglycoside antibiotics and protection may be afforded by the addition of ampicillin or the substitution of a ureido-penicillin such as piperacillin.

The aminoglycosides such as gentamicin, tobramycin and amikacin are no longer recommended for prophylaxis and should be reserved for life threatening aerobic gram negative infections since they are nephrotoxic unless carefully monitored. Furthermore they have no activity against anaerobes. However, considerable synergy between the aminoglycosides and ureido-penicillins has been observed (Kuck & Redin 1978). Patients undergoing extensive surgical procedures and with a history of previous biliary surgery in whom large numbers of bacteria are inevitably present in bile may benefit from combined prophylaxis with these agents. The sulphonamides have been popular in Scandinavia and in combination with trimethoprim (as cotrimoxazole) provide a useful safe agent for prophylaxis in routine elective operations (Morran et al 1978).

Pharmacokinetics

Reference has already been made to certain desirable pharmacokinetic properties such as low protein binding, long half-life, rapid bactericidal activity and good tissue penetration, but the question of biliary excretion has not been considered. Clearly it is desirable, particularly in patients with cholangitis or those undergoing surgery, to have therapeutic level of antibiotic in the bile both to eliminate bacteria from bile and to minimize postoperative sepsis (Bevan & Williams 1971). However, the majority of patients with infected bile have obstructive biliary disease and in these patients it is unlikely that adequate biliary levels of antibiotic can be achieved.

To determine the influence of biliary excretion on prophylactic antibiotic therapy we performed a controlled trial in 150 consecutive patients undergoing biliary operations (Keighley et al 1976a). Patients were allocated to one of three antibiotic groups: gentamicin (an antibiotic with high plasma but low bile levels), no antibiotic or rifamide (an antibiotic excreted almost entirely into the bile). Samples of the bile and blood were collected at operation for antibiotic assay and the concentration of gentamicin or rifamide necessary to inhibit each biliary isolate was determined. The concentration of gentamicin sufficient to inhibit over 80% of organisms in the bile was 2 mg/l. Therefore, twice this figure (4 mg/l) was considered to provide 'adequate' levels of gentamicin in patients with biliary disease. 'Adequate' levels of gentamicin were found in the bile in only two cases (4%) whereas 'adequate' plasma concentrations were present in almost 90% of patients.

Conversely over 80% of the organisms in the bile were inhibited by 31 mg/l rifamide. For this reason twice the level (62 mg/l) was regarded as an 'adequate' concentration for patients with biliary disease. Plasma levels of rifamide were invariably too low to be of therapeutic value and although extremely high bile levels were achieved in most patients in whom there was no evidence of obstruction to the biliary tract, 'adequate' levels were present in only two out of 12 patients with obstructive biliary disease (17%). Hence although high concentrations of rifamide are normally achieved in the bile, for patients with biliary obstruction in whom there is a high risk of infection, both plasma and bile levels of the antibiotic were too low to be of therapeutic value. It is hardly surprising therefore that recovery of organisms in bile was not influenced by either antibiotic and that a significant reduction in postoperative sepsis was demonstrated only in the patients receiving the antibiotic (gentamicin) with satisfactory plasma level (Table 11.6). Hence antibiotics which achieve satisfactory plasma levels are more reliable in patients with obstructive biliary disease than those which are excreted almost entirely into the bile. Similar observations have been recorded with all pharmacokinetic studies of antibiotic excretion in bile. The high risk patients are those with obstruction and, even if the antibiotic in question is normally excreted in high concentration in bile, insufficient biliary levels are always reported when there is obstructive biliary disease (Sales et al 1972, Morris et al 1983). For most clinical situations it is desirable to use an antibiotic which provides both high plasma as well as high bile levels. Cephazolin and piperacillin are good examples of such agents (Table 11.7) and ones which clinical trials have confirmed for their efficacy (Strachan et al 1977, Morris et al 1983).

Table 11.6 The relative importance of adequate plasma levels rather than bile levels of antibiotic in biliary surgery

	Control (n=50)	Gentamicin (n=50)	Rifamide (n=50)
Wound sepsis	11	3*	5
Bacteraemia	7	1*	

* $p < 0.05$

Selection of patients requiring antibiotics in biliary surgery

It has been argued that it is both inappropriate and undisciplined to give antibiotics to all patients having a biliary tract operation since the bile contains organisms in only a third of patients. Abuse of antibiotics will inevitably lead to the emergence of resistant strains. These arguments seemed appropriate until it became clear that a single dose of antibiotic is sufficient for prophylaxis. The problem of emergence of resistance using only a single high dose of antibiotic seems remote and a case could therefore be made for the use of a single dose antibiotic regimen for all patients. Nevertheless there are those who would wish to confine prophylaxis to patients with bacteria in the bile.

The clinical risk factors associated with infected bile have been well described. When we undertook a multi-

Table 11.7 Aetiology of postoperative sepsis following biliary surgery despite prophylactic antibiotics

	Control (n=100)	Gentamicin (n=50)	Rifamide (n=50)	Cephazolin (n=50)	Mecillinam (n=50)	Piperacillin (n=50)
Streptococcus faecalis	4	2	—	—	3	—
Viridans streptococci	1	—	—	—	2	—
Staphylococci	6	—	2	1	4	1
Escherichia coli	18	—	3	1	4	—
Klebsiella species	8	2	1	—	1	—
Proteus species	2	1	1	—	—	—
Pseudomonas aeruginosa	1	—	—	—	—	—
Acinetobacter species	—	—	—	1	—	—
Anaerobes	4	—	—	1	—	—
TOTAL	44	5	7	4	14	1

Table 11.8 Factors significantly associated with infection in bile: results of a multivariate analysis

Preoperative:	Patients over 70 years
	Obstructive jaundice
	Recent cholangitis
	Re-operation on the biliary tract
	Emergency operation
	Operation within one month of acute cholecystitis
Operative:	Bile duct obstruction
	Choledocholithiasis

variate analysis (Keighley et al 1976b) eight factors were found to be significantly more common in the patients with infected bile than in patients with a sterile biliary tract; these factors are listed in Table 11.8. Methods of detecting the presence and type of organisms in the bile include gram stains on material aspirated from the gallbladder at the beginning of the operation or preoperative duodenal aspirates after cholecystokinin. Gram stains on bile may be accurate in 77% of patients (McLeish et al 1980) but it is technically demanding and if an antibiotic policy is based upon these findings most patients will receive their first dose of antibiotic near the completion of the operation which is after potential bacterial inoculation and therefore too late. Murray & Bradley (1983) have recently compared routine preoperative prophylaxis with selective practice based on gram stain results of bile and found that wound sepsis rates were higher in the gram stain groups probably because the antibiotic was generally given near the end of the operation when the results of the gram stain were first known.

A study is currently in progress to compare the use of a single dose of mezlocillin in all patients with the selective use of mezlocillin given only to patients with one or more of the following preoperative criteria: emergency operation; jaundice; age over 70 years; recent cholangitis; re-operation; known bile duct calculi. To date 151 patients have entered the study. There have been two episodes of septicaemia in each group and the rate of wound sepsis has been 4% when mezlocillin has been given to all patients compared with 16% when selective prophylaxis with mezlocillin has been used. Similarly duodenal aspirates (Keighley & Burdon 1978) or bile collected during ERCP (Hatfield et al 1982) may be used to detect patients with organisms in bile who may require subsequent antibiotic prophylaxis. These procedures carry their own risk, are unpleasant for the patient and results may be confused by the normal flora of the duodenum.

Prophylactic antibiotics and radiological techniques

Patients undergoing certain endoscopic and invasive radiological diagnostic procedures will benefit from the prophylactic administration of antibiotics immediately prior to the procedure. Endoscopic retrograde cholangiopancreatography is not frequently associated with proven bacteraemic episodes (Low et al 1980), the greater hazard appearing to be due to nosocomial infection from contaminated endoscopes. However cholangitis was recorded in 72 of 8681 patients (0.8%) reported by Bilbao et al (1976) and was significantly more common in patients with obstruction. The administration of a single dose of an appropriate antibiotic to these patients immediately prior to the procedure seems advisable.

Percutaneous transhepatic cholangiography (PTC) is associated with occasionally severe septic complications and the routine use of prophylactic antibiotics has been recommended (Flemma & Shingleton 1966). In the Hammersmith Hospital Hepatobiliary Unit a single dose of antibiotic has proved successful in most cases although occasionally therapeutic antibiotic administration has been required for up to five days. Many of the septic complications of PTC are related to increased intrabiliary pressure following the introduction of contrast material (Huang et al 1969). This is also seen during T-tube cholangiography in the postoperative period (Dellinger et al 1980) and prophylaxis should be used even if contrast is injected with manometric control. The removal of T-tubes may be associated with extravasation of infected bile into the tissues surrounding the tube tract and, since minor septic episodes are common, all patients should be afforded the protection of a single dose of antibiotic.

Therapeutic hepatic artery embolisation or ligation in the treatment of irresectable malignancy is often followed by a period of pyrexia. This is rarely associated with proven sepsis although the possible presence of ischaemic or frankly necrotic liver tissue represents a considerable risk and necessitates prolonged administration of antibiotics for up to 10 days.

Results of controlled trials

It would be an impossible task to review all of the antibiotic trials in biliary surgery (Chetlin & Eliott 1973, Keighley et al 1975) but a variety of studies confined to patients having biliary surgery are reviewed in Table 11.9. The cephalosporins have been universally successful provided they are given preoperatively although consideration must be given to the relative resistance of pseudomonas and faecal streptococci which may be important pathogens in patients with more complex biliary pathology. It is beyond the scope of this chapter to discuss the relative merits of all available antimicrobial agents, since the choice of agents changes each year and their relative merits become apparent only after extensive usage. Clinicians are bombarded by detailed in vitro microbiological data claiming advantages of one drug against another but with little clinical support for claims of superiority. Fortunately the choice of a prophylactic agent is not crucial provided that the drug is active against the organ-

Table 11.9 Antibiotic prophylaxis in biliary operations (results of controlled trials)

Agent	Reference	Patients	Duration	Administration	Number	% Sepsis Treated	Control
Rifamide	Bevan & Williams 1971	All	3 days	Preop IM	61	3	19
Cephaloridine	Chetlin & Elliott 1973	All	5 days	Preop IM	84	4	27
Gentamicin	Keighley et al 1975	All	5 days	Preop IM	98	7	22
Cephazolin	Stone et al 1976	All	1 dose	12 hours preop IM		5	
				1 hour preop IM	131	4	22
				1–4 hours postop IM		17	
Cephazolin	Strachan et al 1977	All	1 dose	Preop IM		3	
			5 days	Preop IM	201	5	17
Cotrimoxazole	Morran et al 1978	All	1 dose	Preop IV	95	4	21

isms likely to be encountered in bile. However care must be exercised in the choice of therapeutic agents. A failure to respond indicates an incorrect choice of antibiotic or the need for surgical drainage of pus or decompression of an obstructed biliary tract.

FUTURE PROBLEMS OF INFECTION IN BILIARY SURGERY

It is appropriate to review the persistent morbidity and mortality from infection found in a consecutive group of 118 patients having an operation for obstructive jaundice (Keighley et al 1984), all of whom had received single dose antibiotic prophylaxis with cephazolin and oral mannitol as an osmotic diuretic during their operation (Table 11.10). It was surprising to find a high rate of wound sepsis particularly in patients with malignant obstructive jaundice (13%). Many of these patients were diabetic and developed staphylococcal infections. More alarming was the 7% incidence of septicaemia with three fatal cases, two of whom were having an operation for common bile duct stones. It would seem that in jaundiced patients and particularly in the compromised host (such as the patient with diabetes or malignant disease) it is wise to prolong antibiotic cover for up to five days. The clinical trials quoted earlier (Table 11.9) consist largely of patients having elective cholecystectomy and for whom single dose prophylaxis appears to be eminently satisfactory.

Table 11.10 Morbidity of biliary surgery in jaundiced patients all of whom received pre-operative cephazolin and mannitol (1975–1979)

	Total (n=118)	Malignant (n=55)	Non-malignant (n=63)
Wound sepsis	12	7 (13%)	5 (9%)
Septicaemia	7	3 (6%)	4 (7%)
Abscess	2	0	2 (3%)
Mortality (all causes)	10	6 (11%)	4 (7%
Mortality from sepsis	3	1	2

CONCLUSIONS

Sepsis is an important complication of operations and interventional endoscopic or radiographic procedures in biliary disease. The majority of infections originate from organisms in the bile and the predominant pathogens are *E. coli*, *Klebsiella* species and staphylococci. However *Proteus* species, *Peptostreptococcus* species, *C. perfringens* and occasionally *B. fragilis* may be identified in patients with acute cholecystitis, cholangitis or after previous biliary operations. For routine elective biliary surgery, systemic administration of a single dose of cephazolin or a ureidopenicillin such as piperacillin, to all patients before operation has been shown to reduce morbidity. For patients with established infection five-day antibiotic therapy should be employed using a ureidopenicillin or a newer broad spectrum cephalosporin such as moxalactam or cefotaxime. Jaundiced patients without established infection might also benefit from this approach of extended administration of antibiotics.

REFERENCES

Anderson R E, Priestley J T 1951 Observations on the bacteriology of choledochal bile. Annals of Surgery 133: 486–489

Arabi Y, Dimock F, Burden D W, Alexander-Williams J, Keighley M R B 1978 Influence of bowel preparation and antimicrobials on colonic microflora. British Journal of Surgery 65: 555–559

Armstrong C P, Taylor T V, Reeves D S 1982 Pre-incisional intraparietal injection of cephamandole: a new approach to wound infection prophylaxis. British Journal of Surgery 69: 459–460

Bailey M E 1976 Endotoxin, bile salts and renal function in obstructive jaundice. British Journal of Surgery 63: 774–778

Bevan P G, Williams J D 1971 Rifamide in acute cholecystitis and biliary surgery. British Medical Journal 3: 284–287

Bilbao M K, Dotter C T, Lee G T, Katon R M 1976 Complications of endoscopic retrograde cholangiopancreatography (ERCP). Gastroenterology 70: 314–320

Blenkharn J I, Blumgart L H 1985 Streptococcal bacteraemia in

hepatobiliary surgery: implications for prophylaxis. Surgery, Gynecology and Obstetrics 160: 139–141
Blenkharn J I, McPherson G A D; Blumgart L H 1981 An improved system for external biliary drainage. Lancet 2: 781–782
Blenkharn J I, McPherson G A D, Blumgart L H 1984 Septic complications of percutaneous transhepatic biliary drainage: evaluation of a new closed drainage system. American Journal of Surgery 147: 318–321
Chetlin S H, Elliott D W 1973 Pre-operative antibiotics in biliary surgery. Archives of Surgery 107: 319–232
Dellinger E P, Kirschenbaum G, Weinstein M, Steer M 1980 Determinants of adverse reaction following post-operative T-tube cholangiogram. Annals of Surgery 191: 397–403
Edlund Y A, Mollstedt B O, Ouchterlony O 1959 Bacteriological investigations of the biliary system and liver in biliary tract disease correlated to clinical data and microstructure of the gallbladder and liver. Acta Chirurgica Scandanavica 116: 461–476
Elkeles G, Mirrizzi P L 1942 A study of the bacteriology of the common bile duct in comparison with other extrahepatic segments of the biliary tract. Annals of Surgery 116: 306–366
Elliott D W 1980 Prevention of sepsis in biliary surgery. In: Karran S (ed) Controversies in surgical sepsis. Praeger, Sussex p 285–291
Engstrom J, Hellstrom K, Hogman L, Lonngvist B 1971 Microorganisms of the liver, biliary tract and duodenal aspirates in biliary diseases. Scandinavian Journal of Gastroenterology 6: 177–182
Ericsson C D, Duke J, Pickering L K 1978 Clinical pharmacology of intravenous and intraperitoneal aminoglycoside antibiotics in prevention of wound infection. Annals of Surgery 188: 66–69
Evans H J R, Torrealba V, Hudd C, Knight M 1982 The effect of pre-operative bile salt administration on post-operative renal function in patients with obstructive jaundice. British Journal of Surgery 69: 706–708
Finch D R A, Taylor L, Morris P J 1979 Wound sepsis following gastrointestinal surgery: A comparison of topical and two dose systemic cephradine. British Journal of Surgery 66: 580–582
Flemma R J, Shingleton W W 1966 Clinical experience with percutaneous transhepatic cholangiography. American Journal of Surgery 111: 13–19
Flemma R J, Flint L M, Osterhunt S, Shingleton W W 1967 Bacteriological studies of biliary tract infection. Annals of Surgery 116: 563–572
Hares M M, Hegarty M A, Warlow J et al 1981 A controlled trial to compare systemic and intraincisional cefuroxime prophylaxis in high risk gastric surgery. British Journal of Surgery 68: 276–280
Hatfield A R W, Leung T, Ahmet Z, Williams J D 1982 the microbiology of direct bile sampling at the time of endoscopic retrograde cholangiopancreatography. Journal of Hospital Infection 4: 119–125
Huang T, Bass J A, Williams R D 1969 The significance of biliary pressures in cholangitis. Archives of Surgery 98: 629–632
Ingoldby C J H 1980 The value of polymixin B in endotoxaemia due to experimental obstructive jaundice and mesenteric ischaemia. British Journal of Surgery 67: 565–567
Keighley M R B 1977 Micro-organisms in the bile. Annals of the Royal College of Surgeons of England 59: 329–334
Keighley M R B, Graham N G 1971 Infective complications of choledochotomy with T-tube drainage. British Journal of Surgery 58: 764–769
Keighley M R B, Baddeley R M, Burdon D W et al 1975 A controlled trial of parenteral prophylactic gentamicin therapy in biliary surgery. British Journal of Surgery 62: 275–179
Keighley M R B, Drysdale R B, Quoraishi A H, Burdon D W, Alexander-Williams J 1976a Antibiotics in biliary disease: The relative importance of antibiotic concentrations in the bile and serum. Gut 17: 495–500
Keighley M R B, Flinn R, Alexander-Williams J 1976b Multivariate analysis of clinical and operative findings associated with biliary sepsis. British Journal of Surgery 63: 528–531
Keighley M R B, Burdon D W 1978 Identification of bacteria in the bile by duodenal aspiration. World Journal of Surgery 2: 255–259
Keighley M R B, Burdon D W 1979 Antimicrobial prophylaxis in surgery. Pitman Medical, London
Keighley M R B, Razay G, Fitzgerald M 1984 Influence of diabetes on mortality and morbidity following operations for obstructive jaundice. Annals of the Royal College of Surgeons of England 66: 49–51
Kuck N A, Redin G S 1978 In vitro and in vivo activity of piperacillin, a new broad spectrum semisynthetic penicillin. Journal of Antibiotics 31: 1175–1182
Low D E, Micflikier A B, Kennedy J K, Stiver H G 1980 Infectious complications of endoscopic retrograde cholangiopancreatography: A prospective assessment. Archives of Internal Medicine 140: 1076–1077
McLeish A R, Keighley M R B, Bishop H M et al 1980 Selecting patients requiring antibiotics in biliary surgery by immediate Gram stains of bile at operation. Surgery 81: 473–477
McPherson G A D, Blenkharn J I, Nathanson B, Bowley N B, Benjamin I S, Blumgart L H 1982 The significance of bacteria in external biliary drainage systems: A possible role for antisepsis. Journal of Clinical Surgery 1: 22–26
Maddocks A C, Hilson G R F, Taylor R 1973 The bacteriology of the obstructed biliary tract. Annals of the Royal College of Surgeons of England 52: 316–319
Mason G R 1968 Bacteriology and antibiotic selection in biliary surgery. Archives of Surgery 97: 533N–537
Morran G, McNaught W, McArdle C S 1978 Prophylactic cotrimoxazole in biliary surgery. British Medical Journal 2: 462–464
Morris D L, Mojaddedi Z J, Burdon D W, Keighley M R B 1983 Clinical and microbiological evaluation of piperacillin in elective biliary surgery. Journal of Hospital Infection 4: 159–164
Murray W R, Bradley J A 1983 Antibiotic prophylaxis in elective biliary tract surgery. Research and Clinical Forums 5: 97–101
Peska D N 1980 The role of percutaneous transhepatic cannulation in pre-operative and intra-operative evaluation of biliary flora. Journal of the American Osteopathic Association 79: 479–481
Sales J E L, Sutcliffe M, O'Grady F 1972 Cephalexin levels in human bile in the presence of biliary tract disease. British Medical Journal 3: 441–443
Stone H H, Hooper C A, Kolb L D, Geheber C E, Dawkins E J 1976 Antibiotic prophylaxis in gastric, biliary and colonic surgery. Annals of Surgery 184: 443–450
Strachan C J, Black J, Powis S J et al 1977 Prophylactic use of cephazolin against wound sepsis after cholecystectomy. British Medical Journal 1: 1245–1256
Taylor T V, Walker W S, Mason R C, Richmond J, Lee D 1982 Pre-operative intraparietal (intra-incisional) cefoxitin in abdominal surgery. British Journal of Surgery 69: 461–462
Watson J F 1969 The role of bacterial infection in acute cholecystitis, a prospective clinical study. Military Medicine 134: 416–426
Wise R 1981 Pharmacokinetics and tissue fluid penetration: The relevance to elective surgical prophylaxis. In: Herfarth C, Horn J, Daschner F (eds) Aktuelle Probleme in Chirurgie und Orthopadie. Verlag Hans Huber, Berne, p. 15–20

Endotoxins, the liver and haemostasis

In this chapter the importance of endotoxin in the development of liver and biliary tract disease and its complications is reviewed with particular reference to surgical practice. The nature, effects and measurement of endotoxin and the results of experimental and clinical studies of endotoxaemia in liver disease are described. The pathophysiology of endotoxaemia and the possible methods for prevention and treatment are discussed. In the second part of the chapter the current concepts of the normal haemostatic mechanisms and their disturbance in liver disease are reviewed. This is followed by a discussion of the role of endotoxin in the development of these abnormalities of haemostasis and the diagnosis and management of these conditions in clinical practice.

ENDOTOXIN IN LIVER AND BILIARY TRACT DISEASE

Endotoxin — structure and biological activity

Since the early experiments of Parnum in the 19th century demonstrated the toxic properties of a boiled extract of putrid material injected into dogs (Parnas 1976) a vast amount of work has been devoted to the characterization of endotoxin and the study of its biological properties. Despite this extensive effort and the demonstration of a wide range of harmful biological activities, the exact role of endotoxin in the pathogenesis of human disease remains uncertain.

Endotoxin forms the major component of the outer cell wall of gram-negative bacteria and is released spontaneously as well as on bacterial death. Endotoxin is ubiquitous in the external environment and found in high concentrations in the gastrointestinal tract. It is a complex lipopolysaccharide (Morrison & Ulevitch 1978) consisting of three major components: the inner Lipid A portion, an intermediate R-core oligosaccharide, and the outer O-polysaccharide portion (Fig. 12.1). The structure of the O-polysaccharide portion is unique for each strain of organism and forms the strongly immunogenic 'O' antigen. The R-core oligosaccharide is exposed in 'rough' mutant strains, it is often identical for several groups of bacteria and is less antigenic than the O-polysaccharide. The composition of the Lipid A portion varies little between bacterial species. The toxic properties of endotoxin appear largely confined to the Lipid A portion which is poorly antigenic (Morrison & Ulevitch 1978).

The major biological actions of endotoxin are listed in Table 12.1. The multiple experimental observations on which these actions are based require cautious interpretation because of the considerable variation in the toxicity of endotoxin with different methods of extraction, the gram-negative bacteria of origin, the animal model used, the in vivo or in vitro nature of the experiment and the development of endotoxin tolerance. Because of this wide range of biological activities there is often difficulty in separating the direct and indirect effects of endotoxin, and many of the observed biological responses are probably

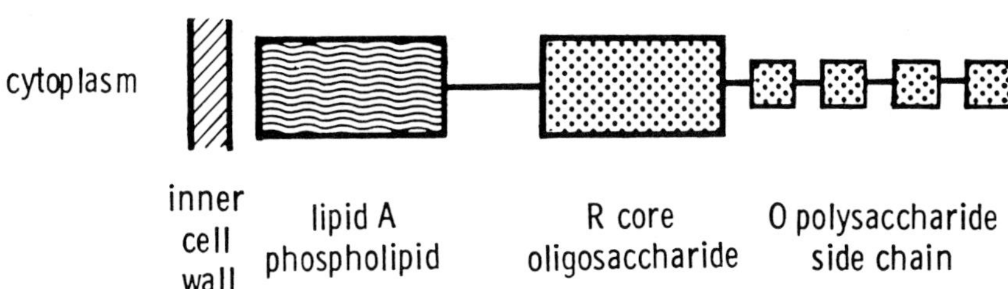

Fig. 12.1 A schematic diagram of the structure of endotoxin, which forms the outer cell wall of gram-negative bacteria

Table 12.1 Biological actions of endotoxin

1. Fever
   indirect effect via endogenous pyrogen release from leucocytes
   direct effect on hypothalamus
2. Haemodynamic effects
   a. vasoconstriction
      direct effect
      secondary sympathetic neurogenic
      catecholamine release
   b. vasodilatation
      secondary to tissue hypoperfusion caused by vasoconstriction, endothelial injury and reduced cardiac output produces pooling of blood in pulmonary and splanchnic vascular beds with hypotensive shock
3. Endothelial cell injury
   probable direct cell membrane damage
4. Intravascular coagulation
   direct intrinsic and extrinsic pathway activation
   two sequential injections in rabbits produce generalized Sanarelli-Shwartzman reaction with disseminated intravascular coagulation and bilateral renal cortical necrosis
5. Complement activation (antibody independent)
   classical pathway activation (Lipid A)
   alternative pathway activation (polysaccharide)
6. White blood cell effects
   transient leucocytopaenia followed by leucocytosis
   neutrophil activation
   monocyte stimulation and release of mediators
   basophil/mast cell release of vasoactive substances, e.g. histamine, serotonin, kinins (probably indirect)
7. Platelet effects
   platelet aggregation and release of active constituents (species dependent — probably not in man)
   thrombocytopaenia, probably secondary to platelet aggregation and intravascular coagulation
8. Activation of reticulo-endothelial system
   probably direct effect on tissue macrophages
9. Immunological effects
   specific B cell antibody response to endotoxin antigens especially potent 'O antigen'
   non-specific polyclonal B cell stimulation
   T cell/macrophage regulation of antibody responses
10. Endocrine & metabolic responses
    raised plasma growth hormone, ACTH, and cortisol
    increased lipolysis with raised plasma free fatty acid levels
    alterations in carbohydrate metabolism
11. Organ specific injury
    especially lung and liver
    probably largely secondary to vascular effects

secondary phenomena. A direct toxic effect on cell membranes may underlie many of the multiple effects of endotoxin. Man is particularly sensitive to endotoxin and observations in human subjects have been limited (Wolff 1973). Experimental models using intravascular injections of endotoxin have produced a variety of end organ injuries which were probably caused by a combination of direct parenchymal toxicity and secondary anoxic damage following vascular injury and haemodynamic responses. The liver and lung have shown particular vulnerability to endotoxin injury, possibly because of their large reticulo-endothelial functional capacity, which appears to play an important role in the uptake and detoxification of endotoxin (Mori et al 1973). Morphological studies of endotoxin induced liver damage in Rhesus monkeys have shown early margination of neutrophils and mononuclear cells in the microcirculation, followed by phagocytosis of endotoxin by sequestered leucocytes and Kupffer cells. Degranulation of neutrophils and fragmentation of sequestered leucocytes and Kupffer cells later occurred. The hepatic sinusoids and spaces of Disse showed extensive fibrinous deposits and subsequent centrilobular and mid-zonal necrosis was seen (Balis et al 1978). Using an isolated perfused rat liver model, endotoxin has been shown to reduce hepatic flow when perfused with plasma and buffy coat cells (Filkins 1969) and to reduce bile flow and bromsulphthalein excretion probably by affecting hepatocyte excretory mechanisms (Utili et al 1976). Endotoxin acts as a stimulant of reticulo-endothelial function. There is evidence that endotoxin absorbed from the gastrointestinal tract plays a role in the development of cirrhosis in animal models (Nolan 1975) although little convincing evidence exists for a role in the development of human cirrhosis (Lancet 1982).

While extrapolation of these experimental observations

to various clinical conditions associated with hepatic disease or bacteraemic shock produces attractive hypotheses, the relevance of these observations remains uncertain largely because of the difficulties in reliably assaying endotoxaemia and the lack of an effective specific anti-endotoxin therapy

Measurement of endotoxin

The development of the sensitive Limulus amoebocyte lysate assay (Levin & Bang 1968), which is based on the activation of a proenzyme in the coagulation system of the horseshoe crab (*Limulus polyphemus*), has facilitated routine testing for endotoxin. This assay has now largely replaced the previous bioassays which used a variety of end points but particularly the febrile response produced in rabbits following endotoxin injection.

The specificity of the Limulus amoebocyte lysate assay has been challenged and activation and inhibition by a variety of agents have been reported (Stumacher et al 1973, Suzaki 1977). However the assay appears a reliable and reproducible measure of endotoxin contamination of products intended for clinical use (Weiss 1979). It has proved clinically reliable in the detection of endotoxin from gram-negative organisms in biological fluids other than plasma. The assay of endotoxin in blood using this method has been complicated by the presence of plasma inhibitors which have been only partially defined but include esterases, protease inhibitors and immunoglobulins and there are conflicting reports of its use in the assessment of clinical endotoxaemia (Elin & Wolff 1976). These discrepancies may also be in part due to the, at best, semiquantitative nature of the gelation end point used in the original Limulus assays. Modifications of this assay including acid treatment and chloroform extraction (Yin 1975) have been reported but combinations of heating and dilution of plasma are now favoured to limit the effects of plasma inhibitors. The use of a chromogenic substrate has increased the sensitivity of these assays which can now measure endotoxin quantitatively into the range of picograms per millilitre (Webster 1980, Harris et al 1983, Cohen & McConnell 1984). The variable activation of Limulus amoebocyte lysate by gravimetrically equal amounts of endotoxin from different bacterial species and residual difficulties with plasma inhibitors and activators, which vary considerably between individual patients (Cohen & McConnell 1984), still pose problems and make direct comparisons between different patients, or even different bacteraemic or endotoxaemic episodes in the same patient, somewhat unreliable. The use of a standard reference endotoxin may overcome some of these difficulties. However, despite these problems, the newer Limulus assays are providing the opportunity for a further and more accurate assessment of the importance of endotoxaemia in many clinical situations (Harris et al 1984) including hepatic and biliary disease.

Alternative methods for assessing endotoxin are available but are generally limited to experimental work. Attempts to develop a radio-immunoassay for endotoxin have been disappointing, mainly because of the high variability of the potent 'O' antigens and the poor antigenicity of the less variable Lipid A portion. The use of immunofluorescent and immunoperoxidase techniques to follow the time distribution of administered endotoxin using a specific bacterial preparation has been described (Freudenberg et al 1982). Radioactively labelled endotoxin (Braude et al 1955) has also been used experimentally to show endotoxin distribution after intravenous injection and following absorption from the gastrointestinal tract. In addition a characteristic electron microscopic appearance for endotoxin has been described allowing study of its cellular localization in animal models of endotoxic shock (Balis et al 1978). The core polysaccharides of endotoxin contain a unique deoxy-sugar (2-keto, 2-deoxy, octulosonate — KDO) and the Lipid A portion an unique fatty acid (beta-hydroxymyristic acid), and this allows biochemical determination of endotoxin in relatively high concentrations (Maitra et al 1981).

Endotoxaemia in human liver disease

Despite the difficulties in measuring endotoxin in plasma specimens using the Limulus amoebocyte lysate assay, there is considerable evidence to suggest that systemic endotoxaemia is a common phenomenon in patients with cirrhosis, acute hepatic failure, severe viral hepatitis and obstructive jaundice (Lancet 1982, Liehr & Jacob 1983). The incidence of endotoxaemia in fulminant hepatic failure appears to correlate with the severity of the disease, and the development of renal failure and intravascular coagulation (Wilkinson et al 1974). In patients with cirrhosis the incidence of endotoxaemia is higher in those with ascites, renal impairment, portal-systemic collaterals and following LeVeen shunting (Tarao et al 1977, Wilkinson et al 1976, Liehr & Jacob 1983), and endotoxaemia is associated with a reduced survival (Tarao et al 1977). The presence of raised levels of antibodies against endotoxin and gram-negative bacteria in the sera of patients with cirrhosis has been regarded as supportive evidence for endotoxaemia, although this may not necessarily be the case (Lancet 1982). These antibodies may not only be protective but also reduce the sensitivity of the Limulus assay (Leihr & Jacob 1983).

Endotoxaemia in patients with obstructive jaundice is particularly relevant to surgical practice. The high post-operative morbidity and mortality still seen in these patients (Blamey et al 1983, Dixon et al 1983) may be, at least in part, related to perioperative portal and systemic endotoxaemia (Bailey 1976). Several clinical studies have been reported using different Limulus assay methods and they are detailed in Table 12.2. There is a large variation in the incidence of preoperative systemic endotoxaemia ranging from 15% to 70% in different series, but peroperative portal and per- and postoperative systemic endotoxaemia appears to occur in a majority of patients with obstructive jaundice. Four of these series have compared jaundiced and non-jaundiced control patients and found a significantly lower incidence of systemic endotoxaemia in all control groups, with the exception of the series reported by Hunt et al (1982). Bailey (1976) found that endotoxaemia was associated with a serum bilirubin above 144 μmol/l, but Ingoldby et al (1984) found no correlation with the depth of jaundice. Wilkinson et al (1976), Bailey (1976) and Cahill (1983) have found perioperative endotoxaemia to be significantly associated with postoperative renal impairment, although this was not so in the series reported by Ingoldby et al (1984). Preoperative systemic endotoxaemia alone was significantly associated with postoperative mortality in one series (Ingoldby et al 1984) and in a second (Hunt et al 1982) when combined with the presence of raised preoperative serum fibrin degradation products. Hunt et al (1982) found a significant association between endotoxaemia and raised serum fibrin degradation products in jaundiced and non-jaundiced patients but this finding was not confirmed by Ingoldby et al (1984).

Taken together these series show that systemic endotoxaemia is common in patients with major liver disease and suggest that this may play an important role in morbidity and mortality. The relevance of endotoxaemia to the coagulopathy and the renal impairment seen in these patients is discussed further in this chapter and in Chapter 31.

Pathophysiology of endotoxaemia in liver disease

There is considerable experimental and clinical evidence to support the theory that the systemic endotoxaemia seen in liver disease is caused by an increased absorption of enteric endotoxin into the portal venous system and a reduced hepatic reticulo-endothelial clearance.

While the incidence of portal endotoxaemia may be increased in patients with hepatic disease it also occurs in patients with normal liver function (Prytz et al 1976, Jacob et al 1977) and indeed low grade portal endotoxaemia without bacteraemia is probably a normal occurrence. Experimental evidence has shown that increased endotoxaemia resulting from absorption of enteric endotoxin occurs in a variety of animal models including superior mesenteric artery occlusion (Cuevas & Fine 1971), intravenous infusion of vasoactive amines (Cuevas & Find 1973), haemorrhagic shock (Ravin et al 1960), obstructive jaundice (Bailey 1976) and total biliary fistula (Kocsar et al 1969). The reduced secretion of bile salts into the intestine may contribute to the endotoxaemia of liver disease, particularly obstructive jaundice (Kocsar et al 1969, Bailey 1976, Iwasaki 1982). The importance of other factors effecting enteric endotoxin absorption including the local amount of anti-endotoxin IgA secretion from liver and intestine, non-specific changes in mucosal permeability and alterations in the enteric content of endotoxin is unknown. Endotoxin in blood undergoes a series of reactions

Table 12.2 Endotoxaemia in obstructive jaundice

Series	serum bilirubin (μmol/l)	% malignant cases	jaundiced patients: peripheral venous endotoxaemia	jaundiced patients: peroperative portal endotoxaemia	non-jaundiced control patients: peripheral venous endotoxaemia	non-jaundiced control patients: peroperative portal endotoxaemia
Wilkinson et al 1974	>340	—	0/7(0%)	—	—	—
Wardle 1974	—	—	4/16(25%)preop 11/15(73%)postop	—	— —	—
Wilkinson et al 1976 +	>150	50%	6/12(50%)	—	—	—
Bailey 1976 *	> 50	79%	13/24(54%)	16/24(67%)	0/16(0%)	0/16(0%)
Iwasaki et al 1980	—	—	9/27(33%)	—	—	—
Iwasaki et al 1982â	—	—	15/53(28%)	—	—	—
Hunt ét al 1982	> 40	61%	4/27(15%)preop	—	2/14(14%)preop	—
Cahill 1983	—	75%	14/22(64%)	12/22(55%)	2/24(8%)	5/24(21%)
Ingoldby et al 1984	> 75	70%	19/27(70%)preop 23/26(88%)postop	19/26(73%)	1/12(8%)preop 1/12(8%)postop	1/12(8%)

\+ Selected series, all 6 patients with endotoxaemia had renal failure and 4 had gram-negative infection
* 3 patients with endotoxaemia had gram-negative infection
^Samples from 37 patients

involving ill-defined plasma factors and high density lipoprotein which results in partial inactivation (Ulevitch et al 1979) and alterations of these reactions may occur in liver disease.

The liver is the major site of endotoxin uptake and detoxification after intravenous injection in animals with normal liver function (Freudenberg et al 1982, Mori et al 1973, Filkins 1971) and Wolter et al (1978) have shown experimentally a much greater clearance from the portal vein than the hepatic artery. In patients with obstructive jaundice there is reduced hepatic reticulo-endothelial function (Drivas et al 1976) and Ingoldby has shown reduced liver but significantly increased splenic and renal uptake of radioactively labelled endotoxin after enteric administration to rats following four weeks of obstructive jaundice. Reduced hepatic reticulo-endothelial function has been associated with endotoxaemia in patients with cirrhosis (Tarao et al 1977). Obstructive jaundice increases sensitivity to intravenous endotoxin (Wardle & Wright 1970) and there is some evidence of increased hepatic toxicity following endotoxin administration in cirrhosis (Liehr et al 1975). This and other data support the contention that an increased portal endotoxaemia of enteric origin and reduced hepatic clearance allows detectable systemic endotoxaemia. While the majority of patients with liver disease and systemic endotoxaemia have no clinical or microbiological evidence of gram-negative bacterial infection, this may be the origin of the endotoxaemia in some of these patients, who have impaired immunity as well as reduced hepatic reticulo-endothelial function.

Prevention and treatment of endotoxaemia

A variety of treatments have been tested experimentally and a few tried clinically in an attempt to reduce the incidence of endotoxaemia or to protect against its toxic effects. These attempts may be divided into those measures aimed at preventing the development of endotoxaemia, those designed to neutralize endotoxin within the circulation and others used to prevent its secondary damaging effects.

The use of prophylactic antibiotics in patients with liver and biliary tract disease is effective in reducing postoperative gram-negative sepsis and thus the development of potential sources of endotoxaemia. Early antibiotic and surgical treatment of established infections is similarly desirable. Specific measures to reduce the amount of endotoxin available for absorption from the gastrointestinal tract have been tried in patients with obstructive jaundice following early encouraging experimental work (Kocsar et al 1969, Cuevas & Fine 1973, Bailey 1976). In a randomized controlled trial Hunt et al (1982) showed no benefit from careful mechanical bowel preparation and oral neomycin for three days prior to surgery in patients with obstructive jaundice when assessed by perioperative endotoxaemia, coagulation disturbance, or mortality. However Cahill (1983) has reported benefit in terms of endotoxaemia and postoperative renal function in eight patients with obstructive jaundice treated for 48 hours preoperatively with oral sodium deoxycholate, which is thought to directly bind endotoxin in the bowel lumen preventing absorption. A similar approach using bentonite and other adsorbents to reduce endotoxaemia following serotonin injection in mice by binding enteric endotoxin has been reported (Ditter et al 1983).

Neutralization of endotoxin in the blood has been attempted with limited success. Immune therapy against endotoxin is complicated by the wide range of O antigens. Some success has been claimed using the J5 anticore antiserum (Ziegler et al 1982) but this is not yet widely available for the treatment of gram-negative bacteraemia or endotoxic shock. Polymixin B, an antibiotic which appears to have an additional direct anti-endotoxin effect, has been shown experimentally to protect against endotoxin (From et al 1979, Ingoldby 1980) but a recent trial of perioperative polymixin B infusion in patients with obstructive jaundice failed to show any benefit (Ingoldby et al 1984). The prospect of successful removal of plasma endotoxin by haemoperfusion appears limited (Maitra et al 1981).

A variety of drugs have been shown to protect against endotoxic damage in different animal models. These agents generally act against the secondary mediators of endotoxic shock and there is at present particular interest in the possible role of steroids, opiate antagonists and modification of the prostaglandin and thromboxane systems (Holaday & Reynolds 1983, Coker et al 1983). Their relevance to clinical practice is as yet not clear.

Although several groups have described encouraging results it may be concluded that at present there is no specific therapy of established efficacy against the endotoxaemia seen in patients with liver disease.

HAEMOSTASIS IN LIVER DISEASE

A general view of haemostasis

Impairment of haemostasis is common in liver disease. Haemorrhage may cause clinical problems in these patients, and is sometimes life-threatening. More frequently, haemostatic abnormalities are monitored to assess liver function. For these reasons disturbances of haemostasis are of great interest to surgeons and physicians managing patients with hepatic disease. The remainder of this chapter is devoted to a summary of these disturbances and the role of endotoxin in their development.

Haemostasis can be regarded as a complex system of sequential interactions among various functional components, as follows:

1. vascular/endothelial phenomena
2. platelet activation

3. plasma enzyme reactions leading to fibrin formation
4. fibrin stabilization
5. fibrinolysis.

These steps will not be analyzed here in detail as they are fully described in standard text books. Rather, we shall briefly review events normally occurring in vivo following a minor vascular lesion, emphasizing a few aspects that are often disregarded when haemostasis is considered as a sequence of separated events.

The first phenonemon that occurs when blood escapes from a vessel is platelet adhesion to subendothelial collagen. A single layer of platelets is rapidly formed. The platelets are immediately 'activated' (i.e. their membrane exposes acidic phospholipids on its outer surface) and the arachidonic acid pathway is triggered, leading to endoperoxide formation, and to the local release of vasoactive, aggregating and procoagulant substances. Moreover, at an early stage tiny amounts of thrombin are formed on the platelet surface, where all the coagulation factors are bound and topographically arranged in an optimal conformation for coagulation to take place.

The adherent platelet layer causes vasoconstriction and platelet aggregation which is mediated by endoperoxide and thrombin. Platelet aggregation amplifies all the above events, since aggregation is always associated with 'activation'. Thus, more endoperoxide and thrombin are formed. When the amount of thrombin produced reaches the critical point, fibrin is formed and is immediately stabilized by platelet-released factor XIII. A clot forms, and bleeding stops. Inside the vessel, excessive extension of platelet aggregation and of fibrin formation are prevented by blood flow and by inhibiting substances (e.g. prostacyclin, alpha-2-macroglobulin).

In this simplified view of haemostasis, many details have been neglected. However, a number of the dynamic aspects of haemostasis will now be emphasized.

The central role of platelets

Although plasma coagulation can be studied in vitro in the absence of platelets, in vivo platelets play a central role in every step of haemostasis (Walsh 1974) (Table 12.3). Indeed, in addition to the better known platelet functions (adhesion, aggregation and release), platelets contribute in an important way to plasma coagulation in vivo. In the presence of ADP, platelets are able to activate factors XII and XI (contact product forming activity — Walsh 1972a); if collagen is present, platelets can directly activate factor XI (collagen-induced coagulant activity — Walsh 1972b). However, the most important platelet procoagulant activity has been termed PF3. It is possible that this activity is entirely due to membrane acidic phospholipids that are exposed on the outer part of the platelet surface through a membrane modification following platelet 'activation' by a non-endothelial surface (Jackson 1981). Platelet activated membrane offers an ideal surface for enzyme reactions to occur, since there are specific receptors on the membrane for all coagulation factors. This produces a number of consequences:

1. Plasma coagulation factors are tenaciously bound to the lesion site, and cannot be washed out by blood flow.

2. Coagulation factors are concentrated at the lesion site by virtue of being bound to platelets and the amount of individual factors bound to the aggregated platelets bears little relationship to their respective plasma levels (which may be as low as 5%–10% of normal without causing excessive bleeding).

3. When bound to the platelet surface, coagulation factors are in their optimal conformation for interacting with all other reactants. It has been calculated, for instance, that the activity of platelet-bound factor Xa is increased by about 50 000 times when compared to its activity in a platelet-free medium (Miletich et al 1978).

4. Binding to platelets protects most factors from plasma inactivators. For instance, factor Xa cannot be inactivated by the complex heparin-antithrombin III if it is bound to the platelet surface (Walsh & Biggs 1972) or to a phospholipid-factor V complex (Marciniak 1973).

5. Some factors are also released from platelet internal granules (e.g. factor V, fibrinogen, factor XIII), thus further increasing their local concentration.

6. Finally, the strength of the fibrin network is considerably increased when platelets are present at nodal points. In the clot, fibrin interacts preferentially with platelets, compared with red and white cells (Doolittle 1981).

Table 12.3 Functions of platelets in haemostasis in vivo

Adhesion to the injured vessel wall
Aggregation
Release of aggregating and vasoactive substances
Synthesis of endoperoxides
Factors XII and XI activation, in the presence of ADP
Direct factor XI activation, in the presence of collagen
Supply of acidic phospholipids (PF3)
Supply of coagulation factors, bound to the surface or released from internal granules
Release of factor XIII, to stabilize fibrin meshwork
Promotion of clot retraction
Production and release of fibroblast growth factor(s)

The importance of platelet function in haemostasis is best manifested in extreme thrombocytopaenia, which is eventually fatal even if all plasma coagulation factors are normal. This is in contrast to extreme reduction of one or more plasma coagulation factors, which does not necessarily carry increased mortality.

Balancing mechanisms

The correct balance of haemostatic activity to prevent excessive haemorrhage on the one hand but to avoid intravascular thrombosis on the other requires precise and complex regulatory mechanisms. The paired factors with opposing actions which contribute to this balance include:

platelet versus endothelium activities;
production of aggregating and antiaggregating substances;
active enzyme production from inactive precursors;
production and clearance of activating and inhibiting factors;
fibrin formation and fibrin degradation (fibrinolysis).

In several instances, opposing factors are produced or activated by the same enzyme. For example thromboxane and prostacyclin are both produced by cyclo-oxygenase, coagulation and fibrinolysis are triggered by factor XII activation, a number of clotting factors and Protein C (which has anticoagulant activity) are produced through a common mechanism involving vitamin K-dependent hepatic enzymes. These complex interrelated regulatory systems defy perturbation of the haemostatic balance by simple means. For instance, it appears that aspirin is largely ineffective as an in vivo antiaggregating agent since, while it inhibits endoperoxide formation within platelets, it also inhibits prostacyclin production by endothelial cells.

Reactions with accessory components

Coagulation factors act in a sequence and according to a hierarchical order of functions that do not follow — unfortunately! — the sequence of Roman numerals by which they are identified. While most factors are serine-proteinases, some are not (e.g. factors VIII and V). The most enzymatically active factors are Xa and thrombin. As shown in Figure 12.2, each of them is produced by a complex reaction which, in vivo, probably occurs only on the platelet surface and involves the following components: 1. a proteolytic enzyme precursor (the zymogen substrate); 2. an active proteolytic enzyme; 3. a protein cofactor; 4. platelet membrane phospholipids (PF3); 5. calcium ions.

The role of the protein cofactor is to accelerate enormously the reaction rate, especially when it occurs on the platelet surface in the presence of calcium ions (Jackson & Nemerson 1980).

Figure 12.2 summarizes the sequence of events leading to fibrin formation. If tissue factors are present, factor X can be activated via factor VII (extrinsic pathway).

Intrinsic/extrinsic pathway bypasses

Classically, the activation of factor X via factor IXa has been called the 'intrinsic pathway', since all the factors involved are present in the plasma as inactive profactors, as opposed to factor X activation via factor VII, which requires factors from tissues outside the vessel, and is thus termed the 'extrinsic pathway'.

Whether the two pathways are really unconnected has been questioned recently. Indeed crossover reactions coupling the intrinsic and extrinsic pathways have been discovered: factor VII can be activated by factor XIIa and IXa, while factor VIIa participates in the activation of factor IX to IXa (Jackson & Nemerson 1980). It is not certain whether these crosslinks are physiologically significant. Nevertheless, whichever pathway is primarily involved, both are ultimately responsible for fibrin formation in vivo.

Relevance of in vitro tests to in vivo haemostasis

Having divided haemostasis into several discrete events, we can evaluate each step by a specific test. However, we must always keep in mind that this is an oversimplification, because: 1. some interactions between the various steps may be abolished in conventional laboratory tests, whereas in vivo almost all these steps occur simultaneously and several positive and negative feedback mechanisms are activated; 2. platelets, endothelial cells and perivascular collagen, which have an important role in haemostatic reactions in vivo, are usually not involved in vitro; 3. experimental procedures may not reflect other in vivo conditions. Some of these deficiencies of in vitro testing are seen in the following examples.

Platelet aggregation profiles are usually studied upon addition of ADP, adrenaline, non-human collagen and ristocetin. However, the most physiological aggregating agents, thrombin and thromboxane A2 (TBX), which are active at extremely low concentrations (Majerus & Miletich 1978), are not used in in vitro tests for technical reasons. (Thrombin causes clotting of platelet-rich-plasma and TBX is an extremely unstable molecule.) Failure of platelets to respond to thrombin or to TBX may not be detected using ADP, adrenaline or collagen.

The most popular coagulation tests, namely prothrombin time (PT) and the partial thromboplastin time (PTT) are carried out in platelet-poor-plasma (i.e. in the absence of intact platelets, endothelial cells, or perivascular collagen), by the use of unphysiological amounts of unusual phospholipids (usually not even of human origin). These tests do measure accurately the plasma concentration of certain coagulation factors, but their correlation with in vivo

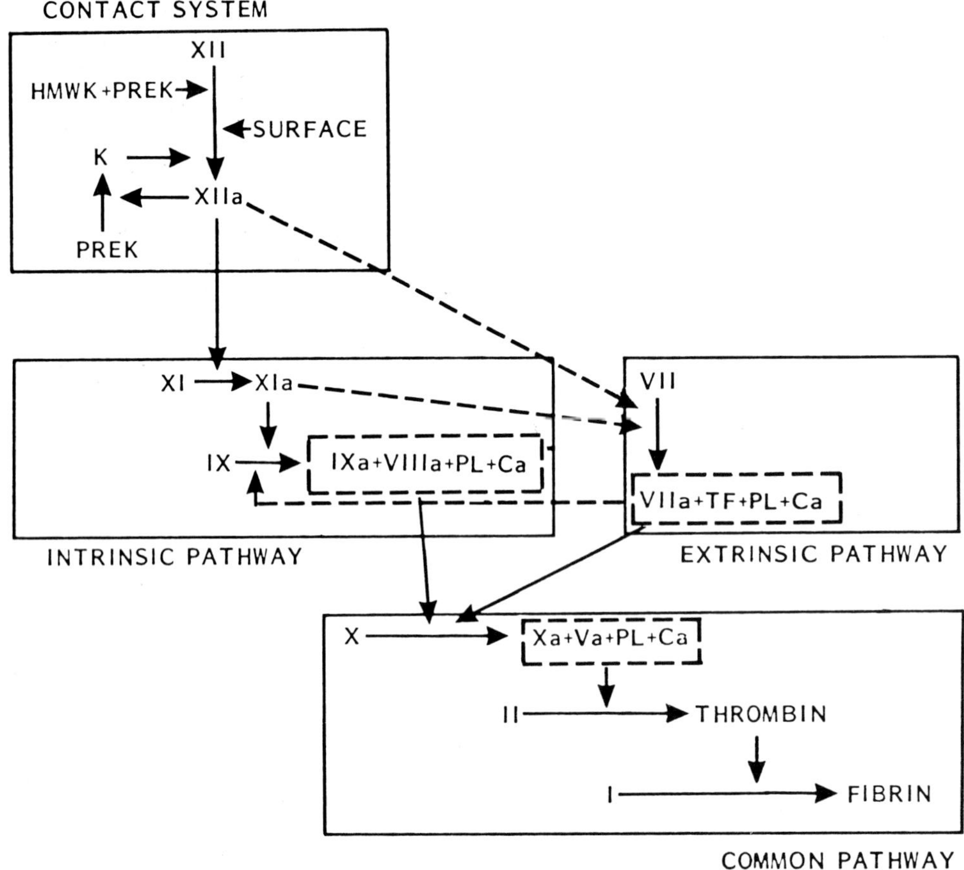

Fig. 12.2 The coagulation system. Apart from the numbered factors, abbreviations are as follows: HMWK = high molecular weight kininogen; PREK = prekallikrein; K = kallikrein; PL = platelet phospholipids; Ca = calcium ions; TF = tissue factor. The postscript 'a' indicates the active form of a factor. The four large boxes outline the four major functional stages of the clotting process. Full arrows indicate precursor-product relationships (e.g. XI → XIa) or enzyme activities (e.g. XIIa catalyzes the conversion of XI to XIa). Broken line boxes enclose an active enzyme with a set of accessory components that accelerate the activity of the main factor involved (e.g. Va, PL and Ca are activators of the enzyme reaction of Xa on II). Broken-line arrows indicate 'cross reactions', i.e. interactions across the boundaries of the main stages. Factors XI, IX, X, VII and II in their 'a' form are all serine proteases. The so-called coagulation 'cascade' runs from XI to thrombin (which is IIa)

haemostasis is imperfect. Indeed, the only firm correlation between these tests and a bleeding tendency occurs in patients with a very prolonged PT or PTT, when one or more plasma coagulation factors are reduced to less than 5%.

Finally, the presence of red blood cells should not be neglected. Millions of living particles with a negatively charged surface modify plasma ionic strength to such an extent that, at a haematocrit of 0.45, whole blood electrical conductivity is halved compared to plasma. Some enzyme reactions are extremely sensitive to ionic strength modifications, e.g. the interaction between platelets and thrombin (Rotoli et al 1978).

In conclusion, in vitro tests of haemostasis bear a limited relationship to in vivo phenomena. A few tests such as capillary fragility tests and bleeding time can be carried out in vivo, but they are difficult to standardize and they are sensitive only to severe vascular or platelet abnormalities. All tests performed using plasma, even the most sophisticated or expensive ones (e.g. those using chromogenic substrates), can only measure the plasma concentration of one or more factors. A personal view (Rotoli et al 1983), is that the plasma should be considered as a reservoir for coagulation factors, which are taken up by platelets as required. This would explain why the plasma level of a coagulation factor is only relevant to haemostatic failure when it is extremely low.

Platelets in liver disease

Both thrombocytopenia and platelet functional impairment may occur in liver disease.

Thrombocytopenia

Decreased numbers of platelets may be found particularly in cirrhosis, when portal hypertension produces congestive splenic enlargement. This results in increased sequestration and destruction of platelets (and white cells) in the spleen. The bone marrow usually shows signs of active platelet regeneration, with increased numbers of megakaryocytes. Rarely, a more marked thrombocytopenia is due to anti-platelet auto-antibodies associated with liver disease (Karpatkin et al 1972). Reduced numbers of platelets may also be caused by intravascular coagulation or, exceptionally, by associated thrombotic thrombocytopenic purpura (Nally & Metz 1979).

Occasionally the transfusion of large volumes of blood after gastrointestinal or operative bleeding results in a 'dilutional' thrombocytopenia (Ratnoff 1984). Finally, platelet production by the bone marrow may be impaired in specific disorders associated with liver disease. Examples are acute alcoholism, via folate deficiency or by a direct effect of heavy alcohol intake itself (Cowen 1980); and severe aplastic anaemia which occasionally follows acute viral hepatitis by B or non A, non B viruses (Ajloumi & Doeblin 1974).

Platelet functional impairment

Abnormalities of platelet function, although strongly suspected in some patients with liver disease, have been largely unexplored. The haemorrhagic phenomena that occur in cryoglobulinaemia are probably the clearest example of a platelet membrane lesion caused by immune complexes. However, circulating immune complexes are present in several other liver diseases, and they may be responsible for some degree of thrombocytopathy.

The normal function of platelets relies in part on clotting factors bound to their surface. Therefore, reduced synthesis and, perhaps more important, the production of abnormal coagulation factors due to hepatocyte metabolic derangement, may be additional causes of altered platelet procoagulant activity. The role of endotoxin in producing platelet functional impairment is discussed later.

Thus, there are both theoretical reasons and clinical observations to suggest that alterations in platelet function occur in some patients with liver disease. However, laboratory work on platelet aggregation and adhesion to glass beads has produced conflicting results (Kumar & Deykin 1979). As already discussed, these discrepancies are probably due to the lack of tests sensitive enough to detect a physiologically significant impairment of platelet function.

Liver disease and coagulation

Production of clotting factors

The liver is the primary site of production of all coagulation factors, except factor VIII. Indeed the plasma levels of fibrinogen, prothrombin, factors V, VII, X, IX, XI, XII, prekallikrein, high molecular weight kininogen and factor XIII, may all be decreased in severe hepatic disease. For many of these factors, evidence that they are produced in the liver is based not only on the finding of reduced levels in liver disease but also on their production by isolated perfused rat liver, by liver slices in vitro and by hepatocytes in culture (Kumar & Deykin 1979).

To express full biological activity, vitamin K-dependent factors (factors II, VII, X and IX) require post-translational modification by a hepatic microsomal K-dependent enzyme. Indeed, in order to bind calcium ions, these factors need gamma-carboxylation of certain glutamic acid residues, and this unique reaction requires the presence of vitamin K. Since both synthesis and post-synthetic carboxylation occur in hepatocytes, and vitamin K requires bile salts to be absorbed, both reduced and abnormal production of clotting factors may be found in liver disease. However, while the prolonged PT in obstructive jaundice is correctable by parenteral vitamin K, this is not possible in patients with hepatocellular damage. Vitamin K deficiency is common in patients with liver and biliary tract disease who require surgery. Oral antibiotics (which impair vitamin K synthesis by intestinal flora), reduced dietary intake, abnormal lipid absorption and total parenteral nutrition without adequate vitamin K supplements may all be causes of hepatocyte vitamin K deficiency. In these situations coagulation abnormalities may not be due solely to shortage of the vitamin K-dependent factors. Abnormal (non gamma-carboxylated) molecules may also compete with the normal coagulation factors for reaction sites (as demonstrated in vitro by the anticoagulant activity of proteins induced by vitamin K antagonists) and thus cause further disturbance of haemostasis.

The sensitivity of the plasma levels of K-dependent factors to vitamin K deficiency depends upon the biological life span of each factor. Factor VII, which has the shortest half-life (3–5 h), is the most appropriate monitor of hepatic protein synthesis in acute liver failure. Factor IX is usually the least affected, while prothrombin and factor X are moderately sensitive. As far as K-independent factors are concerned, the level of factor V may be increased in the early stages of inflammatory disease, while it is decreased in acute and chronic non-inflammatory liver disease. Fibrinogen, at least 50% of which is normally produced by the liver (Kumar & Deykin 1979), is reduced only in severe acute liver failure, such as fulminant hepatitis. Since fibrinogen is the molecule most prominently involved in erythrocyte rouleaux formation, a paradoxical reduction of erythrocyte sedimentation rate may be seen in progressive liver failure.

Abnormal fibrinogen activity has been found in several liver diseases (acute failure, primary hepatoma, cirrhosis, chronic aggressive hepatitis) and leads to abnormal fibrin monomer aggregation (Green et al 1976). It remains uncertain whether this is due to production of an abnormal molecule or to the presence of inhibitors (Kumar & Deykin 1979).

In contrast to all the other clotting factors, factor VIII is often increased in the plasma of patients with liver disease (Van Outryie et al 1973). This raised level could be caused either by increased production (similar to an acute phase reactant protein) or by reduced hepatic clearance.

Anticoagulant and fibrinolytic substances

The liver is also the main site for the production and clearance of physiological anticoagulants. Indeed, antithrombin III (AT III), alpha-2-macroglobulin, and alpha-l-antitrypsin are all synthesized in the liver. Protein C, a K-dependent molecule with anticoagulant activity which inactivates Va and VIIIa (Kisiel et al 1977), is also produced by hepatocytes. Plasminogen is thought to be synthesized in the liver; but the liver is also the primary site for clearance of plasminogen activators and production of antiplasmins.

Thus, the complex involvement of the liver in the production and clearance of both procoagulant, anticoagulant and fibrinolytic substances may be the basis for both the preserved final haemostatic balance in most patients with liver disease, and for the tendency to bleeding or intravascular coagulation in a minority of them.

Disseminated intravascular coagulation (DIC)

Reduced production of naturally occurring coagulation inhibitors and impaired hepatic clearance of active procoagulant molecules may trigger DIC in liver disease. However, true DIC is difficult to prove in these cases because most of the abnormalities considered typical of DIC (hyperfibrinolysis, reduced or abnormal synthesis of clotting factors, reduced clearance of fibrinogen degradation products, and non-specific proteolytic activity by hepatic lysosomal enzymes) can be ascribed to other mechanisms when liver function is impaired. The main finding of accelerated fibrinogen catabolism may be interpreted as a consequence of dysfibrinogenaemia, fibrinogenolysis, loss of fibrinogen into the extravascular space or haemorrhage (Ratnoff 1984). In addition factor VIII, which is reduced in true DIC, is normal or even elevated in liver disease, and intravascular thrombi are not usually seen on liver biopsy or at necropsy. Thus, most recent reviewers are sceptical about the clinical importance of DIC in liver disease (Kumar & Deykin 1979, Mannucci & Mari 1981, Ratnoff 1984). If it does exist, DIC in patients with hepatic impairment could be triggered by endotoxin (see below).

Endotoxaemia as a cause of haemostatic abnormalities

The Lipid A part of endotoxin (see above) is considered to be the major toxic moiety and it may be responsible for some of the haemostatic abnormalities seen in patients with liver disease and endotoxaemia. Although there is little correlation between human and horseshoe crab coagulation enyzme systems, it is of interest that the most sensitive assay for endotoxin is based on the activation of a proenzyme in the coagulation system of the Limulus amoebocyte. In man, Lipid A exerts its toxic effect on cell membranes, including platelets and endothelium, and may activate procoagulant factors.

Platelet and endothelial cell impairment

Receptor sites for bacterial lipopolysaccharide have been found on the surface of platelets (Hawinger et al 1975, 1977). Binding of endotoxin to platelets has two major consequences. On one hand, platelets may help to clear endotoxin. Indeed, removal of a variety of substances from the circulation may be a hitherto unrecognized function of platelets. Immunoglobulins and immune complexes have been found non-specifically adsorbed on platelets, and this may be a way of disposing of such molecules. If such a mechanism has a role in endotoxin clearance from plasma, thrombocytopaenia might be a further cause of raised plasma endotoxin in patients with liver disease.

On the other hand, endotoxin Lipid A may activate or damage platelets, thus triggering intravascular coagulation, which may become disseminated. There is in vitro evidence of platelet modifications following exposure to endotoxin (Lewis & Dixon 1971, Ausprunk & Das 1978). Trace metal (copper) seems to be required for endotoxin-induced changes. However, such damage has been observed in vitro only with washed platelets, suggesting that plasma inactivators of endotoxin may exert some protective effect in vivo. Thus, by altering the platelet membrane, endotoxin may reduce platelet survival. In addition, activation of the reticulo-endothelial system by endotoxin may further accelerate removal of platelets and contribute to thrombocytopaenia.

Endothelial damage by endotoxin has been poorly investigated. Like any other cell, the endothelial cell membrane may be affected by Lipid A. Endothelial cell functional damage may cause reduced local release of protective substances (e.g. prostacyclin), while endothelial cell destruction and exposure of subendothelial collagen would result in local platelet activation and fibrin formation.

Activation of clotting factors

The unusual fatty acid composition of bacterial lipopolysaccharide may be responsible for contact-sensitive plasma system activation (factor XII, high molecular weight kininogen, prekallikrein), and this may cause intravascular coagulation. However, while factor XII activation can be demonstrated in vitro (Pitney 1971), it is unlikely that this mechanism occurs in vivo, where potent inactivators would quickly stop pro-enzyme activation in the circulation.

Increased activation of factor X on the surface of washed platelets by endotoxin has been reported (Semeraro et al 1978).

Consumption coagulopathy

Endotoxaemia has been considered as one of the mechanisms leading to disseminated intravascular coagulation in patients with liver disease (Wilkinson et al 1974). Indeed, intravascular clotting might be triggered by platelet and/or procoagulant factor activation. However, while platelet activation is followed by clotting reactions on the platelet surface itself up to the stage of fibrin formation and stabilization, it is unlikely that circulating activated clotting enzymes will reach the concentration needed to prime the whole clotting system inside intact vessels, since they will be diluted by the blood flow and inactivated by potent inhibitors. Thus, if DIC does occur in liver disease, it must be triggered by platelet membrane damage.

Rarely is the number of activated platelets high enough to cause small vessel embolization, as seen in thrombotic thrombocytopaenic purpura. More often, platelet activation causes utilization of clotting factors and reduced platelet life span, findings which are typical of moderate consumption coagulopathy. However, as already stated, reduced plasma fibrinogen, the presence of fibrin-fibrinogen degradation products and abnormal fibrin polymerization may also occur for reasons other than DIC in liver disease.

Conclusions

In conclusion, endotoxaemia is likely to affect haemostasis but its mechanism of action has not been fully explained. In vitro tests must be viewed cautiously, since many of them do not reflect events taking place within the circulation. The presence of plasma inactivators, and the coexistence in patients with liver disease of reduced or abnormal coagulation factors and thrombocytopaenia, make the evaluation of endotoxin-induced haemostatic abnormalities even more difficult. However, it is known that patients with endotoxaemia have a high risk of bleeding during and after surgery (Wilkinson et al 1974, Hunt et al 1982). Since the bleeding tendency in these patients is seen during or after operation rather than before, it appears that a factor additional to endotoxaemia is necessary, and this is presumably related to surgery itself. Possible factors include a further increase in endotoxaemia, hormonal changes and the effect of the surgical procedure on platelets or on the reticulo-endothelial system.

Diagnosis and treatment of haemostatic abnormalities in liver disease and endotoxaemia

Diagnostic aspects

As discussed above the purpose of investigating haemostatic abnormalities in liver disease may be twofold: to detect patients at risk from haemostatic disturbances and to pinpoint possible causes; to monitor liver function. Most of the tests available at present are only useful for the latter purpose.

The conventional tests for screening of haemostatic abnormalities include: PT, PTT, platelet count, bleeding time and capillary fragility tests (e.g. the Hess test). While PT, PTT and platelet count are part of the routine (usually automated) battery of haematological tests and are readily available, the bleeding time and the Hess test are often neglected because they are relatively time consuming. Moreover, although they are easy to learn, great care must be taken in their execution if results are to be reliable and comparable. Although a haematologist should ideally perform these tests, any member of the clinical staff may carry them out if adequately trained. Despite these problems, the bleeding time and the Hess test are the most important tests for clinical purposes, since they measure platelet function in vivo.

PT correlates well with the plasma level of clotting factors synthesized by the liver, and therefore it can be used as a measure of protein synthesis by the liver, provided severe haemorrhage, consumption coagulopathy and the presence of inhibitors are excluded. Except in the case of fulminant hepatitis, where the plasma level of factor VII can be used as an early marker of disease progression or recovery, there is usually no reason to use single factor measurements in preference to a global test such as PT.

As already mentioned, vitamin K-dependent factors are particularly sensitive to liver failure, while factor V and fibrinogen are more resistant, and factor VIII is often normal or raised even in severe liver disease. Prolonged PT with a normal or raised factor V suggests vitamin K deficiency, as in biliary tract obstruction. Dysfibrinogenaemia, which may be revealed by the thrombin time, is not clinically relevant in liver disease; indeed, it was first described in patients without any bleeding problem (Soria et al 1968, Von Felten et al 1969).

Tests for DIC and for hyperfibrinolysis are often abnormal in patients with liver disease, but they are difficult to interpret. Indeed, it remains uncertain whether these abnormalities are evidence of a true consumption coagulopathy (Mannucci & Mari 1981). However, it is possible that occasional patients may have true DIC, especially when endotoxaemia is present.

Platelet functional studies might be helpful, both in general and especially in conditions such as cryoglobulinaemia. Unfortunately, as we have already stated, none of the many tests available (conventional aggregometry, adhesion to glass beads, PF3, PF4, beta-thromboglobulin etc.) provides a reliable correlation with clinical bleeding problems. It is possible that the recently developed 'aggregometry on whole blood' will provide information on platelet function closer to in vivo conditions. In addition to the screening of haemostasis, every patient with chronic liver disease should be assessed for cryoglobulins. If these are detected, the patient is at risk of heavy post-traumatic bleeding and the necessity of any invasive procedure (e.g. biopsy, angiography, surgery) should be considered carefully.

Treatment

Abnormal clotting tests, especially PT, in patients with obstructive jaundice require parenteral vitamin K administration. However, since vitamin K deficiency may occur in liver diseases other than biliary obstruction (such as in very sick, malnourished patients, and after prolonged oral antibiotic administration) a trial of vitamin K (3 mg i.v.) is reasonable in any patient with liver disease and a prolonged PT. Failure to correct the PT within 48 hours of vitamin K administration suggests that vitamin K deficiency is not the cause. Patients receiving total parenteral nutrition need regular vitamin K supplements.

Haemostatic abnormalities due to causes other than vitamin K deficiency in patients with liver disease usually do not require specific replacement therapy, unless there is active bleeding, a high risk of bleeding (e.g. fulminant hepatitis), or an invasive procedure is to be performed (e.g. liver biopsy, surgery).

In thrombocytopaenic patients, platelet concentrate transfusion may be indicated but several problems including platelet availability, immunization and rapid sequestration by a large spleen remain unsolved. Platelet transfusion is necessary when bleeding occurs in a patient with a platelet count of less than 30 000/μl, but this is not common in liver disease. At least 5 × 10^9 platelets/kg should be given, that is 8–10 single units for an adult of average weight. If available, platelets may also be used for bleeding episodes in patients with a platelet count between 30 000 and 80 000/μl. However, because of frequent production of anti-platelet antibodies (mainly H-LA related), the haemostatic effectiveness of platelet transfusion tends to decrease with repeated administration. In any case, the life span of transfused platelets rarely exceeds 48 hours; therefore, their administration must be repeated every 24–48 hours if bleeding continues. It is possible that small doses of prednisone (10–15 mg/day) may induce better tolerance of thrombocytopaenia, probably by decreasing prostacyclin production by endothelial cells.

Replacement therapy for decreased clotting factor synthesis is common practice, although there is little evidence that this approach is of real value (Cash 1981). Either fresh frozen plasma (FFP), frozen plasma (FP) or prothrombin complex concentrates may be used. FP has reduced or absent levels of unstable factors (V and VIII) compared to FFP. The main advantage of prothrombin complex concentrate is that correction can be achieved by infusing small volumes; but concentrates are expensive, they do not supply factor V, do not contain antithrombin III (which is desirable if DIC is suspected) and may cause complications (embolization, transmission of viruses).

From a practical point of view, treatment of bleeding or prophylaxis against haemorrhage in patients with liver disease can be achieved in an adult by 800–1800 ml of plasma (all FFP or half FFP and half FP), or by two units of prothrombin complex concentrate with 500 ml of FFP. If surgery must be performed and packed red cells are to be transfused, it is reasonable to administer one unit of FFP for each unit of packed cells (Kumar & Deykin 1979).

The use of aminocaproic acid or tranexamic acid (which compete with fibrin for the lysine-binding sites of plasmin) is crucial in the rare cases of primary hyperfibrinolysis, while they can be dangerous in cases of secondary hyperfibrinolysis (e.g. when DIC is present).

Finally, heparin treatment for DIC is seldom considered in patients with liver disease; low doses are probably ineffective while high doses may be harmful and should be cautiously used only in cases of well documented DIC.

SUMMARY

The role of endotoxin in diseases of the liver and biliary tract remains uncertain despite extensive clinical and experimental study. Difficulties with the assay of endotoxin in blood and the lack of an established specific safe anti-endotoxin therapy are responsible for much of this uncertainty. Recent improvements in endotoxin assay technique and sensitivity should lead to an increased understanding of the importance of endotoxaemia in hepatic disease, and to a more accurate assessment of the results of therapeutic efforts.

Bleeding problems are not uncommon in patients with liver and biliary tract disease, and coagulation tests are frequently used as a measure of hepatic function. The disturbances of haemostasis seen in these patients are the result of many complex changes. The central role of platelets in haemostasis in vivo suggests that alterations in platelet function occur in liver disease in addition to the widely recognized changes in coagulation factor production. Endotoxin may play a role in these haemostatic disturbances. The diagnosis and management of these problems in clinical practice has been described.

REFERENCES

Ajloumi K, Doeblin T D 1974 The syndrome of hepatitis and aplastic anaemia. British Journal of Haematology 27: 345–355

Ausprunk D H, Das J 1978 Endotoxin-induced changes in human platelet membrane: morphologic evidence. Blood 51: 487–495

Bailey M E 1976 Endotoxin, bile salts and renal function in obstructive jaundice. British Journal of Surgery 63: 774–778

Balis J U, Rappaport E S, Gerber L, Fareed J, Buddingh F, Messmore H L 1978 A primate model for prolonged endotoxin shock: blood-vascular reactions and effects of glucocorticoid treatment. Laboratory Investigation 38: 511–523

Blamey S L, Fearon K C H, Gilmour W H, Osborne D H, Carter D C 1983 Prediction of risk in biliary surgery. British Journal of Surgery 70: 535–538

Braude A I, Carey F J, Sutherland D, Zalesky M 1955 Studies with radioactive endotoxin. Journal of Clinical Investigation 34: 850–864

Cahill C J 1983 Prevention of postoperative renal failure in patients with obstructive jaundice — the role of bile salts. British Journal of Surgery 70: 590–595

Cash J 1981 Blood replacement therapy. In: Bloom A L, Thomas D P (eds) Haemostasis and thrombosis. Churchill Livingstone, Edinburgh, Ch. 27

Cederblad G, Korstan-Bengsten K, Olsson R 1976 Observation of increased levels of blood coagulation factors and other plasma proteins in cholestatic liver disease. Scandinavian Journal of Gastroenterology 11: 391–396

Cohen J, McConnell J S 1984 Observations on the measurement and interpretation of endotoxaemia using a quantitative Limulus lysate microassay. Journal of Infectious Diseases 150: 916–924

Coker S J, Hughes B, Parratt J R, Roger I W, Zeitlin I J 1983 The release of prostanoids during the acute pulmonary response to E. coli endotoxin in anaesthetised cats. British Journal of Pharmacology 78: 561–570

Cowen D M 1980 Effect of alcoholism on hemostasis. Seminars in Hematology 17: 137–147

Cuevas P, Fine J 1971 Demonstration of a lethal endotoxaemia in experimental occlusion of the superior mesenteric artery. Surgery, Gynecology and Obstetrics 133: 81–83

Cuevas P, Fine J 1973 Production of fatal endotoxic shock by vasoactive substances. Gastroenterology 64: 285–291

Ditter B, Urbaschek R, Urbaschek B 1983 Ability of various adsorbents to bind endotoxins in vitro and to prevent orally induced endotoxaemia in mice. Gastroenterology 84: 1547–1552

Dixon J M, Armstrong C P, Duffy S W, Davies G C 1983 Factors affecting morbidity and mortality after surgery for obstructive jaundice : a review of 373 patients. Gut 24: 845–852

Doolittle R F 1981 Fibrinogen and fibrin. In: Bloom A L, Thomas D P (eds) Haemostasis and thrombosis. Churchill Livingstone, Edinburgh, Ch. 11

Drivas G, James O, Wardle N 1976 Study of reticuloendothelial phagocytic capacity in patients with cholestasis. British Medical Journal 1: 1568–1569

Elin R J, Wolff S M 1976 Biology of endotoxin. Annual Review of Medicine 27: 127–141

Filkins J P 1969 Hepatic vascular responses to endotoxin. Proceedings of the Society for Experimental Biology and Medicine 131: 1235–1238

Filkins J P 1971 Hepatic lysosomes and the inactivation of endotoxin. Journal of the Reticuloendothelial Society 9: 480–490

Freudenberg M A, Freudenberg N, Galanos C 1982 Time course of cellular distribution of endotoxin in liver, lungs and kidneys of rats. British Journal of Experimental Pathology 63: 56–65

From A H L, Fong J S C, Good R A 1979 Polymixin B sulphate modification of bacterial endotoxin: Effects on the development of endotoxin shock in dogs. Infection and Immunity 23: 660–664

Green G, Thomson J M, Dymock I W, Poller L 1976 Abnormal fibrin polymerisation in liver disease. British Journal of Haematology 34: 427–439

Harris R I, Stone P C W, Stuart J 1983 An improved chromogenic substrate endotoxin assay for clinical use. Journal of Clinical Pathology 36: 1145–1149

Harris R I, Stone P C W, Evans G R, Stuart J 1984 Endotoxaemia as a cause of fever in immunosuppressed patients. Journal of Clinical Pathology 37: 467–470

Hawiger J, Hawiger A, Timmons S 1975 Endotoxin-sensitive membrane component of human platelets. Nature 256: 125–127

Hawiger J, Hawiger A, Steckley S, Timmons S, Cheng C 1977 Membrane change in human platelet induced by lipopolysaccharide endotoxin. British Journal of Haematology 35: 285–299

Holaday J W, Reynolds D G 1983 The role of endogenous opiates in shock: introductory comments. Advances in Shock Research 10: 53–5

Hunt D R, Allison M E M, Prentice C R M, Blumgart L H 1982 Endotoxaemia, disturbance of coagulation, and obstructive jaundice. American Journal of Surgery 144: 325–329

Ingoldby C J 1980 The value of Polymixin B in endotoxaemia due to experimental obstructive jaundice and mesenteric ischaemia. British Journal of Surgery 67: 565–567

Ingoldby C J, McPherson G A D, Blumgart L H 1984 Endotoxaemia in human obstructive jaundice : Effect of Polymixin B. American Journal of Surgery 144: 766–771

Iwasaki M 1982 Liver diseases and endotoxin — Part II — clinical study about effect of bile acid on endotoxin. Nippon Shokakibyo Gakkai Zasshi 79: 1424–1434

Iwasaki M, Maruyama I, Ikeziri N, Abe M, Maeyama T, Nagata E, Abe H, Tanikawa K. 1980 Endotoxin in severe liver diseases. Nippon Shokakibyo Gakkai Zasshi 77: 386–394

Jackson C M 1981 Biochemistry of prothrombin activation. In: Bloom A L, Thomas D P (eds) Haemostasis and thrombosis. Churchill Livingstone, Edinburgh, Ch. 10

Jackson C M, Nemerson Y 1980 Blood coagulation. Annual Review of Biochemistry 49: 765–811

Jacob A I, Goldberg P K, Bloom N, Degenshein G A, Kozinn P J 1977 Endotoxin and bacteria in portal blood. Gastroenterology 72: 1268–1270

Karpatkin S, Strick M, Karpatkin M B, Siskind G W 1972 Cumulative experience in the detection of antiplatelet antibody in 234 patients with idiopathic thrombocytopenia purpura, systemic lupus erythematosus and other clinical disorders. American Journal of Medicine 52: 776–785

Kisiel W, Canfield W, Ericsson L, Davie E W 1977 Anticoagulant properties of bovine plasma protein C following activation by thrombin. Biochemistry 16: 5824–5831

Kocsar L T, Bertok L, Varteresz V 1969 Effect of bile acids on the intestinal absorption of endotoxin in rats. Journal of Bacteriology 100: 220–223

Kumar R, Deykin D 1979 Pathogenesis and practical management of coagulopathy of liver disease. In: Davidson C S (ed) Problems in liver diseases. G. Thiene, Stuttgart. Lancet (editorial) 1982 Endotoxin and cirrhosis. Lancet 1: 318–319

Levin J, Bang F B 1968 Clottable protein in Limulus: its localisation and kinetics of its coagulation by endotoxin. Thrombosis et Diathesis Haemorrhagica 19: 186–197

Lewis A F, Dixon R C 1971 Platelet aggregation: induction by means of a complex between endotoxin and copper. Canadian Journal of Biochemistry 49: 1236–1244

Liehr H, Jacob A I 1983 Endotoxin and renal failure in liver disease. In: Epstein M (ed) The kidney in liver disease, 2nd edn. Elsevier Science Publishing Co, New York

Liehr H, Grun M, Thiel H, Brunswig D, Rasenack V 1975 Endotoxin-induced liver necrosis and intravascular coagulation in rats enhanced by portacaval collateral circulation. Gut 16: 429–436

Maitra S K, Yoshikawa T T, Guze L B, Schotz M C 1981 Properties of binding of *Escherichia coli* endotoxin to various matrices. Journal of Clinical Microbiology 13: 49–53

Majerus P W, Miletich J P 1978 Relationship between platelets and coagulation factors in hemostasis. Annual Review of Medicine 29: 41–49

Mannucci P M, Mari D 1981 Hemostasis and liver disease. Haematologica 76: 233–248

Marciniak E 1973 Factor Xa inactivation by antithrombin III: evidence for biological stabilisation of factor Xa by factor V-phospholipid complex. British Journal of Haematology 24: 391–400

Miletich J P, Jackson C M, Majerus P W 1978 Properties of the factor Xa binding site on human platelets. Journal of Biological Chemistry 253: 6908–6916

Mori K, Matsumoto K, Gans H 1973 On the in vivo clearance and detoxification of endotoxin by lung and liver. Annals of Surgery 177: 159–163

Morrison D C, Ulevitch R J 1978 The effects of bacterial endotoxins on host mediation systems. American Journal of Pathology 93: 526–617

Nally S V, Metz E N 1979 Acute thrombotic thrombocytopenic

purpura. Another cause for hemolytic anemia and thrombocytopenia in cirrhosis. Archives of Internal Medicine 139: 711–712
Nolan J P 1975 The role of endotoxin in liver injury. Gastroenterology 69: 1346–1356
Parnas J 1976 Peter Ludwig Parnum: Great Danish pathologist and discoverer of endotoxin. Danish Medical Bulletin 23: 143–146
Pitney W R 1971 Disseminated intravascular coagulation. Seminars in Hematology 8: 65–83
Prytz H, Holst-Christensen J, Korner B, Liehr H 1976 Portal venous and systemic endotoxaemia in patients without liver disease and systemic endotoxaemia in patients with cirrhosis. Scandinavian Journal of Gastroenterology 11: 857–863
Ratnoff O D 1984 Haemostatic defects in liver and biliary tract disease and disorders of vitamin K metabolism. In: Ratnoff O D, Forbes C D (eds) Disorders of hemostasis. Grune and Stratton, New York
Ravin H A, Rowley D, Jenkins C, Fine J 1960 On the absorption of bacterial endotoxin from the gastrointestinal tract of the normal and shocked animal. Journal of Experimental Medicine 112: 783–792
Rotoli B, Miletich J P, Majerus P W 1978 The relation of conductivity to the binding of thrombin to human platelets. Thrombosis Research 13: 1103–1109
Rotoli B, D'Avino R, Chiurazzi F 1983 Combined factor V and factor VII deficiency. Acta Haematologica 69: 117–122
Semeraro N, Fumarola D, Mertens F, Vermylen J 1978 Evidence that endotoxin enhances the factor X activator activity of washed human platelets. British Journal of Haematology 38: 243–249
Soria J, Coupier J, Samama M 1968 Dysfibrinogenemia without bleeding tendency with abnormal polymerisation of fibrin monomers in a case of severe hepatitis. XII Congress of International Society of Hematology, New York, p 180
Stumacher R J, Kovnax M J, McCabe W R 1973 Limitations of the usefulness of the Limulus assay for endotoxin. New England Journal of Medicine 258: 1261–1264
Suzuki M, Mikami T, Matsumoto T, Suzuki S 1977 Gelation of Limulus lysate by synthetic dextran derivatives. Microbiology and Immunology 21: 419–425
Tarao K, So K, Moroi T, Ikeuchi T, Suyama T, Endo O, Fukushima K. 1977 Detection of endotoxin in plasma and ascitic fluid of patients with cirrhosis: its clinical significance. Gastroenterology 73: 539–542
Ulevitch R J, Johnston A R, Weinstein D B 1979 New function for high density lipoproteins. Journal of Clinical Investigation 64: 1516–1524
Utili R, Abernathy C O, Zimmerman H J 1976 Cholestatic effects of *Escherichia coli* endotoxin on the isolated perfused rat liver. Gastroenterology 70: 248–253
Van Outryie M, Baele G, DeWerdt G A, Barbier F. 1973 Antihaemophilic factor A (factor VIII) and serum fibrin-fibrinogen degradation products in hepatic cirrhosis. Scandinavian Journal of Haematology 11: 148–152
Von Felten A, Straub P W, Frick P G 1969 Dysfibrinogenemia in a patient with primary hepatoma. New England Journal of Medicine 280: 405–409
Walsh P N 1972a The role of platelets in the contact phase of blood coagulation. British Journal of Haematology 22: 237–254
Walsh P N 1972b The effect of collagen and kaolin on the intrinsic coagulant activity of platelets. Evidence for an alternative pathway in intrinsic coagulation not requiring factor XII. British Journal of Haematology 22: 393–405
Walsh P N 1974 The platelet coagulant activity and hemostasis: a hypothesis. Blood 43: 597–603
Walsh P N, Biggs R 1972 The role of platelets in intrinsic factor Xa formation. British Journal of Haematology 22: 743–760
Wardle E N 1974 Fibrinogen in liver disease. Archives of Surgery 109: 741–746
Wardle E N, Wright N A 1970 Endotoxin and acute renal failure associated with obstructive jaundice. British Medical Journal 4: 472–474
Webster C J 1980 Principles of a quantitative assay for bacterial endotoxins in blood that uses Limulus lysate and a chromogenic substrate. Journal of Clinical Microbiology 12: 644–650
Weiss P J 1979 Views on the reliability of the Limulus test. Progress in Clinical and Biological Research 29: 507–512
Wilkinson S P, Arroyo V, Gazzard B G, Moodie H, Williams R 1974 Relation of renal impairment and haemorrhagic diathesis to endotoxaemia in fulminant hepatic failure. Lancet 1: 521–524
Wilkinson S P, Moodie H, Stamatakis J D, Kakkar V V, Williams R 1976 Endotoxaemia and renal failure in cirrhosis and obstructive jaundice. British Medical Journal 2: 1415–1418
Wolff SM 1973 Biological effects of bacterial endotoxins in man. Journal of Infectious Diseases 128 (suppl): S259–S264
Wolter J, Liehr H, Grun M 1978 Hepatic clearance of endotoxins: Differences in arterial and portal venous infusions. Journal of the Reticuloendothelial Society 23: 145–152
Yin E T 1975 Endotoxin, thrombin, and the Limulus amoebocyte lysate test. Journal of Laboratory and Clinical Medicine 86: 430–434
Ziegler E J, McCutchan J A, Fierer J, Glauser M P, Sasoff J C, Douglas H, Bidude A I 1982 Treatment of gram-negative bacteraemia and shock with human antiserum to a mutant *Escherichia coli*. New England Journal of Medicine 307: 1225–1230

SECTION 2

Diagnostic techniques

13

I. Taylor, R. Wright

Clinical examination and investigation

With the enormous expansion of investigations (both non-invasive and invasive), which are now at the disposal of the clinician dealing with liver disorders, there is a temptation to ignore the need for a detailed overall clinical assessment of the patient. In this chapter relevant aspects of the history and examination of patients with liver and biliary disease will be considered and general views on specific investigations discussed.

CLINICAL HISTORY

Jaundice is the predominant feature in the majority of patients with liver disease presenting to a surgical department. The following are important questions which may be of value in determining the diagnosis:

Is the jaundice due to obstruction of the biliary tree?
Is the jaundice drug-induced or infective?
Is there any evidence of haemolysis?

Typically, a patient with cholestatic jaundice has dark urine, pale stools and pruritus of varying severity. Information regarding the initial onset, and whether the clinical course is intermittent and associated with pain, fever or rigors must be sought. A long history of biliary symptoms with episodes of colic may clarify the diagnosis. Similarly, attacks precipitated by fat intake can be relevant. Episodes of cholangitis are recognized if the jaundice is associated with pain, rigors and pyrexia. Jaundice without significant pain or pain predominantly radiating to the back may indicate pancreatic pathology. However, this is by no means certain and patients with gallstones can present with back pain whereas patients with an extensive carcinoma of the head of the pancreas may present with a typical history of biliary colic.

A fluctuating depth of jaundice is suggestive of intermittent obstruction, e.g. temporary retention of a stone in the ampulla of Vater or a periampullary carcinoma. It is only rarely present in pancreatic cancer or cholangiocarcinoma. It can also occur with intrahepatic cholestasis or, when mild, with Gilbert's Syndrome.

Weight loss, anorexia and anaemia suggest associated malignancy particularly when of short duration. If these symptoms occur with painless jaundice then neoplasia of the head of the pancreas is likely.

Pruritus may be present in all forms of jaundice and may either be progressive or fluctuate in intensity. If excessive in middle–aged women, then primary biliary cirrhosis should be considered.

A careful history of foreign travel is important, not only because of the possibility of viral hepatitis but also because of exposure to unusual diseases such as malaria and other parasitic infections. A history of previous contact with jaundiced patients, of needle stick exposure, tattooing or homosexuality may also provide the clue to a diagnosis of viral hepatitis.

Various occupations may be relevant, particularly those which result in exposure to particular infections or to hepatotoxins. A careful drug history including the use of the contraceptive pill must be obtained. An increasing number of pharmacological preparations are now recognized to be associated with hepatocellular dysfunction. Excessive alcohol intake is of special relevance and this information must be sought not only from the patient but also from the relatives and general practitioner.

Some forms of liver disease and jaundice are known to be familial, e.g. Wilson's Disease, α-1-antitrypsin deficiency, haemolysis and Gilbert's syndrome. A history of auto-immune disease in the patient or family suggests chronic active hepatitis or primary biliary cirrhosis.

PHYSICAL EXAMINATION

General inspection

The familiar stigmata of liver disease should be looked for. They are all indicators of hepatocellular dysfunction:

Jaundice is due to the staining of the tissues with bilirubin and possibly other pigments such as biliverdin. It is usually detected initially in the sclera. As jaundice progresses the skin becomes progressively more pigmented. *Spider naevi* (Fig. 13.1) are vascular skin lesions supplied by a central arteriole. They can be recognized by noting blanching when the central arteriole is occluded with a pin head. Spider naevi usually occur in the distribution of the superior vena cava; the chest above the nipples, face, arms and hands. It is not unusual to see spider naevi in normal subjects, for example during pregnancy or childhood. However, if they increase in size or appear in later life they are suggestive of liver disease. *Palmar erythema* (Fig. 13.2) is an obvious and pronounced red flushing of the palms. It particularly affects the thenar and hypothenar eminences and the bases of the fingers. It should be remembered that similar changes can be recognized on the soles of the feet. Typical *changes in the nails* are recognized in many patients with cirrhosis. These consist of either clubbing or white nails (leuconychia) (Fig. 13.3). The latter is seen particularly in primary biliary cirrhosis. *Dupuytrens contracture* may also be found commonly in patients with alcoholic cirrhosis and may be related to excess alcohol intake rather than cirrhosis (Fig. 13.4). *Parotid enlargement*, usually bilateral and painless, also occurs in alcoholic liver disease.

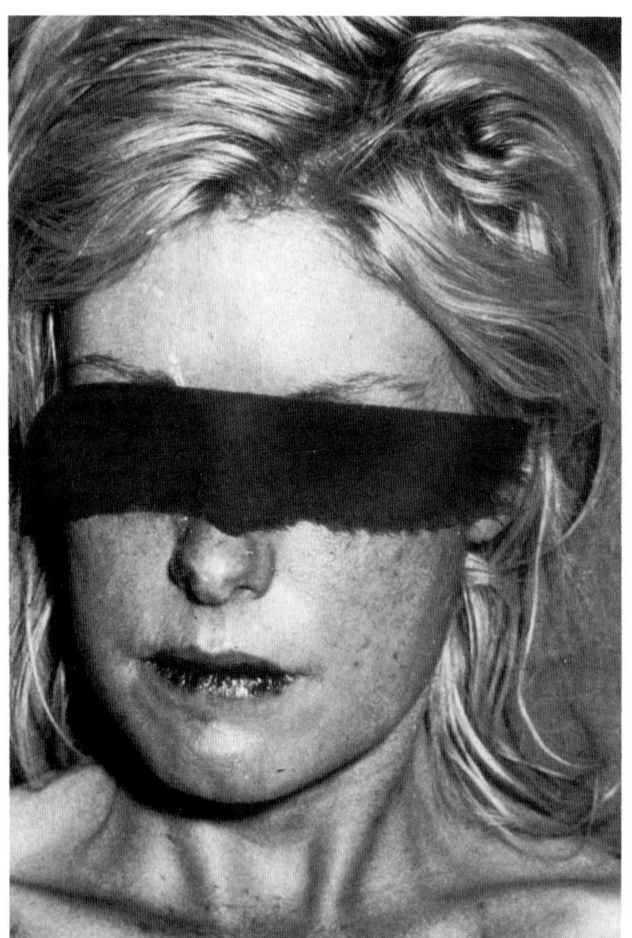

Fig. 13.1 Spider naevi affecting the face and chest wall

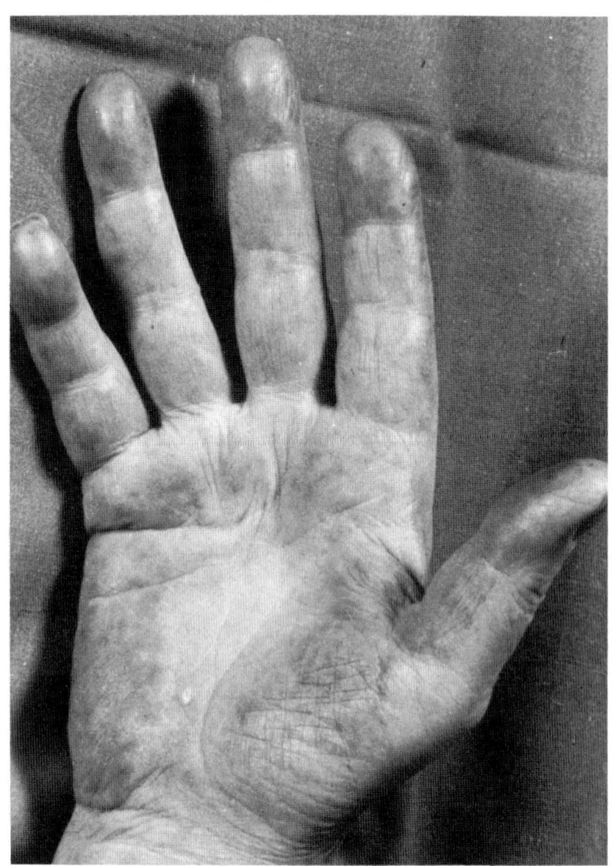

Fig. 13.2 Palmar erythema affecting the thenar and hypothenar eminences

Gynaecomastia is usually a bilateral enlargement of the breast tissue which may be tender and associated with areolar pigmentation (Fig. 13.5). In association with gynaecomastia reduced libido and testicular atrophy are

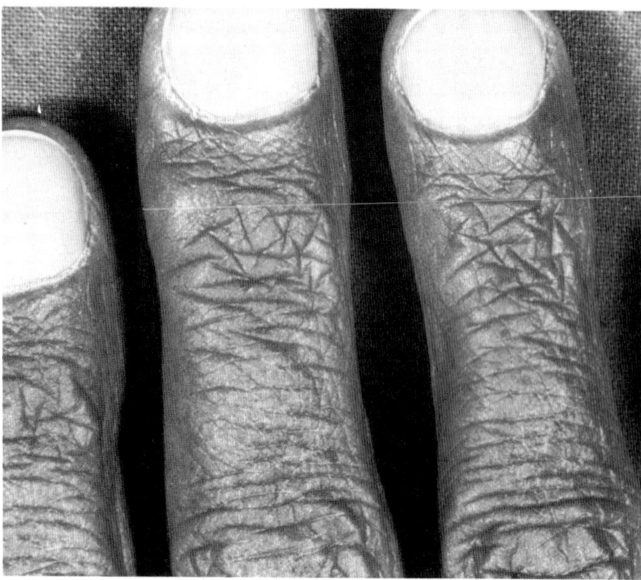

Fig. 13.3 Leuconychia (white nails) in a patient with cirrhosis

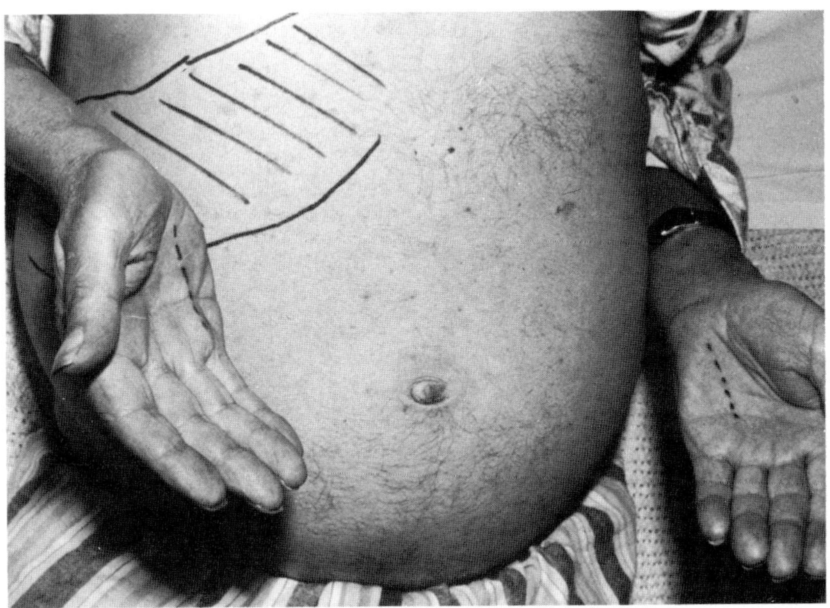

Fig. 13.4 Hepatomegaly and Dupuytren's contracture in a patient with extensive cirrhosis

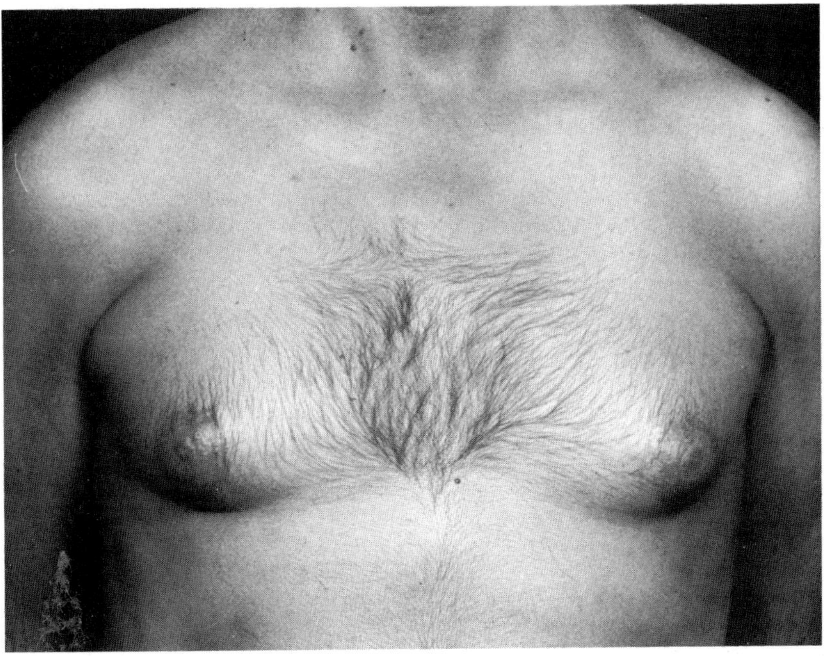

Fig. 13.5 Bilateral gynaecomastia in a patient with alcoholic liver disease

frequent complaints. It should be noted, however, that a number of diuretics (e.g. spironolactone) used in the treatment of ascites are themselves known to be associated with gynaecomastia. Spontaneous *bruising*, ecchymoses and bleeding around venepuncture sites are all well recognized features of liver disease. This is due to abnormal coagulation associated with failure to synthesize clotting factors. *Pruritus* occurs in cholestatic liver disease in association with jaundice. It can be particularly distressing for the patient and often intolerable. The itching is usually generalized but the palms and soles seem most affected. Xanthomas also may be found usually around the eye but may spread to other parts. They are associated with long-standing cholestasis. *Kayser-Fleischer rings* are found in Wilson's disease and are caused by copper deposition on the surface of the cornea.

Examination of the liver

Palpation of the liver should be combined with percussion to determine the upper and lower borders. The upper border of the liver is defined by percussion and dullness normally extends as far as the fifth intercostal space. In addition auscultation for arterial bruits in an enlarged liver is most important and may be associated with hepatocellular carcinoma. A venous hum can occur in portal hypertension.

The liver may be reduced in size in cirrhosis and certain types of hepatitis and this should be noted. The right lobe of the liver can be enlarged due to a tongue-like extension, Riedel's lobe. This anatomical variation is of no significance but can be mistaken for a tumour.

The overall consistency of an enlarged liver may help to determine its aetiology. For example an irregular (knobbly), hard liver is likely to be due to metastases, whereas a diffusely enlarged smooth liver may be cirrhotic in nature (Fig. 13.4).

Sometimes an hypertrophic liver lobe is palpable reflecting an atrophic but diseased yet impalpable lobe (Ch. 6).

Splenic enlargement

Splenomegaly can be detected by palpation commencing in the right iliac fossa and progressing upwards and to the left. In difficult cases, rotation of the patient 45° to the right allows the spleen to fall onto the clinician's right hand. The left hand should support the rib cage and relax the skin and abdominal musculature by drawing these down and to the right. Percussion may be useful and, in the presence of ascites, the spleen may be ballotable.

The splenic notch can sometimes be recognized on the anterior border of a grossly enlarged spleen and may be helpful in distinguishing it from other organs.

Ascites

In a patient with liver disease and a distended abdomen the presence of ascites should be seriously considered. On a lateral view of the patient the maximum circumference is noted above the umbilicus which may be everted (Fig. 13.6). Clinical confirmation of ascites is achieved by eliciting shifting dullness on percussion and a fluid 'thrill' on gently tapping the flanks. There is frequently associated muscle wasting and gynaecomastia.

The ascites may be specifically related to liver disease, e.g. hypoalbuminaemia associated with portal hypertension or alternatively a manifestation of generalized malignancy (malignant ascites) with multiple liver metastases.

Gallbladder signs

Tenderness on palpation over the gallbladder exacerbated by inspiration suggests acute cholecystitis (positive Murphy's sign). The finding of a palpable gallbladder in the presence of obstructive jaundice suggests malignant obstruction to the biliary tree (Courvoisier's law) and is most commonly due to a carcinoma of the head of the pancreas. However, failure to palpate the gallbladder does not necessarily exclude malignant disease. In addition it is possible to have a palpable distended gallbladder in the presence of gallstones where one obstructs the common bile duct and another is impacted in Hartmann's pouch or cystic duct resulting in an empyema (or mucocele) of the gallbladder.

An intermittently palpable gallbladder is suggestive of periampullary carcinoma.

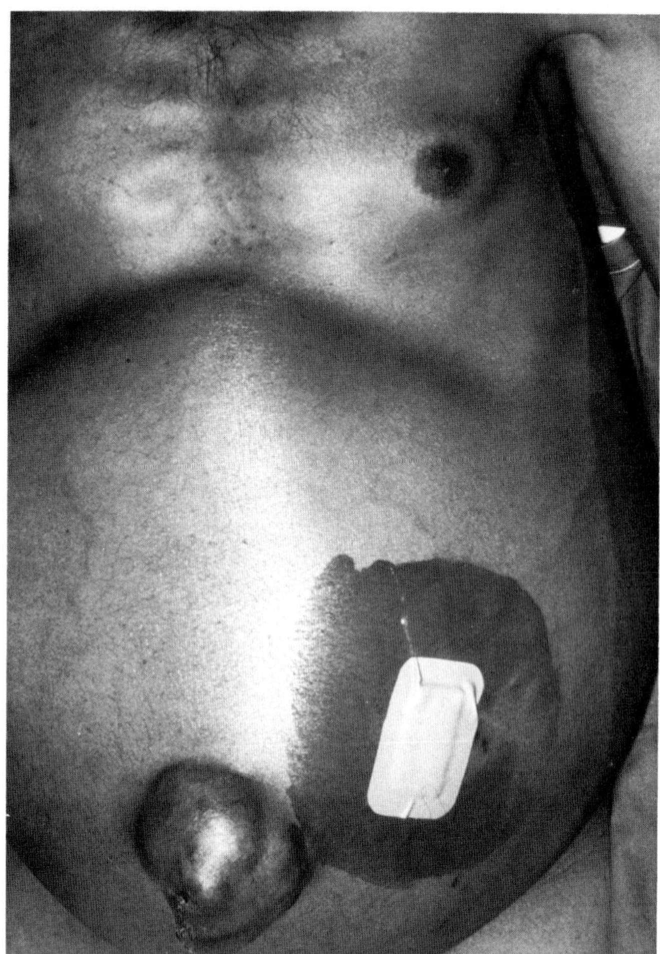

Fig. 13.6 Ascites with an everted umbilicus and venous distension in a patient with cirrhosis

EVIDENCE OF PORTAL HYPERTENSION

Obstruction to the portal system results in portal hypertension. The obstruction may be either intrahepatic or extrahepatic.

Intrahepatic portal hypertension is frequently, but not

always, associated with hepatomegaly. Other features are splenomegaly and ascites. Large dilated abdominal wall veins (Fig. 13.6) occur due to a collateral circulation between the portal system (umbilical vein joining the left branch of the portal vein) and the systemic veins. The direction of blood flow is away from the umbilicus. Patients with portal hypertension most frequently present with bleeding from oesophageal varices. These are best diagnosed by endoscopy and are discussed in Chapter 101. Haemorrhoidal varices may develop around the anus but are extremely rare.

Extrahepatic portal hypertension is most often due to thrombosis of the portal vein. A history of neonatal infection around the umbilicus, major intra-abdominal sepsis (e.g. perforated duodenal ulcer or appendicitis), pancreatic cancer or blood disorders resulting in hypercoagulability will indicate a possible aetiology.

Gross splenomegaly is almost invariably found (often associated with a pancytopenia). The liver appears normal but ascites may be elicited.

EVIDENCE OF ALCOHOLIC LIVER DISEASE

The clinical features associated with alcoholic liver disease may be related to alcoholism itself or to the manifestations of hepatocellular dysfunction.

Trauma and bruising are often evident and related to repeated falls whilst drunk. Multiple fractured ribs — often recognized as multiple 'old' fractures on a chest X-ray — may also be found. Similarly, alcoholic neuropathy is a frequent accompaniment in poorly nourished alcoholics. Paraesthesia, loss of sensation to pin prick and light touch with absent ankle jerks are recognized. There is frequently a poor general state of nutrition with vitamin deficiency.

Specific liver disease

Acute alcoholic hepatitis usually follows a particularly extensive drinking bout. The liver is tender, jaundice may occur and a pyrexia with leucocytosis is often present. Alcoholic cirrhosis may be accompanied by any of the manifestations of extensive liver disease, e.g. portal hypertension, ascites and eventual liver failure.

EVIDENCE OF OTHER TYPES OF CIRRHOSIS

Primary biliary cirrhosis

This condition usually affects middle–aged women. Specific clinical factors are pruritus, which is usually the first symptom and may occur many months before the onset of jaundice. Mild jaundice, pigmentation, vitiligo and arthritis may also be found.

The C.R.S.T. syndrome (Calcinosis, Raynaud's phenomenon, sclerodactyly and telangiectasia) has been described in patients with primary biliary cirrhosis.

Ulcerative colitis & Crohn's disease

Both of these inflammatory bowel diseases can be associated with hepatobiliary disorders, particularly primary sclerosing cholangitis. It is important to exclude these diseases in any patients with an unusual or poorly explained liver disease.

LABORATORY INVESTIGATIONS

Laboratory investigations may be of some value in helping to distinguish intrahepatic cholestatic jaundice from extrahepatic obstruction though the liver function tests themselves are of limited value (Ch. 25). A list of the investigations which should be undertaken appear in Table 13.1 and include tests such as anti-mitochondrial antibody, which is indicative of primary biliary cirrhosis, and hepatitis B surface antigen or IgM antibody to hepatitis A, which make the specific diagnosis of these forms of hepatitis. As yet there is no serological test available for the non-A and non-B forms of hepatitis.

Table 13.1 Laboratory investigations in the jaundiced patient

Haematological tests:
- full blood count; erythrocyte sedimentation rate; reticulocyte count; haptoglobin levels; Coomb's test

Liver function tests:
- conjugated and unconjugated bilirubin levels; aspartate amino transferase (AST); alanine aminotransferase (ALT); γ-glutamyl transferase; alkaline phosphatase

Proteins:
- albumin; globulin; prothrombin time

Immunological and serological tests:
- mitochondrial antibodies
- smooth muscle and antinuclear antibody
- immunoglobulins: IgG, IgM, IgA
- hepatitis B surface antigen (HBsAg)
- IgM antibody to hepatitis A
- cytomegalovirus antibody
- EB virus antibody (monospot)
- leptospiral agglutinins
- fasciola complement fixation test
- amoebic complement fixation test
- hydatid complement fixation test
- Wassermann reaction and other serological tests for syphilis

Alpha-l-antitrypsin levels
Alpha-foetoprotein levels
Serum amylase

Plasma caeruloplasmin levels
Iron and iron binding capacity
Spot blood alcohol
Urine: urobilinogen, haemosiderin
Stools: ova and parasites

Other specific investigations of value are alpha foetoprotein levels in hepatocellular carcinoma, spot blood alcohol and plasma caeruloplasmin levels.

IMAGING

All modalities of imaging have been utilized in the diagnosis of liver disease. Certain investigations have particular indications and some are superior both in terms of specificity and sensitivity. Other chapters in this book will deal in detail with each investigation but in this brief review the different studies will be mentioned with their chief indications.

Plain abdominal and chest X-rays (Ch. 18)

Calcification within the gallbladder will indicate opaque gallstones; similarly multiple areas of calcification in the pancreas are helpful in diagnosing chronic pancreatitis. The presence of gas in the biliary tree should be looked for particularly if subacute small bowel obstruction is present (gallstone ileus) (Ch. 61). Multiple fractured ribs on a chest X-ray or bone scan may indicate that the patient is an alcoholic and suffering from alcoholic hepatitis or decompensated cirrhosis. The presence of primary or secondary tumour and pleural effusions may be relevant.

Ultrasound (Ch. 14)

With its increasing availability, ultrasonography is now established as the major imaging investigation in hepatobiliary disease and particularly in the jaundiced patient. The technique is non-invasive and quick to perform but requires experience in technique and interpretation. It appears as accurate as cholecystography in diagnosing gallstones and a thickened gallbladder wall.

Its chief and most important use, however, is in the jaundiced patient. Extrahepatic obstruction can be diagnosed by the demonstration of dilated biliary radicles (Taylor & Rosenfield 1977). In experienced hands the accuracy in detecting ductal dilatation is over 95%.

A jaundiced patient without dilated ducts on ultrasound is suffering from non-obstructive jaundice unless, rarely, the investigation has been undertaken before the ducts have dilated. Patients with dilated ducts have obstructive jaundice and in some cases a definitive diagnosis can be obtained, e.g. gallstones in gallbladder, common bile duct stones or enlargement of the head of the pancreas suggestive of carcinoma. In extrahepatic obstruction ultrasound imaging will establish the level of the block in approximately 80% of cases (Malini & Sabel 1977). Difficulties in achieving a definitive diagnosis arise principally with small lesions at the lower end of the common bile duct which is often obscured by gas in the duodenum or colon.

In patients without dilated ducts hepatocellular disease is likely. Further information on the underlying aetiology may be obtained from the echo pattern. In multiple liver metastases an irregular echo appearance is present. In colorectal cancer liver metastases are frequently echogenic (Lamb & Taylor 1982). In cirrhosis or chronic active hepatitis the most commonly observed abnormality is a bright, tightly packed echo pattern. However, in several liver disorders a normal echo pattern is recognized. Most frequently in a jaundiced patient without duct dilatation liver biopsy is required to establish a definitive diagnosis.

Isotope scanning (Ch. 15)

99m Technetium Sulphur Colloid imaging gives useful information on liver texture. Patchy uptake in the liver with uptake in the spleen and bone marrow suggests cirrhosis. The presence of multiple liver metastases or primary liver tumour can be diagnosed.

Other more recently introduced hepatobiliary agents such as pyridexylaydine glutamate (PGA) and 2 : 6 dimethylphenylcarbamylmethyl iminochacetic acid (HIDA) outline the biliary ducts and common bile duct even in the presence of moderately raised bilirubin levels. Similar studies have been used as a diagnostic aid in patients presenting with acute cholecystitis where urgent confirmation of diagnosis is required.

Endoscopic retrograde cholangiopancreatography (ERCP) (Ch. 20)

In the hands of experienced endoscopists this is a particularly valuable investigation. In patients with a dilated duct on ultrasound visualization of the biliary tree not only confirms the diagnosis but gives information on the site and cause of obstruction. In the diagnosis of pancreatic pathology this is a particularly important means of recognizing disease of the main pancreatic duct.

Percutaneous transhepatic cholangiogram (PTC) (Ch. 19)

This investigation is also frequently used in the jaundiced patient with dilated ducts on ultrasound to obtain information on the site and cause of obstruction. Following entry into a dilated duct, aspiration of bile can be performed for bacteriology. Contrast is injected but overfilling of the ducts should be avoided. Successful opacification of the bile ducts has been reported in 99% of patients with dilated bile ducts and 82% of normal or sclerosed ducts (Felluci & Wittenburg 1977).

Computerized axial tomography (CT scans) (Ch. 16)

This investigation yields information on liver texture, gallbladder pathology and pancreatic disease. It is particularly valuable for the recognition of small space-occupying lesions in either the liver or the pancreas. As with ultrasound scan it can recognize the presence of dilated intrahepatic ducts in patients with jaundice.

Cholecystography (Ch. 18)

This investigation is of no value and should not be attempted in the presence of jaundice. In non-jaundiced patients gallstones can be recognized in the gallbladder and occasionally common bile duct. Non-opacification of the gallbladder in the absence of either jaundice, chronic diarrhoea or malabsorption indicates gallbladder pathology. The possible mechanisms of this are either a non-functioning gallbladder or a stone impacted in the cystic duct or Hartmann's pouch.

Intravenous cholangiogram (Ch. 18)

This investigation is infrequently performed nowadays. Following intravenous administration, the iodine-containing contrast medium binds to the plasma protein and is excreted by the liver cells. Bile ducts can thus be outlined and these are optimally demonstrated by tomography. Gallbladder opacification will be demonstrated if the cystic duct is patent. Other investigations are, however, more accurate for diagnosis in both the non-jaundiced as well as the jaundiced patient (Osnes et al 1978). Even when successfully performed, the diagnostic yield of this investigation is low (Blumgart et al 1974).

Operative and postoperative T-tube cholangiography

Operative cholangiography, as an accompaniment to cholecystectomy, is performed to ensure that the common bile duct is free of stones and that unhindered flow occurs into the duodenum. It may also have a role during laparotomy in the jaundiced patient when the underlying cause for obstruction to the common bile duct is not apparent.

Angiography (Ch. 21)

A number of angiographic investigations are available and have specific uses and indications.

Hepatic artery angiography may be indicated in the diagnosis of liver tumours, e.g. hepatoma or multiple metastases to ensure that a tumour is truly solitary prior to consideration of surgical excision. In patients considered for surgical excision of a major lobe of liver, important anatomical information can be obtained and is of value to the surgeon. Liver abscess and cyst can also be diagnosed by this technique when other investigations are equivocal. Embolisation of the artery may be performed for symptomatic endocrine tumours (Ch. 94).

Splenoportography is a valuable investigation in patients with oesophageal varices who are being considered for shunt surgery. Of particular importance is whether the portal vein is patent and information on the relevant anatomy is helpful. Portal pressures can also be obtained.

Inferior venacavography is occasionally performed prior to consideration of a major hepatic resection to determine the anatomy of the hepatic veins and to establish whether the inferior vena cava is being compressed or invaded (Ch. 97).

Liver biopsy (Ch. 22)

In the absence of dilated ducts a liver biopsy is often required and should be performed with care. This histology will determine the presence, severity and often the aetiology of acute or chronic liver disease and will help to differentiate the causes of cholestasis.

Laparoscopy (Ch. 23)

This investigation is occasionally performed to enable liver biopsy to be carried out under direct vision. It has also been advocated for use in patients with obstructive jaundice to enable a specific diagnosis before definitive laparotomy. Laparoscopic cholangiography is also feasible and in certain circumstances may reveal useful information.

REFERENCES

Blumgart L H, Salmon P R, Cotton P B 1974 Endoscopic retrograde cholangiopancreatography in the diagnosis of the patient with jaundice. Surgery, Gynecology and Obstetrics 138: 565–570

Felluci J T, Wittenburg J 1977 Refinements in Chiba needle transhepatic cholangiography. American Journal of Roentgenology 129: 11–16

Lamb G, Taylor I 1982 An assessment of ultrasound scanning in the recognition of colorectal liver metastases. Annals of the Royal College of Surgeons 64: 391–393

Malini S, Sabel J 1977 Ultrasonography in obstructive jaundice. Radiology 123: 429–433

Osnes M, Larsen S, Lowe P 1978 Comparison of endoscopic retrograde and intravenous cholangiography in diagnosis of biliary calculli. Lancet ii:230

Taylor K J, Rosenfield A T 1977 Greyscale ultrasonography in the differential diagnosis of jaundice. Archives of Surgery 112: 820–825

14

D. O. Cosgrove

The applications of ultrasound in surgery of the liver

INTRODUCTION

Ultrasound is a tomographic imaging technique capable of providing anatomical information with high resolution and great flexibility at low cost. Structural detail down to around a millimetre, e.g. for intrahepatic ducts, is available without administration of contrast agents. The high intrinsic contrast is due to the tissues' structure at a sub-millimetre level, chiefly the differences in rigidity and density between fluids, watery tissue, collagen fibres and fatty tissue. The tomograms are formed very rapidly, so that imaging in real time is standard. The studies are therefore quick and interactive. Immediate viewing of changing situations is a characteristic feature of routine ultrasound; examples include the effects of respiration or palpation on the organ and the direct real time observation of a biopsy needle. The tomograms can be taken in any plane allowing optimal display of critical anatomy. Since many scanners are small and self-contained, they may readily be wheeled to the ward, theatre or recovery room, a major asset for the surgical patient. Minimal preparation, or none at all, is required so that the procedure is well tolerated, the only practical problem being abdominal tenderness making probe contact painful. Ionizing radiation hazards do not exist.

However, the picture painted by this description omits some important limitations to the use of ultrasound. The variable quality of the images obtained is a problem. Slim patients give the best images, for resolution deteriorates with depth; children are excellent subjects. Bone and gas are impenetrable and also may degrade the image quality of regions of interest lying close to them. In practical terms for the liver this is only an occasional problem since the intercostal spaces allow adequate access in almost all cases where the preferred subcostal route is difficult. But for the pancreas and the lower end of the common bile duct adequate imaging may be impossible in some 10 to 20% of cases, especially where the patient is hospitalized or has an ileus.

The small field of view of an individual ultrasound image, especially with real time scanners, makes the image difficult to review. This can also lead to difficulty in repeating the same tomogram for follow up purposes. It also makes explanation difficult for referring physicians and surgeons who, understandably, find the more complete tomographic images of CT or NMR more believable. If they attend the actual scanning they will readily appreciate the completeness of the study and the added value of the real time display. The fact that the bony skeleton is not displayed, apart from causing difficulty in interpretation, poses a problem when it is necessary to compare ultrasound tomograms with CT or with radiographs.

The interactive nature of ultrasound renders it very operator-dependent: a skilled and motivated operator will produce good results, but lack of experience and lack of essential clinical background information severely devalue the study.

TECHNOLOGY

Ultrasound is a high frequency, mechanical vibration where alternate waves of compression and rarefaction travel through the tissue (McDicken 1981, Kremkau 1980). The waves are generated by a piezo-electric crystal element shaped into a transducer ceramic which focuses the ultrasound waves into a beam. The frequency of the ultrasound used is determined by the thickness of the crystal. A commonly used frequency is 3.5 Megahertz with a wavelength of 0.5 mm.

A small proportion of the ultrasound is absorbed by the tissue and appears as heat. The remainder is reflected as the ultrasound crosses between tissues of different acoustic properties, known as acoustic impedance, a complex of tissue density and rigidity. While both these components are familiar in that they are palpable in bulk, the ultrasound pulse responds to tissue structure in the sub-millimetre range. The smallest structure that can be resolved in practice depends on the contrast in reflectivity: well defined structures such as ducts can be traced down to a millimetre or so in calibre but ill-defined lesions such as liver metastases must be much larger, in the range of 5–10 mm.

The portion of the reflected sound beam returning to the transducer is used to form the image. The depth (range) of a reflecting interface is calculated from the delay between the sending of the pulse and the detection of the returning echo, and the direction from the angle at which the transducer faces, exactly as with RADAR or SONAR. The velocity of ultrasound in different tissues is not quite constant but varies so little that the depth errors amount to only a few percent.

The strength of the echoes is proportional to the change in acoustic impedance at the interface. At risk of oversimplifying a complex phenomenon, it may be said that impedance correlates with tissue rigidity. In the body rigidity ranges from gases at the one extreme through liquids and soft tissue to bone and calcified tissue at the other. For soft tissues the collagen content is usually the main contributor and this occurs in condensed form in fasciae and in diffuse form as the micro-skeleton of the parenchyma, mostly found surrounding blood vessels. It is probably the characteristic vascular pattern as reflected in the ultrasound image that lends tissue-specific texture to sonograms. Fatty tissue is strongly echogenic because of the lipid/watery interfaces at cellular or lobular level.

The real time scanner is now the standard instrument (Fukuda & Cosgrove 1985). In one form a single transducer emits a beam of ultrasound and is oscillated through 90° to form a triangular image. The movement is repeated 20–30 times a second to give a moving image, as with a cine film (cine-sonar). This system has the great advantage that good exposures can be obtained through small access ports, e.g. of the liver intercostally. However, the triangular field of view gives a poor display of superficial structures and the linear array is more convenient in this respect. Here the ultrasound beam is swept electronically along a block of piezo material some 2 cm wide and 5–10 cm long. Electronic versions of the sector system are also available.

To take a scan, the transducer is contacted with the skin using a coupling fluid (usually a jelly), and the examination consists of stroking the probe gently across the surface of the abdomen. For the liver, subcostal views in the transverse and longitudinal sections are convenient and access may be improved with the patient in held inspiration. The gastro-oesophageal junction can also be imaged in this way. If the upper abdomen is gassy, intercostal views give more limited access, but usually allow adequate assessment. Angled views can be useful, e.g. to line up the common bile duct. No preparation is needed for the liver, but the gallbladder is easier to assess when full, so a six-hour fast (clear fluids allowed) is useful, but not obligatory.

For the pancreas, views in the transverse plane give the best anatomical display and usually can be obtained without preparation and in the supine position. When overlying gas obstructs the ultrasound beam, scanning in the erect position can help by allowing bowel loops to drop away as well as by bringing the left lobe of the liver down over the pancreas thus providing a window. In difficult cases access can be improved further by filling the stomach with water before scanning. Using these approaches, the head of the pancreas can be imaged adequately in over 75% of subjects. Patients with ileus (e.g. in acute pancreatitis) and the very obese are usually persistently difficult, and here CT is better able to provide a diagnosis. Though not germane to hepato-biliary surgery, it should be noted that imaging the tail of pancreas with ultrasound is more difficult, though access can often be obtained through the spleen in the coronal plane. The spleen itself, together with the splenic vein and left kidney, may be imaged in the coronal plane through the left intercostal spaces, or subcostally.

NORMAL FINDINGS

The liver

A series of sagittal tomograms (Lyons 1978, McGrath & Mills 1984, Wagner & Lawson 1982) reveals the left lobe (Couinaud 1982) as an almond-shaped structure extending inferiorly from the fibrous portion of the diaphragm (Fig. 14.1) (Cosgrove & McCready 1982). Its inferior border is normally sharp. Its visceral surface is related to the aorta and the oesophago-gastric junction superiorly and to the stomach, lesser sac and body of pancreas inferiorly. Moving to the right the dorsal segment (caudate lobe) is detected superiorly overlying the inferior vena cava. The fissure for the ligamentum venosum, separating it from the left liver, is clearly seen and may pose an interpretative problem by partially shadowing the caudate itself. The ligamentum teres may be encountered here and longitudinal sections further to the right reveal the quadrate lobe (segment IV) before the porta is encountered, where the portal vein and its left and right main branches predominate. Superiorly, the groove for the inferior vena cava is seen, though this and the hepatic veins are better displayed on transverse section. Further to the right, the right liver (segments V–VIII) is visible up against the right hemidiaphragm. Its visceral surface contacts the right kidney, the hepatic flexure of colon and the duodenum, often with the gallbladder intervening. Again, the free edge of the liver has a sharp contour (Hollinshead 1982, Netter 1964, Schneck 1983).

Transverse sections high in the liver cut the terminal inferior vena cava as it penetrates the diaphragm to empty into the right atrium (Fig 14.2). A little below this the point of emptying of the hepatic veins is seen; usually the left and middle form a common trunk which joins the

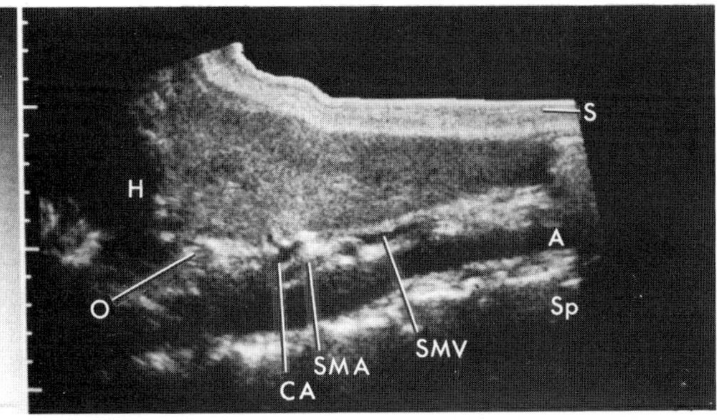

(a)

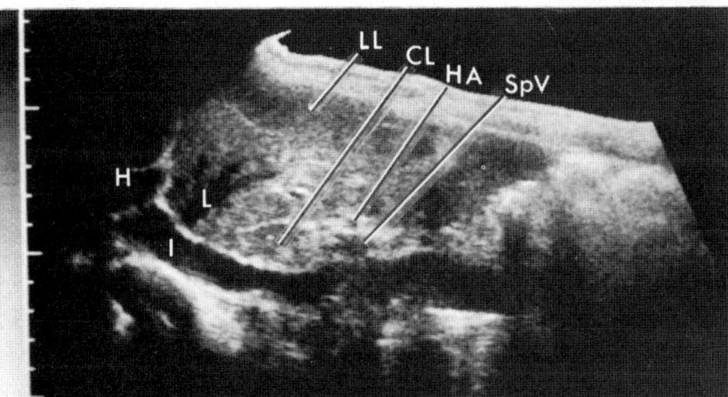

(b)

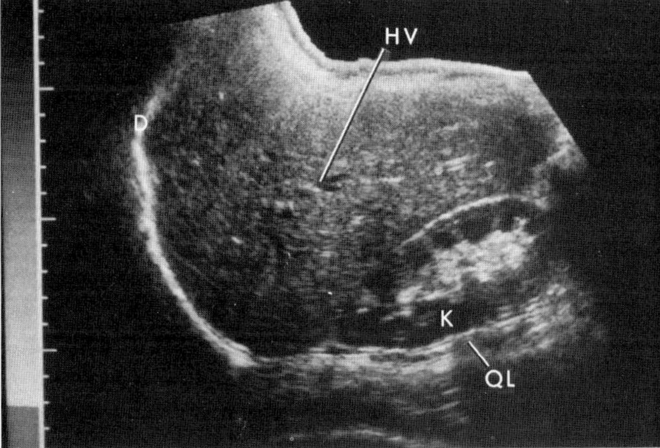

(c)

Fig. 14.1 Normal liver — sagittal sections.

The liver's uniform stippled texture of mid-grey level is shown together with the contiguous organs. Veins are seen as echo-free tubular structures; those with prominent walls are portal veins while the thin walls of the hepatic veins are not apparent. The echo-poor structures centrally placed in the renal parenchyma in (c) are medullary pyramids.

In this and subsequent sagittal tomograms the slices are displayed in the conventional orientation with the patient supine and viewed from the right, as be would be during an examination. Thus the patient's head is to the left of the image, with the feet to the right and the anterior skin line is uppermost. In all the ultrasound images, the small scale divisions are one centimetre apart.

(A = aorta, D = diaphragm, CA = coeliac axis, H = heart, HV = hepatic vein, I = inferior vena cava, LL = left liver, K = kidney, O = oesophagus, QL = quadratus lumborum, S = skin line, SMA = superior mesenteric artery, SMV = superior mesenteric vein, Sp = spine)

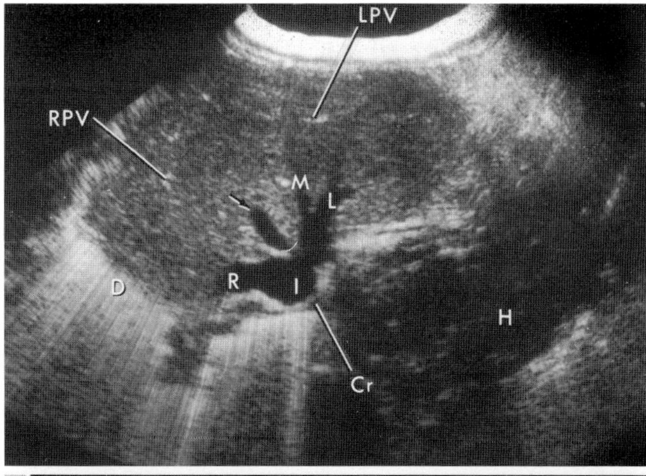

(a)

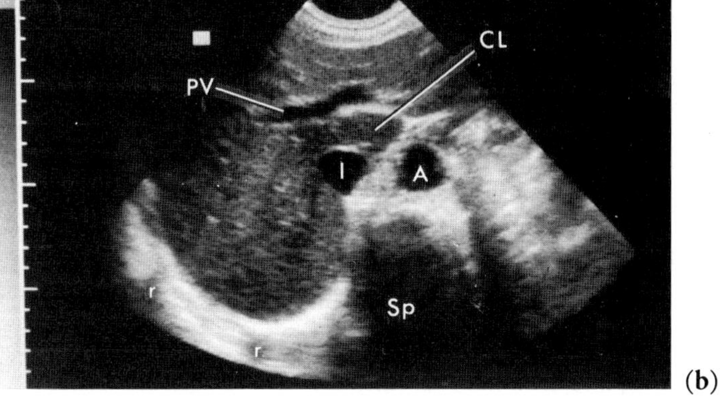

(b)

Fig. 14.2 Normal liver — transverse sections.

High transverse sections show (a) the terminal portions of the hepatic veins, the left and middle usually forming a short common trunk before discharging into the upper inferior vena cava. The middle hepatic vein separates the left and right livers; the terminal branches of the portal veins that supply them can be discerned. A separate vein (arrow) often drains the supero-anterior segment of the right lobe (segment VIII). Further inferiorly (b) the caudate lobe (segment I) and the portal vein are imaged.

Transverse sonograms are displayed as viewed from the patient's feet in the supine position. Thus they correspond with the orientation of conventional X-rays, with the patient's right on the left.

(A = aorta, CL = caudate lobe, Cr = crus, D = diaphragm, H = heart, I = inferior vena cava, L = left hepatic vein, LPV = left portal vein, M = middle hepatic vein, PV = portal vein, R = right hepatic vein, r = ribs, RPV = right portal vein, Sp = spine)

inferior vena cava anteriorly. The right hepatic vein empties into the lateral part of the IVC, often a centimetre or so below. Simply by sliding the transducer inferiorly, the course of these major veins can be traced to define the sector to which structures belong. The smaller inferior hepatic veins are only rarely visualized on ultrasound.

The dorsal segment (segment I) and its process, lying in contact with the left liver, is often apparent in sections a little inferiorly. Segment VII may form a surprising appearance posterior to the inferior vena cava as it partially enfolds it.

The ligamentum teres is well seen cut in cross section; normally solid, a thread-like remnant of the umbilical vein is normal. At this level the gallbladder is often visualized with the right kidney posteriorly. The pancreas may be visualized here also.

The liver parenchyma appears as a sponge-like texture representing the interaction of the echoes from the liver lobules with the ultrasound beam. The texture therefore varies both with equipment parameters (especially the transducer) and with pathology. Distinguishing these influences at present is largely a matter of experience, though more quantitative methods are likely to be developed in the near future (so-called 'tissue characterization', Nicholas 1984).

The uniform liver texture is interrupted by vessels. The hepatic veins, with their thin walls, appear as branching, tubular defects converging to the upper IVC. The portal tracts have strongly reflective walls due to the associated vessels and to the enveloping fat and fibrous tissue. The left portal vein curves anteriorly from the main portal vein to supply the more anteriorly situated left liver. The right portal vein runs in about the same coronal plane as the porta, passing to the right before dividing into anterior and posterior branches. Within the liver the bile ducts and arterial branches are too small to be resolved on ultrasound though both are seen at the porta (see below).

Also disturbing the homogeneous texture of the liver is the echogenic ligamentum teres passing from the free edge of the liver close to the midline, superiorly and to the right to end in the left portal vein. Superiorly the residual sinus venosus is represented by the limit of the echogenic line separating the caudate from the left liver. It passes superiorly to end at the inferior vena cava and contains the attachment of the lesser omentum whose fat accounts for the high reflectivity of this fissure. The fissure between the quadrate (segment IV) and the right liver can often also be visualized as an oblique band stretching from the origin of the right portal vein to the neck of the gallbladder (Fried et al 1984).

The liver capsule is seen as a fine echogenic line. It is not normally well marked though in ascites is readily detected when the ultrasound beam is aligned across it.

The segmental anatomy of the liver is best appreciated in transverse section. Superiorly the easily demonstrated hepatic veins provide obvious landmarks with the middle hepatic veins, running from the gall bladder fossa, separating the left and right livers. The left hepatic vein runs in the plane between the posterior (segment II) and anterior (segment IV) of the left liver. The separation between segments III and IV is easily demonstrated a few centimetres inferiorly where the ligamentum teres is cut across. The falciform ligament cannot be imaged except in the presence of ascites when it appears as a thin sheet attaching the anterior surface of the liver to the anterior abdominal wall. The fissure between the quadrate (segment IV) and the anterior portion of the right lobe (segment V) is often clearly seen, though its oblique or near-coronal orientation may surprise until it is remembered that the quadrate lies anterior to the right liver in the true anatomical orientation of the liver. The right hepatic vein, running in the coronal plane, separates the anterior from the posterior sectors of the right lobe (segment V and VIII from segment VI & VII).

The interdigitating pattern of the portal vein branches, running into the centre of the segments, is also readily demonstrated. The division of the right portal vein into anterior and posterior sectoral branches is usually apparent. The division of the left portal vein may also be demonstrated.

The great variation in shape to which the liver is subject markedly affects its appearance on tomography. A Reidel extension of the right lobe is seen as a tongue passing across the right kidney: a valuable practical application of ultrasound is the demonstration that an apparent right upper quadrant mass is actually a Reidel lobe. The diaphragmatic surface of the right liver is usually smooth, but prominent or hypertrophic diaphragmatic leaflets produce 'cough furrows' that may be seen on ultrasound as indentations, or, if the intervening parts of the liver catch the eye, as lobulations that are easily mistaken for mass lesions.

The caudate lobe (segment I) is very variable in size and shape. Measured transversely to the deepest part of the fissure for the sinus venosus, it is usually 1/3 to 1/2 the width of the right liver: an upper limit of 2/3 defines the hypertrophy seen in cirrhosis and the Budd-Chiari syndrome. The caudate lobe may extend inferiorly as a tongue to below the level of the porta. It can then masquerade as precaval or preaortic lymphadenopathy or even be confused with a pancreatic mass.

The left lobe is very variable in size, occasionally being absent or replaced by a fibrous remnant. It has been suggested that this is due to an extension of the neonatal spasm of the umbilical vein into the left portal vein. This variation in size can also be demonstrated on ultrasound.

Due to the great variations in proportion of the liver, an estimation of its size cannot be made from any single tomogram (Fritschy et al 1983, Niederau et al 1983). A complete series can be measured to determine the liver volume accurately. Both CT and ultrasound are suitable for this but the comparative ease with which the liver's margins can be traced on a CT scan makes this the preferred technique. Linear measurements, such as the span of the liver in the mid-clavicular line or its antero-posterior thickness at the left border of the spine, are easily made on ultrasound but are inaccurate as volume estimates, though useful for serial assessment.

The biliary tree

The filled gallbladder is usually a very obvious structure on sonography of the right upper quadrant because the echo-free bile shows up in strong contrast to the fine echogenic line of the wall (Fig. 14.3a) (Cosgrove & McCready 1982). Classically the gallbladder has a pear shape, though it is so variable that this description can be misleading. Folds in the body or at the fundus can often be effaced by changing the patient's position or by continued filling. The position of the gallbladder is also very variable, since it may possess its own mesentery and wander from its fossa on the visceral surface of the liver. However the position of the neck of the gallbladder is relatively fixed below and to the right of the porta; the fissure separating segment IV (quadrate) from the antero-lateral segment of the right liver (segment V) passes from the porta to the neck of the gallbladder and can act as a useful landmark for its position when there is difficulty in identification such as a contracted or tumour-filled gallbladder (Fried et al 1983). The initial portion of the cystic duct may be imaged as a tortuous tubular structure continuous with the neck of the gallbladder, but this is only possible when it is filled with bile. When empty, it produces strong echoes (due to the fibro-muscular wall) and there may be shadowing of deeper structures. This pattern is confusing since it simulates an impacted gallstone.

(a)

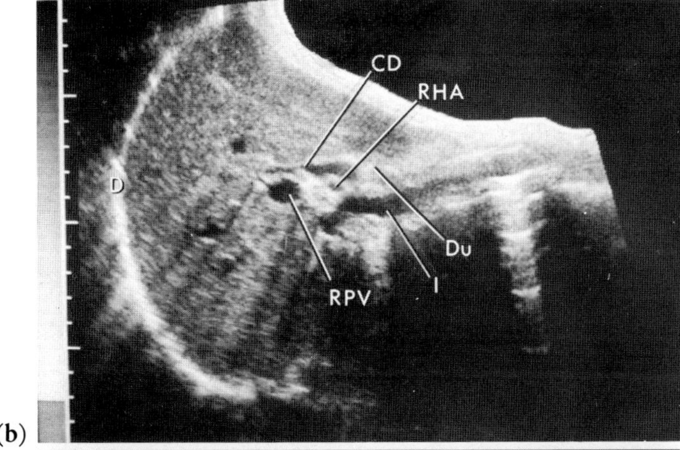

(b)

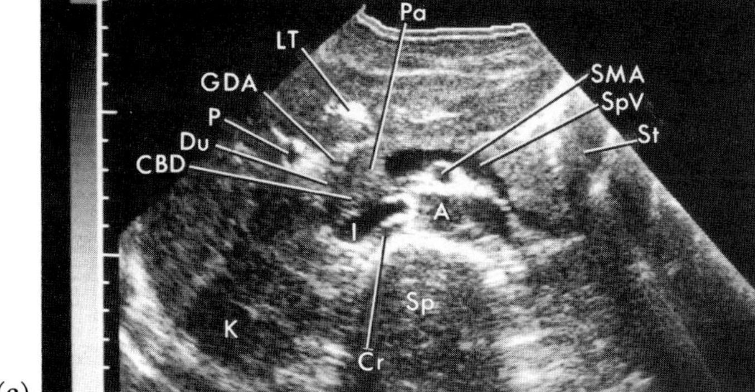

(c)

Fig. 14.3 The biliary tree.
The pear-shape and thin wall of the filled gallbladder are seen in (a).
The upper portion of the bile duct is shown in the oblique tomogram (b) lying anterior to the right portal vein and right hepatic artery. It can be traced down to the level where it passes posterior to the first part of the duodenum. The retroduodenal portion is usually obscured by gas. The terminal portion can be detected again in the head of the pancreas (c).
A = aorta, Du = duodenum, CBD = common bile duct, CD = common duct, G = gall bladder, GDA = gastro-duodenal artery, I = inferior vena cava, K = kidney, LT = ligamentum teres, P = porta (here the neck of the gallbladder), RPV = right portal vein, SMA = superior mesenteric artery, Sp = spine, SpV = splenic vein, St = stomach)

Identification of the biliary tree on ultrasound depends on an awareness of its relationships with the portal vein. Starting high in the porta, portions can be identified lying anterior to the right portal vein; the best view is obtained in an oblique section approximately at right angles to the costal margin, either intercostally or subcostally (Fig. 14.3b). In this plane the right portal vein is cut across and so is seen as a ring; the duct is cut lengthwise or obliquely and is seen as a tube lying anteriorly across the right portal vein. An exact identification of this portion of the duct may be difficult, but probably this represents the right hepatic duct. Traced inferiorly it expands as it is joined sequentially by the left hepatic duct and the cystic duct forming the common hepatic and common bile ducts, respectively. Since the junctions themselves cannot usually be imaged, the imprecise term 'common duct' is often deliberately employed. Further inferiorly the duct passes posterior to the first part of the duodenum; when this contains gas, as is usual, the ultrasound beam is obstructed and the middle third of the duct cannot be imaged. It can be picked up again in the head of the pancreas; transverse sections are usually best for this, with careful study of the pancreas and adjacent duodenum (Fig. 14.3c).

The lumen of the duct measures up to some 4 mm within the porta and some 7 mm inferiorly (common bile duct). A precise upper limit cannot be set because of the spread of the normal range. There is also some overlap with the size in minimal dilatation, the suggested figures allowing approximately 95% discrimination. The duct calibre may also increase with age and following cholecystectomy, either due to instrumentation or to the residual effects of obstruction. The duct diameter as measured on ultrasound is considerably smaller than measured on contrast radiology. The smearing of strong echoes on ultrasound serves to minimize the apparent lumen while tube magnification and choleretic or pressure effects on cholangiography enlarge it (Sauerbrei et al 1980).

ULTRASOUND IN LIVER PATHOLOGY

Ultrasound can be useful to the liver surgeon in both focal and diffuse disorders. Its application may be in diagnosis, preoperative evaluation and in postoperative assessment. Intraoperative uses are becoming increasingly important.

Cystic lesions

Congenital cysts are easily detected on ultrasound as well-defined, rounded, echo-free spaces which show apparent enhancement of the distal echoes, due to the low attenuation of the cyst fluid (Fig. 14.4a & b) (Bruneton et al 1983b). While ultrasound cannot differentiate between the true congenital cyst and post-infective or post-traumatic cysts, complicated cysts (necrotic tumour, superinfection) are obviously different since they have internal echoes and irregular walls. Their segmental location can be determined. Giant cysts so distort the local anatomy that even their organ of origin may be difficult to determine.

Polycystic disease (Fig. 14.4c) has a more complex appearance with numerous cystic spaces which become polygonal where they are contiguous. The complex pattern and the marked distal enhancement make complications difficult to assess: an abscess or tumour deposit in the affected region would probably be missed.

Haemangioma

Haemangiomas are common and can be troublesome on ultrasound since they have a range of appearances which overlaps those of more serious lesions, especially secondary tumour deposits. The pattern on ultrasound depends on whether the condition is localized or diffuse and on their structure. Cavernous haemangiomas are echo-poor unless there is thrombosis or calcification, both of which produce high lever echoes (Bruneton et al 1983a). This is also the appearance in the commoner capillary type (Fig. 14.5). When focal they produce the typical pattern of a highly reflective rounded lesion, often lying in a subcapsular position (Bree 1983). The diffuse type, commoner in neonates, gives an irregular pattern to the affected portion of the liver, with confluent, ill-defined echo-poor regions. Definitive diagnosis requires angiography, either in the form of conventional hepatic arteriography or using CT with dynamic studies to demonstrate the vascular pattern (Freeny et al 1979).

Ultrasound can be useful in assessing progress in the neonate presenting with high-output heart failure, since it is a simple matter to repeat the scans. For the focal lesions, ironically, the ease with which ultrasound can detect them poses a problem since further investigation is usually required for a condition that is of no clinical importance (Gandolfi et al 1983).

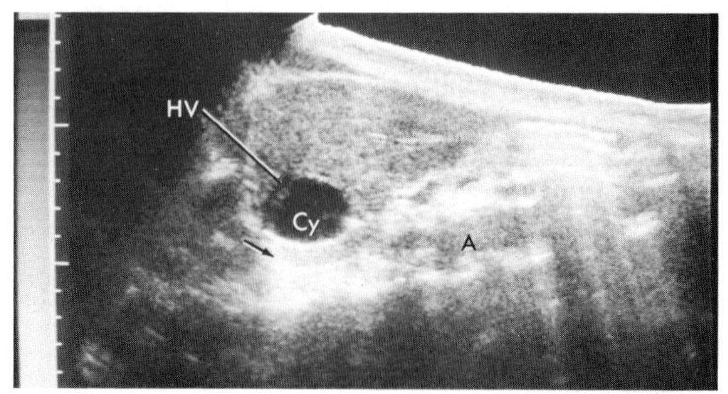

(a)

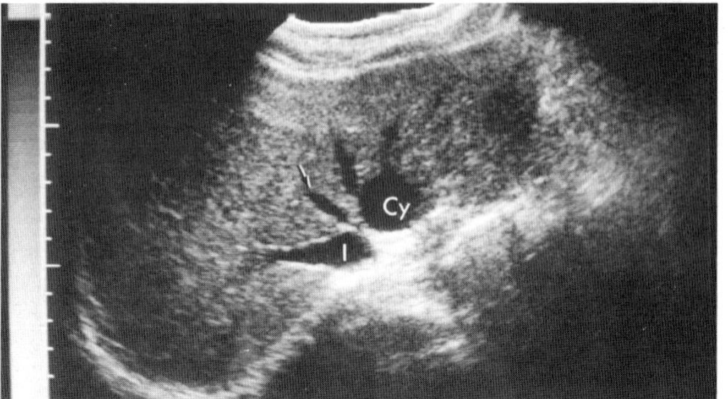

(b)

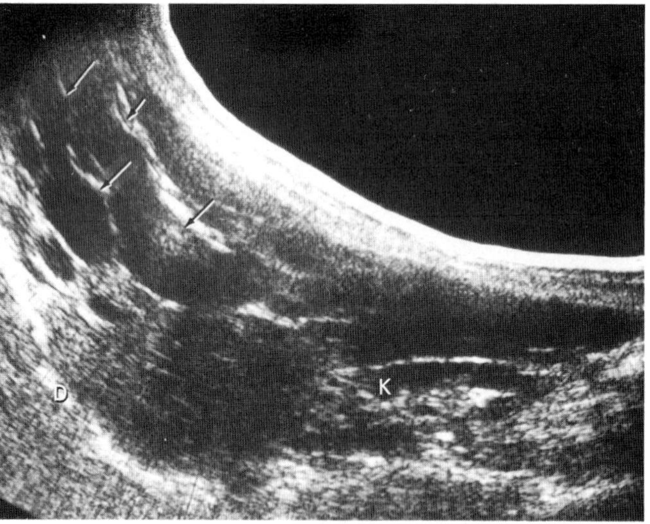

(c)

Fig. 14.4 Liver cysts.

Cysts show the distal echo enhancement (arrow in a) that is the ultrasonic clue that they are fluid filled. This benign cyst also has the characteristic features of smooth walls and absent internal echoes. The hepatic vein that lies immediately superior to it can be identified in the transverse section (b) as the left hepatic vein, and the middle hepatic vein runs to its right. Thus this cyst lies in the left liver but involves both segments II & IV. Note the separate vein (arrow) draining segment VIII.

In polycystic disease the cysts have the same features but their contiguous surfaces tend to be flattened (arrows in c). Assessment of the remaining liver may be difficult because the cysts disturb the ultrasonic texture.

(A = aorta, Cy = cyst, D = diaphragm, HV = hepatic vein, I = inferior vena cava, K = kidney)

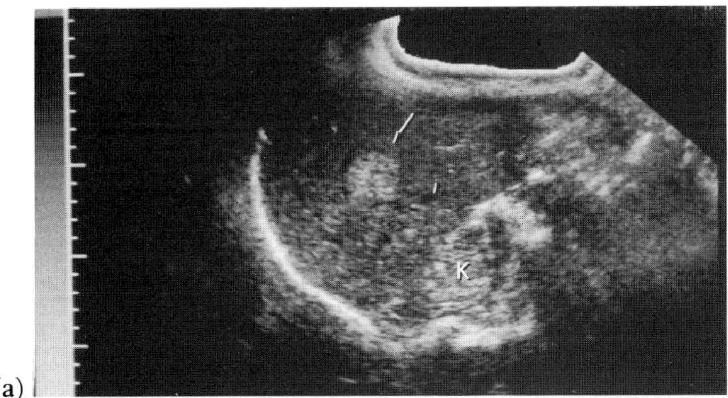

(a)

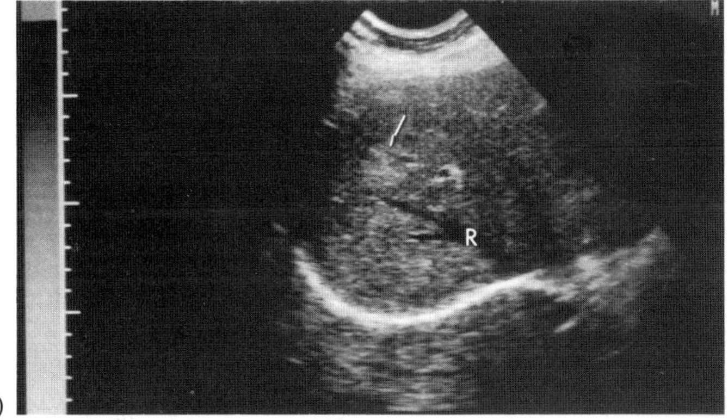

(b)

Fig. 14.5 Haemangioma.
The strong echoes and clear margins of this lesion are typical of the common capillary haemangioma (arrows). It lies in segment VIII, just anterior to the right hepatic vein (arrow-head in a).
(K = kidney, R = right hepatic vein)

Infective conditions

Because of its sensitivity to fluid spaces ultrasound is highly reliable in the detection of liver abscess cavities (Kuligowska & Noble 1983, Rubinson et al 1980). The typical pattern, with an irregular, shaggy margin and debris-containing fluid is easily recognized (Fig. 14.6 a & b). Ultrasound may be used to guide fine needle aspiration for culture and if necessary this may be performed at the patient's bedside using a portable scanner. Adequate sampling both from the wall of the abscess as well as from the fluid region and correct handling for culture (aerobic, anaerobic, TB, fungal) are important for successful diagnosis. In selected cases a drain can be inserted under ultrasound control for definitive treatment. However insertion of a sufficiently large drain may be difficult under local anaesthesia and for abscesses lying high in the right lobe (and similarly for sub-phrenic collections) the extrapleural route may be difficult to achieve. A formal approach under general anaesthetic is preferred unless the patient's condition precludes this.

Abscesses do not always have the typical features. Early on, before a cavity has developed, they form an inflammatory mass (Dewbury et al 1980). This appears as a focal lesion, often poorly defined, with low or high level echoes. The changes may be very subtle, so that a negative ultrasound early in the course of a febrile illness should not be taken to exclude an abscess; an isotope scan may be more revealing and a repeat ultrasound after a few days may show typical changes as pus accumulates.

Gas formation alters the ultrasound appearance markedly since the gas pocket returns very strong echoes and prevents penetration of the ultrasound beam so that deeper structures are obliterated. Detection of such a lesion within the liver is straightforward, though its size may be underestimated. For the abdomen in general, however, the gas pocket is difficult to distinguish from gas in bowel loops and an abscess may escape detection altogether; here CT scanning is more reliable. Because of the way gas collects in the upper part of a cavity, a gas-containing subphrenic collection on the right can usually be detected without special difficulty (Terrier et al 1983). However, on the left, where gut loops often occupy the subphrenic space, especially following splenectomy, the abnormality may be very difficult to detect.

Eventually an abscess cavity may shrink and disappear or it may leave a linear scar. In some cases a fluid space may persist indefinitely as a post-infective cyst (Ralls et al 1983).

The different types of abscess are indistinguishable on ultrasound. Amoebic abscesses have the same pattern as pyogenic and a tuberculous abscess can also take this form (Ralls et al 1979).

Ultrasound can often provide clues to the aetiology of an abscess. For example there may be features of cholecystitis possibly with a pericholecystitic abscess. A mass in the right iliac fossa suggests an appendix abscess or a pelvic scan may demonstrate a tubovarian abscess.

Hydatid disease (*Echinococcus granulosus*) of the liver is readily detected on ultrasound as a cystic cavity, most commonly in the right lobe (Abdel-Latief et al 1982, Hadidi 1983). The presence of daughter cysts (some 50% show this) gives a pathognomonic appearance of one or many cysts within the mother cyst (Beggs 1983). In the mature form the lesion is packed with polygonal cysts which may even show third generation daughters within them (Fig. 14.6c). In earlier cases a careful search may be needed to demonstrate the beginnings of daughter cyst formation. Before this budding begins or when the hydatid is sterile, the lesion is indistinguishable from a simple cyst. Careful general and serological assessment is then required to make the diagnosis. Hydatids often show a sediment of debris, representing the shed scolices (hydatid sand) and they frequently calcify, a change that may be detected on ultrasound as strong echoes but one that is more obvious on plain X-ray. Superinfection with pyogenic organisms may occur; in that event the lesion has the same appearance as an abscess.

The question of aspiration of hydatid cysts is a vexed

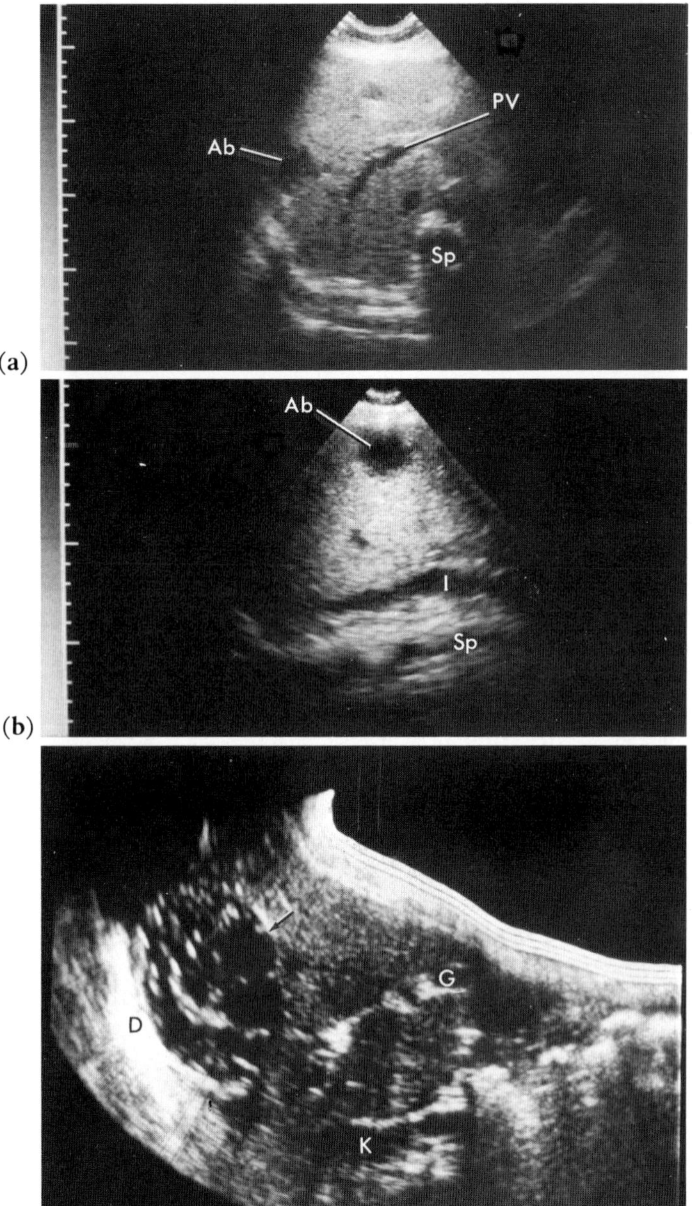

Fig. 14.6 Abscess.
The shaggy, thick walls of this fluid-filled lesion are typical of an abscess though a haematoma or a necrotic tumour deposit would be indistinguishable. This lesion is situated very laterally in the right lobe of the liver.
A rounded cystic mass containing numerous smaller cysts is the typical pattern of a hydatid (arrow in c). Daughter cysts are not always present and in this case the hydatid simulates a simple cyst.
(Ab = abscess, D = diaphragm, G = gall bladder, I = inferior vena cava, K = kidney, PV = portal vein, Sp = spine)

one. Experienced workers in the Middle East have reported this to be devoid of complications. However anaphylactic reactions and peritoneal dissemination are fearful complications. Aspiration would not seem to be a very useful procedure in most cases, excision being the correct management. In patients with multiple lesions that cannot be excised and those with peritoneal disease, aspiration may be considered, possibly under appropriate anti-helminthic cover.

Trauma

In liver trauma ultrasound can be most useful since not only may the extent of liver injury be assessed (Fig. 14.7) but also haemoperitoneum may be detected (Froelich et al 1982, Viscomi et al 1980). Injured liver tissue gives low level echoes, together with a fluid space if there is intra hepatic haematoma (Van Sonnenberg et al 1983). The ruptured liver surface may be represented as an irregularity of the capsule. Blood in the peritoneum has the same appearance as ascites: the clinical background suggests its true nature and a directed tap will confirm this. The fact that the scanner can be brought to the patient's bedside enhances the value of ultrasound, but if the chest or abdominal wall has been injured, the probe contact required for scanning may be difficult. It is impossible to scan through dressings; if these need to be removed, sterility can be maintained by using sterile contact jelly and covering the probe with the latex sleeve used for biopsies. Similar considerations apply for scanning postoperative patients.

Tumours

Benign tumours of the liver are usually apparent as well-circumscribed masses with irregular internal echoes. However, the distinction between focal nodular hyperplasia and oestrogen adenoma is not possible though the Kupffer cells that are often present in focal nodular hyper-

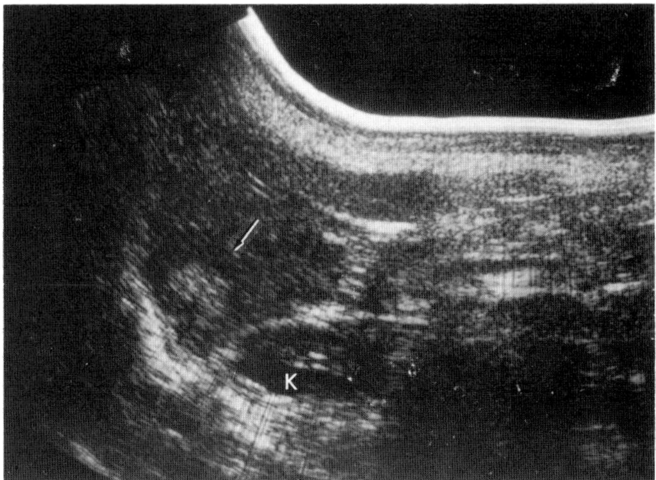

Fig. 14.7 Trauma.
This mixed echo-poor and echogenic lesion in the lateral part of the right lobe (arrow) is a haematoma following a Trucut liver biopsy.
(K = kidney)

plasia phagocytose colloids (Casarella et al 1978). In this case the lesions do not show as a defect on the isotope scan; the combination of a lesion seen on ultrasound or CT and a negative isotope scan is characteristic of this condition (Rogers et al 1981) (Ch. 87). Biopsy of oestrogen adenomas should be approached with caution because of the risk of major haemorrhage.

Hepato-cellular carcinoma has two forms, focal and diffuse (Fig. 14.8) (Atomi et al 1984, La Berge et al 1984, Tanaka et al 1983). The focal type appears as a mass lesion, rounded or lobular and often multiple, with high or low level echoes. Necrotic or haemorrhagic regions are common. Invasion of hepatic veins or the portal vein can be demonstrated. Often they occur on the background of cirrhotic changes (see below), but since cirrhotic nodules are only rarely apparent on ultrasound, any well-defined focus must be regarded as highly suspicious. If excision is considered ultrasound can provide useful information of the segmental distribution of the lesion, but should be used in conjunction with CT and arteriography since each modality may detect lesions missed by the others.

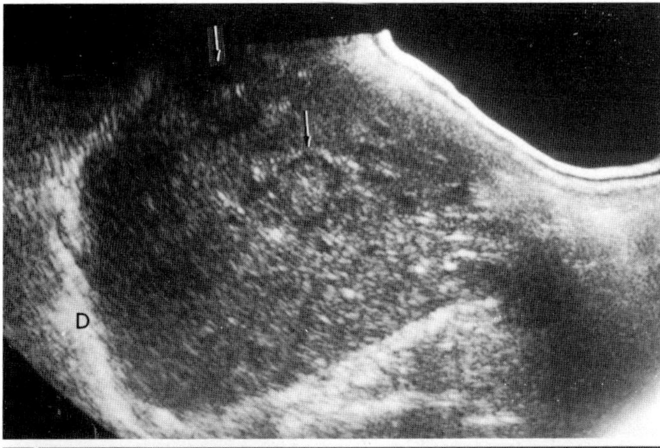

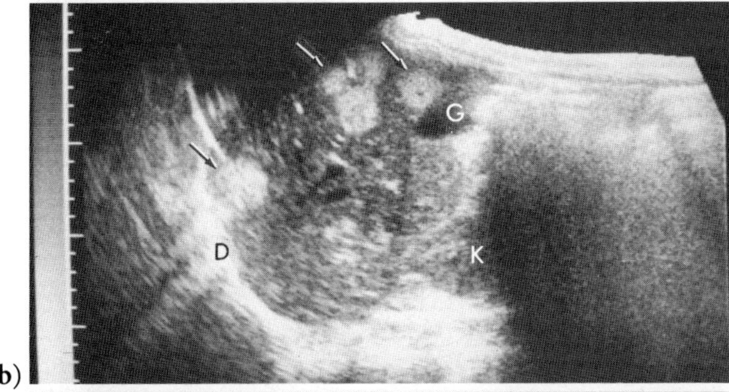

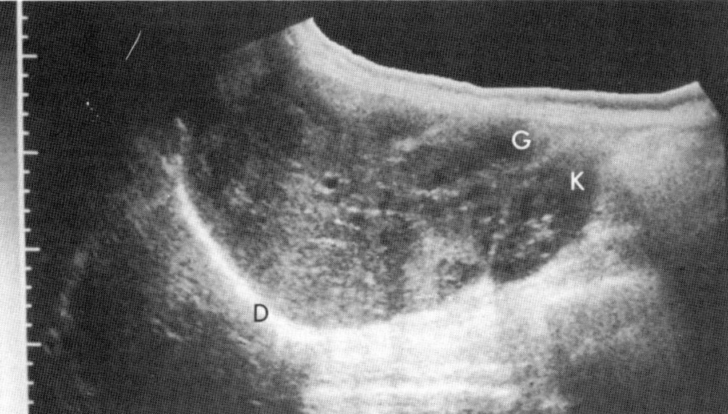

Fig. 14.8 Malignant tumours.
Tumour in the liver is commonly seen as focal masses, either echopoor (arrows in a) or echogenic (arrows in b). Diffuse patterns also occur (c) and all of these forms are found in both metastatic disease and in primary hepatoma.
(D = diaphragm, G = gall bladder, K = kidney)

The diffuse form is a much more difficult problem since the changes may be subtle and indistinguishable from many other diffuse diseases such as cirrhosis and chronic active hepatitis.

In populations at risk from primary hepatoma, ultrasound forms a useful screening tool, being more readily available and quicker than CT and more sensitive than scintigraphy.

Screening for liver metastases forms a major part of the use of ultrasound in many hospitals. Focal metastases appear as space occupying lesions, distorting the liver surface or internal anatomy (Fig. 14.8) (Mayes & Bernardino 1981). Like hepatoma they may be echopoor or echogenic; mixed patterns as well as necrosis also occur. Sometimes a clue to the origin may be obtained since the echogenic types are typically secondary to urogenital and gastrointestinal tract tumours.

Some important limitations of ultrasound need to be born in mind in this application (Scheibel 1982). False positive results for metastases are rare, haemangioma mistaken for tumour being the only significant problem. False negatives occur in up to 15% of cases. Some are lesions too small to be detected reliably (<1 cm), while others lie in portions of the liver that are relatively inaccessible (anterior and extreme lateral portions). Some are missed despite being large and well-placed; here the problem would seem to be lack of contrast between the lesion and the liver, both having the same reflectivity. CT will often reveal these deposits; on the other hand ultrasound can easily detect some that are missed on CT. These considerations dictate the investigative policy in critical cases, i.e. where exclusion of metastases is essential to management, such as patients under consideration for excision of a supposed solitary deposit or where arduous chemotherapy is proposed. Since it is the simplest investigation, ultrasound should be used first, but CT employed when the ultrasound is negative.

Liver metastases also occur in diffuse form (miliary metastases) where only a subtle texture change results. Detection of this type may be very difficult. Perversely also, extensive metastatic replacement, where the lesions have become confluent, can be difficult to recognize since the internal contrast that allows the detection of a discrete lesion is lost (Fig. 14.8c). Ultrasound can usefully monitor progress of metastases by serial assessment of size. To be satisfactory this requires the identification of an individual lesion that can be located and measured again at subsequent examinations.

A potentially valuable development in liver surgery is intraoperative ultrasound scanning (Ch. 98). A small hand-held real time probe that can be draped or gas sterilized and used directly on the liver surface after laparotomy, can demonstrate even minute lesions, far smaller than detectable by conventional ultrasound or by CT scanning. Bismuth has used intraoperative ultrasound as an extension to the inspection and palpation of the liver at laparotomy and found that it altered the surgical management in 22 out of 31 cases of cancer of the gastrointestinal tract (Bismuth et al 1984). Confirmation of the true nature of a lesion detected by ultrasound can be obtained by directed biopsy and frozen section. If a solitary liver metastasis is discovered, it may be resected as a part of the radical excision of the primary while the demonstration of multiple metastases may dictate a limited, palliative resection of the primary (Angelini 1984). Similarly in hepatoma, intraoperative ultrasound can be used to confirm the extent of liver involvement (Makuuchi et al 1982). The ultrasound images can be used to direct injection of a dye into the vessels feeding a tumour to stain the involved segment for excision.

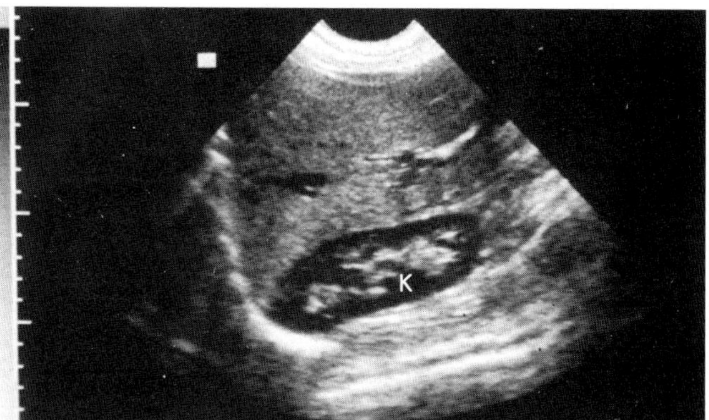

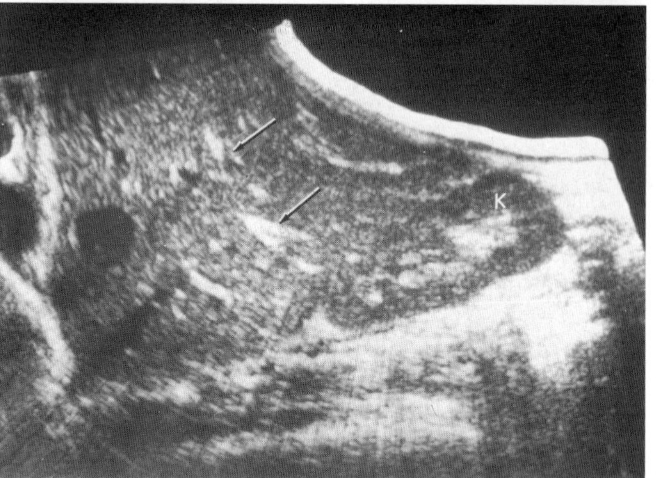

Fig. 14.9 Diffuse liver diseases.
The even texture of the liver parenchyma in (a) is due to the increased echo levels of the 'bright liver' of this patient with fatty infiltration. The hepato-renal contrast is also exaggerated. Cirrhosis and chronic hepatitis are other common causes.
When the liver echo intensity is reduced, the peri-portal echoes seem accentuated (arrows in b) and hepato-renal contrast is reversed. This 'dark liver' pattern is seen in acute hepatitis and congestive changes.
(K = kidney)

Diffuse liver diseases

The changes on ultrasound may be divided into those affecting the liver uniformly and those showing patchy changes. Two main patterns can be identified, known as the bright and the dark liver patterns (Joseph et al 1979, Kurtz et al 1980).

An overall increase in liver parenchymal echoes is the basic change in the bright liver (Fig. 14.9a). The increase may be so marked as to be obvious, but in less gross cases, comparison of the echo level with internal landmarks is required (Dewbury & Clark 1980). The renal cortex is normally only slightly less reflective than the liver (Fig. 14.9b); in the bright liver the liver/kidney contrast is exaggerated so that the kidney appears relatively dark. Similarly the normal contrast between the liver parenchyma and the reflective cuff around the portal vein branches is lost when the liver is strongly reflective. The liver then acquires a uniform appearance (ground-glass pattern) with apparent loss of internal structure. Fat and fibrous tissue are the common causes, fat probably being the predominant factor. Thus the bright pattern occurs in fatty change and in cirrhosis and also in hepatic fibrosis, lipid, glycogen and iron storage diseases. The finding is therefore non-specific but such a liver is always abnormal on biopsy (Foster et al 1980). However ultrasound is not sensitive in this group of disorders and the scan may be quite normal, especially in less severe cases (Gosink et al 1979).

In cirrhosis there may be other changes such as irregularity of the surface, hypertrophy of the caudate lobe, segment I (Fig. 14.10a) (Harbin et al 1980), and features of portal hypertension (Kane & Katz 1982). Ultrasound is very sensitive to ascites, quantities down to 25 ml being detectable (Gefter et al 1982). Recanalization of the umbilical vein is readily demonstrated on ultrasound (Fig. 14.10b, Glazer et al 1981) and varicosities at the splenic hilum (Fig. 14.10c) and around the pancreas can also be detected (Juttner et al 1982). Varices at the oesophago-gastric junction can be demonstrated but, because ultrasound visualizes the serosal vessels, the bleeding submucosal varices viewed on oesophagoscopy are not detected. The calibre of the extrahepatic portal vein is often increased in portal hypertension but this does not seem to form a useful index of pressure. Doppler studies of the portal system are promising since they determine the flow direction and may quantitate the flow rate. Thrombosis of the portal vein is

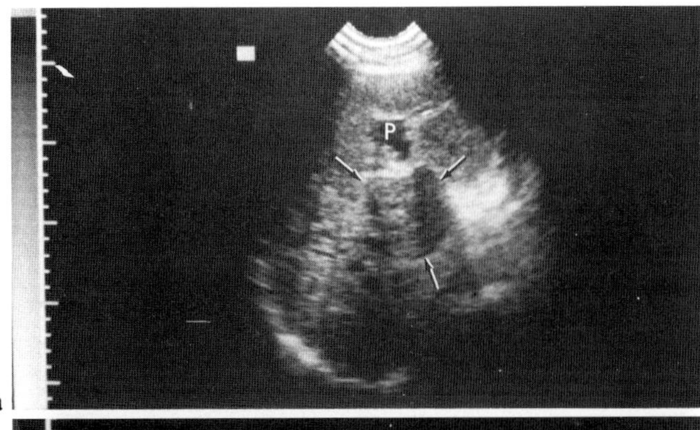

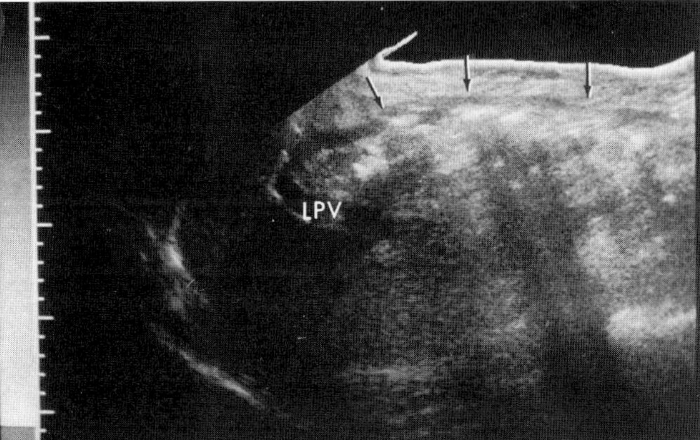

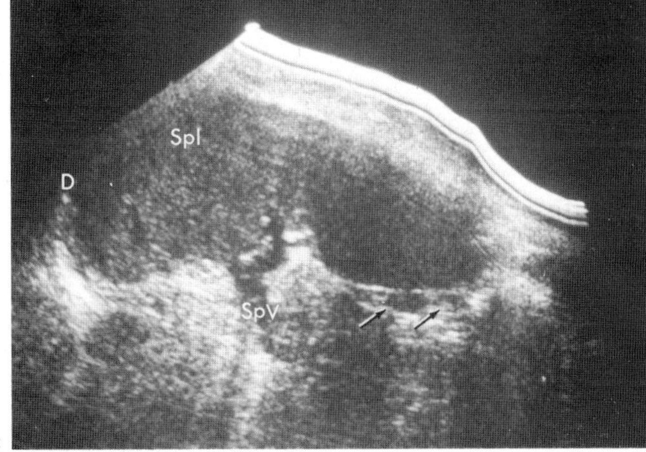

Fig. 14.10 Cirrhosis.
Cirrhosis can only be distinguished from other causes of the bright liver when specific features are present. These include enlargement of the caudate lobe (arrow in a), ascites and signs of portal hypertension such as a recanalized umbilical vein (b), dilated splenic vein (c) or varices (arrows in c). In about half the cases, the ultrasound examination is normal.
(D = diaphragm, LPV = left portal vein, P = porta, Spl = spleen)

readily demonstrated on conventional ultrasound imaging as is the 'cavernous transformation' when recanalization follows (Fig. 14.11c, Kauzlaric et al 1984).

Ultrasound can also be useful in the follow-up assessment of porto-systemic shunts, depending on the anastamotic site (Forsberg & Holmin 1983). Porto-caval and lieno-renal shunts can be evaluated (Fig. 14.11d) but meso-caval shunts are usually obscured by overlying gut and portography is required. Doppler evaluation of the direction (and possibly magnitude) of flow in the portal vessels and the cava forms a rapid, non-invasive method for assessing shunts. For pre-shunt evaluation, ultrasound does not usually provide sufficient detailed information to plan the procedure.

In the 'dark liver' (Kurtz et al 1980) the low intensity echoes from the liver parenchyma throw the peri-portal echoes into relief so that the texture shows accentuation of the vascular markings (Fig. 14.9b). Similarly the liver becomes less reflective than the kidney. This change is seen in inflammatory and congestive conditions where the increase in water content seems to be responsible. In a jaundiced patient, the finding of a dark liver with normal bile ducts suggests a cholestatic hepatitis. The dark pattern also occurs in lymphoreticular malignancies but here does not distinguish between malignant infiltration and reactive lymphocytic infiltration.

In many diseases that affect the whole liver, the process is patchy in its severity and so the ultrasound scan shows an irregular texture. Many infiltrative conditions fall into this category, the commonest examples being focal fatty change and the irregular necrosis in paracetamol or alcoholic toxicity (Scott et al 1980). The scan appearances are confusingly similar to multiple metastases. Serial studies or biopsy are required.

ULTRASOUND IN DISEASES OF THE BILIARY TREE

The bile ducts

The exquisite sensitivity of ultrasound to dilatation of the bile ducts has made it the imaging technique of choice in jaundice problems (Sample et al 1978, Mueller 1984) (Ch. 25). The normal intrahepatic biliary tree is too small to be imaged but when dilated the ducts are seen as tubules lying alongside the portal vein branches (Fig. 14.12a). The pattern is characteristic and specific. The diameters of the common hepatic and bile ducts can be measured and this forms an often more sensitive index of dilatation of the biliary tree (Fig. 14.12b).

Ultrasound has proved to be thoroughly reliable in this application, though obviously it displays anatomy and not duct pressure and will be misleading in the rare cases where these do not correspond. An important instance is when a patient has been referred within a few days of the onset of obstruction, before dilatation has developed. The scan should be repeated in a few days if the diagnostic problem persists. Once dilated, the biliary tree may remain distended for long periods after relief of the obstruction. Thus the duct system may be prominent in patients with gallstone disease or following duct instrumentation at

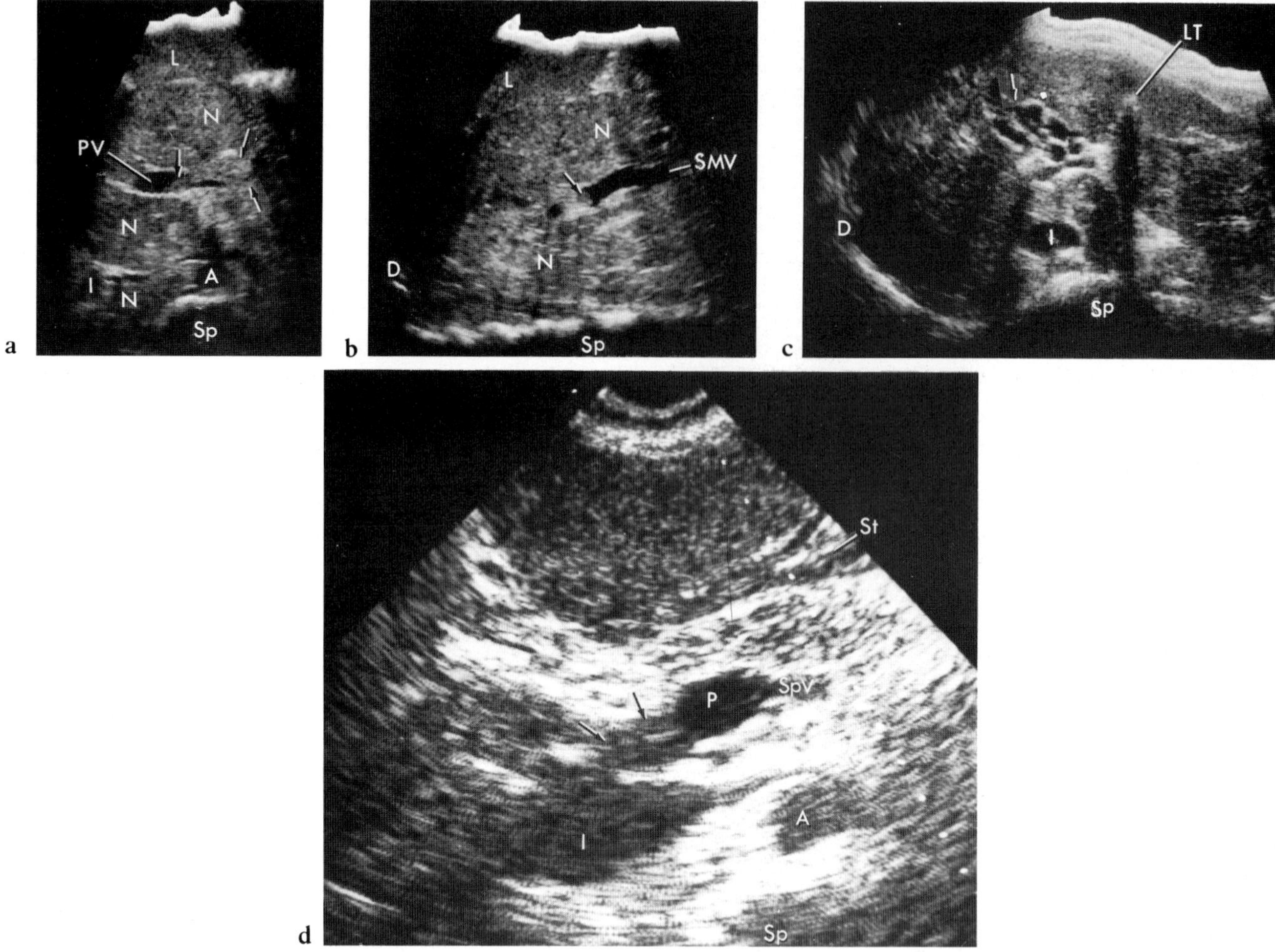

Fig. 14.11 Abnormalities of the portal venous system.

Thrombus is seen in the splenic vein (arrows in a and b) extending up to its junction with the superior mesenteric vein in this patient with massive lymphadenopathy due to lymphoma. The portal vein itself is spared.

In this patient the portal vein is replaced by tortuous vascular channels (arrow in c). This is the appearance of 'cavernous transformation' of the portal vein. It was an incidental finding and presumably represents recanalization following thrombosis in infancy.

A porto-caval shunt is imaged (arrows) in (d); the continuity between the portal vein and the inferior vena cava is evidence of patency but more definite proof is the demonstration of flow using Doppler. (Supplied by Dr. Lillemore Forsberg and reproduced with permission of Acta Radiologica).

(A = aorta, D diaphragm, I = inferior vena cava, L = left hepatic vein, LTT = ligamentum teres, N = nodes, SMV = superior mesenteric vein, Sp = spine)

cholecystectomy. A ball-valve calculus can produce spectacular dilatation of the common bile duct without jaundice.

Definition of the level of obstruction is usually possible on ultrasound by tracing the duct system down to the obstruction (Taylor & Rosenfield 1977). The commonest site is the lower end (Fig. 14.12c); obstruction at the porta gives dilatation of the ducts in one or both of the lobes, but with a normal common bile duct. Lesions in the retroduodenal portion of the duct may be more difficult to image because it is often shadowed here by duodenal gas. Nevertheless the level is accurately predicted in some 80% of cases.

Ultrasound is able to determine the aetiology in a number of cases. The demonstration of stones in the common bile duct depends on their size and position. Larger stones (>5 mm) in the pancreatic portion of the common bile duct are readily demonstrated unless excessive intestinal gas precludes adequate imaging. Smaller stones may not cast an acoustic shadow (for this the stone must be large enough to block the ultrasound beam) and since it is the shadow that draws attention to the stone, they are more difficult to detect. In addition, since smaller stones lodge further down the duct, they tend to lie close to the duodenum whose gas may degrade that part of the image. Gas in the first part of the duodenum also obscures the retro-duodenal portion of the duct and even large stones here may be missed; the operator will know that the study was incomplete and proceed to another investigation. The tell-tale shadowing is often missing, even with large stones,

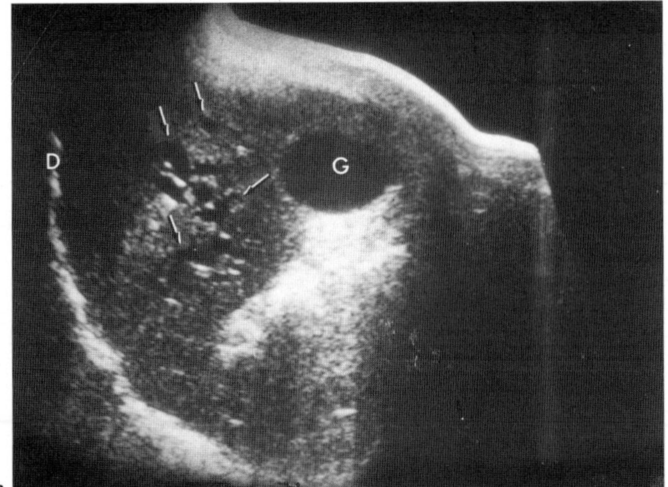

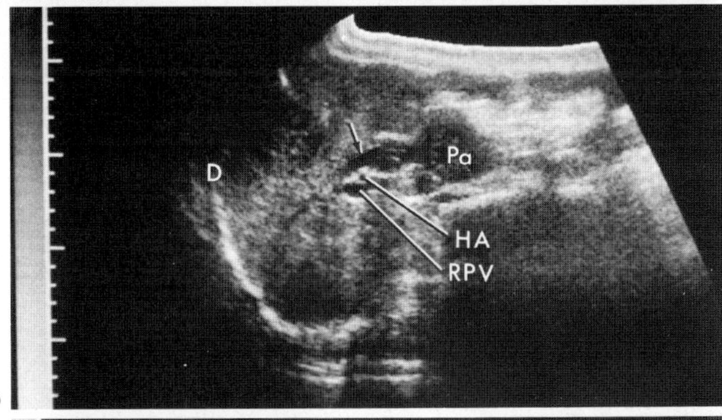

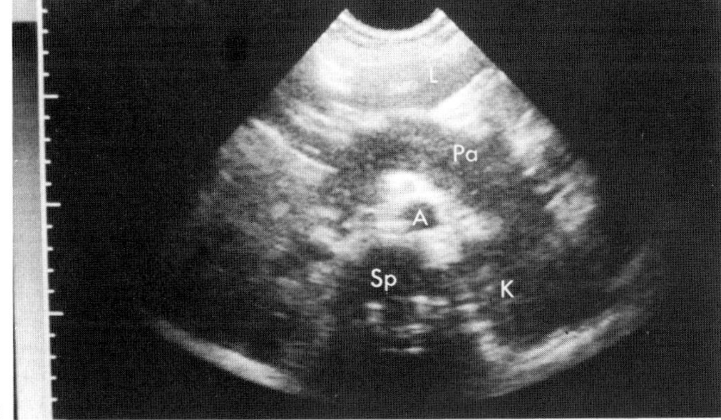

Fig. 14.12 Dilated bile ducts.

Normally the intrahepatic bile ducts cannot be discerned on ultrasound but when dilated they appear as vessels lying parallel to the portal vein branches (arrows in a).

The common duct can be measured as it crosses the right portal vein (arrow in b). In this patient it could be traced through its whole length to an enlarged pancreas which proved to be due to acute pancreatitis. The ultrasound picture is typical, with low level echoes and generalized enlargement.

(A = aorta, D = diaphragm, G = gallbladder, HA = hepatic artery, K = kidney, Pa = pancreas, RPV = right portal vein, Sp = spine)

presumably the crumbly, semi-solid variety (Dewbury & Smith 1984). They appear as intraductal soft tissue masses and simulate tumour. A region of inflammation often develops around a stone impacted at the lower end of the common bile duct. This focal pancreatitis is indistinguishable from a tumour on ultrasound; guided fine-needle aspiration may be helpful.

Pancreatic tumours are usually large enough to be detected as a lesion with irregular, predominantly low level echoes. In some instances the changes may be recognized before the lesion has produced the mass effects of expansion and distortion of the pancreatic contour that are characteristic of more advanced tumours. On the other hand, ampullary carcinomas are too small to be detected though their presence may be inferred by the combination of dilated pancreatic and biliary ducts. ERCP is the method of choice for this problem. Cholangio-carcinoma produces a soft tissue mass that may be demonstrated extending along the biliary tree. Strictures are very difficult to demonstrate on ultrasound, the duct seeming to disappear at the site of narrowing with no characteristic features. Rarer causes that can also be imaged include choledochal cysts and ascaris worms.

Overall it may be seen that ultrasound is highly reliable in the detection of biliary tree dilatation and will usually indicate the level if not the precise site of obstruction. It is less good at determining the aetiology, though in some cases the precise cause can be defined with confidence. Thus ultrasound is most useful as a screening test and should be the first imaging study for jaundiced patients. Where an obstructing stone is demonstrated, the study can provide all the information required to plan surgery. When a pancreatic mass is demonstrated, fine-needle aspiration may be performed under ultrasound control to confirm malignancy. The demonstration of local extension (nodes, tumour in the splenic/portal vein) or liver metastases suggests that palliative surgery is appropriate. Where radical surgery is proposed, further investigation with CT and/or arteriography is required to evaluate local spread more completely. In cases of obstructive jaundice where no causative lesion is seen on ultrasound, some further imaging is required; ERCP or PTC may be used, the selection depending on the probable level of obstruction and on available expertise (Mueller 1984).

The intraoperative applications of ultrasound for the biliary tree are promising (Ch. 30). As with its uses for hepatic surgery, a sterilized hand-held real time probe is applied directly to the surface of the bile duct. Even stones of a millimetre or so in diameter can be detected. The examination is simpler than an operative cholangiogram and should be performed first because air bubbles have a confusing appearance. The detection rate of the two techniques is identical (predictive value of a negative test is 99%) but ultrasound gives fewer false positives, so that unnecessary duct explorations can be avoided (Sigel et al 1983). However ultrasound does not display the overall anatomy of the duct system so that variations and anomalies are not detectable (Angelini 1984). The tomographic display is an unfamiliar one to the surgeon, undermining confidence in the findings and slowing the acceptance of this fast and convenient technique (Sigel 1982).

Ultrasound is also valuable in postoperative evaluation. Chiefly this will be for the biliary tree itself, but bilomas, haematomas and abscesses can be detected and aspirated (diagnostically or therapeutically) under ultrasound control. The speed and flexibility of ultrasound here makes it the method of choice especially for ill patients, because the scanner can be taken to the bedside. Evaluation of the biliary tree consists mainly in assessing calibre; the duct system often does not return to completely normal dimensions but a second increase in calibre following the postoperative reduction suggests drainage failure. An additional and often striking feature is the presence of gas in the biliary tree, including the gallbladder; it demonstrates that the anastomosis is patent (Chu et al 1978). Prostheses and stents can be visualized on ultrasound but contrast X-ray studies give much more useful detailed information on their position.

Ultrasound may also be useful in other biliary disorders. Intrahepatic cholelithiasis is seen as echogenic foci accompanied by shadowing that lies in the distribution of the biliary tree. However, since the stones are often small, they are easily missed on ultrasound so that cholangiography forms a much more useful test (Itai et al 1980). Intrahepatic stones can also be imaged intraoperatively. Intrahepatic stones are also a feature of Caroli's disease and of sclerosing cholangitis. In Caroli's the intrahepatic duct ectasia produces cystic spaces in the liver, often containing stones (Mittlestaed et al 1980). In sclerosing cholangitis there is irregular dilatation of the ducts giving a beaded appearance on the ultrasound scan with the stones giving focal intense echoes accompanied by bands of acoustic shadowing. Complicating cholangiocarcinoma is difficult to detect on ultrasound before it becomes extensive.

In biliary atresia ultrasound may occasionally be useful in that the demonstration of any part of the biliary tree indicates that surgical correction may be possible. Apart from this there are no specific ultrasonic features that allow differentiation between atresia and neonatal hepatitis.

The gallbladder

Ultrasound is the simplest and most reliable method for demonstrating gallstones (Mogensen et al 1984) (Ch. 25). They appear as strongly reflective foci in the gallbladder and cast a well-marked acoustic shadow (Fig. 14.13). Unless impacted, they move with changes in posture. The demonstration of all of these features is almost totally reliable down to stones of a millimetre or so in size. Confusion can occasionally be caused by polyps, especially when they are calcified.

Difficulties arise when the gallbladder is contracted, for contained stones may then simulate gas in a bowel loop; in this situation stones may escape detection and occasional over enthusiastic reporting of stones when the real gallbladder has been missed altogether has occurred. Since the gallbladder neck returns very strong echoes, a stone impacted here may be very difficult to detect. Usually other stones are present in these cases and there may be additional features of cholecystitis. Debris or sludge in the gallbladder should not cause confusion since it does not shadow.

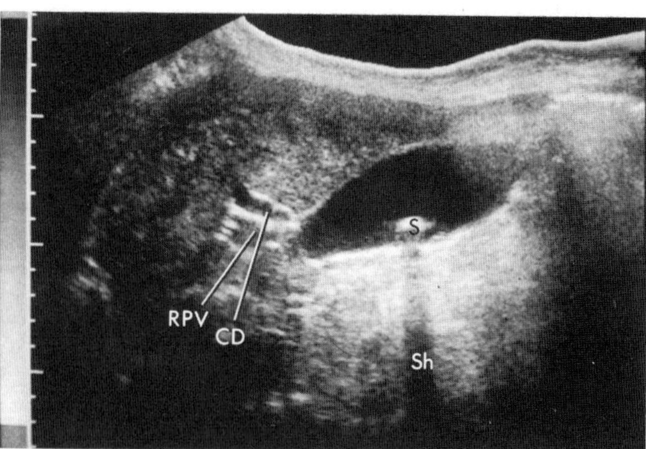

Fig. 14.13 Gallstone.
A small echogenic focus with acoustic shadowing is the characteristic ultrasound appearance of a gallstone.
(CD = common duct, RPV = right portal vein, Sh = acoustic shadow)

The limitations of ultrasound in stone detection, apart from very small stones, are the difficulty in estimating the size and number of stones and in detecting whether or not they are calcified. These are important considerations in the selection of cases for medical treatment of stones. Here X-ray cholecystography is preferred.

Cholecystitis is manifest as wall thickening above 5 mm (Fig. 14.14a) (Croce et al 1981, Dillon & Parkin 1980). This seemingly generous limit makes allowance for the thickening of the wall of the normal gallbladder when it is contracted. Lower limits are appropriate when the gallbladder is well filled. In acute cholecystitis the sub-serosal oedema often gives a laminated configuration to the wall with an echo-poor layer surrounding the gallbladder. Stones are usually present though the causal stone impacted in the neck of the gallbladder may be difficult to demonstrate. Typically there is tenderness elicited by pressing the ultrasound probe over the gallbladder, the ultrasound Murphy's sign (Laing et al 1981). Complications may also be demonstrated, especially perforation with peri-cholecystitic abscess formation. In empyema the bile acquires echoes due to the pus and debris. Gas formation produces intramural foci of intense reflectivity, often with reverberation artefacts. Emphysematous cholecystitis is a sinister development. Ultrasound is a valuable confir-

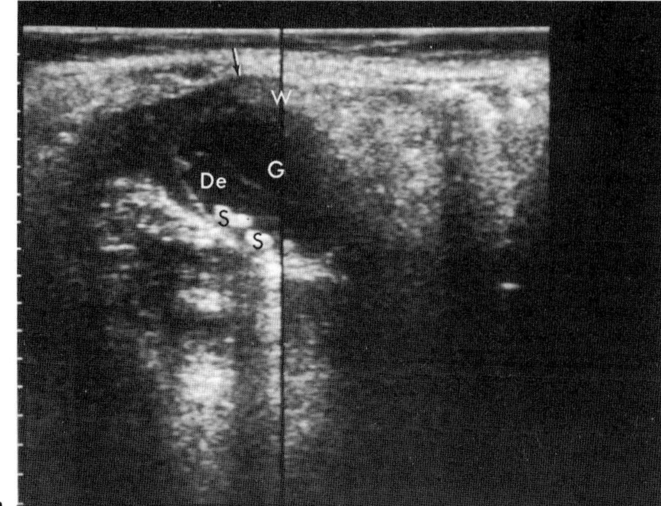

a

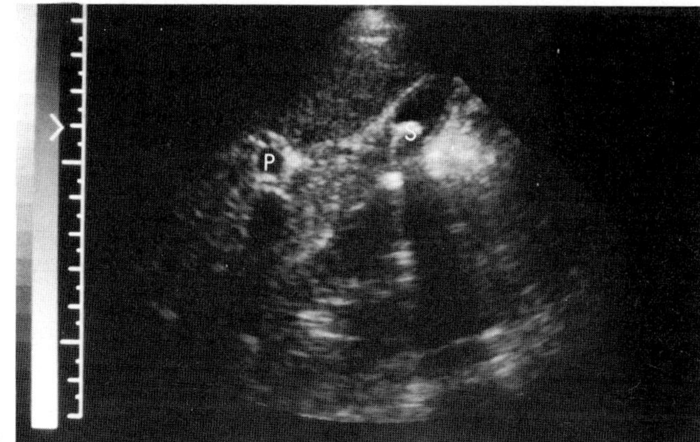

b

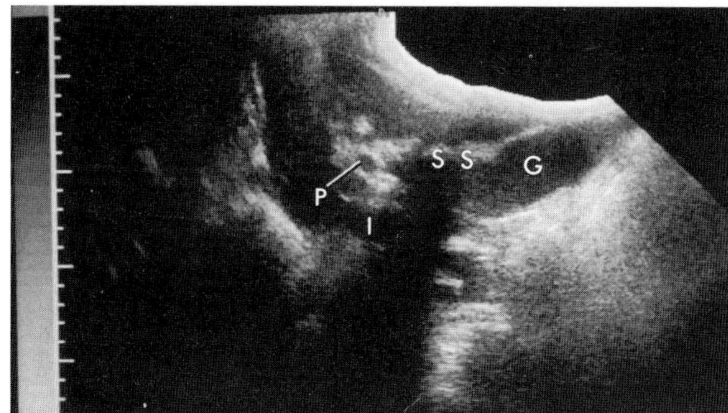

c

Fig. 14.14 Cholecystitis.
In acute cholecystitis (a) thickening of the wall is usually apparent, together with an echo-poor halo (arrow) representing subserosal oedema. Stones and debris were present in this case and there was marked tenderness when the probe was pressed over the gallbladder (ultrasound Murphy's sign).
In chronic cholecystitis (b) the wall thickening is often less obvious and the echo-poor halo is absent.
Mucocele of the gallbladder (c) is often an incidental finding; this patient presented with a right sided mass that proved to be a grossly dilated gallbladder containing stones. (De = debris, G = gallbladder, I = inferior vena cava, P = porta, S = stones, W = wall).

mation of a clinical suspicion of acute cholecystitis though in a proportion of cases the typical features are absent. It may also reveal another cause for the pain and tenderness such as renal or hepatic pathology or a subhepatic abscess (Ralls et al 1984).

In chronic cholecystitis the wall is also thickened but lacks the echo-poor halo and there is no local tenderness (Fig. 14.14b). Stones are usually present. Less common allied problems are also demonstrable on ultrasound. A mucocele appears as a large, sometimes enormous gallbladder which is non-tender and thin-walled (Fig. 14.14c). The contents are usually echo-free apart from stones, though debris may form. In adenomyomatosis there is gross wall thickening, usually segmental in distribution or affecting the fundus predominantly. When large, the Aschoff-Rokitansky sinuses can be visualized as intramural 'cysts'. Cholecystography is more specific in this problem. The porcelain gallbladder has a striking appearance: the gallbladder wall is replaced by a curvilinear band of intense echoes with shadowing. The pattern is similar to gas in the gallbladder lumen and X-ray will differentiate. Apparent thickening of the gallbladder wall is also encountered in a variety of unrelated conditions. It is a common feature of viral hepatitis probably representing direct extension of the inflammatory process. It is also seen in most patients with ascites and here may be a real finding or a scanner artefact.

Adenomas of the gallbladder appear as polypoid increscences into the lumen (Fig. 14.15a). They may have strong echoes and even cast acoustic shadows and so simulate stones. However, their position remains fixed with changes in posture. Cholecystography may be required for confirmation.

Carcinoma in the early stages is indistinguishable from adenoma or cholecystitis (Fig. 14.15b & c). Usually it is a late discovery when there is a gross mass involving the gallbladder wall, sometimes filling the lumen and enveloping the commonly associated stones and often extending into the porta to produce features of obstructive jaundice (Takehara 1984) (Ch. 64). The abnormality is readily demonstrated by ultrasound, though a specific diagnosis is not always possible since chronic cholecystitis and adenomyomatosis can have a similar appearance. Unfortunately, because of the late onset of symptoms in this tumour, improvements in imaging have not improved the prognosis (Klamer & Max 1983). The best chance of successful treatment is in those cases where the tumour is fortuitously detected at a stage when excision is still possible (Collier et al 1984). Ultrasound offers the best prospect since it is so widely used for the gallbladder; the ultrasonologist should have a low threshold for raising the possibility of gallbladder cancer whenever irregular thickening or focal masses are demonstrated, especially in the over-50s and even when no stones are present.

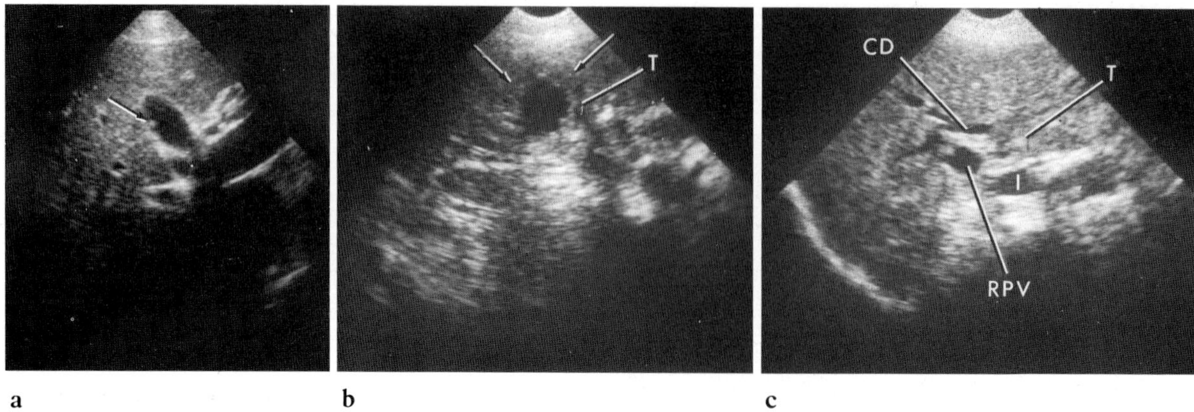

Fig. 14.5 Gallbladder tumours.
A gallbladder polyp is seen as a small mass (arrow in a) attached to the gallbladder wall. Malignancy cannot be excluded but the small size and localized nature of this lesion are reassuring.
Generalized thickening of the gallbladder wall (arrows in b) was due to a carcinoma that was inoperable due to spread to the porta (c) with bile duct involvement. No gallstones were present.
(CD = common duct, I = inferior vena cava, P = portal vein, R = right portal vein, T = tumour)

REFERENCES

Abdel-Latif Z, Abdel-Mahab M F, El-Kady N M 1982 Evaluation of portal hypertension in cases of hepatosplenic schistosomiasis using ultrasound (ab). Radiology 144: 216

Angelini L 1984 Intraoperative diagnostic ultrasonography. In: Angelini L, Fegiz G, Wells P N T (eds) Emerging technologies in surgery. Masson Italia, Milano

Atomi Y, Inoue S, Kawano N, Morioki Y 1984 Hepatocellular carcinoma. In: Kossoff G, Fukuda M (eds) Ultrasonic differential diagnosis of tumors. Igaku-Shoin, New York, ch. 8

Beggs I 1983 The radiological appearance of hydatid disease of the liver. Clinical Radiology 34: 555–563

Bismuth H 1982 Surgical anatomy and anatomical surgery of the liver. World Journal of Surgery 6: 3–9

Bismuth H, Castaing D, Kunstlinger F 1984, L'echographie per-operative en chirugie hepato-biliaire. La Presse Medicale 13: 1819–1822

Bree R L 1983 Schwabb R E, Neiman H L 1983 Solitary echogenic spot in the liver, is it diagnostic of a hemangioma? American Journal of Roentgenology 140: 41–44

Bruneton J N, Drouillard J, Fenart D, et al 1983a Ultrasonography of hepatic cavernous haemangioma. British Journal of Radiology 56: 783–79

Bruneton J N, Eresue J, Caramella E et al 1983b Congenital cysts of the liver in echography. Journal de Radiologie 64: 471–476

Casarella W, Knowles D, Wolff M, Johnson P 1978 Focal nodular hyperplasia and liver cell adenoma. American Journal of Radiology 131: 393–402

Chu J, Husband J E, Cosgrove D O, McCready V R M 1978 The B-scan appearance of gas in the biliary tree. British Journal of Radiology 51: 728–730

Collier N A, Carr D, Hemingway A, Blumgart L H 1984 Preoperative diagnosis and its effect on the treatment of carcinoma of the gallbladder. Surgery, Gynecology and Obstetrics 159: 465–470

Cosgrove D O, McCready V R M 1982 Ultrasonic imaging, liver spleen and pancreas. Wiley, Chichester

Couinaud C L 1957 Le Foie. Etude anatomiques et chirugicales. Masson, Paris

Croce F, Montali G, Solbiati L, et al 1981 Ultrasonography in acute cholecystitis. British Journal of Radiology 54: 927–931

Dewbury K C, Clark B E 1980 The accuracy of ultrasound in the detection of cirrhosis of the liver. British Journal of Radiology 52: 945–950

Dewbury K C, Joseph A E A, Sadler G H M, et al 1980 Ultrasound in the diagnosis of early liver abscess. British Journal of Radiology 53: 1160–1167

Dewbury K C, Smith C L 1984 The misdiagnosis of common bile duct stones with ultrasound. British Journal of Radiology 56: 625–630

Dillon N, Parkin G J S 1980 The role of upper abdominal ultrasonography in suspected acute cholecystitis. Clinical Radiology 31: 175–179

Forsberg L, Holmin T 1983 Pulsed Doppler and B-mode ultrasound features of interposition meso-caval and porto-caval shunts. Acta Radiologica 24: 353–357

Foster K J, Dewbury K C, Griffith A H et al 1980 Accuracy of ultrasound in the detection of fatty infiltration of the liver. British Journal of Radiology 53: 440–448

Freeny P C, Vimont T R, Barnett D C 1979 Cavernous hemangioma of the liver: ultrasonography, arteriography, and computed tomography. Radiology 132: 143–150

Fried A M, Kreel L, Cosgrove D O 1984 The hepatic interlobar fissure. American Journal of Roentgenology 143: 561–563

Fritschy P, Robotti G, Schneekloth G, et al 1983 Measurement of liver volume by ultrasound and computed tomography. Journal of Clinical Ultrasound 11: 299–303

Froelich J W, Simeone J F, McKusick K A, et al 1982 Radionuclide imaging and ultrasound in liver/spleen trauma. Radiology 145: 457–461

Fukuda M, Cosgrove D O 1985 Real time ultrasound in the abdomen. Igaku-Shoin, Tokyo

Gandolfi L, Solmi L, Bolondi L et al 1983 The value of ultrasonography in the diagnosis of hepatic haemangiomas. European Journal of Radiology 3: 222–232

Gefter W B, Arger P H, Edell S I 1982 Sonographic patterns of ascites. Seminars in Ultrasound 2: 226–241

Glazer G M, Laing F C, Braun T W, et al 1981 Sonographic demonstration of portal hypertension: patent umbilical vein. Radiology 136: 161–169

Gosink B B, Lemon S K, Scheible W, et al 1979 Accuracy of ultrasonography in diagnosis of hepatocellular disease. American Journal of Roentgenology 133: 19–25

Hadidi A 1983 Sonography of hepatic echinococcal cysts. Radiology 147: 913–927

Harbin W P, Robert N J, Ferrucci J 1980 Diagnosis of cirrhosis based on regional changes in hepatic morphology: radiological and pathological analysis. Radiology 135: 273–288

Hollinshead W H 1982 Anatomy for surgeons, 3rd Edn, Vol 2: Thorax, abdomen and pelvis. Harper and Row, New York

Itai Y, Araki T, Furui S, et al 1980 Computed tomography and ultrasound in the diagnosis of intrahepatic calculi. Radiology 136: 399–412

Joseph A E A, Dewbury K C, McGuire P G 1979 Ultrasound detection of chronic liver disease. British Journal of Radiology 5: 184–188

Juttner H-U, Jenney J M, Ralls P W, et al 1982 Ultrasound demonstration of porto-systemic collaterals in cirrhosis. Radiology 142: 459–466

Kane R A, Katz S G 1982 Spectrum of sonographic findings in portal hypertension. Radiology 142: 453–458
Kauzlaric D, Petrovic M, Barmeir E 1984 Sonography of cavernous transformation of the portal vein. American Journal of Roentgenology 142: 383–385
Klamer T W, Max M H 1983 Carcinoma of the gallbladder. Surgery, Gynecology and Obstetrics 156: 641–645
Kremkau F W 1980 Diagnostic ultrasound, physical principles. Grune and Stratton, New York
Kuligowska E, Noble J 1983 Sonography of hepatic abscesses. Seminars in Ultrasound 4: 102–112
Kurtz A L, Rubin C S, Cooper H S et al 1980 Ultrasound findings in hepatitis. Radiology 136: 717–725
La Berge J M, Laing F C, Federle M P, Jeffrey R B, Lim R C 1984 Hepatocellular carcinoma: assessment of resectability by computed tomography and ultrasound. Radiology 152: 485–490
Laing F C, Federle M P, Jeffrey R B et al 1981 Ultrasonic evaluation of patients with acute right upper quadrant pain. Radiology 140: 449–455
Lyons E A 1978 A color atlas of sectional anatomy. Mosby, St. Louis
McDicken W N 1980 Diagnostic ultrasound, physical principles and use of instruments, 2nd edn. Wiley, New York
McGrath P, Mills P 1984 Atlas of sectional anatomy. Karger, Basel
Makuuchi M, Hasegawa H, Yamazaki S 1982 Intraoperative ultrasonographic examination for hepatectomy. In: Lerski R A, Morley P (eds) Ultrasound '82. Pergamon Press, Oxford, p 493–497
Mayes G B, Bernardino M E 1981 Role of ultrasound in the evaluation of hepatic neoplasms. Seminars in Ultrasound 2: 212–228
Mittlestaed C, Volberg, Fischer G et al 1980 Caroli's disease: sonographic findings. American Journal of Roentgenology 134: 585–587
Mogensen N B, Madsen M, Stage P et al 1984 Ultrasonography versus roentgenography in suspected instances of cholecystolithiasis. Surgery, Gynecology and Obstetrics 159: 353–356
Mueller P R 1984 Jaundice. In: Simeone J (ed) Coordinated diagnostic imaging (Clinics in diagnostic ultrasound, vol 14) Churchill Livingstone, New York, ch. 2
Netter F H 1964 Ciba collection of medical illustrations vol 3. Digestive tract (2nd edn), part III. Liver, biliary tract and pancreas. Ciba-Geigy, Summit, New Jersey
Nicholas D 1984 Present status of ultrasound tissue characterisation. In: Kossoff G, Fukuda M (eds) Ultrasonic differential diagnosis of tumors. Igaku-Shoin, New York, ch.3
Niederau C, Sonnenberg A, Muller J E, et al 1983 Sonographic measurements of the normal liver, spleen, pancreas and portal vein. Radiology 149: 537–540
Ralls P W, Meyers H I, Lapin S A, et al 1979 Grey-scale ultrasonography of hepatic amoebic abscesses. Radiology 132: 125–137
Ralls P W, Quinn M F, Boswell W D, et al 1983 Patterns of resolution in successfully treated hepatic amoebic abscess: sonographic evaluation. Radiology 149: 541–543
Ralls P W, Colletti P M, Boswell W D, Halls J M 1984 Right upper quadrant pain. In: Simeone J (ed) Coordinated diagnostic imaging. Churchill Livingstone, New York, ch. 1
Rogers J V, Mack L A, Freeny P C, et al 1981 Hepatic focal nodular hyperplasia: angiography, CT, sonography, and scintigraphy. American Journal of Roentgenology 137: 983–991
Rubinson H A, Isikoff M B, Hill M C 1980 Diagnostic imaging of hepatic abscesses: a retrospective analysis. American Journal of Roentgenology 135: 735–740
Sample W F, Sarti D A, Goldshein L I et al 1978 Grey-scale ultrasonography of the jaundiced patient. Radiology 128: 719–725
Sauerbrei E E, Cooperberg P L, Gordon P et al 1980 The discrepancy between radiographic and sonographic bile duct measurements. Radiology 137: 751–755
Scheibel W 1982 Diagnostic algorithm for liver masses. Seminars in Roentgenology 18: 84–97
Schneck C 1983 Tomographic anatomy. In: Joseph A E A, Cosgrove D O (eds) Ultrasound in inflammatory diseases (Clinics in diagnostic ultrasound vol. 11) Churchill Livingstone, New York, ch. 2
Scott W W, Sanders R C, Siegelman S S 1980 Irregular fatty infiltration of the liver. American Journal of Roentgenology 135: 67–75
Sigel B 1982 Operative ultrasonography. Lea and Febiger, Philadelphia
Sigel B, Machi J, Beitler J C, et al 1983 Comparative accuracy of operative ultrasonography and cholangiography in detecting common duct calculi. Surgery 92: 715–719
Sigel B, Coelo J C U, Machi J et al The application of real time ultrasound imaging during surgical procedures. Surgery, Gynecology and Obstetrics 157: 33–37
Takehara Y 1984 Ultrasonic diagnosis of gallbladder cancer. In: Kossoff G, Fukuda M (eds) Ultrasonic differential diagnosis of tumors. Igaku-Shoin, New York, ch. 10
Tanaka S, Kitamura T, Imaoka S, et al 1983 Hepatocellular carcinoma: sonographic and histologic correlations. American Journal of Roentgenology 140: 701–710
Taylor K J W, Rosenfield A 1977 Grey-scale ultrasonography in the differential diagnosis of jaundice. Archives of Surgery 112: 820–825
Terrier F, Becker C D, Triller J K 1983 Morphologic aspects of hepatic abscesses at computed tomography and ultrasound. Acta Radiologica 24: 129–737
Van Sonnenberg E, Simeone J F, Mueller P R, et al 1983 Sonographic appearance of hematoma in liver, spleen and kidney. Radiology 147: 507–512
Viscomi G N, Gonzalez R, Taylor K J W, Crade M 1980 Ultrasonic evaluation of hepatic and splenic trauma. Archives of Surgery 115: 320–331
Wagner M W, Lawson T L 1982 Segmental anatomy. Macmillan, New York

15

J. P. Lavender

Isotopic studies

INTRODUCTION

Until the 1950s imaging of the liver was restricted to a radiological examination of the biliary tract and a very limited use of angiography. The first liver scan, using radioactive gold, was performed in 1954 by Stirret et al and was the first non-invasive way of creating an image of this organ. The emergence of ultrasound and computerized tomography (CT) in the last 15 years, with magnetic resonance appearing more recently, now offers a sometimes confusing choice. Radio-isotope images have a poorer resolution than either ultrasound or CT and therefore, if regarded as images of anatomy, might be deemed superseded. Radioactive tracers are however primarily physiological tools; thus the static image only represents one part of the information. The dynamics of the various tracers used can illustrate flow, reticulo–endothelial function and biliary excretion. The other powerful advantage of radioactive tracers is their flexibility. Tracers can be created for specific purposes: to label proteins, cells or substrates. For the surgeon this is probably best illustrated by the development of a number of different biliary agents for use in jaundiced patients; and a further example is the use of labelled autologous granulocytes for detecting inflammatory disease.

Increasingly sophisticated tracers are being developed which hold out hopes of imaging cell types through the use of monoclonal antibodies and so increasing the specificity of liver imaging.

This chapter attempts to review the place of isotopic scanning of the liver and to discuss briefly some of the more recent developments in this field.

RADIOACTIVE COLLOID SCINTIGRAPHY OF THE LIVER

Any colloidal particles administered intravenously are rapidly cleared from the circulation by cells of the reticulo–endothelial system in the liver, spleen and bone marrow. The clearance into these organs is affected by particle size, small colloidal particles tending to accumulate to a greater extent in bone marrow while larger particles are trapped more readily by the spleen. The choice of colloidal preparation, however, is not of very great importance. Perhaps the most important aspect is that the preparation should be both stable and reproducible so that the relative uptake in liver and spleen can be assessed in a reliable way. The standard preparation used over many years is technetium^{99m} labelled sulphur colloid with a particle size of approximately 1μ. It has the disadvantage of requiring a boiling water bath during preparation but shows a relatively greater uptake by the liver than tin colloid which has a tendency to produce very large particles. Technetium antimony colloid has a particle size which is smaller and therefore more suited for examining the bone marrow than liver and spleen. Mini microspheres of human serum albumin have a particle size which can be described in precise terms but for normal clinical imaging this is not a matter of any importance.

Colloidal preparations are labelled with technetium^{99m} with an activity of 40–80 MBq (1–2mCi).

Physiology

Following an intravenous bolus, colloids are cleared from the circulation by the reticulo–endothelial system, that is the Kupffer cells lining the liver sinusoids, the macrophages in the spleen and bone marrow. Since there is a high extraction of colloids from blood by the liver and spleen (and probably by the bone marrow) the distribution of radioactivity throughout the body represents a relative blood flow to these organs. Approximately 85% of particles are normally trapped by the liver, 10% in the spleen and 5% in the bone marrow. Blood clearance is normally complete in 10 min.

Any radioactive colloid reaching the liver following an intravenous bolus will arrive there by two different routes. The first is the colloid delivered by the hepatic artery followed some ten seconds later by colloid which has tra-

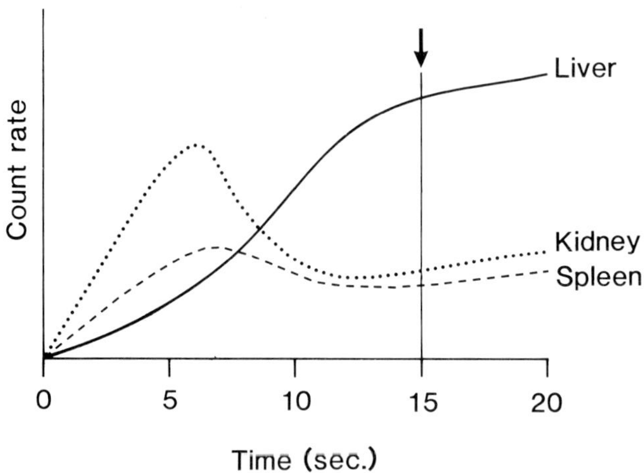

Fig. 15.1 Colloid uptake into liver. Time activity curves over the liver, spleen and kidney following an intravenous bolus of radioactive colloid. The curve over the kidneys shows the bolus passing through the renal vasculature, corresponding to a rising curve over the liver due to hepatic artery supply. The inflection (arrow) shows change from arterial to portal inflow (curves adapted from Fleming et al 1983 with permission)

versed the mesenteric circulation and arrives from the portal vein. This double vascular supply can be investigated by looking at the uptake curve of the liver and analyzing the two components (see Fig. 15.1) (Fleming et al 1983).

Imaging and normal appearances

Imaging is carried out 15 minutes after the intravenous injection of the radioactive colloid using either a large field of view gamma camera or small field of view with diverging collimator. In general, views can be taken either erect or supine with a minimum total count collected in each image of 350 K counts. Four standard views should be taken: anterior, posterior and both laterals with markers to outline the subcostal margin. Oblique views can occasionally be useful. Blurring due to respiratory movement is a cause of degradation of the image. Though not in general use, respiratory gating has been shown to improve the quality of the pictures.

Dynamic acquisition during the injection of the bolus can demonstrate areas of increased vascularity within the liver and may be of use in patients with suspected AV malformations or highly vascular lesions. Patients with possible Budd-Chiari Syndrome may be injected with tracer in the leg to examine the inferior vena cava.

Single photon emission tomography can also be used as a supplement to standard views (see below).

Normal appearances, planar views (see Fig. 15.2, 15.3)

The shape of the liver is very variable and a cause of considerable confusion. In the anterior view the right lobe is usually larger than the left and the position of the porta hepatis and the insertion of the ligamentum teres can usually be delineated. The right lobe is frequently indented by the costal margin and the diaphragmatic surface of the right lobe undergoes attenuation by the breast and the same artefact may also be seen in the right lateral views. This appearance should not be mistaken for pathological replacement. The superior surface is indented by the heart. The position of the left lobe is very variable. In the right lateral view the junction of the liver to the right and left of the gallbladder fossa is represented by a notch on the anterior aspect of the image which again should not be mistaken for a pathological appearance. The posterior view will demonstrate the posterior aspect of the right lobe of the liver, the spleen and also allows a comparison of the count rates of these two organs and thus an estimate of the relative uptake of colloid. The left lateral view is mainly dominated by the spleen with usually a small portion of the left lobe of the liver appearing anteriorly.

Emission tomography

Because of its large size and complex anatomy, the liver is an organ well suited to tomographic reconstruction. There are a number of different techniques for acquiring data needed for emission tomography including tomographic scanners, rotating banks of detectors or the rotating gamma camera. It is the last mentioned which is now in most common use and has the advantage of employing a standard instrument which can be used for both planar views and tomography. The rotating gamma camera also has the advantage of allowing multiple slices covering the whole organ to be acquired in one rotational movement of the instrument around the patient.

Data acquisition and reconstruction using a rotating gamma camera

This is performed with the patient supine and the camera rotating through 360° around the patient. Before data acquisition begins, alignment and uniformity of the camera is checked. A series of 64 frames is then acquired to the computer with a frame time of 10–15 seconds, data being stored and processed either during or after acquisition. The body outline can also be supplied to the computer thus allowing for attenuation corrections to be applied. Processing of data involves filtration applied to each line array followed by back projection and image creation.

Normal appearances of emission tomography of the liver (see Fig. 15.4)

Due to its complex shape and internal structure, emission tomography of the liver shows anatomical structures which can be misinterpreted as pathological replacement.

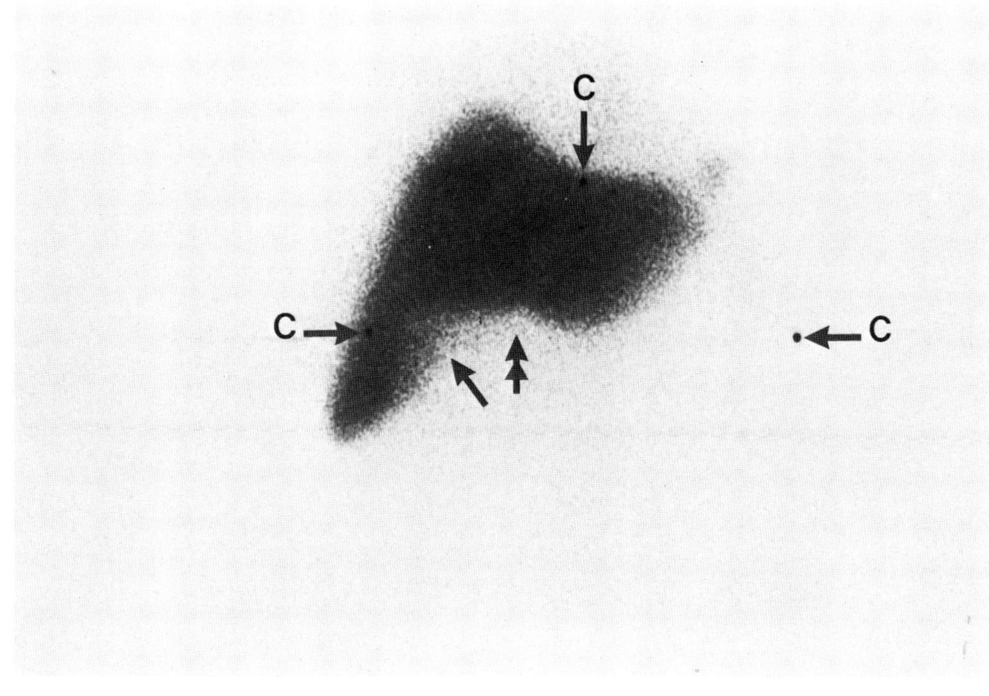

a

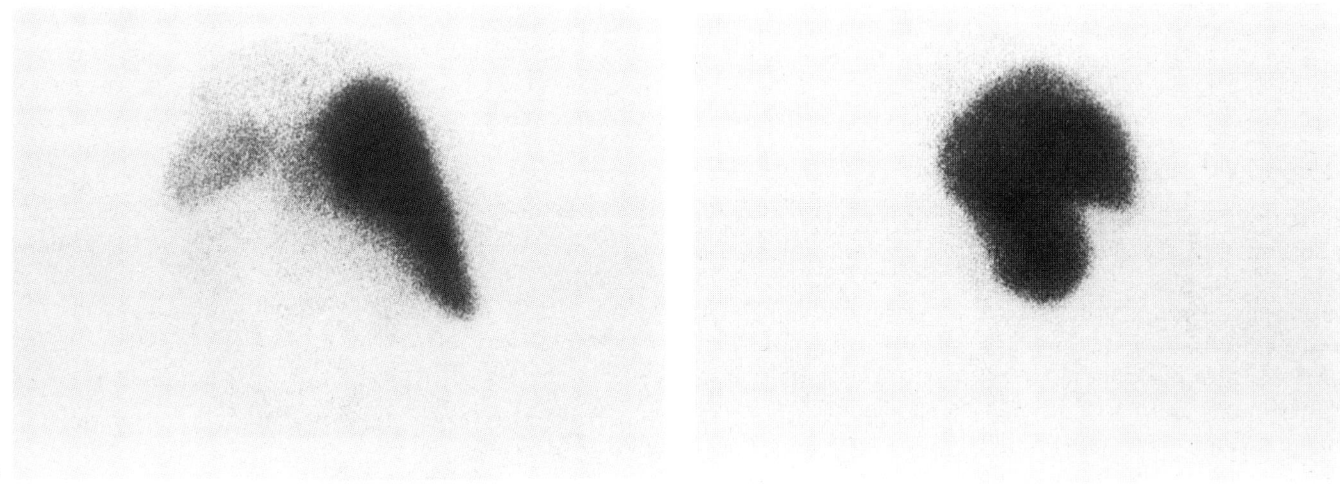

b

c

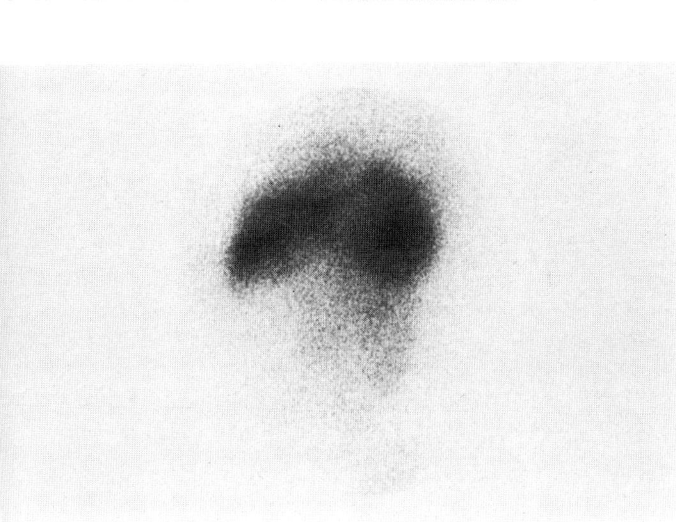

Fig. 15.2 Normal colloid scan. a. Anterior view showing gallbladder bed (single arrow) between rather large right lobe and quadrate lobe. Notch of ligamentum teres (double arrow) shows junction of quadrate and left lobe. Spleen is just visible above and lateral to the left lobe. Black dots (C) mark the costal margins. b. Posterior view shows spleen and posterior aspect of right lobe of liver. c. Right lateral view. Elongated right lobe is visible with a notch separating it from the quadrate and left lobes. d. Left lateral view. Spleen lies posteriorly and the left lobe of liver anteriorly

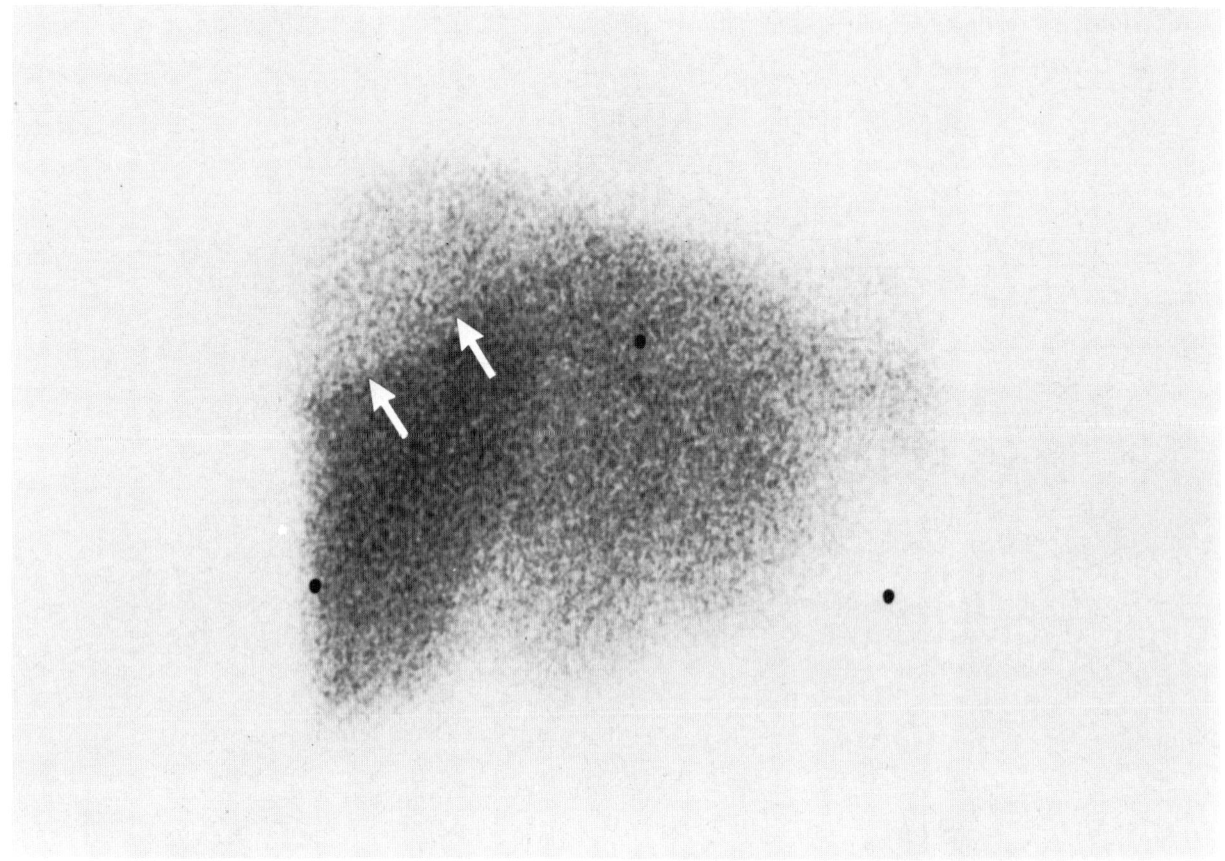

a

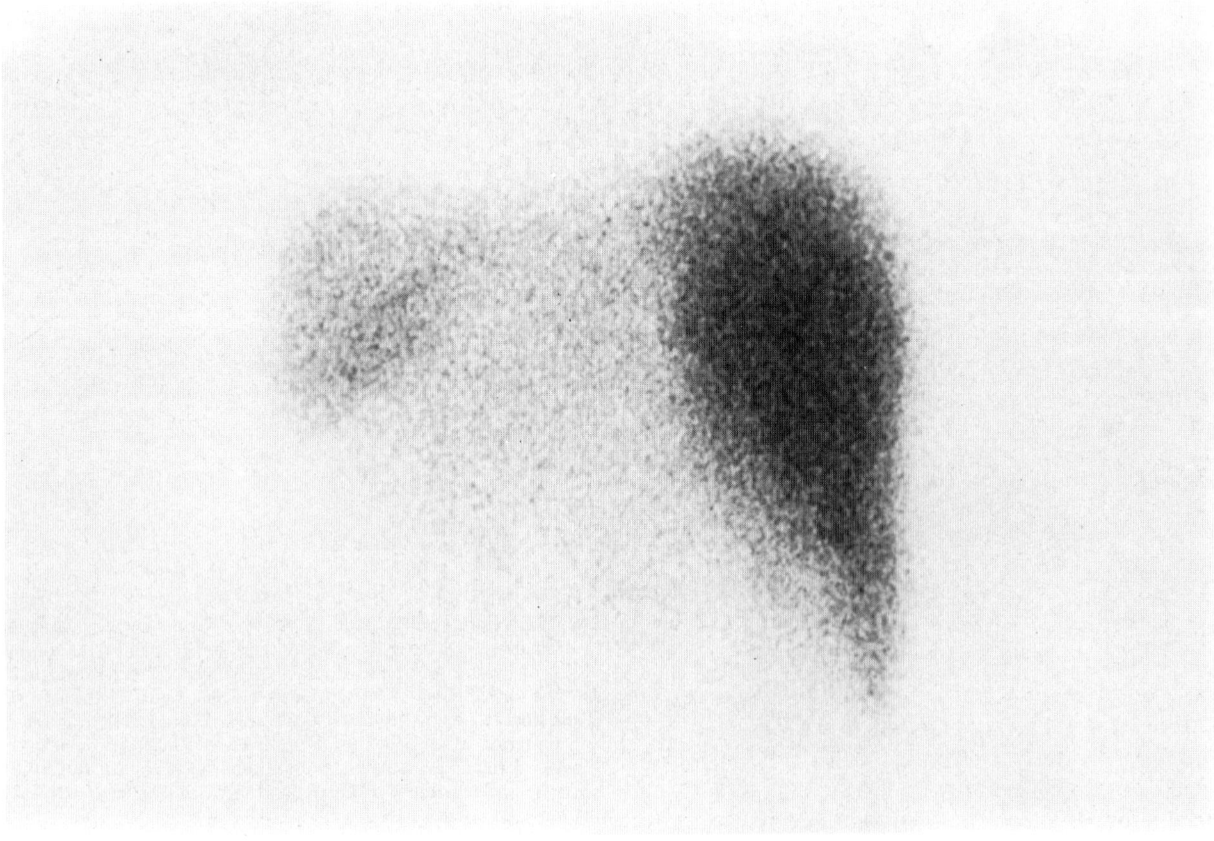

b

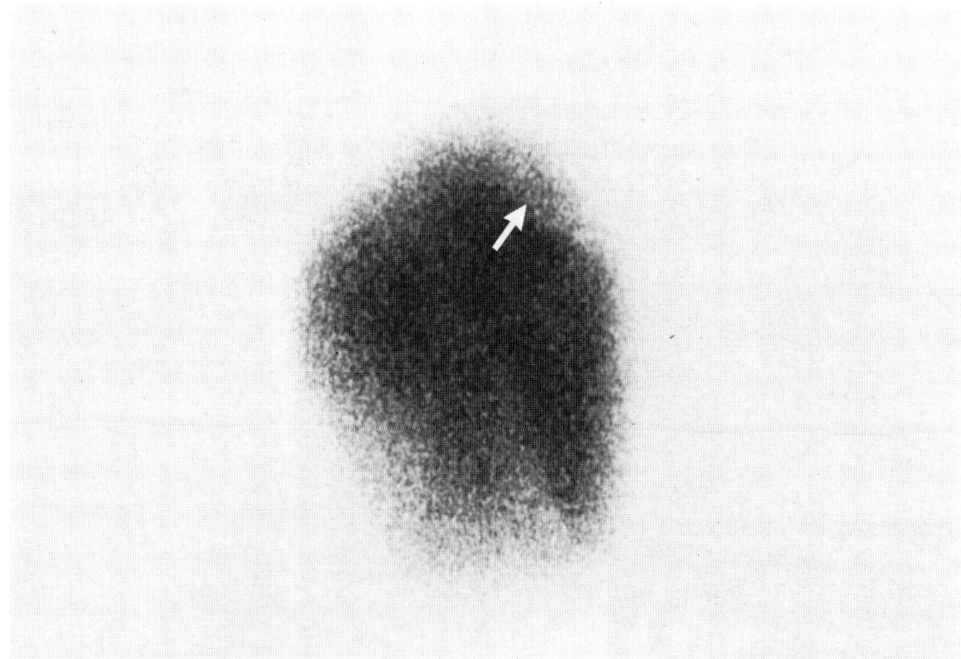

c

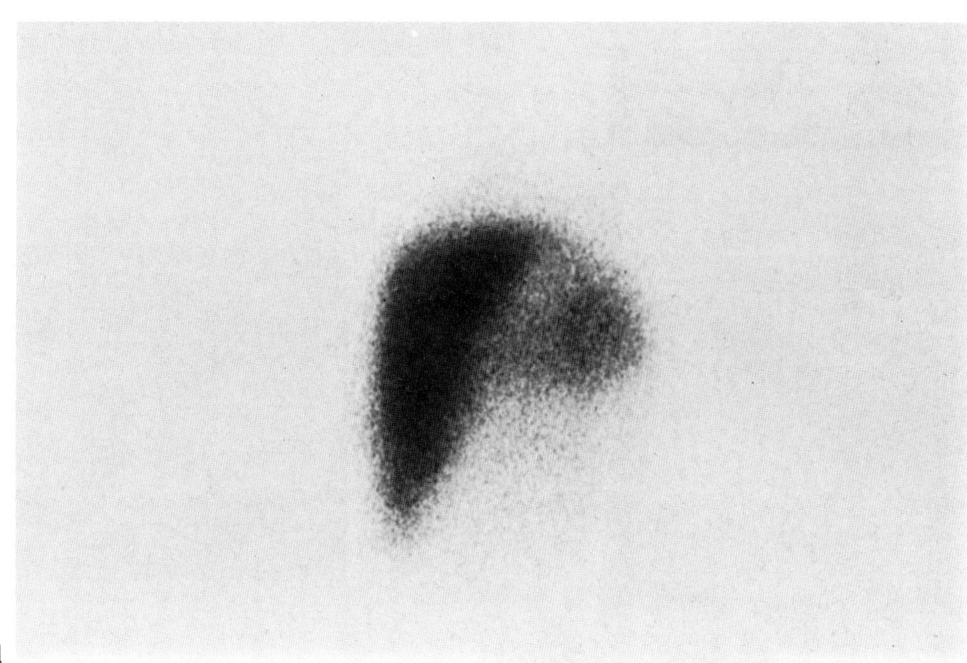

d

Fig. 15.3 Normal colloid scan showing breast artefact (arrows)

The axial slices at the diaphragmatic surface are straightforward with the two domes of the liver and spleen visualized (Fig. 15.4a). Below this the ligamentum teres is frequently visible dividing the left lobe from the quadrate lobe and the upper porta created by the portal and biliary tracts can be usually identified. The gallbladder fossa may be a very deep cleft or relatively shallow but usually recognizable by its shape and position.

COLLOID LIVER SCINTISCAN — ABNORMAL

The abnormal image can be described under three general situations:

the Kupffer cells have been focally replaced by other tissue or have been destroyed;

diffuse infiltration causes generalized enlargement which may be accompanied by non-uniform colloid uptake;

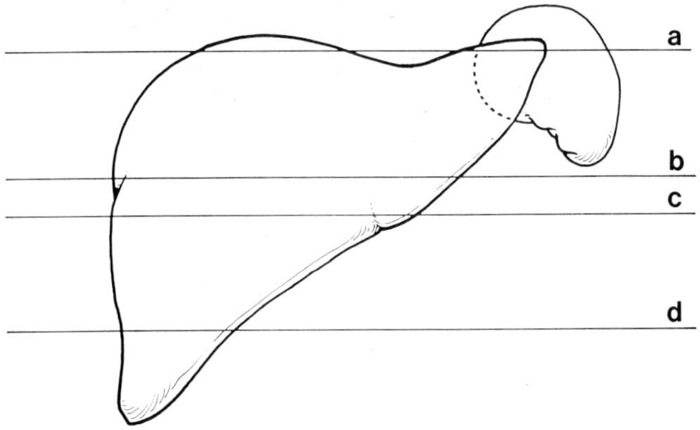

a
b
c
d

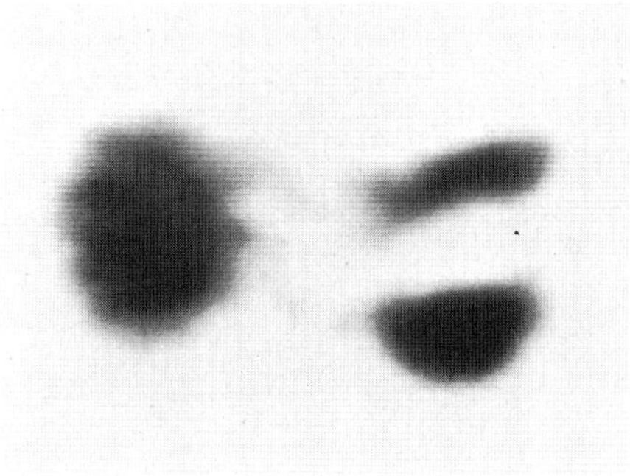

a

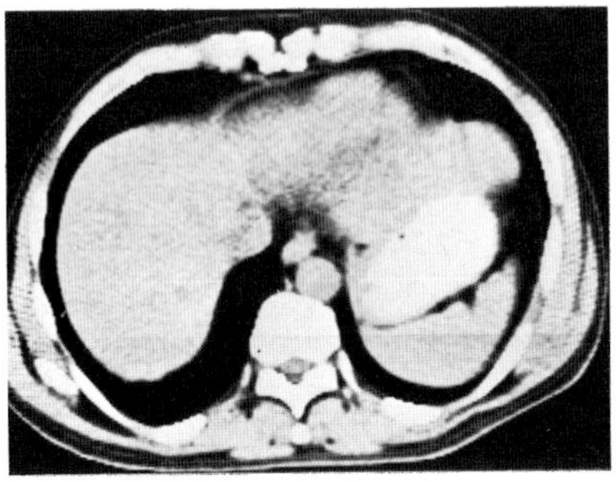

Left Lobe Liver
Right Lobe Liver
Spleen

a1

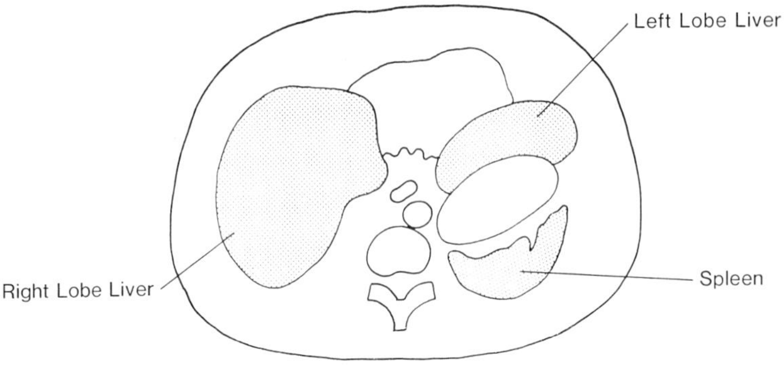

a2

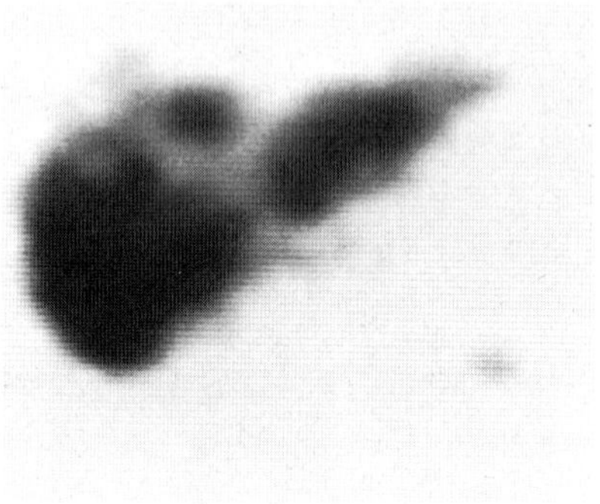

b

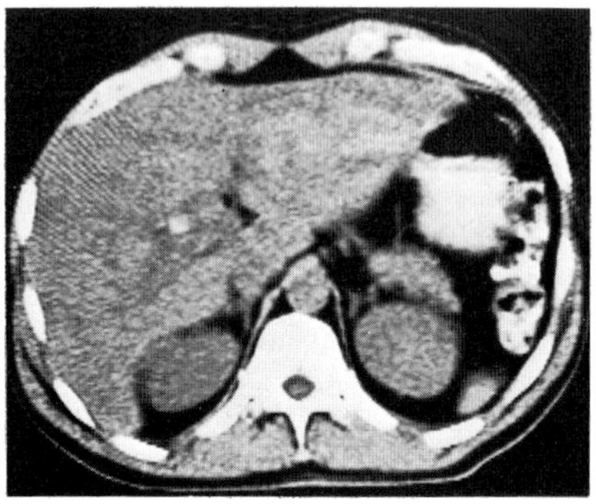

b1

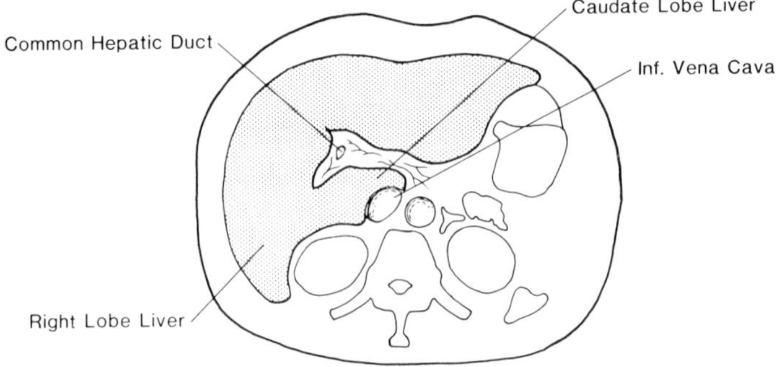

b2

Fig. 15.4 Normal colloid scan emission tomography. CT scan and related emission tomographic slices in a 44-year-old man with obstructive jaundice. a. Section through diaphragmatic portion of right and left lobes. b. Section at upper pole of kidneys showing relationship of caudate lobe and porta hepatis. c. Section at level of Hartmann's pouch. Note the gallbladder fossa is seen on the emission tomography dividing right from quadrate lobe but not seen on this CT, section. d. Section passing through inferior borders of right and left lobes.

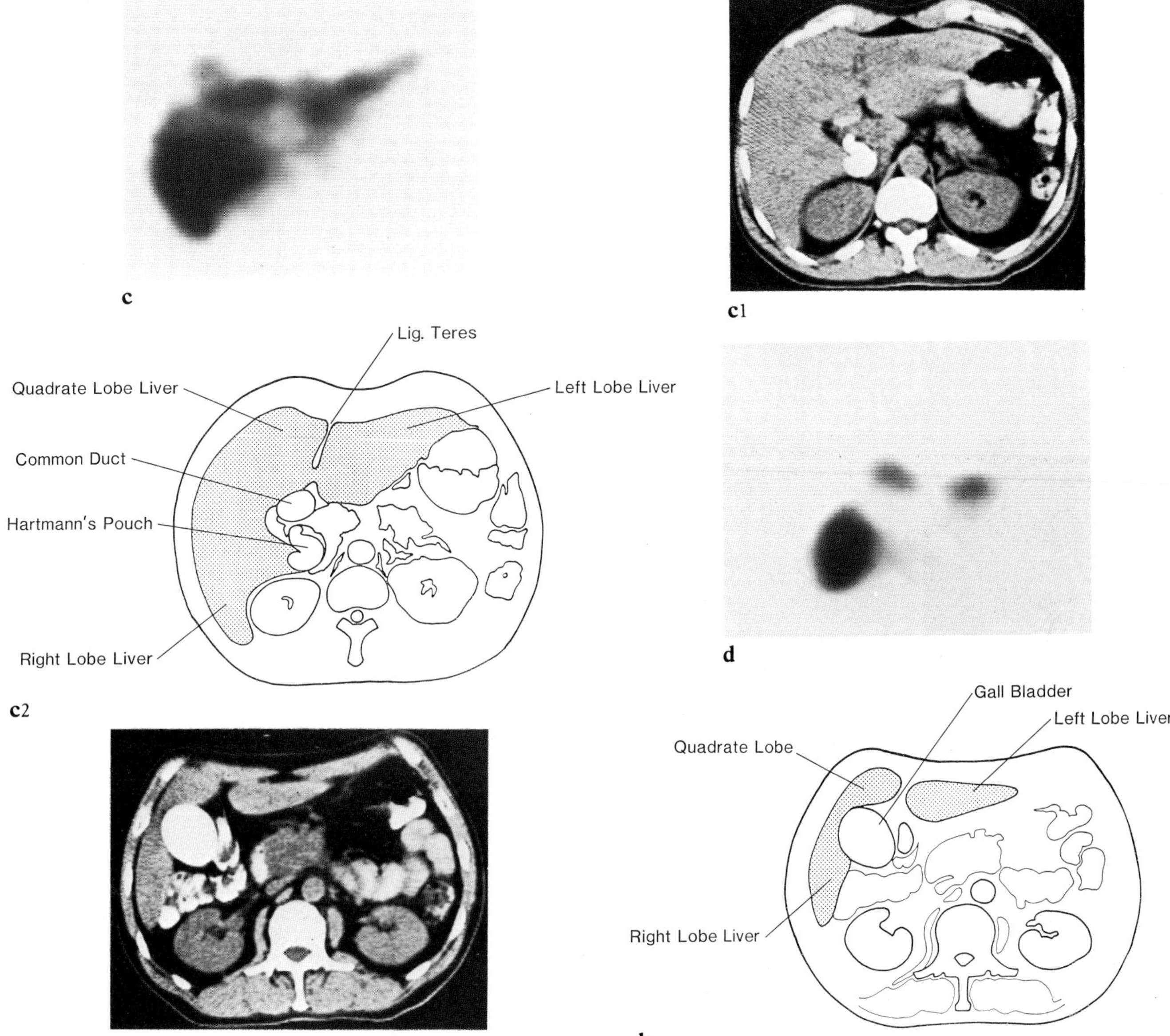

changes in the relative distribution of colloid reflect changes in the flow or extraction of colloid.

Focal defects — metastatic (Fig. 15.5)

Scintigraphy of the liver with radioactive colloid is the simplest method of survey for metastatic disease, representing a series of four images taking 10–15 min in total, and with the advantage of not requiring either skilled operator or expensive machine time.

Resolution at the surface of the liver approaches 1 cm but with respiratory movement and depth may fall to as low as 3 and 4 cm deep within the right lobe. In general, lesions of 2 cm upwards should be detected by modern apparatus. Emission tomography will improve the ability to detect lesions marginally (Ell & Khan 1981, Brendel et al 1983) but probably has its greatest advantage in defining more clearly the normal from the abnormal.

Metastatic carcinomas of the colon and kidney usually result in large well defined defects in an otherwise normal liver. In secondary hepatic carcinoma the incidence of 15% of positive scans has been reported, and a scan accuracy of 85% (Harbert 1984). In the case of carcinoma of the breast, the incidence of an abnormal liver scan at the time of diagnosis is low (1–3%). In advanced disease the accuracy of the isotope scan is lower than in colorectal cancer (67%) due to the tendency to smaller or more diffuse lesions (Drum & Beard, 1976). In the case of bronchogenic carcinoma, the incidence of metastatic disease is approximately 7% but here, as in the case of other primary tumours, there are few confirmed metastases in the liver which are not associated with a rise in alkaline phosphatase or other indication of liver dysfunction. If therefore liver

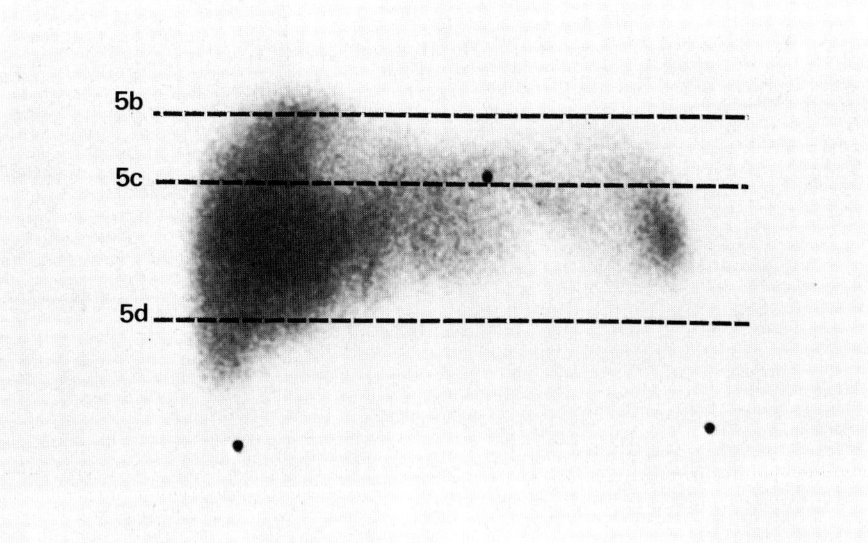

a

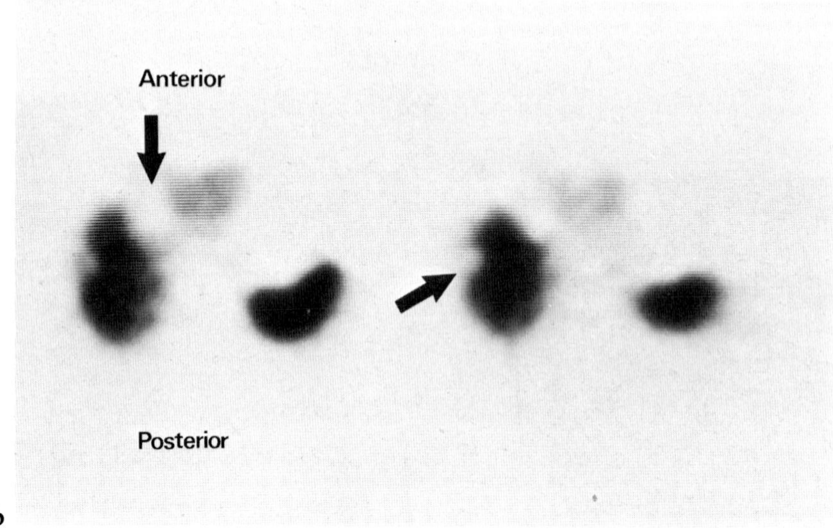

b

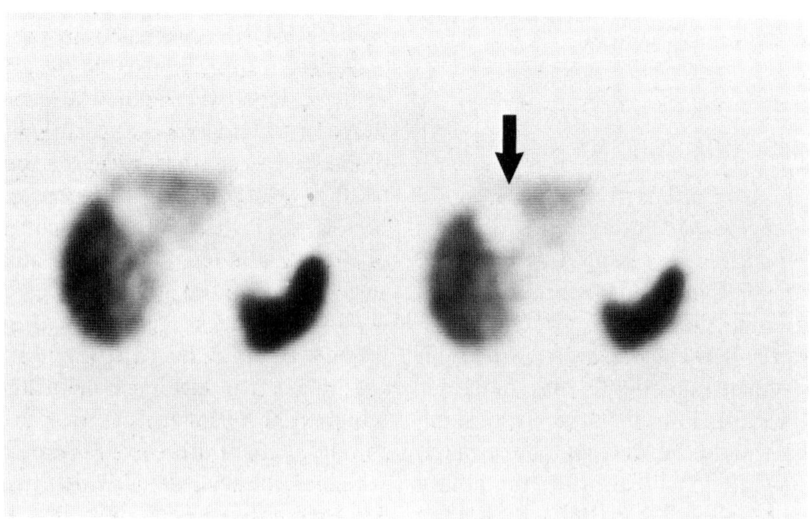

c

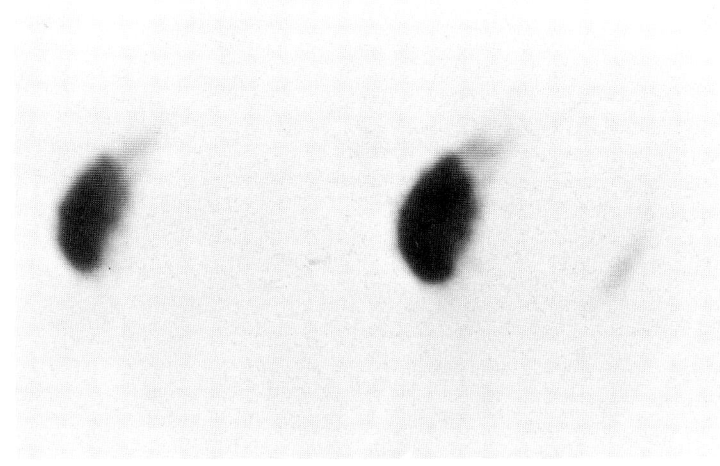

Fig. 15.5 73-year-old patient with carcinoma of breast. Metastases were seen at laparotomy. A single focal defect is seen on the anterior view (a) and transverse tomographic images (b,c,d). Note multiple lesions seen on emission tomography (arrows)

function tests are quite normal there is probably little indication for liver imaging and conversely where the liver biochemistry is abnormal serial follow-up scans are justified.

Comparison with ultrasound and computerized tomography

For reasons outlined above the relative accuracy will vary with the pathology. Modern CT scanning provides a sensitive and accurate image which allows not only the examination of the liver but also surrounding structures. Ultrasound has intrinsically better resolution than scintigraphy but is operator dependent and also influenced by echogenicity of lesions. Comparison of CT and radionuclide scanning with the previous generation of scanners showed figures of accuracy between 80 and 90% with comparable results for all the techniques. Thus a prospective study published in 1982 by Smith et al showed an accuracy of 80% for both the liver scintigraphy and ultrasound with a figure of 84% for CT. A more recent study from the same centre (Miller et al 1983) showed that CT will detect smaller lesions than scintigraphy when enhancement with iodized oil was added although in this small series of patients, the overall detection did not vary statistically between the two techniques.

Diffuse infiltration

This can result from a large number of disease processes none of which are specific in their appearance. These include infiltration with abnormal cells as, e.g. in chronic leukaemias and storage disease. Fatty infiltration of the liver will usually cause an increase in size, sometimes non-homogenous in distribution.

Hodgkin's Disease usually manifests itself as a generalized enlargement of liver and spleen but may more rarely cause focal defects.

Cirrhosis of the liver In the early stages of alcoholic cirrhosis, the liver is enlarged and may show a non-homogenous distribution of colloid. As the portal venous pressure increases, the spleen enlarges and there is relative increased uptake of colloid by that organ and the bone marrow. These changes are recognized most clearly on the posterior view (see Fig. 15.6). The irregular pattern within the liver and areas of nodular hyperplasia may create focal defects which may resemble metastatic deposits. These changes in pattern correlate fairly well with the histological findings (Geslien et al 1976).

PRIMARY TUMOURS OF THE LIVER

Hepatocellular carcinoma This usually presents as a large defect on the colloid scan and has no specific features. It may be multicentric and may co-exist with changes suggesting cirrhosis (Broderick et al 1980). Hepatocellular carcinomas are often highly vascular and have a high metabolic activity and for this reason in suspected cases blood pool and dynamic scanning may give extra information. The tumour frequently shows uptake of the labelled amino acid, selenium labelled methionine (see Fig. 15.7). This is not a specific feature for hepatocellular carcinoma but may occur in other tumours with a rapid turnover. Most metastases however fail to show uptake of selenium labelled methionine. Hepatocellular carcinomas also show uptake of gallium citrate in most cases (see below) and uptake of hepatobiliary agents may be demonstrated but this is seen in only a proportion and therefore is not of diagnostic value (Savitch et al 1983).

Cholangiocarcinoma This may appear as a cold defect in the region of the porta but has no specific features.

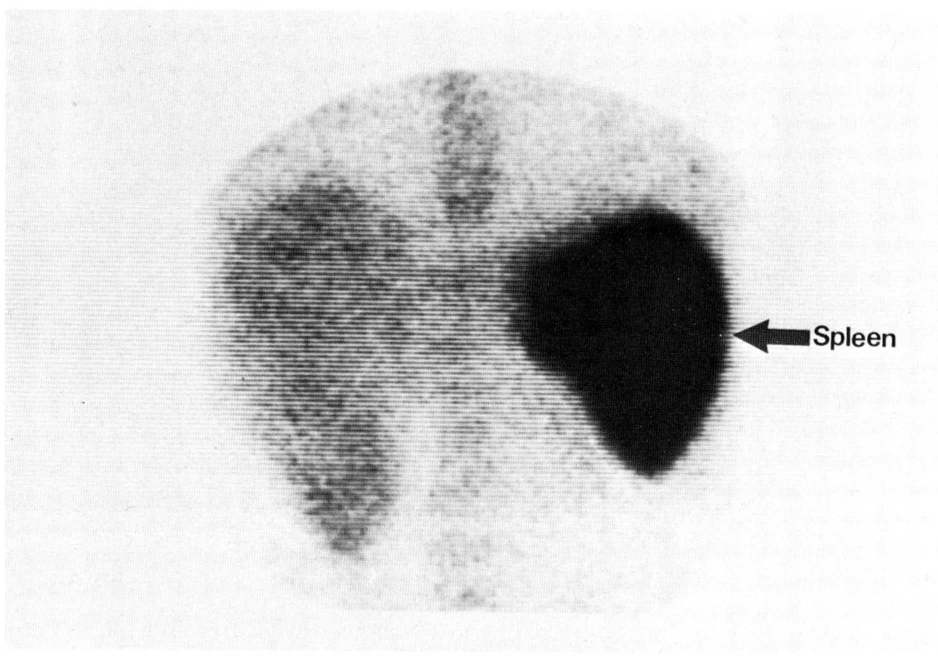

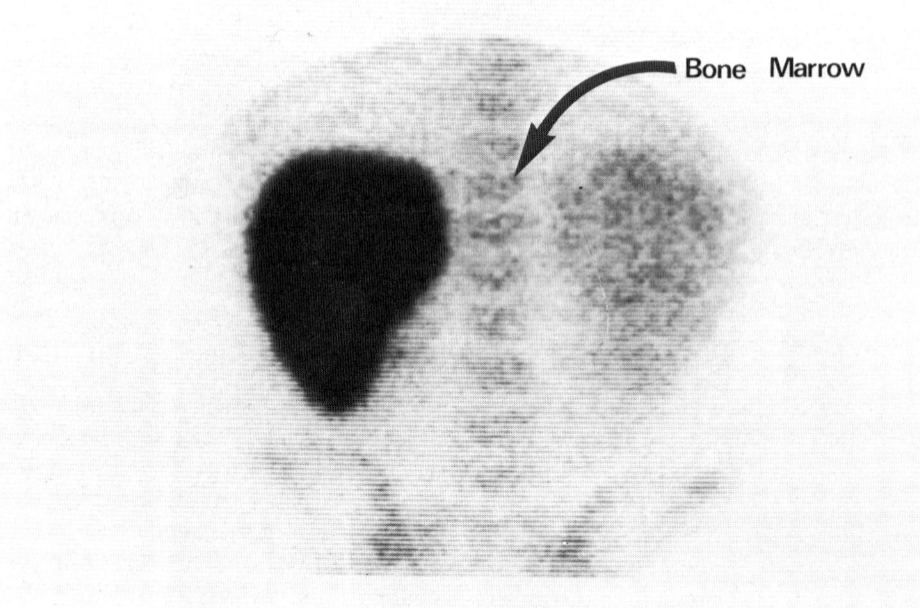

Fig. 15.6 Anterior and posterior colloid scans of patient suffering from alcoholic cirrhosis. Note increased localization in spleen (arrow) and bone marrow (curved arrow)

Hepatic cysts and multicystic disease show defects on the colloid scan. This diagnosis is readily made by CT or ultrasound. Multicystic liver may appear identical to multiple metastatic deposits and should not be misinterpreted.

Haemangiomas appear as defects on the colloid scan. However because of their vascular pattern, they can be shown to 'fill in', when imaging using technetium red cells is employed. This phenomenon can be compared to the characteristic enhancement of these lesions during computerized tomography with contrast.

Focal nodular hyperplasia These islands of parenchymal cells occurring usually in patients on oestrogens, are usually first detected by ultrasound. They may show low, normal or high relative uptake of colloid and usually show uptake of biliary tracers such as HIDA. The patient, often

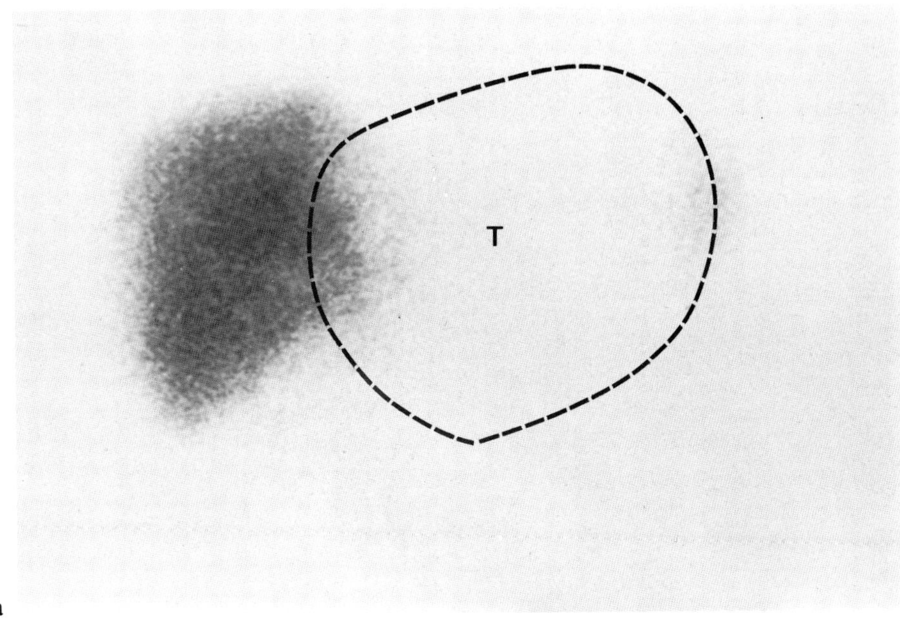

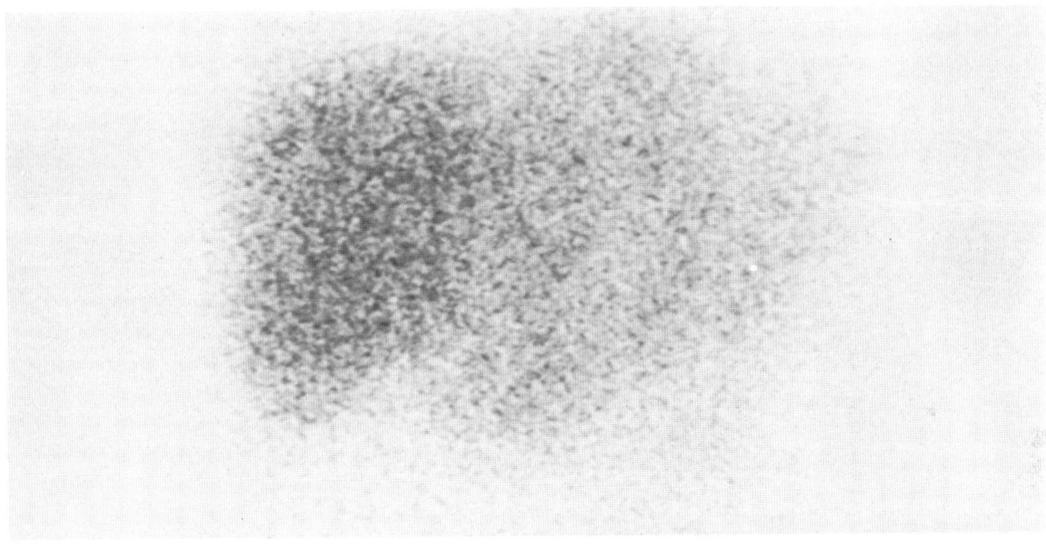

Fig. 15.7 a. Anterior colloid scan showing defect in left lobe of liver due to a hepatoma (T). b. A repeat scan of same patient using 75 Se methionine showing uptake by tumour

with minimal symptoms, who is discovered to have a tumour on ultrasound and CT, should have liver scanning performed. This is probably best done using a biliary agent. These lesions can thus be shown to contain liver parenchymal cells and the patient may well be saved from biopsy or laparotomy (Rogers et al 1981).

Liver abscess In the West the main cause of liver abscess is pyogenic infection, usually arising in the abdomen, but worldwide *entamoeba histolytica* remains the most common cause.

The appearance on the colloid scintigram is that of a rounded focal defect. Its necrotic or fluid contents may be determined by ultrasound. The use of alternative tracers particularly labelled autologous white blood cells can make a specific diagnosis (see Fig. 15.14).

Miscellaneous lesions Trauma to the liver may produce focal defects due to an intra-hepatic haematoma. More commonly a combination of intra-hepatic defect with displacement may be seen.

Irradiation of the liver will produce a defect of colloid uptake. This is usually recognizable for what it is by the sharply demarcated field.

Hepatic venous occlusion — Budd-Chiari Syndrome In total occlusion of the hepatic veins colloid uptake may be markedly reduced to the majority of the liver with preservation of the caudate lobe due to its independent venous

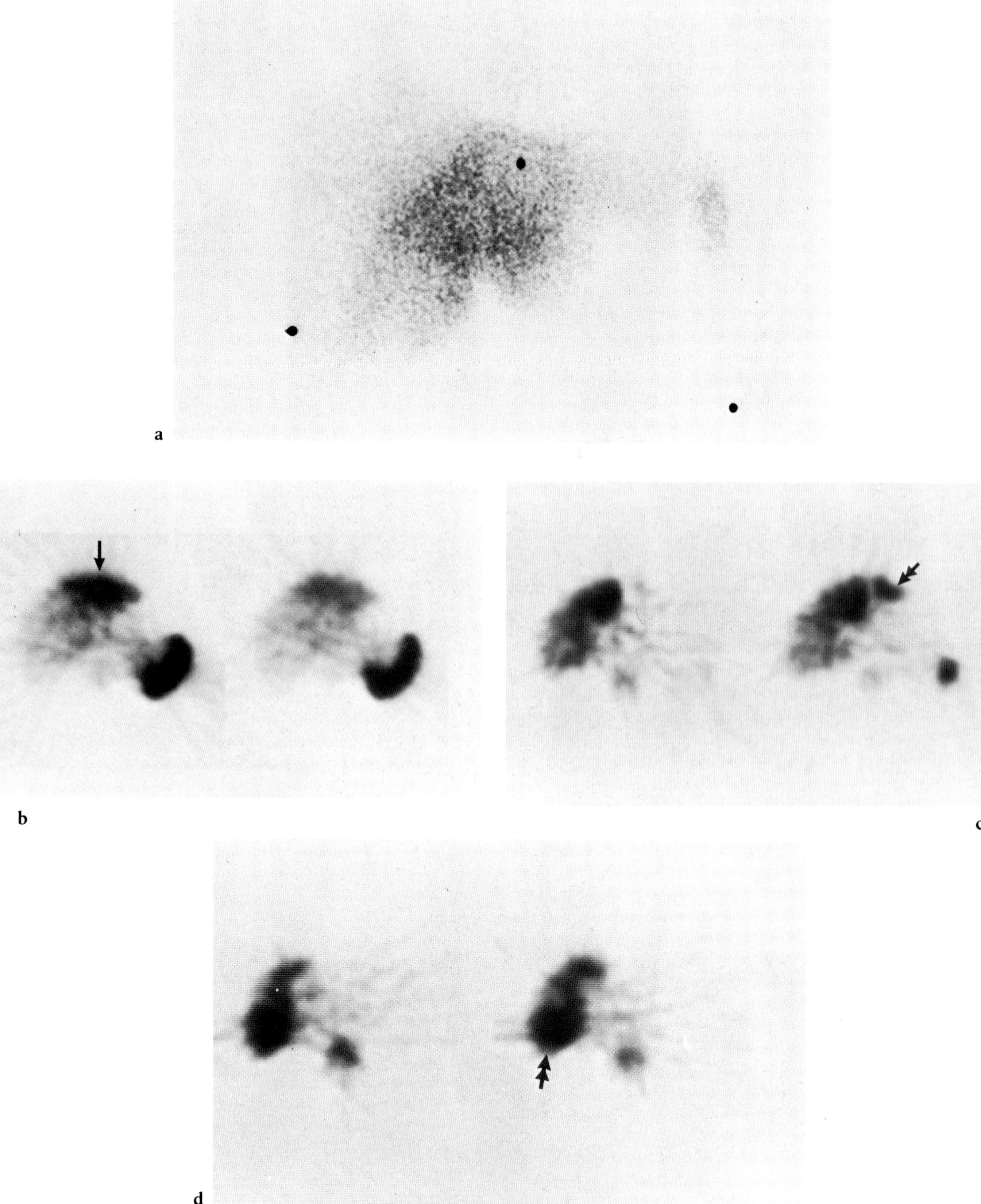

Fig. 15.8 Anterior colloid scan and emission tomography in Budd-Chiari syndrome. Note colloid uptake centrally (a). Tomography (b, c, d) shows that this represents caudate lobe (single arrow), quadrate and left lobes (double arrow)

drainage (Meindok et al 1976) (see Fig. 15.8). However this picture is not by any means invariable. Irregular uptake of colloid may be seen and venous occlusion may be a cause of 'hot spots', that is, areas of increased colloid uptake. This phenomenon is also seen in haemangiomas, focal nodular hyperplasia and veno-occlusive disease (Coel et al 1972).

HEPATOBILIARY SCANNING

Radiopharmaceuticals

The first agent for this purpose was iodinated Rose Bengal originally developed by Taplin et al (1955). However although still in use fairly recently its uptake is slower, imaging poorer, and radiation greater than the technetium labelled agents which were developed in the mid 1970s. Several technetium labelled agents have been developed but the ones now in general use are derivatives of imido diacetic acid. A number of different molecules are available which differ to some extent in their behaviour, all under the general term of HIDA. The diisopropyl derivative is less affected by high serum levels of bilirubin than the dimethyl while the Parabutyl derivative, although rapidly cleared from the blood, has a slower transport through the liver than other compounds. The

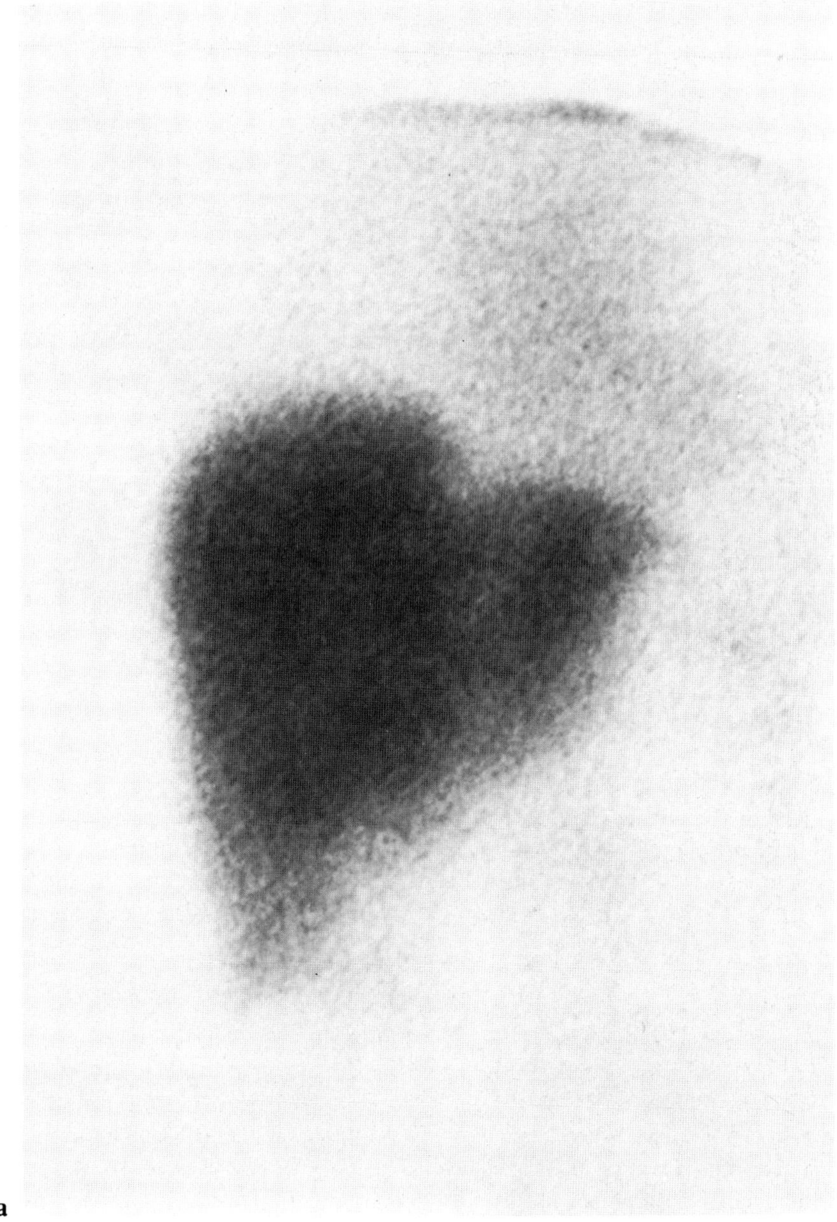

Fig. 15.9 Normal biliary scan. Anterior sequential views at 5(a), 10(b), 20(c) and 40(d) min using HIDA showing tracer in common duct (single arrow) and gallbladder (double arrow). e. Time activity curve over liver and abdomen showing a maximal peak at 12 min with subsequent clearance from liver and rising activity over the gut

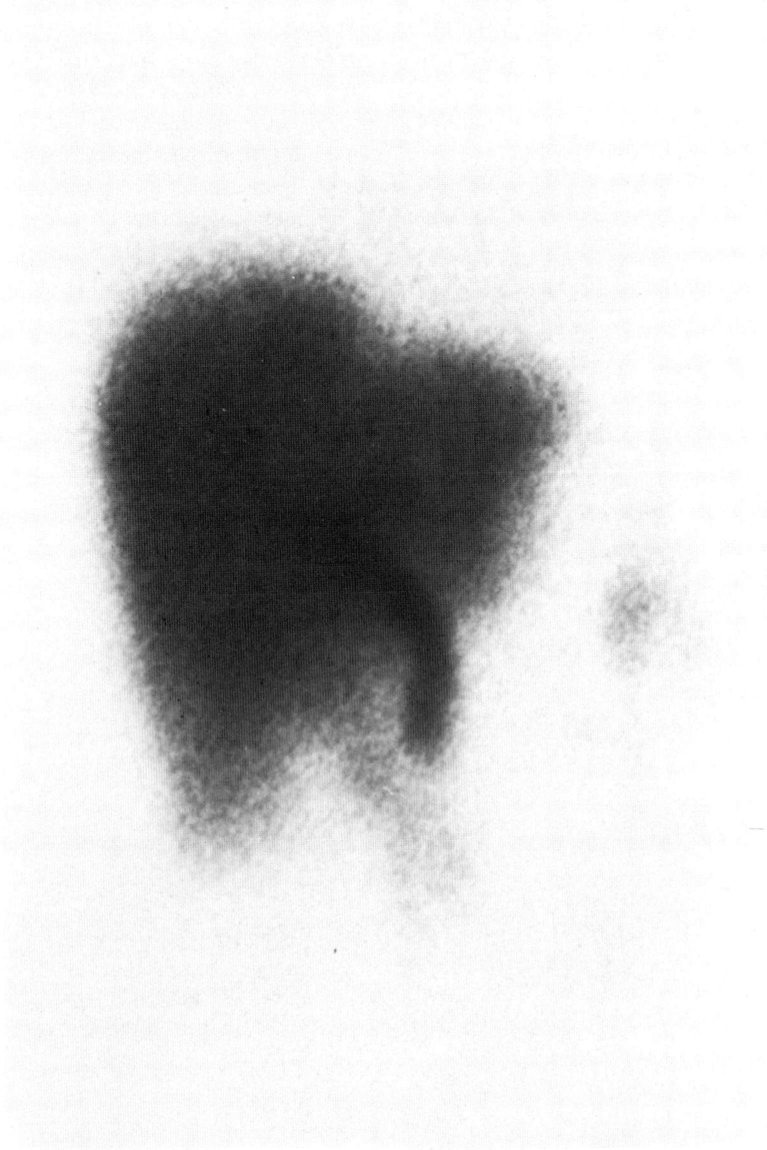

Fig. 15.9b

agent therefore in most general use in patients with relatively normal liver function is the dimethyl IDA; but one of the alternative compounds should be used for the patient with jaundice.

Imaging

(40–80 MBq) 1–2mCi technetium labelled HIDA is injected intravenously. The patient should preferably be fasting. Sequential static anterior images at 5, 10, 15 and 20 min can be recorded with later views where required. An alternative which has certain advantages is a slow dynamic recording over the liver of 1 frame per minute for 40 min. This recording has the advantage of allowing time activity curves to be created to examine hepatic and biliary function. Patients with suspected fistulas or abnormal anatomy may require posterior and lateral views. Where acute cholecystitis is under investigation, delayed views up to 4 h are necessary and in the differential diagnosis of jaundice again delayed views are needed.

Normal appearances (see Fig. 15.9)

Following the intravenous injection of dimethyl HIDA there is a rapid uptake of tracer into the liver. In the patient with normal liver function no other organ shows significant concentration and renal excretion is minimal. The peak of liver activity is at approximately 10 min with clearance of tracer following this. Defects due to liver replacement can be identified by recording standard views during the first 10 min. Biliary ducts can usually be identified from 10 to 15 min and activity rapidly appears in the

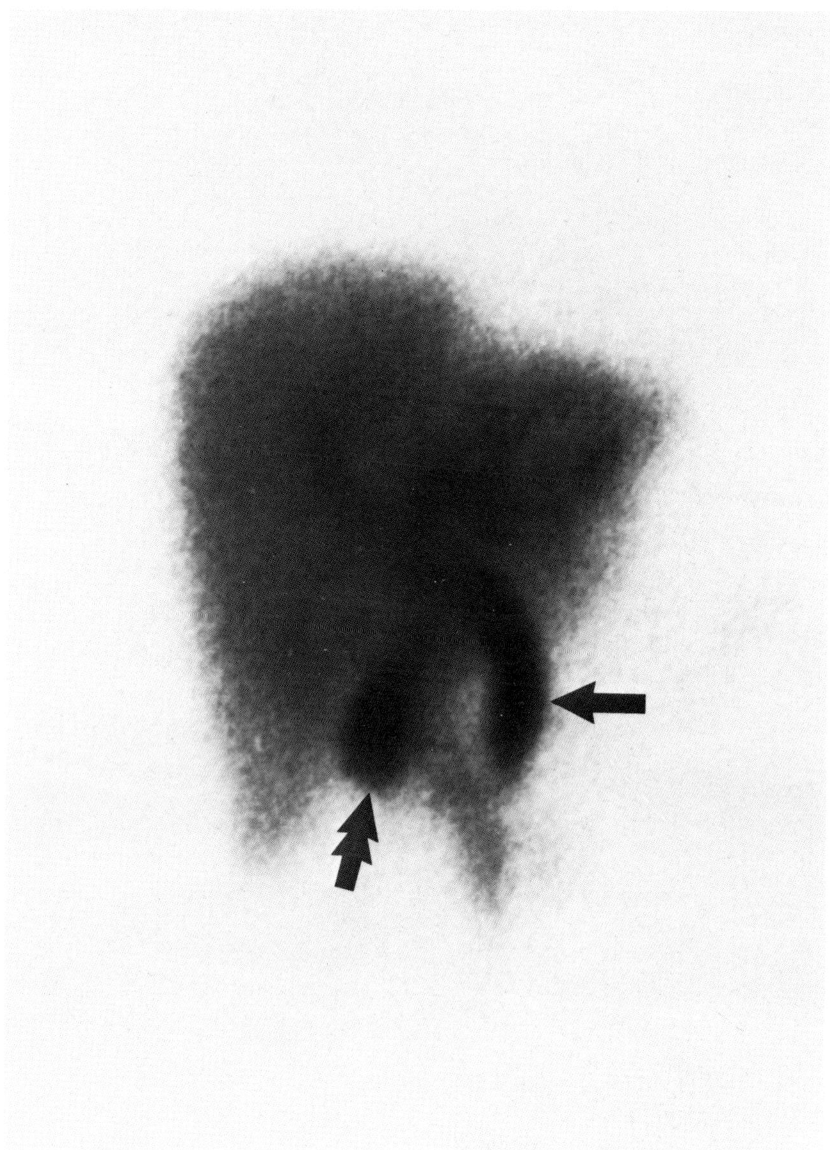

Fig. 15.9c

common duct, gallbladder and duodenum. In fasting subjects the gallbladder should be clearly visualized within 60 min but in the non-fasting patient filling may be delayed. A right lateral view may be advisable to differentiate renal from gallbladder activity.

The time activity curve over the liver rises steeply and becomes maximal at 10 min. This curve represents hepatic blood flow and hepatocyte function. Delays in uptake correlate with other evidence of abnormal liver function. The disappearance of tracer from the liver is a reflection of biliary drainage (see Fig. 15.9).

Acute cholecystitis

The patient with acute cholecystitis will almost invariably have a functional or organic obstruction of the cystic duct. Although this may rarely occur in the normal population and may occur in chronic cholecystitis, the combination of a characteristic clinical picture and evidence of cystic duct obstruction is highly diagnostic (Ch. 41). Thus in a series of 296 patients, examined by biliary scintigraphy, there was one false positive and six false negatives, giving an overall accuracy of 97.6% (Weissman et al 1981).

Investigation by ultrasound is less specific. Ultrasound will accurately identify stones but these may be absent. Evidence of inflammatory change in the wall of the gallbladder may be seen.

The appearances on biliary scanning will usually show normal uptake of tracer into the liver and excretion in the common duct with non-visualization of the gallbladder. It is important to continue to image for 4 hours, since delayed filling of the gallbladder can occur particularly in

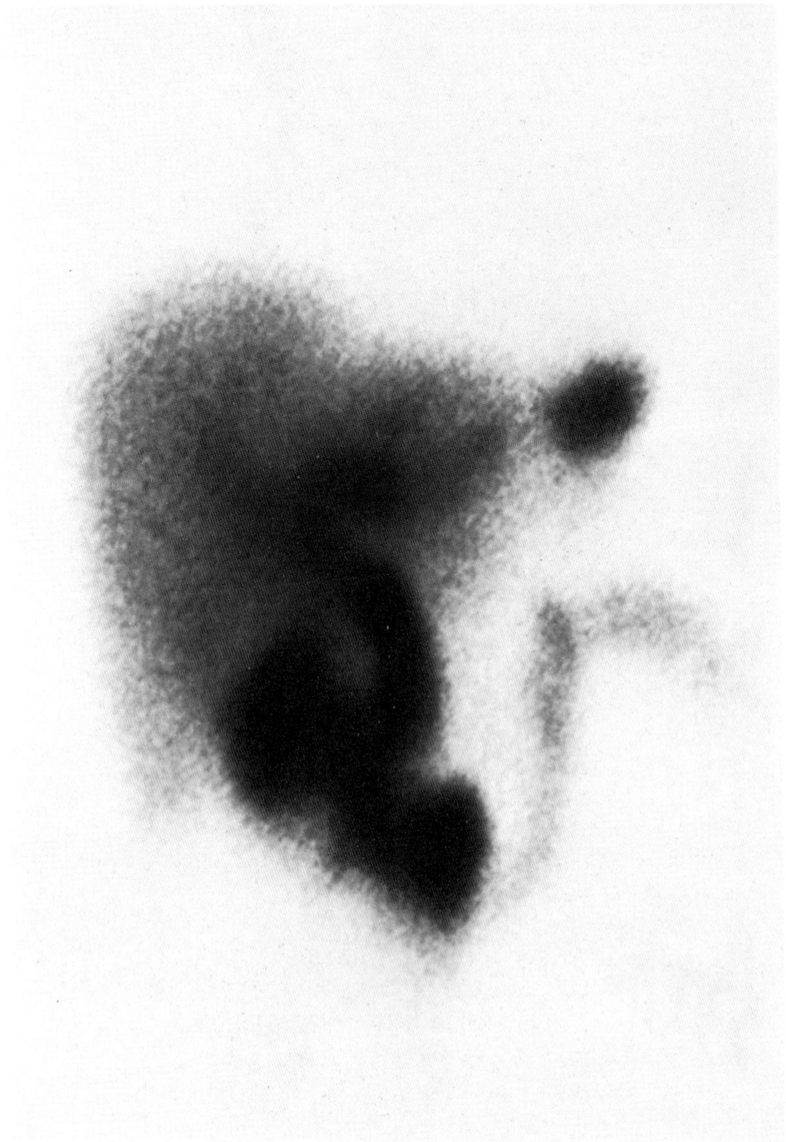

Fig. 15.9d

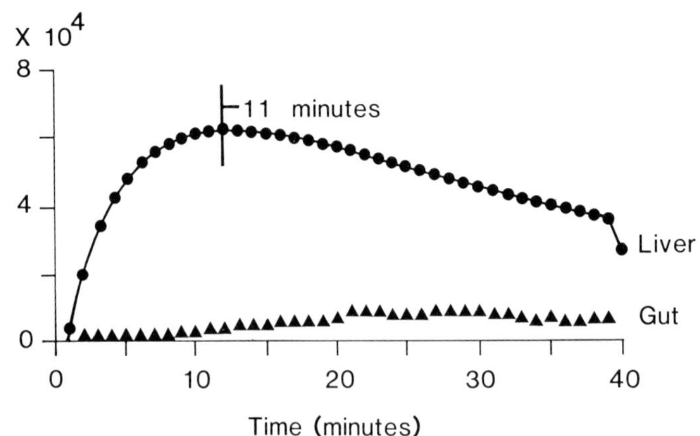

Fig. 15.9e

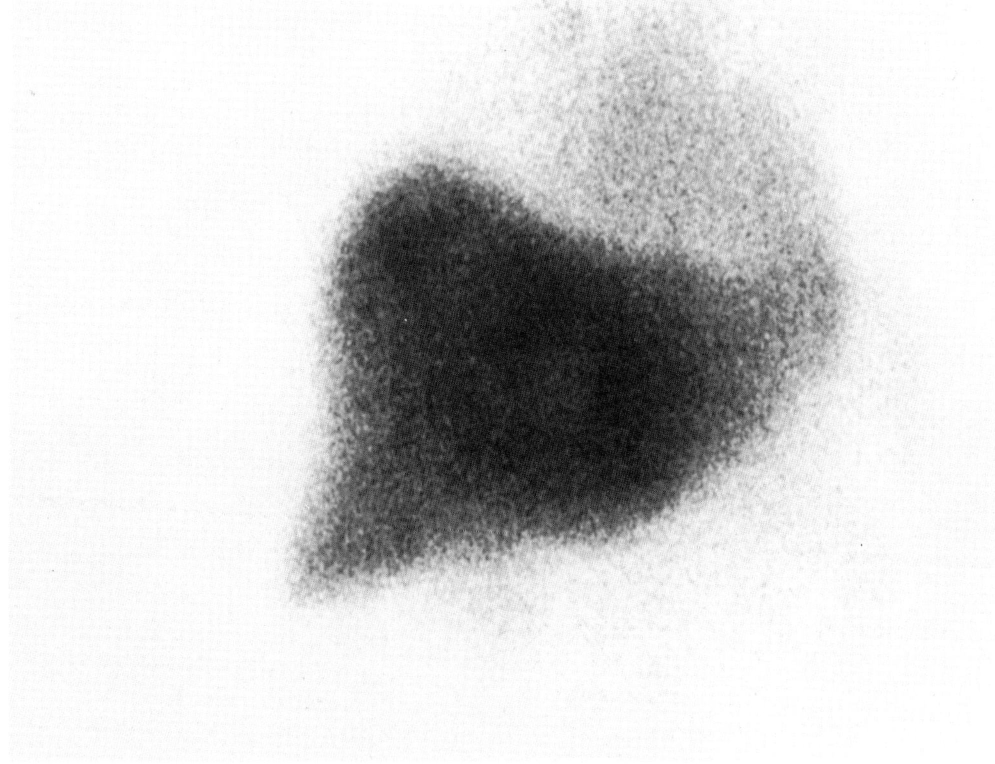

a

b

Fig. 15.10 Biliary scan in 46-year-old diabetic with gallstones and chronic cholecystitis. Time sequence as for Fig. 15.9 showing non-filling gallblader

chronic cholecystitis. A failure to see the common duct, and bile activity, but normal visualization of the liver indicates common duct obstruction.

Occasionally perforation of the gallbladder may be identified as a complication of acute cholecystitis demonstrating a fistulous tract from the cystic duct or gallbladder bed (Selby & Glasman 1983).

Chronic cholecystitis

The most suitable investigation of this group of patients is by ultrasound since the hallmark is the presence of stones with wall thickening, not necessarily associated with cystic duct obstruction. However delayed filling of the gallbladder or partial, and in some cases, complete obstruction of cystic duct, is quite common (see Fig. 15.10).

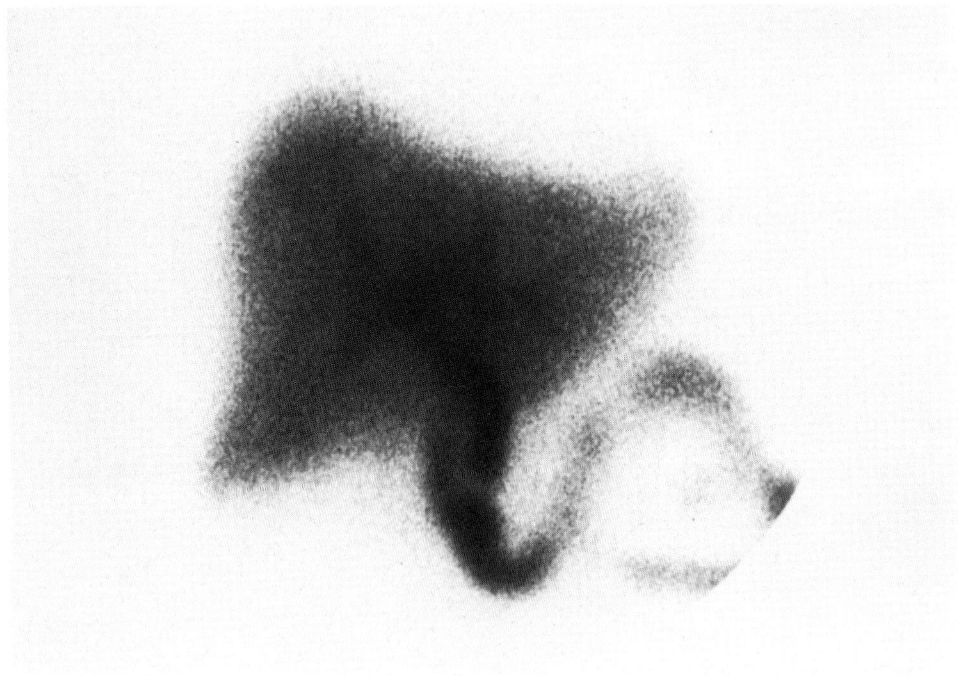

Fig. 15.10c

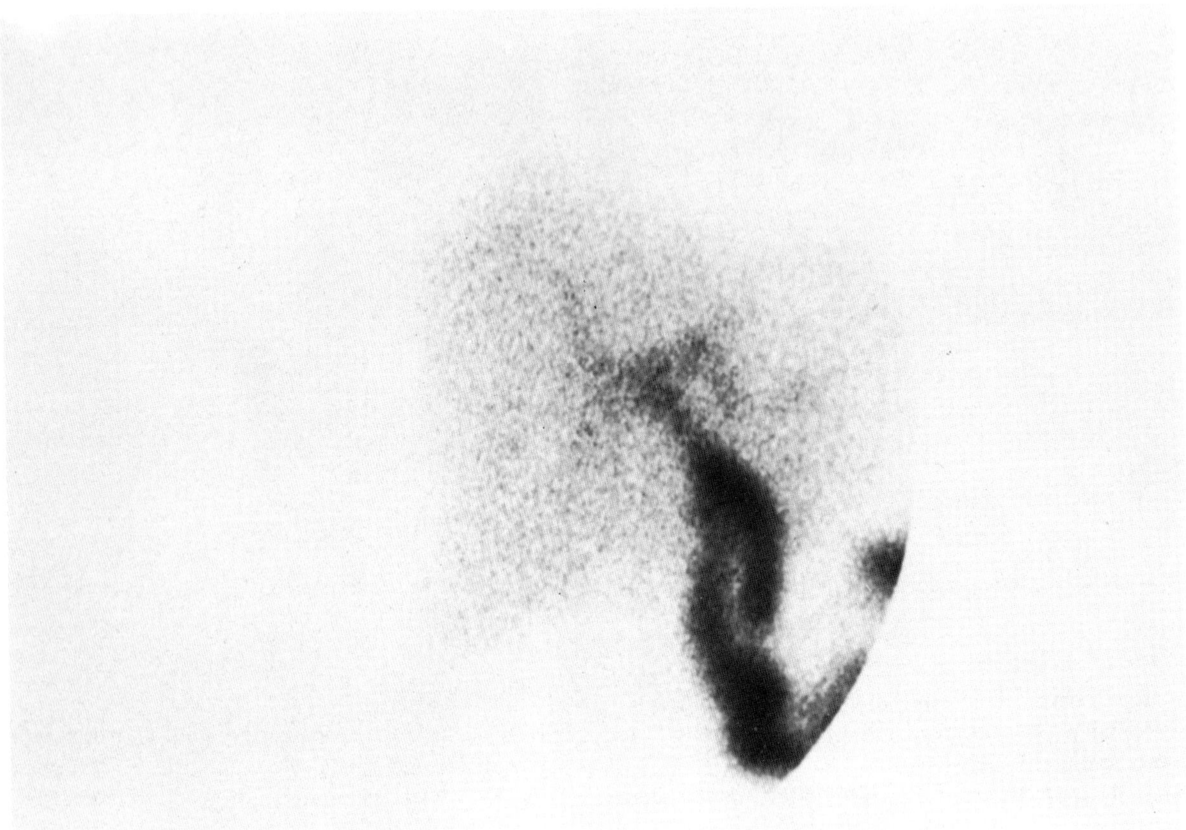

Fig. 15.10d

Liver disease

Hepatic cell failure due to any cause is associated with marked delay or absent uptake of tracer by the liver. This uptake mirrors other indicators of hepatic cell dysfunction. In ascending cholangitis the uptake curve is usually delayed but frequently there is very poor clearance of tracer from the liver, presumably representing partial intrahepatic cholestasis. This same appearance may also be seen in viral hepatitis or biliary cirrhosis as well as drug induced jaundice.

Partial obstruction can produce again evidence of some

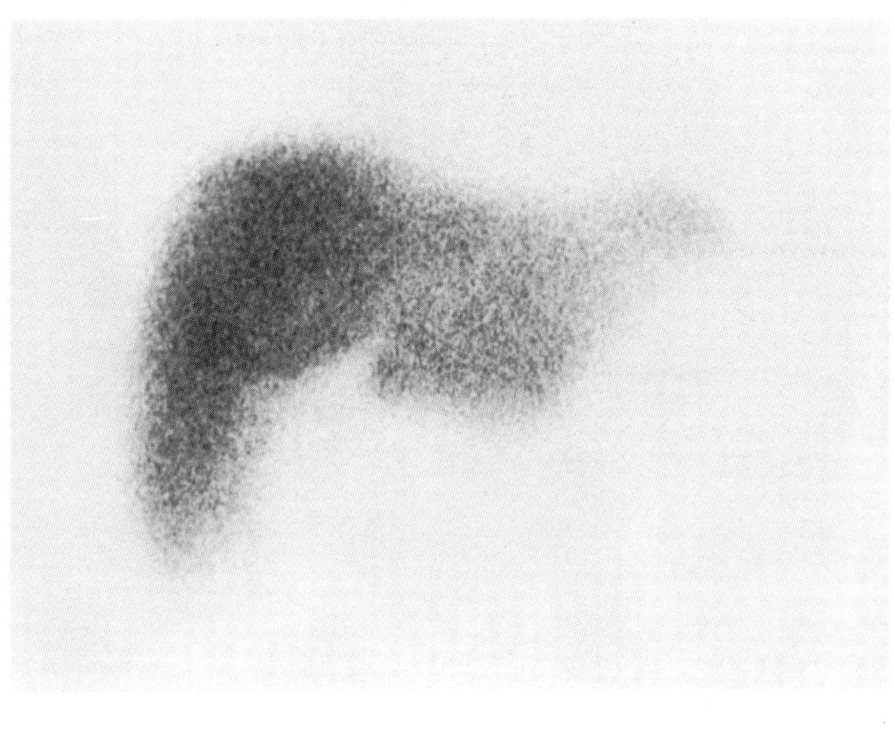

a

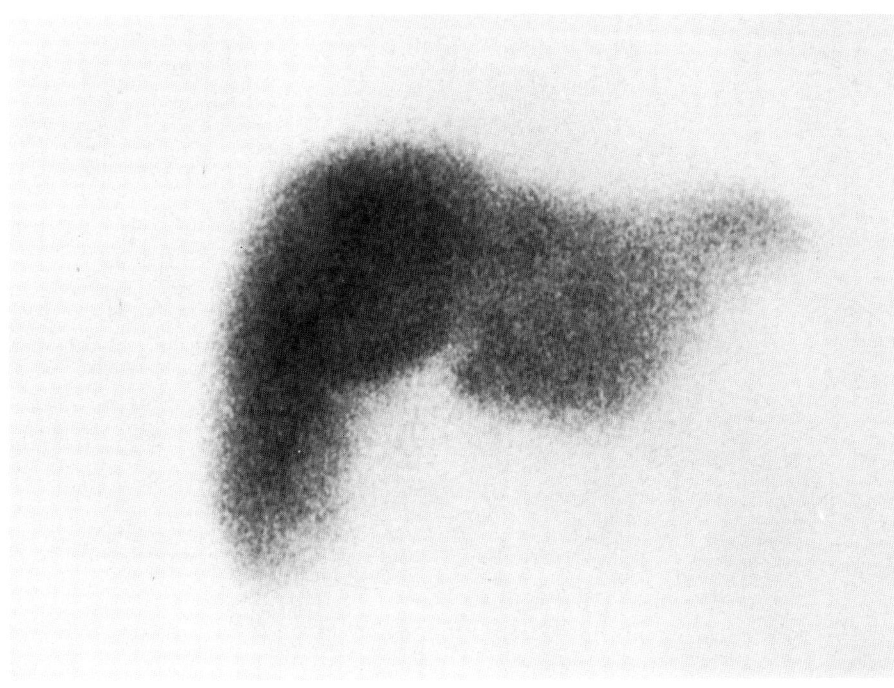

b

Fig. 15.11 Biliary scan and partial obstruction due to choledochal cyst. Images at 10, 15, 35 and 50 min show delayed appearance of tracer in dilated ducts and stretched common duct. Pattern of slow uptake of tracer into the liver indicates some hepatic cell damage and no clearance over 40 min

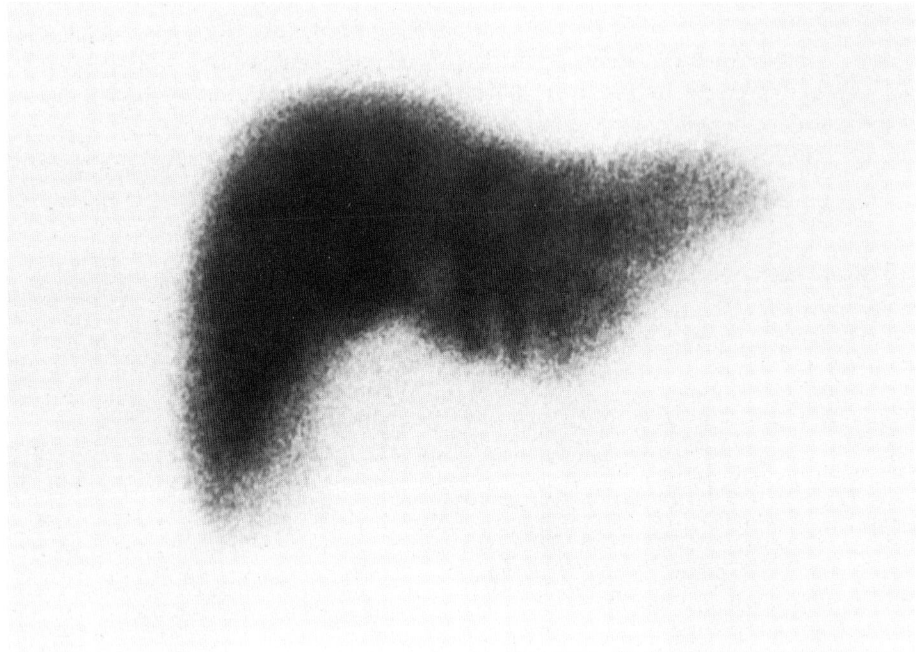

Fig. 15.11c

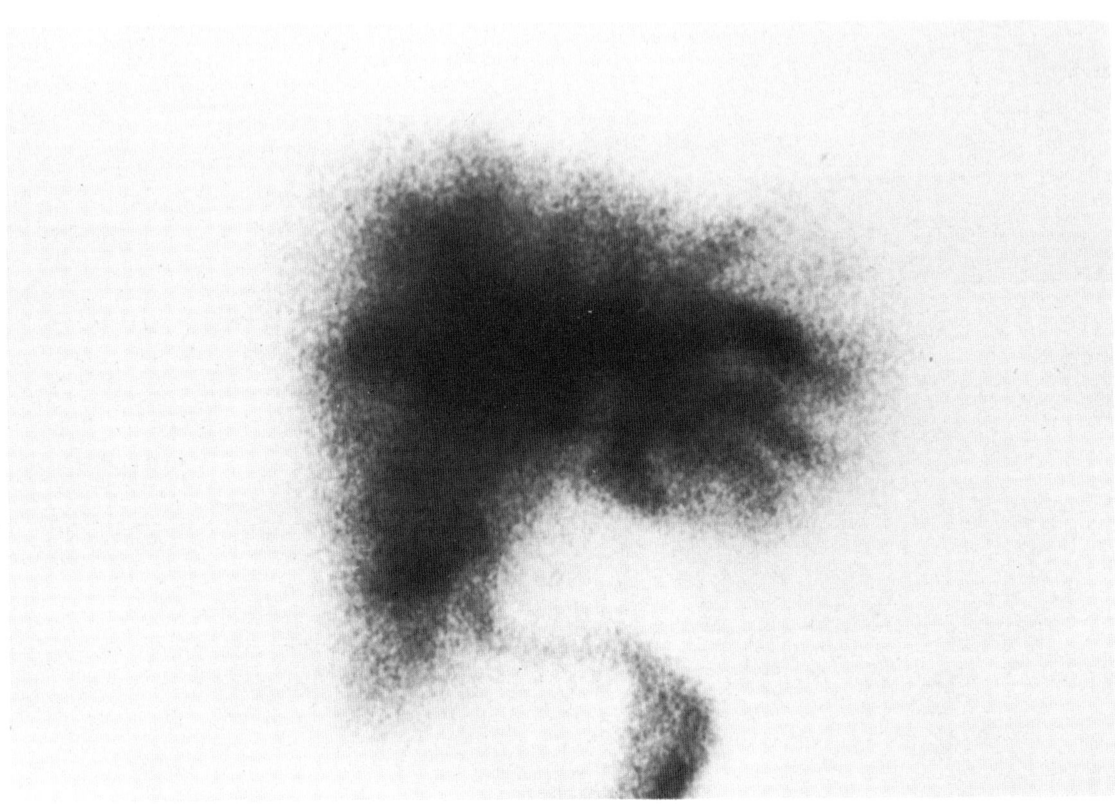

Fig. 15.11d

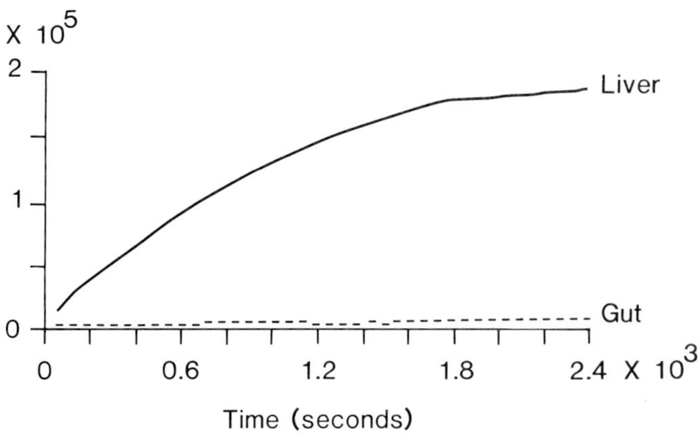

Fig. 15.11e

liver damage showing mildly delayed uptake curves but usually is associated with evidence of dilated ducts and slow clearance of tracer (Fig. 15.11).

Total obstruction in its early stages may appear as uptake of tracer with no clearance. However with the passage of time, hepatic function and tracer uptake diminishes.

Lobar obstruction and atrophy The behaviour of tracer uptake and clearance by the liver as a whole can also be seen segmentally (Ch. 6). Thus a partial obstruction to a duct is associated initially with delayed clearance of tracer; this may be followed by atrophy manifested by poor or delayed uptake of tracer in the segment which also shows loss of volume (Fig. 15.12).

Jaundice The differentiation of obstruction from hepatocellular jaundice should start with ultrasound (Ch. 14) which may give evidence of dilated ducts and this may in turn be followed by percutaneous cholangiography to identify the cause.

The use of hepatobiliary agents may differentiate between hepatic failure and obstructive jaundice with a fairly high degree of accuracy. Characteristically the tracer shows poor uptake into the liver in patients who are suffering from hepatocyte failure, whereas in the early stages of obstructive jaundice, uptake into the liver parenchyma is normal but no activity is seen in the gut. Delayed views should always be taken.

Jaundice in infancy

The use of biliary scanning to differentiate between the diagnosis of neonatal hepatitis and biliary atresia is controversial. The characteristic findings are those of a poor uptake of tracer in cases of hepatitis with activity appearing in the gut on delayed views. In contrast to this, in biliary atresia hepatic cell function is usually preserved but no activity appears in the bowel. However, where there is extensive hepatic cell damage, the findings may be equivocal and this may occur in long-standing jaundice (Gerhold et al 1981).

Sequelae of surgery. Biliary strictures and fistula

Biliary strictures, benign or malignant, usually associated with bile duct dilatation proximally can be investigated by ultrasound. Such patients may undergo surgery with anastomoses between small bowel and hepatic ducts. These anastomoses may undergo narrowing which may be total or segmental. It is a useful policy in such patients to perform periodic biliary scans to assess hepatic cell function and biliary drainage. (Ch. 58) It can be shown that both the uptake and the clearance rates are sensitive indicators which parallel changes in alkaline phosphatase levels. As outlined above, segmental obstruction and atrophy may be shown by focal changes in the images and curves (Zeman et al 1982).

Post-traumatic and post-surgical biliary leaks and fistulas are readily identified. (Ch. 60). A local pool of activity is usually seen to connect with the biliary tract. In suspected cases, biliary scanning is the most convenient and accurate way of identifying such leakage using multiple views to identify the anatomy and delayed views are frequently valuable in these patients. The exact anatomy of any pooling can also be checked by ultrasound examination.

Biliary scanning can also be used to investigate bile reflux into the stomach. In most cases this can be identified by sequential imaging of bile ducts and duodenum but the diagnosis may be made more secure by administering further tracer of technetium labelled colloid by mouth in order to outline the stomach.

ALTERNATIVE RADIOACTIVE TRACERS

Gallium-67 citrate

Gallium-67 is a tracer with a 67 h half-life which can be used for the localization of both inflammatory and neoplastic lesions throughout the body. Its mechanism is not understood and this lack of a clear scientific rationale limits its usefulness. Following intravenous injection, gallium shows protein binding mainly to transferrin. Transferrin is present in tumours, and the related globulin, lactoferrin, is present in and around inflammatory cells, and this may be in part the mechanism which results in local accumulation of the tracer.

The technique employed is the intravenous injection of 80–200 MBq (2–5 mCi). Early views at 4 h are sometimes useful but usually imaging is carried out at 48 to 72 h. The imaging is preceded by bowel preparation to eliminate colonic activity. The normal distribution shows activity in the liver, to a minor extent in the spleen, the bone marrow and some excretion in bowel. Activity may also appear in lactating breasts and in lacrymal glands.

Tumours of the liver show variable uptake. In most hepatocellular carcinomas increase of gallium is seen and in a fairly high proportion of lymphomas. Metastatic

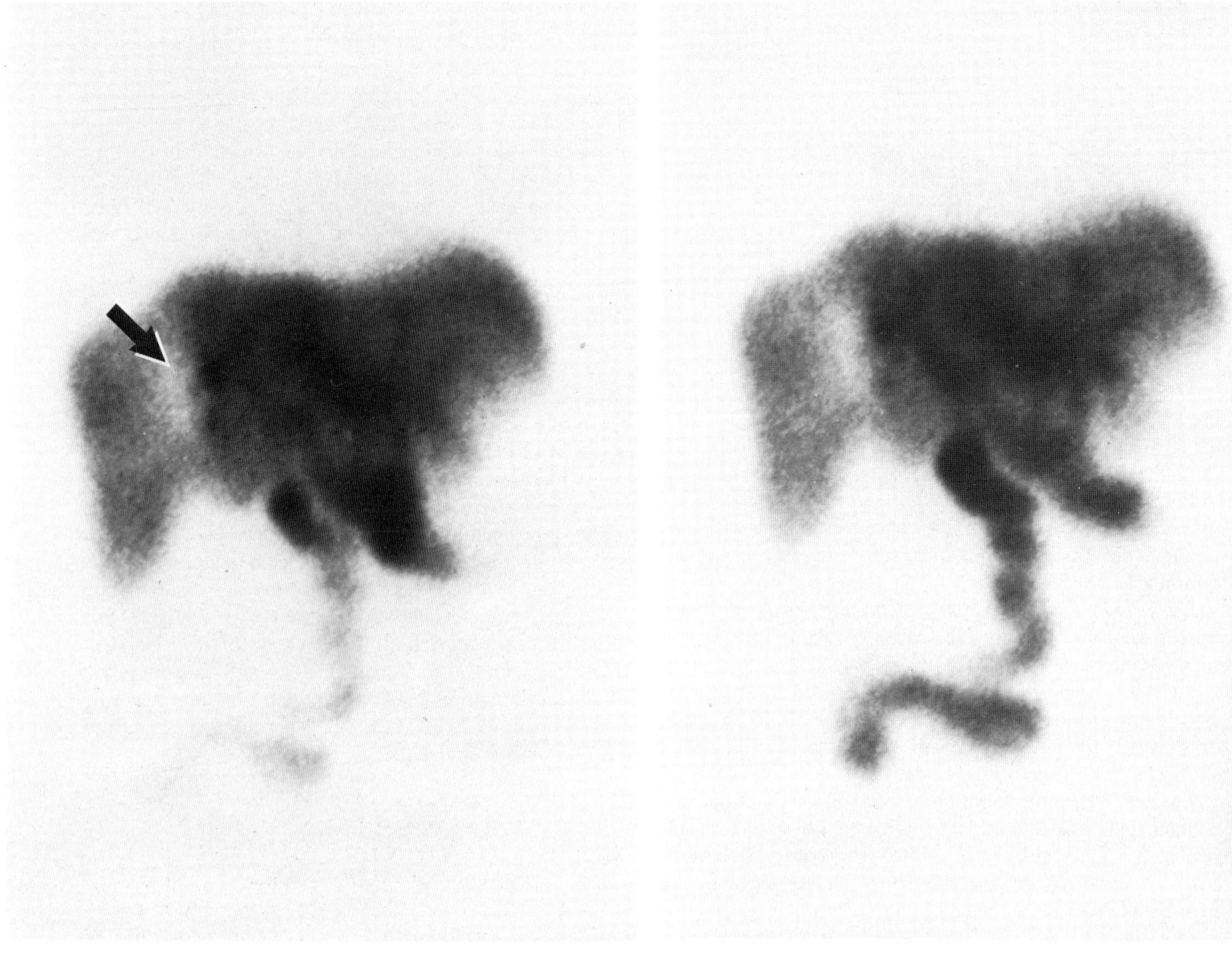

Fig. 15.12 Biliary scan and partial obstruction with lobar atrophy due to cholangiocarcinoma. Post hepatojejunostomy showing focal defect in porta (arrow) with atrophic right lobe, enlarged left lobe with dilated ducts. Activity is seen in small bowel.

carcinoma is unpredictable in its behaviour, showing some increase in perhaps 50%. Inflammatory lesions, either abscess or granulomas, almost always show increased uptake. Multiple small (less than 5 mm) granulomata will not be seen due to the increased background activity in hepatocytes.

The main indication for the use of gallium lies in its ability to locate a site of pathology where this is unknown, as, for instance, in the patient with occult sepsis or tumour suffering from generalized symptoms and signs. It is also used in the staging of disease, as, for instance, in the patient known to have granulomatous disease in one site but who may also have occult granulomata elsewhere. The staging of lymphoma has also utilized gallium although its reliability in the primary staging of such patients is not very great and probably its best use in lymphomas is to identify recurrent disease in a patient whose tumour is known to take up gallium (see Fig. 15.13).

Selenium labelled methionine

Selenium-75 labelled methionine is an amino acid with selenium, a tracer with a relatively long half-life (121 d), incorporated into the molecule. The agent has been available since its first synthesis by Blau & Bender in 1962 and in the past has had as its main use pancreatic scanning where its incorporation and excretion by the pancreas has been used for imaging. Uptake of the tracer is also seen by hepatic cells and this property has been used in looking at hepatocellular carcinoma, which in most cases shows a metabolism of this amino acid to a fairly marked extent. However currently other agents, in particular, the biliary

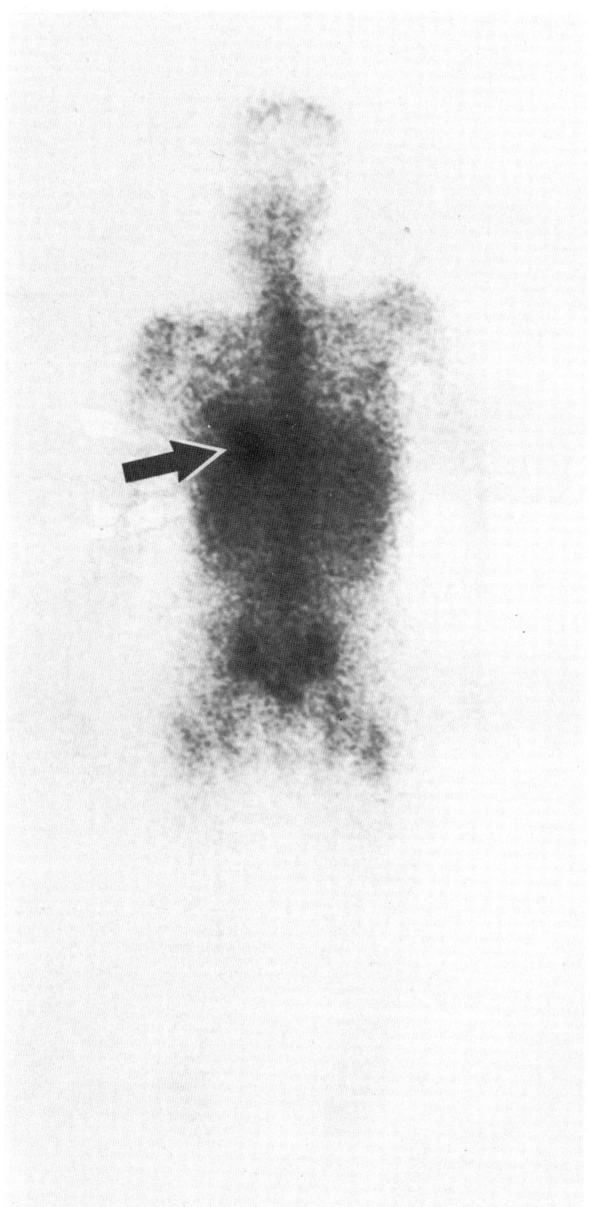

a

b

Fig. 15.13 Gallium-67 citrate scan in patient with Hodgkin's disease involving the liver. a. Posterior whole body image showing area of increased activity on the posterior aspect of the liver (arrow). b. Longitudinal ultrasound showing abnormal region with diminished echoes on the posterior aspect of the liver (arrows)

tracers, behave in a similar fashion and the use of selenium labelled methionine is diminishing.

Indium-III labelled white blood cells

The use of radioactive labelled granulocytes to identify inflammatory lesions is a technique which is more complex technically but more specific than gallium scintigraphy referred to above. The method requires cell separation. This starts with a blood sedimentation, the supernatant cell-rich plasma then being centrifuged to harvest white cells. The cells are labelled in buffer or small volumes of plasma with an indium-111 chelate and the resuspended cells are then injected back into the patient (Thakur et al 1977, Danpure 1982). Imaging is normally carried out at 3 h and 24 h. The normal distribution of cells shows activity in the liver, spleen and bone marrow. If the technique is carried out correctly there are no false positives since abnormal sites of activity will indicate migrating cells. Thus in a group of 50 patients examined for suspected intra-abdominal sepsis, sensitivity and specificity of labelled granulocytes was 95 and 99% compared with 60% and 83% for ultrasound in the same group (Saverymuttu et al 1983). However this migration may be seen in healing wounds particularly bowel anastomoses; white cells may also be swallowed by patients with intercurrent chest infections and these possibilities must be allowed in interpreting images.

Since the liver is a normal site of cell pooling and destruction it may be advisable to outline the liver with radioactive colloid and compare the two images. Liver abscesses are usually identifiable as areas of increased activity above that of surrounding parenchyma (Fig. 15.14). Sub-phrenic, perinephric and splenic abscesses are usually readily identified but again it is advisable to outline the liver with colloid since the abscess may show a similar count rate to surrounding normal parenchyma.

THE USE OF RADIOLABELLED MONOCLONAL ANTIBODIES

The diagnostic use of radiolabelled monoclonal antibodies is being explored in a number of centres and has not been fully assessed. The principle lies in the development of monoclonal antibodies directed against a cell type or a characteristic which a number of cells may have in common. Most effort is directed to applying this to malignant tumours and antibodies have been produced which show localization on a number of epithelial tumours but may show a cross reaction with normal epithelial surfaces to a minor extent. Such antibodies can be labelled with Iodine-131 or Iodine-123, or probably most effectively with Indium-111 and their localization identified by means of imaging with a gamma camera. Within the liver itself

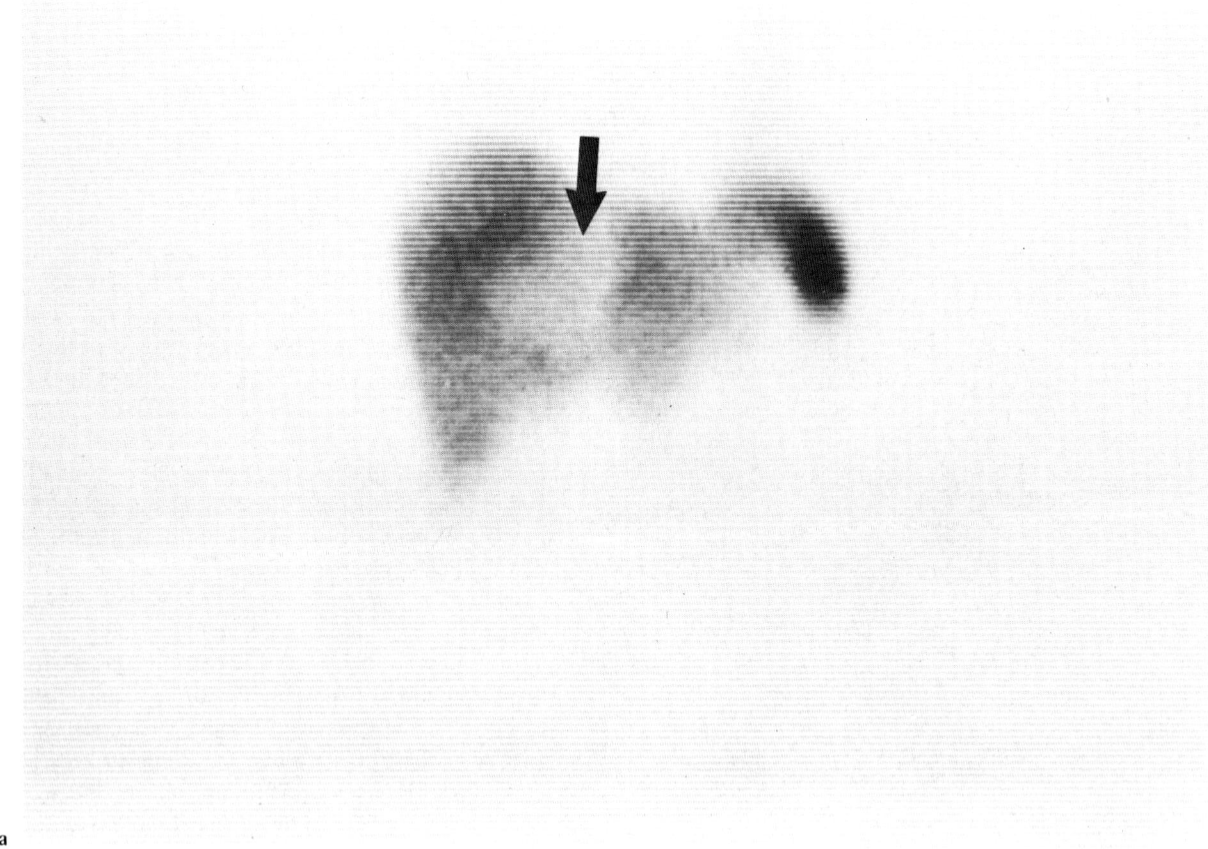

Fig. 15.14a

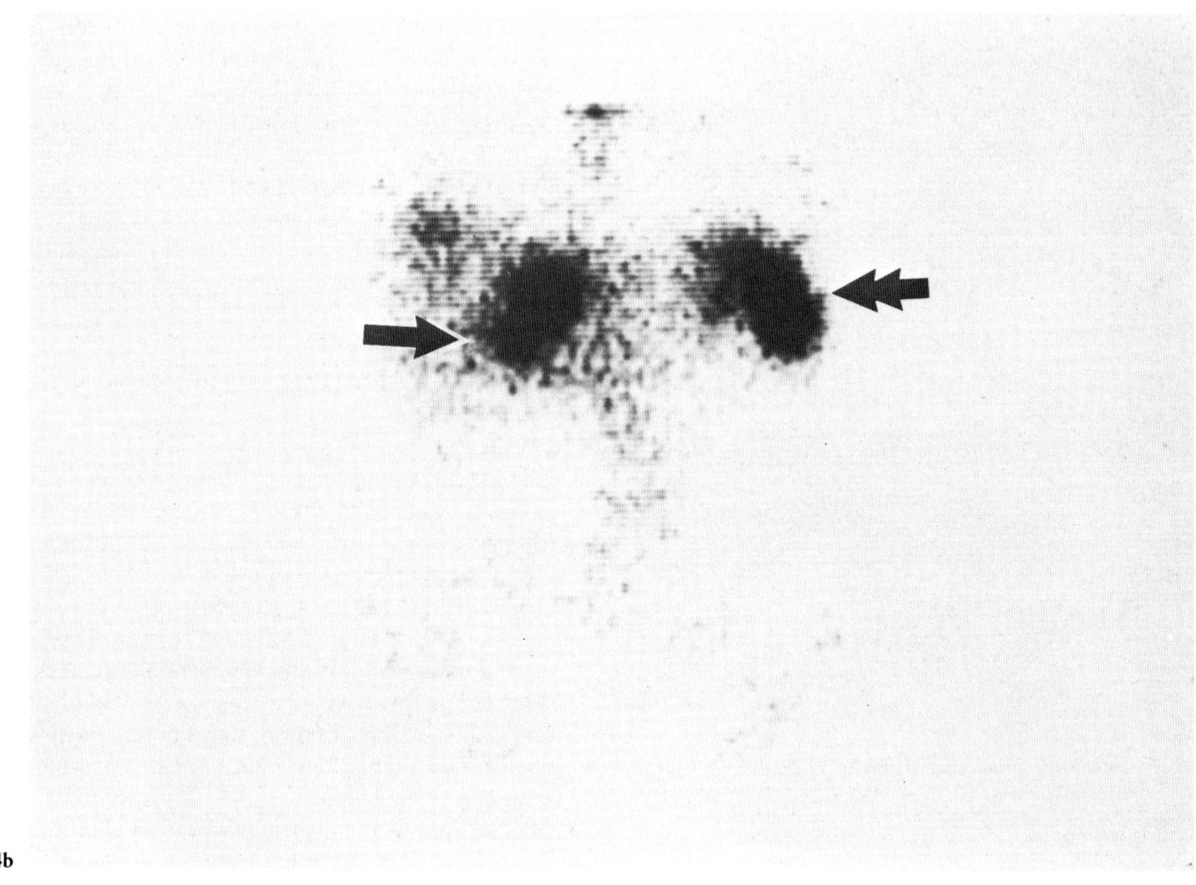

Fig. 15.14b

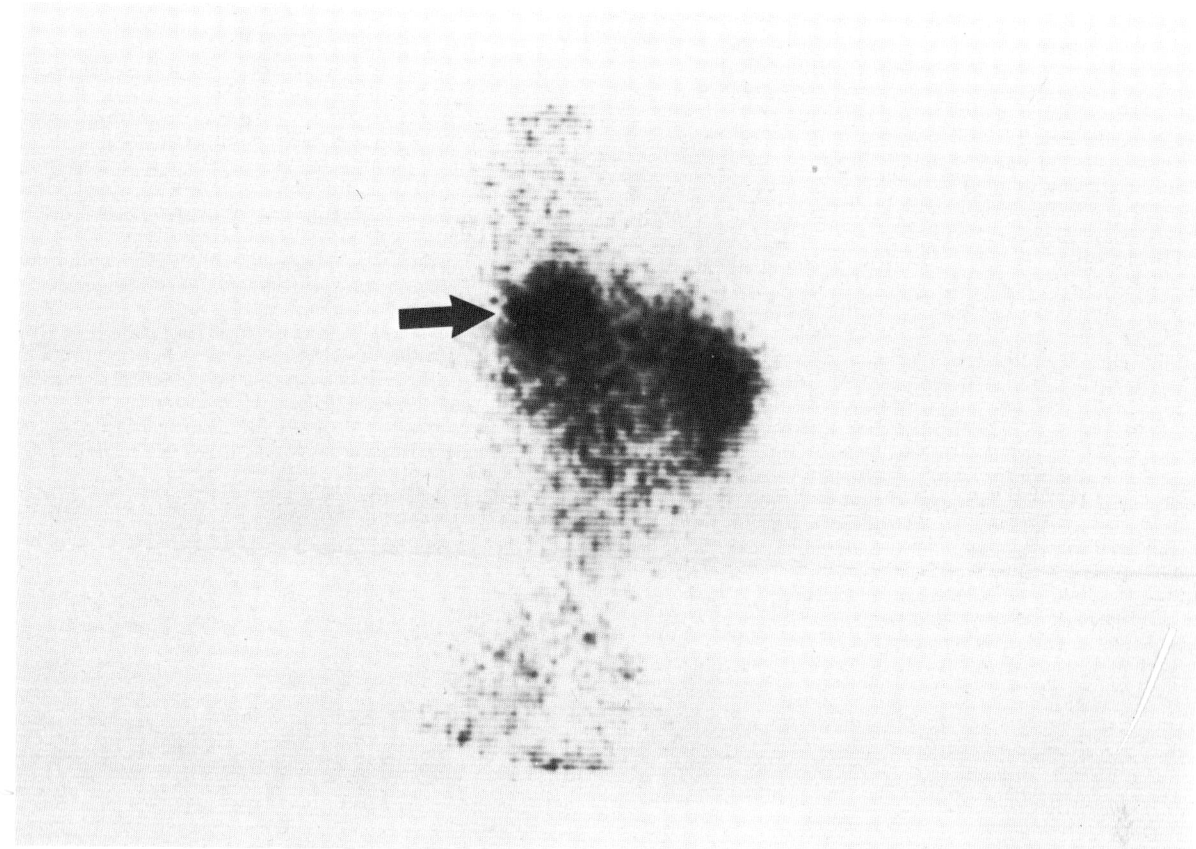

Fig. 15.14c

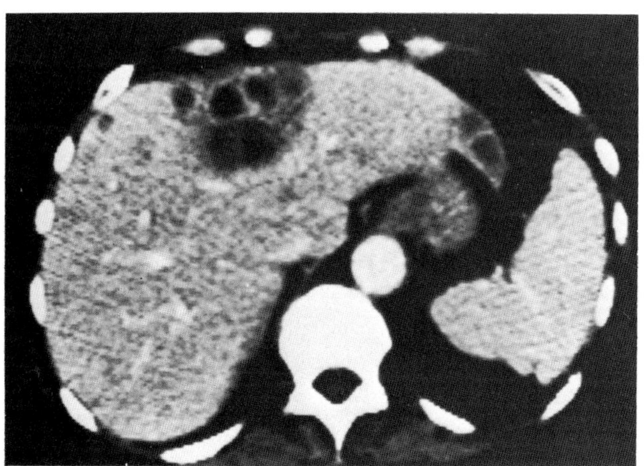

Fig. 15.14d

Fig. 15.14 Colloid liver scan using Indium labelled autologous granulocytes in a patient with liver abscess. a. anterior colloid scan showing defect in region of quadrate lobe (arrow). b & c. Anterior and right lateral views showing labelled white cells in two abscesses (single arrows); double arrows show cells in normal spleen. d. CT showing abscess cavities within the liver

there is a high background count particularly with the use of Indium-111 which seriously interferes with identifying lesions. However a number of avenues can be explored, such as the antibody fragment which may improve the accuracy and sensitivity of this ingenious method (Goldenberg et al 1978, Larson et al 1983, Rayburn 1978).

REFERENCES

Blau M, Bender M A 1962 Se-75 selenomethionine for visualisation of the pancreas by isotope scanning. Radiology 78:974

Brendel A J, Leccia F, Phillippe J C, Lacroix F, Barat J L, Ducassou D 1983 Comparison of single photon emission computed tomography with planar scintigraphy and transmission computed tomography in focal hepatic disease. Journal of Nuclear Medicine 24: P 37

Broderick T W, Gosink B, Menuck L, Harris R, Wilcox J 1980 Echographic and radionuclide detection of hepatoma. Radiology 135: 149–151

Coel M, Halpern S, Alazraki N, Ashburn W, Leopold G 1972 Intrahepatic lesions presenting as an area of increased radiocolloid uptake on a liver scan. Journal of Nuclear Medicine 13: 221–222

Danpure H J, Osman S O, Brady F 1982 The labelling of blood cells in plasma with indium-111 tropolonate. British Journal of Radiology 55: 247–249

Drum D E, Beard J M 1976 Scintigraphic criteria for hepatic metastases from cancer of the colon and breast. Journal of Nuclear Medicine 17: 677–680

Ell P J, Kahn O 1981 Emission computerised tomography, clinical applications. Seminars in Nuclear Medicine 11: 50–60

Fleming J S, Ackery D M, Walmsley B H, Karran S J 1983 Scintigraphic estimation of arterial and portal blood supplies to the liver. Journal of Nuclear Medicine 24: 1108–1113

Gerhold J P, Klingensmith W C, Kuni C C, Lilly J R, Silverman A, Fritzberg A R, Nixt T 1981 Diagnosis of biliary atresia with hepatobiliary imaging (abst). Journal of Nuclear Medicine 22: P 91

Geslien G E, Pinsky S M, Poth R K, Johnson M C 1976 The sensitivity and specificity of 99m technetium suphur colloid liver imaging in diffuse hepatocellular disease. Radiology 118: 115–119
Goldenberg D M, DeLand F, Kim E, Bennett S, Primus F J, Van Nagell J R, Estes N, Desimone P, Rayburn P 1978 Use of radiolabelled antibodies to carcinoembryonic antigen for the detection and localisation of diverse cancers by external photoscanning. New England Journal of Medicine 298: 1384–1388
Harbert J C 1984 Efficacy of liver scanning in malignant diseases. Seminars in Nuclear Medicine 14: 287–295
Larson S M, Carrasquillo J A, Krohn A 1983 Localisation of I-131 labelled specific FAB fragments in human melanoma as a basis for radiotherapy. Journal of Clinical Investigation 72: 2101–2114
Meindok H, Langer B 1976 Liver scan in Budd-Chiari syndrome. Journal of Nuclear Medicine 17: 365–368
Miller D L, Rosenbaum R C, Sugarbaker P H, Vermess M, Willis M, Doppman J L 1983 Detection of hepatic metastases: comparison of EOE 13 computed tomography and scintigraphy. American Journal of Roentgenology 141: 931–935
Rogers J V, Mack L A, Freeny P C, Johnson M L, Sones P J 1981 Hepatic focal nodular hyperplasia. Angiography, CT, sonography and scintigraphy. American Journal of Roentgenology 137: 983–990
Saverymuttu S H, Crofton M E, Peters A M, Lavender J P 1983 Indium-111 tropolonate leucocyte scanning in the detection of intra abdominal abscesses Clinical Radiology 34: 593–596
Savitch I, Kew M C, Paterson A, Esser J D, Levin J 1983 Uptake of technetium 99m di-isopropyl iminodiacetic acid by hepatocellular carcinoma. Journal of Nuclear Medicine 24: 1119–1122
Selby J B, Glasman A B 1983 Cholescintigraphic diagnosis of gall-bladder rupture. Clinical Nuclear Medicine 8: 64–65
Smith T J, Kemeny M M, Sugarbaker P H, Jones A E, Vermess M, Shawker T H, Edwards B K 1982 A prospective study of hepatic imaging in the detection of metastatic disease. Annals of Surgery 195: 486–491
Stirrett L A, Yeuhl E T, Cassen B 1954 Clinical applications of hepatic radioactivity surveys. American Journal of Gastroenterology 21: 310–315
Taplin G V, Meredith O M, Kade H 1955 The radioactive (I–131-tagged) Rose Bengal uptake-excretion test for liver function using external gamma ray scintillation counting techniques. Journal of Laboratory and Clinical Medicine 45: 665–678
Thakur M L, Lavender J P, Arnot R N, Silvester D J, Segal A W 1977 Indium-111 labelled autologous leukocytes in man. Journal of Nuclear Medicine 18: 1014–1021
Weissman H S, Badia J, Sugarman L A, Kluger L, Rosenblatt R, Freeman L M 1981 The spectrum of cholesintigraphic patterns in acute cholecystitis Radiology 138: 167–175
Zeman R K, Lee C, Stahl R S, Cahow C E, Viscomi G N, Neumann R D, Gold J A, Burrell M I 1982 Ultrasonography and hepatobiliary scintigraphy in the assessment of biliary enteric anastomoses. Radiology 145: 109–115

16

D. M. Balfe, J. K. Lee

CT of the liver and biliary tract

INTRODUCTION

In the early 1970s, non-invasive imaging of the liver was essentially limited to liver-spleen scintigraphy, a method with only modest spatial resolution, and, therefore, poor sensitivity to space-occupying lesions less than 3 cm in size. Now, the clinician has at his disposal computerized tomography (CT), grey-scale ultrasonography, and magnetic resonance imaging (MRI); each of these imaging methods combines good contrast resolution with excellent spatial resolution.

The search for intrahepatic mass lesions prompts radiological studies in a large number of patients. While computed tomography is only slightly more accurate than ultrasonography in the detection of focal hepatic lesions (Bernardino et al 1982, Biello et al 1978, Bryan et al 1977, Grossman et al 1977), there are a few additional advantages to CT. Firstly, CT is less operator-dependent and, therefore, more reproducible; secondly, the CT image displays all of the upper abdominal anatomy, providing information about extrahepatic processes important to scan interpretation; thirdly, administration of water-soluble intravenous contrast material provides information regarding the regional blood flow characteristics of focal lesions, and increases the detection rate of 1–2 cm masses, provided their contrast response differs from that of normal liver.

When the liver is the organ of interest, scans are performed with 8 mm–1 cm beam collimation, at 1 cm intervals throughout the liver parenchyma. The radiologist should review the scans on the video monitor while the examination is in progress; narrowing the window width and varying the window level allows the interpreter to detect lesions that differ in density only slightly from that of normal liver parenchyma. Controversy exists among radiologists regarding the necessity of obtaining images both before and after administration of intravenous contrast. In a study by Moss et al (1979), 16% of space-occupying lesions were better seen prior to contrast administration, and in 13% were only visible before contrast enhancement. However, a later study (Berland et al 1982) on newer-generation equipment using higher volumes of rapidly infused contrast showed that no lesion was obscured because of contrast administration. A rapid infusion of contrast material quickly produces an 'arterial' phase, in which there is a density difference of 10 or more Hounsfield units between the aorta and the inferior vena cava. This allows direct demonstration of portal and hepatic veins and is followed by a prolonged display of the liver in the capillary or parenchymal phase. Very rapid (bolus) contrast administration may be useful to show the vascular response of the liver and its contents at a specific level of interest; therefore, it is best utilized when a previous examination has pinpointed a focal lesion. As a routine screening examination, multiple bolus administration is somewhat unwieldy. The major advantage of the bolus technique is in demonstrating lesions with rapid contrast turnover, such as arteriovenous shunts (Fig. 16.1) or highly vascular tumours; and in characterizing lesions with specific vascular patterns, e.g. cavernous haemangioma or portal venous thrombosis. Analysis of the reconstructed images obtained at six-second intervals after rapid contrast administration yields time-density curves which allow predictions regarding the proportion of arterial vascular supply to the target lesion.

More invasive methods may be useful in selected cases. Direct contrast infusion into a catheter selectively placed in a superior mesenteric or coeliac artery is a means of prolonging the arterial phase and provides the highest possible sustained arteriovenous contrast difference (Nakao et al 1983). This may be the best method for detecting small hypervascular lesions; however, it requires arterial puncture and selective catheterization, and is therefore best reserved for patients in whom radical therapy such as partial hepatectomy is being considered. Ethiodized oil emulsion (EOE-13) (Miller et al 1984b, Vermess et al 1977, 1982) is an experimental agent which, being colloidal material, is rapidly distributed within the reticulo-endothelial system, providing selective enhancement of those portions of the liver and spleen which contain Kupffer cells. Preliminary data from several insti-

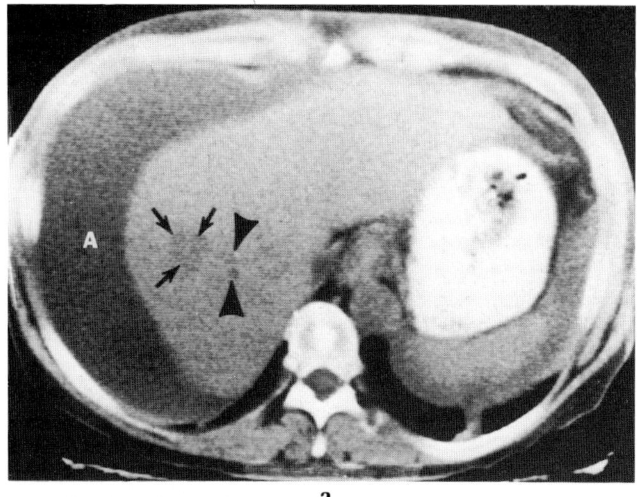

a

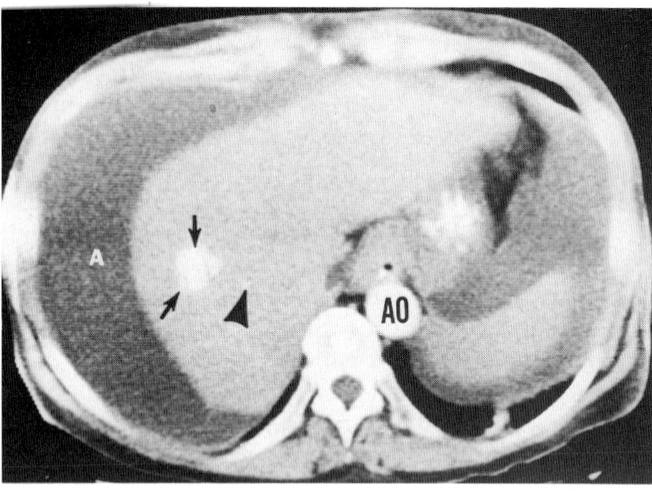

b

Fig. 16.1 Arteriovenous malformation caused by prior biopsy. a. Precontrast CT near dome of liver shows irregular low attenuation defect (arrows) in right hepatic lobe. Small hepatic venous structures (arrowheads) drain the structure. b. Fifteen seconds after rapid administration of intravenous contrast, there is dense opacification of the aorta (AO) and simultaneous equal opacification in the lesion (arrows). Note rapid opacification of nearby hepatic veins (arrowheads). A = ascites

tutions show that more hepatic lesions can be detected by EOE-13 than by other conventional contrast media. The frequent incidence of fever, headaches and rigors after injection of EOE-13 has prevented this specific agent from gaining widespread acceptance, but similarly composed contrast materials are being developed and may ultimately prove useful.

NORMAL ANATOMY

Morphological Anatomy

The largest abdominal structure, the liver, occupies most of the right upper quadrant. Liver attenuation on computed tomography averages approximately 50 Hounsfield units; in normal subjects there is an appreciable density difference between the liver and the spleen (Piekarski et al 1980). Except in cases of diffuse fatty infiltration, the liver is the densest structure in the abdomen.

The diaphragmatic surface of the liver is smoothly convex and in apposition to the diaphragm. The visceral, or inferior, margin of the liver is generally somewhat concave. Three large fissures interrupt the surface of the liver. Slightly to the right of midline, the anterior inferior portion of the diaphragmatic surface of the liver is notched by the fissure for the ligamentum teres. A deeper fissure on the superior margin of the visceral surface is the fisssure for the ligamentum venosum, which is continuous with the porta hepatis, a large cleft containing the portal vein, common hepatic duct and hepatic artery. Immediately inferior and slightly lateral to the porta hepatis is the fossa for the gallbladder.

Segmental anatomy

Many systems dividing the liver into segments have been described. A functional anatomical system, designed to correlate with surgical technique, has been described by Bismuth (1982), (Ch. 1). In this system, the three main hepatic veins divide the liver into four sectors, each of which is independent in that it receives a separate portal venous and hepatic arterial supply, and is drained by a separate bile duct. The middle hepatic vein lies within the main portal fissure (scissura), and divides the liver into right and left portions. The right hemiliver is divided into two sectors by the right hepatic vein and the left similarly by the left hepatic vein. Since computed tomography readily demonstrates the course of all three major hepatic veins on contrast-enhanced scans obtained near the diaphragm, the major hepatic sectors are easy to identify at this level (Fig. 16.2). However, on scans obtained more caudally, the hepatic veins are difficult to differentiate from portal radicles, and may occupy a plane oblique to the transverse axis of the scan. Despite this difficulty, Pagani (1983) attempted to classify appropriately the distribution of tumour in 24 consecutive patients. Of the 13 patents in whom operative proof was available, CT was correct in 11. Errors were due to metastases measuring under 1 cm in both cases. In this limited series, CT was as accurate as angiography in evaluating patients prior to partial hepatectomy.

The interlobar fissure is continuous inferiorly with the galbladder fossa and medially opens into the porta hepatis. Immediately anterior to the porta hepatis and lateral to the fissure for the ligamentum teres is the quadrate lobe, representing the medial segment of the left liver. Posterior to the porta hepatis and anterior to the inferior vena cava is the caudate lobe, which has an independent venous

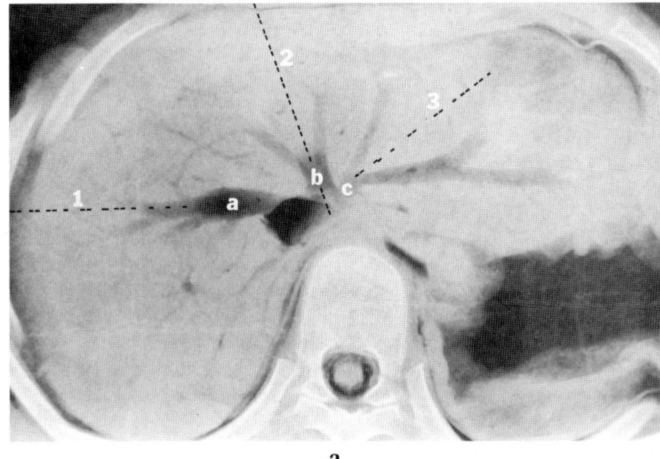

a

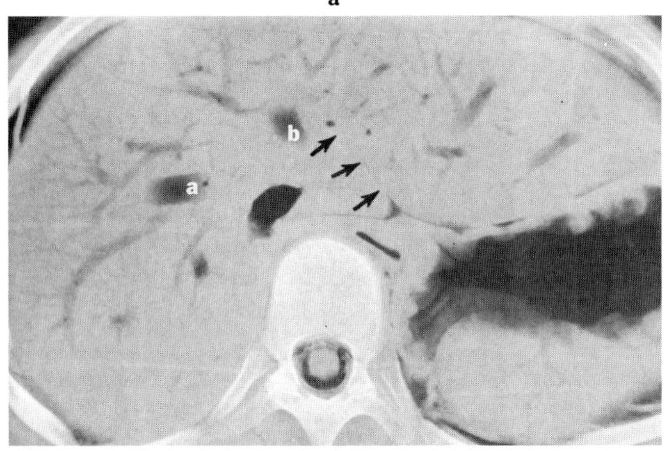

b

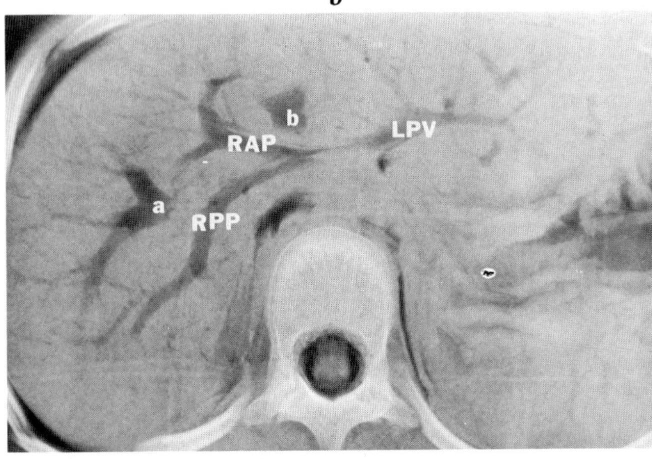

c

Fig. 16.2 Portal sectors in the liver are defined by the course of the major hepatic veins. a. Anatomical section near the dome of diaphragm. At this level, the hepatic venous trunks are easily defined. The middle hepatic vein ('b') lies in the interlobar fissure (dotted line 2), dividing the right liver from the left. b. Section above the porta hepatis. The right ('a') and middle ('b') hepatic veins are well-defined trunks, while the main left hepatic trunk has divided and is not definable at this level. Arrows point to the fissure for the ligamentum venosum. c. Section at the porta hepatis demonstrating the interdigitation of the portal system and the main hepatic trunks. RAP = right anterior portal vein; RPP = right posterior portal vein; LPV = left portal vein. a = right hepatic vein; b = middle hepatic vein; c :eq left hepatic vein; 1 = right portal scissura, 2 = interhepatic fissure; 3 = left portal scissura. See also Ch. 1.

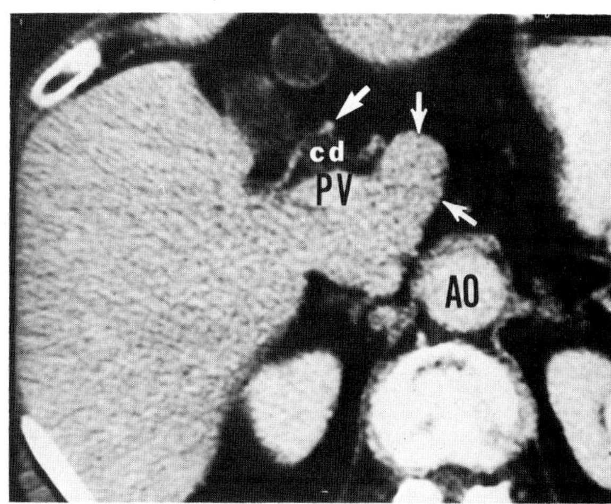

Fig. 16.3 Large papillary process of the caudate lobe (arrows) projects anteriorly and leftwards into the superior recess of the lesser sac. Note proper hepatic artery coursing anterior to the common hepatic duct (cd) which in turn lies on the right anterior surface of the portal vein (PV). AO = aorta

drainage into the vena cava. Medially this lobe gives rise to the papillary process, which protrudes to the left and anteriorly and invaginates the superior recess of the lesser sac. When large, the papillary process may be mistaken for an extrahepatic mass (Auh et al 1984) (Fig. 16.3).

The gallbladder, which is readily recognized on computed tomography as an oval water-dense structure, lies in the main interhepatic fissure on the inferior surface of the liver.

Vascular anatomy

The portal vein begins at the junction of the splenic and superior mesenteric vein, immediately posterior to the neck of the pancreas. It then courses towards the right and cephalad as it enters the hepatoduodenal ligament. Within the ligament, it runs a course parallel to the proper hepatic artery, which lies on its anteromedial surface, and the common bile duct which lies on its anterolateral surface. After entering the hepatic parenchyma, the portal vein branches in a predictable fashion to supply each portal sector. The branching patterns of the hepatic artery and bile ducts are identical with those of the portal vein (Fig. 16.4) (Ch. 1).

A common normal variant which can be recognized on CT is an anomalous origin of the right hepatic artery, generally from the superior mesenteric artery. This vessel nearly always courses between the inferior vena cava and the portal vein to supply the right lobe of the liver.

PATHOLOGICAL PROCESSES

Neoplasms

The ability of computed tomography to display precise

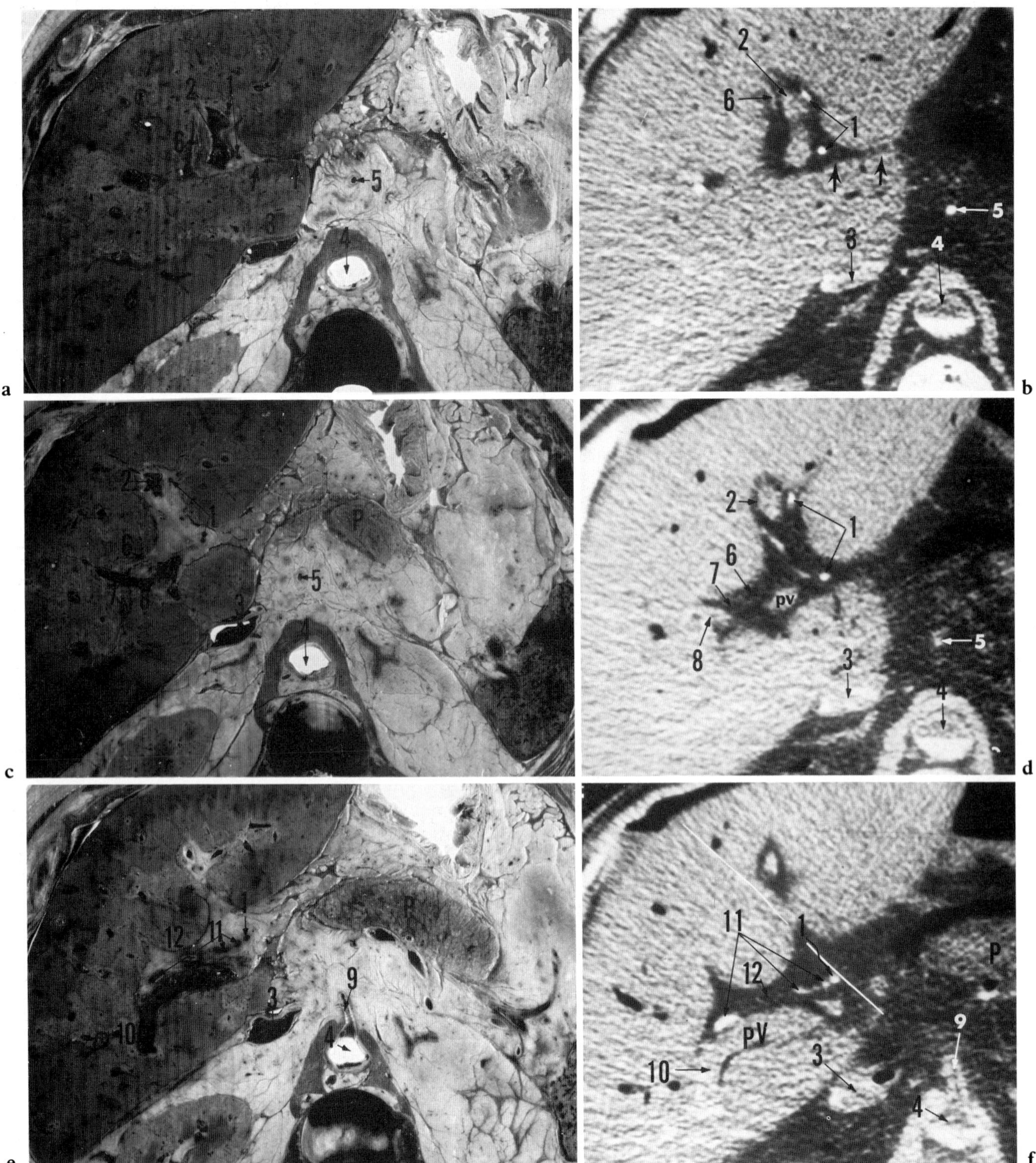

Fig. 16.4 Gross anatomy of the porta hepatis in cross section (a,c,e — cadaver slice; b,d,f — CT scan). a,b Section above porta hepatis shows the caudate lobe of the liver separating the fissure for the ligamentum venosum (arrows) from the inferior vena cava (3). The left portal vein (2) occupies a central position in the left portal triad; the hepatic arterial branches (1) lie on its left side, whereas the left hepatic duct (6) lies on its right. c,d In a scan plane 2 cm caudal, the left hepatic duct (6) has coursed posteriorly to join the right hepatic duct (7) immediately anterior and slightly to the right of the portal vein (PV). e,f On a cross-sectional slice 1 cm more caudal, the common hepatic duct (12) lies on the anterior surface of the porta vein, joined by segments of the right hepatic artery (11). 1 = left hepatic artery; 2 = left portal vein; 3 = inferior vena cava; 4 = aorta; 5 = left gastric artery; 6 = left hepatic duct; 7 = right hepatic duct; 8 = right anterior portal vein; 9 = coeliac trunk; 10 = right posterior portal vein; 11 = right hepatic artery; 12 = common hepatic duct; P = pancreas; PV = portal vein

anatomical information has made it a cornerstone in the evaluation of focal hepatic lesions. However, the ability of CT to characterize an hepatic mass is limited to defining its size and location and displaying its response to contrast administration. No set of CT-derived criteria is capable of unequivocally distinguishing between a benign and a malignant lesion. It is, therefore, often necessary to perform a CT-guided percutaneous biopsy to obtain tissue for histological examination.

Malignant lesions

Hepatocellular carcinoma

Hepatocellular carcinoma, while not as prevalent in the United States as it is in Africa and Asia, is still the most common primary hepatic tumour. There is a distinct correlation between hepatocellular carcinoma and chronic liver disease, most often cirrhosis. Only 5% of patients are candidates for surgical resection at the time of their diagnosis. The characteristics that generally contraindicate surgical resection are:

1. Distribution of tumour in both major sectors of the liver;
2. Main portal vein or inferior vena cava invasion by the tumour;
3. Extrahepatic spread via lymph nodes or direct invasion (Ch. 97).

The CT findings in hepatocellular carcinoma are best observed on scans obtained before and after rapid administration of water-soluble contrast material (Kunstlinger et al 1980) (Fig. 16.5). Three distinct categories have been described based upon the CT findings (Hosoki et al 1982). In a tumour which pathologically proves to be diffusely hypovascular, or which has moderate vascularity but central necrosis, the tumour appears on precontrast scans as a low-attenuation structure which increases in attenuation during the arterial phase of the examination; however, its overall enhancement by contrast is less than that of the surrounding normal parenchyma. A moderately vascular tumour also displays a rapid increase in attenuation during the arterial phase; during this initial response, its density is greater than the surrounding normal parenchyma. During the portal phase a rapid decrease in attenuation occurs, so that in equilibrium the overall tumour density may be the same as or lower than the surrounding liver (Hosoki et al 1984). Highly vascular tumours containing no central necrosis display an initial rapid increase in density during the arterial phase which persists during the portal phase.

The major pitfall in assessing a primary carcinoma is missing a small lesion (Inamoto et al 1983a). In a study of 18 patients with hepatocellular carcinoma measuring under 5 cm in size (Takashima et al 1982), CT detected 56% of all lesions; only angiography demonstrated lesions under

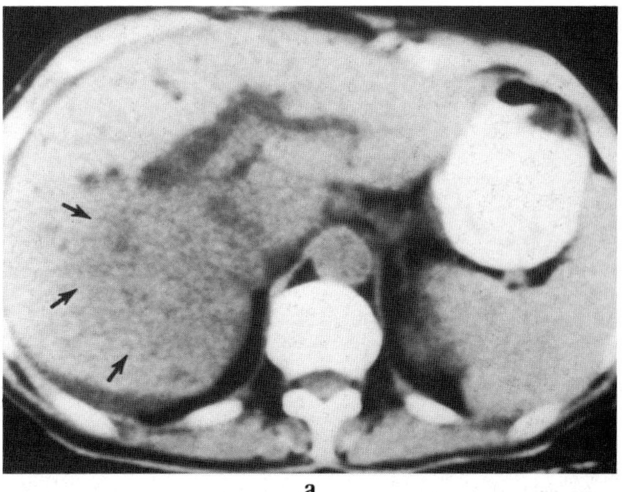

a

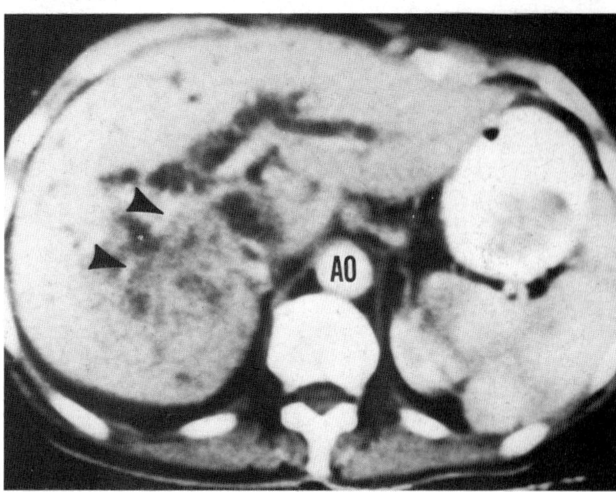

b

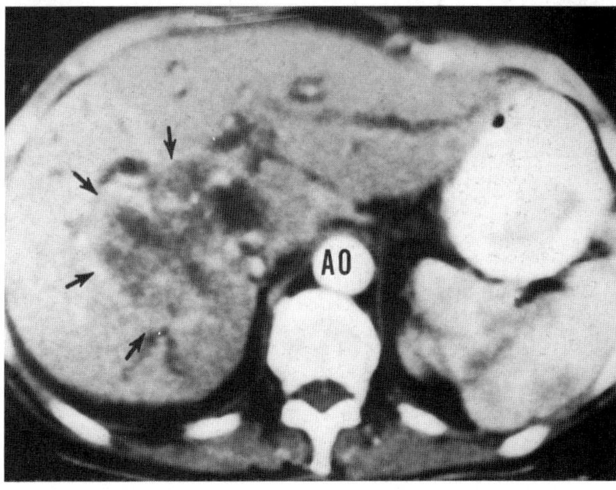

c

Fig. 16.5 Hepatoma producing biliary obstruction. a. Non-enhanced scan just above porta hepatis shows an ill-defined low density mass (arrows) present in the posterior sector of the right hepatic lobe. b. Same level, after bolus infusion of intravenous contrast. Dilated left, right and common hepatic ducts are imaged. A highly vascular tumour periphery surrounds lower attenuation, heterogeneous interior (arrowheads). c. Slightly cephalad to b, the intense tumour vessel stain (arrows) is easily seen. AO = aorta

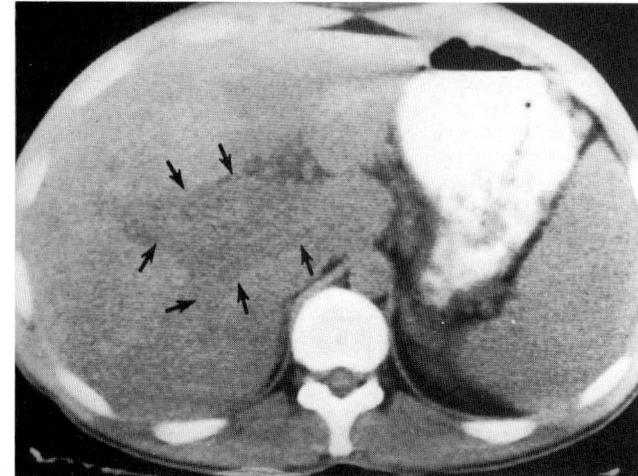
a

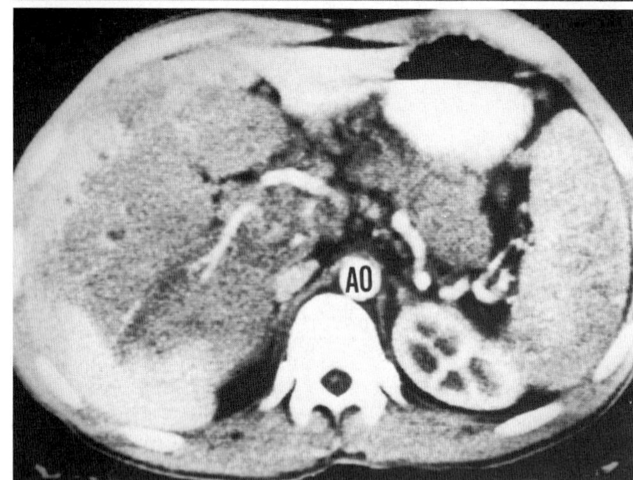

b

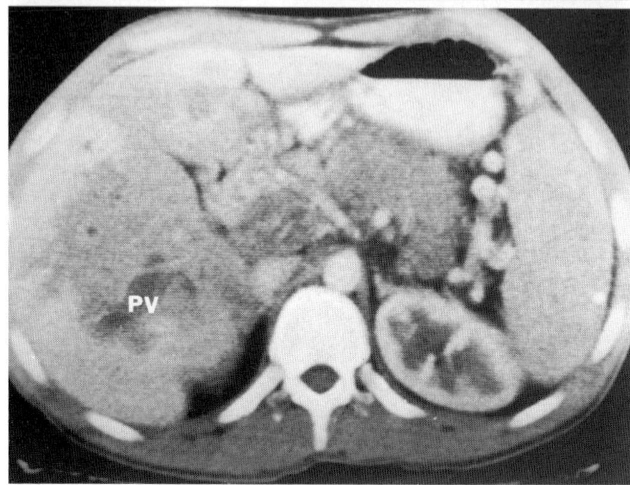

c

Fig. 16.6 Undifferentiated tumour producing portal vein thrombosis. a. Unenhanced scan near the top of the porta hepatis shows low attenuation tumour (arrows) enlarging the right portal vein and its major tributaries. b. Fifteen seconds after bolus administration of intravenous contrast, there is dense opacification of the aorta (AO), proper hepatic and splenic arteries. Note the unusual pattern of peripheral hepatic enhancement. There is no opacification of portal vein. c. Thirty seconds after bolus administration of contrast, multiple serpentine collateral vessels are present in the region of the main portal vein. A distended, clot-filled right posterior portal vein (PV) remains unenhanced. The peripheral pattern of liver enhancement persists, although it is less pronounced than on the previous scan.

1 cm. A somewhat later study, performed with dynamic CT scanning, successfully detected 7 out of 10 primary hepatocellular carcinomas that were under 2 cm in size. A possible way to improve the detection of small primary lesions is CT-angiography (Nakao 1983), with a catheter positioned in the superior mesenteric artery or hepatic artery, as described in the previous section.

The demonstration of portal vein invasion by the tumour on CT has been regarded as a contraindication to surgical resection (Inamoto et al 1981) (Fig. 16.6). However, tumours may cause abnormalities in segmental or lobar distribution without actually invading the portal vein. Both Doppman et al (Doppman et al 1984) and Inamoto et al (Inamoto et al 1981) observed low attenuation hepatic defects occurring in segmental or lobar distribution adjacent to hepatomas, in lobes with occluded hepatic veins, adjacent to parenchymal injuries, and in lobes compressed by extrahepatic masses. Doppman speculates that this phenomenon is due to compression of the hepatic veins with a concomitant rise in segmental pressure and diversion of portal blood away from the segment involved. This produces a compensatory increase in hepatic arterial flow; on CT, this is reflected by a dense enhancement during the arterial phase followed by retrograde portal flow away from the site of compression. With time, the liver within this area of diminished portal supply suspends its normal metabolic activity, giving rise to a decrease in glycogen stores and a recognizable increase in fat. Itai et al (1982) reported a similar phenomenon, in which less transient lobar or segmental attenuation difference within the liver was noted by dynamic CT. This segmental decrease in lobar attenuation may be due to arterial siphonage from an adjacent vascular tumour. Thus, simple demonstration of attenuation differences in the distribution of a portal vein does not imply portal vein invasion.

CT findings of portal venous invasion by hepatocellular carcinoma include arterio-portal fistulas (Nakayama et al 1983), periportal streaks of high attenuation, or dilatation of the main portal vein or its major branches (Mathieu et al 1984). While the finding of portal venous enlargement is suggestive, it is not specific. Arterial opacification of tumour thrombus within a portal vein or direct arterio-portal shunting (Inamoto et al 1983b) are more specific signs of invasion. That CT may not be the most sensitive means of detecting portal tumour invasion is borne out in a study by LaBerge et al (1984), in which ultrasound demonstrated portal venous thrombus in 11 cases, while CT findings of portal thrombus were only present in two.

Extrahepatic metastatic disease from hepatocellular carcinoma is best displayed by computed tomography, and was seen in 70% of patients in LaBerge's series. Nodes in the hepatoduodenal ligament are the commonest site of lymphatic spread; hematogeneous metastases may be encountered in the lungs or adrenal glands.

Other primary malignancies

Angiosarcomas of the liver occur in patients after exposure to polyvinylchloride, arsenicals, or thorium dioxide. This last compound was a widely-used contrast agent in the late 1920s and early 1930s. It is an alpha-emittor with a biological half-life of 400 years and a physical half-life of 1.4×10^{10} years. The mean latent period between Thoratrast administration and the subsequent development of malignancy is 29 years; most patients develop angiosarcoma, but both hepatocellular carcinoma and cholangiocarcinoma have been described. Because Thoratrast accumulates in the reticulo-endothelial system, both the liver and spleen are densely opacified on CT. An angiosarcoma appears as a mass of lower attenuation, with peripheral hypervascularity on dynamic CT (Mahony et al 1982, Silverman et al 1983).

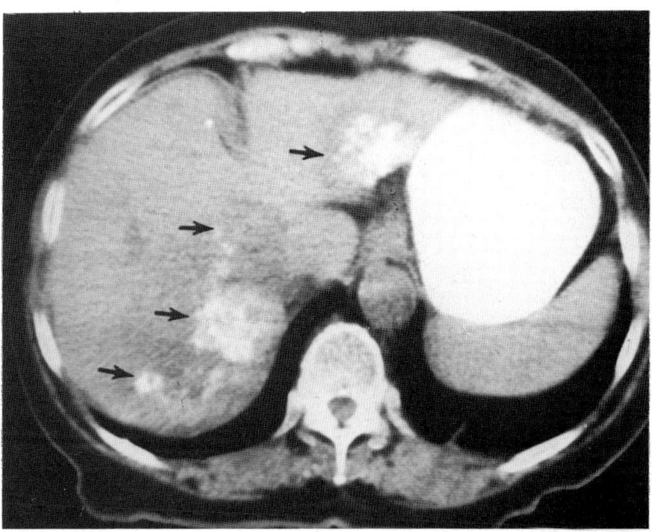

Fig. 16.7 Mucinous adenocarcinoma of the colon produces metastases (arrows) which typically calcify in this amorphous pattern.

Hepatic metastases

The approach to a patient with metastases to the liver is becoming more aggressive. A recent review (Adson et al 1984) of 141 patients with colorectal cancer who underwent resection of their hepatic metastases showed an overall five-year survival of 25% (Ch. 92). This study suggests that in selected patients surgical resection may be of value; correct preoperative identification of patients with well-circumscribed lesions amenable to resection is therefore of paramount importance.

Most metastatic deposits are detectable on CT, with low-attenuation and rounded areas which undergo minimal contrast enhancement after rapid administration of intravenous iodinated contrast material (Marchal et al 1980). Since metastases are largely supplied by the hepatic artery (although some portal supply is also present) (Lin et al 1984a, 1984b), enhanced tumour detection is expected in patients studied with intra-arterial contrast material (Matsui et al 1983, Prando et al 1979). Indeed, in patients studied by Moss et al (1982), arterial delivery via a percutaneous catheter resulted in more lesions being detected. The same investigators also demonstrated that contrast uptake by metastatic lesions was extremely rapid so that the contrast enhancement characteristics observed after arterial delivery were markedly different from those seen after slower peripheral contrast infusion. Similarly, when a rapid bolus was administered, the maximum detection of metastases occurred prior to the equilibrium phase (Burgener & Hamlin 1983a).

Unfortunately, the behaviour of a specific space-occupying lesion cannot be correlated with its histology (Burgener & Hamlin 1983b). Enhancement characteristics depend upon the relative size of the vascular and interstitial compartments within the tumour. Early in the scanning sequence (arterial phase), the size of the vascular space is dominant. Later, the relative contribution of the interstitial space within the tumour to the total contrast accumulation increases (Araki et al 1980a). The relatively common finding of delayed entrance of administered contrast into metastatic tumours and delayed washout of contrast from those tumours probably relates to the fact that tumour capillaries are much larger in diameter than normal liver capillaries, so that a reduced surface for permeation is present.

While there are no pathognomonic CT features to separate metastatic disease from primary malignant or even benign tumours, observations favouring the diagnosis of metastases include multiplicity, variation in size, punctate, amorphous or branching calcification (Hughes et al 1984) (Fig. 16.7) and peripheral contrast enhancement on dynamic CT scans (Lin et al 1984b).

Overall, the detection rate of contrast-enhanced CT in metastatic disease compares favourably with other non-operative methods such as sonography or scintigraphy (Lunderquist & Ouman 1983). Moreover, in a report (Danielson et al 1983) comparing CT with peritoneoscopy in the detection of liver metastases, the sensitivity of computed tomography was 89%, while its specificity was 94%.

Administration of a substance such as EOE-13, which is preferentially taken up by the reticulo-endothelial system, increases the detection of small deposits (Miller et al 1983).

CT can be helpful in recording the clinical course of patients with hepatic malignancy following the institution of therapeutic manoeuvres such as hepatic infusion pumps, therapeutic infarctions or hepatic resection.

Pitfalls in diagnosing metastases

Although cystic metastases may be confused with simple benign cysts (Barnes et al 1981), the two entities can

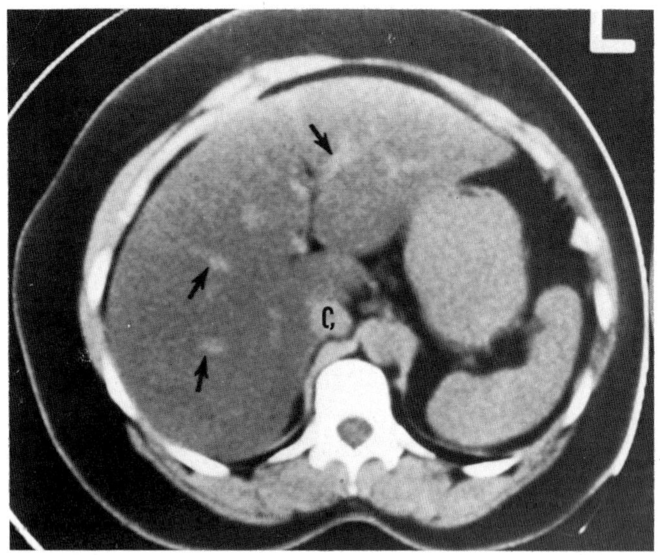

Fig. 16.8 Fatty infiltration of the liver. Note that the liver morphology is normal in appearance, and that the portal venous structures (arrows) are undisturbed. C = inferior vena cava

usually be differentiated since cystic metastases often contain mural nodules, fluid-fluid levels or septations. These features are sometimes better demonstrated by ultrasonography (Federle et al 1981) (Ch. 14).

Fatty infiltration may occur in a geographical distribution that resembles multiple hepatic metastases (Halversen et al 1982, Lewis et al 1983, Nishikawa Tasaka 1981, Patel et al 1982). Observation of normal distribution of portal venous radicles throughout the affected region may be helpful in recognizing this potential pitfall (Gale et al 1983) (Fig. 16.8). In addition, focal fatty infiltration can mask coexisting metastatic deposits (Fig. 16.9).

The axial anatomy displayed by CT may not be the best imaging plane to show the origin of a lesion; thus extra-hepatic processes may mimic intrahepatic lesions. Frick & Feinberg 1982b) reported 11 patients in whom the CT scan strongly suggested liver disease; each proved to have an extrahepatic mass, usually arising from the adrenal gland or the perirenal region. In questionable cases, sonography and/or arteriography may be helpful in making this distinction.

Benign tumours and tumour-like conditions

Cysts

Hepatic cysts may be either congenital or acquired. Congenital cysts are more common than the acquired type, which are secondary to inflammation, trauma or parasitic disease. Benign cysts, usually solitary (Fig. 16.10), are not uncommon and are a frequent cause of an unexpected focal lesion detected by radionuclide liver-spleen scan. Multiple hepatic cysts are seen usually with polycystic renal disease, but may occur without renal lesions.

On CT scans, hepatic cysts are sharply defined, homogeneous areas of near-water attenuation, which do not enhance after administration of an intravenous contrast agent. Generally, the CT appearance of a simple cyst is so characteristic that no further evaluation is indicated. If the clinical history strongly suggests the possibility of a cystic neoplasm or abscess or if the CT appearance is atypical

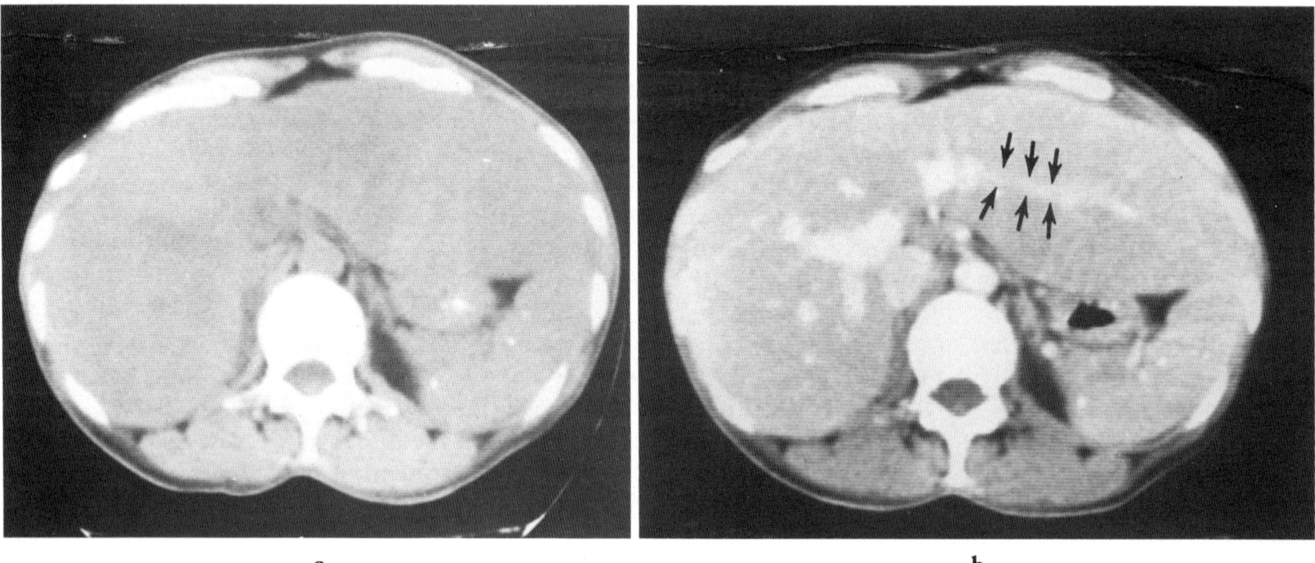

Fig. 16.9 Metastatic melanoma mimicking fatty infiltration. a. Unenhanced scan through the region of the porta hepatis demonstrates a large left hepatic lobe with a diffusely diminished attenuation compared to the normal right lobe. b. After rapid administration of intravenous contrast, there is subtle stretching and attenuation of a segment of the left portal vein (arrows). Biopsy in this region disclosed metastatic melanoma.

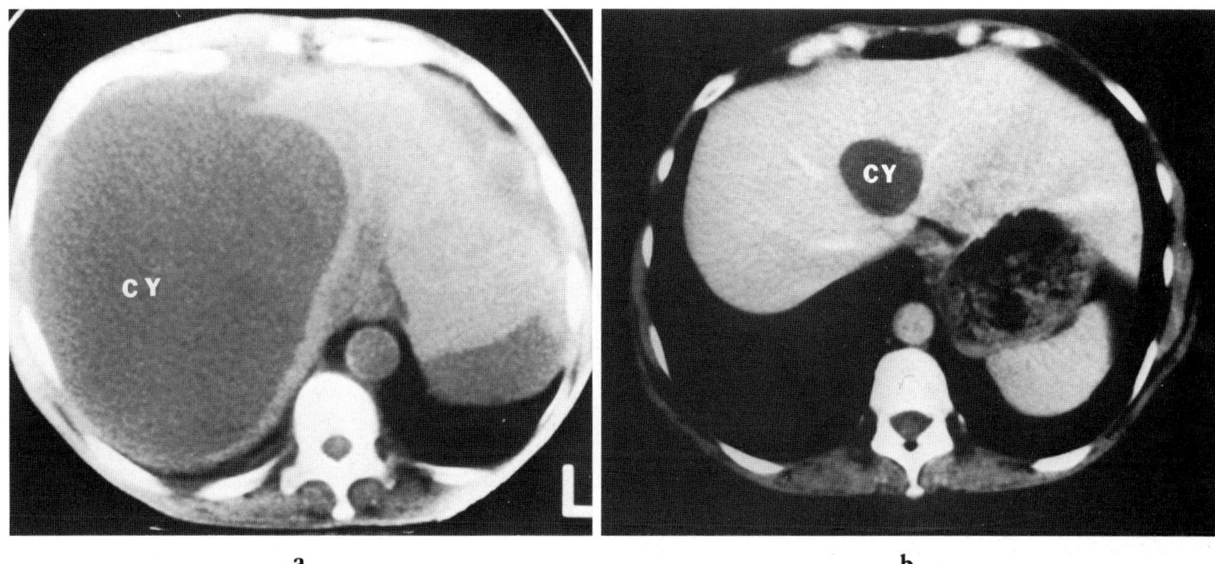

a b

Fig. 16.10 a. This simple hepatic cyst (CY) occupies almost the entire right hepatic lobe. b. Smaller simple cyst takes origin between the middle and left hepatic veins. Note the homogeneous, near-water attenuation contents and the sharp boundary between the cyst and the normal liver parenchyma.

(e.g fluid–fluid level, septa, etc.), percutaneous CT-guided needle aspiration of the lesion should be performed.

Cavernous haemangiomas

The single tumour which responds in so characteristic a fashion to intravenous contrast that its histology can be confidently predicted by CT criteria is the cavernous haemangioma (Barnett et al 1980; Freeny et al 1979; Itai et al 1980a; 1983, Johnson et al 1981). Because of its extensive vascular compartment, intense peripheral enhancement occurs after a bolus of contrast is administered, followed by slow diffusion from the periphery toward the centre (Fig. 16.11). The contrast enhancement often lasts up to 10 or more minutes. Cavernous haemangioma predominantly occurs in females, and tends to occur in the posterior segment of the right lobe. 10% of patients have multiple angiomata. With the exception of small tumours (less than 2 cm) which do not exhibit these typical enhancement patterns, the combination of the clinical and radiographic features are usually diagnostic of this entity.

Benign hepatic adenomas were at one time a curiosity. Recently, however, there has been an increase in prevalence of this benign tumour, a fact which has been related to the widespread use of oral contraceptives. Adenomata usually appear as well-circumscribed, low-attenuation lesions which enhance homogeneously after administration of contrast material (Angres et al 1980; Fishman et al 1982, Rehnava & Rothenberg 1981, Salvo et al 1977). Larger ones may contain areas of necrosis, and their enhancement pattern is less homogeneous. Since the larger subcapsular adenomata may present with massive intraperitoneal bleeding, surgery may be contemplated in individual cases. The ability of CT to render precise anatomical information may thus be clinically useful.

Focal nodular hyperplasia is not a true neoplasm; rather it reflects a hyperplastic response to hepatic injury (Atkinson et al 1980, Fishman et al 1982, Rogers et al 1981, Salvo et al 1977). Such lesions usually arise on the surface of the liver and most large nodules have a central, somewhat stellate, scar of low attenuation. After contrast administration there is generally intense homogeneous enhancement of all but the central portion (Fig. 16.12). When doubt exists about the diagnosis, a radionuclide scan (Piers et al 1980) may be helpful since focal nodular hyperplasia, unlike other liver tumours, contains Kupffer cells (Ch. 15).

Peliosis hepatis is an unusual condition occurring in patients suffering from chronic debilitating diseases, such as tuberculosis or malignancy and in those receiving androgenic steroids. In this condition, multiple blood-filled cystic spaces occur within the liver, and generally range in size between a few millimetres and 1 cm. Some may be as large as 4–5 cm in diameter and there is danger of exsanguinating haemorrhage (Tsukamoto et al 1984). CT directly displays the multiple blood-dense irregular spaces; contrast administration provides rapid increase in density during the arterial and capillary phase.

Inflammatory diseases

Pyogenic abscess

Due to the widespread use of broad spectrum antibiotics, there has been a change in the clinical presentation of pyogenic hepatic abscesses. Rather than a fulminating,

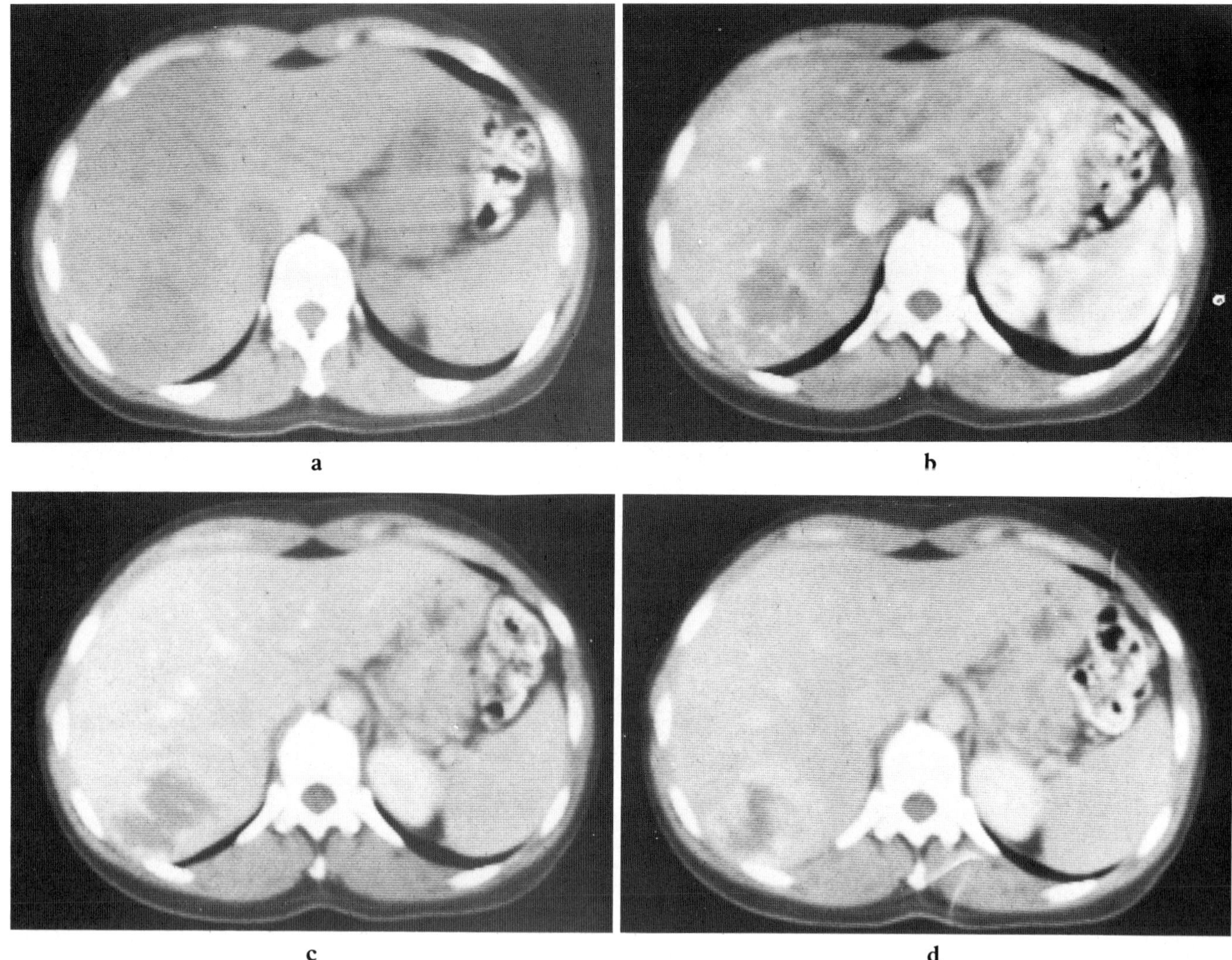

Fig. 16.11 Cavernous haemangioma. a. Precontrast scan demonstrates a hypodense mass in the posterior aspect of the right lobe. b–d. Serial scans obtained 15 sec (b), 1 min (c) and 5 min (d) after a bolus injection of iodinated contrast material show initial intense peripheral enhancement followed by centripetal migration of contrast material. After 5 minutes, only the central portion of the mass remains unenhanced.

toxic process, it is not unusual for an hepatic abscess to present as a well-defined space-occupying lesion discovered incidentally in a patient with only vague systemic symptoms; both clinically and radiographically, abscesses may mimic primary or metastatic neoplasm (Halversen et al 1984).

The majority of pyogenic abscesses occur in the posterior portion of the right lobe, and are observed on computed tomography as a well-defined mass of low attenuation with a thick, irregular wall (Fig. 16.13). The central portion of such abscesses is purulent material without vascularity, but the periphery is frequently hypervascular and will enhance strongly on dynamic CT. The major contribution of computed tomography in the diagnosis is to direct percutaneous puncture with aspiration of the contents. When the diagnosis of abscess is established in this way, the same route may be used for placement of a percutaneous drainage catheter (Ch. 37, 73). While most pyogenic abscesses are solitary, up to one-third are multiple; however, it is rare for more than two pyogenic abscesses to be present.

Fungal abscesses

Patients immunosuppressed because of organ transplantation or due to an underlying haematological disorder may become infected by unusual organisms. In contrast to pyogenic abscesses, fungal hepatic abscesses are usually multiple and are distributed throughout the liver (Berlow 1984) (Fig. 16.14.) The value of computed tomography in identifying and subsequently aspirating such collections has been emphasized; since broad-spectrum antibiotic coverage is ineffective, a specific antifungal agent must be administered. Sampling the purulent cavity is mandatory,

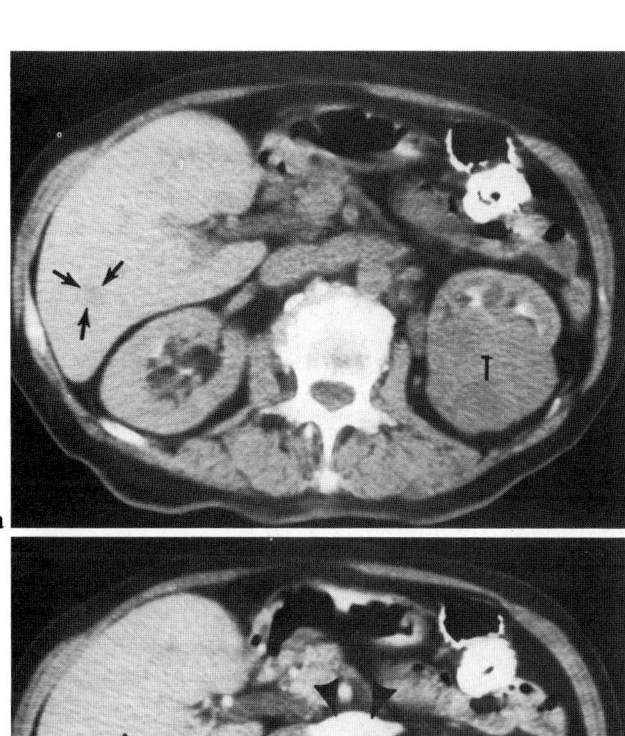

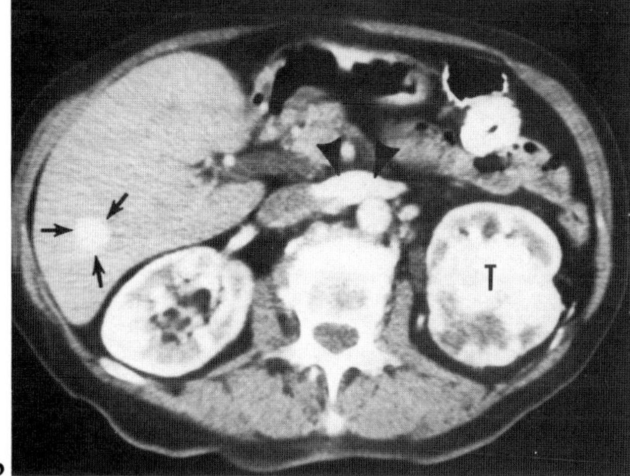

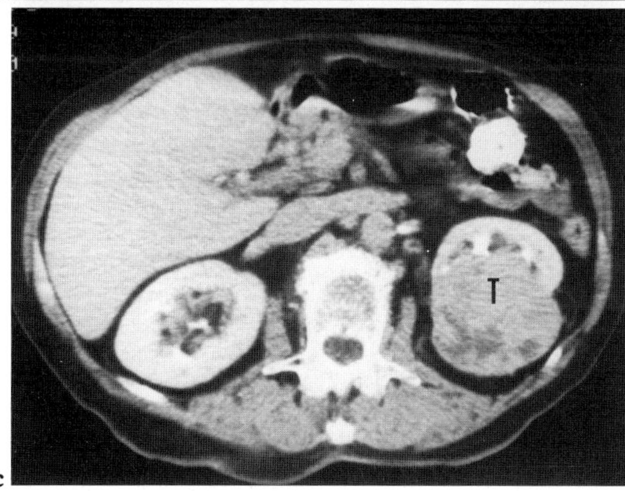

Fig. 16.12 Focal nodular hyperplasia. a. Unenhanced scan through the region of the main portal vein illustrates a large left renal tumour (T). Also noted is a 2.5 cm round area of lower attenuation (arrows) in the posterior right hepatic segment. The CT study was performed after an excretory urogram accounting for the opacified renal collecting system. b. Same level 15 seconds after rapid intravenous administration of water-soluble contrast. There is dense opacification of the renal tumour (T) and the left renal vein (arrowheads). Simultaneously, there is uniform enhancement of the liver lesion (arrows). c. Scan obtained after equilibrium phase shows less pronounced enhancement of renal tumour (T). The hepatic tumour is now completely invisible.

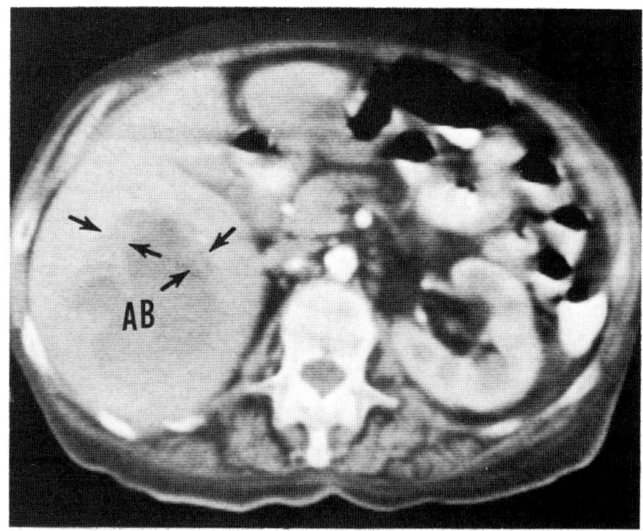

Fig. 16.13 Typical pyogenic abscess. Scan through the posterior right lobe of the liver 15 seconds after intravenous administration of contrast material demonstrates slight enhancement of the wall of the abscess (arrows). No enhancement of the internal contents is demonstrated.

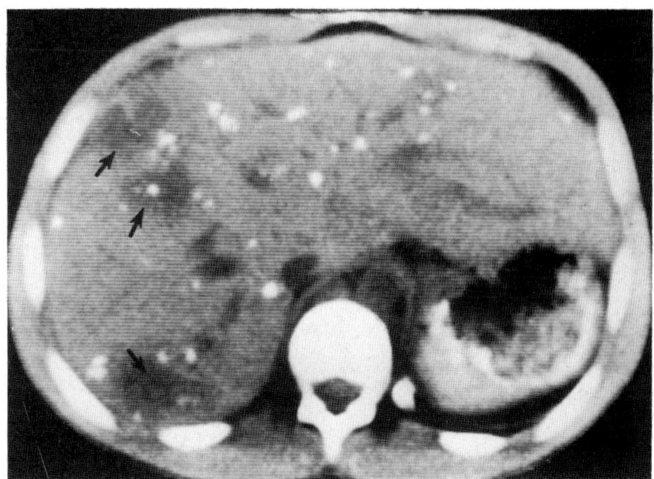

Fig. 16.14 Fungal abscesses. Scan obtained near the dome of the diaphragm in this chronically immunosuppressed renal transplant patient demonstrates multiple low attenuation areas (arrows) in addition to obvious punctate calcifications. Aspiration of one of these locules retrieved *candida albicans*.

since blood cultures may be unrevealing. Organisms such as Candida, Aspergillus, or Cryptococcus have been retrieved from these cavities.

Echinococcus (Ch. 75)

In endemic areas, involvement of the liver by hydatid disease is a common finding. *Echinococcus granulosus* presents with large single mass or multiple well-defined cystic lesions, which often contain internal 'daughter' cysts

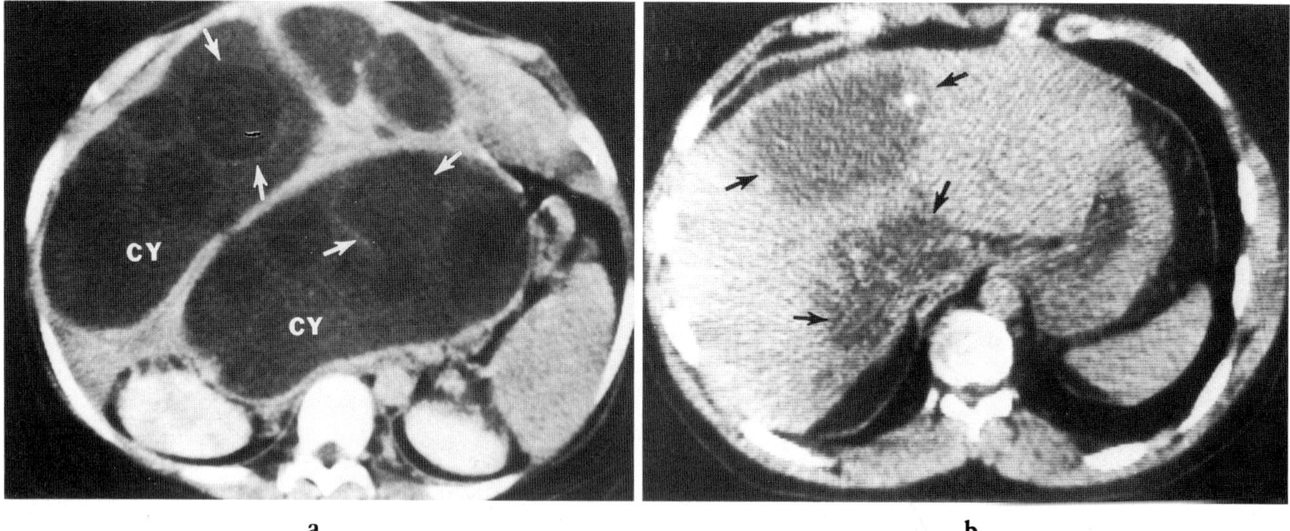

Fig. 16.15 Abscesses due to echinococcosis. a. *E. granulosus* typically demonstrates multiple, well-circumscribed cysts (CY) in which smaller daughter cysts, some with peripheral calcification (arrows), are situated. b. *E. alveolaris*, in contrast, typically involves the region of the porta hepatis and presents radiographically as low attenuation areas with poorly-defined margins (arrows). These may be confused with metastases. (Fig. 16.15a courtesy of Dr M A Rudwan, Ibn Sina Hospital, Kuwait; Fig. 16.15b courtesy of Dr M Cayle, Providence Hospital, Anchorage, Alaska.)

(Fig. 16.15a). Calcification in the wall of the large or internal cysts occurs in most patients. There is communication between the cysts and the biliary tree in approximately 25% of cases (Choli et al 1982), and frank rupture of cyst contents into the bile ducts occurs in 5–10%, accompanied by clinical features of cholangitis. *Echinococcus alveolaris*, in contrast, resembles both clinically and radiographically an infiltrating hepatic tumour (Fig. 16.15b)

Amoebic abscess

On computed tomographic scans, amoebic abscesses appear as well-defined masses of near-water attenuation with a thick enhancing rim (Fig. 16.16). The CT findings are not specific and serological tests are necessary to confirm the diagnosis.

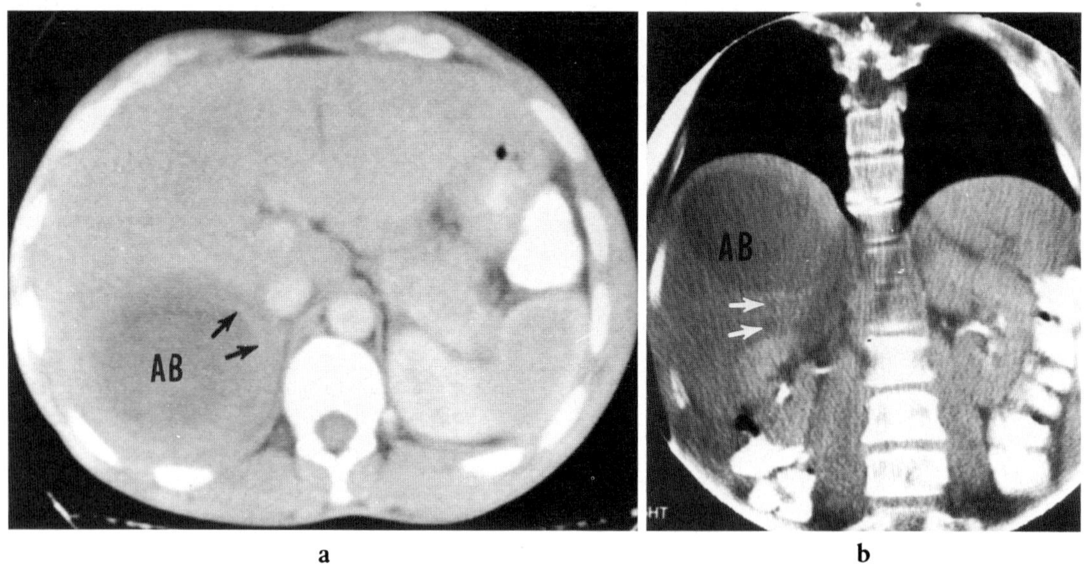

Fig. 16.16 Amoebic abscess. a. Axial scan demonstrates a large abscess cavity (AB) in the posterior segment of the right hepatic lobe. During infusion of water soluble contrast, a portion of the wall of the abscess cavity (arrows) is seen to enhance. b. Direct coronal scan obtained in the same patient demonstrates the major portion of the abscess (AB) under the dome of the diaphragm, with several smaller cavities (white arrows) extending inferiorly toward the superior renal margin. These proved to be amoebic abscesses.

Diffuse hepatocellular diseases

In general, CT is of less value in assessing diffuse parenchymal disease than in the evaluation of focal lesions. The CT appearance of diffuse parenchymal disease is quite variable, depending upon the aetiology of the process and the severity of its involvement. Acute hepatitis, for example, will not produce any change in the density or contour of the liver. While excess iron deposition and glycogen storage disease lead to increased hepatic density, fatty infiltration causes generalized decrease in hepatic attenuation.

Fatty infiltration

Fatty infiltration, whether associated with cirrhosis or in a variety of other systemic disorders, including diabetes mellitus, cystic fibrosis, or malnourishment, results in a decrease in hepatic density. Mild degrees of fatty change may be subtle unless liver density is carefully compared to that of the spleen. The liver is normally 6–12 Hounsfield units higher in attenuation than the spleen; reversal of this relationship is the earliest CT indication of fatty infiltration. With more advanced changes, the hepatic parenchyma becomes less dense than intrahepatic vessels.

In most instances, fatty infiltration is diffuse and uniform, but non-uniform focal distribution can also occur (Scott et al 1980). As mentioned previously, focal fatty infiltration should not be confused with a neoplastic process.

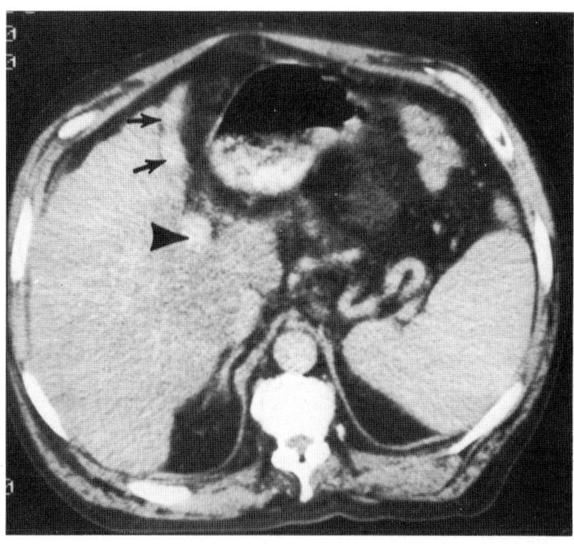

a

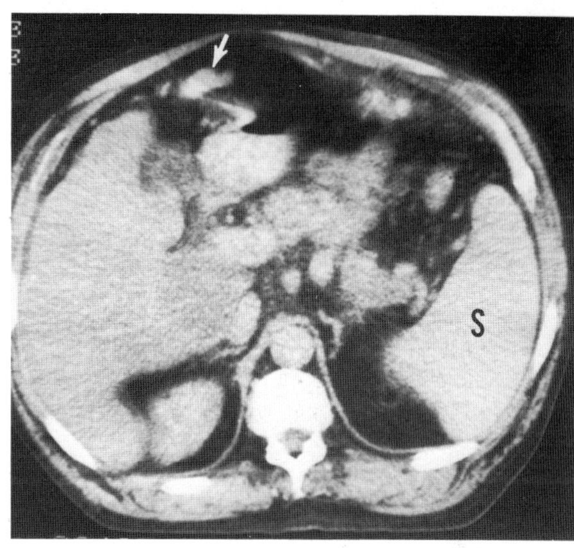

b

Fig. 16.17 Morphological changes in a patient with cirrhosis. a. CT scan through the porta hepatis demonstrates enlargement of the spleen (S) and wavy irregularity of the margin of the liver. The caudate lobe and papillary process are low in attenuation and enlarged. In addition, a large vein (arrows) in the region for the fissure ligamentum teres is part of a network of porta-systemic shunting. Arrowhead points to the left portal vein. b. On a slightly lower scan, the large collateral vein (arrow) follows the exact course of the obliterated umbilical vein. Other retroperitoneal collaterals are present posterior to the pancreas.

Cirrhosis

CT is capable of demonstrating morphological changes associated with advanced hepatic cirrhosis. Due to the disturbance in normal portal flow, the right lobe undergoes shrinkage, while the caudate lobe increases in volume (Harbin et al 1980). Diffuse or focal decrease in liver attenuation may be observed, and is probably due to fatty infiltration (Mulhern et al 1979) resulting from disturbance in hepatic metabolism. When portal flow is reversed, porta–systemic shunts form through numerous potential collateral systems. Splenomegaly and splenic venous enlargement are readily apparent on CT scans, as is collateral flow through the ligamentum teres towards the umbilicus (Ishikawa et al 1980) (Fig. 16.17). Paraoesophageal and gastrohepatic ligament varices are also readily observed, particularly after contrast medium is administered.

Budd-Chiari syndrome (Ch. 111)

Budd-Chiari syndrome is a rare disorder characterized by upper abdominal pain, marked enlargement of the liver and rapid accumulation of ascites. It is caused by partial or complete thrombosis of the hepatic veins or the inferior vena cava adjacent to the hepatic venous drainage. In over half the cases, the instigating cause is unknown. CT scans demonstrate patchy postcontrast enhancement of the uninvolved segments of liver (Rossi et al 1981, Yang et al 1983) and no visualization of the hepatic veins. One reported case (Yang et al 1983) demonstrated enlargement of the caudate lobe similar to that seen in cirrhosis; after contrast administration the caudate lobe enhanced normally, while the rest of the liver exhibited diminished contrast response.

Hepatic infarction

Hepatic infarction is rare, and implies compromise to both the arterial and portal venous supply to a segment or lobe of the liver. CT findings include a well-defined wedge-shaped area of low attenuation in segmental or subsegmental distribution, extending to the liver surface. After contrast administration, the affected zone enhances minimally; a peripheral, thin subcapsular rim often contains enhancing hepatic tissue (Adler et al 1984). A late complication of hepatic infarction is formation of bile lakes in the affected segments (Peterson & Neumann 1984), a pathologic feature similar to that of Caroli's disease.

Miscellaneous diseases

Increase in overall liver attenuation is seen in cases of Wilson's disease (Mayer et al 1983), β-thalassaemia (Mitnick et al 1981) and sickle-cell disease (Magid et al 1984). Patients with haemosiderosis due to haemochromatosis or multiple blood transfusions also exhibit increased liver attenuation (Fig. 16.18).

Patients who have received radiation therapy are often observed to have sharply-defined areas of low attenuation within the radiation portal (Jeffrey et al 1980, Kolbenstvedt et al 1980). This appears to reflect an acute form of radiation hepatitis and is most commonly observed in patients who have received dosages greater than 35 Gy. Sporadic cases of identical changes in patients who have received lower doses of radiation are, however, reported.

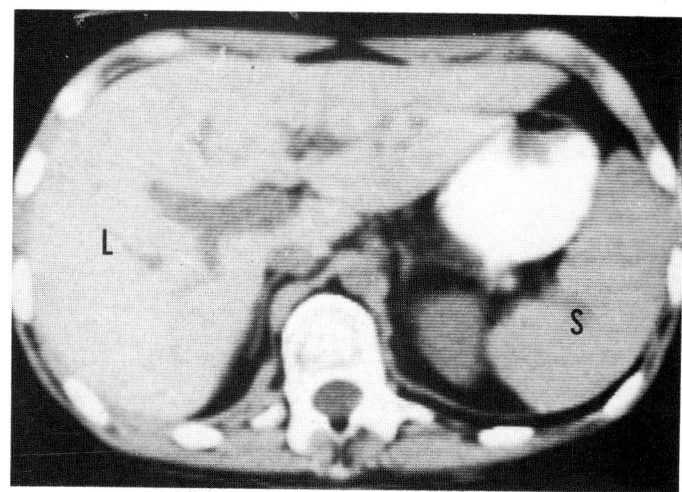

Fig. 16.18 There is dense increase in attenuation of the parenchyma of the liver (L) compared to the normal attenuation of the spleen (S) in this patient with hemochromatosis due to multiple blood transfusions.

THE BILIARY SYSTEM

INTRODUCTION

The characteristics of biliary tract disease which can be assessed by computed tomography are biliary dilatation, either focal or diffuse, and intrabiliary calcification. Since both of these primary characteristics can be assessed very well with ultrasound examination, CT is not used routinely as a screening examination for biliary disease. The major contribution of computed tomography towards the understanding of biliary processes lies in its ability to depict the extrahepatic course of the biliary duct, and define those extrahepatic viscera adjacent to it. Information provided by CT is often critical in selecting an appropriate group of patients for surgical intervention to relieve obstructive jaundice (Harell et al 1977, Levitt et al 1977).

TECHNIQUE

The attenuation difference between blood flowing in the portal veins and bile in the biliary tree is appreciable, but minimal intrahepatic ductal dilatation may go undetected if intravenous contrast material is not used. We, therefore, routinely administer iodinated urographic contrast material when evaluating the biliary tree. Oral contrast material is also helpful in defining portions of the extrahepatic biliary tree, particularly in the region of the head of the pancreas. If a calcified common duct stone is suspected, it may be helpful, although not absolutely necessary, to perform scans in the region of the ampulla of Vater prior to the administration of oral contrast, so that a small calcified stone is not obscured.

Oral (Greenberg et al 1982) or intravenous (Pretorius et al 1982) biliary contrast agents can be administered, and may be useful in evaluating the region of the head of the pancreas. However, since most patients who are undergoing CT examination of the biliary tract are jaundiced, biliary contrast agents are not excreted into bile in visible concentration; thus, such agents serve no useful purpose.

ANATOMY

The intrahepatic biliary tree branches in a fashion nearly identical to the portal system. The left and right hepatic ducts form the common hepatic duct near the lateral margin of the main portal vein near its junction with the right portal vein (Ch. 2). The common hepatic duct then continues inferiorly, towards the left and somewhat posteriorly, and maintains its anterolateral position with respect to the portal vein throughout its course within the hepatoduodenal ligament (Fig. 16.19). It becomes retroperitoneal at the level of the head of the pancreas and occupies a position on the posterolateral surface of the pancreas until it joins the pancreatic duct immediately before entering the ampulla of Vater. Numerous variations

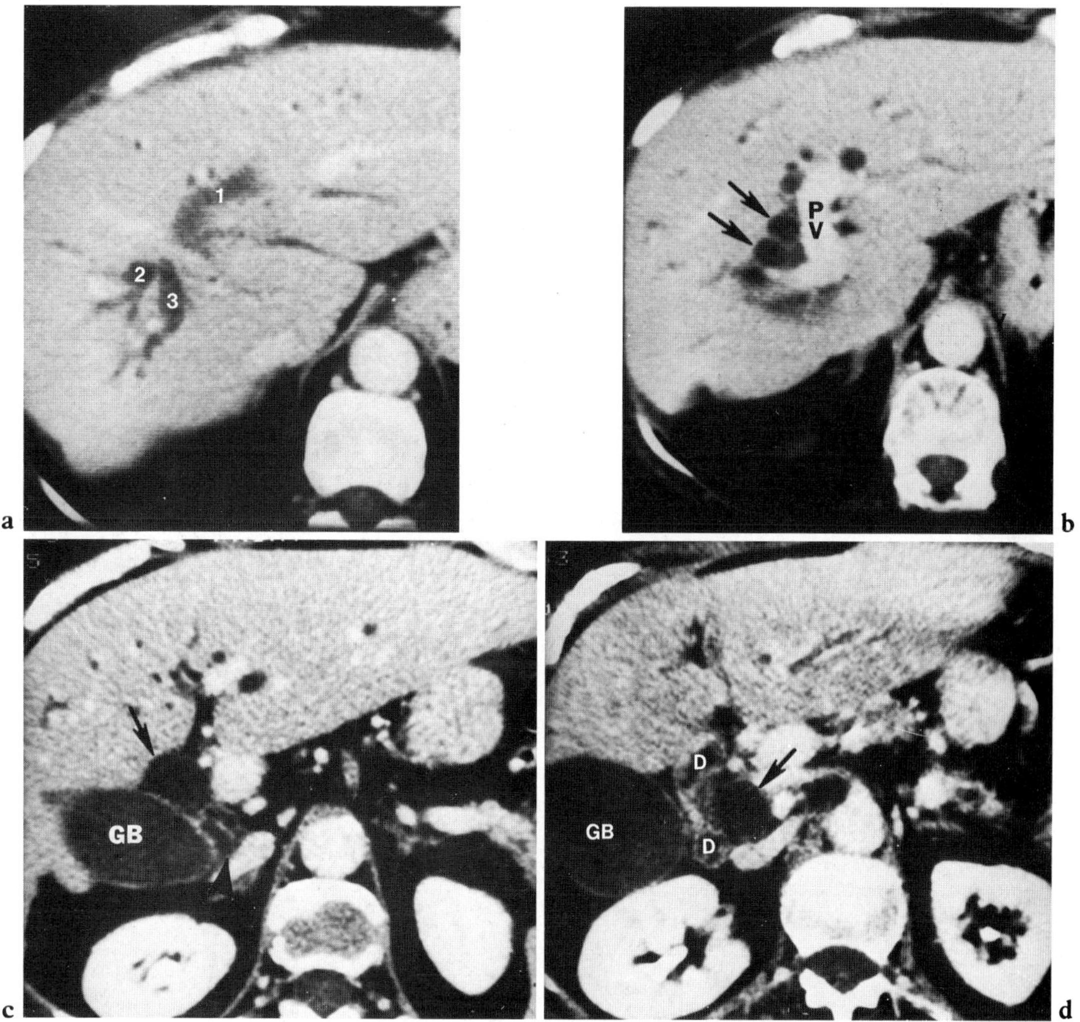

Fig. 16.19 Normal biliary anatomy illustrated in a patient with dilatation of the intrahepatic biliary system. a. Scan above the porta hepatis demonstrates dilated segments of the left hepatic duct (1), and both anterior (2) and posterior segments (3) of the right hepatic duct. Note the opacified major divisions of the portal vein which follow the branching pattern of the biliary system. b. Scan through the main portal vein (PV) shows the junction of dilated right and left hepatic duct (arrows). c. Scan caudal to the porta hepatis reveals a dilated extrahepatic duct (arrow) near its junction with the cystic duct (arrowhead). GB = gallbladder d. Scan at the level of the body of the pancreas demonstrates the dilated common bile duct (arrow) to lie medial to the descending duodenum (DD). GB = gallbladder

in the distribution of the common bile duct exist. It had been suggested that a transverse segment of the proximal common hepatic duct as it exits the porta hepatis was a sign of malignant biliary obstruction. However, a study by Jacobson & Brodey (1981) demonstrates the presence of a transverse segment in 18% of dilated ducts and 6% of normal ducts, with no relationship between the cause of dilatation and the presence of a transverse segment.

Normal intrahepatic biliary radicles are not visible on CT. However, the extrahepatic duct, which measures 3–6 mm in cross-sectional diameter, can often be seen as a circular structure of near-water density posterolateral to the head of the pancreas on a post-contrast scan.

The site of entry of the cystic duct into the common hepatic duct to form the common bile duct is quite variable and is often impossible to detect on CT images. When the cystic duct and common hepatic duct have a common wall and course in parallel, they may be detected as separate entities by a thin septum separating the two water-density structures (Goldberg 1982).

PATHOLOGICAL PROCESSES

Gallbladder

Cholecystitis

Sonography has proved to be extremely effective in screening patients for gallbladder disease. Occasionally, however, patients with cholecystitis will present with a confusing clinical picture and may undergo CT examination before the precise nature of the disease is clear. It is helpful, therefore, to recognize the appearance of

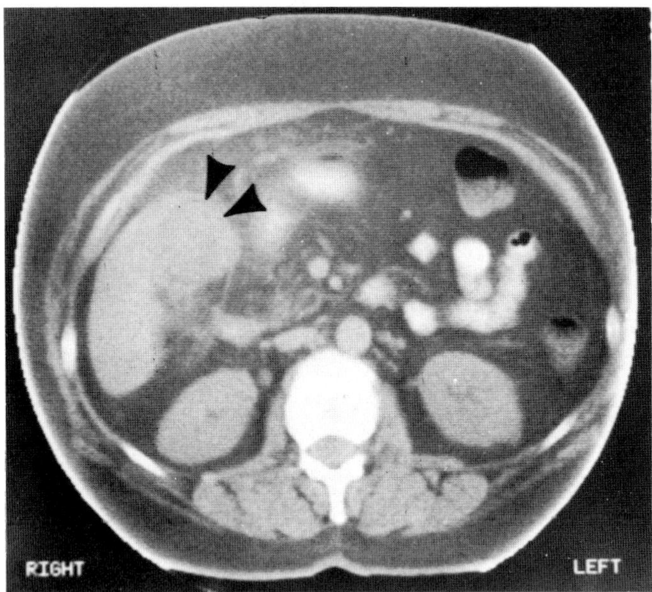

Fig. 16.20 Complicated cholecystitis. Scan through the gallbladder fossa in this acutely ill female demonstrates wispy serpigenous soft tissue densities within the perihepatic and pericholecystic fat. A 'halo' of low attenuation (arrowheads) surrounds the gallbladder partially, and there is focal thickening of the gallbladder wall medially which corresponded surgically to a small abscess.

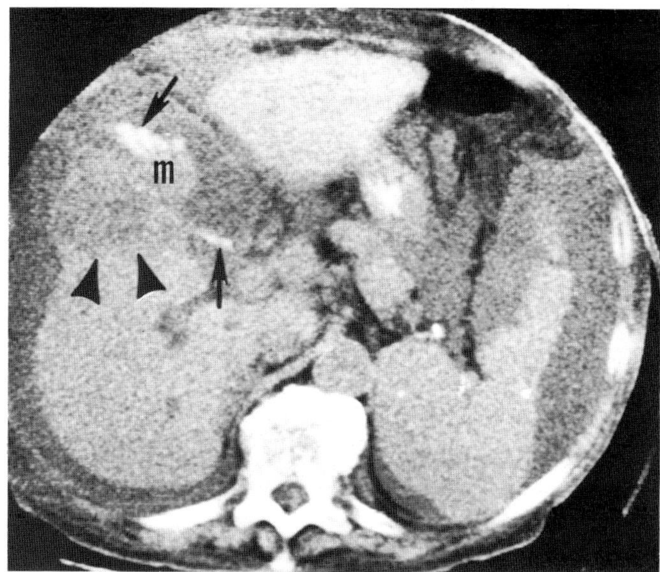

Fig. 16.21 Carcinoma of the gallbladder. A soft tissue mass (m) is seen projecting into the lumen of the gallbladder and extending posterolaterally to involve the liver (arrowheads). Multiple calcified gallstones (arrows) are also noted.

complicated cholecystitis on computed tomography. An enlarged gallbladder, with a thickened enhancing wall and an increased attenuation of the bile contained within it, are suggestive findings, but not specific for intrinsic gallbladder disease (Havrilla et al 1978, Kane et al 1983). Pericholecystic abscesses are readily recognized on computed tomography and may be useful for surgical planning (Tenier et al 1984). A pericholecystic halo of low attenuation material is seen in patients with complicated cholecystitis, and is not a feature of gallbladder malignancy (Smathers et al 1984) (Fig. 16.20). Extremely high attenuation of gallbladder contents can be seen in patients with haemorrhagic cholecystitis, a rare complication of cholelithiasis (Jenkins et al 1983). In the majority of patients with acute pancreatitis, the gallbladder appears abnormal on CT (Somer et al 1984). The overall density of the contained bile is approximately twice that of normal, and a thickened, intensely enhancing wall is displayed. This may be due to lymphatic obstruction caused by the pancreatitis.

Gallbladder cancer

Carcinoma of the gallbladder is the fifth most common gastrointestinal malignancy but is extremely difficult to diagnose preoperatively. Cholelithiasis is often present in patients with gallbladder cancer, and it may be difficult to distinguish between complicated cholecystitis and gallbladder cancer (Itai et al 1980c; Weiner et al 1984). As mentioned, the presence of a low attenuation pericholecystic halo suggests benign disease, whereas the presence of irregular soft tissue lesions within the liver parenchyma adjacent to the gallbladder is a feature only of carcinoma (Smathers et al 1984) (Fig. 16.21) (Ch. 64). There is a marked propensity for gallbladder carcinoma to spread directly through the hepatoduodenal ligament into the porta hepatis producing high extrahepatic biliary obstruction. Obstruction may also be caused by intraductal spread of the malignancy, which occurs in 4% of patients.

Biliary tree

Obstruction: general considerations

Sonography is well established as the preferred initial screening examination for patients with suspected biliary obstruction because of its ease of performance, lower cost, lack of ionizing radiation, and wide availability (Ch. 14). However, false-negative sonograms may occur in patients with extrahepatic biliary obstruction with minimal or no dilatation of the intrahepatic system. Computed tomography may also add information about structures adjacent to the extrahepatic course of the biliary tree, particularly the pancreas and the lymph nodes contained within the hepatoduodenal ligament (Goldberg et al 1978, Pedrosa et al 1981, Shimizu et al 1981). In one prospective study of jaundiced patients (Baron et al 1982), CT correctly predicted the level of obstruction in 88%, compared with 60% by ultrasound; the precise cause of the obstruction was correctly identified by computed tomography in 70%, while sonography predicted only 38% of aetiologies.

The CT diagnosis of biliary obstruction is based on the demonstration of dilated intrahepatic or extrahepatic bile ducts. Dilated intrahepatic ducts appear on CT as linear branching, or circular structures of near-water density, enlarging as they approach the junction of the left and right hepatic ducts in the porta hepatis. The extrahepatic bile duct is considered unequivocally dilated if it is 9 mm or more in diameter and definitely normal if it is less than 7 mm.

Although CT has proved to be accurate in establishing a diagnosis of biliary obstruction, there is not always a direct correlation between the calibre of the biliary tree and the presence of clinically significant obstruction. In patients with significant dilatation of the biliary tree in whom the obstruction is later relieved surgically or by spontaneous passage of a calculus, the bile duct may remain somewhat more dilated than normal for the remainder of the patient's life. In such patients, the CT findings may falsely suggest the presence of biliary obstruction. Likewise, a normal calibre bile duct can be observed in the presence of a surgically correctable cause of jaundice. Intermittently obstructing calculi and subtle strictures of the extrahepatic duct may be present when the overall duct calibre is normal. In situations where there is discrepancy between clinical or biochemical evidence and the CT findings, direct cholangiography by the percutaneous or endoscopic route should be performed to resolve the problem (Ch. 19, 20).

In addition to its ability to detect the presence or absence of biliary obstruction, CT is also able to predict the cause of obstruction in a majority of cases. While abrupt termination of the extrahepatic duct with a mass effect and enlargement of the pancreatic duct is indicative of a malignant process, smooth gradual tapering of bile ducts favours benign disease (Baron et al 1983).

One major pitfall in CT diagnosis of biliary disease is in the detection of cholesterol stones, which have an attenuation exactly the same as that of surrounding bile. Jeffrey et al (1983) have suggested that an abrupt termination of the common bile duct without a mass effect or a rim of increased attenuation along the peripheral margin of the duct at its lower end suggest choledocholithiasis.

Obstruction: specific causes

Biliary calculi

The insensitivity of sonography in detecting choledocholithiasis has been documented in studies by Einstein et al (1984) and Mitchell & Clark (1984), both of which report a detection rate in the range of 18–22%. In Mitchell's study, the sensitivity of CT was 87%, and its accuracy 84%. Obviously, calcified stones lying within an obstructed duct present no challenge to the radiologist (Suzuki et al 1983) (Fig. 16.22); most errors in diagnosis are due to cholesterol stones, which may blend imperceptibly with the surrounding bile. Nevertheless, the overall accuracy of

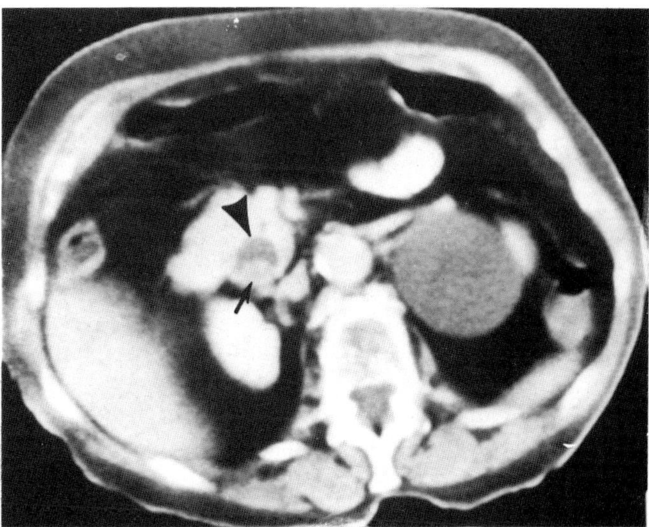

Fig. 16.22 Two calcified common bile duct stones (arrow) lie in the dependent portion of a dilated, obstructed common bile duct (arrowhead).

CT in the diagnosis of choledocholithiasis is in the range of 80%.

Intrahepatic choledocholithiasis may present a bizarre appearance (Itai et al 1980b, Myracle et al 1981), due to segmental or subsegmental biliary radicles filled with calculi (Fig. 16.23). In Asian immigrants with recurrent pyogenic cholangitis (Federle et al 1982) who subsequently form intra- and extrahepatic bile pigment stones, the debris filling the biliary system is generally of higher attenuation than that of normal bile, which should allow the correct diagnosis.

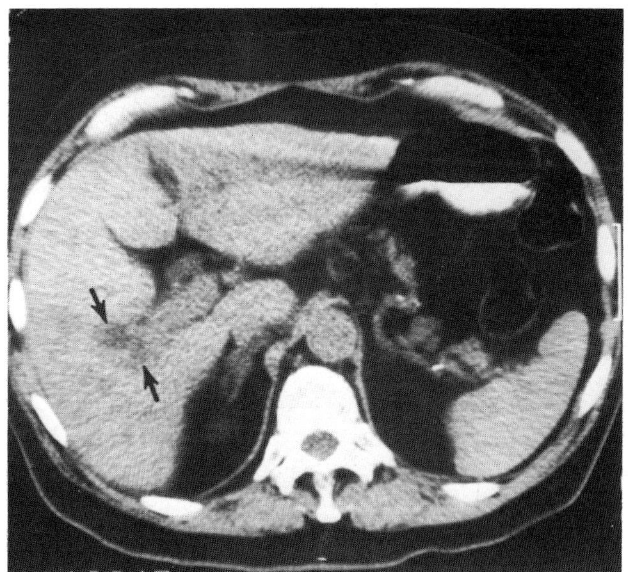

Fig. 16.23 Two cholesterol stones (arrows) dilate the intrahepatic portion of the right hepatic duct in this febrile patient.

Mirizzi's syndrome

Mirizzi's syndrome is an uncommon condition in which the common hepatic duct is obstructed due to stones in or extruded from the cystic duct, the cystic duct remnant or the gallbladder. Cholecystobiliary or cholecystoenteric fistulas are common complications (Ch. 58, 61). The typical CT features of Mirizzi's syndrome are dilatation of the biliary system above the level of the neck of the gallbladder with a normal system below, and a gallstone impacted in a cystic duct (Pedrosa et al 1983) or gallbladder neck (Becker et al 1984, Berland et al 1984). An irregular cavity adjacent to the gallbladder neck was reported by Pedrosa (Pedrosa et al 1983) in five out of six cases, and represented stone penetration outside the gallbladder. Since not all of the findings may be present on CT, direct cholangiography is recommended to document the nature of the obstruction and the presence or absence of a biliary fistula.

Acalculous obstruction

Several other conditions may cause segmental or diffuse obstruction of the biliary tree. In patients with echinococcosis, rupture of the hydatid cyst into the biliary tree occurs in 5–10% of cases and may produce biliary obstruction (Subramanyam et al 1983). Chronic pancreatitis with biliary stricture may produce high grade obstruction, and is difficult to distinguish by any means from pancreatic carcinoma (Fig. 16.24, 16.25). Localized intrahepatic dilatation has been reported in patients with choledochal cyst (Araki et al 1980a, 1981) (Fig. 16.26). In the commonest form of this entity, only the central portions of the left and right hepatic ducts are dilated, and the periphery of the biliary tree appears normal.

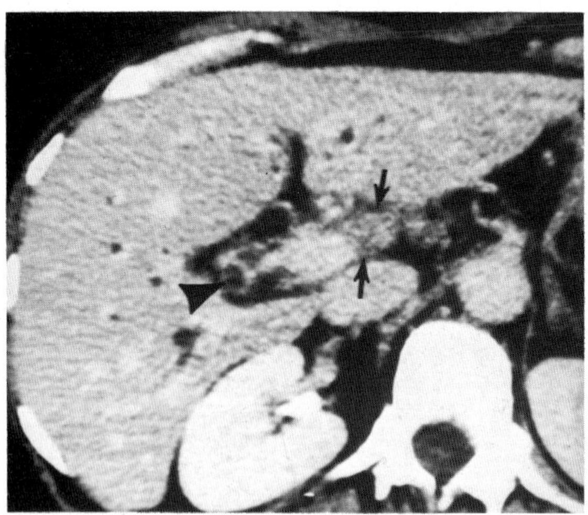

Fig. 16.24 Scan through the porta hepatis demonstrates enlargement of the common hepatic duct (arrowhead) because of a stricture in the pancreatic segment. In addition, matted lymph nodes (arrows) are present in the hepatoduodenal ligament, a result of pancreatic inflammation.

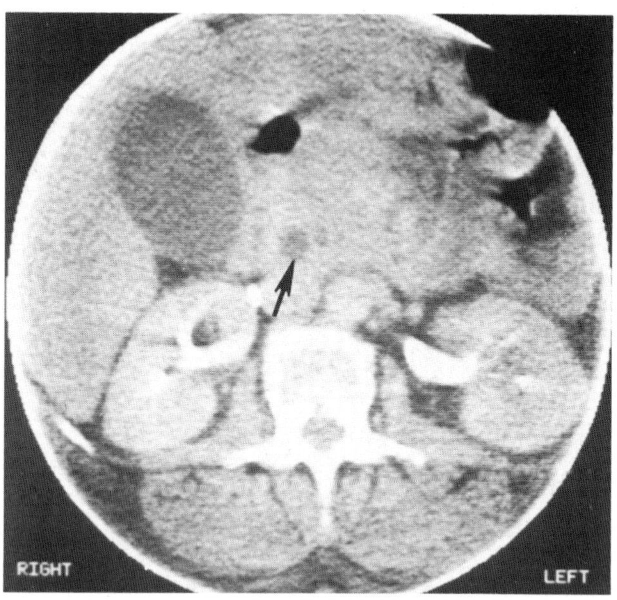

a

RIGHT LEFT

b

Fig. 16.25 Young patient with chronic relapsing pancreatitis. a. Scan through the mid-portion of the pancreas demonstrates an enlarged common bile duct (arrow) and bulbous enlargement of the body and tail of the pancreas.The margins of the anterior wall of the pancreas with the left hepatic lobe are blurred because of repeated episodes of pancreatitis. b. Four millimetres caudal, there is narrowing but not obliteration of the pancreatic segment of the common bile duct in the midst of the inflammatory enlargement. This was surgically proven to be a benign stricture.

Sclerosing cholangitis is an unusual entity consisting of progressive diffuse cicatrization of the intra- and extrahepatic biliary tree. It is often associated with inflammatory bowel disease. The CT appearance (Ament et al 1983,

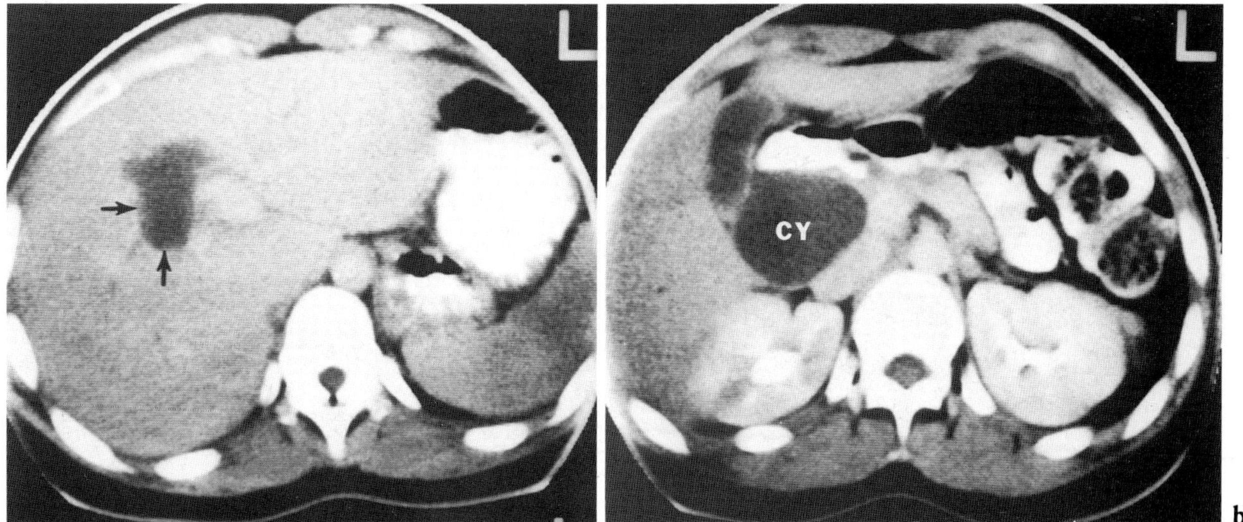

Fig. 16.26 Choledochal cyst. a. Scan through the top of the porta hepatis demonstrates a large, irregular, low attenuation structure (arrows), representing dilated distal segments of the left and right hepatic ducts. Peripheral ductal dilatation is not present. b. Several centimetres caudal, a large cystic dilatation (CY) of the extrahepatic common bile duct displaces the duodenum superiorly and laterally. This was surgically proved to be an Alonso-Lej type I choledochal cyst.

Rahn et al 1983) is that of focal, discontinuous areas of minimal intrahepatic biliary dilatation without a mass lesion (Fig. 16.27).

Caroli's disease is cystic dilatation of intrahepatic biliary radicles. It is often associated with congenital hepatic fibrosis (Ch. 80). The areas of bile lake formation appear spherical on CT, as distinct from the more serpentine appearance of other forms of focal obstruction (Doppman et al 1979, Sorenson et al 1982) (Fig. 16.28). Cholangiographic contrast may be administered to demonstrate communication of the cystic structures with the main biliary radicles. Patients with intrahepatic arterial emboli with subsequent focal areas of liver infarction may also develop bile lakes which pathologically resemble Caroli's disease (Doppman et al 1979).

Tumours

Cholangiocarcinoma is uncommon compared with hepatocellular carcinoma, but is an important cause of painless

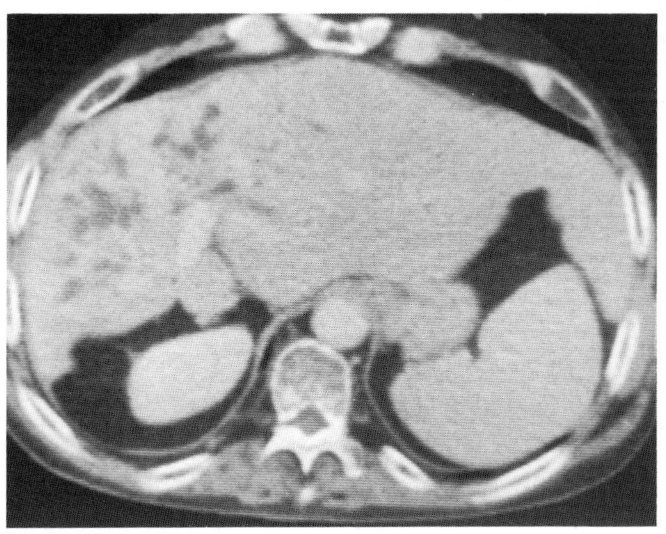

a

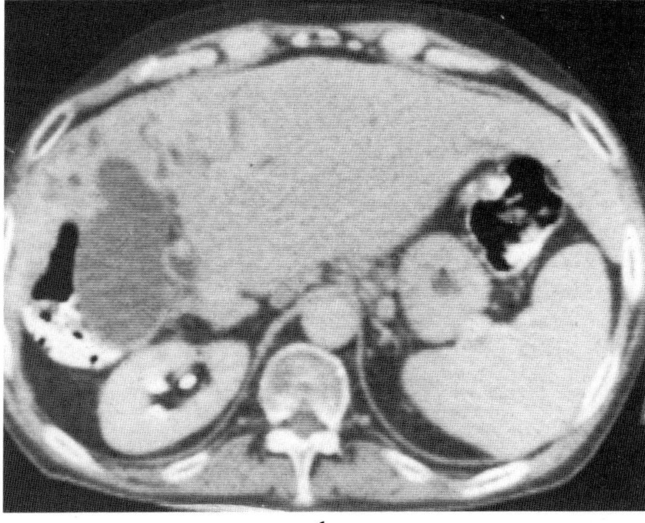

b

Fig. 16.27 Sclerosing cholangitis. a. Contrast enhanced CT scan through the gastro-oesophageal junction demonstrates marked enlargement of the lateral segment of the left hepatic lobe, with corresponding diminution in size of the right lobe. There are multiple segmentally dilated ducts in both hepatic segments, but no evidence of central dilatation. b. Scan more caudal demonstrates enlargement of the gallbladder due to involvement of the distal portion of the cystic duct.

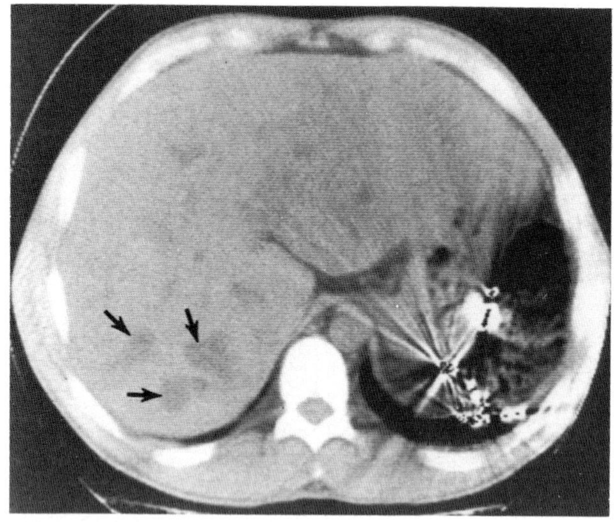

Fig. 16.28 Caroli's disease with congenital hepatic fibrosis. This 20-year-old male with an unclassified cystic disease of the kidneys presented at 10 years of age with variceal bleeding due to congenital hepatic fibrosis. CT scan through the gastroesophageal junction demonstrates multiple low attenuation areas in the posterior segment of the right hepatic lobe which were shown to communicate with the biliary tree by a subsequent cholangiogram.

jaundice. In the majority of patients, the tumour arises centrally either at the junction of the left and right hepatic ducts, or more distally in the common hepatic and common bile duct (Itai et al 1983a, Thorsen et al 1984) (Fig. 16.29) (Ch. 65). Gross dilatation of the intrahepatic biliary tree in the absence of an obvious mass at the site of obstruction is the most common finding. Some patients, however, exhibit sizeable masses with infiltration into the surrounding liver parenchyma. Even in patients without an obvious mass, careful attention to the wall of the duct at the site of obstruction will generally demonstrate diffuse mural thickening. This appearance is not, however, pathognomonic and direct cholangiography with directed biopsy is necessary to confirm the diagnosis.

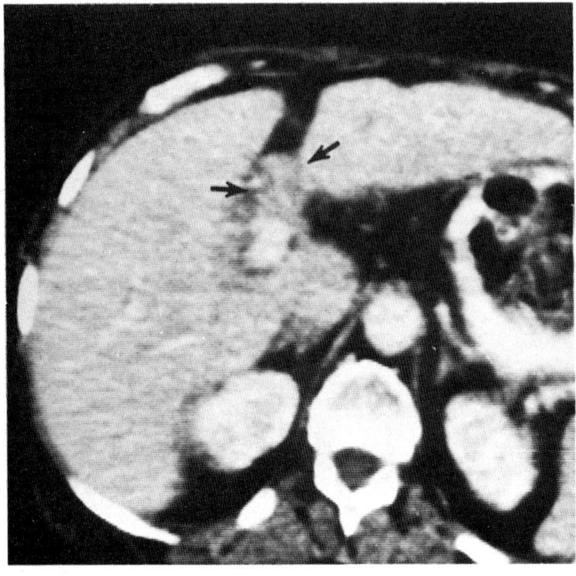

Fig. 16.29 Cholangiocarcinoma. Scan through the porta hepatis in a patient with painless jaundice demonstrates a 2 cm mass immediately anterior to the main portal vein in the expected position of the common hepatic duct. This proved to be cholangiocarcinoma.

Cancer of the pancreas

Pancreatic carcinoma is the most common cause of malignant extrahepatic biliary obstruction. Neoplasms situated in the head of the pancreas directly invade or surround the intrapancreatic portion of the common bile duct, producing characteristic findings on CT:

1. a mass in the pancreatic head
2. abrupt termination of the common bile duct in this region
3. dilatation of the intra- and extrahepatic biliary tree proximal to the mass
4. dilatation of the pancreatic duct (Fig. 16.30).

Occasionally, distal pancreatitis may occur. As the tumour spreads posteriorly, it characteristically obliterates the fat margin around the superior mesenteric artery, a finding rarely seen in inflammatory conditions.

Spread via the hepatoduodenal ligament from cancer in the pancreatic body or head may produce extrahepatic biliary obstruction high in the porta hepatis (Fig. 16.31).

Metastatic deposits within the liver will not infrequently cause segmental intrahepatic dilatation, and cause no difficulty in interpretation. Occasionally, particularly in patients with diffuse intrahepatic metastases due to colon carcinoma, lymphatic metastases will occur in the porta hepatis, producing high-grade biliary obstruction at the level of the proximal common hepatic duct (Fig. 16.32). Similarly, lymphoma may involve nodes in the hepatoduodenal ligament, producing obstruction of the intrahepatic biliary tree.

Primary biliary cystadenoma (Ch. 63) (Frick & Feinberg 1982) is a rare cause of intrahepatic biliary ductal dilatation. CT demonstrates a large, chiefly cystic mass with septa and often mural nodules.

RECOMMENDATIONS FOR THE USE OF CT IN BILIARY DISEASE

In most cases, the combination of sonography and direct cholangiography is sufficient to solve the problem of clinical jaundice (Ch. 25). Thus, use of CT in the biliary tree is limited to the following clinical situations:

1. Patients in whom previous biliary surgery has been performed (thus precluding adequate sonographic evaluation).

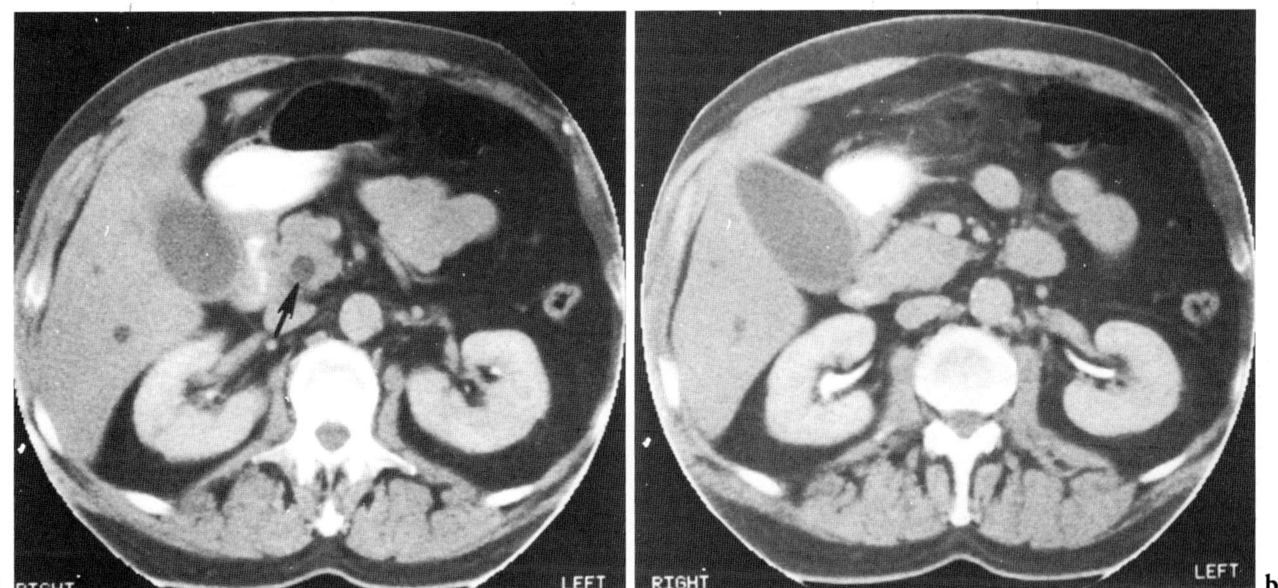

Fig. 16.30 Small pancreatic carcinoma. a. Contrast-enhanced scan through the uncinate process demonstrates an enlarged common bile duct (arrow), and dilated intrahepatic biliary radicles (arrowheads). b. Five millimetres caudal, there is abrupt termination of the common bile duct and slight enlargement of the uncinate process which has convex posterior and right margins. This proved to be an adenocarcinoma of the pancreas.

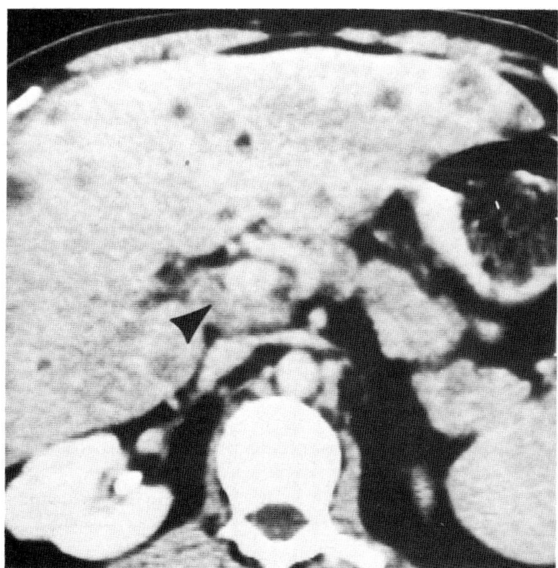

Fig. 16.31 Biliary obstruction at the level of the porta hepatis by carcinoma of the pancreas occurred because of direct extension of the carcinoma along the hepatoduodenal ligament (arrowhead).

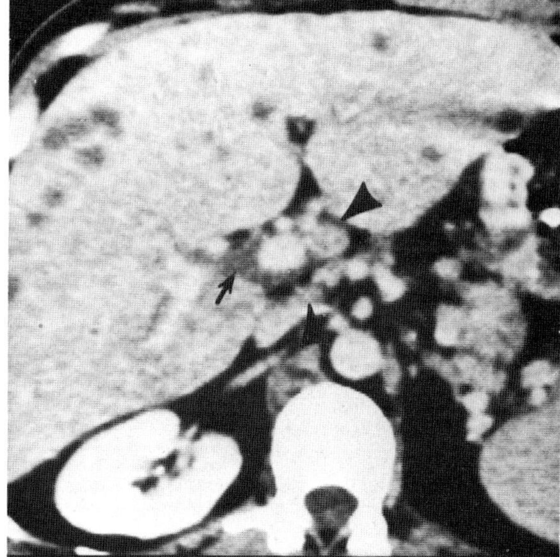

Fig. 16.32 54-year-old man with metastatic colon cancer. CT scan demonstrates multiple low attenuation metastases in the periphery of the liver as well as an obstructed common hepatic duct (arrow). Multiple large lymph nodes in the porta hepatis (arrowheads) are demonstrated and were surgically found to cause the obstruction.

2. Obese patients in whom ultrasound examination is often suboptimal.
3. Patients in whom a malignant process is known or suspected, and in whom staging is warranted to choose between surgery and a percutaneous drainage procedure.
4. Patients in whom extrahepatic inflammatory disease is known or suspected, in whom a percutaneous drainage procedure is entertained.

Moreover, CT may be useful in patients with complex problems in whom biliary disease is not an obvious feature, and in whom CT scanning is performed for other reasons; in these individuals, CT may significantly guide management by providing clues to an unsuspected biliary process.

REFERENCES

Adler D D, Glazer G M, Silver T M 1984 CT of liver infarction. American Journal of Roentgenology 142: 315–318

Adson M A, Van Heerden J A, Adson M H, Wagner J S, Ilstrup D M 1984 Resection of hepatic metastases from colorectal cancer. Archives of Surgery 119: 647–651

Ament H E, Haaga J R, Wiedemann S D, et al: 1983 Primary sclerosing cholangitis. Journal of Computer Assisted Tomography 7: 795–800

Angres G, Carter J B, Velasco J M 1980 Unusual ring in liver cell adenoma. American Journal of Roentgenology 135: 172–174

Araki T, Itai Y, Furui S, Tasaka A 1980a Dynamic CT densitometry of hepatic tumors. American Journal of Roentgenology 135: 1037–1043

Araki T, Itai Y, Tasaka A 1980b CT of choledochal cyst. American Journal of Roentgenology 135: 729–734

Araki T, Itai Y, Tasaka A 1981 CT of localized dilatation of the intrahepatic bile ducts. Radiology 141:733

Atkinson G O, Kodroff M, Sones P J, Gay B B 1980 Focal nodular hyperplasia of the liver in children: a report of 3 new cases. Radiology 137: 171–174

Auh Y H, Rosen A, Rubenstein W A, Engel I A, Whalen J B, Kazam E 1984 CT of the papillary process of the caudate lobe of the liver. American Journal of Roentgenology 142: 535–538

Barnes P A, Thomas J L, Bernadino M E 1981 Pitfalls in the diagnosis of hepatic cysts by CT. Radiology 141: 129–133

Barnett P H, Zerhouni E A, White R I, Siegelman S S 1980 CT in the diagnosis of cavernous hemaniomas of the liver. American Journal of Roentgenology 134: 439–447

Baron R L, Stanley R J, Lee J K T, Koehler R E, Melson G L, Balfe D M, Weyman P J 1982 Prospective comparison of the evaluation of biliary obstruction using computed tomography and ultrasonography. Radiology 145: 91–98

Baron R L, Stanley R J, Lee J K T, Koehler R E, Levitt R G 1983 CT features of biliary obstruction. American Journal of Roentgenology 140: 1173–1178

Becker C D, Hassler H, Terrier F 1984 Preoperative diagnosis of the Mirizzi syndrome: limitations of sonography and CT. American Journal of Roentgenology 143: 591–596

Berland L L, Lawson T L, Foley W D, Melrose B L, Chintapalli K N, Taylor A J 1982 Comparison of pre- and post-contrast CT in hepatic masses. American Journal of Roentgenology 138: 853–858

Berland L L, Lawson T L, Stanley R J 1984 CT appearance of Mirizzi syndrome. Journal of Computer Assisted Tomography 8: 165–166

Berlow M E 1984 Hepatic and splenic fungal microabscesses. Journal of Computer Assisted Tomography 8: 42–45

Bernardino M E, Thomas J L, Barnes P A, Lewis E 1982 Diagnostic approaches to liver and spleen metastases. Radiologic Clinics of North America 20: 469–485

Biello D R, Levitt R G, Siegel B A, Sagel S S, Stanley R J 1978 CT and RN imaging of the liver: a comparative evaluation. Radiology 127: 159–163

Bismuth H 1982 Surgical anatomy and anatomic surgery of the liver. World Journal of Surgery 6: 3–9

Bryan P J, Dinn W M, Grossman Z D, Wistow B W, McAfee J E, Kieffer S A 1977 Correlation of CT, gray scale ultrasonography and radionuclide imaging of the liver in detecting space occupying processes. Radiology 124: 387–393

Burgener F A, Hamlin D J 1983a Contrast enhancement of hepatic tumors in CT: comparison between bolus infusion techniques. American Journal of Roentgenology 140: 291–295

Burgener F A, Hamlin D J 1983b Contrast enhancement of focal hepatic lesions in CT: effect of size and histology. American Journal of Roentgenology 140: 297–301

Choli J D, Olaveni F J L, Casas T F, Zubieta S O 1982 CT in hepatic echinococcosis. American Journal of Roentgenology 139: 699–702

Danielson K S, Sheedy P F, Stephens D H, Hattery R R, LaRusso N F 1983 CT and peritoneoscopy for detection of liver metastases: review of Mayo Clinic experience. Journal of Computer Assisted Tomography 7: 230–240

Doppman J L, Dunnick N R, Girton M, Fauci A S, Popovsky M A 1979 Bile duct cysts secondary to liver infarcts: Report of a case and experimental production by small vessel hepatic artery occlusion. Radiology 130: 1–5

Doppman J L, Dwyer A, Vermess M, Girton M, Sugarbaker P, Miller D, Cornblath M 1984 Segmental hyperlucent defects in the liver. Journal of Computer Assisted Tomography 8: 50–57

Einstein D M, Lapin S A, Ralls P W, Halls J M 1984 Insensitivity of sonography in the detection of choledocholithiasis. American Journal of Roentgenology 142: 725–728

Federle M P, Filly R A, Moss A A 1981 Cystic hepatic neoplasms: complementary role of CT and sonography. American Journal of Roentgenology 136: 345–348

Federle M P, Cello J P, Laing F C, Jeffrey R B 1982 Recurrent pyogenic cholangitis in Asian immigrants. Radiology 143: 151–156

Fishman E K, Farmlett E, Kadiz S, Siegelman S S 1982 CT of benign hepatic tumors. Journal of Computer Assisted Tomography 6: 472–481

Freeny P C, Vimont T R, Barnett D C 1979 Cavernous hemangioma: ultrasonography, arteriography, and CT. Radiology 132: 143–148

Frick M P, Feinberg S B 1982a Biliary cystadenoma. American Journal of Roentgenology 139: 393–395

Frick M, Feinberg S B 1982b Deceptions in localizing extrahepatic right upper quadrant abdominal masses by CT. American Journal of Roentgenology 139: 501–504

Gale M E, Gerzof S G, Robbins A H 1983 Portal architecture: a differential guide to fatty infiltration of the liver on CT. Gastrointestinal Radiology 8: 231–236

Goldberg H I, Filly R A, Korobkin M, Moss A A, Kressel H Y, Callen P W 1978 Capabilities of CT body scanning and ultrasound to demonstrate status of biliary ductal system in patients with jaundice. Radiology 129: 731–73

Goldberg R P 1982 Distal bile duct 'septum'. Radiology 143:142

Greenberg M, Greenberg B M, Rubin P R, Greenberg I M 1982 CT cholangiography. Radiology 144: 363–368

Grossman Z D, Wistow B W, Bryan J P, Dinn W M, McAfee J G, Kieffer S A 1977 RN imaging, CT and gray-scale ultrasonography of the liver: a comparative study. Journal of Nuclear Medicine 18: 327–332

Halversen R A, Korobkin M, Ram P C, Thompson W M 1982 CT appearance of focal fatty infiltration of the liver. American Journal of Roentgenology 139: 277–281

Halversen R A, Korobkin M, Foster W L, Silverman P M, Thompson W M 1984 The variable CT appearance of hepatic abscesses. American Journal of Roentgenology 141: 941–946

Harbin W P, Robert N J, Ferucci J T 1980 Diagnosis of cirrhosis based on regional changes in hepatic morphology. Radiology 135: 273–283

Harell G S, Marshall W H, Breiman R S, Seppi E J 1977 Early experience with the Varian six second body scanner in the diagnosis of hepatobiliary tract disease. Radiology 123: 355–360

Havrilla T R, Reich N E, Haaga J R, Seidelmann E E, Cooperman A M, Alfidi R J 1978 Computed tomography of the gallbladder. American Journal of Roentgenology 130: 1059–1067

Hosoki T, Chatani M, Mori S 1982 Dynamic CT of hepatocellular carcinoma. American Journal of Roentgenology 139: 1099–1106

Hosoki T, Toyonaga Y, Araki Y, Mori S 1984 Dynamic CT of isodense hepatocellular carcinoma. Journal of Computer Assisted Tomography 8: 263–268

Hughes J H, Pollock W J, Schworm C P 1984 Branching pattern in CT scan of mucin producing carcinoma metastasis of the liver. Journal of Computer Assisted Tomography 8: 553–555

Inamoto K, Sagiki K, Yamasaki H, Miura T 1981 CT of hepatoma: effects of portal vein obstruction. American Journal of Roentgenology 136: 349–353

Inamoto K, Tanaka S, Yanakazi H, Okarmoto E 1983a CT in the detection of small hepatocellular carcinomas. Gastrointestinal Radiology 8: 321–326

Inamoto K, Tanaka S, Yamakazi H, Hayashi T, Hidaka H, Miura K 1983b Arterioportal fistula in hepatocellular carcinoma. Journal of Computer Assisted Tomography 7: 151–153

Ishikawa T, Tsukune Y, Ohyama Y, Fujikawa M, Sakiyama K, Fujii M 1980 Venous abnormalities in portal hypertension demonstrated by CT. American Journal of Roentgenology 134: 271–276

Itai Y, Furui S, Araki S, Yashiro N, Tasaka A 1980a CT of cavernous hemangioma of the liver. Radiology 137: 149–155, 1980a.

Itai Y, Araki T, Furai S, Tasaki A, Atomi Y, Kuroda A 1980b CT and ultrasonography in the diagnosis of intrahepatic calculi. Radiology 136: 399–405

Itai Y, Araki T, Yoshikawa K, Furui S, Yashiro N, Tasaka A 1980c CT of gallbladder carcinoma. Radiology 137: 713–718

Itai Y, Moss A A, Goldberg H I 1982 Transient hepatic attenuation difference of lobar or segmental distribution detected by dynamic CT. Radiology 144: 835–839

Itai Y, Araki T, Furui S, Yashiro N, Ohtomo K, Ito M 1983a CT of primary intrahepatic biliary malignancy. Radiology 147: 485–490

Itai Y, Ohtomo K, Araki T, Furiu S, Ico M, Atomi Y 1983b CT and sonography of cavernous hemangioma of the liver. American Journal of Roentgenology 141: 315–320

Jacobson J B, Brodey P A 1981 The tranverse common duct. American Journal of Roentgenology 136: 91–95

Jeffrey R B, Moss A A, Quivey J M, Federle M P, Wara W M 1980 CT of radiation-induced hepatic injury. American Journal of Roentgenology 135: 445–448

Jeffrey R B, Federle M P, Laing F C, Wall S, Rego J, Moss A A 1983 CT of choledocholithiasis. American Journal of Roentgenology 140: 1179–1183

Jenkins M, Golding R H, Cooperberg P L 1983 Sonography and CT of hemorrhage in cholecystitis. American Journal of Roentgenology 140: 1197–1198

Johnson C M, Sheedy P F, Stanson A W, Stephens D H, Hattery R R, Adson M A 1981 CT and angiography of cavernous hemangiomas of the liver. Radiology 138: 115–121

Kane R A, Costello P, Duszlak E 1983 CT in acute cholecystitis: new observations. American Journal of Roentgenology 141: 697–701

Kolbenstvedt A, Kjolseth I, Klepp O, Kolmannskog F 1980 Postirradiation changes of the liver demonstrated by CT. Radiology 135:391

Kunstlinger F, Federle M P, Moss A A, Marks W 1980 CT of hepatocellular carcinoma. American Journal of Roentgenology 134: 431–437

LaBerge J M, Laing F C, Federle M P, Jeffrey R B, Levin R C 1984 Hepatocellular carcinoma: assessment of resectability by CT and ultrasound. Radiology 152: 485–490

Levitt R G, Sagel S S, Stanley R J, Jost R G 1977 Accuracy of computed tomography in the evaluation of the liver and biliary tract. Radiology 124: 123–128

Lewis E, Bernadino M E, Barnes P A, Parvey H R, Soo C-S, Chuang V P 1983 The fatty liver: pitfalls in the CT and angiographic evaluation of metastatic disease. Journal of Computer Assisted Tomography 7: 235–241

Lin G, Hagerstrand I, Lunderquist A 1984a Portal blood supply of liver metastases. American Journal of Roentgenology 143: 53–59

Lin G, Gustafson T, Hagerstrang I, Lunderquist A 1984b CT demonstration of low density ring in liver metastases. Journal of Computer Assisted Tomography 8: 450–452

Lunderquist A, Owman T 1983 Preoperative diagnosis and evaluation of hepatic tumor resectability. Gastrointestinal Radiology 8: 227–230

Magid D, Fishman E K, Siegelman S S 1984 CT of the spleen and liver in sickle cell disease. American Journal of Roentgenology 143: 245–249

Mahony B, Jeffrey R B, Federle M 1982 Spontaneous rupture of hepatic and splenic angiosarcoma demonstrated by CT. American Journal of Roentgenology 138: 965–966

Marchal G J, Baert A L, Wilms G E 1980 CT of noncystic liver lesions: bolus enhancement. American Journal of Roentgenology 135: 57–65

Mathieu D, Grenier P, Larde D, Vasile N 1984 Portal vein involvement in hepatocellular carcinoma: dynamic CT features. Radiology 152: 127–132

Matsui O, Kadoya M, Suzuki M, Inoue K, Itoh H, Ida M, Takashima T 1983 Dynamic sequential CT during arterial portography in the detection of hepatic neoplasms. Radiology 146: 721–727

Mayer D P, Kressel H Y, Soloway R S 1983 Asymptomatic carrier state in Wilson disease. Journal of Computer Assisted Tomography 7: 146–147

Miller D L, Rosenbaum R C, Sugarbaker P H, Vermess M, Willis M, Doppman J L 1983 Detection of hepatic metastases: comparison of EOE-13 CT and scintigraphy. American Journal of Roentgenology 141: 931–951

Miller D L, Schneider P D, Willis M, Vermess M, Doppman J L 1984a Intraarterial administration of EOE-13 for the CT evaluation of hepatic artery infusion chemotherapy. Journal of Computer Assisted Tomography 8: 332–334

Miller D L, Vermess M, Doppman J L, Simon R M, Sugarbaker P H, O'Leary T J, Grimes G, Chatterji D G, Willis M 1984b CT of the liver and spleen with EOE-13. American Journal of Roentgenology 143: 235–243

Mitchell S E, Clark R A 1984 A comparison of CT and sonography in choledocholithiasis. American Journal of Roentgenology 142: 729–733

Mitnick J S, Bosniak M A, Megibow A J, Karpatkin M, Feiner H D, Kertin N, VanNatta F, Pionelli S 1981 CT in B-Thalassemia: iron deposition in the liver, spleen and lymph nodes. American Journal of Roentgenology 36: 1191–1194

Moss A A, Schrump F J, Shnyder P, Korobkin M, Shimshak R R 1979 CT of focal hepatic lesions: a blind clinical evaluation of the effect of contrast enhancement. Radiology 131: 427–430

Moss A A, Dean P B, Axel L, Goldberg H T, Glazer G M, Friedman M A 1982 Dynamic CT of hepatic masses with intravenous and intraarterial contrast material. American Journal of Roentgenology 138: 847–852

Mulhern C B, Arger P H, Coleman B G, Stein G N 1979 Nonuniform attenuation in CT study of the cirrhotic liver. Radiology 132: 399–402

Myracle M R, Stadalhik R C, Blaisdell F W, Farkan J P, Martin P 1981 Segmental biliary obstruction: diagnostic significance of bile duct crowding. American Journal of Roentgenology 137: 169–171

Nakao N, Miura K, Takayasu Y, Wada Y, Miura T 1983 CT angiography in hepatocellular carcinoma. Journal of Computer Assisted Tomography 7: 780–787

Nakayama T, Hiyama Y, Ohnishi K, Tsuchiwa S, Kohno K, Kakajima Y, Okuda K 1983 Arterioportal shunts on dynamic CT. American Journal of Roentgenology 140: 953–957

Nishikawa J, Tasaka A 1981 Lobar attenuation difference of the liver on CT. Radiology 141: 725–728

Pagani J J 1983 Intrahepatic vascular territories shown by CT. Radiology 147: 173–178

Patel S, Sandler C M, Rauschkolb E N, McConnell B J 1982 ^{133}Xe uptake in focal hepatic fat accumulation: CT correlation. American Journal of Roentgenology 138: 541–544

Pedrosa C S, Casanova R, Rodriguez R 1981a CT in jaundice. I: Level. Radiology 139: 627–634

Pedrosa C S, Casanova R, Lezena A H, Fernandez M C 1981b CT in jaundice. II: Cause. Radiology 139: 635–645

Pedrosa C S, Casanova R, de la Torre S, Villacorta J 1983 CT findings in Mirizzi syndrome. Journal of Computer Assisted Tomography 7: 419–425

Peterson I M, Neumann C H 1984 Focal hepatic infarction with bile lake formation. American Journal of Roentgenology 142: 1155–1156

Piekarski J, Goldberg H I, Royal S A, Axel L, Moss A A 1980 Difference between liver and spleen CT numbers in the normal adult. Radiology 137: 727–729

Piers D A, Houthoff H J, Krom R A F, Schuer K H, Sikkeus H, Wites J 1980 Hot spot liver scan in FNH. American Journal of Roentgenology 135: 1289–1292

Prando A, Wallace S, Bernardino M E, Lindell M M 1979 CT arteriography of the liver. Radiology 130: 697–701

Pretorius D H, Gosink B B, Olson L K 1982 CT of the opacified biliary tract: use of calcium Ipodate. American Journal of Roentgenology 138: 1073–1075

Rahn N H, Koehler R E, Weyman P J, Truss C D, Sagel S S, Stanley R J 1983 CT appearance of sclerosing cholangitis. American Journal of Roentgenology 141: 549–552

Renhava R R, Rothenberg J 1981 Spontaneous resolution of oral-contraceptive-associated liver tumor. Journal of Computer Assisted Tomography 5: 102–103

Rogers J V, Mack L A, Freeny P C, Johnson M L, Sones P J 1981 Hepatic focal nodular hyperplasia: angiography, CT, sonography and scintigraphy. American Journal of Roentgenology 137: 983–990

Rossi P, Sposito M, Sumonetti G, Eposato S, Cusimano G 1981 CT diagnosis of Budd-Chiari syndrome. Journal of Computer Assisted Tomography 5: 366–369

Salvo A F, Schiller A, Athanasoulis C, Galdabini J, McKusick K A 1977 Hepatoadenoma and focal nodular hyperplasia: pitfalls in radionuclide imaging. Radiology 125: 451–455

Scott W W, Sanders R C, Siegelman S S 1980 Irregular fatty infiltration of the liver: diagnostic dilemmas. American Journal of Roentgenology 135: 67–71

Shimizu H, Ida M, Takayama S, Seki T, Yoneda M, Nakaya S, Yanago T, Bando B, Sato H, Uchiyama M, Okumura T, Miura S, Fujisawa M 1981 CT in obstructive biliary disease. Radiology 138: 411–416

Silverman P M, Ram P C, Korobkin M 1983 CT appearance of abdominal thorotrast deposition and thorotrast-induced angiosarcoma of the liver. Journal of Computer Assisted Tomography 7: 655–658

Smathers R L, Lee J K T, Heiken J P 1984 Differentiation of complicated cholecystitis from gallbladder carcinoma by CT. American Journal of Roentgenology 143: 255–259

Somer K, Kivisaari L, Standertkjold-Nordenstam C G et al 1984 Contrast-enhanced CT of the gallbladder in acute pancreatitis. Gastrointestinal Radiology 9: 31–34

Sorenson K W, Glazer G M, Francis I R 1982 Diagnosis of cystic ectasia of intrahepatic bile ducts by CT. Journal of Computer Assisted Tomography 6: 486–489

Subramanyam B R, Balthozar E J, Naidich D P 1983 Ruptured hydrated cyst with biliary obstruction: diagnosis by sonography and CT. Gastrointestinal Radiology 8: 341–343

Suzuki M, Takashima T, Kunaki H, Uogishi M, Isobi T, Matsuda Y, Kamno S, Ushitami K, Fuchuh K 1983 CT diagnosis of common bile duct stone. Gastrointestinal Radiology 8: 327–331

Takashima T, Matsui O, Suguki M, Ida M 1982 Diagnosis and screening of small hepatocellular carcinomas. Radiology 145: 635–638

Tenier F, Becker C D, Stoller C, Triller J K 1984 CT in complicated cholecystitis. Journal of Computer Assisted Tomography 8: 58–62

Thorsen M K, Quiroz F, Lawson T L, Smith D F, Foley W D, Stewart E T 1984 Primary biliary carcinoma: CT evaluation. Radiology 152: 479–483

Tsukamoto Y, Nakata H, Kimoto T, Noda T, Kuroda Y, Harataki J 1984 CT and angiography of peliosis hepatis. American Journal of Roentgenology 142: 539–540

Vermess M, Adamson R H, Doppman J L, Girton M 1977 CT demonstration of hepatic tumor with the aid of intravenous iodinated fat emulsion. Radiology 135: 711–715

Vermess M, Doppman J L, Sugarbaker P H, Fisher R I, O'Leary T J, Chatterji D C, Grimes G, Adamson R H, Willis M, Edwards B K 1982 CT of the liver and spleen with intravenous lipoid contrast material. American Journal of Roentgenology 138: 1063–1071

Weiner S N, Koenigsberg M, Morehouse H, Hoffman J 1984 Sonography and CT in the diagnosis of carcinoma of the gallbladder. American Journal of Roentgenology 142: 735–739

Yang P J, Glazer G M, Baverman R A 1983 Budd-Chiari syndrome: CT and ultrasonographic findings. Journal of Computer Assisted Tomography 7: 148–150

17

G. M. Bydder

Nuclear magnetic resonance imaging

INTRODUCTION

Nuclear magnetic resonance (NMR) was first demonstrated in 1946 (Bloch et al 1946, Purcell et al 1946). It is a phenomenon whereby certain nuclei emit or absorb electromagnetic radiation when exposed to particular magnetic fields. The technique has been used widely in analytical chemistry because the spectrum of the absorbed or emitted electromagnetic radiation provides information about molecular structure.

The medical application of NMR was developed in the 1950s and 1960s by Erik Odeblad, a Swedish physicist and gynaecologist, who used NMR spectroscopy to study human red cells, mucus myometrium and other tissues (Odeblad 1966, Odeblad & Lindstrom 1955). Subsequent studies in animals revealed abnormal NMR properties in malignant tumours (Damadian 1971, Weisman et al 1972).

The production of images with NMR required the use of graduated magnetic fields, a technique which was suggested by Damadian (1972), Mansfield & Gannell (1973) and Lauterbur (1973). The first published image was produced by Lauterbur in 1973. Human images were first produced in 1977 (Damadian et al 1977, Hinshaw et al 1977, Mansfield et al 1977). In 1980 workers at the University of Aberdeen (Mallard 1981), the University of Nottingham (Hawkes et al 1980) and the Central Research Laboratories of EMI (Hounsfield 1980) had functioning imaging systems in the laboratory phase and by 1981 these groups had each placed systems in clinically accessible sites and begun programmes of clinical evaluation. Soon after other groups in Boston (Buonanno et al 1980), Cleveland (Alfidi et al 1982), San Francisco (Crooks et al 1982) and Eindhoven (Luiten 1981) began clinical programmes and now there are over 150 NMR machines installed or ordered worldwide.

The initial clinical results indicate that NMR is likely to play a useful role in the diagnosis of neurological disorders but its role in the body is much less certain.

TECHNIQUE

All NMR machines are constructed around a large magnet which provides a uniform static magnetic field (Fig. 17.1). In the presence of this field hydrogen nuclei behave like tiny bar magnets. Their magnetization is aligned with the static magnetic field producing a net proton magnetization in the long axis of the patient. Additional perpendicular magnetic pulses are used to rotate the nuclear magnetization into the transverse plane following which it recovers or relaxes back to its original position.

During this recovery or relaxation phase the component of the magnetization in the long axis of the patient recovers to its original magnitude exponentially. This recovery is called longitudinal or 'spin-lattice' relaxation and is characterized by the time constant T_1. Relaxation of the magnetization in the transverse direction back to its original value of zero is termed transverse relaxation or 'spin-spin' relaxation and is characterized by the time constant T_2.

As the magnetization relaxes it induces an electrical signal in a receiver coil which surrounds the patient. It is this signal which is used to reconstruct the image.

Both T_1 and T_2 are sensitive indices of the local nuclear and magnetic environment. By using a variety of pulse sequences it is possible to produce images with varying dependence on T_1 and T_2.

There are two major types of pulse sequence: inversion-recovery (IR) where the image contrast largely depends on changes in T_1 and spin-echo (SE) where the image contrast largely depends on changes in T_2.

IMAGE INTERPRETATION

This has been largely empirical. Lesion identification has depended on the fact that in many pathological processes both T_1 and T_2 are increased. The increase in T_1 generally

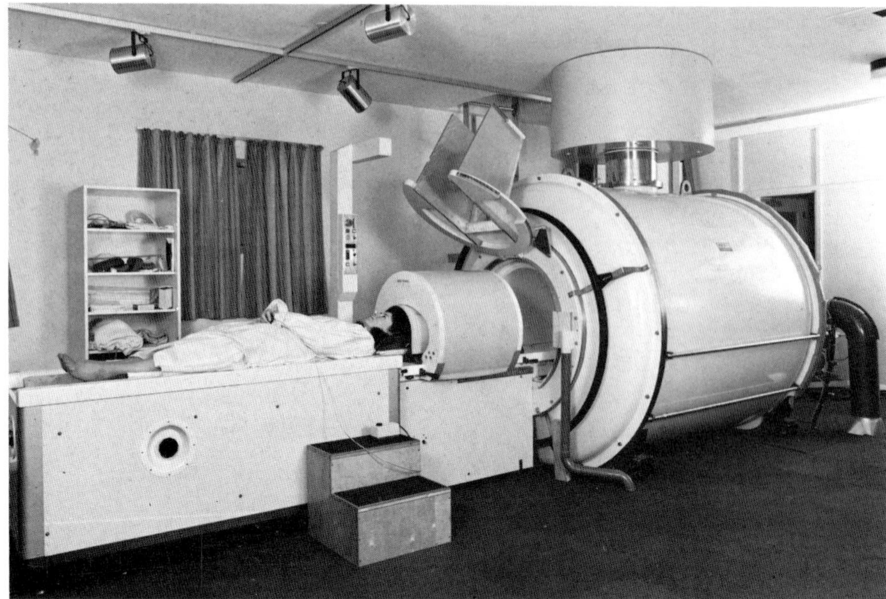

Fig. 17.1 An NMR imaging machine. The patient is placed within the large cylindrical magnet

produces a dark appearance on IR images and the increase in T_2 produces a light appearance on SE images.

The change in T_1 and T_2 may be 200% or 300% but is relatively non-specific. Specificity is usually derived from localization, associated radiological features and the clinical context.

THE LIVER

In routine practice IR and SE images are used. These take several minutes to produce (although it is possible to obtain 8 to 16 of them simultaneously) resulting in blurring or loss of definition due to respiratory motion. This movement can also be regarded as an effective increase in slice thickness with the result that tissue planes are often not as clearly defined as with X-ray computerized tomography (CT).

Inversion recovery images of the liver display the parenchyma as light with blood vessels and bile ducts dark. Spin-echo images show the liver parenchyma as darker.

Metastases are identified either by their dark appearance (due to an increase in T_1) on IR images (Fig. 17.2a) or as a lighter area on SE images due to an increase in T_2 (Fig. 17.2b). It is often necessary to refer to more than one type of image to ensure that an apparent lesion is not a normal vascular structure.

Several groups have reported accuracy of detection of metastases with NMR as similar to that with CT and ultrasound (Smith et al 1981, Doyle et al 1982, Margulis et al 1983) although these results have been more in the nature of pilot studies than rigorous comparisons. In four

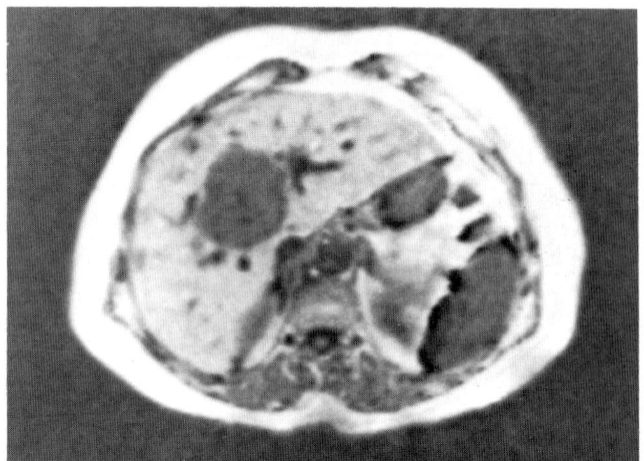

a

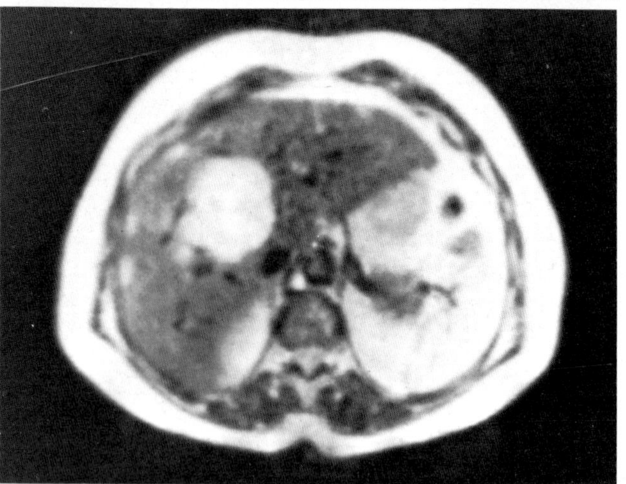

b

Fig. 17.2 Metastasis of the liver: inversion recovery (a) and spin echo (b) images. The liver parenchyma is light in (a) with the tumour dark. The reverse is seen in (b).

instances we have identified metastases not seen with X-ray CT. The lack of artefact from the air/fluid interface in the stomach is an advantage over CT in detecting metastases within the left lobe of the liver.

Primary tumours are also readily detected (Fig. 17.3) although the increase in T_1 and T_2 is generally less than that seen with metastases. The situation may also be complicated by the fact that many hepatomas occur in the liver of patients who also have cirrhosis. Since both these diseases tend to increase T_1 and T_2, contrast between the tumour and the surrounding parenchyma may be small.

Hepatic and subphrenic abscesses are readily identified (Fig. 17.4). Although the features are not specific, generalized changes have been seen in infective hepatitis.

Increasing iron content within the liver results in a decrease in T_1 and T_2 as a result of its paramagnetic effect. With very large increases in iron the relaxation times of the liver may become so short that signal is no longer detectable giving a dark appearance with both IR and SE sequences (Fig. 17.5).

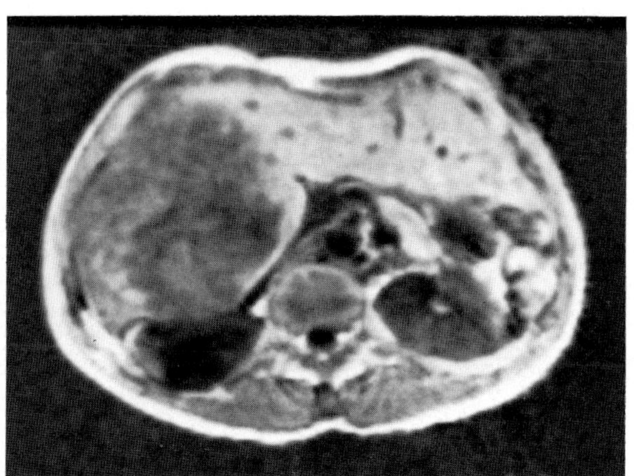

Fig. 17.3 Hepatoma: inversion recovery image. The tumour appears dark

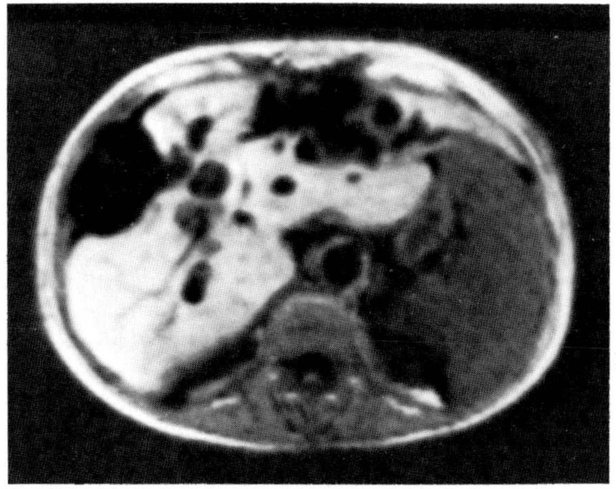

Fig. 17.4 Subphrenic and hepatic abscesses: inversion recovery image. The abscesses appear dark

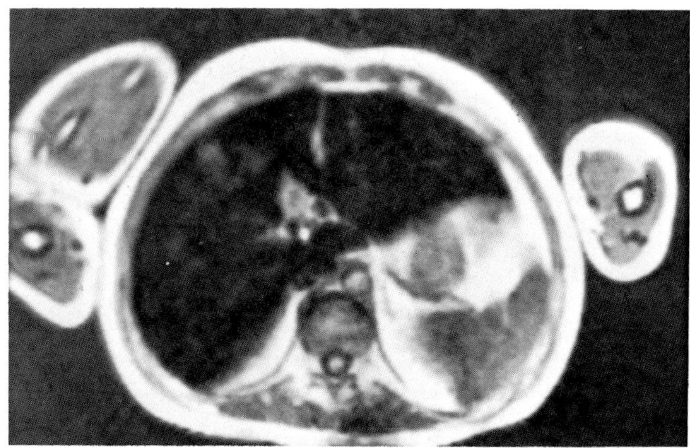

Fig. 17.5 Iron overload: spin echo image. The liver appears unusually dark

In a variety of other conditions the T_1 of the liver may be non-specifically measured. These include chronic active hepatitis and the Budd-Chiari syndrome.

It is fair to say that after the initial wave of enthusiasm progress in imaging the liver has reached a plateau and is unlikely to evolve further without new approaches to the technical problems caused by motion, the NMR properties of fat, the unusual NMR properties of the liver and other factors (see later).

GALLBLADDER

The gallbladder and biliary system are readily seen. In the fasting state, layering is seen within the gallbladder as a result of the accumulation of bile salts and it has been suggested that this may form the basis for a test of biliary function (Hricak et al 1983).

THE PANCREAS

The normal pancreas has a relatively short T_1 and appears light on IR images.

Large pancreatic tumours have been identified with NMR (Smith et al 1982). Problems are experienced in distinguishing pancreatic tumours from the duodenum and other loops of bowel which usually have a long T_1 and T_2. There are also difficulties in distinguishing tumours from fat with the usual SE sequences. It is likely that oral contrast agents will be necessary in NMR in a way analogous to CT in order to circumvent the problem of distinguishing tumours from loops of bowel.

Acute pancreatitis and pseudocysts have also been identified in a similar way to X-ray CT (Fig. 17.6).

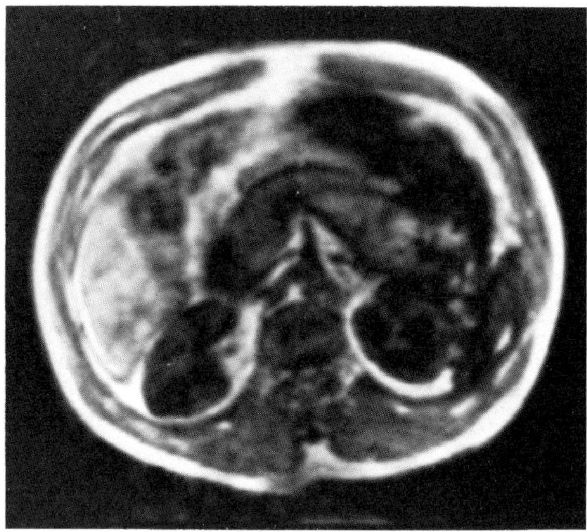

Fig. 17.6 Acute pancreatitis: inversion recovery image. The pancreas and adjacent tissue appear dark

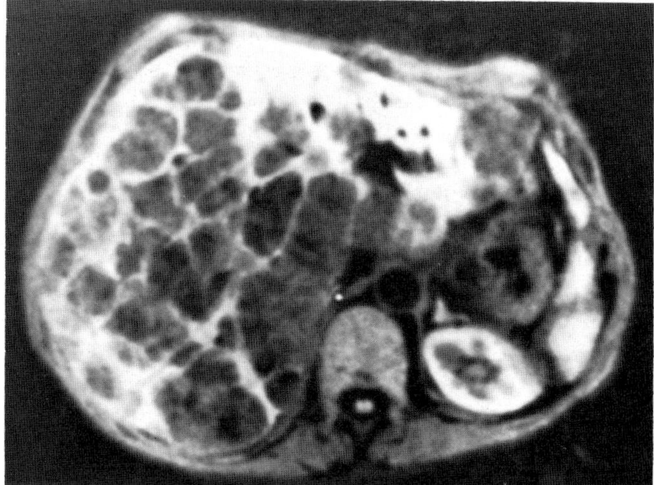

a

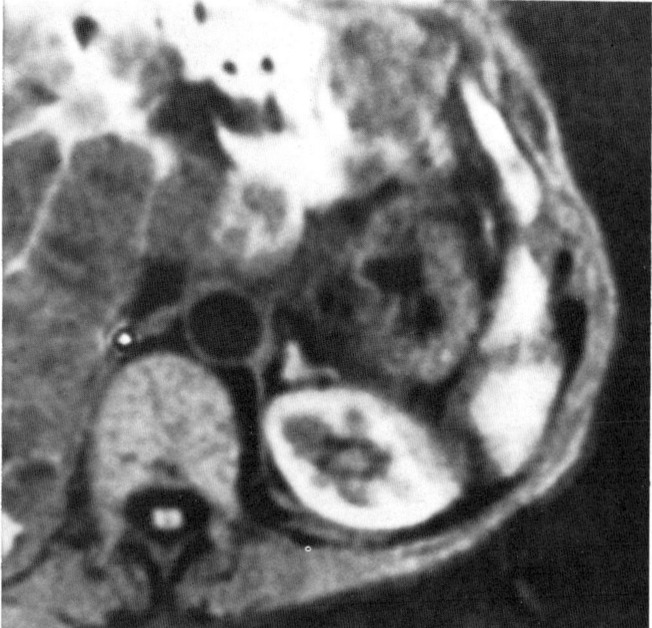

b

Fig. 17.7 Multiple metastases: inversion recovery image on high resolution matrix. The tumours appear dark (a) and the left adrenal gland is seen in the enlargement (b)

ADRENAL GLAND

The normal adrenal gland can be seen without difficulty and hypertrophy, benign tumours and metastases have been recognized (Moon et al 1983). No systematic studies have yet been conducted to compare the accuracy of CT and NMR in diagnosis.

PRESENT DEVELOPMENTS

There are major technical problems yet to be resolved before NMR makes a major contribution to imaging within the abdomen and the problems which are listed below are the principal focus of attention for current research.

The need for higher resolution imaging

To date imaging of the abdomen has been performed with a low resolution (64 × 64 or 128 × 128) matrix which is a limitation in relation to X-ray CT which is basically a 256 × 256 matrix (Fig. 17.7). In order to obtain this with NMR, machine performance must be improved and the principal technique we have employed is improved receiver coil design (Bydder et al 1985). Higher resolution imaging produces constraints on other facets of machine performance and in particular increases the T_2 dependence of sequences which renders conventional IR pulse sequences less useful.

The development of sensitive pulse sequences for body imaging

The T_2 of the liver and other body soft tissues is about half that of the brain. As a result pulse sequences which are useful in the brain may produce ambiguous results when used in the abdomen and care is required to avoid this (Fig. 17.8). One approach to this problem has been the use of short T_1 inversion recovery (STIR) sequences where the T_1 dependent and T_2 dependent phases of the sequence add to image contrast (Bydder & Young 1985). With this type of sequence the signal from fat may be completely suppressed which avoids ambiguity with lesions which also have an increased T_2. It is also possible to use the double inversion recovery sequence to simultaneously suppress the signal from fat and other fluids such as bile ducts, bowel contents and urine.

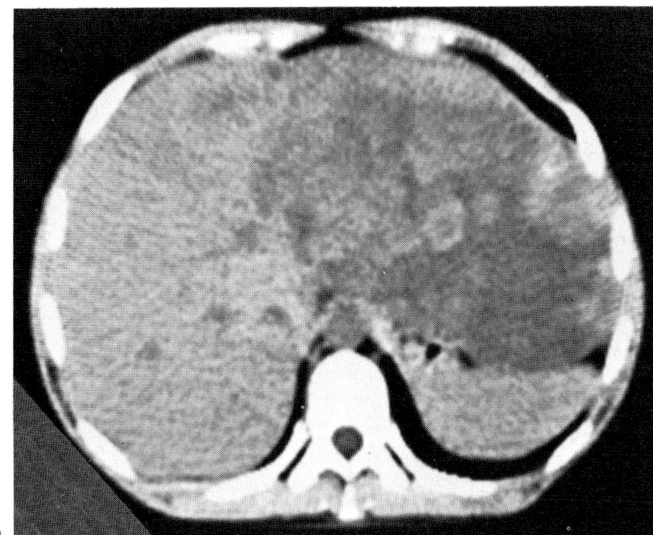

Fig. 17.8 Hepatoma: CT (a) and spin echo (b) images (high resolution). The tumour appears more extensive in (b)

The need for control of movement artefact

The STIR sequence mentioned above has the advantage of reducing the signal from fat and thus decreasing the characteristic ghost artefact commonly seen on NMR images. It also reduces the echo times for equivalent soft tissue contrast which has the result of reducing the vulnerability of the sequence to motion.

Two other techniques are also important; one is using an alternating 90° pulse in the spin-echo sequence and the second is respiratory ordered phase encoding (ROPE) (Bailes et al 1985). This latter technique partially controls respiratory ghost artefacts and respiratory blur without requiring extra time for the examination.

The need for bowel labelling

The STIR sequence has the advantage that bowel signal is high and may be increased by the ingestion of water. This is probably the simplest approach to identifying bowel. Paramagnetic contrast agents have also been used but they have not so far proved to be consistently effective.

Intravenous contrast agents

While most lesions produce an increase in T_1 and T_2, paramagnetic contrast agents produce the reverse effect and this may lead to difficulty since the lesions are detected by virtue of their prolonged relaxation times (Fig. 17.9) (Carr et al 1984). It is possible to use rapid saturation recovery sequences to overcome this difficulty and there may well be a useful role for contrast agents.

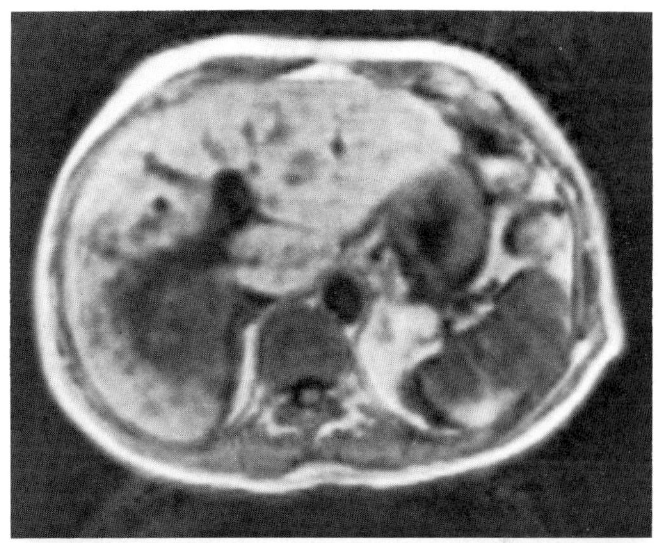

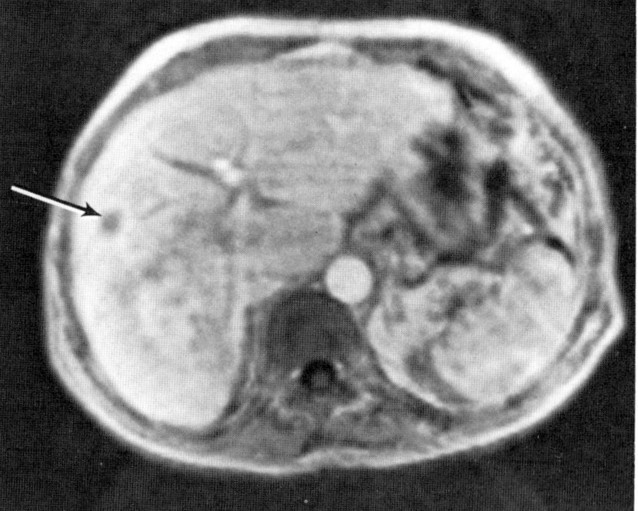

Fig. 17.9 Multiple metastases: inversion recovery image before (a) and after (b) intravenous contrast enhancement. One metastasis (arrow) is better seen after enhancement

CONCLUSIONS

Insufficient clinical results are yet available to determine the likely clinical role of NMR in imaging of the abdomen, and its role may well be determined by the degree of success with which the various technical problems are overcome. As with CT, the implications of this new technique in studies of the brain are more obvious than in those of the abdomen.

There are other new NMR techniques which have reached the laboratory stage but have not yet been implimented in clinical practice which may be important. These include sodium imaging of the body and spectroscopy.

Whether NMR will remain largely of research interest or will play a useful role in clinical practice remains to be seen but it will certainly be the subject of active investigation in the next few years.

REFERENCES

Alfidi R J, Haaga J R, El Yousef S J et al 1982 Preliminary experimental results in humans and animals with a superconducting, whole-body nuclear magnetic resonance scanner. Radiology 143: 1175–1181

Bailes D R, Gilderdale D J, Bydder G M, Collins A G, Firmin D N 1985 Respiratory ordered phase encoding (ROPE): a method for reducing respiratory motion artefact in magnetic resonance imaging. Journal of Computer Assisted Tomography 9: 835–838

Bloch F, Hansen W W, Packard H 1946 The nuclear induction experiment. Physical Review 70: 474–485

Buonanno F S, Pykett I L, Kistler J P, et al 1982 Cranial anatomy and detection of ischaemic stroke in the cat by nuclear magnetic resonance imaging. Radiology 143: 187–193

Bydder G M, Young I R 1985 MRI: Clinical use of the inversion recovery sequence. Journal of Computer Assisted Tomography (in 9: 659–675

Bydder G M, Curati W L, Gadian D G, et al 1985 Use of closely coupled receiver coils in MRI: practical aspects. Journal of Computer Assisted Tomography 9: 987–996

Carr D H, Brown J, Bydder G M, et al 1984 Gadolinium-DTPA as a contrast agent in MRI: initial clinical experience in 20 patients. American Journal of Roentgenology 143: 215–224

Crooks L, Arakawa M, Hoenninger J, et al 1982 Nuclear magnetic resonance whole-body imager operating at 3.5 K gauss. Radiology 143: 169–174

Damadian R 1971 Tumor detection by nuclear magnetic resonance. Science 171: 1151–1153

Damadian R 1972 Apparatus and method for detecting cancer in tissue. US Patent No. 3789832

Damadian R, Goldsmith M, Minkoff L 1977 NMR in cancer: XVI. Sonar image of the liver in the human body. Physiological Chemistry and Physics 9: 97–100

Doyle F H, Pennock J M, Banks L M, et al 1982 Nuclear magnetic resonance (NMR) imaging of the liver: initial experience. American Journal of Roentgenology 138: 193–200

Hawkes R C, Holland G N, Moore W S, Worthington B S 1980 Nuclear magnetic resonance (NMR) tomography of the brain: a preliminary clinical assessment with demonstration of pathology. Journal of Computer Assisted Tomography 4: 577–586

Hinshaw W S, Bottomley P A, Holland G N 1977 Radiographic thin section image of the human wrist by nuclear magnetic resonance. Nature 270: 722–723

Hounsfield G N 1980 Computed medical imaging. Journal of Computer Assisted Tomography 4: 665–674

Hricak H, Gilly R A, Margulis A R, et al 1983 Nuclear magnetic resonance imaging of the gall bladder. Radiology 147: 481–484

Lauterbur P C 1973 Image formation by induced local interactions: examples employing nuclear magnetic resonance. Nature 242: 190–191

Luiten A L 1981 Nuclear magnetic resonance: an introduction. Medica Mundi 26: 98–101

Mallard J 1981 The noes have it! Do they? British Journal of Radiology 54: 831–849

Mansfield P, Maudsley A A 1971 Medical imaging by nuclear magnetic resonance. British Journal of Radiology 60: 188–194

Mansfield P, Grannell P K 1973 NMR 'diffraction' in solids. Journal of Physics C: Solid State Physics 6: L422

Margulis A R, Moss A A, Crooks L E, Kaufman L 1983 Nuclear magnetic resonance in the diagnosis of tumors of the liver. Seminars of Roentgenology 18: 123–126

Moon K L, Hricak H, Crooks L E, et al 1983 Nuclear magnetic resonance of the adrenal gland: a preliminary report. Radiology 147: 155–160

Moore W S, Holland G N, Kreel L 1980 The NMR CAT scanner: a new look at the brain. Computed Tomography 4: 1–7

Odeblad E 1966 Micro-NMR in high permanent magnetic fields. Acta Obstetrica et Gynecologica Scandinavica 45 (Suppl 2): 1–188

Odeblad E, Lindstrom G 1955 Some preliminary observations on the proton magnetic resonance in biologic samples. Acta Radiologica (Stockholm) 43: 469–476

Purcell E M, Torrey H C, Pound R V 1946 Resonance absorption by nuclear magnetic moments in a solid. Physical Review 69:37

Smith F W, Mallard J R, Reid A, Hutchison J M S 1981 Nuclear magnetic resonance tomographic imaging of liver disease. Lancet i: 963–966

Smith F W, Reid A, Hutchison J M S, Mallard J R 1982 Nuclear magnetic resonance imaging of the pancreas. Radiology 142: 677–680

Weisman I D, Bennett L H, Maxwell L R, et al 1972 Recognition of cancer in vivo by nuclear magnetic resonance. Science 179: 1288–1290

18

D. J. Nolan

Plain radiographs, oral cholecystography and intravenous cholangiography

The more widespread use of ultrasound, endoscopic retrograde cholangiopancreatography (ERCP), radionuclide studies and computerized tomography (CT) has resulted in a significant decrease in the number of requests for conventional oral cholecystography and intravenous cholangiography. Plain radiographic examination remains, however, very important in the investigation of patients presenting acutely with suspected biliary tract disease. Even in centres where the newer imaging techniques are available, investigation by oral cholecystography and intravenous cholangiography is still indicated in certain circumstances. The techniques are, of course, widely used in departments and hospitals with little or no access to the newer imaging modalities.

PLAIN RADIOGRAPHS

The initial investigation for patients presenting acutely with suspected biliary tract disease should be plain abdominal radiographs. Radio-opaque calculi may be shown in the gallbladder area. The presence of opacities consistent with radio-opaque gallstones is not always proof of biliary tract disease but it helps focus attention on the biliary tract. Identification of calculi in the common bile duct in a patient with biliary colic or jaundice makes the diagnosis fairly certain and appropriate further investigations and treatment can be planned.

Acute emphysematous cholecystitis is an uncommon disease of the gallbladder (Fig. 18.1) characterized by the presence of intraluminal or intramural gas, often with associated gas in the pericholecystic tissues (Esguerra-Gomez & Arango 1963, Baddeley, Nolan & Salmon 1978). Early radiological examination is desirable as plain radiographs remain the most reliable method of confirming the diagnosis. The signs vary according to the stage of the disease. The presence of gas in the lumen of the gallbladder is shown as a homogeneous gas shadow in the right upper quadrant, conforming to the shape of the gallbladder in the supine view (Blum & Stagg 1963, Esguerra-Gomez & Arango 1963, Baddeley et al 1978). The intraluminal gas may be seen as a gas/fluid level in the upright view (May & Strong 1971, Baddeley et al 1978). Calculi may also be seen in the gallbladder. In the second stage of the disease, intramural gas may be seen as a thin, concentric well-demarcated ring or gaseous collar surrounding part or all of the gallbladder. There may be gas in both the lumen and the wall of the gallbladder. Pericholecystic abscesses may have developed and appear as multiple small radiolucent gas shadows disseminated in the perivesicular tissues (Esguerra-Gomez & Arango 1963).

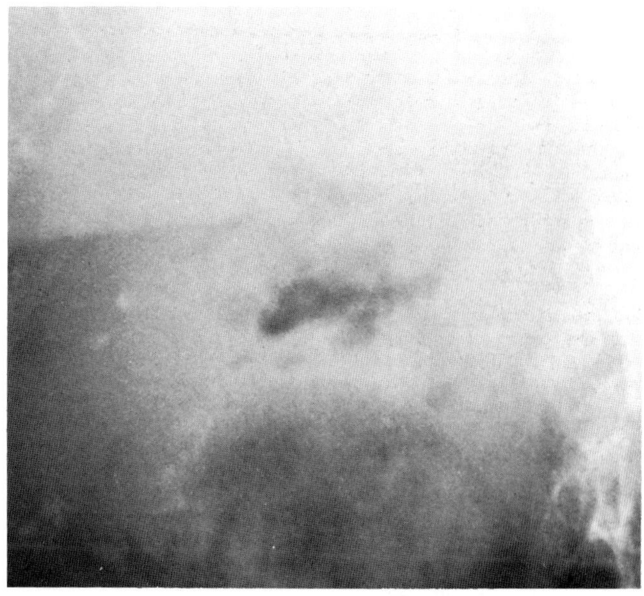

Fig. 18.1 Acute emphysematous cholecystitis. Multiple small round radiolucent gas shadows are seen in the gallbladder area

Gallstone ileus (Ch. 61), mechanical intestinal obstruction caused by impaction of a gallstone in the lumen of the intestine, shows characteristic radiological appearances (Fig. 18.2). Plain abdominal radiographs are of major importance in establishing the diagnosis (Day & Marks 1975). Obstruction results from a gallstone entering the gastrointestinal tract, usually through a cholecystenteric

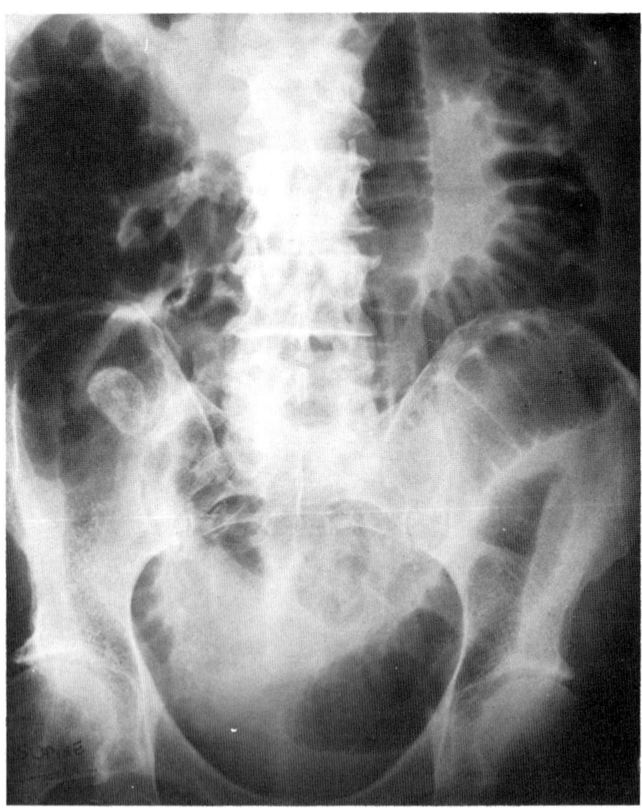

Fig. 18.2 Gallstone ileus. A plain radiograph shows dilated gas-filled loops of small intestine with a calculus in the terminal ileum. Gas is also seen outlining much of the colon. There was no evidence of gas in the biliary tree. A barium enema, performed about 12 hours later, showed the calculus to have passed as far as the transverse colon. The patient subsequently passed the calculus

fistula between the gallbladder and duodenum. The usual site of impaction is the terminal ileum. Calculi less than 2.5 cm pass spontaneously in most cases. One or all of the following signs may be seen: air in the biliary tree, visualization of the obstructing calculus, change in position of a previously observed calculus, or possibly evidence of intestinal obstruction (Rigler, Borman & Noble 1941). The signs are not always present; air in the biliary tree was reported in 30% and evidence of intestinal obstruction in 50% of 34 patients reviewed by Day and Marks (1975). Barium studies may demonstrate the cholecystenteric fistula or the obstructing calculus may be visualized directly or indirectly in about 35% of cases (Day & Marks 1975). If there is doubt about the presence of air in the biliary tree, a localized plain radiograph centred on the right upper quadrant of the abdomen should be taken (Rigler et al 1941).

When air is seen in the biliary tree in a patient who has not presented with emphysematous cholecystitis or gallstone ileus and has no history of previous sphincterotomy or choledochoenterostomy other possible causes have to be considered (McSherry, Stubenbord & Glen, 1969) (Ch. 61). Cholecystocolic fistulae may develop due to calculous disease of the gallbladder. Primary carcinoma of the biliary tract, stomach, duodenum and colon may lead to fistulous communication with the gallbladder (McSherry et al 1969). Peptic ulcers of the anterior wall of the duodenum and Crohn's disease may invade the biliary tract and result in fistula formation. Choledochobronchial fistulae may result from trauma, and amoebic or hydatid disease of the liver (McSherry et al 1969). Gas contrast studies, performed following the ingestion of carbonated drinks, may be used to assess the anastomosis in patients with biliary-intestinal anastomoses (Williams, Wilding & Kay 1976).

Plain radiographs and radiographs of the abdomen taken during urographic and gastrointestinal contrast examinations may reveal unsuspected biliary tract abnormalities, such as gallbladder calculi. Extensive calcification of the gallbladder wall, known as the 'porcelain gallbladder', is an uncommon but easily recognized finding (Fig. 18.3). The aetiology is unknown but possibly is related to chronic cystic duct obstruction causing large quantities of calcium carbonate to pass from the wall of the gallbladder into its lumen (Phemister, Rowbridge & Rudisill 1931, Cornell & Clarke 1959). Calcification of the gallbladder wall results and there is also an increase of calcium salts in the luminal contents of the gallbladder. Calculi are usually present in the gallbladder, often with a calculus obstructing the cystic duct. Radiologically the calcification is seen as a linear, flaky or plaque-like calcification taking the shape of the gallbladder (Ochsner & Carrera 1963, Baddeley, Nolan

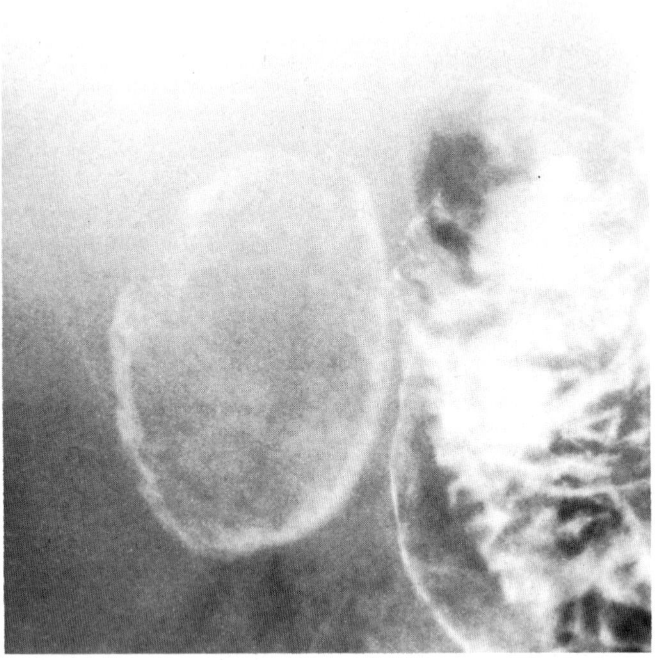

Fig. 18.3 Calcification of the gallbladder. The typical appearances of the so-called 'porcelain gallbladder' are seen on a radiograph taken during a barium meal examination.

& Salmon 1978). Occasionally the calcification may form a round shadow similar to a calcified renal mass (Baddeley et al 1978). Carcinoma of the gallbladder occurs so frequently in association with calcification of the gallbladder wall that it warrants a prophylactic cholecystectomy even when the patient is asymptomatic (Berk, Armbuster & Saltzstein 1973) (Ch. 64).

The presence of radio-opaque bile, 'limy bile' or 'milk of calcium bile', is another condition which may be recognized on plain abdominal radiographs (Fig. 18.4). This results from obstruction of the cystic duct, usually by a calculus, causing large quantities of calcium carbonate to pass into the lumen of the gallbladder. Limy bile is nearly always associated with gallbladder calculi. Spontaneous passage of limy bile and associated gallstones is not uncommon and the limy bile may disappear completely (Holden & Turner 1972).

ORAL CHOLECYSTOGRAPHY

Indications

The main indication for performing oral cholecystography in the past was in the detection of gallbladder calculi and this remains the case in centres where ultrasound is not available. Even in large centres with ultrasound facilities it may be more efficient to use oral cholecystography as the initial procedure to detect gallbladder calculi. Good ultrasound examinations are very operator dependent while oral cholecystography can be performed satisfactorily by radiographers or radiologists-in-training and the images are easily interpreted. In centres with very limited facilities, oral cholecystography may be performed satisfactorily using basic radiographic equipment. Oral cholecystography remains invaluable for investigating patients following unsatisfactory or equivocal ultrasound examination.

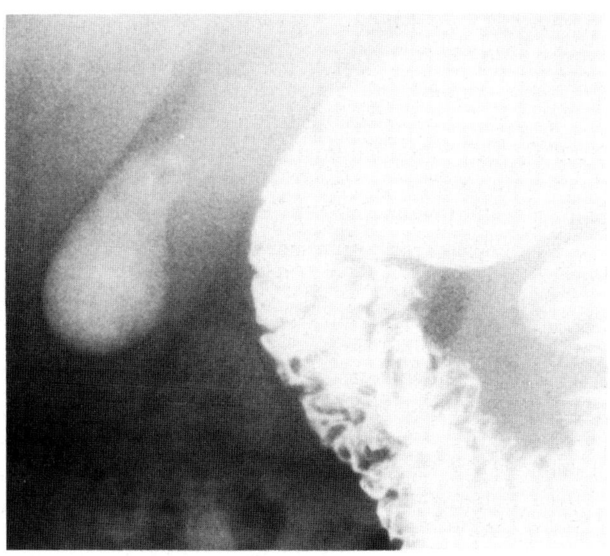

Fig. 18.4 Limy bile. The gallbladder is opaque and contains calculi. Barium is seen outlining the duodenal loop

Contrast medium

Biliary contrast agents are, like urographic contrast media, basically substituted triiodobenzoic acid compounds (Lasser 1966). The biliary contrast media differ in that they are primarily excreted by the liver, tend to have a higher molecular weight and do not contain a side chain at the number 5 position on the benzene ring. They bind strongly to serum albumin enabling them to be excreted by the liver while the urographic contrast media have completely substituted rings with little or no conductive binding to albumin. The oral contrast media are lipid soluble and absorbed by diffusion across the intestinal mucosa. An active transport process transfers the media from the blood through the liver to the bile. In the gallbladder the contrast medium becomes concentrated due to reabsorption of water by the gallbladder mucosa (Berk et al 1974). Oral contrast media in current use include iopanoic acid (Telepaque®), sodium ipodate (Biloptin®; Oragrafin Sodium®), calcium ipodate (Solu-Biloptin®; Oragrafin Calcium®), sodium tyropanoate (Bilopaque®) and iocetamic acid (Cholebrin®).

Nausea, diarrhoea, abdominal pain and dysuria may be side-effects of oral cholecystographic agents; skin reaction and vomiting occur infrequently (White & Fisher 1962). Mudge in 1971 stated that there had been about 50 cases of renal failure following the use of oral cholecystographic contrast media, a large number of whom had bunamiodyl (Orabilex®), a contrast agent no longer in use. Renal failure resulting from contrast agents in current use occurred after large doses of iopanoic acid (Telepaque) (Canales et al 1969). This side effect is more likely if the patient is dehydrated, if there is hepatobiliary disease of increasing severity or if there has been a recent intravenous cholangiogram.

Contraindications

Contraindications to oral cholecystography include sensitivity to iodine, combined severe liver and renal disease and pregnancy. The examination should not be performed within seven days of an intravenous cholangiographic examination.

Examination technique

Contrast ingestion

Ideally, a plain radiograph of the gallbladder area should be taken prior to ingestion of the contrast medium but, as this would require an extra visit by the patient to the department, it is usually impractical. If a preliminary plain radiograph is not taken it is possible that gallbladder calculi of the same density as the contrast medium may be missed at oral cholecystography (Gough 1977).

The oral contrast medium, a dose of 3.0 gm, is taken on the evening preceding the examination. A meal containing fat taken before the contrast medium significantly increases the subsequent gallbladder opacification and the diagnostic yield of the examination (Stanley et al 1974). No further solid food is taken until after the examination on the following day. The patient should avoid smoking before oral cholecystography (Owen 1983). Fluids that do not contain fat are encouraged to prevent nephrotoxicity from the uricouric action of the oral cholecystographic agents (Mudge 1971). Water can be taken in large quantities without any reduction in the quality of gallbladder opacification (Bainton et al 1973).

Radiographic examination

The patient attends the radiology department for the examination; optimum visualization of the gallbladder occurs 14–19 hours after contrast ingestion. Good radiographic technique with careful centring and collimation is essential. The first view taken is usually a prone oblique to show the gallbladder clear of the spine. This is followed by views taken with the patient erect. All radiographic views, but particularly the erect ones, may be taken using fluoroscopy for positioning and also compression to obtain views of the gallbladder free from overlying gas shadows. When the initial radiographs have been viewed a fatty meal is ingested by the patient and 20–40 minutes later a final radiograph is taken. The after-fat radiograph is essential for the diagnosis of adenomyomatosis and cholesterolosis and it is sometimes helpful for detecting small calculi (Harvey, Thwe & Low-Beer 1976). Cholecystokinin, given as an intravenous injection, may be used instead of fat to make the gallbladder contract. In most cases, however, this is of no advantage as there is marked variation in the degree of contraction making it unreliable for indicating the presence of acalculus cholecystitis (Davis et al 1982). If the gallbladder is poorly opacified it may be necessary to perform tomography. Opacification of the bile ducts with non-filling of the gallbladder indicates the presence of gallbladder disease (McNulty 1975). Tomography may prove useful for demonstrating the bile ducts in such cases.

The gallbladder may fail to opacify because the contrast medium is trapped in a pharyngeal or oesophageal diverticulum. Obstructive lesions such as achalasia of the cardia, carcinoma of the oesophagus, pyloric stenosis and vomiting may prevent the contrast medium from reaching the small intestine. Malabsorption and diarrhoea are sometimes mentioned as reasons for non-opacification of the gallbladder at oral cholecystography. It has been shown, however, that such patients absorb sufficient contrast medium to produce gallbladder opacification (Low-Beer, Heaton & Roylance 1972). Failure of visualization may be caused by poor liver function or bile duct obstruction. A radiograph of the whole abdomen should always be taken if the gallbladder is not visualized on radiographs of the right upper quadrant. In the past, patients with non-visualization of the gallbladder were investigated again following a double dose of contrast medium. A double dose rarely results in gallbladder visualization if a single dose has failed (Wise 1966, Achkar et al 1969) and it is more likely to cause renal insufficiency (Grainger 1972, Berk 1973).

Conditions shown as oral cholecystography

Cholelithiasis

Gallbladder calculi are far the most common abnormal finding at oral cholecystography (Fig. 18.5a & b). They are usually seen as radiolucent filling defects in the contrast filled gallbladder. Some may be calcified and prove to be of greater density than the contrast medium. In the erect position gallstones may form a horizontal layer in the radiopaque bile (Fig. 18.5b).

Developmental anomalies

Oral cholecystography is particularly useful for demonstrating developmental anomalies such as the so-called intrahepatic gallbladder, double-gallbladder, or transverse septa of the body of the gallbladder 'Phrygian cap' deformity. Occasionally the gallbladder may lie under the left lobe of the liver.

Adenomyomatosis

Adenomyomatosis can be diagnosed best by oral cholecystography. Three main varieties of adenomyomatosis are recognized: generalized, segmental and fundal (Jutras & Levesque 1966). In the generalized type a ring of dilated Rokitansky-Aschoff sinuses is seen surrounding the gallbladder (Fig. 18.6). These 'intramural diverticula' may be the only evidence of adenomyomatosis and are often shown well on radiographs taken after fat. Segmental adenomyomatosis may produce gallbladder strictures which are often single (Fig. 18.7), but may be multiple (Colquhoun 1961). A combination of Rokitansky-Aschoff sinuses and stricture formation may occur at the same site. The fundal type of adenomyomatosis is less common and is shown as a small filling defect caused by a sessile mass. An irregular outline and multiple parallel or interlacing translucent lines may be seen due to intramural projections of the thickened gallbladder wall (Cynn, Forbes & Schreiber 1974). Tiny marginal indentations and transverse striations have also been described (Jutras & Levesque 1966). Calculi are frequently present in the gallbladder in association with adenomyomatosis.

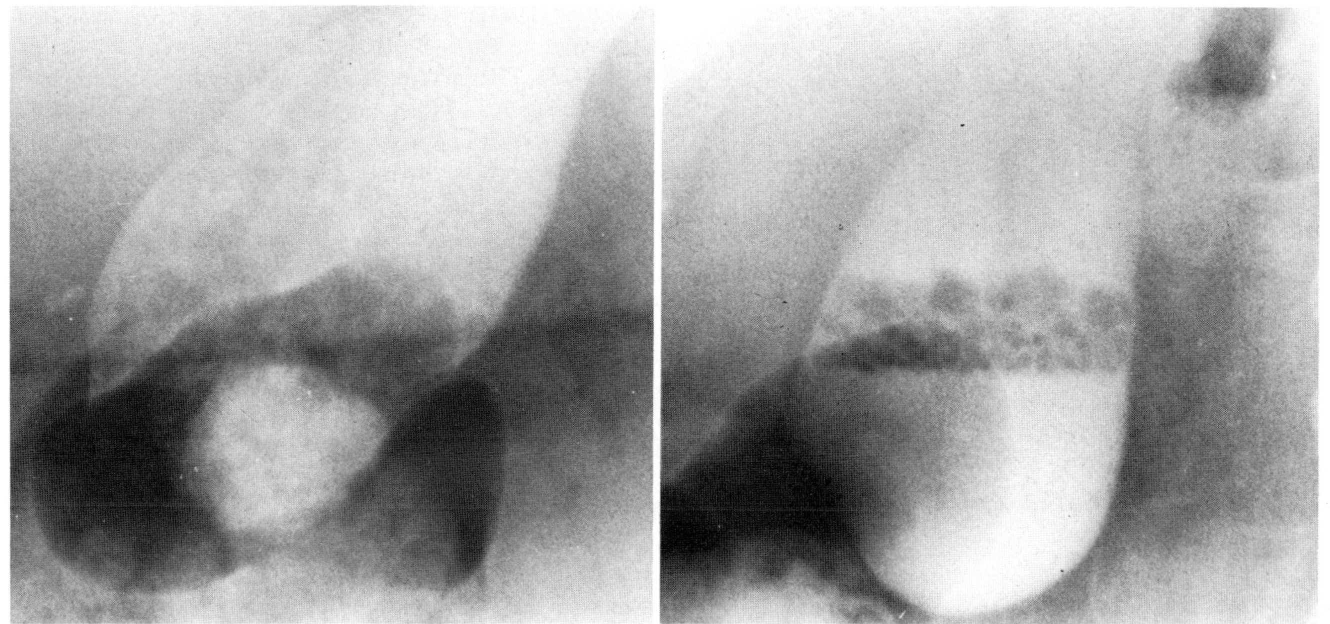

Fig. 18.5 Cholelithiasis. a. Multiple faint radiolucent filling defects are seen in the gallbladder in a view taken with the patient horizontal. b. An upright view clearly shows the calculi forming a layer in the contrast-filled gallbladder

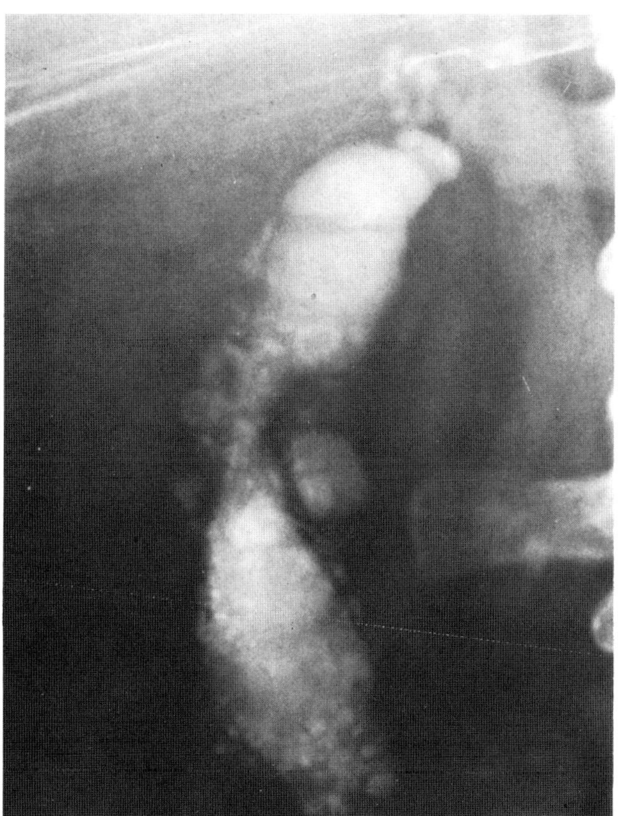

Fig. 18.6 Adenomyomatosis. Dilated Rokitansky-Aschoff sinuses are outlined with contrast medium at oral cholecystography on a radiograph taken after fat. Reproduced with permission from Mr M H Gough and Dr J C MacLarnon

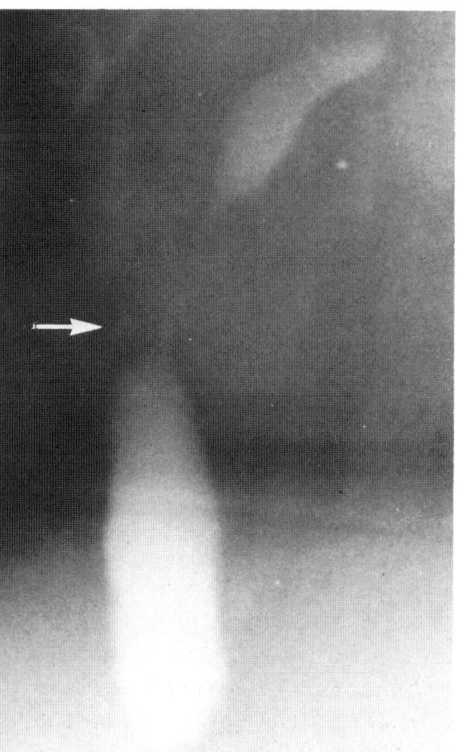

Fig. 18.7 Adenomyomatosis. A stricture of the body of the gallbladder is seen at oral cholecystography. A Rokitansky-Aschoff sinus is seen outlined with contrast medium (arrow)

Cholesterosis

Two types of cholesterosis of the gallbladder may be seen at oral cholecystography: diffuse and localized (Feldman & Feldman 1954). In the diffuse forms radiographs of the gallbladder appear normal and oral cholecystography is usually unhelpful. The localized form, however, shows lipid deposits heaped up to form small polypoid filling defects, usually around the neck of the gallbladder.

Polyps

Benign gallbladder polyps are seen as single or multiple small filling defects in the gallbladder (Fig. 18.8). Unlike calculi they do not change position during the examination. Ultrasound is also reliable for diagnosing benign gallbladder polyps and should be used if there is doubt about the diagnosis.

INTRAVENOUS CHOLANGIOGRAPHY

Intravenous cholangiography plays a lesser role in the investigation of the biliary tract since the introduction of fine-needle percutaneous transhepatic cholangiography (PTC), endoscopic retrograde cholangiography (ERCP), ultrasound and radionuclide studies. Good quality intravenous cholangiography, however, still has a definite role to play in the investigation of suspected bile duct disease.

Contrast medium

The contrast agents available include meglumine ioglycamate (Biligram), meglumine iotroxate (Biloscopin) and meglumine iodoxamate (Endobil). The ioglycamate molecule contains two iodinated benzene rings linked by diglycolic acid. These contrast agents are freely soluble in aqueous solution, which enables their use for intravascular injection. Like the oral cholecystographic agents they bind to serum protein and are preferentially excreted in the bile (Lasser et al 1962). Ioglycamate is transferred against the gradient of a low serum level through the liver to a much higher level in the bile by an active transport process (Fisher 1965, Rosati & Schiantarelli 1970).

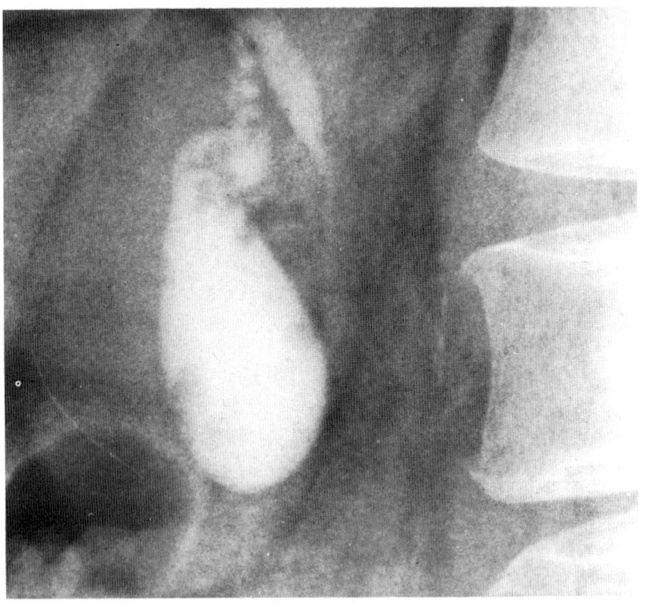

Fig. 18.8 Gallbladder polyps. A view of the gallbladder taken at oral cholecystography shows a number of small filling defects. These did not change position in different projections

Indications

Intravenous cholangiography is indicated in the investigation of patients who have had a previous cholecystectomy and present with symptoms suggestive of recurrent bile duct disease although ERCP is regarded as the best first investigation by Hany (Ch. 25 & 55). In the past, the technique was used in the diagnosis of acute cholecystitis when active surgical intervention was being considered. HIDA radionuclide studies and ultrasound have now replaced it for the investigation of acute cholecystitis in most centres. If these techniques are not available intravenous cholangiography may prove helpful. Biliary obstruction by the roundworm, *Ascaris lumbricoides*, a frequent problem in parts of Europe, Asia, Africa and the Americas, can be diagnosed using intravenous cholangiography with tomography (Cremin 1969). Failed oral cholecystography, a frequent indication for intravenous cholangiography in the past, is no longer an indication unless it is not practical to refer the patient for ultrasound. Likewise, the intravenous contrast examination is no longer indicated in suspected choledochal cyst or in the assessment of bile ducts in patients with chronic pancreatitis.

Contraindications

Combined severe liver and renal disease (Wise 1967), known sensitivity to iodine, and monoclonal IgM paraproteinaemia (Waldenstrom's macroglobulinaemia) (Bauer, Tragl & Bauer, 1974) must be regarded as absolute contraindications for the use of intravenous biliary contrast agents. Relative contraindications include a history of allergy to contrast media or drugs, asthma, pregnancy, and patients in whom hypotension would be dangerous, such as those with ischaemic heart disease (Baddeley, Nolan & Salmon 1978). Intravenous cholangiography should not be carried out within 48 hours of oral cholecystography. Severe reactions are common if this time lapse is not allowed and the biliary tract fails to opacify in a large number of patients (Finby & Blasberg, 1964, Moss, Nelson & Amberg 1973). An interval of at least one week should be allowed between oral cholecystography and intravenous cholangiography.

Examination technique

Preparation

Bowel preparation is recommended on the two days before the examination to ensure that detail of the biliary tree is not obscured by overlying gas and faecal shadows. The patient should be well hydrated and have a light fat-free breakfast on the morning of the examination (Martinez et al 1971, Kreel 1973, Hatfield & Wise 1976).

Radiographic examination

The contrast medium is given as a slow injection over 5–10 minutes or an infusion over 30–60 minutes. Patients experience fewer unpleasant side effects when the contrast medium is given by slow infusion (Darnborough & Geffen 1966, Nolan & Gibson 1970) and the concentration of contrast medium in the bile is increased (Whitney & Bell 1972, Bell et al 1975). The slow infusion technique is the author's method of choice.

Strict attention to radiographic detail is essential in order to obtain consistently good results (Hatfield & Wise 1976), with accurate positioning, centring, collimation and a low kilovoltage (50–70 kV) (Hatfield & Wise 1976). The patient is placed supine and rotated slightly into the right posterior oblique position before a preliminary radiograph of the right upper quadrant is obtained. The contrast medium is then infused. Further radiographs are taken at the end of the infusion and at 15 minute intervals thereafter. Tomography should be performed as soon as the bile ducts are visualized (Fig. 18.9). This completes the examination in patients who have had a previous cholecystectomy.

The examination will take longer in patients with an intact gallbladder as the gallbladder fills slowly with contrast medium over about one to three hours. A technique similar to that for oral cholecystography should then be used to examine the gallbladder. The contrast medium may stratify in the gallbladder at intravenous cholangiography resulting in calculi being missed on views taken after the infusion. When stratification occurs, calculi are identified best on radiographs obtained at 24 hours (Ounjian & Laing 1976).

Delayed visualization of the biliary system occurs in hepatocellular and obstructive jaundice and radiographs may need to be taken for up to eight hours after the infusion (Burgener & Fisher 1975).

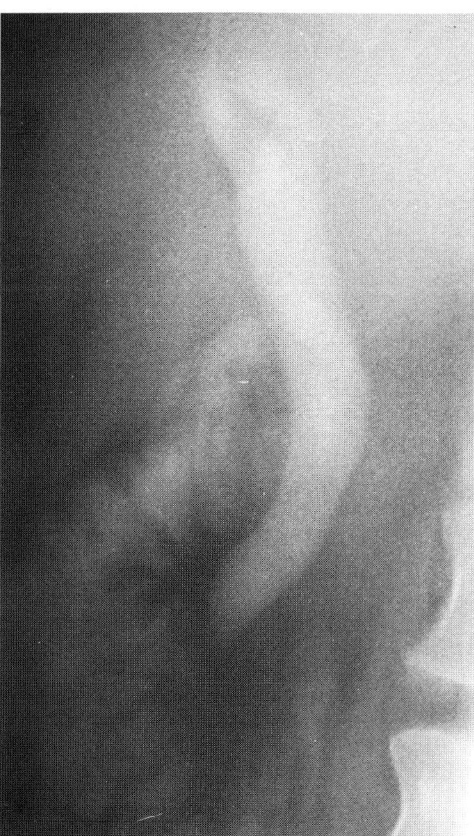

Fig. 18.9 Normal intravenous cholangiogram. A tomographic cut shows the bile ducts slightly dilated in a patient who had a previous cholecystectomy. No filling defects are seen and contrast medium has passed freely into the duodenum. The cystic duct remnant can be identified joining the medial side of the common hepatic duct to form the common bile duct

Conditions shown at intravenous cholangiography

Calculi are by far the most frequent abnormal finding at

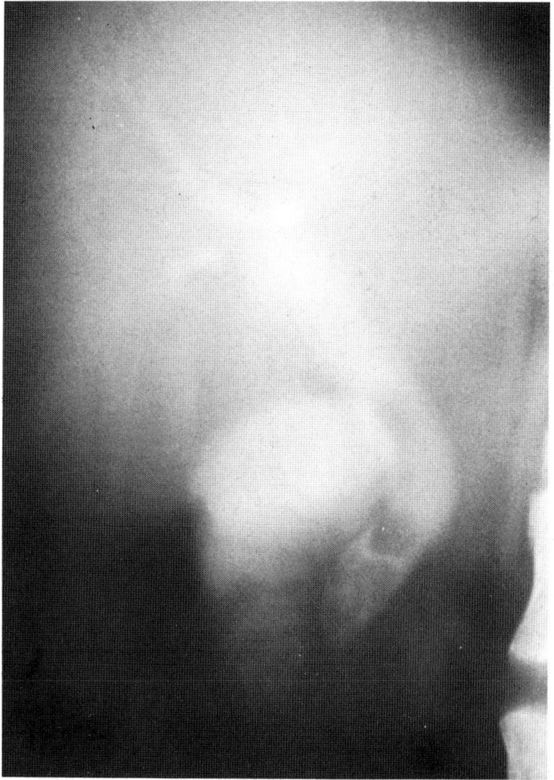

Fig. 18.10 Choledocholithiasis. Intravenous cholangiography with tomography shows a number of calculi in the common bile duct

intravenous cholangiography. They are shown as single or multiple, round or faceted, usually radiolucent, filling defects in the common bile duct (Fig. 18.10). Occasionally there may be a large number of calculi completely filling the common hepatic and common bile duct. Roundworms are a frequent finding in patients who live in tropical countries where infestation is common (Cywes & Krige 1963, Cremin 1969). Foreign bodies such as T-tube remnants may be seen in the bile ducts at intravenous cholangiography.

Cholecystitis can be confirmed or regarded as highly probable when the bile ducts are visualized but the gallbladder is not (Johnson, McLaren & Weens 1960, Becker et al 1970). It is necessary to take a radiograph as late as four hours after the infusion before concluding that no gallbladder filling has occurred. Narrowing with medial and upward displacement of the bile duct by the acutely inflamed gallbladder may be demonstrated at intravenous cholangiography in patients with acute cholecystitis (Wise 1962, Nolan & Espiner 1972). HIDA radionuclide scanning is an easier and less time-consuming procedure than intravenous cholangiography for showing non-filling of the gallbladder in suspected acute cholecystitis. Intravenous cholangiography has been used in the past for clearly demonstrating choledochal cysts (Jones & Olbourne 1973) but most cases can now be confidently diagnosed using ultrasound.

REFERENCES

Achkar E, Norton R A, Siber F J 1969 The fate of the nonvisualised gallbladder. American Journal of Digestive Diseases 14: 80–83

Baddeley H, Nolan D J, Salmon P R 1978 Radiological Atlas of Biliary and Pancreatic Disease. HM+M, Aylesbury

Bainton D, Davies G T, Evans K T, Gravelle I H, Abernathy M 1973 A comparison of two preparation regimens for oral cholecystography. Clinical Radiology 24: 381–384

Bauer K, Tragl K H, Bauer G 1974 Intravasale denaturterung von plasmoproteinen bei einer IgM-paraproteinamie, ausgelost durch ein intravenos verabreichtes lebergangiges Rontgenkontrastmittel. Wiener Klinische Wochenschrift 86: 766–769

Becker J, Borgstrom S, Fajers C-M, Saltzman G-F 1970 Acute Cholegraphy. Acta Chirurgica Scandinavica 136: 197–202

Bell G D, Fayadh M H, Frank J, Smith P L C, Kelsey-Fry I 1975 Intravenous cholangiography, is technique important? Gut 16: 841

Berk R N 1973 Radiology of the gallbladder and bile ducts. Surgical Clinics of North America 53: 973–1005

Berk R N, Armburster T G, Saltzstein S L 1973 Carcinoma in the porcelain gallbladder. Radiology 106: 29–31

Berk R N, Loeb P M, Goldberger L E, Sokoloff J 1974 Oral cholecystography with iopanoic acid. New England Journal of Medicine 290: 204–210

Blum L, Stagg A 1963 Emphysematous cholecystitis. American Journal of Roentgenology 89: 840–846

Burgener F A, Fischer H W 1975 Intravenous cholangiography in jaundice. Letter. Lancet 1: 274–275

Canales C O, Smith G H, Robinson J C, Remmers A R Jr, Sarles H E 1969 Acute renal failure after the administration of iopanoic acid as a cholecystographic agent. New England Journal of Medicine 281: 89–91

Colquhoun J 1961 Adenomyomatosis of the gallbladder. British Journal of Radiology 34: 101–112

Cornell C M, Clarke R 1959 Various calcifications involving the gallbladder. Annals of Surgery 149: 267–272

Cremin B J 1969 Biliary parasites. British Journal of Radiology 42: 506–508

Cynn W S, Forbes T, Schreiber M 1974 Unusual radiographic manifestations of adenomyomatosis of the gallbladder. Radiology 113: 577–579

Cywes S, Krige H 1963 Intravenous cholangiography and tomography in the diagnosis of biliary ascariasis. Radiologia Clinica (Basel) 14: 271–272

Darnborough A, Geffen N 1966 Drip infusion cholangiography. British Journal of Radiology 39: 827–832

Davis G B, Berk R N, Scheible F W et al 1982 Cholecystokinin cholecystography, sonography and scintigraphy; detection of chronic acalculous cholecystitis. American Journal of Roentgenology 139: 1117–1121

Day E A, Marks C 1975 Gallstone ileus. Review of the literature and presentation of thirty-four new cases. American Journal of Surgery 129: 552–558

Esguerra-Gomez G, Arango O 1963 Emphysematous cholecystitis. A report of seven cases. Radiology 80: 369–373

Feldman M, Feldman M Jr 1954 Cholesterosis of gall bladder; autopsy study of 165 cases. Gastroenterology 27: 641–648

Finby N, Blasberg G 1964 A note on the blocking of hepatic excretion during cholangiographic study. Gastroenterology 46: 276–277

Fischer H W 1965 The excretion of iodipamide. Relation of bile and urine outputs to dose. Radiology 84: 483–491

Gough M H 1977 'The cholecystogram is normal', but ---. British Medical Journal 1: 960–962

Grainger R G 1972 Renal toxicity of radiological contrast media. British Medical Bulletin 28: 191–195

Harvey I C, Thwe M, Low-Beer T S 1976 The value of the fatty meal in oral cholecystography. Clinical Radiology 27: 117–121

Hatfield P M, Wise R E 1976 Radiology of the gallbladder and bile ducts. Williams & Wilkins, Baltimore

Holden W S, Turner M J 1972 Disappearing limy bile. Clinical Radiology 23: 500–507

Johnson H C Jr, McLaren J R, Weens H S 1960 Intravenous cholangiography in the differential diagnosis of acute cholecystitis. Radiology 74: 790–797

Jones C A, Olbourne N A 1973 Choledochal cyst with associated cholelithiasis diagnosed by infusion cholangiography and tomography. British Journal of Radiology 46: 711–714

Jutras J A, Levesque H-P 1966 Adenomyoma and adenomyomatosis of the gallbladder. Radiologic Clinics of North America 4: 483–500

Kreel L 1973 Radiology of the biliary system. Clinics in Gastroenterology 2: 185–212

Lasser E C 1966 Pharmacodynamics of biliary contrast media. Radiologic Clinics of North America 4: 511–519

Lasser E C, Farr R S, Fugimagari T, Tripp W N 1962 The significance of protein binding of contrast media in roentgen diagnosis. American Journal of Roentgenology 87: 338–360

Low-Beer T S, Heaton K W, Roylance J 1972 Oral cholecystography in patients with small bowel disease. British Journal of Radiology 45: 427–428

Martinez L O, Viamonte M, Gassman P, Boudet L 1971 Present status of intravenous cholangiography. American Journal of Roentgenology 113: 10–15

May R E, Strong R 1971 Acute emphysematous cholecystitis. British Journal of Surgery 58: 453–458

McNulty J 1975 Oral cholecystography: a sign of gallbladder disease. Letter. British Medical Journal 1: 38–39

McSherry C K, Stubenbord W T, Glenn F 1969 The significance of air in the biliary system and liver. Surgery, Gynecology and Obstetrics 128: 49–61

Moss A A, Nelson J, Amberg J 1973 Intravenous cholangiography. American Journal of Roentgenology 117: 406–411

Mudge G H 1971 Uricouric action of cholecystographic agents. A possible factor in nephrotoxicity. New England Journal of Medicine 284: 929–933

Nolan D J, Gibson M J 1970 Improvements in intravenous cholangiography. British Journal of Radiology 43: 652–657

Nolan D J, Espiner H J 1972 Compression of the common bile duct in acute cholecystitis. British Journal of Radiology 45: 821–824

Ochsner S F, Carrera G M 1963 Calcification of the gallbladder ('Porcelain Gallbladder'). American Journal of Roentgenology 89: 847–853

Ounjian Z J, Laing F C 1976 Stratification in the gallbladder on intravenous cholangiography. Radiology 121: 591–593

Owen J P 1983 The biliary tract. In: Whitehouse G H, Worthington B. Techniques in diagnostic radiology. Blackwell, Oxford 60–86

Phemister D B, Rowbridge A G, Rudisill H Jr 1931 Cholecystitis and cystic duct obstruction; significance in formation of gallstones rich in calcium carbonate and in calcification of the gallbladder wall: preliminary report. Journal of the American Medical Association 97: 1843–1847

Rigler L G, Borman C N, Noble J F 1941 Gallstone obstruction: pathogenesis and roentgen manifestations. Journal of the American Medical Association 117: 1753–1759

Rosati G, Schiantarelli P 1970 Biliary excretion of contrast media. Investigative Radiology 5: 232–243

Stanley R J, Melson G L, Cubillo E, Hesker A E 1974 A comparison of three cholecystographic agents. A double-blind study with and without a prior fatty meal. Radiology 112: 513–517

White W W, Fischer H W 1962 A double blind study of Oragrafin and Telepaque. American Journal of Roentgenology 87: 745–748

Whitney B, Bell G D 1972 Single bolus injection or slow infusion for intravenous cholangiography? — measurement of iodipamide (Biligrafin) excretion using a rhesus monkey model. British Journal of Radiology 45: 891–895

Williams J E, Wilding R P, Kay D N 1976 Gas contrast studies of the biliary tract following reconstructive surgery. Clinical Radiology 27: 249–254

Wise R E 1962 Intravenous cholangiography. Thomas, Springfield, Illinois

Wise R E 1966 Current concepts of intravenous cholangiography. Radiologic Clinics of North America 4: 521–523

Wise R E 1967 Intravenous cholangiography. Postgraduate Medicine 41: 113–117

19

R. N. Gibson

Percutaneous transhepatic cholangiography

The most complete and detailed radiographic demonstration of the biliary system (cholangiography) is obtained when contrast medium is introduced directly into a bile duct (direct cholangiography). This can be performed preoperatively, intraoperatively, or via tubes placed in the biliary tract either surgically, radiologically or endoscopically. The preoperative techniques are percutaneous transhepatic cholangiography (PTC) and endoscopic retrograde cholangiography (ERC) (see Ch. 20).

HISTORY

The first PTC is generally attributed to Huard and Do-Xun-Hop in 1937 (Wechsler & Wechsler 1975). Prior to this cholecysto-cholangiography had been performed by percutaneous puncture of the gallbladder in 1921 by Burckhardt and Muller. Later workers also used gallbladder puncture, either laparoscopically (Lee 1942, Keil & Landis 1951), or percutaneously (Karaki 1956). However, the risk of bile leakage and the limitations of the examination in the presence of cystic duct or common hepatic duct obstruction led to the abandonment of this technique in favour of percutaneous transhepatic puncture of intrahepatic bile ducts (Carter & Saypol 1952, Nurick et al 1953, Kidd 1956). Various techniques were developed using either an anterior, lateral or posterior puncture with a sheathed or unsheathed needle of up to 1.5 mm external diameter. However, the still significant risk of biliary peritonitis and haemorrhage meant that many patients underwent laparotomy immediately following PTC (Seldinger 1966). The incidence of these complications has been substantially reduced by the popularization of the PTC technique developed at Chiba University (Ohto & Tushiya 1969, Okuda et al 1974) and at the same time the rate of duct opacification has significantly improved.

TECHNIQUE

The examination should be performed on a tilting fluoroscopic table as a sterile procedure, using local anaesthesia and usually intravenous sedation and analgesia. A preliminary clotting profile and platelet count should be near normal. Because of the high incidence of bacterial colonization of obstructed biliary systems (Keighley 1977) broad-spectrum antibiotics should be administered before and after the procedure; our current regimen is 2 g piperacillin intra-muscularly one hour before and six hours after PTC. A 22 gauge (0.71 mm) flexible Chiba needle is inserted into the liver usually from the right side, just anterior to the mid-axillary line and inferior to the visible lateral costophrenic recess. The needle is directed medially and slightly craniad (Fig. 19.1) avoiding puncture of the gallbladder and extrahepatic bile ducts. Successful entry of a duct is identified by aspiration of bile or on injection of contrast medium. Ultrasonographic guidance can also be used for duct puncture (Ohto et al 1980) and this is

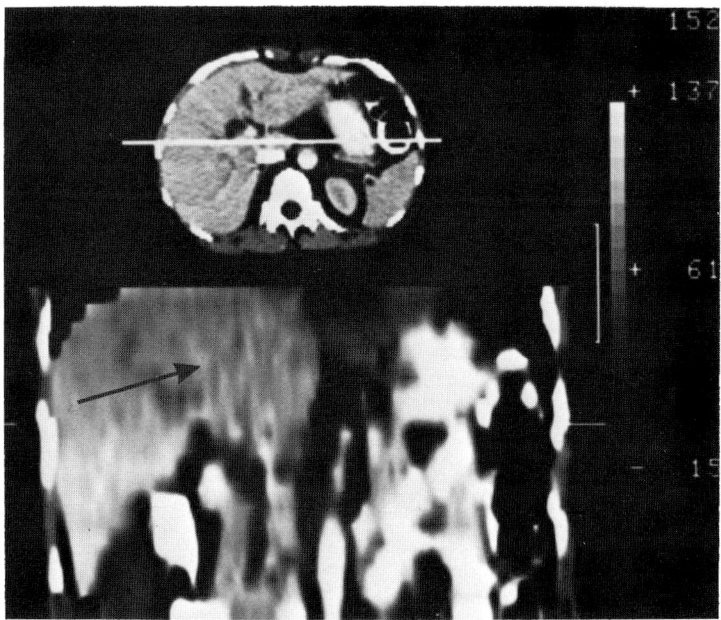

Fig. 19.1 Transverse CT scan and coronal reconstruction through optimal plane for needle entry with needle orientation shown (arrow)

particularly useful if there is marked distortion of normal liver anatomy such as can occur following hepatic resection or in the presence of lobar atrophy. In an obstructed system as much bile as possible is aspirated and in all cases samples should be sent for bacteriology and cytology studies. Water-soluble contrast medium of 200–300 mg/ml iodine concentration is injected to fill as much of the intrahepatic and extrahepatic biliary system as possible without using undue pressure. Contrast has a higher specific gravity than bile and so, by tilting the fluoroscopic table and rotating the patient, more of the biliary system can be opacified with a low injection pressure. Radiographs should then be taken in multiple projections and occasionally tomography will be helpful. In cases of near-complete duct obstruction delayed views may show more distal ducts and determine the length of the stricture or the presence of a second stricture. Delayed views can also be helpful for assessing the degree of obstruction produced by a partial stricture. The patient should be observed closely for 24 hours afterwards as most complications will occur in this time.

COMPLICATONS

Although the incidence of complications of PTC has fallen significantly since the introduction of the fine needle technique (Harbin et al 1980) major complications do occasionally occur (Table 19.1). The commonest significant complications are bile leakage, sepsis and haemorrhage. The first two are almost unknown in the absence of ductal obstruction. Bile leakage is often asymptomatic but can result in peritonitis or subphrenic abscess (Harbin et al 1980). With routine antibiotic cover septic complications are usually minor in the form of transient fever but occasionally this is accompanied by hypotension and, rarely, endotoxic shock. Bacteraemia and, more importantly, endotoxaemia, occur via cholangiovenous reflux (Hultborn et al 1962) or biliary-venous fistulae created by the needle.

When major haemorrhage occurs it is usually either into the bile ducts (haemobilia) or intraperitoneal. Haemobilia may be recognized at the time of cholangiography by the presence of intraductal cast-like filling defects produced by blood clot (Fig. 19.2). Extensive clot should alert one to the possibility of continuing haemorrhage.

Arterioportal fistulae occurred in 3.8% of patients

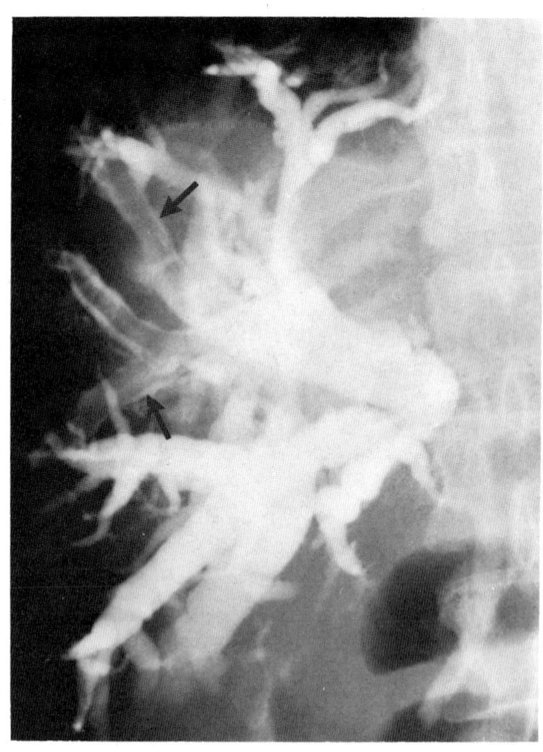

Fig. 19.2 Haemobilia indicated by cast-like filling defects (arrows) in several ducts

Table 19.1

	No. of patients	Bile leak.	Sepsis	Haemorrhage	Miscellaneous	Deaths	Overall complication rate (%)
Ariyama 1983	1149	2	0	0	0	0	0.2
Gibbons et al 1983	123	6	3	0	1	0	9
Harbin et al 1980	2005	29	28	7	5	4	3.6
Kreek & Balint 1980	322	6	10	13	4	3	10.2
Kocher & Mousseau 1979	94	0	2	—	—	0	2.1
Mueller et al 1980	450	2	?	?	?	1	4.8
Michel & Adda 1980	3472	62	24	7	17	4	6
Nagasue & Inokuchi 1979	58	—	2	2	—	0	6.8
Ohto et al 1978	1442	2	10	1	2	0	1.0
TOTAL	9115	109 1.2%	151 1.7%	30 0.3%	59 0.7%	12 0.13%	4.1%

studied angiographically by Okuda (1978) following PTC. These most often are of no consequence but may be accompanied by significant bleeding which can be controlled by angiographic embolization (Sarr et al 1984), or may produce localized 'parenchymal' staining during hepatic arteriography which can mimic a small vascular tumour deposit. Small intrahepatic haematomas not uncommonly occur and produce discrete low attenuation areas on CT scanning (Tylen et al 1981) which should not be confused with tumour.

ANATOMY AND NORMAL VARIATIONS

The anatomy of the bile ducts is covered in Chapters 2 and 3. A knowledge of the common variations of ductal branching is essential for accurate interpretation of cholangiograms and these are shown in Fig. 19.3 and 19.4. Segmental nomenclature is summarized in Table 19.2.

In the right lobe the posterior segments lie more laterally than the anterior segments so that the most lateral ducts on a cholangiogram are usually segments 6 inferiorly and 7 superiorly. The posterior sectoral duct is often recognizable by an arched course close to the confluence (Fig. 19.5, 19.19b).

A right sectoral duct crosses to the left to join the left hepatic duct in 28% of cases according to Healey & Schroy (1953); in 22% this is the posterior sectoral duct (Fig. 19.4b, 19.16, 19.19b) and in 6% the anterior (Fig. 19.4c, 19.19d). Occasionally a right sectoral or segmental duct, posterior more often than anterior, courses inferiorly and enters the common hepatic duct directly (Fig. 19.14) (Hand 1973) (Ch. 2).

The confluence of the right and left ducts takes the form of a 'trifurcation' rather than a 'bifurcation' in 12% of cases according to Couinaud (1957) (Fig. 19.4a).

In the left lobe the superior and inferior lateral segment ducts (segments 2 and 3 respectively) unite in the line of, or to the right of, the umbilical fissure in 92% of cases. In the latter instance the quadrate lobe (segment 4) may drain wholly or partly into the segment 3 duct and less frequently into the segment 2 duct. Rarely, segment 2 and 3 ducts join at or close to the confluence (Fig. 19.4e, 19.19c) and segment 4 drains directly into the common hepatic duct in 1% of cases (Figure 19.4f) (Healey & Schroy 1953).

Table 19.2 Segmental nomenclature, after Couinaud (1957), and Healey & Schroy (1953)

I	Caudate lobe
II	Left lateral superior segment
III	Left lateral inferior segment
IV	Left medial segment or quadrate lobe
V	Right anterior inferior segment
VI	Right posterior inferior segment
VII	Right posterior superior segment
VIII	Right anterior superior segment

Table 19.3 Average duct diameters measured directly from 50 normal PTC examinations (Ohto et al 1978)

Right hepatic duct	4.7 mm
Left hepatic duct	5.2 mm
Common hepatic duct	6.5 mm
Common bile duct	7.6 mm

The caudate ducts are often difficult to identify. There are usually two or three ducts which drain most commonly into the right posterior sectoral duct, right hepatic duct or left hepatic duct (Healey & Schroy 1953). The recognizable caudate ducts are usually a few centimetres long and drain downwards or to the right.

The left hepatic duct (average length 17 mm) is considerably longer than the right (average length 9 mm) and has a longer extrahepatic course (Ch. 2). The normal diameters of the main bile ducts as measured at PTC are shown in Table 19.3. These figures are greater than the true duct dimensions because of some distension produced by direct cholangiography together with considerable magnification occurring on any fluoroscopic 'spot film'. The latter is of the order of 40% (Nichols & Burhenne 1984) and affects all structures in the image including calculi, tubes and strictures.

MALIGNANT DISEASE

Cholangiocarcinoma

Direct cholangiography is an important investigation for

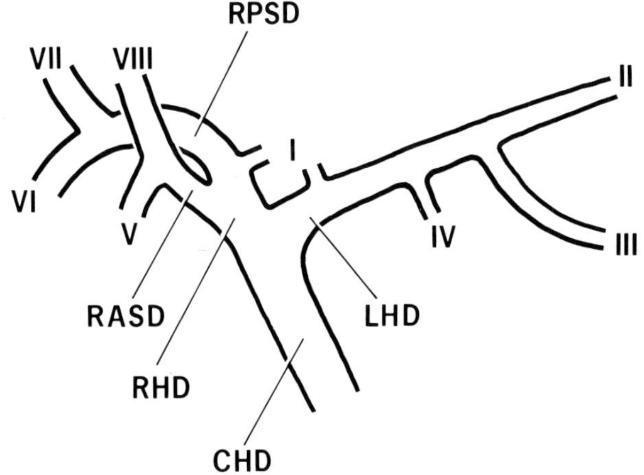

Fig. 19.3 Standard intrahepatic ductal anatomy. Segments numbered according to Couinaud's description (see Table 19.2).
RASD — right anterior sectoral duct
RPSD — right posterior sectoral duct
RHD — right hepatic duct
LHD — left hepatic duct
CHD — common hepatic duct

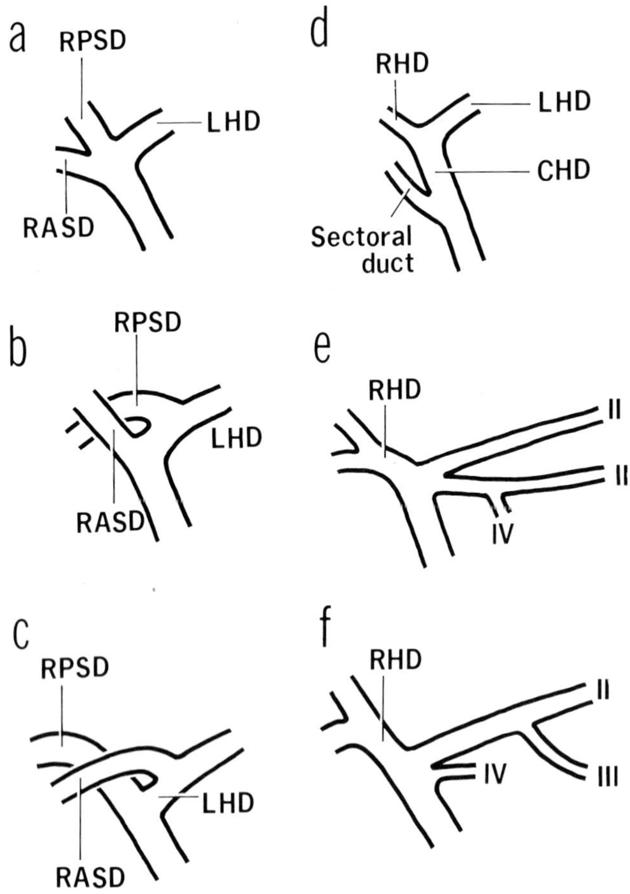

Fig. 19.4 Variations of perihilar ductal anatomy

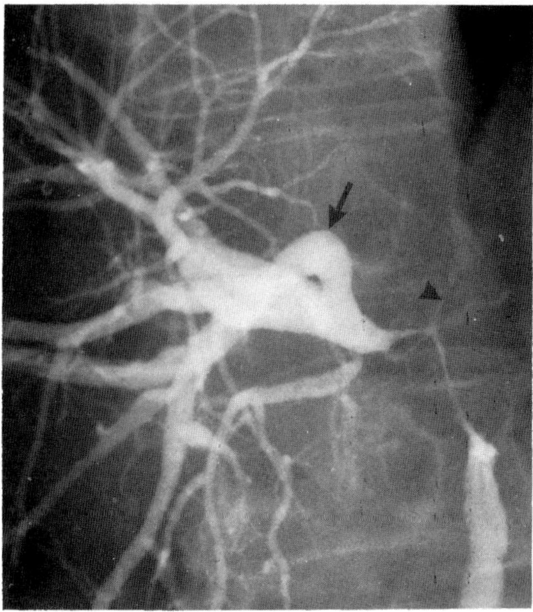

Fig. 19.5 Hilar cholangiocarcinoma involving first order right hepatic duct, proximal common hepatic duct and faintly opacified left hepatic duct (arrowhead). Note the characteristic arched course of the right posterior sectoral duct (arrow)

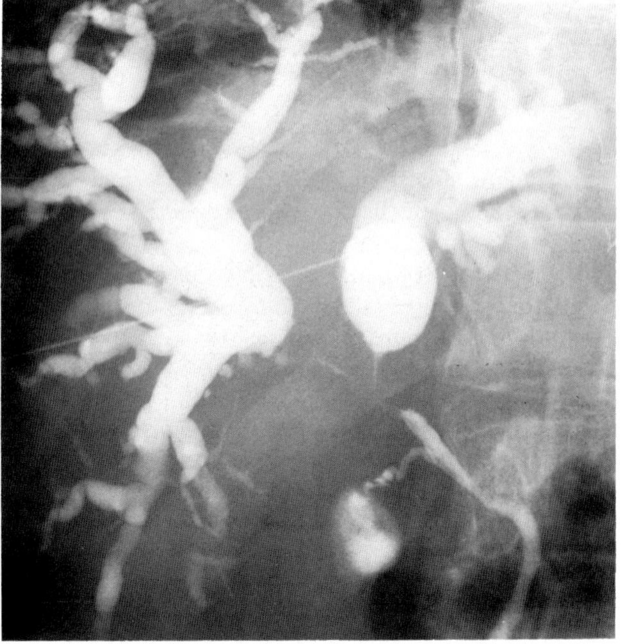

Fig. 19.6 Hilar cholangiocarcinoma involving first order right and left hepatic ducts. Separate needle punctures were required to fill the right and left ducts

both diagnosis and preoperative evaluation of cholangiocarcinoma (Ch. 65).

Although peripheral intrahepatic cholangiocarcinoma does occur, most bile duct cancers encountered on PTC are located either intrahepatically near the hilus or in the extrahepatic bile ducts. The extrahepatic ducts are involved more often proximally than distally with 53–68% of tumours occurring at or above the junction of the common hepatic duct and cystic duct (Warren et al 1972, Longmire et al 1973, Ohto et al 1978, Tompkins et al 1981). Cholangiocarcinoma usually produces concentric stricturing (Fig. 19.5, 19.6) which sometimes appears 'shouldered'; a polypoid appearance is very uncommon (Fig. 19.7).

The length of stricture varies considerably but is usually at least 1 cm (Voyles et al 1983) in contrast to most traumatic strictures. If obstruction is complete even on delayed films then ERC can be used to delineate the lower extent of the stricture. When complete obstruction involves the confluence of the right and left hepatic ducts separate punctures of the right and left ductal systems are necessary (Fig. 19.6). Stricturing may extend peripherally from the confluence on one or both sides to involve 2nd or 3rd order ducts, a feature precluding local resection. Frequently such extension is asymmetrical involving, e.g. second or third order ducts on the right but only the main left hepatic duct (Fig. 19.8).

Cholangiocarcinoma, particularly the uncommon diffuse form, may mimic sclerosing cholangitis and furthermore

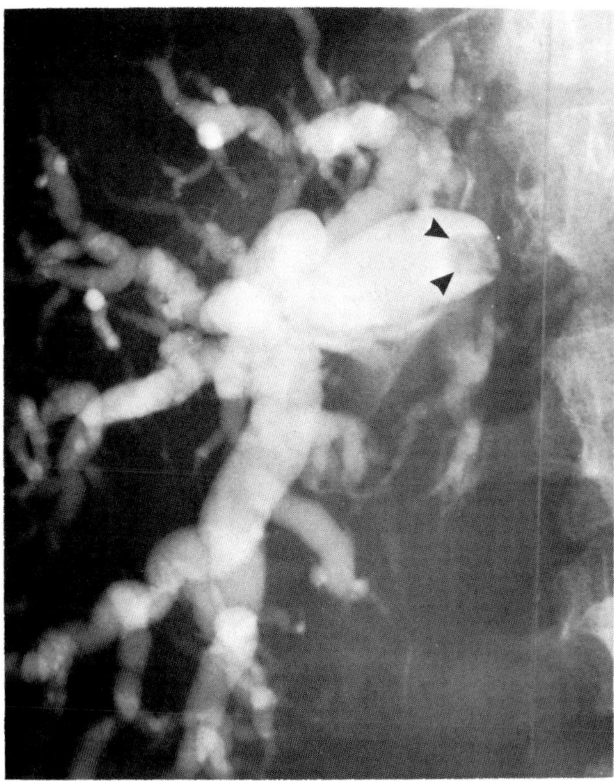

Fig. 19.7 Papillary hilar cholangiocarcinoma (arrowheads). Only the right ducts are opacified

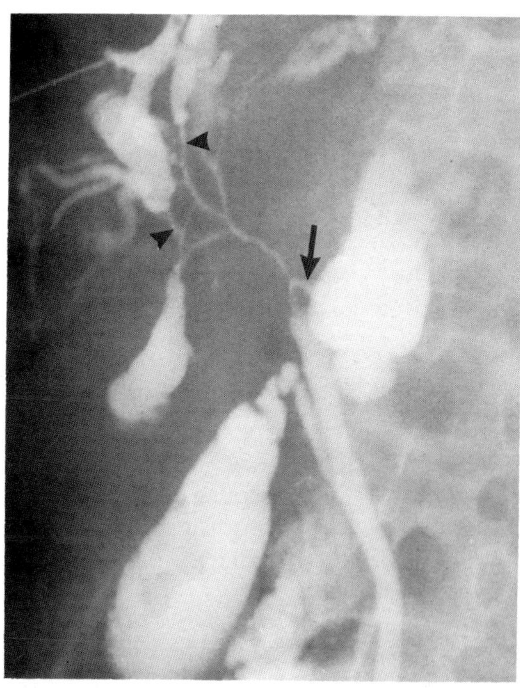

Fig. 19.8 Hilar cholangiocarcinoma with asymmetrical ductal extension: first order duct involvement on the left (arrow) and at least third order involvement on the right (arrowheads)

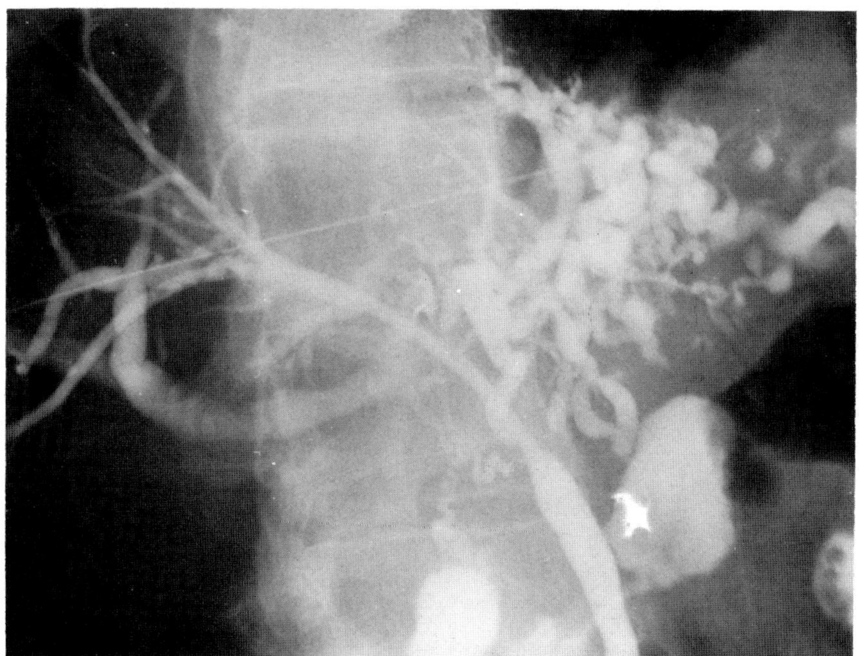

Fig. 19.9 Hilar cholangiocarcinoma with crowded left ducts indicating left lobe atrophy. Right ducts are opacified via a percutaneous transhepatic drainage catheter

the two diseases may co-exist in patients with inflammatory bowel disease (Rohrmann et al 1978).

In a significant number of cases we have found lobar or segmental liver atrophy (Ch. 6) (Fig. 19.9) occurring in association with hilar cholangiocarcinoma due to either prolonged ductal obstruction or portal vein branch occlusion. Atrophy is indicated by crowding of ducts and has important implications when one is considering lobar resection or palliative biliary-enteric anastomosis or intubation.

Multiple strictures are occasionally seen either due to multifocal primary tumours or metastatic disease (Voyles et al 1983).

Carcinoma of the gallbladder

When carcinoma of the gallbladder causes obstructive jaundice, the usual cholangiographic finding is that of tapered stricturing of the common hepatic duct which is characteristically deviated medially (Fig. 19.10). This latter feature is helpful in differentiating it from cholangiocarcinoma but it is important to be aware that such ductal deviation may also be seen in the benign Mirizzi syndrome (Ohto et al 1978). The tumour can extend to involve the right and left hepatic ducts (Fig. 19.10). A more recently described cholangiographic feature suggestive of gallbladder carcinoma is distortion of the intrahepatic bile ducts in segment 5 (Collier et al 1984).

Carcinoma of the pancreas

Carcinoma of the pancreas can involve the intrapancreatic or suprapancreatic portions of the common bile duct. Obstruction is frequently complete and its shape varies between tapered, rounded, square or convex upwards (Ariyama 1983) (Fig. 19.11). Metastatic spread can also

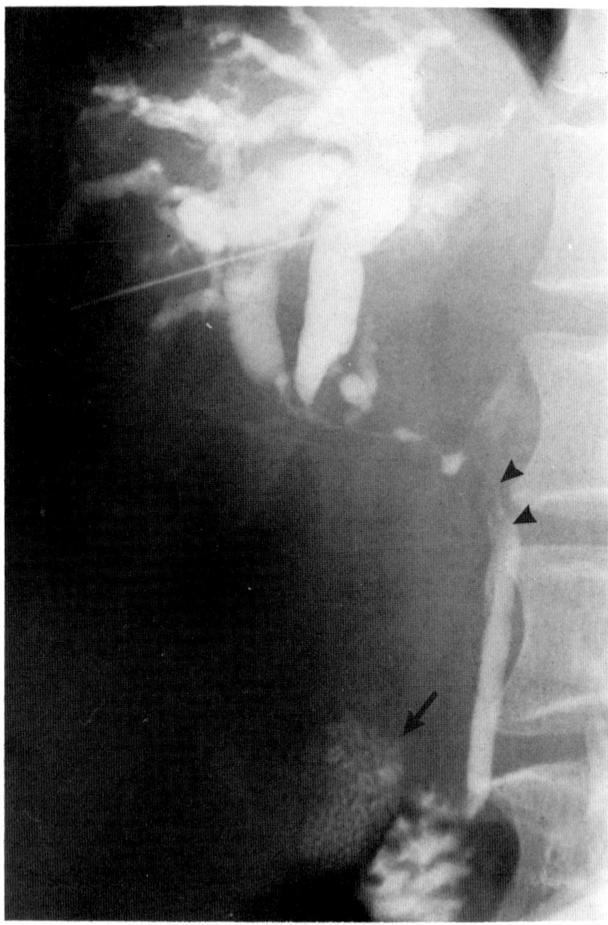

Fig. 19.10 Gallbladder carcinoma involving right third order ducts and deviating upper common hepatic duct medially (arrowheads). There are multiple small calculi in the gallbladder fundus (arrow) which is separated from the strictured ducts by the tumour.

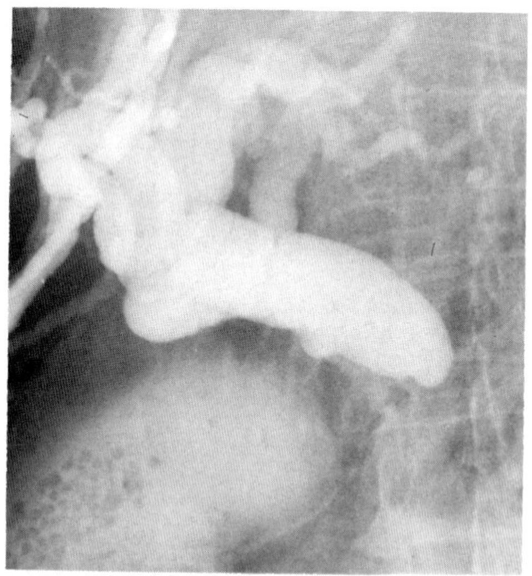

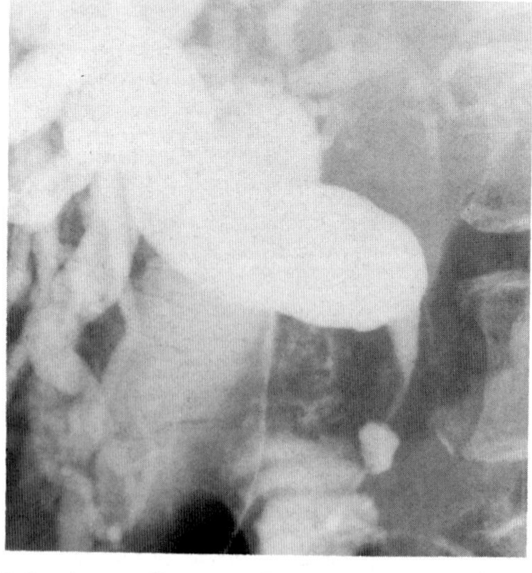

Fig. 19.11 Carcinoma of pancreas. Two of the appearances commonly seen: a. Rounded obstruction with characteristic horizontal common bile duct. Note coincidental stones in distended gallbladder. b. Tapered obstruction with slight shouldering. Compare with pancreatitis (Fig. 19.14) where shouldering tends to be absent

produce ductal narrowing in the porta hepatis (Fig. 19.12) and intrahepatic ductal distortion (Fig. 19.13).

Differentiation from common bile duct narrowing due to pancreatitis is often difficult cholangiographically but pancreatitis typically produces a longer, smooth, incomplete stricturing compared with carcinoma of either the pancreas or the lower common bile duct (Ariyama 1983) (Fig. 19.14). The course of the common bile duct above the obstruction is commonly rather horizontal (Fig. 19.11a) and this appears quite specific for pancreatic carcinoma (Freeny & Lawson 1982).

Carcinoma of the intrapancreatic portion of the common bile duct may be indistinguishable from pancreatic carcinoma. The latter produces displacement of the common bile duct more often than does cholangiocarcinoma. If the pancreatic duct is also involved on ERCP then tumour is usually of pancreatic origin (Freeny & Lawson 1982). Metastases to the region of the pancreatic head tend to produce cholangiographic findings similar to primary pancreatic tumours.

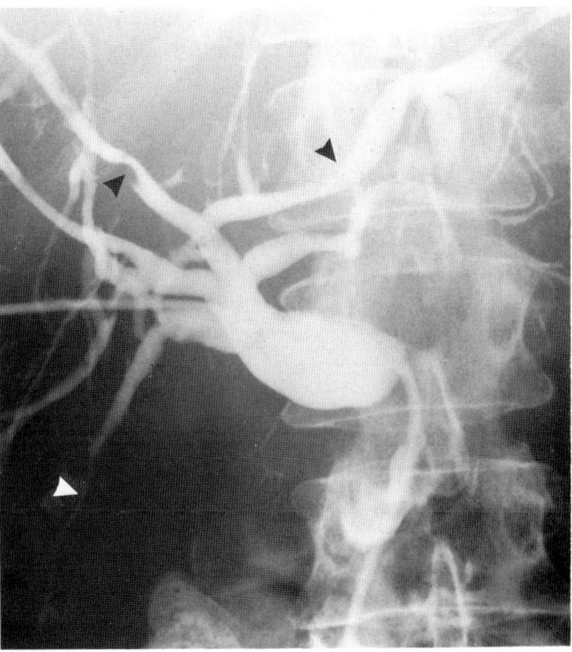

Fig. 19.13 Carcinoma of pancreas managed by percutaneous catheter drainage. Several intrahepatic ducts (arrowheads) are distorted by metastases

Periampullary carcinomas

Tumours of the ampulla, bile duct and pancreas arising from the periampullary region tend to be indistinguishable on PTC. These are discussed in more detail in Ch. 4.

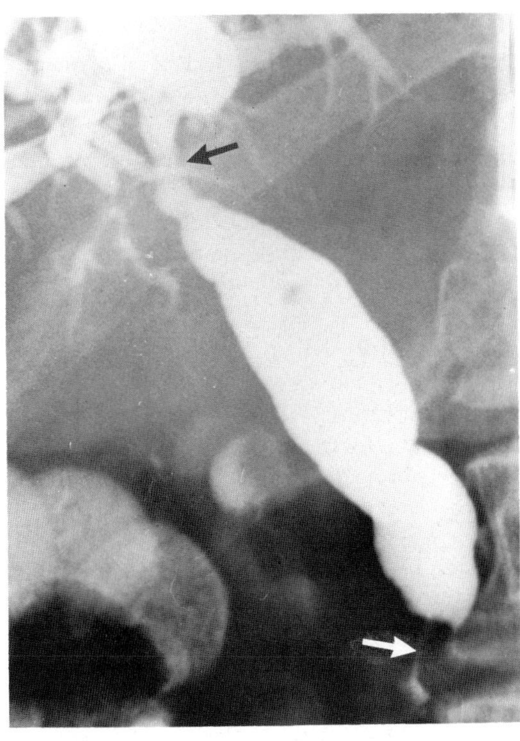

Fig. 19.12 Carcinoma of pancreas producing localized stricture of distal common bile duct (white arrow) indistinguishable from cholangiocarcinoma. Stricturing of the upper common hepatic duct (black arrow) is due to porta hepatis lymphadenopathy

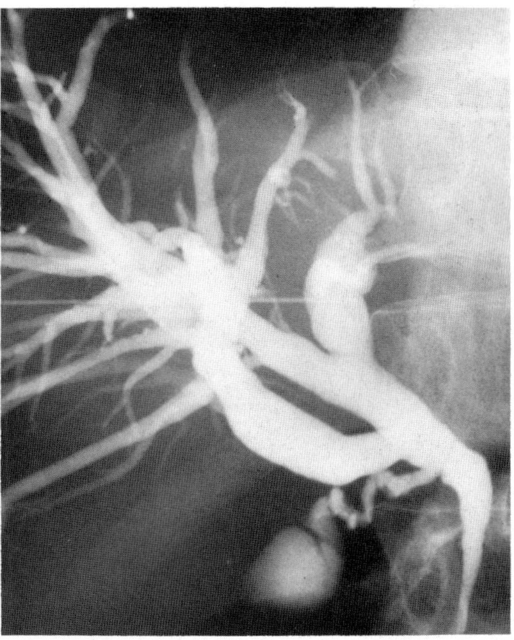

Fig. 19.14 Pancreatitis producing a typical incomplete long stricture of the common bile duct. The right posterior sectoral duct has a low entrance into the common hepatic duct, an uncommon but important normal variant

Other malignancies

Metastatic tumour has a number of cholangiographic manifestations;

1. Intrahepatic duct displacement (Fig. 19.13) or amputation.

2. Intrahepatic ductal obstruction which may affect several ducts resulting in non-communicating obstructed segments.
3. Extrahepatic duct distortion or obstruction in the porta hepatis region caused by lymph node metastases. This may involve the common bile duct, common hepatic duct or the right and left hepatic ducts. Such involvement may be seen in association with a more distal obstructing tumour such as in the pancreatic head (Fig. 19.12). Lymphadenopathy due to lymphoma or even leukaemia may produce very similar cholangiographic findings (Severini et al 1981).

In hepatocellular carcinoma direct cholangiography is seldom indicated but may show ductal displacement or obstruction with intraluminal filling defects if there is intraductal tumour extension (Ariyama 1983) (Fig. 19.15).

Benign versus malignant strictures

Benign strictures occasionally mimic malignant lesions (Hadjis et al 1985). This is particularly true of localized sclerosing cholangitis and the Mirizzi syndrome. Histological or cytological confirmation should therefore be obtained when the cholangiographic appearances suggest malignancy. The PTC can be used to guide a fine needle aspirate for cytological studies if appropriate (Fig. 19.16).

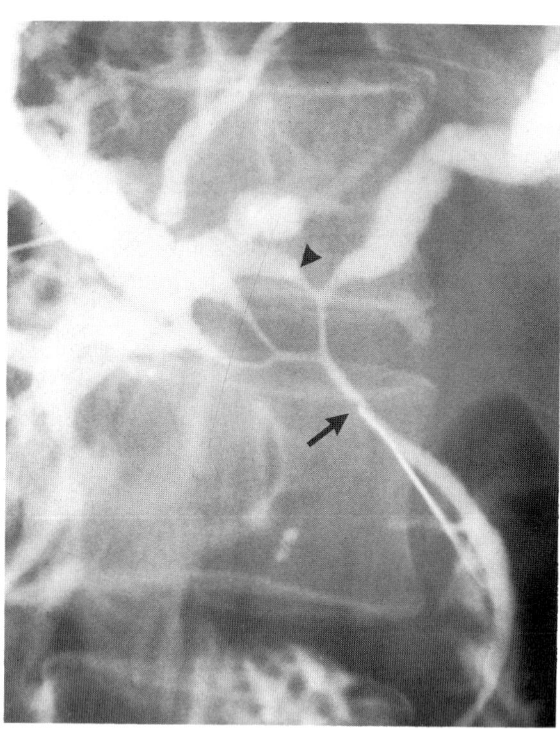

Fig. 19.16 Sclerosing cholangitis producing a stricture of common hepatic duct extending into second order ducts bilaterally. Differentiation from extensive cholangiocarcinoma is aided by fine needle aspiration cytology (arrow). Note the right posterior sectoral duct (arrowhead) entering the left hepatic duct

BENIGN TUMOURS

Benign bile duct tumours (see Ch. 63) are very uncommon but one should be aware of them from the cholangiographic viewpoint as they are frequently not diagnosed preoperatively, indeed may be overlooked at operation and they have a relatively good prognosis following resection (Cattell et al 1962, Dowdy et al 1962). Cholangiographically they can be expected to appear as small intraluminal polypoid or papillary filling defects producing incomplete or complete obstruction (Hossack & Herron 1972, Ohto et al 1978).

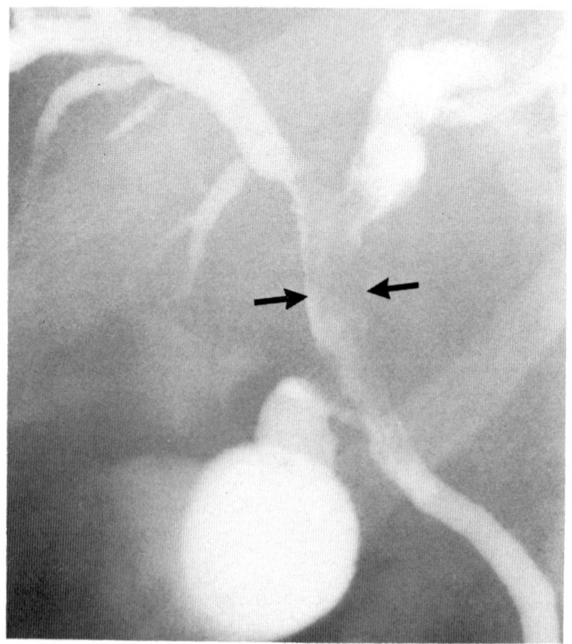

Fig. 19.15 Right lobe hepatoma with intraductal tumour extension manifested by an irregular filling defect in the common hepatic duct (arrows)

CALCULOUS DISEASE

Direct cholangiography (PTC or ERC) is the most accurate imaging technique for the detection of ductal calculi. PTC will more reliably show intrahepatic calculi because of generally better ductal filling while ERC is more appropriate for demonstrating common bile duct calculi. Either technique may fail to demonstrate small calculi if the concentration of the contrast medium is too high. Calculi can usually be differentiated from other causes of intraductal filling defects by using the features listed in Table 19.4.

Occasionally an intraductal tumour will mimic an impacted calculus, e.g. at the lower end of the common bile duct. One should be aware that, rarely, common bile duct calculi may be found in association with a distal tumour.

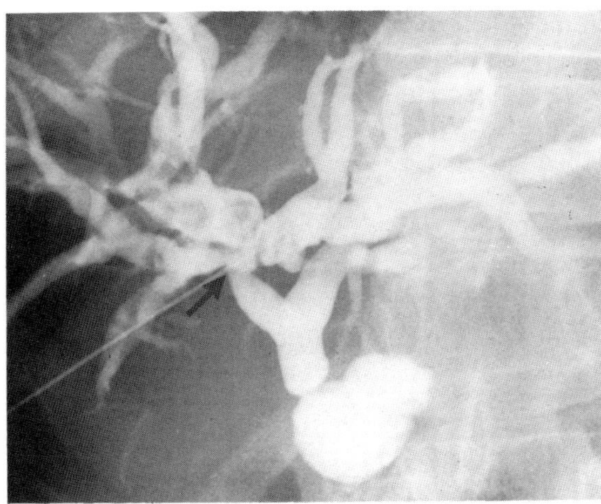

Fig. 19.17 Benign stricture of right hepatic duct (arrow) with multiple ductal calculi proximal to it. The hepatojejunostomy is partially strictured

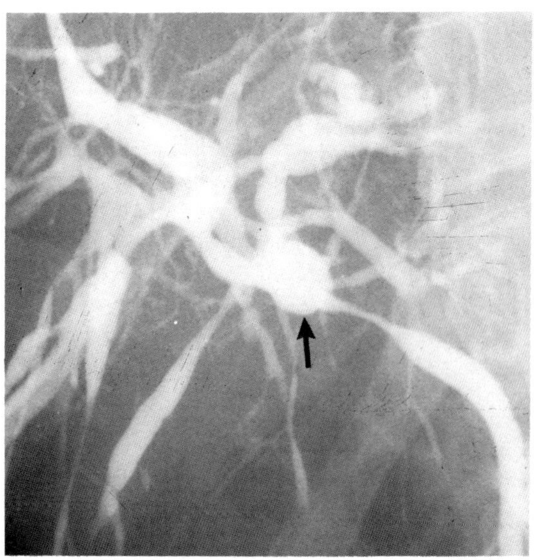

Fig. 19.18 Sclerosing cholangitis with multiple intrahepatic and extrahepatic segments of stricturing. A characteristic 'diverticulum' (arrow) overlies the confluence of the right and left hepatic ducts

Ductal calculi and benign strictures, including biliary-enteric anastomotic strictures, are frequently associated and if one is detected then the other should be carefully sought (Fig. 19.17). In the Far East, at least, there is also an association between intrahepatic calculi and peripheral hilar cholangiocarcinoma (Chen et al 1984) which may manifest itself on PTC as non-filling of a duct, stricture or an intraductal nodular filling defect (Ch. 51, 77).

It should be emphasized that neither PTC nor ERC are optimal modalities for assessment of the gallbladder, as neither technique consistently produces complete gall-bladder opacification.

SCLEROSING CHOLANGITIS

Sclerosing cholangitis (Ch. 59) usually produces cholangiographic changes in both the intra- and extrahepatic biliary tree (La Russo et al 1984), although occasionally one part may be solely affected. The predominant feature is multiple areas of stricturing which may affect short or long segments, tend to be more pronounced at duct 'bifurcations' (Fig. 19.16), and may be associated with duct dilatation, usually of a mild degree, between strictures (Fig. 19.18). Frequently there is peripheral duct pruning and parts of the biliary tree may be impossible to opacify (Li-Yeng & Goldberg 1984). Diverticular outpouchings (Fig. 19.18) of the extrahepatic ducts are reported to be specific for sclerosing cholangitis (La Russo et al 1984).

Similar changes may be seen secondary to choledocholithiasis or post-cholecystectomy strictures and sclerosing cholangitis may be indistinguishable from the diffuse form of cholangiocarcinoma. The more common localized cholangiocarcinomas can usually be differentiated by the presence of proximal uniform duct dilatation which is not a common feature of sclerosing cholangitis (Li-Yeng & Goldberg 1984), but occasionally what appears to be a cholangiocarcinoma on PTC may prove histologically to be a localized change of sclerosing cholangitis (Hadjis et al 1985) (Ch. 65).

MIRIZZI SYNDROME

Impaction of a calculus in the gallbladder neck or cystic duct or even its remnant may produce common hepatic

Table 19.4 Intraductal filling defects and their differentation

	Shape	Mobility	Constancy
Calculi	Rounded or *angulated**	If not impacted *fall** with repositioning	Usually on all films
Bubbles	*Round** unless filling duct	*Rise** on repositioning	Tend not to be on all films
Clot	Forms *casts** of ducts	Limited mobility	Usually absent or less prominent on early films
Intraductal tumour	Round, *irregular** or lobulated	*Immobile**	Should be on all films

*Main differentiating feature

duct stricturing by direct mechanical impression or associated inflammation, the so-called Mirizzi Syndrome (Koehler et al 1979). The affected segment of duct is usually 2–3 cm in length and is usually proximal although it may be distal if the cystic duct has a low insertion. On cholangiography there is partial or complete obstruction of the duct which commonly is deviated medially. A calcified gallstone may be visible adjacent to the stricture or, if the stone has eroded into the common hepatic duct, it may be seen as a filling defect or the resulting fistula may be opacified (Cruz et al 1983).

Awareness of this syndrome is of utmost importance cholangiographically as it may mimic gallbladder carcinoma, cholangiocarcinoma or metastatic tumour at the porta hepatis.

POST-CHOLECYSTECTOMY STRICTURES (Ch. 58)

These strictures are usually short and affect the common hepatic duct although not infrequently they occur very high and involve the right or left hepatic ducts or even

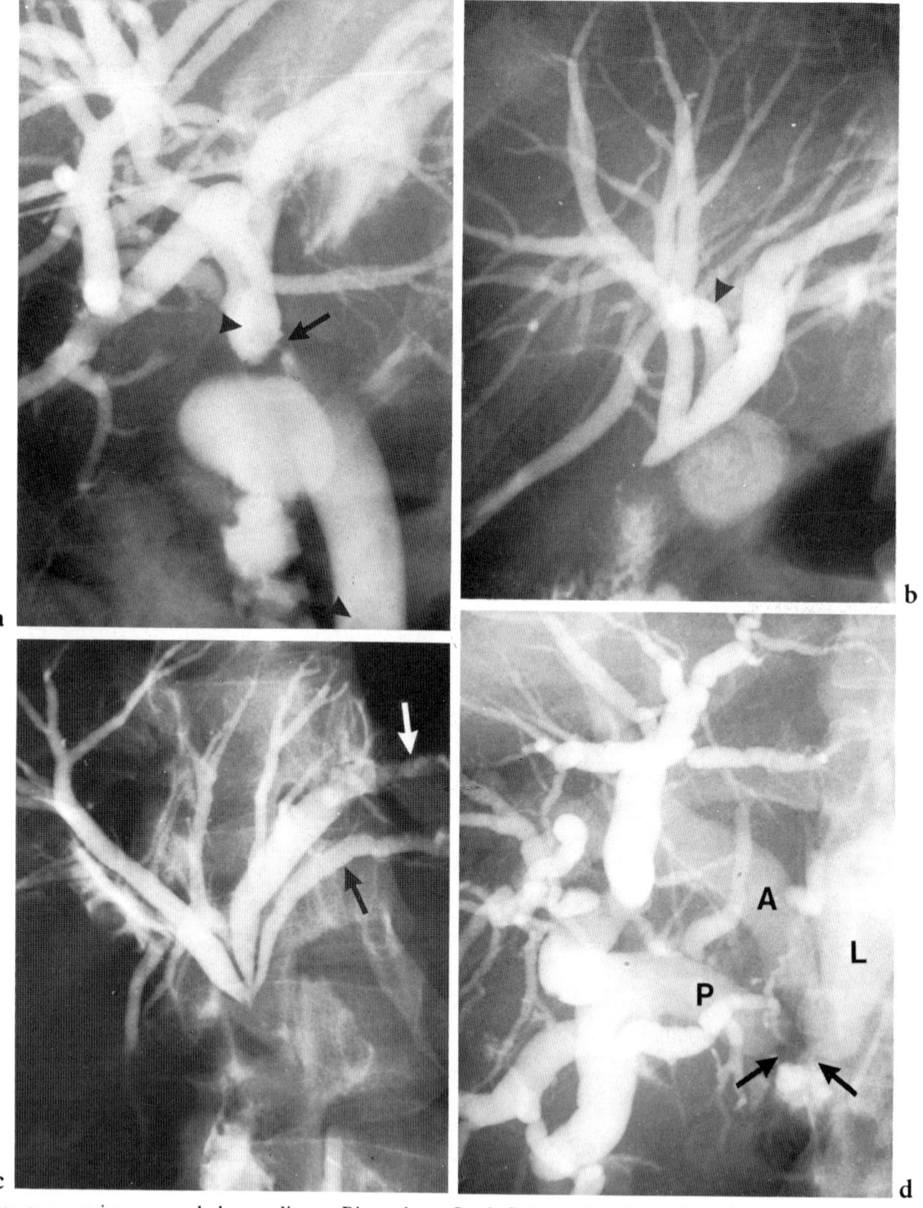

Fig. 19.19 Post-cholecystectomy strictures graded according to Bismuth. a. Grade I (more than 2 cm from the confluence of right and left hepatic ducts). Calculi (arrowheads) lie above and below the stricture (arrow). b. Grade II (less than 2 cm from confluence). There has been a previous hepatojejunostomy. Right posterior sectoral duct (arrowhead) has an exaggerated arched course and enters the left hepatic duct as a normal variant. c. Grade III (confluence involved by stricture but right and left hepatic ducts not completely separated). Ducts of segment 2 (white arrow) and segment 3 (black arrow) join the confluence independently as a normal variant. d. Grade IV (right and left ducts separated by the stricture). Right anterior sectoral duct (A) is draining into the left hepatic duct (L) which is separated from the right posterior sectoral duct (P) by the stricture (arrows)

second order ducts (Fig. 19.19). Associated segmental or lobar atrophy may result from either prolonged ductal obstruction or accompanying vascular injury (Blumgart et al 1984). Irregularity of duct calibre suggests secondary cholangitis. Single or multiple intrahepatic calculi may be seen, sometimes in association with additional strictures (Fig. 19.17).

If there is a biliary fistula associated with bile duct injury then PTC or ERC may fail to delineate the damaged duct particularly if it is a lobar or segmental duct. In this clinical setting the first approach should be to inject contrast directly into the fistulous tract and then proceed to PTC or ERC if necessary.

CYSTIC DISEASE OF THE BILE DUCTS

Direct cholangiography is useful in the diagnosis and preoperative assessment of this complex spectrum of diseases (see Ch. 78, 79, 80).

Intrahepatic cystic biliary dilatation may be demonstrated without associated extrahepatic duct dilatation (Caroli's disease), but is also seen in up to 44% of patients with choledochal cysts (Dayton et al 1983) (Fig. 19.20). In both conditions cholangiography may reveal evidence of complications including calculi, abscesses or cholangiocarcinoma, the latter having an incidence of 7% in Caroli's disease and 4% in choledochal cysts (Bloustein 1977). In patients with choledochal cysts the cholangiogram may also demonstrate an abnormally proximal junction of the common bile duct with the pancreatic duct (Fig. 19.20), which is well documented and suggested to be an aetiological factor (Kimura et al 1977).

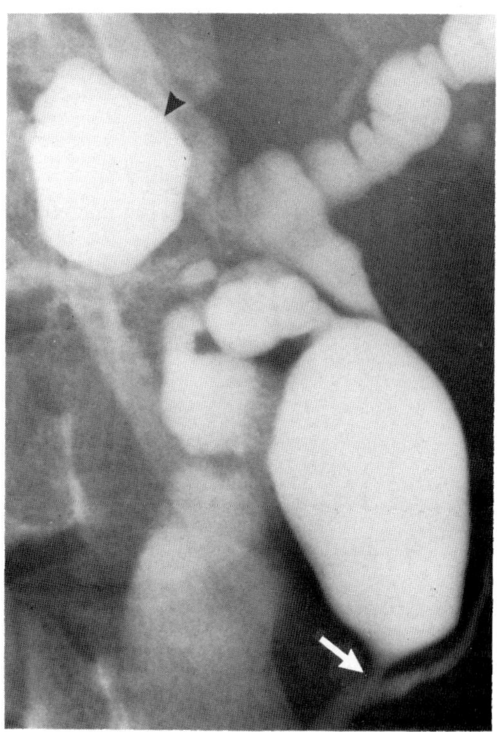

Fig. 19.20 Choledochal cyst with intrahepatic cyst formation (arrowhead). The common bile duct has an abnormally proximal junction with the pancreatic duct (arrow)

ABSCESSES (Ch. 73)

Hepatic abscesses of any cause may communicate with the biliary tree and so be seen on cholangiography. Multiple hepatic abscesses are usually secondary to acute suppurative cholangitis in association with ductal obstruction, and appear as multiple small rounded cavities with slightly indistinct margins (Fig. 19.21). Such an appearance should lead to consideration of urgent biliary decompression, either surgically, percutaneously or endoscopically.

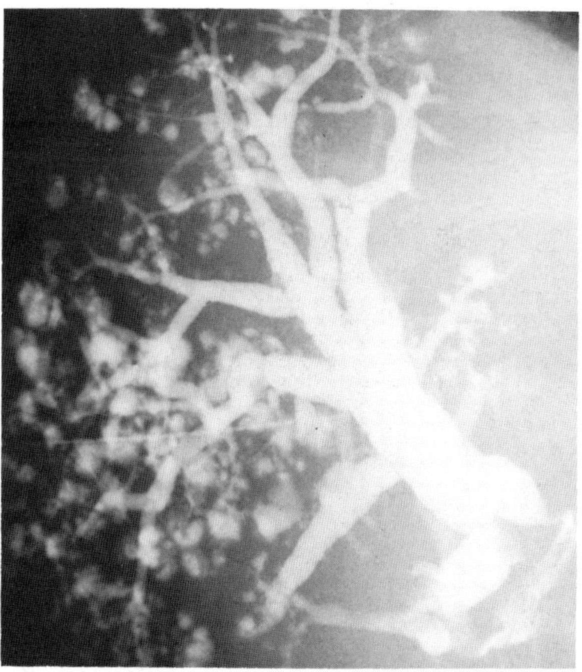

Fig. 19.21 Multiple hepatic abscesses associated with suppurative cholangitis in a patient with hilar duct obstruction

PTC, ERC AND ULTRASOUND

If direct cholangiography is indicated the choice between PTC and ERC will be affected by the local availability and quality of the two services as well as by factors listed in Table 19.5. The authors' practice is to choose ERC if there is no intrahepatic bile duct dilatation on ultrasound, or if a *low* common bile duct obstruction is suspected. PTC is preferable if there is suspected *high* obstruction and intrahepatic duct dilatation or if there has been previous biliary-enteric anastomosis. Both examinations are sometimes necessary to determine the length of a stricture when obstruction is complete.

It is our recent experience in the investigation of bile

Table 19.5 Comparison of PTC and ERC

	PTC	ERC
Advantages	Less expertise needed Less expensive equipment Good duct filling above an obstruction.	Visualization of stomach and duodenum Biopsy of ampullary lesions possible Simultaneous pancreatogram
	Both may be followed by catheter or endoprosthesis insertion for biliary drainage.	
Contraindications	Significant coagulopathy Marked ascites*	Unfavourable anatomy Pseudocyst* Recent acute pancreatitis*
Success rates	98% — dilated ducts 70% — undilated ducts (Harbin et al 1980)	Up to 90% (Cotton 1977)
Major complications	4.1%	2 3% (Cotton 1977)
Mortality	0.13%	0.1–0.2% (Cotton 1977)

*Relative contraindications

duct obstruction that direct cholangiography frequently provides no important additional information over that obtained by detailed ultrasound examination (Gibson et al 1986).

PITFALLS IN INTERPRETATION

False localization of obstruction

Failure to inject adequate volumes of contrast or to position the patient appropriately can lead to false localization of the level of obstruction. This is a problem usually only with complete obstruction and may be recognized by the presence of a 'hazy' margin at the level of the apparent obstruction (Kittredge & Baer 1975) (Fig. 19.22).

Incomplete cholangiogram

Opacification of only the right-sided ducts is often mistaken for a complete cholangiogram leading to a diagnosis of high common hepatic duct obstruction. This is recognizable by the absence of any left hepatic ducts, which should usually be visible overlying the spine. If the left ducts do not fill with further contrast injection in the left lateral decubitus position then a separate puncture and direct opacification of the left system should be performed, either from the right side (Fig. 19.6) or via the epigastrium.

Variations in duct anatomy can also cause some difficulty in interpretation and may result in an incomplete cholangiogram if unrecognized. For example, the relatively common arrangement of a right sectoral or segmental duct entering the left hepatic duct can be particularly confusing in the presence of a hilar lesion (Fig. 19.23).

Extraductal contrast injections

Contrast injected around a portal vein branch may mimic a dilated bile duct but should be recognizable by the central 'filling defect' which represents the portal vein (Fig. 19.24). Opacification of hepatic lymphatics (Fig. 19.25) has no pathological significance in itself and the multi-

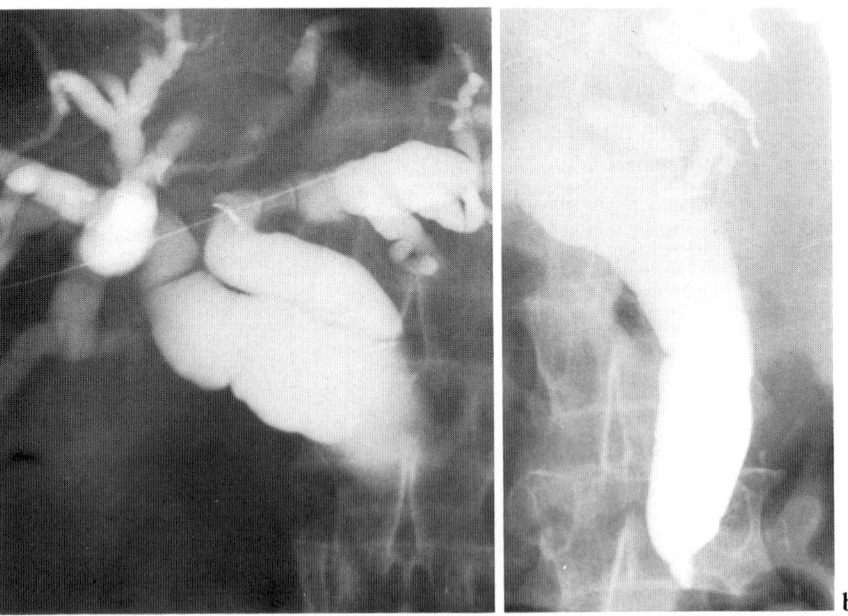

Fig. 19.22 Ampullary carcinoma. a. With patient supine contrast pools proximally giving false impression of a high bile duct obstruction. The spurious nature of the level is suggested by the hazy inferior margin to the contrast column. b. With patient semi-erect contrast pools at true point of obstruction which is sharply defined

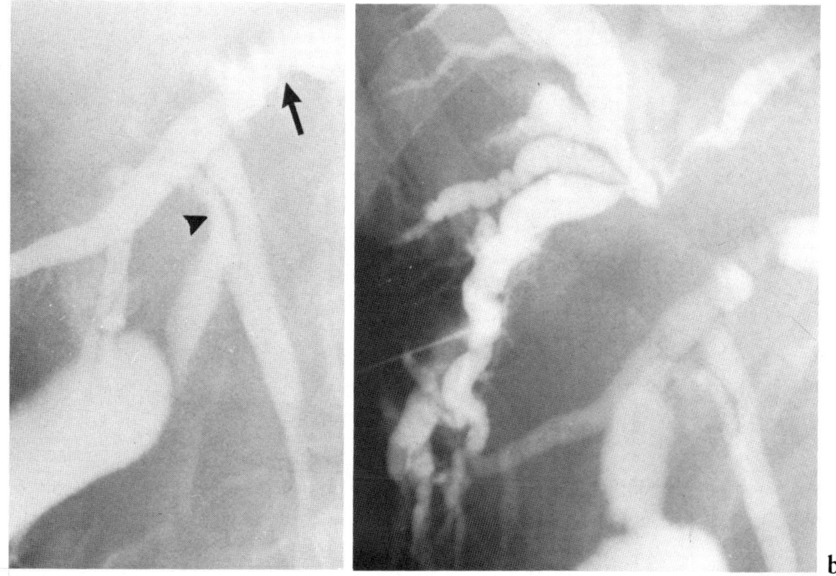

Fig. 19.23 Hilar cholangiocarcinoma. a. Initial injection opacifies segment 5 duct which is crossing to join the left hepatic duct (arrow). Cystic duct indicated by arrowhead. b. Second injection opacifies remaining right ducts which are obstructed adjacent to the hilus.

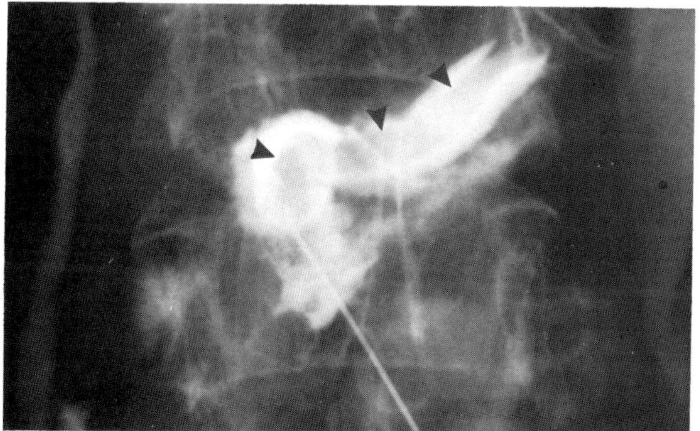

Fig. 19.24 Periportal contrast injection. The 'filling defect' (arrowheads) is a left portal vein branch

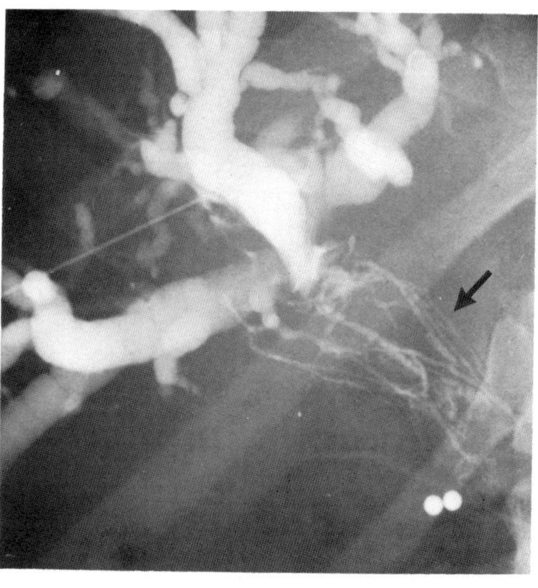

Fig. 19.25 Lymphatic filling (arrow) recognizable by their multiplicity and beaded appearance

plicity of beaded channels should not be mistaken for narrow, irregular bile ducts.

Extraductal contrast injections may obscure information and can compress bile ducts sufficiently to produce an artificial level of obstruction (Fig. 19.26).

Some contrast medium is frequently injected into a portal or hepatic vein branch and this is excreted by the kidney with resulting opacification of the renal pelvis or ureter. The latter should not be mistaken for a bile duct (Fig. 19.27).

Portal vein and hepatic vein branches are frequently visible on screening during the PTC but these are rarely visible on the radiographs. Extrahepatic injection of contrast is usually easily recognizable and tends to produce transient pain and sometimes local peritonitis.

SUCCESS RATE AND ACCURACY OF PTC

The success rate of bile duct opacification depends on the presence of bile duct dilatation and the number of needle passes made. With dilated ducts the opacification rate approaches 100% and at least a 95% success rate should be achieved even if the number of needle passes is limited to six (Jain et al 1977, Jacques et al 1980). If ducts are undilated the chance of success increases with the number of needle passes and in most series is between 60% and 80% (Fraser et al 1978, Jacques et al 1980, Harbin et al

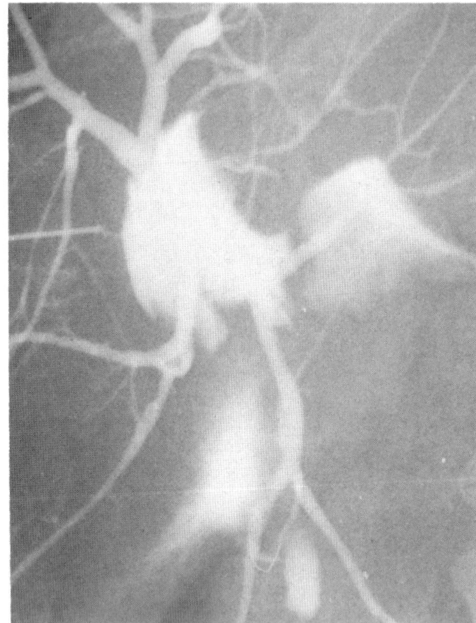

Fig. 19.26 Perihilar extraductal contrast injection in a patient with cirrhosis. Note the narrow slightly distorted intrahepatic ducts. Contrast extravasation obscures ducts and has produced an artificial hilar obstruction

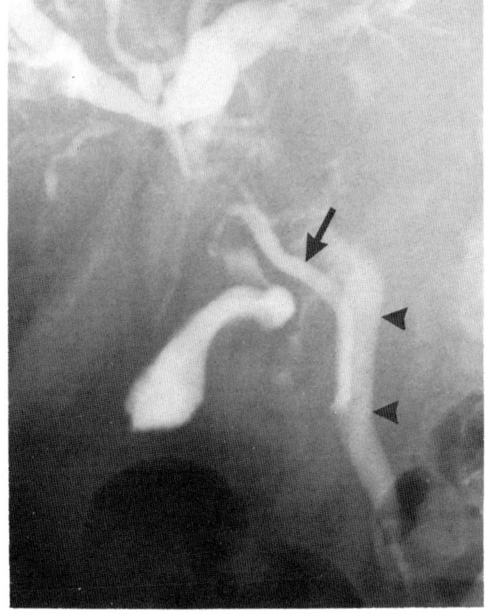

Fig. 19.27 Proximal ureter (arrowheads) opacified by renal excretion of contrast medium. This may be confused with the common bile duct (arrow)

1980). Surprisingly perhaps, no correlation has been shown to exist between the number of needle passes and the incidence of significant complications (Ariyama et al 1978, Harbin et al 1980), and the limiting factor to the number of passes made is usually patient discomfort.

When duct opacification is achieved there is usually no difficulty in deciding whether or not there is duct obstruction. However, the correlation between obstruction and dilatation is not always good, e.g. it is possible to have obstruction as indicated by raised biliary pressure with little or no dilatation (Van Sonnenberg et al 1983). This occurs most often with choledocholithiasis and benign strictures. Secondary cholangitis tends to limit the distensibility of both intrahepatic and extrahepatic bile ducts (Benjamin 1982) and cirrhosis and liver metastases can have the same effect on intrahepatic ducts.

The *level* of duct obstruction will be accurately determined in all cases providing attention is paid to details of technique, in particular, the use of patient rotation and table tilt. The *cause* of obstruction is less accurately determined by PTC and although accuracy rates of over 90% are reported (Mueller et al 1982) there are patients in whom a specific diagnosis cannot be made on PTC grounds alone; indeed differentiation between benign and malignant stricturing is sometimes impossible. It is important to recognize this and take into account clinical features, other radiological findings and, preferably, histological or cytological evidence.

ACKNOWLEDGEMENT

The author would like to thank Dr. E. Yeung for his assistance.

REFERENCES

Ariyama J 1983 Direct cholangiography. In: Herlinger H, Lunderquist A, Wallace S (eds) Clinical Radiology of the Liver. Marcel Dekker, New York, Ch 18 p 471

Ariyama J, Shirakabe H, Ohashi K, Roberts G M 1978 Experience with percutaneous transhepatic cholangiography using the Japanese needle. Gastrointestinal Radiology 2: 359–365

Benjamin I S 1982 The obstructed biliary tract. In: Blumgart L H (ed) The biliary tract. Churchill Livingstone, Edinburgh, Ch 10 p 157

Bloustein P A 1977 Association of carcinoma with congenital cystic conditions of the liver and bile ducts. American Journal of Gastroenterology 67: 40–46

Blumgart L H, Kelley C J, Benjamin I S 1984 Benign bile duct stricture following cholecystectomy: Critical factors in management. British Journal of Surgery 71: 836–843

Burckhardt H, Muller W 1921 Versuche uber die Punktion der Gallenblase und ihre Rontgendarstellung. Deutsche Zeitschrift fur Chirurgie 162: 168–197

Carter R F, Saypol G M 1952 Transabdominal cholangiography. Journal of the American Medical Association 148: 253–255

Cattell R B, Braasch J W, Kahn F 1962 Polypoid epithelial tumours of the bile ducts. New England Journal of Medicine 266: 57–61

Chen P H, Lo H W, Wang C S et al 1984 Cholangiocarcinoma in hepatolithiasis. Journal of Clinical Gastroenterology 6: 539–547 Gastroenterology 6: 539–547

Collier N A, Carr D, Hemingway A, Blumgart L H 1984 Preoperative diagnosis and its effect on the treatment of carcinoma of the gall bladder. Surgery, Gynecology and Obstetrics 159: 465–470

Cotton P B 1977 Progress report: ERCP. Gut 18: 316–341

Couinaud C 1957 Le foie. Etudes anatomiques et chirurgicales. Masson, Paris

Cruz F O, Barriga P, Tocornal J, Burhenne H J 1983 Radiology of the Mirizzi syndrome: Diagnostic importance of the transhepatic cholangiogram. Gastrointestinal Radiology 8: 249–253

Dayton M T, Longmire W P, Tompkins R K 1983 Caroli's disease: A premalignant condition? American Journal of Surgery 145: 41–48

Dowdy G S, Olin W G, Shelton E L, Waldron G W 1962 Benign tumours of the extrahepatic bile ducts. Archives of Surgery 85: 503–513

Fraser G M, Cruikshank J G, Sumerling M D, Buist T A S 1978 Percutaneous transhepatic cholangiography with the Chiba needle. Clinical Radiology 29: 101–112

Freeny P C, Lawson T L 1982 Radiology of the Pancreas. Springer-Verlag, New York

Gibbons C P, Griffiths G J, Cormack A 1983 The role of percutaneous transhepatic cholangiography and grey-scale ultrasound in the investigation and treatment of bile duct obstruction. British Journal of Surgery 70: 494–496

Gibson R N, Yeung E, Thompson J N et al 1986 Radiological evaluation of bile duct obstruction: level, cause and tumour resectability. Radiology 160: 43–47

Hadjis N S, Collier N A, Blumgart L H 1985 Malignant masquerade at the hilum of the liver. British Journal of Surgery 72: 659–661

Hand B H 1973 Anatomy and function of the extrahepatic biliary system. Clinics in Gastroenterology 2: 3–29

Harbin W P, Mueller P R, Ferrucci J T 1980 Transhepatic cholangiography. Complications and use patterns of the fine-needle technique. A multi-institution survey. Radiology 135: 15–22

Healey J E, Schroy P C 1953 Anatomy of the biliary ducts within the human liver. AMA Archives of Surgery 66: 599–616

Hossack K F, Herron J J 1972 Benign tumours of the common bile duct: report of a case and review of the literature. Australian and New Zealand Journal of Surgery 42: 22–26

Hultborn A, Jacobsson B, Rosengren B 1962 Cholangiovenous reflux during cholangiography. An experimental and clinical study. Acta Chirurgica Scandinavica 123: 111–124

Jain S, Long R G, Scott J, Dick R, Sherlock S 1977 Percutaneous transhepatic cholangiography using the 'Chiba' needle — 80 cases. British Journal of Radiology 50: 175–180

Jaques P F, Mauro M A, Scatliff J H 1980 The failed transhepatic cholangiogram. Radiology 134: 33–35

Keighley M R B 1977 Mirco-organisms in the bile. A preventable cause of sepsis after biliary surgery. Annals of the Royal College of Surgeons of England 59: 328–334

Keil P G, Landis S N 1951 Peritoneoscopic cholangiography. Archives of Internal Medicine 88: 36–41

Kidd H A 1956 Percutaneous transhepatic cholangiography. Archives of Surgery 72: 262–268

Kimura K, Ohto M, Ono T et al 1977 Congenital cystic dilatation of the common bile duct: relationship to anomalous pancreaticobiliary ductal union. American Journal of Roentgenology 128: 571–577

Kittredge R D, Baer J W 1975 Percutaneous transhepatic cholangiography. Problems in interpretation. American Journal of Roentgenology 125: 35–46

Kocher F, Mousseau R 1979 Percutaneous transhepatic cholangiography with the Chiba needle. American Journal of Gastroenterology 71: 39–44

Koehler R E, Melson G L, Lee J K T, Long L 1979 Common hepatic duct obstruction by cystic duct stone: Mirizzi syndrome. American Journal of Roentgenology 132:1007

Kreek M J, Balint J A 1980 'Skinny needle' cholangiography — results of a pilot study of a voluntary prospective method for gathering risk data on new procedures. Gastroenterology 78: 598–604

La Russo N F, Wiesner R H, Ludwig J, MacCarty R L 1984 Primary sclerosing cholangitis. New England Journal of Medicine 310: 899–903

Lee W Y 1942 Evaluation of peritoneoscopy in intra-abdominal diagnosis. Review of Gastroenterology 9: 133–141

Li-Yeng C, Goldberg H I 1984 Sclerosing cholangitis: Broad spectrum of radiographic features. Gastrointestinal Radiology 9: 39–47

Longmire W P, McArthur M S, Bastounis E A, Hiatt J 1973 Carcinoma of the extrahepatic biliary tract. Annals of Surgery 178: 333–345

Michel H, Adda M 1980 La cholangiographie transparietale laterale a l'aiguille fine. Gastroenterologie Clinique et Biologique 4: 137–143

Mueller P R, Harbin W P, Ferrucci J T, Wittenberg J, Van Sonnenberg E 1980 Fine needle cholangiography: reflections after 450 cases. American Journal of Roentgenology 136: 85–90

Nagasue N, Inokuchi K 1979 Diagnostic value of percutaneous transhepatic cholangiography judged by personal experience of 58 patients. Clinical Radiology 30: 451–455

Nichols D M, Burhenne H J 1984 Magnification in cholangiography. American Journal of Roentgenology 141: 947–949

Nurick A W, Patey D H, Whiteside D G 1953 Percutaneous transhepatic cholangiography in the diagnosis of obstructive jaundice. British Journal of Surgery 41: 27–30

Ohto M, Tsuchiya Y 1969 Non-surgically available percutaneous transhepatic cholangiography: technique and cases. Medicina (Tokyo) 6: 735–739

Ohto M, Ono T, Tsuchiya Y, Saisho H 1978 Cholangiography and pancreatography. Igaku-Shoin. Tokyo

Ohto M, Karasawa E, Tsuchiya Y, Kimura K, Saisho H, Ono T, Okuda K 1980 Ultrasonically guided percutaneous contrast medium injection and aspiration biopsy using a real-time puncture transducer. Radiology 136: 171–176

Okuda K, Tanikawa T, Emura T, Kuratomi S, Jinnouchi S, Urabe K et al 1974 Non-surgical, percutaneous transhepatic cholangiography-diagnostic significance in medical problems of the liver. American Journal of Digestive Diseases 19: 21–36

Rohrmann C A, Ansel H J, Freeny P C et al 1978 Cholangiographic abnormalities in patients with inflammatory bowel disease. Radiology 127: 635–641

Sarr M G, Kaufmann S L, Zuidema G D, Cameron J L 1984 Management of haemobilia associated with transhepatic biliary drainage catheters. Surgery 95: 603–607

Seldinger S I 1966 Percutaneous transhepatic cholangiography. Acta Radiologica. Supplement 253

Severini A, Bellorni M, Cozzi G, Pizzetti P, Spinelli P 1981 Lymphomatous involvement of intrahepatic and extrahepatic biliary ducts. PTC and ERCP findings. Acta Radiologica Diagnosis 22: 159–163

Tompkins R K, Thomas D, Wile A, Longmire W P 1981 Prognostic factors in bile duct carcinoma. Annals of Surgery 194: 447–457

Tylen U, Hoevels J, Nilsson U 1981 Computed tomography of iatrogenic hepatic lesions following percutaneous transhepatic cholangiography and portography. Journal of Computer Assisted Tomography 5: 15–18

Van Sonnenberg E, Ferrucci J T, Neff C C, Mueller P R, Simeone J F, Wittenberg J 1983 Biliary pressure: Manometric and perfusion studies at percutaneous cholangiography and percutaneous biliary drainage. Radiology 148: 41–50

Voyles C R, Bowley N J, Allison D J, Benjamin I S, Blumgart L H 1983 Carcinoma of the proximal extrahepatic biliary tree. Radiologic assessment and therapeutic alternatives. Annals of Surgery 197: 188–194

Warren K W, Mountain J C, Lloyd-Jones W 1972 Malignant tumours of the bile ducts. British Journal of Surgery 59: 501–505

Weschsler R L, Wechsler L 1975 The first application of transhepatic cholangiography to the localization of liver or biliary tract pathology: Hanoi, 1937. American Journal of Digestive Diseases 20: 699–700

Endoscopic retrograde choledochopancreatography

INTRODUCTION

Endoscopic cannulation of the papilla of Vater with instillation of contrast medium into the pancreas and biliary tract (ERCP) was first described by McCune et al (1968) and was brought to maturity as a clinical method by the early 1970s in Japan (Oi et al 1970), Europe (Demling & Classen 1970, Jean Pierre & Leger 1971, Cotton et al 1972) and North America (Vennes & Silvis 1972).

In spite of the increase in refined non-invasive methods such as sonography and computerized tomography, it has maintained its place among the methods of diagnosis of disorders of the biliary tract and pancreas and is nowadays used all over the world. Mastery of ERCP is, moreover, the basis for carrying out a large number of endoscopic therapeutic procedures, especially endoscopic papillotomy (Classen & Demling 1974) and the various methods of biliary drainage (Nagai et al 1976, Wurbs & Classen 1977, Soehendra & Reynders-Fredericks 1980) (Ch. 35, 45, 47, 69).

The technique of ERCP

Instrumentation ERCP is a combined endoscopic/radiological method which requires a high-performance radiograph with a TV image intensifier system. Long, lateral viewing instruments are usually used for the endoscopy. In patients who have undergone a Billroth II operation, it is occasionally easier to intubate the afferent loop and visualize the papilla of Vater when a thinner instrument with prograde optic is used. A wide variety of companies now have available numerous models of catheters for the intubation of the papilla. The differences from standard catheters, which go as far as catheters with dirigible tips, are meant to facilitate intubation in special cases. However, two or three different types usually suffice for experienced investigators. Conventional biopsy forceps are used for differentiation between pathological findings. The concentration of contrast medium used for visualization of the biliopancreatic system is 60%. Lower concentrations of contrast medium carry the risk of overfilling of the pancreatic duct but they are occasionally useful for detecting smaller bile duct concrements.

The staff required for ERCP are a physician and a nurse trained in endoscopy. A radiologist in attendance is only necessary if the radiograph cannot be operated simultaneously by the endoscopist. The general precautions for radiation protection must be observed.

Information, preparation and premedication of the patient

The patient is informed about the investigation and provides his written consent on the preceding day. The premedication is not standardized (Tolksdorf et al 1985). Its object is to bring about sedation and a raising of the pain threshold of the patient and it should be individualized. We prefer local anaesthesia of the pharynx with xylocaine and intravenous administration of 5–10 mg diazepam or 1–2 ml medimazole. To relax the duodenum, we administer 2–5 ml hyoscine N-butylbromide (Buscopan®). The intubation can occasionally be facilitated by ceruletide or hymecromone which relax the sphincter of Oddi. Lingual administration of 1.2 mg glycerol trinitrate, corresponding to three actuations of a Nitrolingual spray, has a similar effect (Staritz et al 1985).

There have been virtually no changes in the technique of investigation since the introduction of ERCP, and it has been described many times (Cotton 1977). The optimal position of the instrument is reached when the papilla is located in the centre of the field of view and the tip of the catheter can be directed frontally towards the orifice. To reach this position, it is occasionally necessary to increase the compression or extension of the instrument. It is frequently necessary for selective visualization of the duct, because of the variations in the openings of the ducts, to make a small correction in the angle of the catheter tip.

Radiography

The findings are documented by radiography and this is most reliably carried out in accordance with a set scheme: preliminary films of the papillary region, survey radiographs of the filled duct systems, spot films of the pathological or suspicious regions and observation of the outflow phase and motility of the papilla. The screening times depend on the particular problem and normally vary within the limits required for conventional examinations of the gastrointestinal tract. The mean screening time for diagnostic ERCP was found in the investigations of van Husen et al (1984) in 2439 consecutive examinations to be 5 min, and ERP alone took a mean of 3.8 min, which meant a significantly shorter exposure to radiation than ERC which took a mean of 5.3 min.

Indications and contraindications

Division of the examination into retrograde cholangiography and pancreatography is possible to only a limited extent. After all, one of the main grounds for carrying out this examination is to obtain additional information on the immediately adjacent organ. This is particularly evident where there are lesions in the bile duct resulting from chronic pancreatitis or carcinoma of the head of the pancreas. In this context, the indications for ERC are summarized in a table in which particular problems are specified (Table 20.1).

There are virtually no contraindications to ERCP when the procedure is indicated. It may be a life-saving measure even for extremely ill patients with septic cholangitis or biliary pancreatitis. However, this is only true when it is ensured that the cause of the disorder can be eliminated at the same session by subsequent endoscopic therapeutic measures (e.g. by EPT, stone extraction or insertion of a bile drain) (Ch. 35).

Table 20.1 Indications for ERC

Main indications
1. Differentiation between obstructive jaundice and unexplained cholestasis
2. Suspected biliary disorder where
   — a conventional cholangiogram is ambiguous
   — there is excretory hepatic insufficiency with elevated bilirubin
   — there is allergy to contrast medium
3. Post-choledochoduodenostomy (sump syndrome)
4. Post-cholecystectomy syndromes
5. Suspected papillary stenosis; where appropriate combined with manometry
6. Suspected carcinoma of the pancreas and chronic pancreatitis
7. Chronic inflammatory intestinal disorders with elevated alkaline phosphatase

Secondary indications
1. Suspected Caroli syndrome
2. Suspected parasitic infestation
3. Suspected tumours, metastases and abscesses of the liver

Success rate

Practised investigators find the papilla in 98–99% of cases. There may be difficulties with extensive papillary tumours and duodenal stenoses or if the papilla is located inside a duodenal diverticulum. The success rate is not more than 60–85% in patients who have undergone Billroth II gastrectomy (Katon et al 1975, Osnes & Myren 1975), since the papilla cannot always be reached owing to the postoperative formation of loops.

The success rate with cannulation increases with increasing experience of the investigator. However, even experienced investigators succeed with retrograde cholangiography in only 90–95% of cases (Rösch 1985). Suprapapillary stab incision (Caletti et al 1980) is particularly successful when the bile duct is dilated. Another way of increasing the success rate of cannulation is previously to intubate the papilla using a guide wire with a diameter of 0.035 in, over which the definitive catheter can then be advanced (Siegel et al 1985).

Complications and their prevention

In the matter of complications of ERCP, the inexperienced investigator is again the most significant risk factor (Bilbao et al 1976). Statistics on complication rates vary accordingly. The most important complications and their frequency are listed in Table 20.2 (Rösch 1981).

Knowledge of the possible complications is the most important prerequisite for their prevention. Necrotizing pancreatitis, which is a serious problem, is observed in about 0.1% of pancreatographies. In our patients, the rate of iatrogenic pancreatitis requiring treatment is about 1% in 1600 operations a year (ERCP, papillotomy, stone extraction, insertion of drains). There was no case of necrotizing pancreatitis (Phillip et al 1985).

Acute pancreatitis following ERCP should be distinguished from transient hyperamylasaemia which occurs in 40–75% of cases (Classen & Demling 1975, Staritz & Ewe 1984. However, this gives rise to no symptoms and disappears within 1–2 days, as do hypertrypsinaemia (Phillip et al 1983) and elevation of lipase and elastase 1 (Okuno et al 1985). The use of a non-ionic contrast medium of low osmolarity has no convincing advantages over an ionic contrast medium (Hannigan et al 1985). The risk of complications is reduced by cautious administration of the contrast medium, avoidance of injec-

Table 20.2 The most important complications of ERCP

Pancreatitis	0.7% – 7.4%
Cholangitis	0.6% – 0.8%
Phlegmon/abscess of the pancreas	0.5% – 1.3%
Side effects of drugs	0.1% – 0.6%
Injury to the gastrointestinal tract	0.07% – 0.4%
Mortality	0.001% – 0.8%

tion of more than the pancreatic duct can take and avoidance of repeated filling of the pancreas when visualization of the bile duct has not succeeded. It is not possible to prevent pancreatitis by prophylactic administration of somatostatin during ERCP (Börsch et al 1984). Nor does additional administration of somatostatin increase the rate of healing once pancreatic complications related to the ERCP have occurred (Phillip et al 1985).

The complication of retrograde choledochography which was the most serious problem for a long time was the development of cholangitis. This may occur when the drainage of the contrast medium takes place only slowly owing to a stenosis in the duct system. The pathogens have been found to be primarily *Enterobacteria* sp. and *Pseudomonas aeruginosa* (Helm et al 1984). For this reason, it is particularly important when carrying out ERCP to ensure that the equipment is adequately disinfected in order to prevent the implantation of hospital bacteria. The most important measure to be taken when an obstruction in the bile duct has been demonstrated is to remove the hindrance to outflow as soon as possible (Classen & Phillip 1982).

It is possible to dispense with systemic or local antibiotic administration for prophylaxis (Jandrzejewski et al 1980) where there is free outflow of the contrast medium. We administer an antibiotic which passes into the bile, e.g. mezlocillin or cefotaxime, only if the outflow of contrast medium is insufficient or zero.

ENDOSCOPIC FINDINGS IN THE DUODENUM AND PAPILLA OF VATER

It is not rare for preliminary examination of the stomach and duodenal cap to provide important principal and secondary findings, especially when preceding upper endoscopy has been dispensed with. Displacement of the antrum or pylorus or constriction of the duodenum frequently indicate the presence of a space-occupying process of the pancreas causing the cholestasis. The diagnosis is confirmed by biopsies taken from an infiltrated duodenal wall.

90% of duodenal diverticula are located on the descending part of the duodenum, principally in the region of the papilla. Large juxtapapillary diverticula are of clinical significance because they are associated with choledocholithiasis significantly more often. On inspection of the papilla, anatomical variants should be looked for even before intubation (Phillip et al 1974). On occasion, two orifices are found and this indicates separate efferent ducts. If there is a smaller papilla it is located about 1–2 cm above the greater papilla. Incarcerated papillary stones give rise to a characteristic distension of the papilla (Plate 20.1). Previous spontaneous discharge of a stone can be recognized by a fissured splitting of the orifice. Previous

Table 20.3 Histological findings in 63 cases of papillary tumours

Adenomatous carcinoma	23 (36 %)
Adenoma	20 (32 %)
Papillary polyp	6 (10 %)
Hypeplasia	4 (6 %) 6
Inflammation	6 (10 %)
Pancreatic carcinoma	4 (6 %)
	63 (100%)

University Hospital, Frankfurt/Main 11.1981 — 01.04.1984

Table 20.4 Papillary carcinoma (n = 23)
Mean age = 70.7 years (49–91 years)
sex ♂ 11, ♀ 12

Therapy	n	Survival time (months)
EPT	7	6–8, mean 9.3
EPT + drainage	6	1–18, mean 6.3
operation	10	mean 12.2
		2 patients died after operation 3 patients still alive

University Hospital Frankfurt/Main 1985

surgical bougienage of the papilla or spontaneous stone perforations above the papilla also produce a characteristic appearance. Occasionally, a fistulous perforation in the roof of the papilla is found, being the consequence of a false passage produced at surgical bougienage (Tanaka 1983). Biliodigestive anastomoses appear as circular or slit-like openings. Diagnosis of a papillary carcinoma when viewed through a duodenoscope is not difficult if the tumour is growing above the surface. However, diagnosis becomes difficult when the expansion of the tumour is predominantly intramural. In such instances, the diagnosis is frequently not confirmed until after papillotomy, by (loop) biopsy from the edges of the tumour which are then exposed. Table 20.3 shows a list of the papillary tumours found by endoscopy at the University Hospital in Frankfurt, their malignancy or otherwise having been determined by biopsy, surgery, autopsy or follow-up. Of the 23 papillary carcinomas, even following EPT forceps biopsies for two patients were not positive until the time of follow-up investigation, in one patient the diagnosis was only made at operation, and in a further two it was confirmed at autopsy (five out of 23). The progress of these carcinoma patients is shown in Table 20.4. Benign papillary stenoses will be dealt with below.

ENDOSCOPIC RETROGRADE CHOLANGIOGRAPHY

The normal cholangiogram, variants and anomalies

The standard lumen widths in the bile ducts are known from conventional radiology. The upper limits for the widths of the extrahepatic bile ducts as measured by ERCP vary between 9 and 14 mm, (Niederau et al 1984). Combined radiological/manometric studies (Poralla et al 1985) have shown that even in the absence of extrahepatic cholestasis the diameter of and the pressure difference in the bile ducts increase with advancing age. It should be noted that the widths of the bile ducts measured by sonography are somewhat less but do strictly correlate with the measurements carried out during ERCP (Meier et al 1984, Niederau et al 1984).

Relevant anatomical abnormalities of the hepatobiliary system are cystic dilatations (Fig. 20.1) of the bile duct or of the intrahepatic bile ducts (Caroli syndrome). Less clinical significance attaches to multiple hepatic ducts. There is also wide variation in the point of junction of the cystic duct; one which is very low down, with a correspondingly long cystic duct (Fig. 20.2), may result in difficulties at surgery.

Stones in the gallbladder and biliary tract

Gallstones are the most frequent disorder affecting the biliary system. About 12% of the population in western Europe and the United States have stones in the gallbladder, and 2–3% have concrements in the bile ducts. About 10–20% of the patients with stones in the gallbladder also have concrements in the bile ducts. Stones which have been left behind or have formed again after cholecystectomy are found in 5–10% of patients (references in Leuschner & Baumgärtel 1984). The incidence of intrahepatic stones (hepatolithiasis) is greater in the Far East than in Western countries. Most of these stones consist of bilirubinate (Ohto et al 1984).

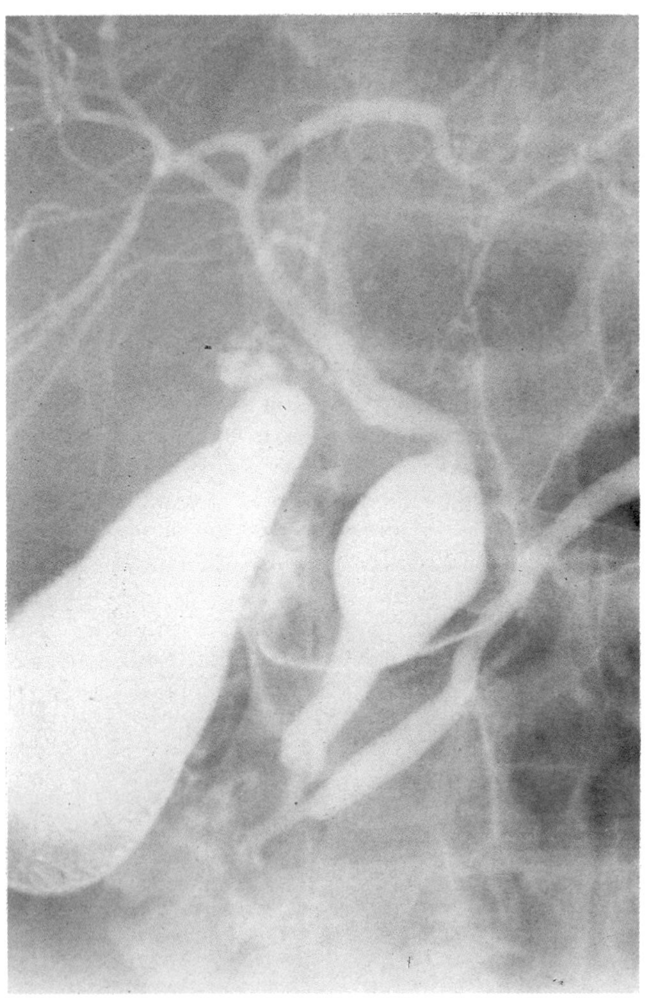

Fig. 20.1 Choledochal cyst

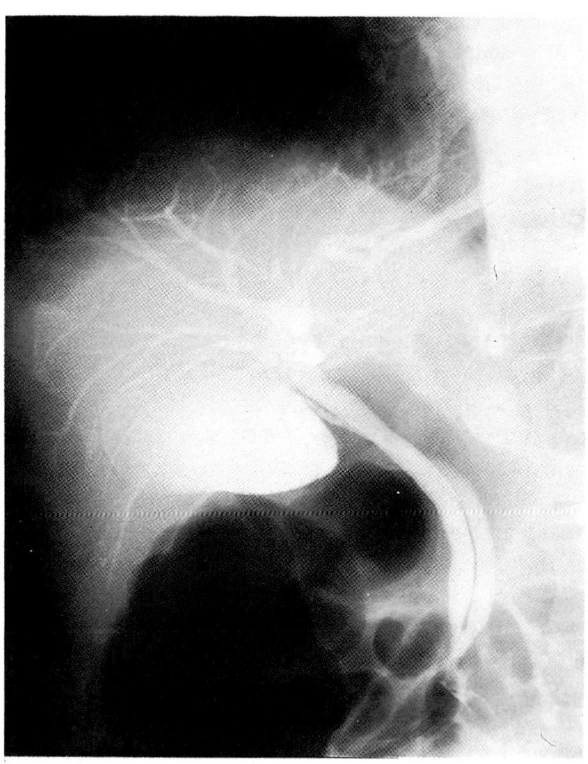

Fig. 20.2 Long cystic duct

Once the bile duct has been cannulated, it is possible to instil sufficient contrast medium to fill the entire biliary system, including the smallest intrahepatic branches. This ensures that stones are visualized (Fig. 20.3). The detection of the concrements must be carried out on the basis of the lack of change in or the characteristic shape of the recess in the contrast medium on several radiographs. The instillation of air bubbles should be avoided since it may give rise to false findings. They can be distinguished from concrements by the fact that when the patient is set upright they migrate upwards in the bile duct, whereas the weight of stones usually means that they sink.

It is frequently the case that initial detection of smaller concrements is only possible during a brief period while the contrast medium is being injected and the bile duct is only faintly shadowed. During this, they are frequently flushed upwards with the contrast medium. They are no longer visualized once the entire system is completely full.

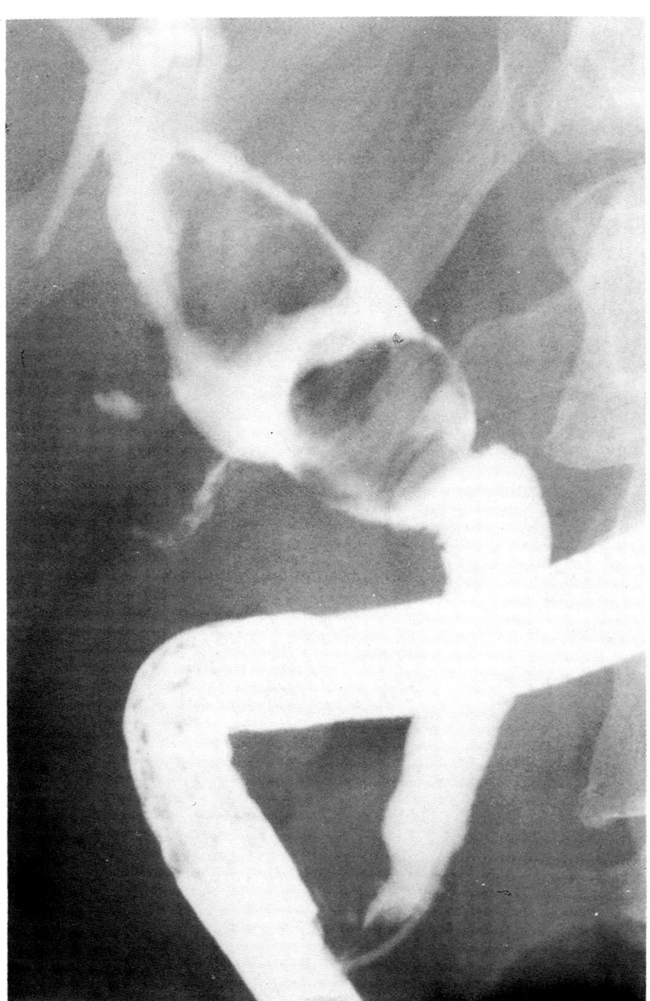

Fig. 20.3 Choledocholithiasis

For this reason, it is always necessary to await the emptying of the bile duct for detection of stones of this type. In some cases, small concrements can only be detected using diluted contrast medium.

The detection of concrements in the gallbladder is in the domain of sonography. Nevertheless accurate visualization of the gallbladder should not be omitted during the ERCP. There is no doubt that ERCP is superior to sonography (Goodman et al 1985). Visualization of stones in the gallbladder demands accurate estimation of the correct degree of filling. Both too little and too much contrast medium can give rise to assessment errors. Even when the findings are initially normal, a picture should always be taken while the gallbladder is emptying. Sometimes the gallbladder does not fill until the patient has been lying on his right side for about 15 min. If filling has not taken place even after this time then the probable diagnosis is cholecystolithiasis, a shrunken gallbladder or a carcinoma and surgery may be assumed to be necessary. However, rapid detection of concrements in the bile duct should not mislead one into premature discontinuation of the investigation. Otherwise it is easy to overlook important secondary findings, such as gallbladder tumours or stenoses (Fig. 20.4). Moreover, with the exception of acute cholecystitis the complications arising from gallstones are in the domain of ERCP. This particularly applies to stenosis, obstruction and penetration.

Stenoses of the biliary tract

Stenoses of the biliary tract result in the biochemical and clinical signs, depending on the severity, of cholestasis. 9% of our patients had stenosis, whereas far more, 55%, had cholangiolithiasis. The other causes of extrahepatic cholestasis were organic papillary stenosis (12%, usually following previous surgery), fistulae between the bile ducts and other abdominal organs in 6%, and carcinoma of the papilla of Vater in 3% (Classen 1977). Mechanical obstructive jaundice can be confirmed with ERCP in 85–90%. For the remaining cases, percutaneous transhepatic cholangiography can be used as a supplementary method (Classen et

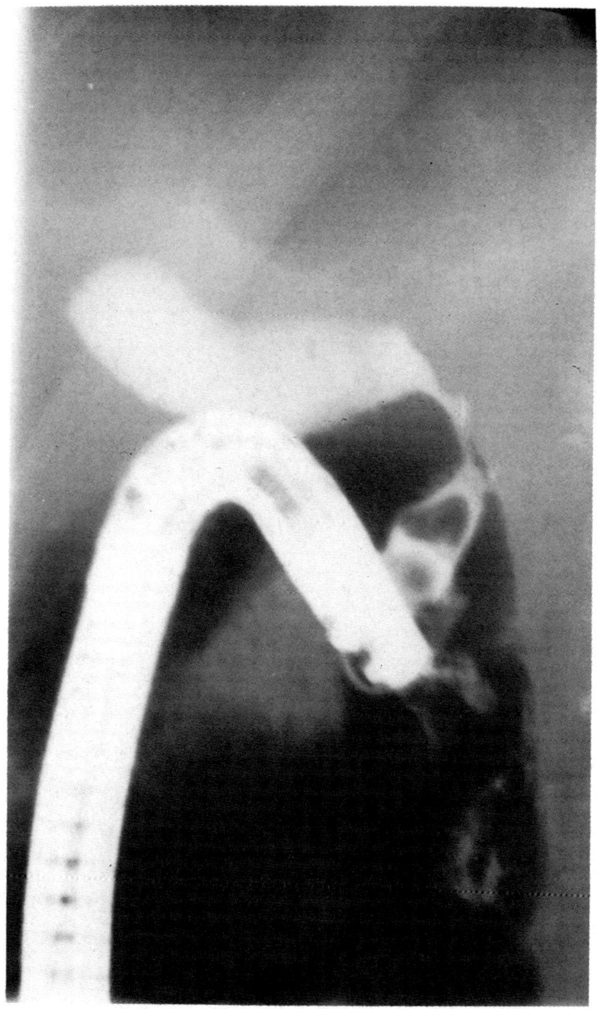

Fig. 20.4 Choledocholithiasis and gallbladder carcinoma (filiform stenosis)

al 1981, Matzen et al 1982). Weissmüller et al (1983) were able to confirm the diagnosis of malignant obstructive jaundice by ERCP or PTC in 122 cases. PTC was the primary diagnostic method in only 7% of the cases.

Malignant stenoses

It is not as a rule possible during ERCP to distinguish primary bile duct carcinomas from stenoses caused by metastases with tumour infiltration. Differentiation is, however, assisted by the history, investigation of the surroundings, direct biopsy and fine-needle biopsy targeted by ultrasound. A carcinoma of the extrahepatic bile ducts is located frequently near the papilla of Vater. Thus a distinction from a primary carcinoma of the pancreas is often impossible (Fig. 20.5).

Two types of malignant stenosis can be distinguished by radiology.

1. Circumscribed stenosis with irregular sharp edges to the wall of the part of the bile duct adjoining the stenosis. There is pronounced congestion of the prestenotic duct system (Seifert et al 1974).
2. Complete occlusion or discontinuity of the duct, with the wall in the region of the obstruction being either sharp-edged or, occasionally, frayed. In such cases the distal part of the bile duct is noticeably thin and delicate (Oi 1973).

It is noteworthy that, in contrast to distal occlusion of the bile duct, when the tumour is located high up, in the region of the hepatic duct and the bifurcation, no pronounced dilatation of the intrahepatic bile ducts is found in about one-fifth of the cases (Weismüller et al 1983).

Benign stenoses

Benign stenoses of the extrahepatic bile ducts are relatively rare. Annular stenosis of the distal part of the bile duct associated with chronic pancreatitis and the generalized strictures and stenoses associated with sclerosing cholan-

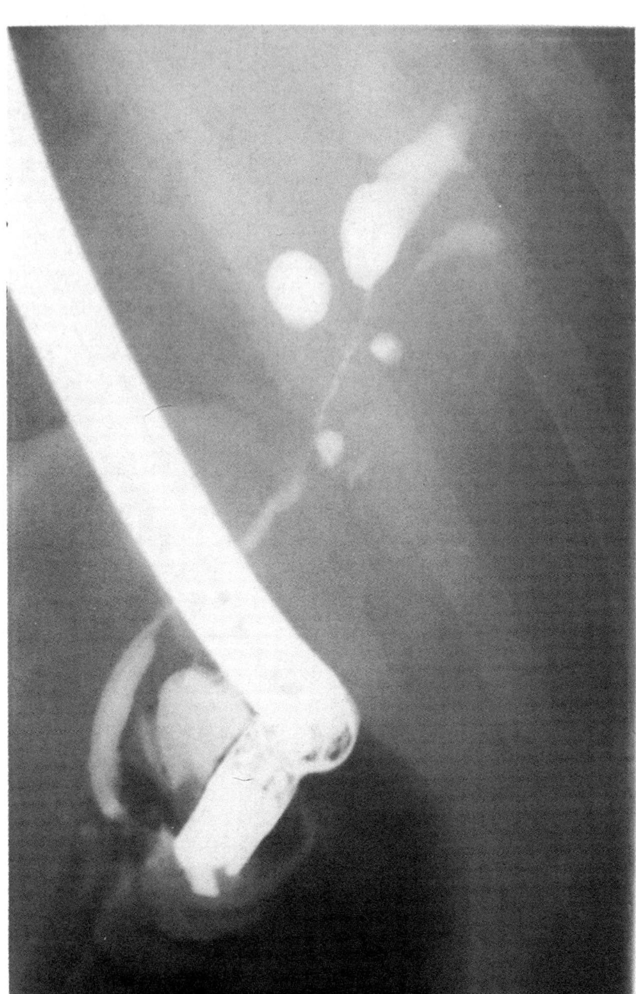

Fig. 20.5 Malignant stenosis of the common bile duct: bile duct carcinoma.

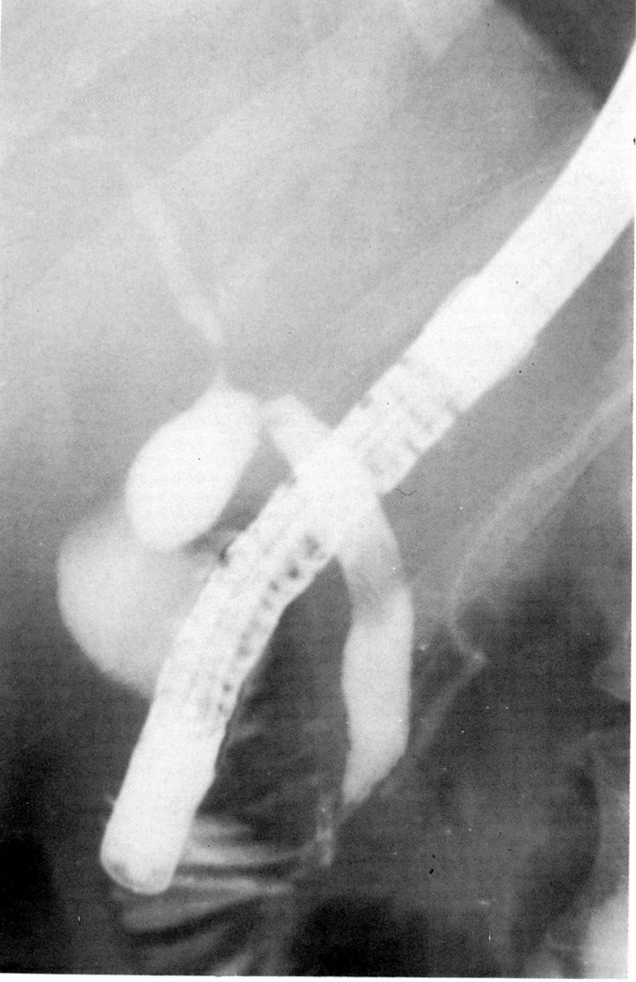

Fig. 20.6 Mirizzi syndrome

gitis will be dealt with below. Stones in the infundibulum of the gallbladder may lead to involvement of the hepatic duct if there is adhesion of the inflamed infundibulum to the hepatic duct and the latter becomes involved in the inflammatory fibrosis. The result is cicatricial stenosis of the hepatic duct with hindrance to outflow of hepatic bile, this being known as the Mirizzi syndrome. There is often difficulty with differentiating this from carcinoma of the biliary confluence or of the gallbladder (Fig. 20.6) (Ch. 64, 65).

Differential diagnosis of bile duct stenoses must include changes brought about by surgery. Iatrogenic injury to the extrahepatic bile ducts following cholecystectomy has been reported not to exceed 1% in a selected group of patients (Femppel et al 1981). In endoscopic practice this affects the common hepatic duct at the level of the junction with the cystic duct (Fig. 20.7, 20.8). The clinical picture of the stenosis is variable and should be viewed in the context of the surgery which has previously taken place. In most cases, the spindle-like nature of the constriction points to the diagnosis. Distinction from carcinoma of the bile duct may be difficult if there has been extensive oversewing of the bile duct followed by T-drainage and corresponding scarring.

Iatrogenic stenoses are part of what is called the post-cholecystectomy syndrome. The results obtained during ERCP have shown that the incidence of those caused by biliary and pancreatic factors is greater than originally assumed (references in Philip & Hagenmüller 1983). The most frequent organic bilio-pancreatic causes of the post-cholecystectomy syndrome are shown in Table 20.5.

A diagnostic problem may result from the cystic duct remnant syndrome, especially when the cystic duct cannot be visualized by endoscopy/radiology owing to occlusion by a stone. There is still controversy about the pathological significance of this syndrome (Grözinger 1984, Aaerima & Maekelae 1981). Nevertheless, Daniels et al (1980) report an incidence of about 5% in more than 4000 cholecystectomies, it being assumed that there was a causal

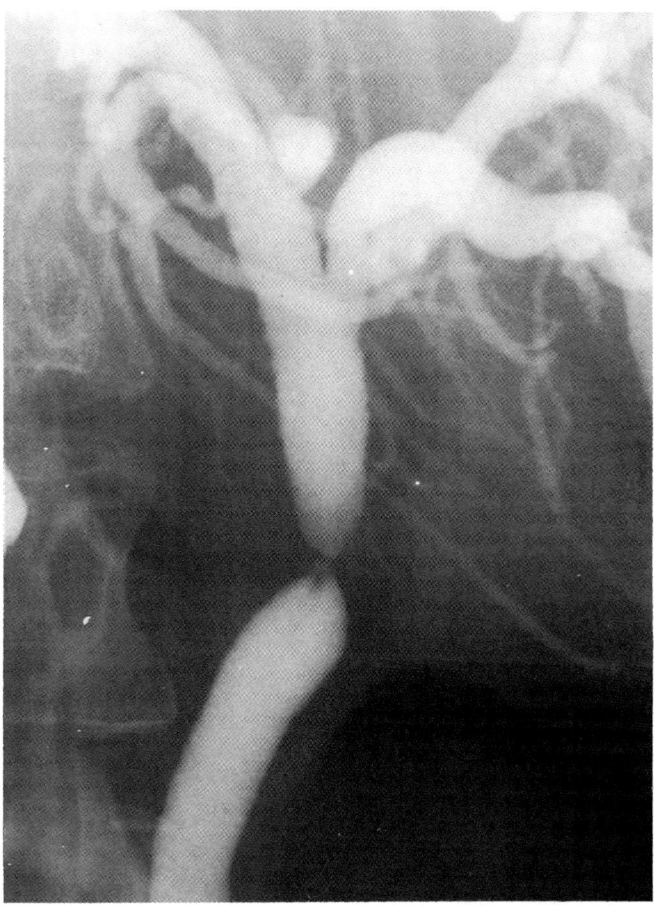

Fig. 20.8 Cicatricial stenosis of the common bile duct following cholecystectomy and biliary drainage via T-tube

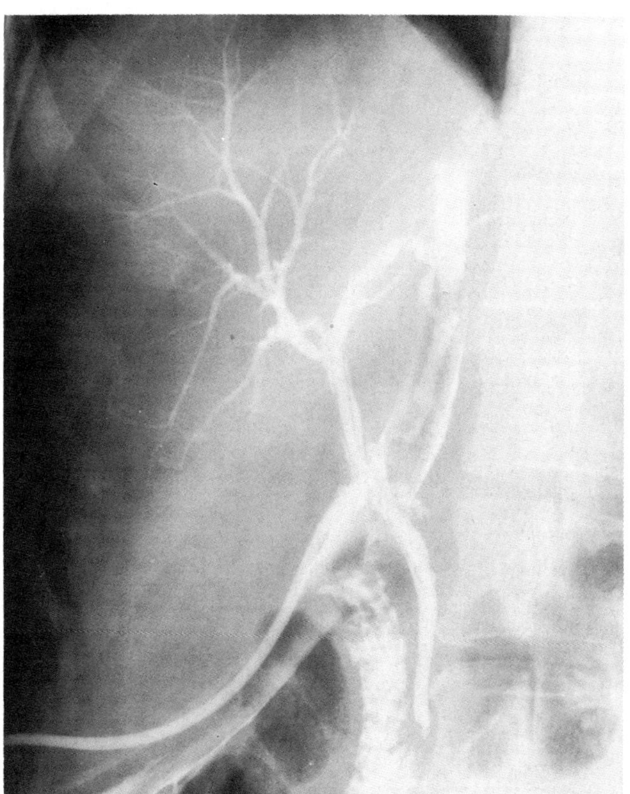

Fig. 20.7 T-tube following cholecystectomy

Table 20.5 Possible causes of the post-cholecystectomy syndrome (PCS)

Choledocholithiasis
Papillary stenosis
Benign iatrogenic stricture of the common bile duct
Long cystic duct
Biliodigestive anastomoses
Duodenal diverticula
Stenosis of the distal bile ducts due to chronic pancreatitis
Malignant tumours (papilla Vateri, bile ducts and pancreas)

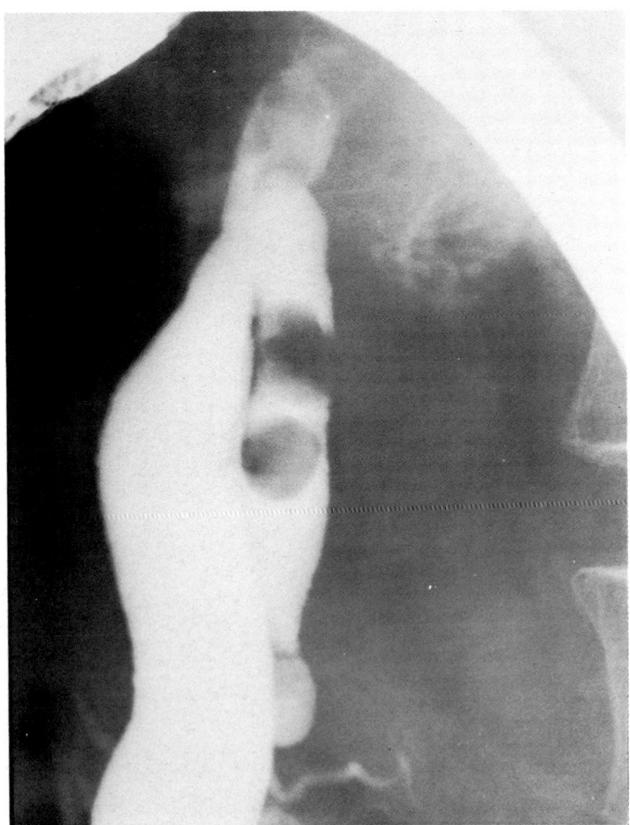

Fig. 20.9 'Cystic duct remnant syndrome': stones in the cystic duct stump following cholecystectomy

connection with the symptoms in about one-third of the patients (Fig. 20.9).

Biliodigestive anastomoses frequently give rise to ascending cholangitis (Plate 20.2).

Cholangitis

Among the various types of cholangitis, particular importance attaches to lesions of the intrahepatic bile ducts. There is no doubt that improvements in the methods of diagnosis will be associated with primary cholangitis, in particular, being diagnosed more frequently and sooner.

Chronic destructive, non-suppurative cholangitis and suppurative primary sclerosing cholangitis

Various stages of chronic destructive, non-suppurative cholangitis, which leads to biliary cirrhosis, can be distinguished by ERCP. However, it is only rarely possible to achieve a genuine correlation between the clinical, radiological, macroscopic and microscopic stagings (Lesch & Weitzel 1981). In the early stage, the 3rd order bile ducts exhibit a wavy course, do not have sharp margins and have stenosing areas with prestenotic dilatations. Subsequently, the 2nd order bile ducts are also affected and show spindly or bulbous changes. The predominant impression given by the radiographs is a deficiency of branching of the intrahepatic bile ducts. In the final stage, that of biliary cirrhosis, all the intrahepatic bile ducts and some of the extrahepatic bile ducts are affected (Fig. 20.10).

Primary sclerosing cholangitis (PSC) (Ch. 59) is characterized by annular, concentric sclerosis of the walls of the bile ducts which is usually multifocal and only rarely unifocal and which affects submucous and subserous sections. The lesions are frequently located intrahepatically and may also affect the hepatic and bile ducts and involve the gallbladder too. The cholangiogram is characterized by alternation between short foci of stenosis and prestenotic dilatations, which leads to the larger ducts having irregularities of the walls (beading) (Rogers et al 1972). An equally characteristic sign is the deficiency in the smallest ducts which leads to reduced branching of the biliary tree (pruned tree) (Fig. 20.11).

It no longer appears justified to distinguish between primary sclerosing cholangitis and the types associated with ulcerative colitis, Crohn's disease or retroperitoneal

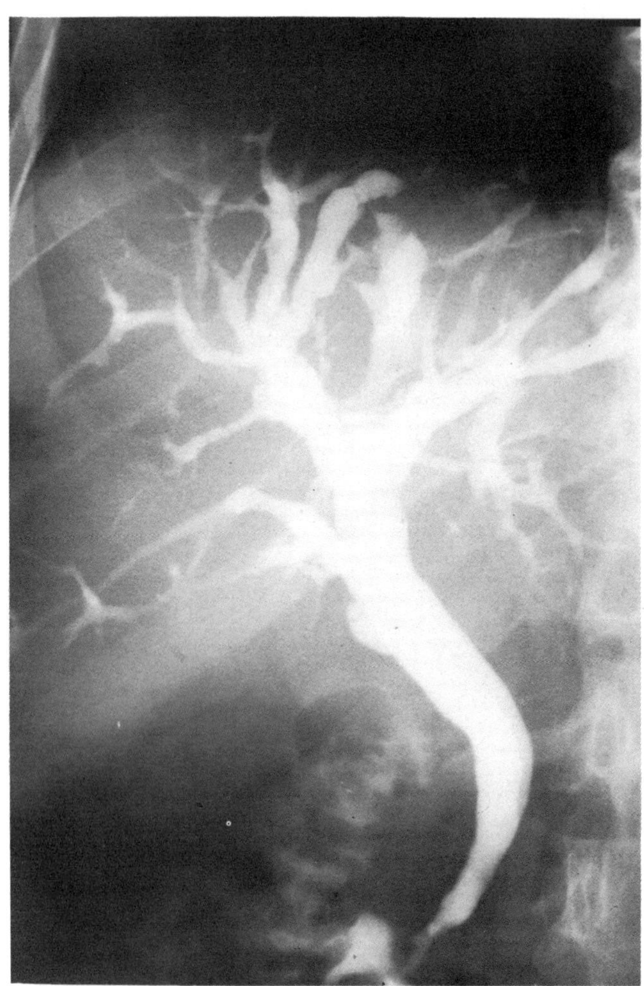

Fig. 20.10 Chronic destructive non-suppurative cholangitis

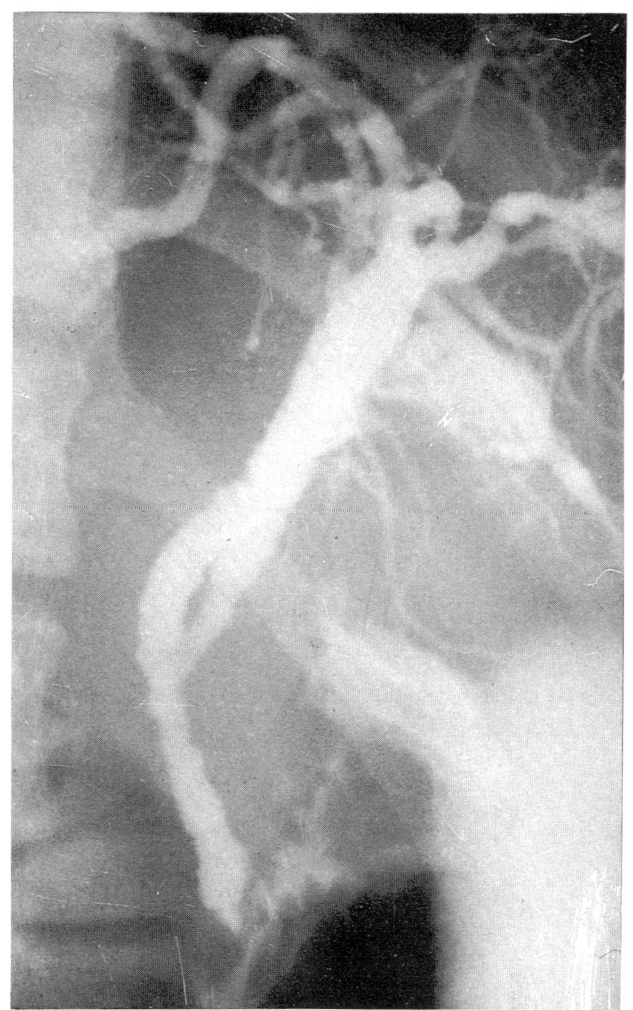

Fig. 20.11 Primary sclerosing cholangitis

fibrosis (Danzi et al 1976). Recent work on patients with ulcerative colitis has shown that the incidence of PSC is 1% (Mihas et al 1978). Conversely, PSC is associated with ulcerative colitis in about one-third of the cases. Likewise, a combination of sclerosing cholangitis, chronic pancreatitis and Sjögren's syndrome appears to be a homogeneous complex of symptoms with an autoimmune basis (Montefusco et al 1984). The differential diagnosis of such cases has to take account of diffusely growing sclerosing carcinoma of the biliary tract which is often in association with chronic inflammatory intestinal disorders (Ch. 65).

It is often very difficult to differentiate between chronic destructive cholangitis and primary sclerosing cholangitis by radiology and, in the final analysis, it is unnecessary. The deciding factors are the biochemical, immunological and histological findings.

Types of secondary cholangitis

Acute suppurative obstructive cholangitis with choledocholithiasis, jaundice and gram-negative septicaemia as a complication of ERCP gave rise to anxiety in the past. However, nowadays it is regarded as an indication for ERCP followed by EPT, where neccessary combined with relieving drainage (Wurbs et al 1980). In contrast to types of primary cholangitis, obstructive cholangitis, which is usually caused by a stone, is characterized by dilatation of the 2nd and 3rd order bile ducts. The appearance of irregularities in the walls, short stenoses and prestenotic dilatation of the intrahepatic bile ducts are reliable evidence of secondary cholangitis only if the clinical circumstances are taken into account (Plate 20.3).

A special type is recurrent pyogenic cholangitis (RPC) (Cook et al 1954) (Ch. 77). The disease occurs predominantly in south-east Asia and is hardly ever seen in Western countries. The infection and inflammation are restricted mainly to the biliary tract and they lead to strictures and the formation of stones. The prime pathogens are *E. coli*, *Klebsiella aerogenes*, *Pseudomonas*, *Proteus* and *Salmonellae*. 80% of the concrements which are usually present (Lam et al 1978) are located in the common bile duct, while 20% are located in the intrahepatic bile ducts. These are predominantly bilirubin stones (Wong and Choi 1984). In the early stage, ERCP shows slight dilatation of the intrahepatic bile ducts with pronounced branching, arrow-head formations or abrupt termination of the ducts (Lam et al 1978). The advanced stage is characterized by strictures of the intrahepatic bile with proximal dilatation and stones. The radiological changes correlate well with the severity of the clinical picture. There may be isolated, segmental or multiple cholangitic liver abscesses. Abnormal pancreatic ducts are found in up to 8% of the cases investigated (Lam et al 1978).

The Caroli syndrome (Ch. 80)

Cases of congenital Caroli syndrome show cystic dilatations of bile ducts in one or more segments of the liver, which are frequently filled with multiple concrements of various sizes (references in Kurtz et al 1980). It is also possible to speak, in an extended sense, of a Caroli syndrome when concrements can be detected in bile ducts which have undergone secondary dilatation.

Parasites

Echinococcal cysts (Ch. 75) do not show a uniform morphological appearance and thus a combination of diagnostic methods is necessary. 5–10% of hepatic hydatid cysts rupture and this may simulate choledocholithiasis. The daughter cysts which are released may lead to biliary obstruction. Calcified cysts are easy to recognize. Where this is not the case, stenoses with their associated hindrance to flow may show considerable irregularities in calibre and, in particular, extensive displacement of the intrahepatic branches, with or without impression effects (Cottone

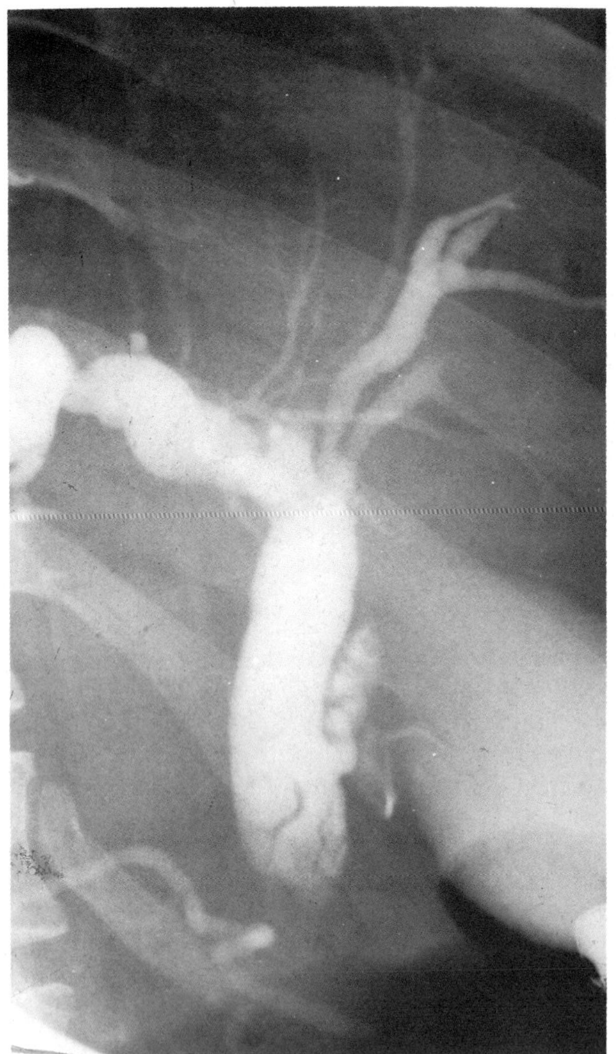

Fig. 20.12 Liver flukes in the distal bile duct presenting as 'biliary sludge'

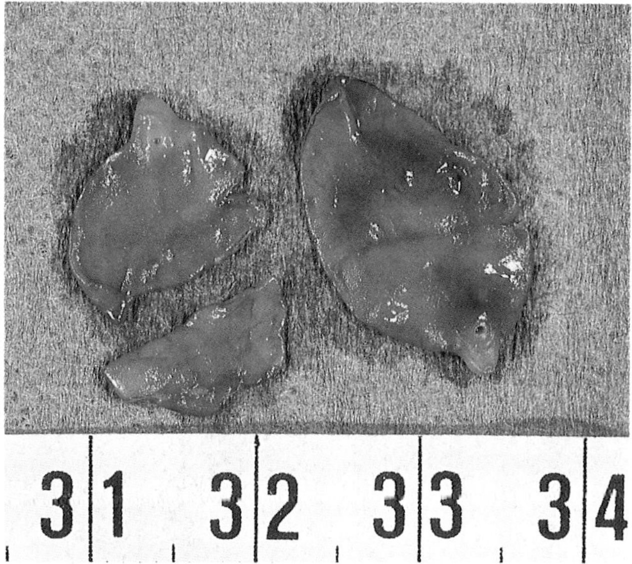

Fig. 20.13 Extracted liver flukes (same patient)

et al 1978, Dyrszka & Sangbavi 1983, Ibrahim & Kawanishi 1981).

Ascaris lumbricoides is a helminth which is among those found most frequently and it has worldwide distribution. Its prevalence is 90% in some parts of Africa and the Far East. If the worm passes through the sphincter of Oddi it may cause acute pancreatitis or a cholestasis syndrome (Winters et al 1984). In the acute stage, the worm may occasionally be found and extracted from the ampulla, and it can be detected in the biliary tract by endoscopy/radiology (Ch. 74).

It is also possible after raw meat has been eaten for *Clonorchis sinensis* to penetrate through the papilla into the bile ducts. The typical endoscopic/radiological appearance is of widely dilated extrahepatic bile ducts which are filled with biliary sludge and stones. It is predominantly the branches of the left hepatic duct where strictures are found (Yellin & Donovan 1981). The eggs of *Cl. sinensis* act as a nucleus of crystallization for the development of the stones (Lam et al 1978). Recently, Naval et al (1984) reported successful endoscopic biliary lavage after preceding choledochoenterostomy.

Invasion of *Fasciola hepatica* into the biliary tract may also cause serious lesions and, in the chronic stage, it can resemble the appearance of sclerosing cholangitis (Hauser & Bynum 1984). We were recently able, following endoscopic papillotomy, to extract two live liver flukes with a Dormia basket from a 35-year-old Turkish woman with obstructive jaundice. The appearance on ERCP was merely of the dilated bile ducts with unexplained sludgy formations in the distal bile duct (Fig. 20.13).

Traumatic intrahepatic lesions

Damage to the parenchyma resulting from blunt abdominal injury may give rise to direct or indirect connections between the blood vessels and bile ducts (Fig. 20.14). Depending on the existing pressure gradient, either blood enters the biliary tract (haemobilia) or bile infiltrates into the circulating blood (cholaemia) (Ch. 85). There have been descriptions of, *inter alia*, endoscopic/radiological detection of a biliary pseudocyst following cholecystectomy (Novis & Adam 1982) and of a fistula, caused by injury, from the right hepatic duct into the subphrenic space with a connection to a catheter placed through the skin (Nelson 1984). Haemobilia may also occur after liver biopsy and percutaneous cholangiography. The authors consider the best method of diagnosing these complications is ERC.

Intrahepatic tumours

It is necessary to differentiate between the syndromes described above and benign and malignant expansile

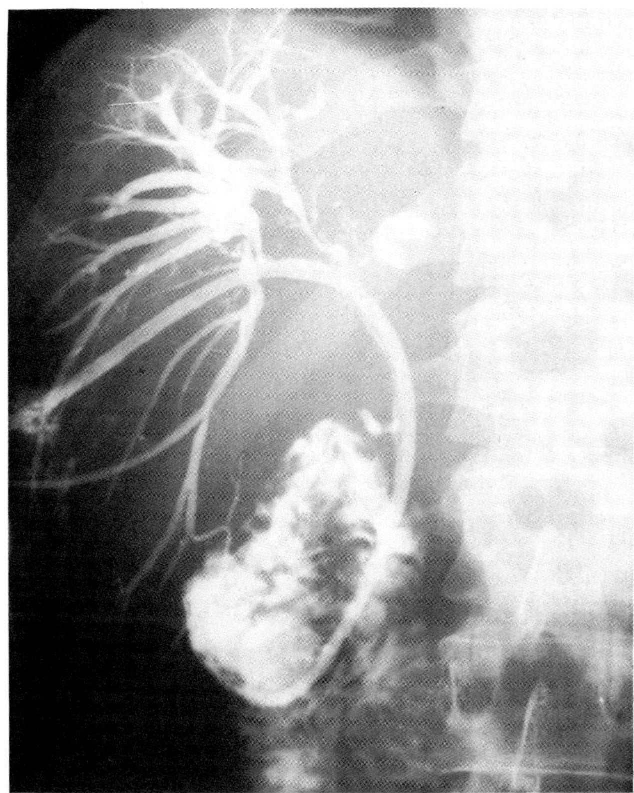

Fig. 20.14 Multiple traumatic stenoses of the intrahepatic bile ducts two years following liver rupture (motor vehicle accident)

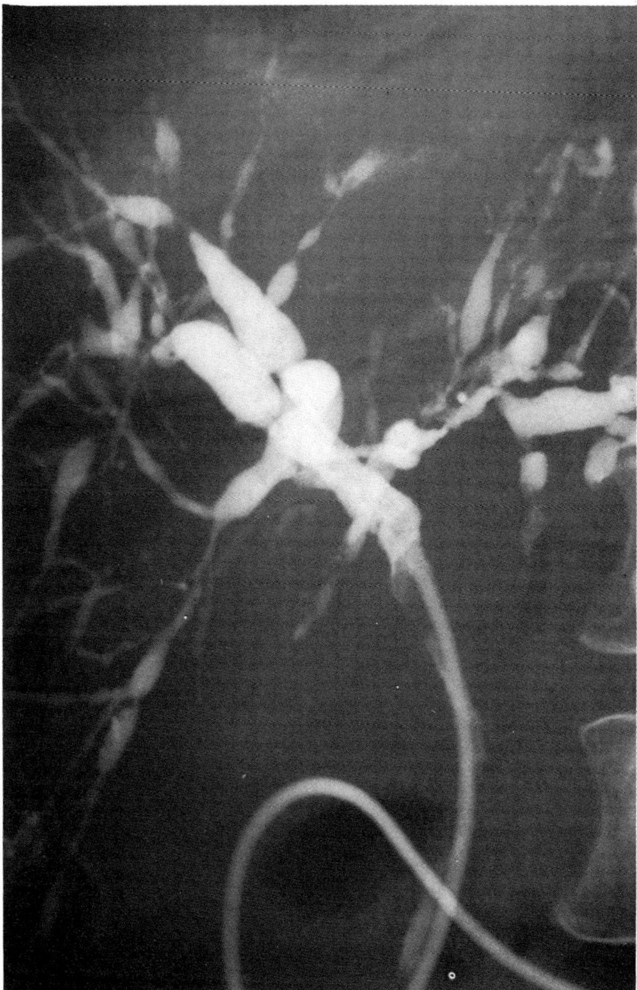

Fig. 20.15 Diffuse intrahepatic metastases of a gallbladder cancer: typical tapering, irregularities and rarefication of the intrahepatic bile ducts

processes of a non-inflammatory nature. Depending on the size, there may be displacement, stenoses and obstructions. Conically tapering occlusions of bile ducts point to intrahepatic metastases (Fig. 20.15). Arched displacements of intrahepatic bile ducts and impression effects do not permit differential diagnosis. They are found with haemangiomas, abscesses and abdominal lymph node enlargements, as with Hodgkin's disease or carcinomas of the adjacent organs. Nowadays, the diagnosis is increasingly being confirmed by fine-needle biopsy targeted by ultrasonography (Greiner 1985).

ERCP has little to contribute to the diagnosis of diffuse liver disorders, such as hepatitis, fatty degeneration and cirrhosis, differentiation of these disorders being better performed with other methods.

The biliary duct system in pancreatic disease

The close topographical relation between the pancreatic part of the bile duct and the head of the pancreas is the reason for the frequent involvement of the bile duct in disorders of the pancreas, especially of its head. Inflammatory swelling, cicatricial fibroses, displacement by cysts and tumours, and invasion of tumours into the bile duct result in a constriction of its distal part, with a variety of types of stenoses and strictures. The clinical consequences are various degrees of cholestasis which may result in secondary cholangitis and stone formation.

Chronic pancreatitis

In about 25% of patients with chronic pancreatitis the terminal part of the bile duct is involved, this depending on the severity of the inflammation. Analysis of 531 patients with chronic pancreatitis showed that 12.3% of them had constriction of the bile duct (Kasugai 1975) grade II and 50% of them had grade III. Signs of cholestasis appeared in 18.1% of the patients (Rösch et al 1981) (Fig. 20.16).

Groove pancreatitis (Stolte et al 1982) occupies a special position. This is a peripancreatic sheet of scarring which is located in the groove between the duodenum, the bile duct and the head of the pancreas, without or with only slight scarring of the latter. In most cases, there are changes to the pancreatic duct system only in the head of

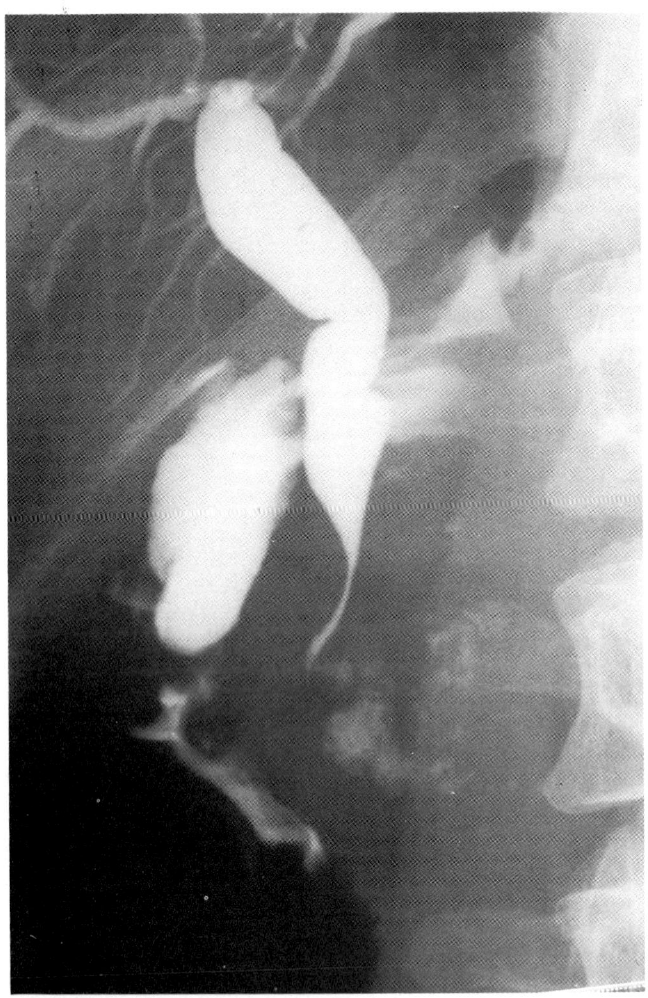

Fig. 20.16 Filiform stenosis caused by chronic pancreatitis

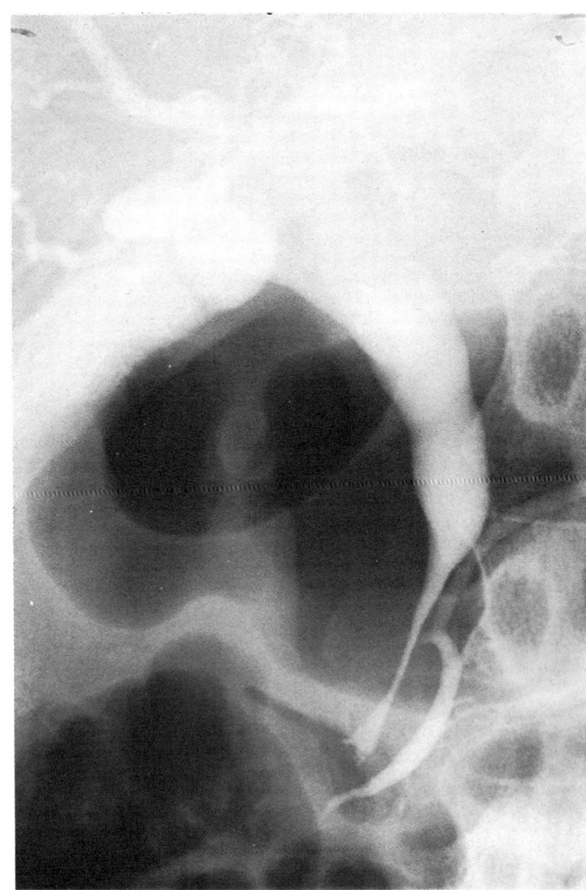

Fig. 20.17 Acute pancreatitis with pseudocyst in the head of the pancreas (verified on operation) leading to cholestasis

the pancreas, and it is occasionally difficult to distinguish this from carcinoma of the latter. The annular stenosis of the bile duct characteristic of chronic pancreatitis is found in 27–58% of these cases, depending on the type (Stolte 1984).

Acute pancreatitis

Pseudocysts which are consequent on acute pancreatitis and are located adjacent to the bile duct may cause, owing to displacement, pronounced symptoms of cholestasis (Fig. 20.17). In acute biliary pancreatitis, which is usually caused by incarceration of a stone in the region of the papilla, the changes in the bile duct caused by the congestion are not the consequence but the cause of the pancreatitis. The authors consider the treatment of choice nowadays to be demonstration using ERCP followed by EPT, and this will be dealt with in a section to itself.

Carcinoma of the pancreas

The preferred location for carcinomas of the pancreas is in the region of the papilla of Vater and of the head of the pancreas (periampullary carcinomas) and, accordingly, the bile duct is frequently also involved. Annular stenosis is not found associated with carcinoma of the pancreas; on the other hand circumscribed stenosis with irregular boundaries, or even occlusion of the bile duct, is found in about two-thirds of the cases (Plumley et al 1982, Stolte 1984) (Fig. 20.18).

BENIGN PAPILLARY STENOSIS

The problems associated with malignant papillary stenosis have already been dealt with (see above). The diagnosis of circumscribed benign papillary stenosis is likewise not always straightforward by endoscopy/radiology. In cases of benign papillary stenosis (Ch. 56), the endoscopic appearance of the papilla varies; it may be completely unremarkable or it may be slightly protruding with a smooth mucosal surface. Occasionally, a small papilla merely shows irregular folds. There appears to be no good correlation between the macroscopic and microscopic findings in benign papillary stenosis (Classen 1981). After filling with contrast medium, the bile duct is frequently found

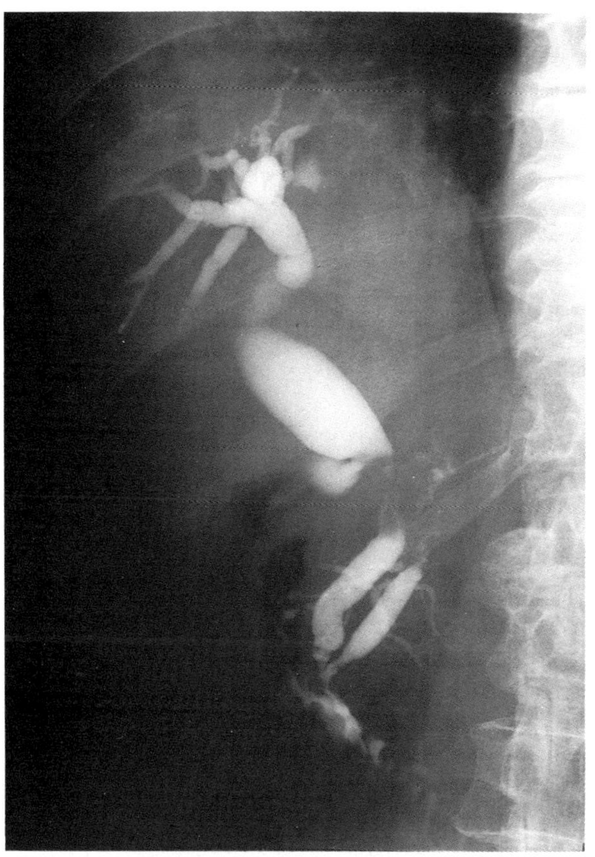

Fig. 20.18 Double duct sign (stenosis of bile duct and pancreatic duct) in a case of pancreatic carcinoma

in such cases to be dilated with a fusiform constriction of its distal end, usually in the intramural part of the duct. The pancreatic duct is, if it can be visualized, usually also slightly dilated (Greenen 1977). The outflow of contrast medium is prolonged to more than 45 min, and as a rule there are biochemical signs of cholestasis. Isolated stenosis of the sphincter ampulla causes in addition a prestenotic dilatation of the ampulla (hydroampulla). A Y-shaped stenosis shows the involvement of all segments of the sphincter. Serial radiographs are necessary in order to demonstrate the deficient contraction and relaxation of the sphincter muscle (Fig. 20.19).

ASSOCIATED METHODS

In recent years, diagnostic ERCP has undergone an expansion owing not only to the endoscopic methods of surgical treatment but also to associated methods, some of which have already been mentioned in passing, which allow confirmation or ruling out of a suspected diagnosis.

Manometry

New information on the motility of the biliary tract, in particular of the sphincter of Oddi, has been obtained since 1975 when endoscopic manometry became available (Rösch et al 1976). This technique of investigation makes use of duodenoscopy to find the papilla of Vater. A triple-

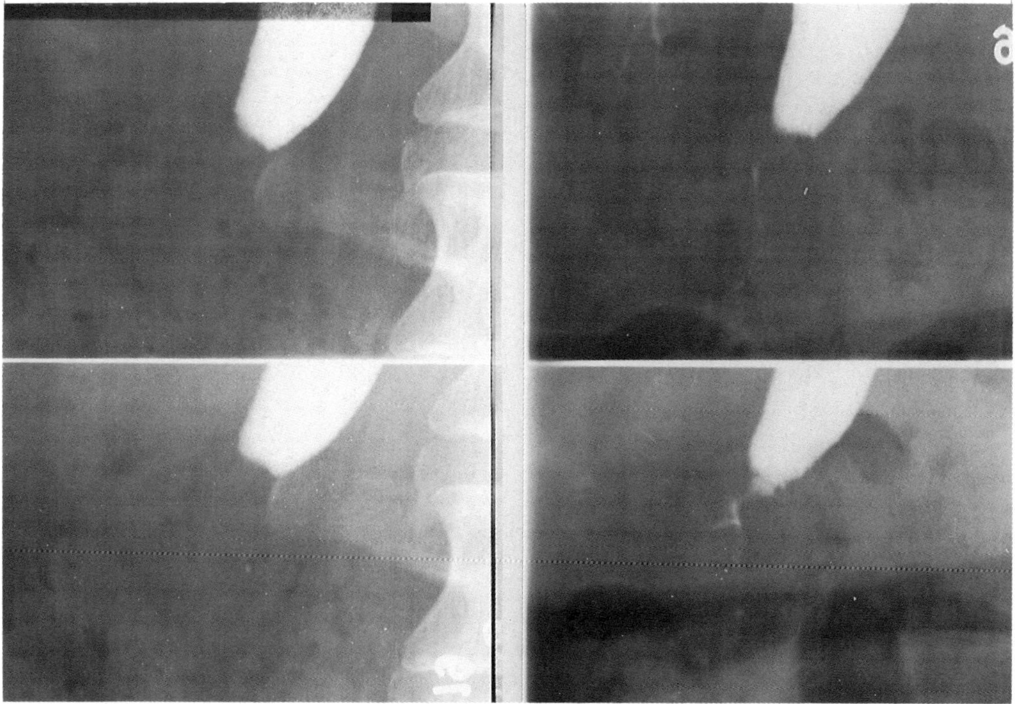

Fig. 20.19 Papillary stenosis

lumen measuring catheter is introduced with visual monitoring into the papilla and the bile duct. It is perfused with fluid by means of a pneumohydraulic pump during the measurement of pressure. The fluid column transmits the pressure from three lateral openings in the catheter, which act as measurement points, to the outside where an electromechanical pressure transducer and pen recorder are used to record the pressure changes (Ch. 9) (Fig. 20.20). For a detailed description of the method see Geenen (1983), and Hagenmüller (1983). Using this

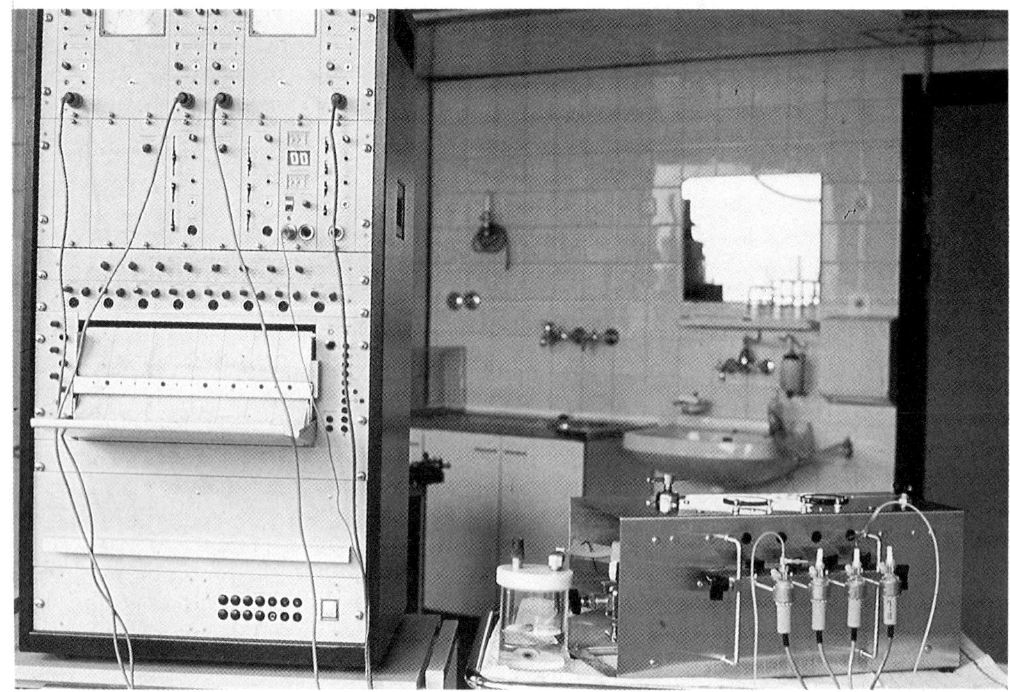

Fig. 20.20 Equipment for manometry: four–channel writing unit (left), pneumo hydraulic perfusion pump (right)

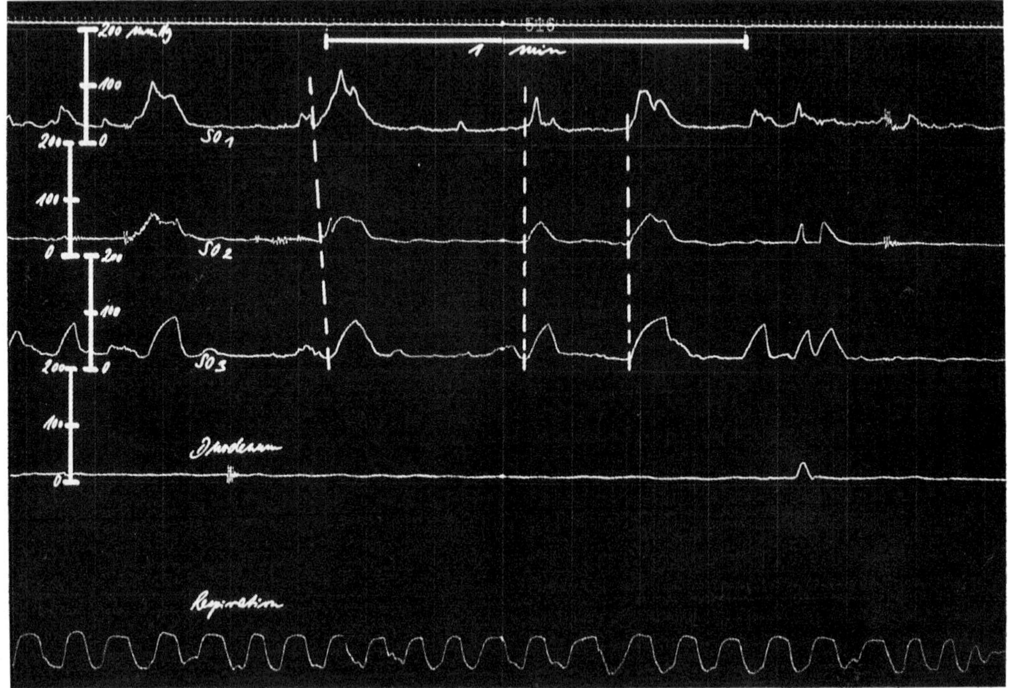

Fig. 20.21 Normal manometric finding of the motor activity of the sphincter of Oddi: The dotted lines show the antegrade propulsion of the motor activity from the upper sphincter region (SO_1) towards the duodenal wall. Channel four shows the pressure within the duodenum. Additionally shown are the respiratory movements

method it is possible to analyze the bilio-duodenal pressure difference, the frequency and amplitude of the contractions of the sphincter of Oddi and the direction of propagation of the contraction waves (Fig. 20.21). Measurements on healthy volunteers have shown that the normal bilio-duodenal pressure difference is 9.6 mmHg, the frequency of the contractions of the sphincter of Oddi is 5/min, and the mean amplitude of these contractions is 100 mmHg. Geenen (1982) deduced from investigations that the basal pressure in the region of the sphincter of Oddi, as measured by endoscopy, is a reliable objective parameter for the presence of dysfunction of the sphincter, but this term does not distinguish between organic papillary stenosis and purely functional dyskinesia. Endoscopic papillotomy was carried out on 29 patients with dysfunction of the sphincter of Oddi detected by endoscopic manometry, and this led to an improvement in the symptoms in 27 cases (93%) (Geenen 1982).

Toouli et al (1982) found, using endoscopic manometry, that patients with bile duct stones have an abnormally high proportion of retrograde contractions of the sphincter (Ch. 9). This finding gave rise to the question of whether this form of dyskinesia might be a pathogenetic mechanism for the stone formation or whether it was the consequence of this. De Masi et al (1984) were unable to confirm a reversal of the peristalsis of the sphincter in patients with bile duct stones. A number of investigators (Guelrud et al 1983, Cuschieri et al 1983) found dysfunction of the papilla which could be measured by manometry only when the bile duct stones were accompanied by recurrent pancreatitis. Endoscopic biliary tract manometry has also pointed to the possibility of paradoxical motor reactions of the sphincter to hormonal stimuli. Thus, intravenous injection of cholecystokinin in some patients with clinically suspected dysfunction of the sphincter resulted in a marked increase in its motility, which is the converse of the normal behaviour (Toouli et al 1985). Abnormally high frequencies of the contractions of the sphincter (tachyoddia) have also been observed and have been interpreted as the pathogenetic mechanism of the biliary tract dyskinesia (Staritz et al 1985a).

Biopsy

A biopsy is indispensable for distinguishing between the various pathological changes in the papilla (see above). Bourgeois et al (1984) have pointed out that papillary biopsies should be undertaken either immediately after EPT or not until about one week has elapsed, since atypical cells may be found within 48 hours even with benign papillary processes, and these then give rise to faulty interpretations.

The development of endoscopic papillotomy has also provided the basis for transpapillary access to the extrahepatic biliary tract for endoscopic biopsy (Nishumura et al 1980, Seifert et al 1980) (Fig. 20.22). The results of 47 biopsies on 16 of our own patients are shown in Table 20.6 (Danzygier & Classen 1985). Moreover, transpapillary bile duct biopsy has established itself as a valuable method of increasing our knowledge about the fine structure and histopathology of the biliary tract (Danzygier et al 1983)

Exfoliative cytology of the bile duct and the periampullary region (Weidenhiller et al 1975) has not fulfilled

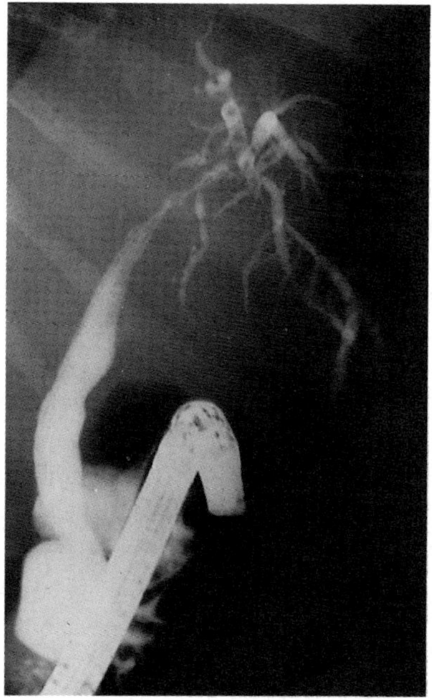

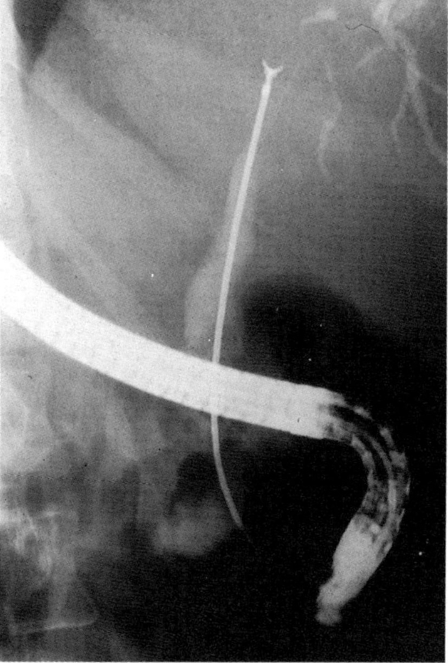

Fig. 20.22 Stenosis of the upper common bile duct. A biopsy forceps is advanced under fluoroscopic control in the region of a suspected malignant stenosis

Table 20.6

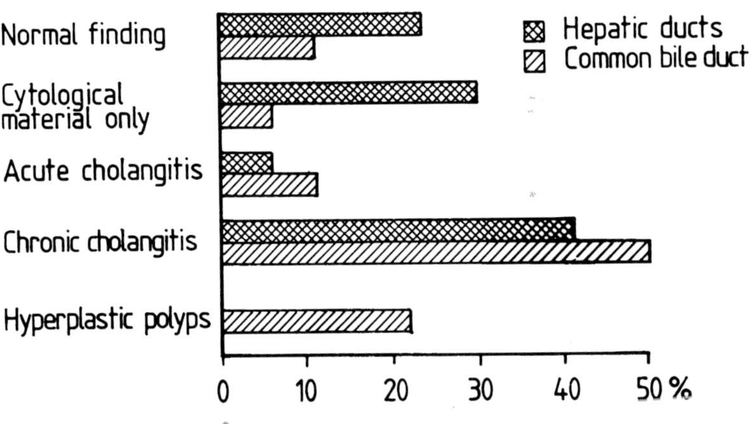

expectations (Gmelin & Weiss 1981) and is now used only rarely.

Direct collection of bile

Collecting bile and pancreatic secretions for diagnostic and scientific purposes is one of the established methods associated with ERCP. A nasobiliary tube has proved satisfactory for prolonged drainage of bile, and it is usually necessary to carry out EPT before insertion of such a tube. It is used both for temporary drainage of bile where there is an obstructive process and for determining the antibiotic sensitivity in cases of cholangitis (Wurbs et al 1980). It is possible to carry out organism-elimination studies for scientific purposes. Physiological and pathophysiological questions relating to the enterohepatic circulation, e.g. of particular drugs, can readily be investigated if the drained bile is reinfused into the duodenum via a feeding pump. For short-term selective collection of bile it is sufficient to intubate the bile duct with a tube through the intact papilla.

DIAGNOSTIC STEPS IN PATIENTS WITH CHOLESTASIS — RELEVANCE OF ERCP

The information to be gained about biliary disorders by direct cholangiography makes it the preferred method. In contrast to percutaneous transhepatic cholangiography (PTC) it provides a multiplicity of additional information about adjacent organs. However, the method of first choice depends primarily on the facilities of the particular hospital. We use PTC only as a complementary method, if ERCP proves impossible, or if the intrahepatic biliary tract cannot be assessed because of complete stenosis by a tumour (Classen et al 1981). However, ERCP or PTC is not the first step in the stepwise diagnosis of biliary disorders. Information is first obtained from the history, the clinical findings, the biochemistry and intravenous

Table 20.7 Diagnostic approach to patients with extrahepatic cholestasis

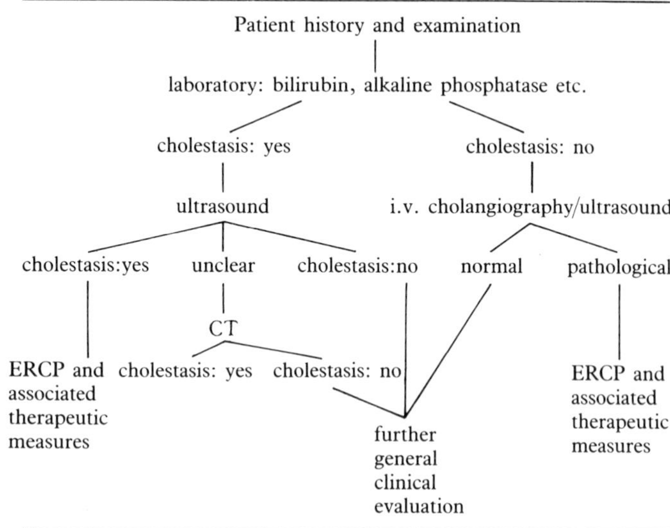

cholangiography (IVC). In order to rank the various methods in the context of a department of gastroenterology, we carried out a prospective blind study with this in mind on 108 consecutive patients referred to us with suspected biliary disorders. In a stepwise programme, the history and physical examination (H+PE), routine serum cholestasis tests (L), ultrasonography (US), IVC and ERCP were compared. The physician reported his findings with respect to the presence of malignancy, biliary obstruction and final diagnosis without knowing the results of the other methods. Additionally, an independent gastroenterologist made his diagnosis for each of the following diagnostic steps: H+PE, H+PE+L, H+PE+L+US, H+PE+L+US+IVC, and H+PE+L+US+IVC+ERCP. 103 patients with 153 biliary diagnoses were evaluated, of whom 46 with serum bilirubin $\leq$ 2 mg/dl had undergone an IVC. Table 20.8 summarizes the diagnostic accuracy for each step (Hagenmüller et al 1984).

Table 20.8 Choledocholithiasis

	UST	IVC	ERCP
SENS. (%)	28.6	85.7	92.9
SPEC. (%)	87.5	93.8	96.2
P.V. + (%)	50.0	85.7	92.9
P.V. − (%)	73.7	93.8	96.2

UST vs IVC: $P<0.01$; IVC vs ERCP: $P>0.05$; UST vs ERCP: $P<0.01$

It emerged that the biochemical findings provided the least information on the malignancy, presence of biliary obstruction and final diagnosis. Ultrasonography and ERCP significantly improved the diagnosis compared with the previous investigations. The value of sonography increases as cholestasis increases. In contrast to other investigators (Goodman et al 1980, Osnes et al 1978), IVC was better than expected, account being taken of the contraindications (bilirubin ≤ 2 mg %), an appropriate investigation technique and use of an up-to-date contrast medium (Table 20.8), especially for the detection of choledocholithiasis. The final diagnosis, which was confirmed by endoscopic surgical treatment, other surgery or follow-up, showed that ERCP was the standard by which the other methods should be measured (Phillip et al 1984). Only in the case of malignant tumours, in which the diagnosis can be confirmed by sonographic fine-needle biopsy, is sonography on the same level as ERCP. Nevertheless, even in these cases it is frequently necessary to carry out ERCP subsequently to determine whether palliative treatment is appropriate.

REFERENCES

Aaerimaa M, Maekelae P 1981 The cystic duct stump and the postcholecystectomy syndrome. An analysis of 54 patients subjected to ERCP. Annales Chirurgicae Gynaecologicae 70: 297–303

Bilbao M K, Dotter C T, Lee R G, Katon R M 1976 Complications of endoscopic retrograde cholangiopancreatography (ERCP). A Study of 1000 cases. Gastroenterology 70: 314–320

Börsch G, Bergbauer M, Nebel W, Sebin G 1984 Der Einfluβ von Somatostatin auf die Amylasespiegel und Pankreatitisrate nach ERCP. Medizinische Welt 35: 102–109

Bourgeois N, Dunham F, Verhest A, Cremer M 1984 Endoscopic biopsies of the papilla of Vater at the time of endoscopic sphincterotomy: difficulties in interpretation. Gastrointestinal Endoscopy 30: 163–166

Caletti G C, Cerucchi G, Bolondi L, Lebo G 1980 Diathermy ERCP. An alternative method for endoscopic retrograde cholangiopancreatography (ERCP) in jaundiced patients. Gastrointestinal Endoscopy 26: 13–15

Classen M 1977 Endoscopic retrograde cholangiopancreatography (ERCP). In: Bianchi L, Gerok W, Sickinger K (eds) Liver and bile. MTP Press, Lancaster, England, 235–241

Classen M 1981 Endoscopic approach to papillary stenosis. Endoscopy 13: 154–156

Classen M, Demling L 1974 Endoskopische Sphinkterotomie der Papilla Vateri und Steinextraktion aus dem Ductus choledochus. Deutsche Medizinische Wochenschrift 99:496

Classen M, Demling L 1975 Hazards of endoscopic retrograde cholangiopancreatography. Acta Hepatogastroenterologica 22: 1–3

Classen M, Phillip J, Wurbs D 1981 Fortschritte der direkten Cholangiographie und Cholangioskopie. In: Tittor W, Schwalbach G (eds) Leberdurch-blutung und Kreislauf. Thieme-Verlag, Stuttgart, 158–161

Classen M, Phillip J 1982 Endoscopic retrograde cholangiopancreatography (ERCP) and endoscopic papillotomy (EPT). Seminars in Liver Disease 2: 67–74

Cook J, Hou P C, Ho H C 1954 Recurrent pyogenic cholangitis. British Journal of Surgery 42: 188–203

Cotton P B 1977 Progress Report ERCP. Gut 18: 316–341

Cotton P B, Salmon P R, Blumgart L H, Burwood R J, Davies G T, Lawrie G T, Pierce J W, Read A E 1972 Cannulation of the papilla of Vater via fiber-duodenoscope. Lancet 1: 53–58

Cottone M, Amuso M, Cotton P 1978 Endoscopic retrograde cholangiography in hepatic hydatid disease. British Journal of Surgery 66:107

Cuschieri A, Cumming J G, Wood R A, Baker P R 1984 Evidence for sphincter dysfunction in patients with gallstone associated pancreatitis. British Journal of Surgery 71: 885–888

Daniels C, Schmidt H D, Lenner V, Brunner H 1980 Langer Zystikusstumpf als Ursache der Restbeschwerden nach Cholezystektomie. Leber Magen Darm 10: 207–212

Danzygier H, Phillip J, Hagenmüller F, Jessen K, Klein U, Hübner K, Leuschner U, Classen M 1983 Forceps biopsy of human bile ducts — light and electron microscopical findings, clinical significance. Gastroenterology 84:1132

Danzygier H, Classen M 1985 Endoskopisch-transpapilläre Biopsie (ETPB) — Morphologische Befunde, klinische Bedeutung. In: Henning H, Volkheimer G (eds) Fortschritte der gastroenterologischen Endoskopie. Demeter-Verlag, Gräfelfing 14: 94–106

Danzi J T, Makipour H, Farmer R G 1976 Primary sclerosing cholangitis. American Journal of Gastroenterology 65:109

De Masi Corazziari E, Habib F I, Fontana B, Gatti V, Fegiz G F, Torsoli A 1984 Manometric study of the sphincter of Oddi in patients with and without common bile duct stones. Gut 25: 275–278

Demling L, Classen M 1970 Duodenojejunoskopie. Deutsche Medizininische Wochenschrift 95: 1427–1428

Dyrszka H, Sanghavi B 1983 Hepatic hydatid disease: findings on endoscopic retrograde cholangiography. Gastrointestinal Endoscopy 29: 248–249

Femppel J, Lux G, Rösch W 1981 Intraoperative Gallenwegsläsionen. Medizinische Welt 32: 111–114

Geenen J E 1977 Endoscopic electrosurgical papillotomy and manometry in biliary tract disease. Journal of the American Medical Association 237:2075

Geenen J E 1982 New diagnostic and treatment modalities involving endoscopic cholangiopancreatography and esophagogastroduodenoscopy. In: Quadriennial Reviews World Congress. Falkenberg, Stockholm, 93–106

Geenen J E 1983 Spincter of Oddi Manometry. In: Classen M, Schreiber W (eds) Clinics in Gastroenterology — biliary tract disorders Saunders, London 12/1: 108–114

Gmelin E, Weiss H D 1981 Tumours in the region of the papilla of Vater. European Journal of Radiology 1: 301–306

Goodman A J, Neoptolemos J P, Carr-Locke D L, Finlay D B L, Fossard D P 1985 Detection of gall stones after acute pancreatitis. Gut 26: 125–132

Goodman M W, Ansel H J, Vennes J A, Lasser R B, Silvis S E 1980 Is intravenous cholangiography still useful? Gastroenterology 79: 642–645

Greiner L 1985 Diagnostische und therapeutische Punktionssonographie in der Gastroenterologie. Thieme, Stuttgart

Grözinger H H 1984 Zur Kritik des sog. Postcholezystektomie-Syndroms. In: Demling L (ed) Klinische Gastroenterologie Part II. 378–386

Guelrud M, Mendoza S, Vicent C, Gomez M, Villalta B 1983 Pressures in the sphincter of Oddi in patients with gallstones, common duct stones, and recurrent pancreatitis. Journal of Clinical Gastroenterology 5: 37–41

Hagenmüller F 1983 Manometrie der Gallenwege. In: Dölle W,

Classen M (eds.) Ergebnisse der Gastroenterologie 1982. Demeter Verlag, Gräfelfing, 130

Hagenmüller F, Ruus B, Phillip J, Strohm W D, Rübesam W, Classen M 1984 A Prospective blinded comparison of diagnostic methods for biliary disease. Gastroenterology 86:1104

Hannigan B F, Keeling P W N, Stavin B, Thompson R P H 1985 Hyperamylasemia after ERCP with ionic and non-ionic contrast media. Gastrointestinal Endoscopy 31: 109–110

Hauser S C, Bynum T E 1984 Abnormalities on ERCP in a case of human fascioliasis. Gastrointestinal Endoscopy 30: 80–81

Helm E B, Bauernfeind A, Frech K, Hagenmüller F 1984 Pseudomonas-Septikämie nach endoskopischen Eingriffen am Gallengangsystem. Deutsche Medizinische Wochenschrift 109: 698–701

Ibrahim M A H, Kawanishi H 1981 Endoscopic retrograde cholangiography in the evaluation of complicated-echinococcus of the liver. Gastrointestinal Endoscopy 27: 20–22

Jeanpierre R, Lèger L 1971 Pancrèatographie transpapillaire sous duodènoscopie. Chirurgie 97:489

Jandrzejewski J W, McAnally T, Jones S R, Katon R M 1980 Antibiotic and ERCP: In vitro activity of aminoglycosides when added to iodinated contrast agents. Gastroenterology 78: 745–748

Kasugai T 1975 Recent advances in the endoscopic retrograde cholangiopancreatography. Digestion 13:76

Katon R M, Bilbao M K, Parent J A, Smitz F W 1975 Endoscopic retrograde cholangio-pancreatography in patients with gastrectomy and gastrojejunostomy (Billroth II), a case for the forward look. Gastrointestinal Endoscopy 21: 164–165

Kurtz W, Strohm W D, Leuschner U, Classen M 1980 Die kongenitale Dilatation der intrahepatischen Gallenwege (Caroli-Syndrom). Innere Medizin 7: 50–56

Lam S K, Wong K P, Chan P K W, Ngan H, Ong G B 1978 Recurrent pyogenic cholangitis: A study by endoscopic retrograde cholangiography. Gastroenterology 74: 1196–1203

Lesch P, Weitzel J 1981 Die primären Cholangitiden. In: Zöckler L E, Lesch P (eds) Die spezielle Diagnostik der Gallenwegserkrankungen. TM-Verlag, Bad Oeynhausen, 227–239

Leuschner U, Baumgärtel H 1984 Chemical dissolution of common bile duct stones. In: Okuda K, Nakajama F, Wong J (eds) Intrahepatic calculi. Alan R, Liss, New York, 193–225

Matzen P, Malchow-Moller A, Lejerstofte J, Stage P, Juhl E 1982 Endoscopic retrograde cholangiopancreatography and transhepatic cholangiography in patients with suspected obstructive jaundice. Scandinavian Journal of Gastroenterology 17: 731–735

McCune W S, Shorb P E, Moscowitz H 1968 Endoscopic cannulation of the ampulla of Vater: a preliminary report. Annales of Surgery 167:752

Meier P, Ansel H, Silvis S, Vennes J 1984 Comparison of ultrasound and ERCP measurements of bile duct size. Gastroenterology 87:615

Mihas A A, Murad T M, Hischowitz B I 1978 Sclerosing cholangitis associated with ulcerative colitis. American Journal of Gastroenterology 70:614

Montefusco P P, Geiss A C, Bronzo R L, Randall S, Kahn E, McKinley M J 1984 Sclerosing cholangitis, chronic pancreatitis and Sjögren's syndrome: a syndrome complex. American Journal of Surgery 147: 822–826

Nagai N, Toki F, Oi J, Suzuki H, Kozu T, Tako T 1976 Continuous endoscopic pancreatocholedochal catheterization. Gastrointestinal Endoscopy 23: 78–80

Naval F, Diner W C, Westbrook K C, Kumpuris D D, Uthman E O 1984 Endoscopic biliary lavage in a case of Clonorchis sinensis. Gastrointestinal Endoscopy 30: 292–294

Nelson A M 1984 Demonstration of a traumatic biliary fistula by ERCP. Gastrointestinal Endoscopy 30: 315–316

Niederau C, Sonnenberg A, Müller J 1984 Comparison of the extrahepatic bile duct size measured by ultrasound and by different radiographic methods. Gastroenterology 87: 615–621

Nishumura A, Otsu H, Hiura T 1980 Forceps biopsy of the bile duct under choledochoscopic control. Endoscopy 12:23

Novis B H, Adam Y G 1982 Endoscopic retrograde cholangiography in a case of biliary pseudocyst. Endoscopy 14:24

Ohto M, Kimura K, Tsuchiya Y, Saisho H, Matsutani S, Kuniyasu Y, Okuda K 1984 Diagnosis of hepatolithiasis. In: Okuda K, Nakayama F, Wong J (eds) Intrahepatic calculi. Alan R, Liss, New York, p 129–148

Oi I, Kobayashi S, Kondo T 1970 Endoscopic pancreato-cholangiography. Endoscopy 2: 103–106

Oi I 1973 Duodenoscopic cholangiography-contouring around the diagnosis of biliary neoplasms. Stomach and Intestine (Japan) 8: 315

Okuno M, Himeno S, Kurakawa M, Shinomura Y, Kuroshima T, Kanayma Sh, Tsuju K, Higashimoto Y, Tarui S 1985 Changes in serum levels of pancreatic isoamylase, lipase, trypsin, and elastase 1^h after endoscopic retrograde pancreatography. Hepato-gastroenterology 32: 87–90

Osnes M, Myren J 1975 Endoscopic retrograde cholangiopancreatography (ERCP) in patients with Billroth II partial gastrectomies. Endoscopy 7:225

Osnes M, Larsen S, Lowe P 1978 Comparison of endoscopic retrograde and intravenous cholangiography in diagnosis of biliary calculi. Lancet 2: 230–231

Phillip J, Koch H, Classen M 1974 Variations and anomalies of the papilla of Vater, the pancreas and the biliary duct system. Endoscopy 6: 70–77

Phillip J, Hagenmüller F 1983 Postoperative Syndrome an den Gallenwegen: das sog. Postcholezystektomie-Syndrom. In: Henning H (ed) Fortschritte der gastroenterologischen Endoskopie. Demeter Verlag, Gräfelfing 12: 47–52

Phillip J, Hagenmüller F, Wildgrube H J, Althoff P H, Rickert S, Schellhaas H, Classen M 1983 Einfluβ des synthetischen Proteaseninhibitors FOY auf die Trypsinkonzentrationen nach ERCP. In: Grötzinger H H, Schrei A, Wabnitz R W (eds) Proteasen-Inhibition. C. Wolf, München, 146–155

Phillip J, Kurtz W, Ruus P, Hagenmüller F, Rübesam D, Strohm W D, Jessen K, Classen M 1984 Does infusion cholangiography still make sense? XII. International congress of Gastroenterology, Lisbon

Phillip J Usadel K H, Porto A, Hagenmüller F, Jessen K, Classen M 1985 Effekt von Somatostatin auf pankreatitische Komplikationen nach ERCP und Eingriffen an der Papilla Vateri. Fortschritte der Gastroenterologischen, Endoskopie 14: 124–129

Plumley T F, Rohrmann C A, Freeny P C, Silverstein F E, Ball T J 1982 Double duct sign: Reassessed significance in ERCP. American Journal of Radiology 183:31

Poralla T, Staritz M, Manns M, Klose K, Hommel G, Meyer zum Büschenfelde K H 1985 Age and sex dependency of bile duct diameter and bile duct pressure — an ERC manometry study. Zeitschrift für Gastroenterologie 23: 235–239

Rogers J V, Copeland A J, Schroder J S, Amerson J R 1972 Sclerosing cholangitis — roentgenographic features. South African Medical Journal 65:587

Rösch W 1981 Report on a symposium '10 years of ERCP': Diagnostic and therapeutic aspects. E.S.G.E. Newsletter 15: 7–9

Rösch W, Koch H, Demling L 1976 Manometric studies during ERCP and endoscopic papillotomy. Endoscopy 8: 30–33

Rösch W, Lux G, Riemann J F, Hoh L 1981 Chronische Pankreatitis und Nachbarorgane. Fortschritte der Medizin 99: 1118–1120

Rösch W 1985 Endoskopische retrograde Gallenwegsdiagnostik (ERC). Krankenhausarzt 58: 27–34

Seifert E, Safrany L, Stender H St, Lesch P, Luska G, Misaki F 1974 Identification of bile duct tumours by means of endoscopic retrograde pancreato-cholangiography (ERCP). Endoscopy 6:156

Seifert E, Urakami Y, Elster K 1980 Duodenoscopic guided biopsy of the biliary and pancreatic duct. Endoscopy 9:154

Siegel J H, Wright G, Snady H, Yarro R P 1985 Catheter and guide wire manipulation of papilla of Vater: A new method to selectively cannulate the bile duct. Gastrointestinal Endoscopy 138:158

Soehendra N, Reynders-Frederix V 1980 Palliative bile duct drainage — a new endoscopic method of introducing a transpapillary drain. Endoscopy 12: 8–11

Staritz M, Poralla Th, Dormeyer K H, Meyer zum Büschenfelde K H 1985 Endoscopic removal of common bile duct stones through the intact papilla after medical sphincter dilatation. Gastroenterology 88: 1807–1811

Staritz M, Porolla T, Ewe K, Meyer zum Büschenfelde K H 1985a Effect of glyceryl trinitrate on the sphincter of Oddi motility and baseline pressure. Gut 26: 194–197

Stolte M, Weiβ W, Volkholz H, Rösch W 1982 A special form of

segmental pancreatitis: 'Groove Pancreatitis'. Hepatogastroenterologica 29: 198–208
Stolte M 1984 Chronische Pankreatitis. Perimed, Erlangen
Tanaka M, Ikeda S 1983 Parapapillary choledochoduodenal fistula: an analysis of 83 consecutive patients diagnosed at ERCP. Gastrointestinal Endoscopy 29: 88–89
Tolksdorf W, Müller H P, Schratzer M, Jung M, Manegold B C, Kappa E 1985 Intravenöse Sedierung vor endoskopischen Eingriffen. Fortschritte der Medizin 9: 249–252
Toouli J, Geenen J E, Hogan W J, Doods W J, Arndorfer R C 1982 Sphincter of Oddi motor activity: A comparison between patients with common bile duct stones and controls. Gastroenterology 82: 111–117
Toouli J, Roberts-Thomson I C, Dent J, Lee J 1985 Manometric disorders in patients with suspected sphincter of Oddi dysfunction. Gastroenterology 88: 1243–1250
van Husen N, Högemann B, Egen V, Mehnert U 1984 Radiation exposure in endoscopic retrograde cholangiopancreatography. Endoscopy 16: 112–114
Vennes J A, Silvis S E 1972 Endoscopic visualization of bile and pancreatic ducts. Gastrointestinal Endoscopy 18:149
Weidenhiller S, Flügel H, Rösch W 1975 Abrasive cytology of the pancreatic and biliary duct in man. Endoscopy 7: 72–74
Weismüller J, Gail K, Seifert E 1983 Maligner extrahepatischer Gallenwegsverschluβ. Diagnostik und palliative Therapie. Deutsche Medizinische Woschenschrift 108:203
Winters C, Chobassian S J, Benjamin S B, Ferguson R K, Cattan E L 1984 Endoscopic documentation of Ascaris-induced acute pancreatitis. Gastroinestinal Endoscopy 30: 83–84
Wong J, Choi T K 1984 Recurrent pyogenic cholangitis. In: Okuda K, Nakayama L, Wong J (eds) Intrahepatic calculi Alan R, Liss, New York, p 175–192
Wurbs D, Classen M 1977 Transpapillary long standing tube for hepato-biliary drainage. Endoscopy 9: 192–193
Wurbs D, Phillip J, Classen M 1980 Experience with the long standing nasobiliary tube in biliary diseases. Endoscopy 12: 219–223
Wurbs D, Phillip J, Classen M 1980 Endoskopische Papillotomie mit Gallenwegsdrainage. Internist 21:617
Yellin A E, Donovan A J 1981 Biliary lithiasis and helminthiasis. American Journal of Surgery 142: 128–135

21

A. P. Hemingway, D. J. Allison

Angiography

INTRODUCTION

The medical and scientific significance of the ability to visualize structures radiographically was recognized from the earliest days of radiology. In January 1896, just two months after Roentgen had delivered his historic manuscript reporting the discovery of X-rays to the Physical Medical Society of Wurzburg, Haschek and Lindenthal produced a radiograph showing the injected vessels of an amputated hand (Haschek & Lindenthal 1896). During the next two decades detailed anatomical X-ray studies were obtained of the vascular systems in animals and man by workers in both Europe and America, and it is astonishing to reflect on the fact that the first X-ray atlas of the arterial tree was published (in England) as long ago as 1920 (Orrin 1920). During the 1920s attention turned to obtaining arteriograms in vivo, and substances such as lipiodol, strontium bromide, sodium iodide, thorotrast, and selectan were used in man to obtain peripheral arteriograms and venograms, aortic and pulmonary arteriograms and even cerebral arteriograms.

Portuguese workers such as Egas Moniz, Reynaldo dos Santos and Lopo de Carvalho were pre-eminent among the pioneers of human arteriography (Veiga-Pires & Grainger 1982), and the extent of their contribution has not been sufficiently acknowledged by many of those who have followed in their footsteps. The significance of the work they did was not lost on their contemporaries, however; when Moniz returned to Portugal after presenting his epoch-making paper entitled, 'Arterial encephalography, its importance in the localization of brain tumours' to the Academy of Medicine in Paris in 1928, he received a salutation from the combined professors of the Medicine Faculty at the railway station! (Goncalves 1982) Another pioneer in the field of arteriography was Forssmann who was particularly interested in techniques for visualizing the heart and pulmonary vessels (Forssmann 1931). In 1928 after practising on a cadaver, he passed a catheter from his own antecubital vein into the right atrium, a procedure that not only paved the way for subsequent development in cardiac catheterization, but must also surely be remembered as one of the most courageous feats of self-experimentation in modern medicine.

In the early days of arteriography, vessel exposure by incision was required for vascular catheterization and though this technique is still used in certain circumstances (see below), percutaneous arterial puncture is the preferred method in most cases. Percutaneous puncture was used at first simply to introduce contrast medium directly through a needle into a vessel, but a major advance came with the introduction of percutaneous techniques for the introduction of catheters into blood vessels (Lindgren 1950, Peirce & Ramey 1953), and the 'percutaneous catheter replacement technique of Seldinger' (Seldinger 1953) introduced in 1953 soon became, and remains, the most widely used method of angiographic catheterization. As vascular puncture and catheterization techniques developed, together with improvements in contrast media and catheters and the introduction of rapid film-changers, it became possible to obtain high quality arteriograms of all the principal vascular beds in the body. Angiography rapidly occupied a vital place in diagnostic medicine and became not only an indispensable investigation in branches such as vascular surgery, cardiac surgery, neurosurgery and more recently gastrointestinal and hepatic surgery, but played no small part in influencing the actual direction of development of these and other specialities.

During the 1970s it seemed that angiography, having reached its apparent zenith, was about to face a slow decline in importance as many of its roles were supplanted by less invasive and, for the most part, easier imaging techniques such as ultrasound, isotope studies, computerized tomography, and more recently magnetic resonance imaging. While it is true that arteriography will probably never regain the dominant position it once held in many fields of diagnosis, there are three recent factors which seem certain to secure it an important place in radiology for many years to come. The first of these is the development of digital vascular imaging (DVI), also known as digital subtraction angiography (DSA) (Meaney & Weinstein 1985). This technique enables high quality vascular images to be obtained using only very small volumes of intra-arterial contrast medium. For many purposes sufficient detail of the arteries can be obtained using only an intravenous injection of contrast medium. The second important factor influencing modern angiographic practice is the introduction of a new generation of contrast media (Grainger 1985). These media do not give the sensation of intense heat or pain that conventional contrast agents induce when injected into vessels. They also cause less damage to the vascular endothelium and have fewer systemic toxic effects than the older agents. Finally, a development which seems certain to assure a place for the angiographer in the management of liver disease is the advent of interventional vascular radiology.

TECHNIQUE

The risks associated with modern angiography are extremely small. Angiography is still nevertheless an invasive procedure and it should never be undertaken unless the radiologist is satisfied that the likely benefits justify the potential risks. An angiogram should never be done simply because it has been scheduled or 'routinely requested' by a clinical team; mistakes inevitably occur and the radiologist responsible for the procedure should be satisfied in every case that proper indications exist for the particular study requested. The angiographer should also be quite clear before starting as to what information is required from the procedure; this ensures that the correct studies and projections are obtained and allows rational decision-making during the procedure if something unexpected is shown or a problem arises.

Patient preparation

Informed consent should be obtained for angiography. A doctor, preferably the responsible radiologist or a member of the radiology department, should see the patient before the procedure to explain what is to be done, check that no contraindications to the study exist, check the appropriate pulses and ensure that adequate premedication is arranged. The groin should be shaved if a femoral approach is to be used. It has been the usual practice for patients to be on 'nil by mouth' for an appropriate period prior to the procedure to avoid the risk of aspiration during a possible contrast reaction or other serious accident. It is now the policy in many departments, however, only to stop solid foods and to permit free oral fluids unless general anaesthesia or heavy premedication is being used. Whatever regimen is adopted adequate measures should be taken to avoid dehydration during the procedure and the recovery period.

Contraindications

There are very few absolute contraindications to angiography but there are many factors which considerably increase the hazards of the technique. Always check that a patient is not *pregnant* before angiography as the radiation dose may be considerable. If angiography is essential in a pregnant patient, the dose to the fetus should be minimized by protection, field collimation and careful choice of filming sequences. Caution should be exercised in patients on *anticoagulant* therapy or with other *bleeding diatheses*, a point of particular relevance in patients with liver disorders. Arteriography should be avoided if possible in such cases; if it is essential then all possible steps should be taken to correct or improve the coagulation defect before and during the procedure if this is clinically acceptable. Other factors which increase the risk of bleeding from an arterial puncture site include systemic hypertension and disorders predisposing to increased fragility of the vessel wall such as Cushing's syndrome, prolonged steroid treatment and rare connective tissue disorders such as certain types of the *Ehlers-Danlos syndrome*. If angiography should prove to be necessary in a patient with suspected or proven previous adverse reaction to contrast medium, appropriate steroid prophylaxis should be administered (Grainger 1985).

Arteriography can require larger doses of contrast medium than any other radiological procedure and particular care must be exercised in: infants, dehydrated or shocked patients, patients with serious cardiac or respiratory disease, patients in hepatic or renal failure and other patients with serious metabolic abnormalities.

Anaesthesia

Most angiography is now performed under local anaesthesia, though general anaesthesia is necessary for babies and young children, confused, difficult or very nervous patients, and some complex interventional procedures Although general anaesthesia can be more pleasant for the patient than local anaesthesia and reduces motion artefact on the radiographs, it nevertheless adds to the risks of angiography. This is not only because of the (small) risks inherent in general anaesthesia, but also because it masks the patient's subjective symptoms and reactions. These may provide the radiologist with immediate warning of a mishap such as the subintimal injection of contrast medium or the inadvertent wedging of the catheter tip in a small artery, a warning which may well prevent more serious injury. A further point to remember is that many patients being investigated for 'surgical' liver disorders may well be operated on within a day or two of angiography and will then require another general anaesthetic within a short period. When local anaesthesia is to be used the patient should be sedated with a suitable premedication. This should contain an analgesic as most procedures cause some discomfort: it is not only kinder to the patient to make the study as painless as possible but it makes for appreciably better angiography. A suitable premedication for a 70 kg adult is papaveretum (Omnopon) 20 mg i.m., and lorezapam 2 mg orally one hour prior to the procedure.

It is also very important that the vascular puncture site is adequately anaesthetized; 5–10 ml of 1–2% lignocaine should be infiltrated around the vein or artery; inadequate initial anaesthesia not only causes patient discomfort but predisposes to arterial spasm and restricts free catheter movement.

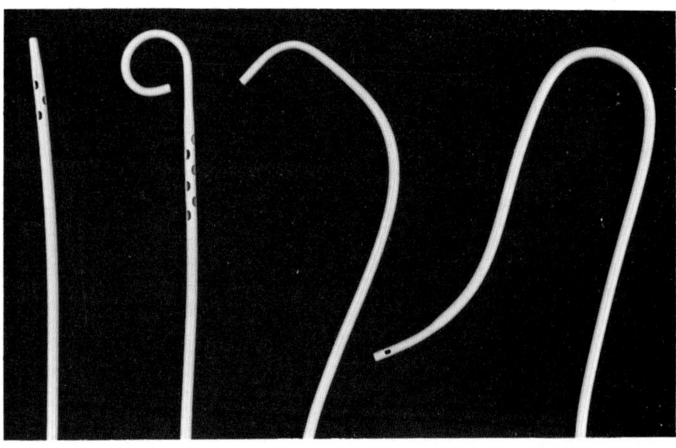

Fig. 21.2 Some of the many different available catheter shapes are illustrated. From left to right: straight 'flush', 'pigtail', 'cobra', and 'side-winder'. Note the side ports on some of the catheters

Arterial puncture and catheterization

The majority of arterial studies are performed percutaneously via the femoral artery in the groin. The vessel is punctured using the Seldinger technique (Seldinger 1953) (Fig. 21.1). Occasionally it is necessary to use other routes of arterial access such as axillary artery puncture, or brachial artery cutdown. By manipulating the catheter under fluoroscopic control it is possible to insert the catheter selectively into various branches of the vascular system such as the renal artery, coeliac axis, superior mesenteric artery. Different catheter shapes are available (Fig. 21.2) each of which is suitable for a particular manoeuvre or for catheterizing certain arterial branches. Superselective (subselective) catheterization of small subsidiary arteries such as the pancreaticoduodenal arteries or intrahepatic branch vessels is being increasingly used for embolization procedures (Ch. 94). Arteriographic anatomy is described in Ch. 3.

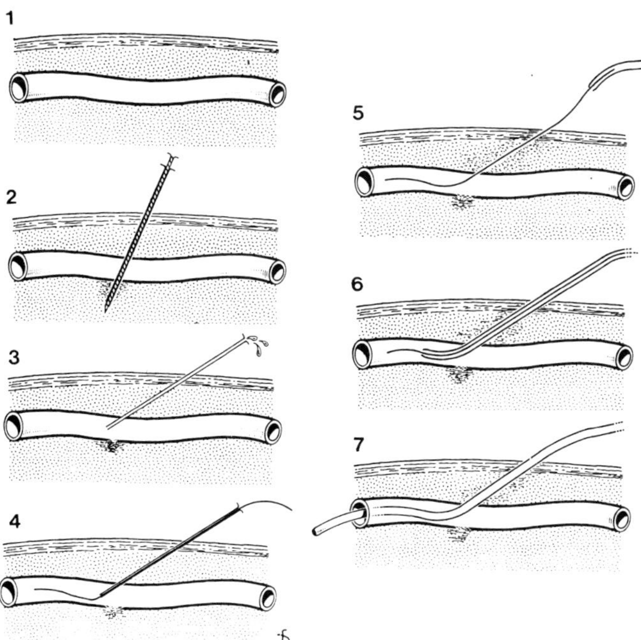

Fig. 21.1 One of the commonly-used techniques of percutaneous arterial catheterization. The artery (1) is transfixed (2). The needle is partially withdrawn and re-angled (3). A guidewire is passed into the needle during free back-flow of blood (3,4); the needle is removed and a catheter or introducer inserted over the wire (5,6). When the catheter is safely within the arterial lumen the wire is withdrawn (7)

In the evaluation of liver disease it is necessary to inject selectively the coeliac axis and the superior mesenteric artery.

The coeliac axis

The coeliac axis (Allison & Hemingway 1983) is the artery of the primitive foregut and through its three branches (left gastric, splenic and common hepatic) it supplies the stomach and upper duodenum, spleen, liver and pancreas (Fig. 21.3 and see Fig. 21.4). The coeliac stem arises from

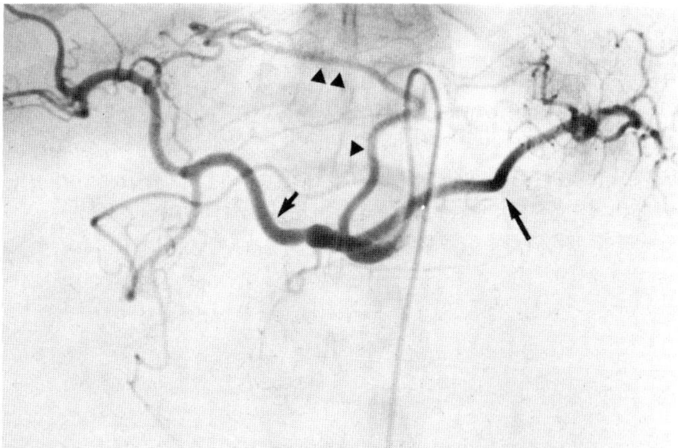

Fig. 21.3 Coeliac axis arteriogram using a side-winder catheter. The splenic (long arrow), left gastric (single arrowhead) and common hepatic arteries (short arrow) are well demonstrated. Note that the left gastric artery also gives rise to an accessory left hepatic artery (double arrowhead)

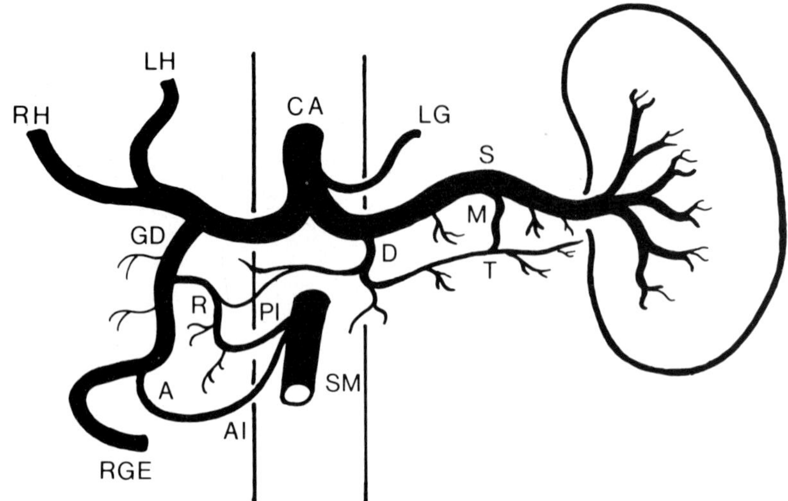

Fig. 21.4 Diagram showing the branches of the coeliac axis. CA = coeliac axis; LG = left gastric artery; S = splenic artery; M = arteria pancreatica magna; D = dorsal pancreatic artery; SM = superior mesenteric artery; T = transverse pancreatic artery; PI = posterior inferior pancreaticoduodenal artery; AI = anterior inferior pancreaticoduodenal artery; A = anterior superior pancreaticoduodenal artery; R = retroduodenal artery (posterior superior pancreaticoduodenal artery); GD = gastroduodenal artery; RH = right hepatic artery; LH = left hepatic artery; RGE = right gastroepiploic artery

the front of the aorta at the level of LI; it can be catheterized with a femoral-visceral catheter but a sidewinder catheter (Fig. 21.2) is preferred by the authors because it is less likely to be dislodged during a pump injection and can be further manipulated into the splenic or hepatic arteries in a high proportion of cases. Superselective studies of the left gastric, gastroduodenal, dorsal pancreatic and hepatic vessels (Fig. 21.5) can be obtained with appropriate catheters.

Distension of the stomach and duodenum with carbon dioxide gas helps to reduce the number of confusing shadows produced by opacification of normal folded mucosa in these organs and oblique views are necessary for the complete demonstration of the duodenum and pancreas.

The coeliac territory can normally be adequately opacified in the average adult by 30–50 ml Urografin 370 or equivalent delivered at 8–10 ml/sec by a mechanical injector. Pump injections are also necessary for splenic or common hepatic arteriograms but hand injections suffice for superselective studies. The radiographic filming sequence should extend sufficiently long to allow visualization of the portal venous system providing an *indirect splenoportogram* (see below). This occurs in 8–14 seconds after injection in most patients but may take longer in the presence of splenomegaly or portal obstruction.

Hepatic arteriography (Ring 1983) is usually performed for the assessment of liver tumours primary or secondary (see Fig. 21.16, 21.20) or hepatic bleeding.

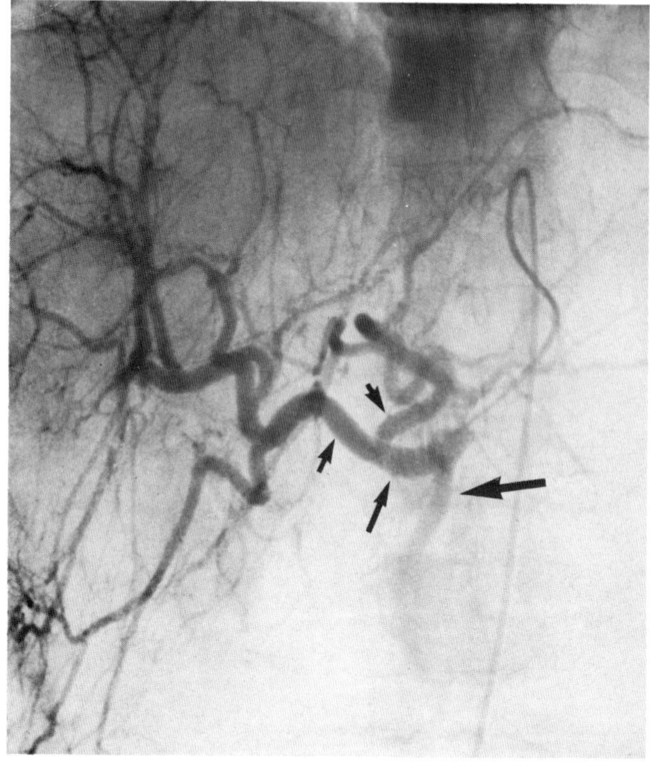

Fig. 21.5 Selective hepatic arteriogram. A sidewinder catheter has been positioned in the common hepatic artery with its tip just proximal to the origin of the gastroduodenal artery which is faintly opacified (large arrow). The proper hepatic artery (mid-sized arrow) divides into the right and left hepatic branches (short arrows)

The superior mesenteric artery

The superior mesenteric artery (SMA) (Allison & Hemingway 1983) supplies the bowel derived from the primitive mid-gut, from the mid-duodenum to the splenic flexure. It arises from the front of the aorta 1 cm below the coeliac axis and is easily catheterized selectively in most individuals with a sidewinder or femoral-visceral catheter. 30–50 ml Urografin 370 or its equivalent injected at 8–10 ml/sec from an automatic injector will opacify the SMA in the average adult (Fig. 21.6a & b). It is important to continue filming up to 20 seconds after the contrast injection. This allows visualization of the superior mesenteric and portal veins. It is also of great importance to

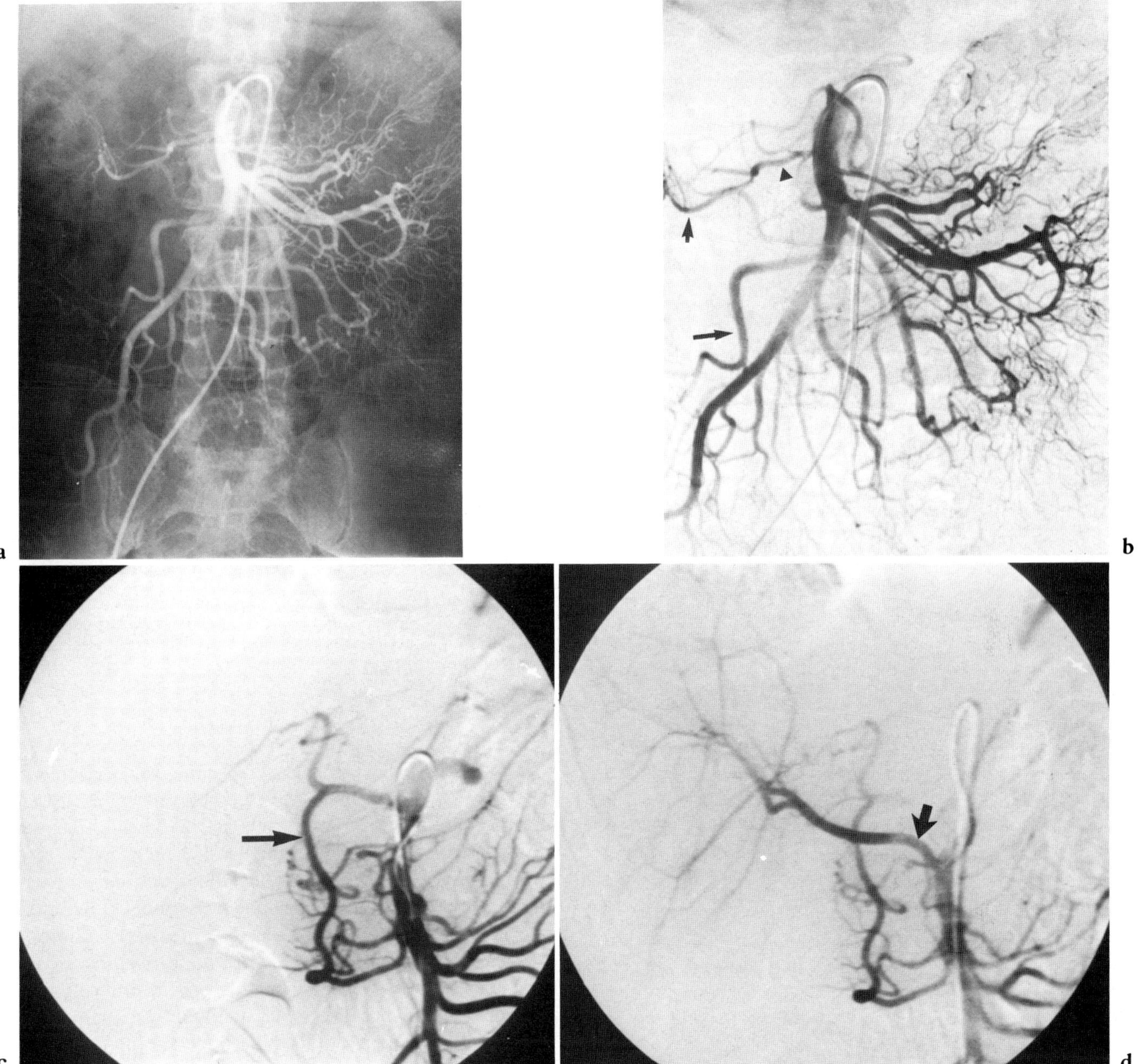

Fig. 21.6 a & b. Superior mesenteric arteriogram. The upper branches on the patient's left supply the jejunum, the lower branches the ileum. On the right are the middle colic artery (arrowhead) the right colic artery (short arrow) and the ileo-colic artery (long arrow). The continuation of the main arterial stem ultimately forms the left-hand limb of the ileo-colic anastomotic loop.
a. shows this angiogram unsubtracted; b. shows the subtraction print of the same study.
c. Superior mesenteric angiogram. The catheter is selectively inserted into the SMA. Following the injection of contrast medium there is filling of the SMA and retrograde filling of the coeliac axis via the gastroduodenal artery (arrow). Note that there is no evidence of a right hepatic artery arising from the coeliac axis
d. Same patient as in c. The catheter has been withdrawn so that the tip lies nearer the orifice. When a further injection of contrast medium is made the accessory right hepatic arising from the SMA is now visualized (arrow)

ensure that the presence of an accessory right hepatic artery (Ch. 3) is not missed by having the tip of the catheter too far into the stem of the SMA (Fig. 21.6c & d).

Venous access

The venous system may be studied either directly by puncturing the vein under investigation with a needle or catheter and injecting contrast medium from an antegrade or retrograde approach, or indirectly by injecting the medium into the arterial system and imaging the venous return. In evaluation of hepatobiliary disease it may be necessary to image both the systemic and portal venous systems. The detailed anatomy of these systems is discussed in Ch. 3.

Systemic venography

The hepatic veins are usually catheterized retrogradely; the catheter may be passed from an arm vein, the jugular vein or femoral vein into the hepatic venous system. It is frequently necessary to measure free and wedged hepatic venous pressures in the investigation of liver disease. Wedged hepatic venous pressure measurement requires that a catheter is impacted in a small branch of an hepatic vein. The catheter position is confirmed by the injection of contrast medium, and a dense stain is produced. Reports have indicated (Casteneda-Zuniga et al 1978) that excess injection pressure may occasionally cause local hepatocellular damage. Venography, with the catheter lying free in the hepatic veins, requires the injection of about 20–30 ml of contrast medium at a rate of 10–15 ml/sec. Filling of the small hepatic venous radicles is assisted if the patient performs a Valsalva manoeuvre (Fig. 21.7)

Occasionally it is not possible to catheterize the hepatic veins retrogradely. In this situation direct transhepatic puncture of the hepatic veins can be performed (Fig. 21.8).

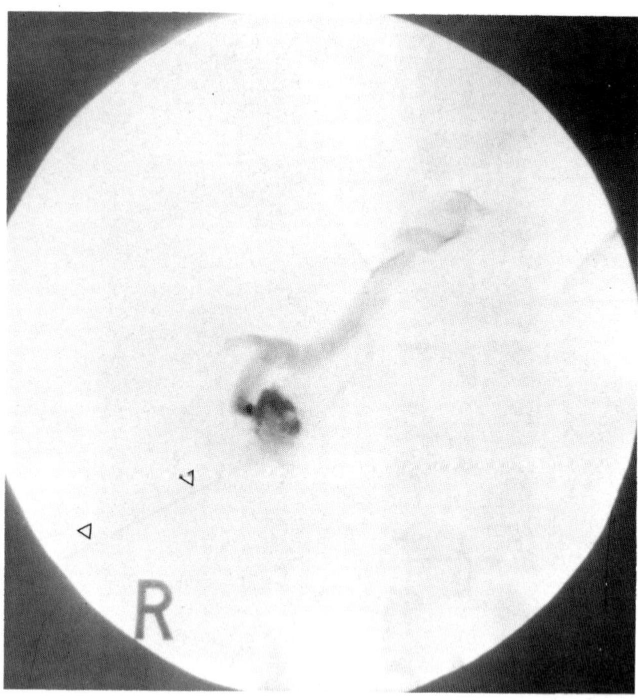

Fig. 21.8 Direct (hepatic) venogram. Retrograde right hepatic venography had been attempted but had failed. A Chiba needle (arrowheads) has been passed through the liver substance into a venous radicle. Contrast has been injected and a right hepatic vein has been opacified. A stenosis was demonstrated at the junction of the vein with the inferior vena cava

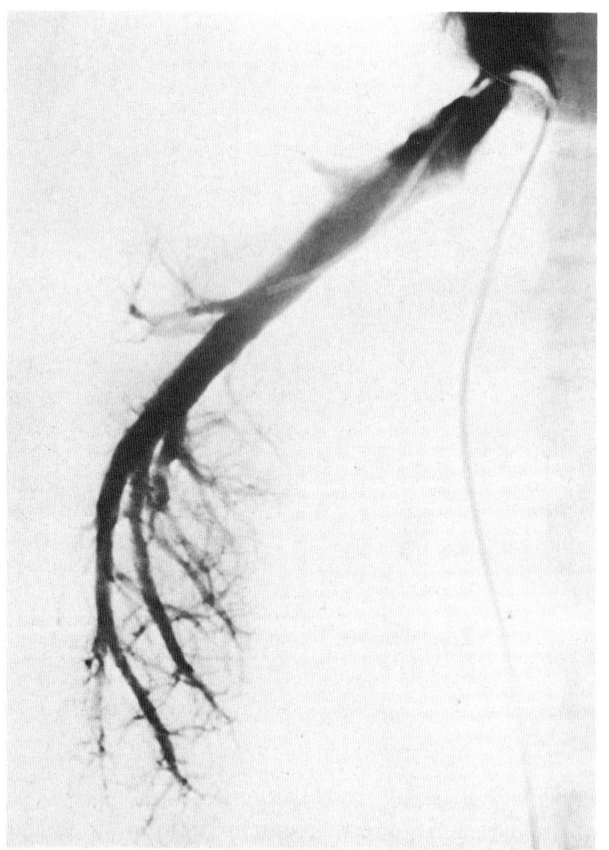

Fig. 21.7 Normal hepatic venogram. A femoral-cerebral III (sidewinder) catheter has been passed from the femoral vein into the inferior vena cava and hence the main right hepatic vein. Contrast medium has been injected into the hepatic vein while the patient performs a Valsalva manoeuvre. Small intrahepatic venous radicles are seen

The first in vivo *inferior venacavogram* was performed by Dos Santos (Dos Santos 1935) in 1935; he injected radio-opaque material via a saphenous vein cutdown. The technique has been greatly modified since then owing to the introduction of the Seldinger technique and developments in catheters, guidewires and imaging systems. The inferior vena cava can be approached antegradely from the femoral veins or retrogradely via the arm or neck veins. The technique employed depends on the indication and area of interest, but the most commonly used approach is the one from the femoral vein. Puncture of the femoral vein has many similarities in technique to puncture of the femoral artery. The vein is not palpable, however, and the operator relies on the fact that the vein is just medial to the artery to achieve a successful puncture. The procedure is usually performed under local anaesthesia. It is useful to ask the patient to perform a Valsalva manoeuvre during the puncture as this temporarily distends the vein. If the presence of caval thrombus is suspected the catheter should be advanced extremely cautiously under fluoroscopic control employing only small injections (2–3 ml) of contrast medium. Once the catheter has been positioned satisfactorily then 45–60 ml of contrast medium, e.g. Urografin 370 or Omnipaque 350, is injected over three seconds. Serial films are taken at two films a second for about five seconds followed by one film a second for 5–10 seconds depending on the indications for the procedure

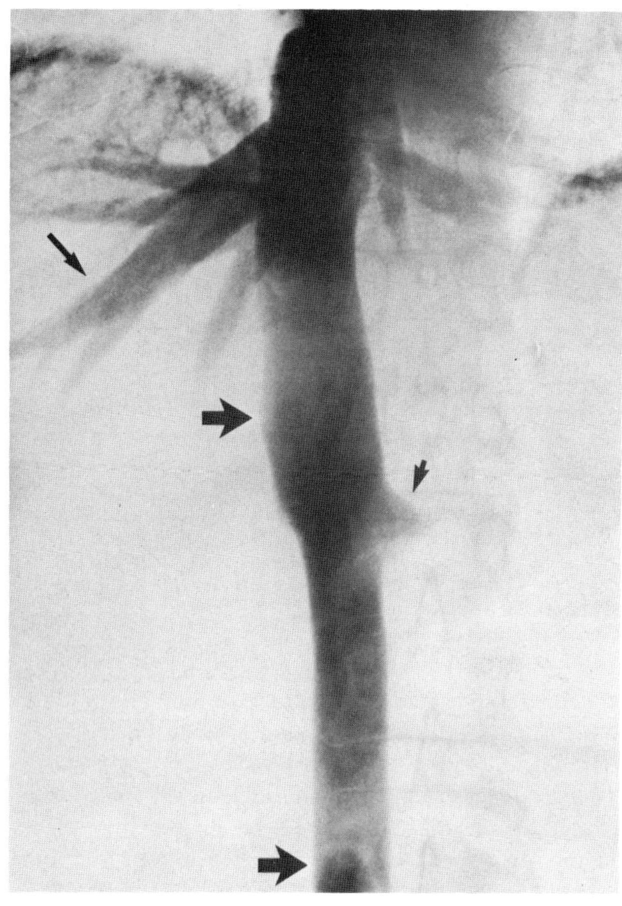

Fig. 21.9 Normal inferior vena cava (broad arrow); anteroposterior projection. Contrast medium has been injected via the right femoral vein. The patient has performed a Valsalva manoeuvre during the contrast injection and reflux has occurred into the hepatic veins (long arrow) and the left renal vein (short arrow)

(Fig. 21.9). The procedure is performed in the anteroposterior and lateral projections. In some cases (e.g. Budd-Chiari syndrome) it may be necessary to record pressure measurements. The advent of digital vascular imaging has meant that much smaller doses of contrast can be injected (20 ml of either Urografin 370 or Omnipaque 350 which has been previously diluted 1 in 4 with normal saline). Indeed it is possible, using DSA, to vizualize the vena cava adequately from injection of contrast medium into a vein on the dorsum of the foot; in the investigation of venous thrombosis, therefore, a cavogram can be performed at the same time as a peripheral venogram.

An approach from the arm may require a small cutdown or may be performed percutaneously. If the jugular vein is utilized, the Seldinger technique is employed and care must be taken to avoid the potentially serious complication of air embolism.

Portal venography

Visualization of the portal venous system may be helpful in the diagnosis of portal hypertension and is essential for its proper management. It may also be of great value in the evaluation of other liver disease and pancreatic disease (see below). The portal vein was first demonstrated by the direct injection of contrast medium into the main vein or one of its tributaries at laparotomy. This technique was devised by Blakemore & Lord (1945). In 1951 Abeatici & Campi demonstrated that contrast medium injected into the spleen flowed into the splenic and portal veins and, in the same year, Leger performed the first successful direct percutaneous splenoportogram in man. It was noted in the early 1950s that the portal vein was occasionally faintly visualized after injection of contrast medium into the aorta (Rigler et al 1953) and in 1958 Odman demonstrated the portal vein after injection of contrast medium into the coeliac axis. In recent years developments in equipment (especially DVI), angiographic techniques and contrast agents have further improved the accuracy and safety of portography.

The portal venous system can be outlined in the following ways:

Direct methods
- percutaneous splenoportography
- transhepatic portography
- perioperative mesenteric portography
- transumbilical portography
- transjugular portography
- direct percutaneous transabdominal portography

Indirect methods
- arterioportography

Direct percutaneous splenoportography

Following the first successful use of this technique in man in 1951 (Leger 1951) it was for many years the most widely used means of demonstrating the portal venous systems following percutaneous puncture of the organ. Splenic pulp pressure can be measured through the cannula and the position of the catheter tip ascertained by injecting a small volume of contrast medium. 30–50 ml of contrast medium is then injected rapidly into the splenic pulp and films of the area of interest are obtained at a rate of 1–2/sec for 10–20 seconds (or longer if necessary). Great variation exists in the timing and film sequences required in different patients. Once satisfactory pictures have been obtained the cannula is removed. It may prove to be beneficial to embolize the cannula track and this is most effectively done by injecting embolic material (e.g. Sterispon) down the cannula as it is withdrawn (Probst et al 1978). The procedure is contraindicated in the presence of markedly deranged coagulation or ascites and is hazardous if the spleen is small (see below).

Complications The most dangerous complications of the procedure are haemorrhage and splenic rupture, though

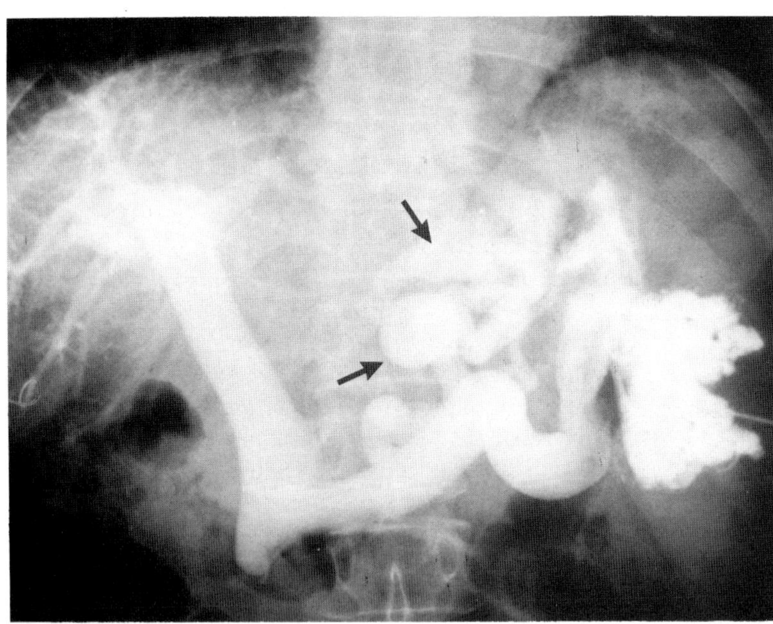

Fig. 21.10 Direct splenoportogram. Contrast medium has been injected via a cannula into the splenic pulp. The splenic vein, portal and intrahepatic portal veins are visualized. Massive variceal dilatation of the left gastric vein is demonstrated (arrows)

the incidence of haemorrhage can be significantly reduced by embolization of the needle track (Probst et al 1978). A review of the literature has shown only four fatalities from haemorrhage in over 1200 studies (Anacker et al 1957). Splenic rupture can occur if the procedure is performed in a very small spleen (Bergstrand 1983). Some subcapsular extravasation of contrast medium is common and may cause pain which can last for a few hours. Injection of contrast medium into the peritoneum may also cause pain but no serious sequelae have been reported.

Indications Splenoportography is used in the investigation of portal hypertension (see below) (Fig. 21.10), in gastrointestinal bleeding of unknown cause and, occasionally, in cases of unexplained splenomegaly. Accurate delineation of the splenic and portal veins may also be needed when assessing the operability of hepatic and pancreatic tumours. The need for direct portography has declined dramatically with the improvements in indirect portography techniques.

Transhepatic portography (Lunderquist et al 1983)

This technique was first described by Bierman et al 1952. Subsequent workers have modified the technique from the original simple needle puncture of an intrahepatic portal venous radicle to sophisticated catheterization techniques. As with direct splenic puncture it is important that the procedure is not performed in patients with deranged blood coagulation. The position of the portal vein can be outlined using either ultrasound or indirect splenoportography. It is also very useful to opacify the gallbladder prior to the procedure by giving oral cholecystographic contrast medium the preceding day (Fig. 21.11). A catheter inserted transhepatically into the portal vein can be used for venography, venous sampling or embolisation techniques. At the end of the procedure the catheter track can be embolized with Sterispon/gelfoam.

Complications (Lunderquist et al 1983) of the procedure include: haemorrhage from a liver surface into the peritoneum or within the liver substance into the biliary system; fistula formation (arterioportal, arteriobiliary); portal vein thrombosis; biliary peritonitis; puncture of the gallbladder or colon (particularly in very sick patients who are unable to suspend their respiration); pneumothorax; intrapleural bleed; pleural effusion and biliary-pleural fistula.

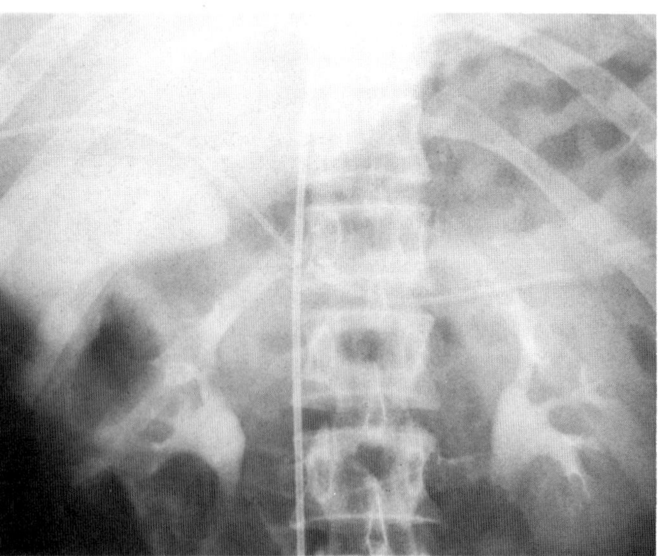

Fig. 21.11 Percutaneous transhepatic portal vein cannulation. An oral cholecystographic contrast agent was given on the day preceding the investigation to minimize the risk of inadvertent puncture of the gallbladder during the procedure

Indications The major indication for this technique is the embolization of gastric and oesophageal varices (Ch. 107), though the role that the method should play in the management of varices is controversial (Lunderquist et al 1977, Sos 1983). Transhepatic cannulation of the portal vein is also used for venous sampling procedures when a pancreatic hormone secreting tumour is suspected clinically, but cannot be localized by less invasive means (Allison 1980). Multiple samples are taken from the splenic, superior and inferior mesenteric veins, and also selectively from pancreatic veins. Simultaneous hepatic venous and arterial samples may also be obtained to assess whether or not functioning hepatic metastases are present and allow arteriovenous hormone gradients to be estimated.

Other direct methods of opacifying the portal venous system include perioperative mesenteric phlebography, transumbilical portography, transjugular portography (via the hepatic vein and liver), and direct transabdominal portography. Improvements in imaging technology and indirect portography have rendered these techniques largely obsolete.

Indirect portography (arterioportography) (Bron 1983)

All the direct methods of opacifying the portal venous system are associated with a small but definite incidence of morbidity. Indirect or arterioportography has not only the advantage of being less hazardous than many of the direct methods, but it can be combined with a study of the arterial system as well. It is also possible, by selective injections into the coeliac axis (or splenic artery), superior mesenteric artery and inferior mesenteric artery, to opacify the splenic and mesenteric veins as well as the portal vein.

Technique The coeliac axis, or superior mesenteric artery (or both) are selectively catheterized and films are exposed for up to 40 seconds following the injection of contrast medium, e.g. 40–50 ml at 7–10 ml/sec (Fig. 21.12a & b). Larger quantities of contrast medium may be required in patients with splenomegaly. The radiographs that are taken following the injection of contrast medium should be centred so that the lower oesophagus is included on the film in order that varices are not missed. Oblique views may be needed to properly visualize the division into right and left intrahepatic branches.

The advent of DSA/DVI has further improved the quality of images obtained using indirect injection methods. 15 ml of diluted (one part contrast '350' or '370' to two parts normal saline) contrast medium can be injected rapidly by hand and the portal vein, if patent, is readily visualized (Fig. 21.13). If the main splenic or portal veins are occluded, large collateral vessels may be demonstrated arising through the abdomen. If only one

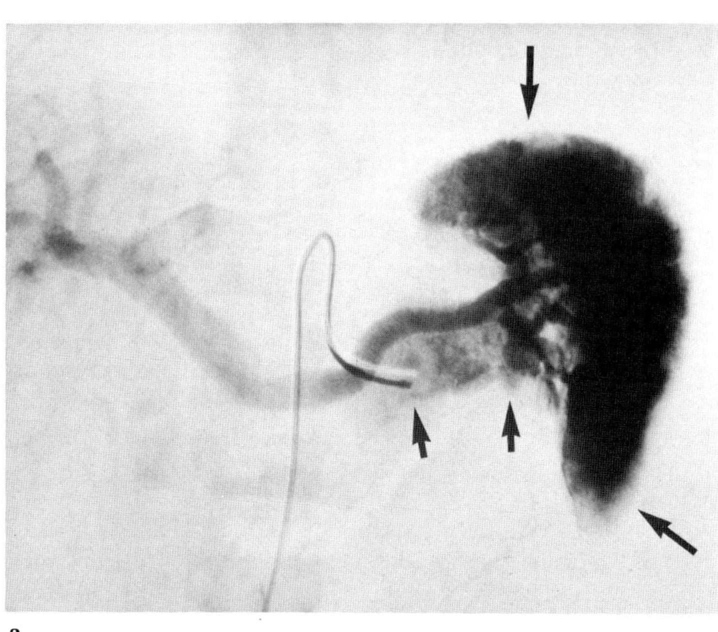

a

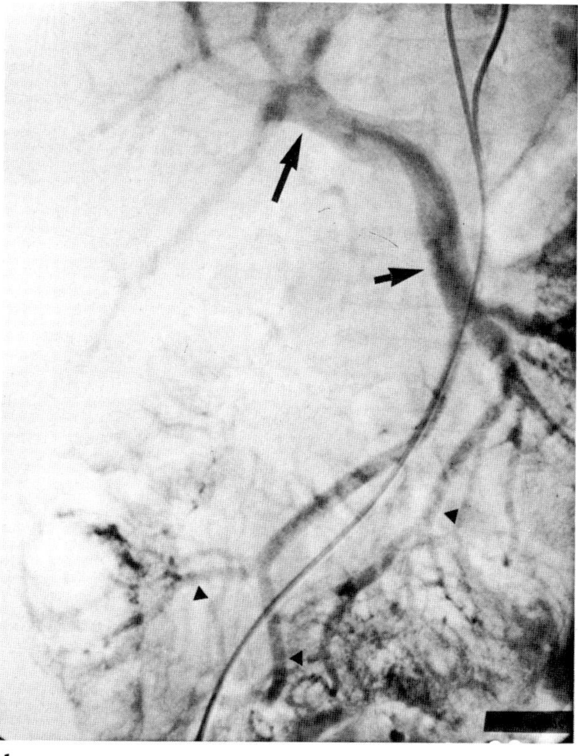

b

Fig. 21.12 (a). Indirect splenoportogram. A catheter has been placed selectively in the splenic artery. Contrast medium has been injected and films taken to 20 seconds. The spleen (long arrows) and tail of the pancreas (short arrows) are both opacified with contrast medium. The splenic vein, main portal vein and intrahepatic portal venous radicles are seen. b. Superior mesenteric venogram. Late films have been taken following an injection of contrast medium into the superior mesenteric artery; the superior mesenteric vein (short arrow) and portal vein (long arrow) are demonstrated

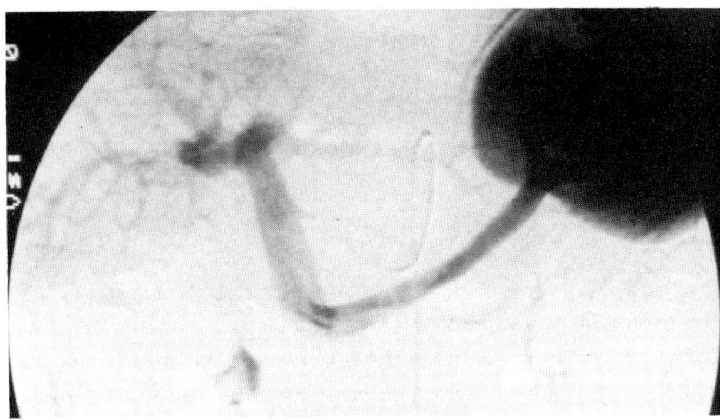

Fig. 21.13 Indirect-splenoportogram using digital subtraction techniques. 15 ml of diluted contrast medium were injected into the splenic artery

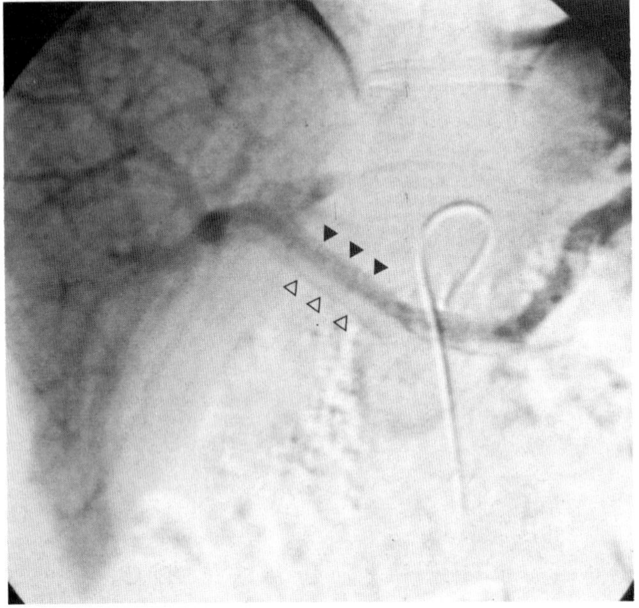

Fig. 21.14 Portal vein 'streaming'. A splenic arterial injection has opacified the splenic blood. In the portal vein the splenic blood (open arrowheads) is seen outlining the upper axial portion of the vein, while unopacified blood from the superior mesenteric system is occupying the lower axial portion of the vessel (solid arrowheads)

visceral artery is injected the portal vein may exhibit quite marked streaming and non-mixing of opacified and non-opacified blood (Fig. 21.14).

Indications The major indications for arterioportography are listed in Table 21.1

Aftercare

When an arteriographic study is completed the catheter is withdrawn and firm manual pressure applied to the puncture site for 5–10 minutes. The radiologist should be absolutely satisfied that bleeding has stopped before the

Table 21.1 Indications for arterioportography

Assessment of portal hypertension
Delineation and extent of varices
Evaluation of porto-systemic shunts
Assessment of operability of hepatic biliary or pancreatic neoplasms
Assessment of feasibility of therapeutic hepatic arterial embolization

patient leaves the angiography suite. The wound site is then checked at regular intervals by the nursing staff who should also record pulse and blood pressure observations for a reasonable period following the procedure and check that distal pulses remain palpable. Pressure pads, sand bags and other accoutrements are generally a waste of time. It is much better to be able to see the puncture site than to cover it up. If bleeding does not stop from a puncture site, press for a longer period! Almost all post-catheterization bleeding can ultimately be controlled by local pressure unless the artery has been torn or there is a serious coagulation abnormality.

An adequate record of the procedure should be entered in the patient's case notes. This should include the date, the name of the operator, the names and doses of anaesthetic agents, the volumes and concentrations of contrast medium and other drugs administered, preliminary findings, any complications during the procedure, the integrity or otherwise of the pulse peripheral to the puncture site at the end of the procedure, and the post-procedural nursing instructions. These notes are important not only for patient care but also as a medico-legal record, and they should be comprehensive and accurate. Arteriography is most safely performed on an in-patient basis, the patient remaining on bed rest overnight following the procedure.

Radiographic considerations

Good radiography is a vital factor in arteriography. A control film should always be obtained so that the correct exposure factors can be established and the film accurately centred. The radiographs should be carefully collimated to the field of interest and exposed during arrested respiration when the study involves regions affected by respiratory movement.

Subtraction films

Subtraction films may help by showing the arteries free of confusing shadows cast by non-vascular structures such as bone. They are particularly useful in the head and neck. A subtraction film is made by exposing a radiograph of the area of interest immediately prior to the injection of contrast medium. A reversed image of this radiograph (the subtraction mask) is then superimposed on subsequent radiographs showing opacified vascular structures so that the mask obscures all non-vascular detail. A final image showing only the opacified vessels can then be obtained (subtraction print) (See Fig. 21.6a & b).

Digital subtraction techniques in which the process is performed electronically are rapidly superseding the manual method described above.

COMPLICATIONS

The principal complications of arteriography are listed in Table 21.2.

Table 21.2 Complications of arteriography

1. *Complications related to contrast medium*
   - Minor adverse reactions
   - Major adverse reactions and death
   - Local vascular changes (effects on blood cells, viscosity, vascular tone; results of extravasation, etc)
   - Systemic vascular changes (effects on blood volume, osmolality, etc).
   - Individual organ toxicity (heart, kidney, brain, etc).
2. *Adverse reactions to local anaesthetic or other drugs*
3. *Puncture site complications*
   - Haemorrhage (external bleeding or haematoma)
   - Intramural or perivascular injection of contrast medium
   - Vascular thrombosis (dissection, local trauma)
   - Peripheral embolization from puncture site
   - Vascular stenosis or occlusion
   - Aneurysm or pseudoaneurysm formation
   - AV fistula
   - Local sepsis
   - Damage to nerves
   - Damage to other local structures
4. *Catheter-related and general complications*
   - Catheter thrombus embolism
   - Air embolism
   - Gauze embolism
   - Dissection, perforation or rupture of vessels
   - Organ ischaemia or infarction secondary to spasm, dissection or embolism
   - Interventional accidents
   - Fracture and loss of guidewire or catheter fragments
   - Knot formation in catheter
   - Inadvertent injection of toxic material (e.g. skin cleansing lotion)
   - Inadvertent over-heparinization
   - Vaso-vagal reaction

INDICATIONS

The indications for vascular studies in hepatobiliary disease can be divided into three broad groups: preoperative angiography, diagnostic angiography and therapeutic angiography.

PREOPERATIVE ANGIOGRAPHY

Angiography is used preoperatively to delineate vascular anatomy, to assess vascular involvement by the disease process and to determine venous patency. Vascular anatomy is dicussed in detail in Ch. 3. It is important to detect the presence of any normal anatomical variants such as an accessory right hepatic artery (Fig. 3.29, 21.6c & d), or an hepatic system arising completely from the SMA (Fig. 3.30).

Preoperative assessment is usually required prior to the resection of hepatic neoplasms whether benign (Fig. 21.15) or malignant (Fig. 21.16). It is important to ascertain whether a tumour is supplied by the right or left hepatic artery or by both, as this may allow determination as to whether or not the lesion is confined to either the right or

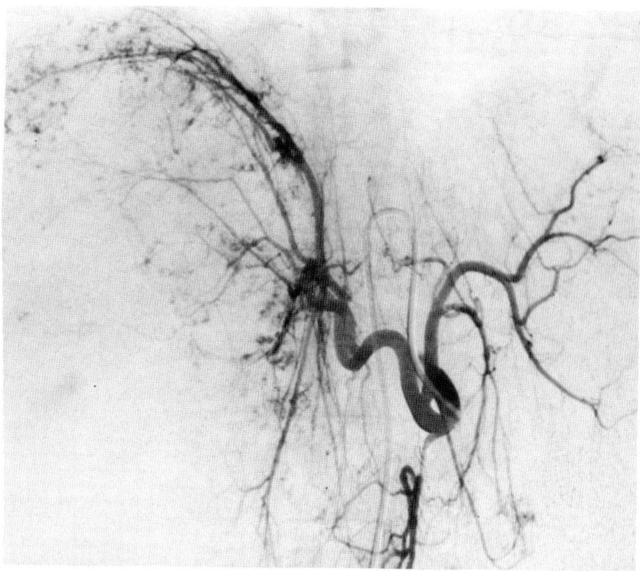

a

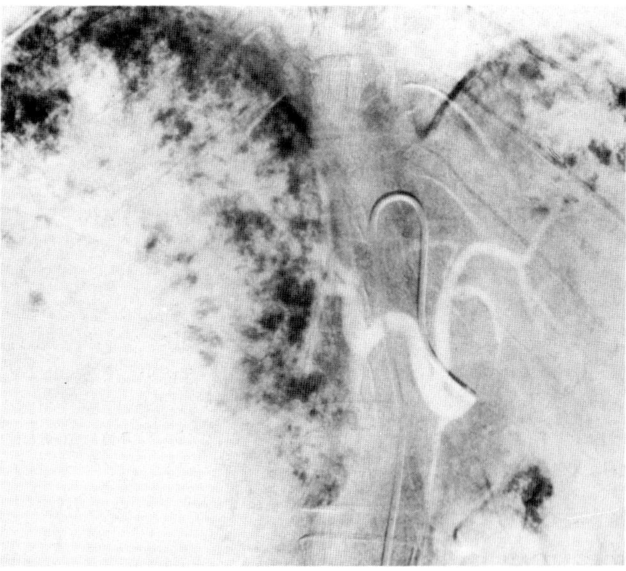

b

Fig. 21.15 Coeliac axis arteriogram in a young woman shows the characteristic features of a massive benign haemangioma. There is filling of abnormal vascular lakes in the arterial phase (a) which retain contrast medium well into the venous phase (b) of the study

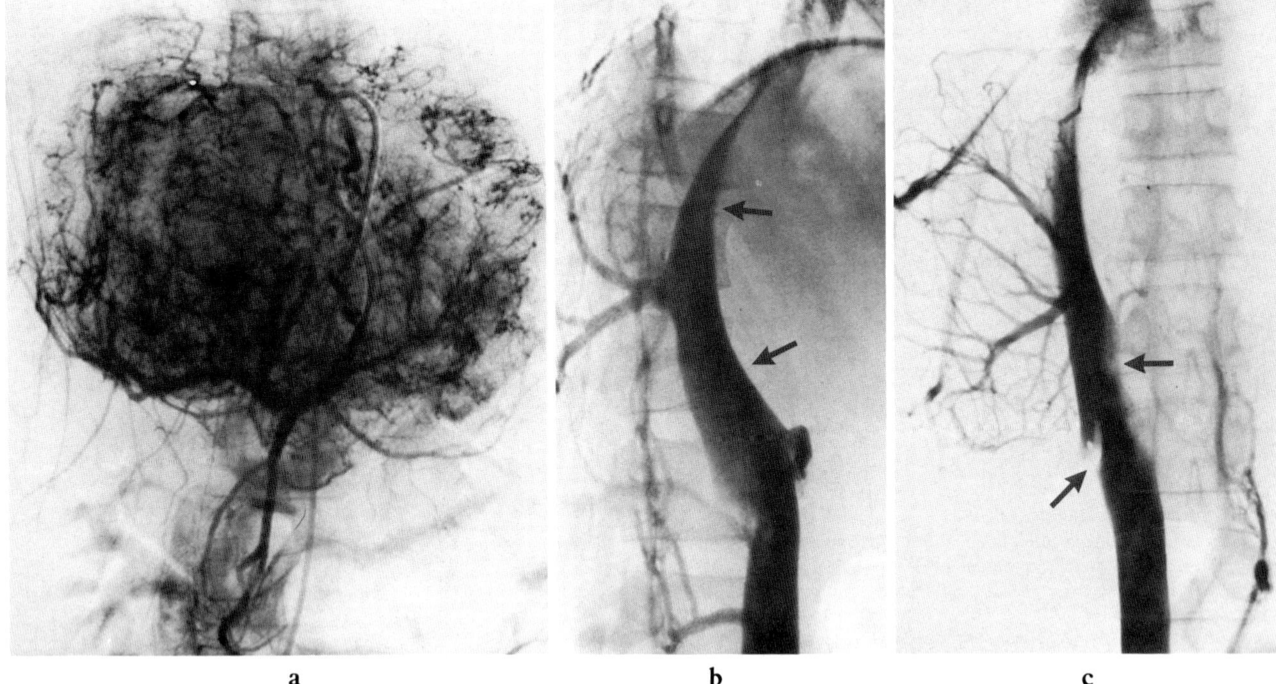

Fig. 21.16 Inferior vena caval compression by a hepatoma. a. Hepatic arteriogram showing the vascular tumour; b. Lateral cavogram showing smooth posterior displacement and compression of cava (arrows); c. AP projection showing abnormal filling of the intrahepatic veins due to compression of the principal veins (note their extensive intercommunication). The filling defects in the caval contrast (arrows) are produced by the influx of unopacified blood from the renal veins. This study suggested the vena cava was compressed and displaced but not invaded and the liver tumour was successfully resected (see Ch. 97)

left liver. In the presence of a relatively avascular tumour vascular encasement or displacement may still be seen (Fig. 21.17). The presence of a patent main portal vein and patent branch to the uninvolved part of the liver is important in determining resectability. When the tumour is very large it is also important to perform an inferior vena cavogram to determine whether there is compression or invasion (see Fig. 21.16b & c). It may also be necessary to exclude invasion of the hepatic veins. In a proportion of patients undergoing surgery for the repair of benign biliary stricture secondary to previous surgery it may be important to determine whether or not the portal vein and/or hepatic artery were also damaged at the time of the biliary tract damage (Ch. 58) (Fig. 21.18).

The other group of patients who require preoperative vascular assessment are those with oesophageal and/or gastric varices (see Fig. 21.10, 21.33). Prior to shunt surgery it may be necessary to determine caval, splenic, superior mesenteric and left renal vein patency.

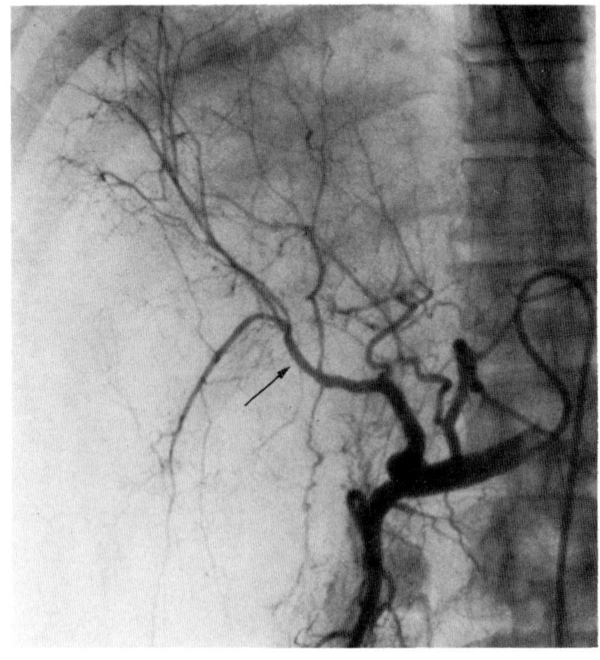

Fig. 21.17 Hepatic arteriogram in a case of cholangiocarcinoma. The tumour is arteriographically avascular but has produced a curved displacement of the right hepatic artery (arrow)

DIAGNOSTIC ANGIOGRAPHY

Congenital lesions

Angiography does not play a major role in the diagnosis of congenital liver anomalies. The diagnosis of the major

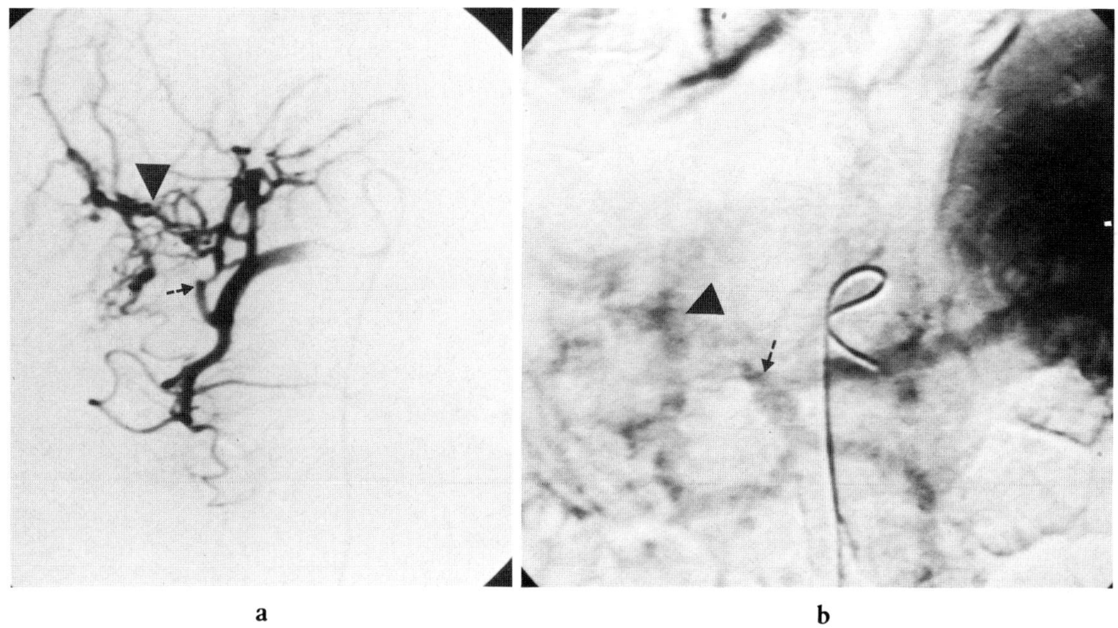

Fig. 21.18 (a). Selective hepatic arteriogram in a woman who had undergone surgery for benign biliary disease, showing disruption of the normal right hepatic artery (arrow), with reconstitution via collateral vessels (arrowhead) (b). Indirect splenoportogram. Same patient showing disruption of the main portal vein (arrow) and cavernous transformation (arrowhead)

congenital lesions such as biliary atresia is made clinically and by other imaging modalities.

Acquired lesions

Vascular studies play a major role in the diagnosis of intrahepatic neoplasms, extrahepatic neoplasms which may involve the liver or mimic liver tumours, vascular lesions, traumatic lesions, cirrhosis, portal hypertension and the effects of infection and infestation.

Intrahepatic neoplasms

Following the detection of an intrahepatic mass lesion or lesions either clinically or by other imaging modalities, angiography may be useful in attempting to characterize the lesions and make a diagnosis. It may be particularly helpful in determining the multiplicity of lesions and whether or not more than one lobe of the liver is involved. Some tumours such as benign haemangiomas have a fairly characteristic arteriographic pattern. Caution must be expressed, however, as other lesions including primary hepatocellular carcinomas and metastases can occasionally produce an identical appearance. Neither size nor multiplicity of lesions *per se* can be used to distinguish benign from malignant or primary from secondary tumours.

Benign tumours (Ch. 87) The most commonly encountered benign intrahepatic tumour is the *haemangioma* (Abrams et al 1969, Alfidi et al 1968, Pantoga 1968). Calcification is occasionally seen within haemangiomas on a plain radiograph.

The characteristic angiographic appearances consist of abnormal vascular lakes which fill in the arterial phase and which retain contrast medium within them well into the venous phase of the study (Fig. 21.15). The lesions may be single, multiple, small or large. Depending on their position and size, giant haemangiomas may cause displacement and/or compression of the portal veins and inferior vena cava. Haemangiomas may bleed spontaneously and if subcapsular in position can result in fatal intraperitoneal haemorrhage (Shearman & Finlayson 1982). Massive haemangio-endotheliomas are occasionally seen in infants when they may cause cardiac failure owing to massive shunting of blood. Angiographically there are abnormal tortuous vessels, large vascular lakes and arteriovenous shunts into hepatic veins.

Adenomas are uncommon tumours. A proportion of these lesions are thought to be associated with the contraceptive pill (Shearman & Finlayson 1982, Baum et al 1973). They may achieve a very large size prior to diagnosis and may rupture and bleed spontaneously; they may regress once the pill is stopped. They are usually intensely vascular and may respond well to therapeutic embolization although they are occasionally partly or wholly avascular. It may be difficult to differentiate these lesions from areas of focal nodular hyperplasia (FNH), but the distinction is important (Casarella et al 1978), as the prognosis and management is different. FNH is multiple in about 20% of cases (Knowless & Wolff 1976). The lesions are hypervascular (Fig. 21.19) and characteristically a dilated branch of the hepatic artery penetrates the lesion and the centre then divides into small radiating

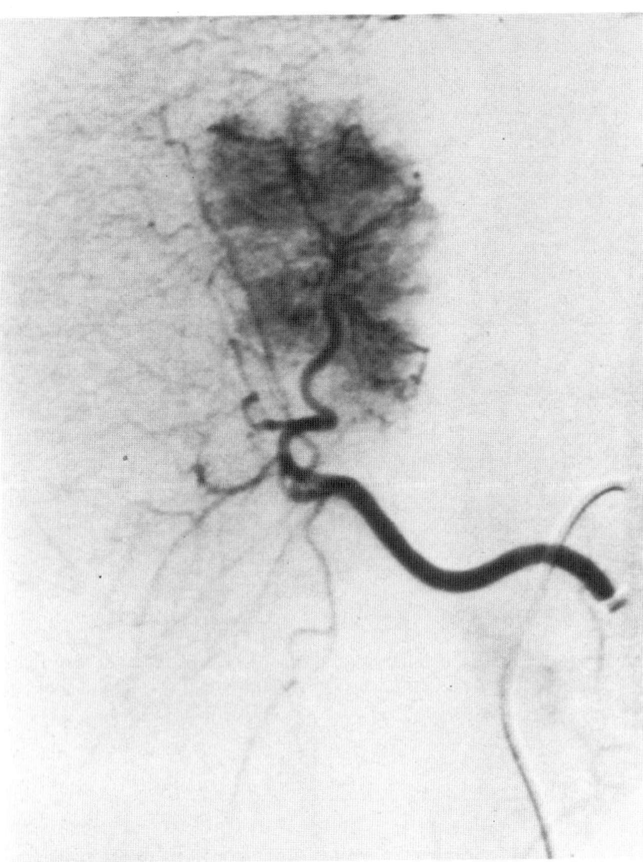

Fig. 21.19 Focal nodular hyperplasia. Selective hepatic arteriogram shows a highly vascular 'tumour', the artery of supply dividing centrally to give stellate pattern of vessels

branches; there is a dense granular stain during the hepatogram phase (Casarella et al 1978). Other benign tumours are rare. Haematomas occur but the angiographic appearances are not specific and these lesions may undergo cystic degeneration.

Primary malignant tumours Primary malignant tumours usually arise from the hepatic parenchyma (hepatocellular carcinoma), the biliary system (cholangiocarcinoma) or the vascular structures (angiosarcoma).

Hepatocellular carcinomas may be solitary but are frequently multifocal. They are characteristically hypervascular, showing a bizarre pathological circulation (Fig. 21.20a & b) but occasionally relatively avascular lesions are encountered (Baum 1983). The tumours may reach enormous size and invade or obtain blood supply from adjacent structures such as the diaphragm (Fig. 21.20c) and kidney. The portal vein is frequently involved in the tumour process and it may be compressed, invaded or

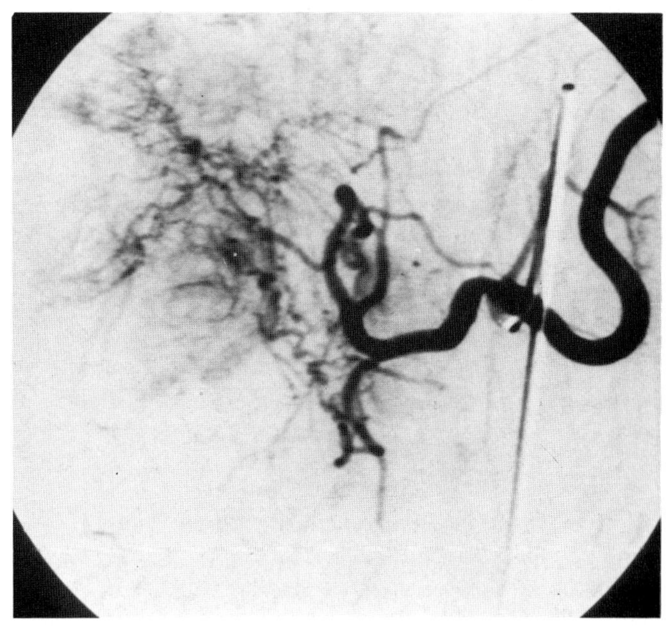

a

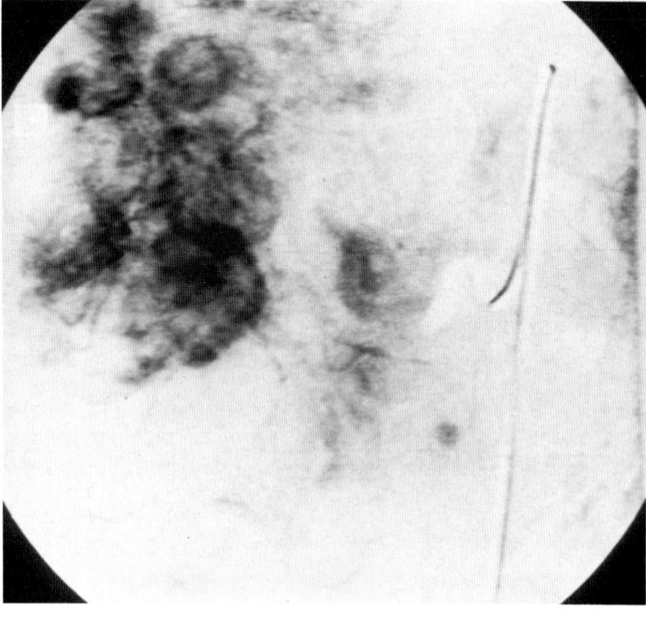

b

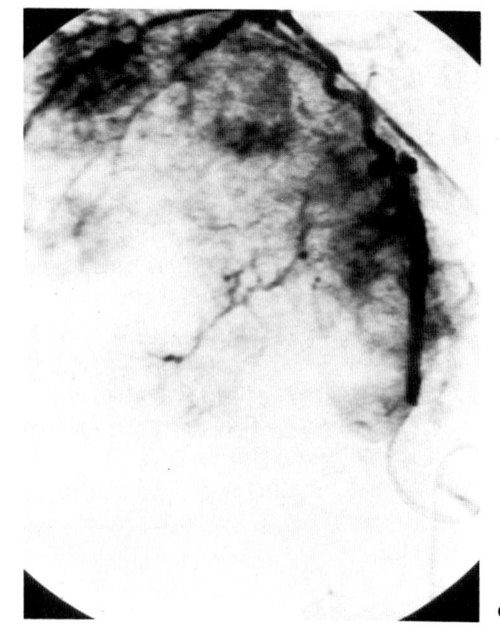

c

Fig. 21.20 Selective hepatic arteriography (a) shows evidence of a bizarre vascular pattern. In the venous phase (b) multiple vascular tumour nodules are seen within the liver parenchyma. The tumour is also being supplied by the phrenic artery (c)

completely obstructed. Marked arteriovenous shunting has been reported in hepatocellular carcinoma and, if the shunting is great enough, angiography may delineate tumour thrombi within the portal vein (Okuda et al 1975). Approximately 75% of hepatocellular tumours occur in patients with pre-existing cirrhosis. It may occasionally be difficult to detect a malignancy within the distorted vascular pattern of advanced cirrhosis. The use of a small dose of intra-arterial vasoconstrictor prior to the angiographic run has been reported as being helpful. This is based on the principle that tumour vessels, unlike normal vessels, do not respond to vasconstrictor drugs (Kaln et al 1967). In the presence of large tumours there may be displacement, compression or invasion of the hepatic veins and/or the inferior vena cava (Okuda et al 1977). Angiography plays an important role in assessing the resectability of hepatomas. Tumours may be amenable to embolization either as a preoperative manoeuvre or as palliative therapy (Ch. 94).

The fibrolamellar variant of hepatoma is also usually hypervascular. These lesions are frequently solitary, very large at diagnosis and may appear on imaging to be quite clearly demarcated from the surrounding normal liver. As this group of tumours may respond favourably to resection, adequate demonstration of their vascular supply and of the systemic and portal venous anatomy is essential (see Fig. 21.16) (Soreide et al 1985).

The major role of angiography in the assessment of *cholangiocarcinoma* is in the evaluation of resectability. The diagnosis is usually made by cholangiography, biopsy cytology and non-invasive imaging. The tumours are usually hypovascular; a faint stain may be seen in the capillary phase, and they frequently cause arterial encasement and portal vein compression, occlusion or invasion (Fig. 21.21) (Walter et al 1976). In the assessment of resectability it is important to determine whether the changes are confined to the vascular supply to the right or left liver and the relationship of the vascular and biliary involvement. Portal venous involvement may occur in the absence of arterial changes and adequate views of both left and right systems should be obtained. Digital subtraction angiography has greatly improved the capability of indirect splenoportographic techniques to visualize not only major portal branches but also their intrahepatic radicles (see Fig. 21.13)

Angiosarcomas are rare primary malignant tumours which may occur *de novo* but in 40% of cases their development is linked to exposure to various substances, including vinyl chloride (Whelan et al 1976), thorotrast, arsenicals and radium (Lecker et al 1979). Angiographically the tumours characteristically show peripheral staining with central hypovascularity (Fig. 21.22)

Metastatic disease The commonest tumours to involve the liver parenchyma are metastases (Van Breda & Waltman 1984), their most frequent site of origin being the gastrointestinal tract, followed by the breast and genitourinary tract. Hepatic metastases are supplied almost exclusively by the hepatic artery. The vascularity of metastases is usually similar to that of the primary tumours, vascular primaries giving rise to vascular metastases and avascular primaries giving rise to relatively avascular metastases. The exception to this is a pancreatic tumour when the metastases may be more vascular than the primary (Baum 1983, Van Breda & Waltman 1984).

Hypervascular metastases frequently arise from endocrine tumours (Fig. 21.23), particularly carcinoid tumours, colonic primaries (Fig. 21.24), chorioncarcinomas, hypernephroma and leiomyosarcomas. Angiography is a sensi-

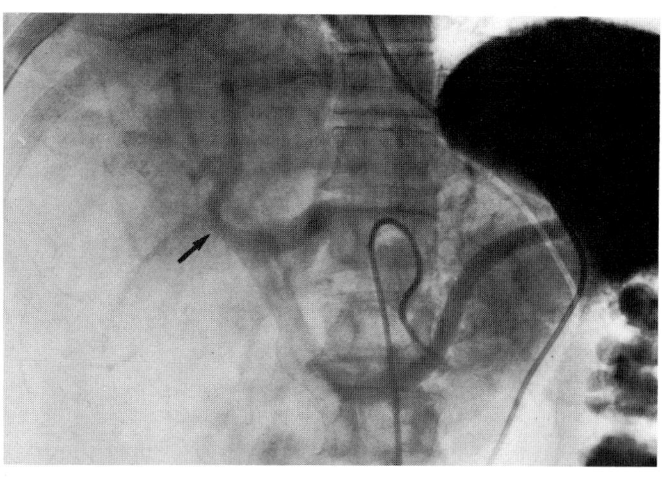

a

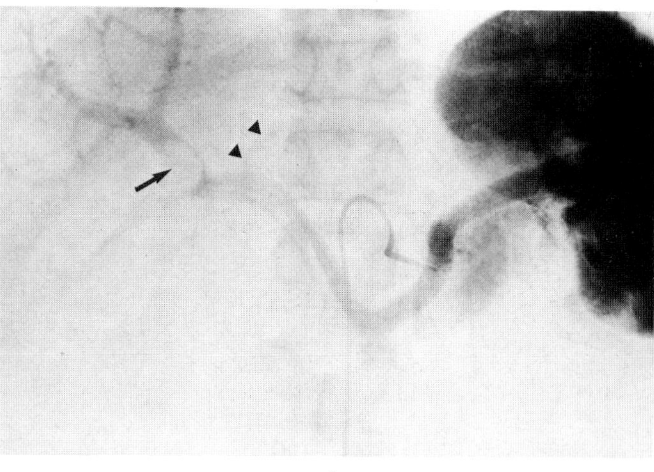

b

Fig. 21.21 (a). An indirect splenoportogram showing narrowing of the right portal vein due to encasement by tumour (arrow). (b). An indirect splenoportogram showing a filling defect in the right portal vein due to invasion of the vein by tumour (arrow). The left portal vein is occluded by tumour (arrowheads)

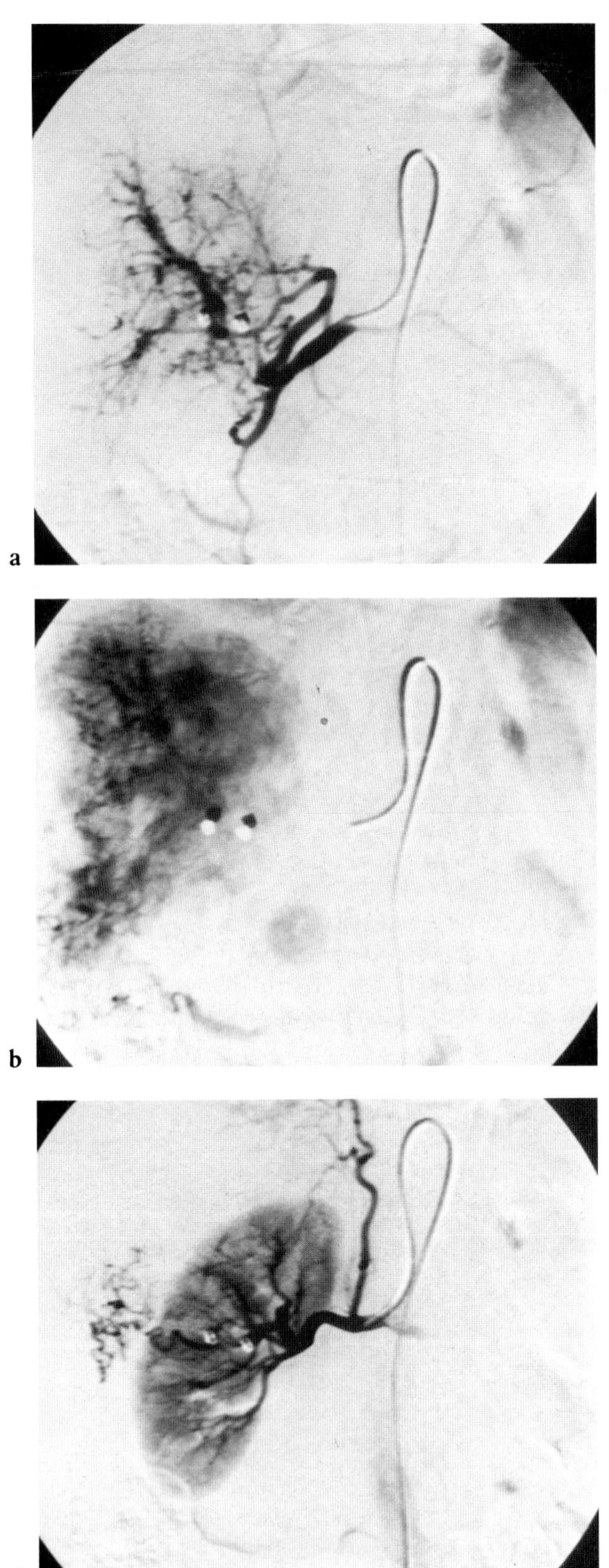

Fig. 21.22 Angiosarcoma. Arterial (a) and venous (b) phases from a hepatic arteriogram showing a highly vascular tumour. The two round, well defined opacities seen on both films represent artefacts caused by the presence of two Gianturco embolisation coils. This tumour is also supplied by the renal artery (c)

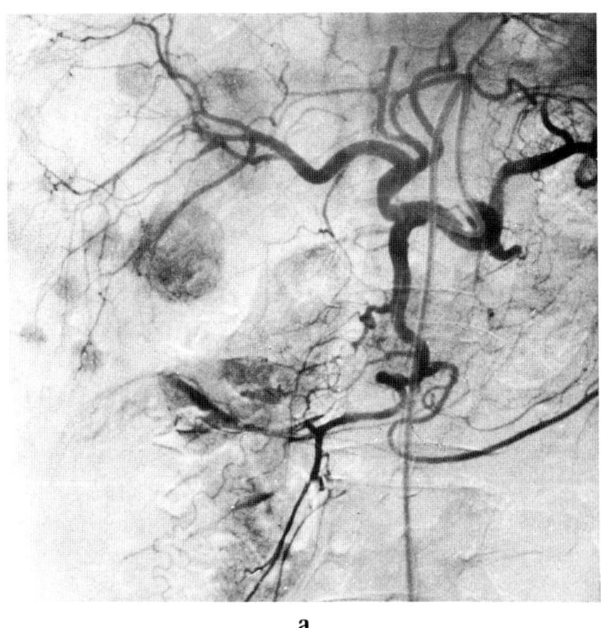

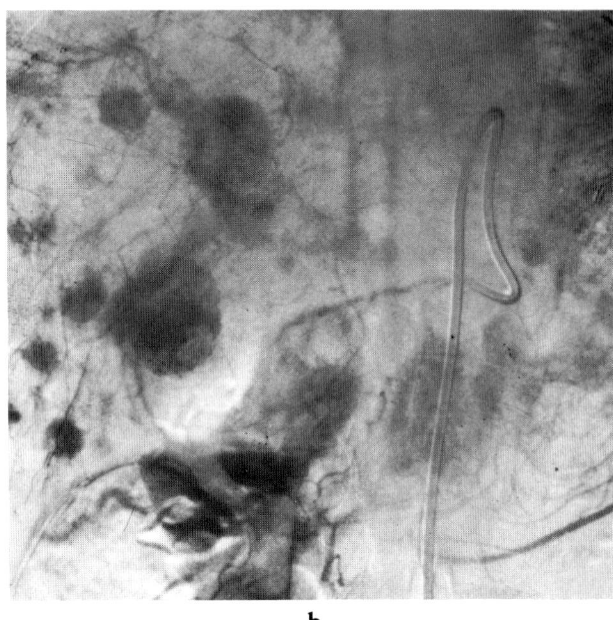

Fig. 21.23 Glucagonoma metastases. Selective hepatic arteriography shows multiple vascular metastases throughout the liver substance in both the arterial (a) and capillary (b) phases

tive tool for diagnosing hypervascular lesions even when quite small, though in most cases the diagnosis of metastatic disease is usually made prior to angiography. Angiography has a role to play, however, in determining the multiplicity and extent of disease, in particular as to whether both lobes of the liver are involved with multicentric disease. It is also important to determine if there is any evidence of portal venous and systemic venous involvement. This is particularly true when assessing the potential resectability of solitary metastases, or whether tumours are suitable for embolization (Ch. 94).

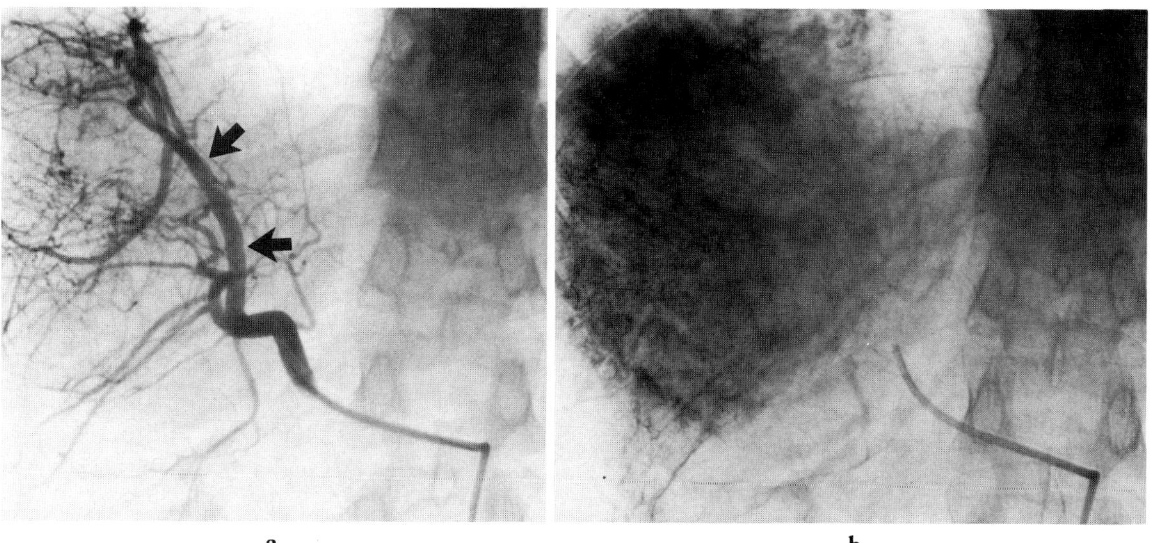

Fig. 21.24 Metastasis from a colonic primary. Hepatic arteriography in a case of massive liver metastasis. (a). Arterial phase: the tumour deposit is displacing the hepatic artery (arrows). (b). Parenchymal phase: there is a dense 'blush' in the large tumour deposit

Hypovascular metastases reveal themselves angiographically by causing displacement and distortion of vessels (arterial and portal venous) and negative filling defects in the hepatogram phase.

When arteriography is performed in the search for intrahepatic mass lesions it is vital that selective hepatic angiography is carried out as well as a general coeliac study. When a large bolus of contrast medium is infused into the hepatic arterial tree even poorly vascularized lesions may be detected more readily (Van Breda & Waltman 1984), particularly if they are metastatic deposits. This is because during coeliac angiography the liver is opacified by both arterial (hepatogram) and portal (portogram) blood. When contrast is injected selectively into the artery, the portogram phase is eliminated and the metastases (which are supplied predominantly by the hepatic artery) are more conspicuous. Arteriography may reveal secondary tumour deposits which previous investigations have failed to demonstrate. This is most likely to happen in the case of liver metastases which, if vascular in nature, can be shown by arteriography when only a few millimetres in diameter (Fig. 21.25)

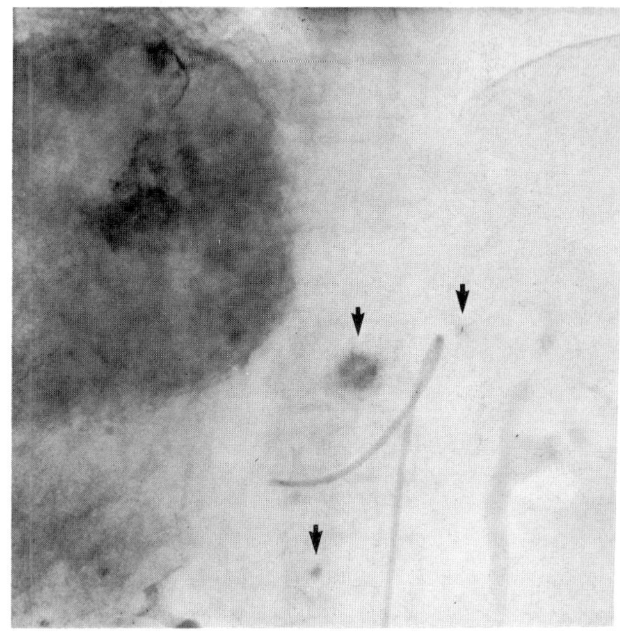

Fig. 21.25 Selective hepatic arteriography in a patient with metastatic tumour deposits in the liver. The large right lobe tumour was shown in CT, but the small deposits in the left lobe (arrows) were only demonstrated on this vascular study

Extrahepatic neoplasms

When performing vascular studies for the investigation of a right upper quadrant mass or jaundice one must remember that some extrahepatic tumours may produce jaundice (pancreatic and gallbladder neoplasms) or mimic intrahepatic tumours (adrenal neoplasms). These lesions may derive a significant proportion of their blood supply from the hepatic arterial system.

Carcinoma of the gallbladder (Abrams et al 1970, Collier et al 1984) Carcinoma of the gallbladder may be found incidentally at cholecystectomy; alternatively it may present as either a mass lesion or from the effects of spread into the liver, extrahepatic biliary system, stomach or duodenum. The gallbladder is supplied by the cystic artery which usually arises from the right hepatic artery although it may occasionally arise from the left hepatic, coeliac axis, common hepatic or gastroduodenal arteries.

The outline of the normal gallbladder is not uncommonly seen on selective hepatic arteriography (Fig. 21.26).

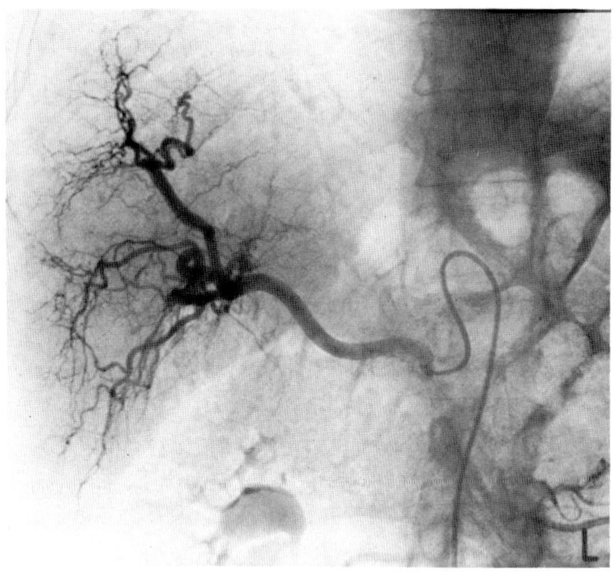

a

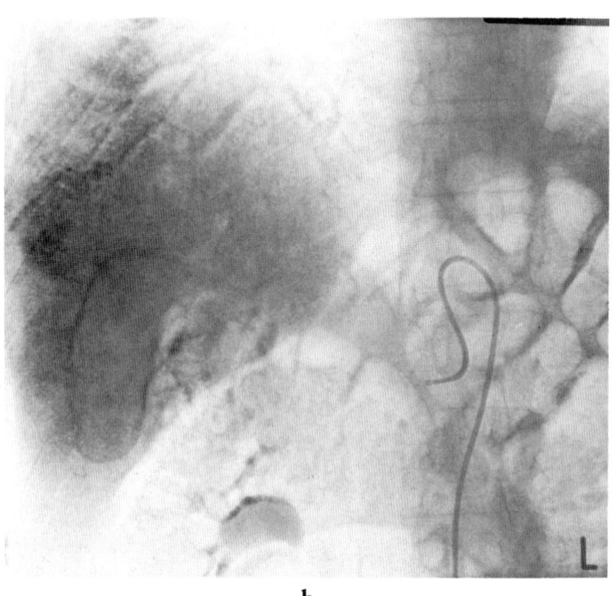

b

Fig. 21.26 Normal gallbladder blush. Following selective hepatic arteriography the wall of the gallbladder is often visualized in the 'hepatogram' phase of the study

In the presence of malignancy the cystic artery may appear enlarged and encasement or occlusion of cystic artery branches has been reported (Abrams et al 1970). In the venous phase the wall of the gallbladder may be seen to be thickened and irregular. Neovascularity in the tumour is frequently detected. If the lesion is large, encasement and amputation of intrahepatic vessels can be seen secondary to invasion of liver substance by the tumour (Fig. 21.27)

Pancreatic neoplasia The diagnosis of pancreatic carcinoma is usually made clinically and by non-invasive imaging techniques. Angiography may be useful preoperatively to assess resectability and to detect intrahepatic metastases. The primary tumour may cause encasement or occlusion of the splenic and portal vein; the gastroduodenal artery and/or the splenic artery may also show evidence of encasement. Adequate visualization of the hepatic circulation is important so that an attempt can be made to exclude or confirm the presence of metastases.

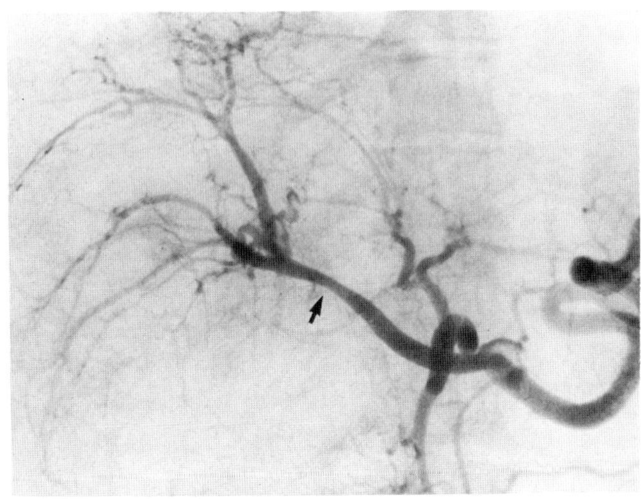

Fig. 21.27 Carcinoma of the gallbladder. The tumour has produced displacement and encasement (arrow) of the right hepatic artery

Pancreatic endocrine tumours (apudomas) present clinically with symptoms of excess hormone production, the hormone being produced by the primary tumour or the secondary deposits or both. Angiography in the assessment of these lesions should include adequate views of the splenic artery, pancreatic arteries, gastroduodenal artery and hepatic arteries as well as views of the splenic and portal vein (Fig. 21.28). Angiography is often performed prior to therapeutic hepatic embolization (Ch. 94).

Adrenal tumours Large right-sided adrenal tumours can cause a serious diagnostic dilemma. These tumours may derive their blood supply not only from the adrenal arteries but also from the renal and hepatic vessels. The malignancy may invade the liver substance and mimic very closely right-sided hepatic neoplasms.

Cystic disease

The advent of ultrasound and computerized tomography has greatly facilitated the diagnosis and assessment of hepatic cystic disease. Angiography is only occasionally required in the evaluation of non-parasitic cysts, the usual indication being prior to operative management of some cysts. The centres of the lesions are avascular and the rims of compressed liver appear hypervascular.

Hydatid cysts (Ch. 75) present as single or multiple intrahepatic lesions. Angiography is rarely performed in the diagnostic work-up of these patients or prior to surgery. As with non-parasitic lesions the cysts may show hypervascularity at the rim with an avascular centre.

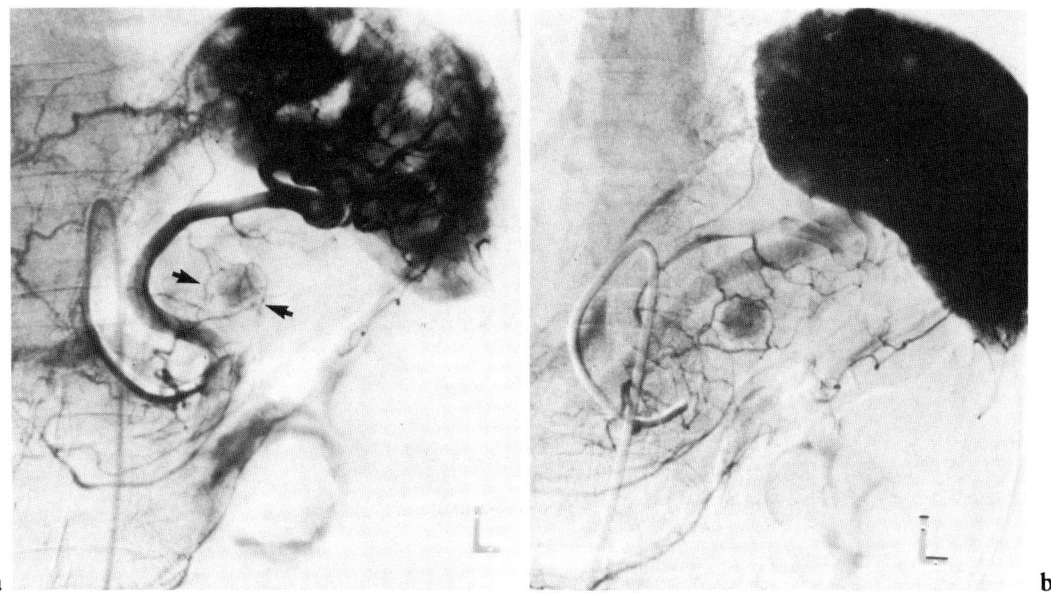

Fig. 21.28 Splenic arteriogram. Early (a) and late (b) radiographs showing the characteristic 'blush' of a pancreatic insulinoma (arrows)

Vascular lesions

Primary venous disorders may involve the liver and show fairly chacracteristic appearances. *Peliosis hepatis* (Pliskin 1975) is a rare condition associated with the ingestion of anabolic steroids. The characteristic angiographic changes in this disorder include areas of contrast accumulation of various sizes which persist through the venous phase. Although the lesions tend to respond to withdrawal of the causative agent, spontaneous rupture and intraperitoneal bleeding has been reported. Other associations of peliosis include angiosarcoma, vinyl chloride exposure and hepatocellular carcinoma.

Polyarteritis nodosa is a necrotizing vasculitis which characteristically involves small- and medium-sized arteries. In a significant proportion of cases this process leads to the formation of microaneurysms and these may rupture spontaneously. Arterial stenoses may also occur. Angiography may be of value in establishing the diagnosis (Fig. 21.29). The renal and hepatic arterial trees should be examined; aneurysms occur in the liver in 40% to 60% of affected individuals and in the kidney in 80% to 100% (Van Breda & Waltman 1984, Travers et al 1979). From a technical point of view it is important to inject contrast selectively into the hepatic artery and to take films for at least fifteen seconds. Similar appearances have been reported in patients suffering from drug abuse, in metastatic atrial myxoma and, rarely, in other collagen diseases, such as systemic lupus erythematosus.

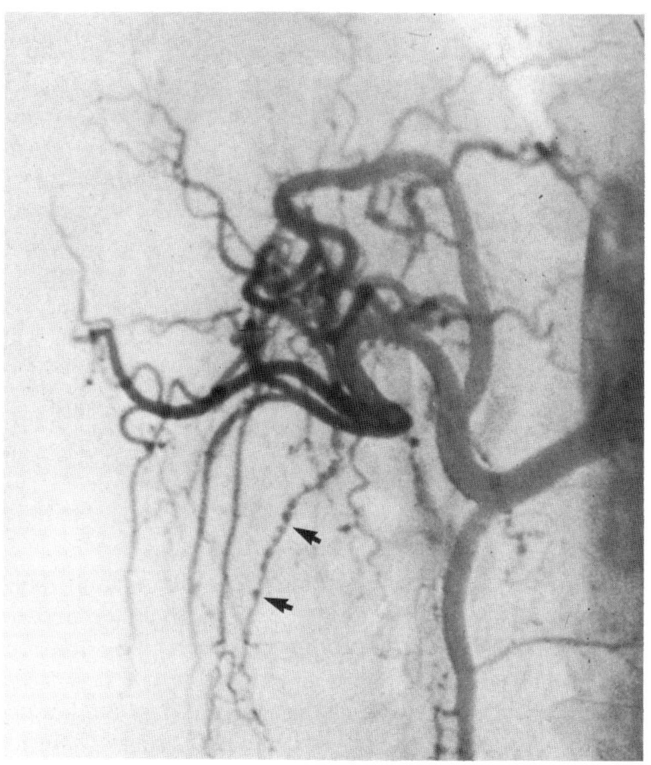

Fig. 21.29 Polyarteritis nodosa (PAN). The classic microaneurysms are seen in this hepatic arteriogram (arrows)

Aneurysms Aneurysms of the hepatic and splenic arteries and their branches may be atherosclerotic, traumatic, mycotic or inflammatory in nature; they have also been reported following intra-arterial cytotoxic agents (Forsberg et al 1978). Aneurysms may be multiple and may attain a very large size. Large hepatic artery aneurysms may present with jaundice and/or an epigastric mass. Spontaneous rupture and fistulation into the biliary system can prove to be life-threatening. Angiography is invaluable in detecting and accurately delineating these abnormalities and therapeutic embolization of the vessel of supply is

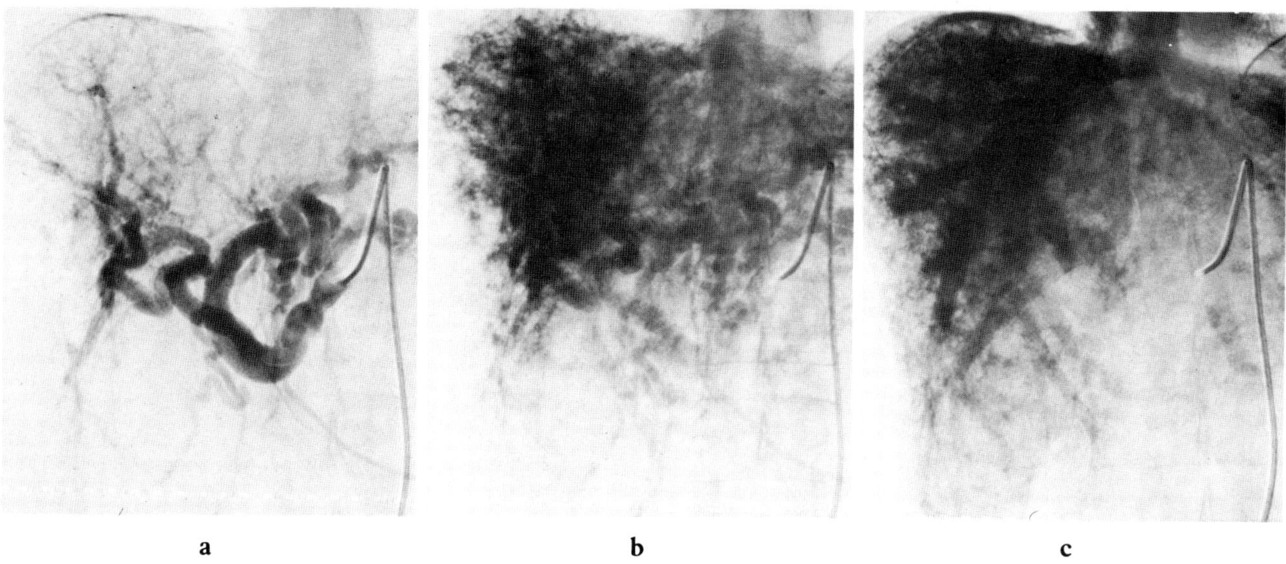

Fig. 21.30 Osler-Weber-Rendu disease. Selective hepatic arteriography, arterial a, capillary b and venous c phases show abnormal vascularity, multiple small angiomas and hepatic artery to hepatic vein fistulae. Such dense opacification of the hepatic vein following injection of contrast into the hepatic artery is highly suggestive of pathology

frequently the most appropriate therapy (Ch. 85).

Hereditary haemorrhagic telangiectasia. This condition (also known as Osler-Weber-Rendu disease) is a familial disease characterized by telangiectasia of the skin and mucous membranes. It is a multisystem disease and the liver is frequently involved. The typical appearances seen at angiography include multiple, small arteriovenous (hepatic artery to hepatic vein) fistulae (Fig. 21.30) and multiple discrete angiomas. The appearances may mimic a vascular neoplasm (hepatocellular carcinoma) but the presence of hepatic artery to hepatic vein fistulae is only rarely seen in other types of liver pathology (Halpern et al 1968). Occasionally the condition gives rise to haemobilia.

Hepatic trauma (see Ch. 82–84)

Angiography may prove invaluable in investigating both the immediate and delayed effects of trauma. Hepatic vascular damage can be caused by either blunt or penetrating injury.

Blunt trauma. The commonest causes of blunt hepatic injuries are road traffic accidents and sports injuries (including horse riding, parachuting, skiing). Major liver injury has also occurred following external cardiac massage and in some areas of the world blast injury is an important cause. When angiography is performed following blunt trauma, several important points need to be considered. The operator needs to be aware if any arterial branches have not been filled, a finding suggestive of either transection or spasm: in this situation active bleeding may also be demonstrated in some cases. The hepatogram phase may show the lateral margin of the liver to be displaced medially by an extrahepatic or subcapsular haematoma (Fig. 21.31). It is also of great importance to determine portal vein patency and to take radiographs in the portogram phase as well as the arterial phase. Any area of the liver which appears avascular in both the arterial and portogram phases is non-viable and will usually require surgical intervention at some stage (usually earlier rather than later). Aneurysms of the hepatic artery and arterioportal fistulae may occur, often as late complications of

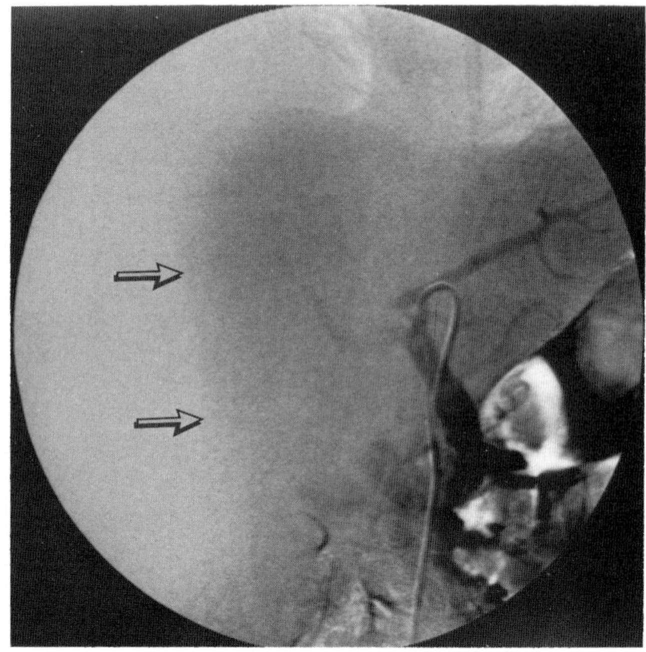

Fig. 21.31 Liver trauma. The late phase of a superior mesenteric arteriogram shows that the left portal vein is patent, the right portal vein is poorly seen and the liver is displaced medially (arrows) by a large haematoma

injury. These lesions may give rise to haemobilia which can be life-threatening (see below).

Penetrating injury. Penetrating liver injury may be self-inflicted, violent, accidental or iatrogenic in nature. Self-inflicted and violent injuries are usually due to stabbings, gunshot or shrapnel. Accidental injury such as may occur following road traffic accidents may be a mixture of blunt and penetrating trauma. The advent of more aggressive and invasive investigation of liver pathology has engendered its own complications. Biliary and hepatic surgery of all grades of complexity can also give rise to some specific vascular problems.

The finding of *arterioportal fistulae* following penetrating injury such as stabbing, liver biopsy and percutaneous biliary drainage is not uncommon. Small fistulae may resolve spontaneously but larger lesions cause a rise in portal pressure and if left may give rise to portal hypertension (Sones & Oliver 1984). These lesions can also involve the biliary tract and bleed giving rise to haemobilia. Embolization may be the treatment of choice for these lesions (Ch. 85). Intrahepatic arterial aneurysms are not infrequently seen following liver injury (Fig. 21.32). The aneurysms often develop late and are usually asymptomatic until they rupture causing life-threatening haemorrhage. Rupture usually occurs into either the peritoneal cavity or the biliary system (Guida & Moore 1966). Transcatheter embolization is now the treatment of choice for many of these lesions, but consultation between surgeon and radiologist is important. It is important that the interventional radiologist occludes the aneurysm itself and does not just block the feeding vessel. The rich collateral network to the liver renders simple ligation or occlusion of the feeding vessel ineffectual. Surgical ligation of the main hepatic arterial trunk feeding such a lesion is often ineffective and compromises interventional radiological therapy. The fact that injudicious surgical ligation may render embolization impossible should always be kept in mind.

Cirrhosis and portal hypertension (see Section 16)

The diagnosis of cirrhosis and portal hypertension is usually made by means other than angiography. The role of vascular studies in the investigation of portal hypertension is summarized in Table 21.3.

The aetiology and classification of portal hypertension will not be discussed in this section. The angiographer should be acquainted with the general principles of investigation and management and the working diagnosis in each case, as this significantly affects the type of vascular study that should be performed.

Table 21.3 Angiography in portal hypertension

1. Direct/indirect measurement of portal pressure
2. Assessment of portal vein patency
3. Delineation of arterial system
4. Demonstration of systemic venous anatomy and patency
5. Visualization of portal venous collaterals
6. Transhepatic embolization of varices

Measurement of portal pressure. The normal portal venous pressure ranges from 5 to 10 mm Hg. Pressure may be measured by either direct or indirect means. Direct measurements are performed either by recording splenic pulp pressure prior to performing a direct splenoportogram, or following direct transhepatic catheterization of the portal venous system prior to an embolization procedure for variceal bleeding.

Assessment of portal vein patency. Ultrasound has become so sophisticated that a vast amount of information about both the extra- and intrahepatic portal venous systems may be obtained by this non-invasive technique (Ch. 14).

Angiographic techniques however will continue to be the mainstay of portal vein imaging in many units. In the majority of cases adequate information is obtained from indirect splenoportographic techniques and the advent of DVI/DSA has further improved the accuracy of these investigations (see above).

The portal vein may be compressed or invaded in its extrahepatic or intrahepatic course. Intrahepatic portal venous abnormalities may be due to cirrhosis where the necrosis and subsequent fibrosis and regeneration gradually impair circulation through the liver. Portal hypertension ensues, and varices may develop. Schistosomiasis is in many countries the most common cause of hepatic fibrosis and portal hypertension. Tumours, either primary intrahepatic or metastastic, may compromise the intrahepatic portal veins. This abnormality may take the form of either invasion of the vein or compression and displacement of the vein. Portosystemic collateral vessels develop when the portal venous system is obstructed resulting in varices but they are usually unable to decompress the system completely.

The portal venous system may also be compressed or invaded in its extrahepatic course. Cavernous transformation of the portal vein usually occurs as a result of neonatal umbilical vein infection, often associated with the use of umbilical vein cannulae. The extrahepatic portal vein is thrombosed and multiple tortuous collateral vessels develop around the thrombosed vessels and drain portal blood into the intrahepatic portal radicles (Fig. 21.33). Abdominal sepsis later in life may also cause portal vein thrombosis and give rise to cavernous transformation. Calcification may occur in the portal vein as a result of previous thrombosis. The extrahepatic portal vein may be compressed or invaded by tumours arising at or near the hilum of the liver.

Delineation of arterial anatomy. It may be important to accurately delineate arterial anatomy, particularly if surgery is contemplated or if an arterioportal fistula is suspected. Arterial changes occur in cirrhosis where the intrahepatic vessels may show a characteristic corkscrew

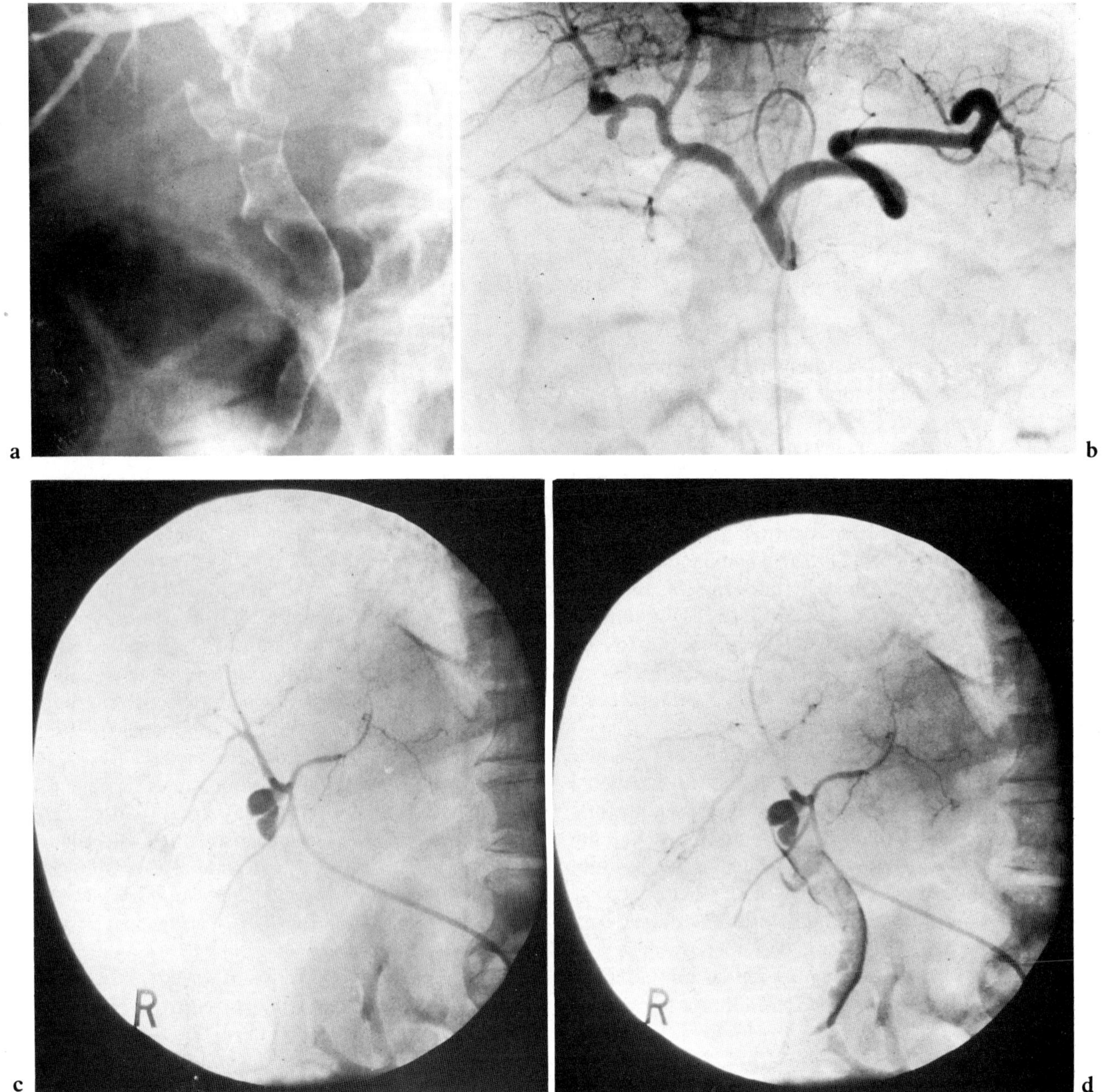

Fig. 21.32 Embolization of an intrahepatic aneurysm. The patient had undergone a difficult cholecystectomy three months earlier and now presented after recent jaundice and malaena with active gastrointestinal bleeding. a. A PTC shows the common bile duct to contain blood clot (filling defects). b. A coeliac arteriogram shows an aneurysm (presumably post-surgical) in the right hepatic artery. c. A selective study shows detail of the aneurysm which is actively bleeding into the biliary tree. d. e. Note the contrast outlining the ampulla and duodenum (arrow) only 12 seconds after the arterial injection of contrast medium. f. The hepatic artery has been embolized (arrow). The patient was discharged from hospital with no further treatment one week after the procedure

pattern. The liver may be noted to be small and, in the hepatogram phase, may be seen to be displaced from the lateral abdominal wall by ascites.

Demonstration of systemic venous anatomy and patency. The angiographer should not forget the hepatic veins when performing pan-angiography in the investigation and management of portal hypertension. Hepatic vein occlusion, the Budd Chiari syndrome, causes 'post-hepatic' portal hypertension. The appearances seen at selective hepatic venography are characteristic, showing a spider's web pattern (Fig. 21.34). Prior to shunt surgery it is important to determine patency of both the inferior vena cava and left renal vein and to measure inferior vena caval and portal pressure.

Visualization of portal venous collaterals. If the main splenic or portal veins become occluded the many potential

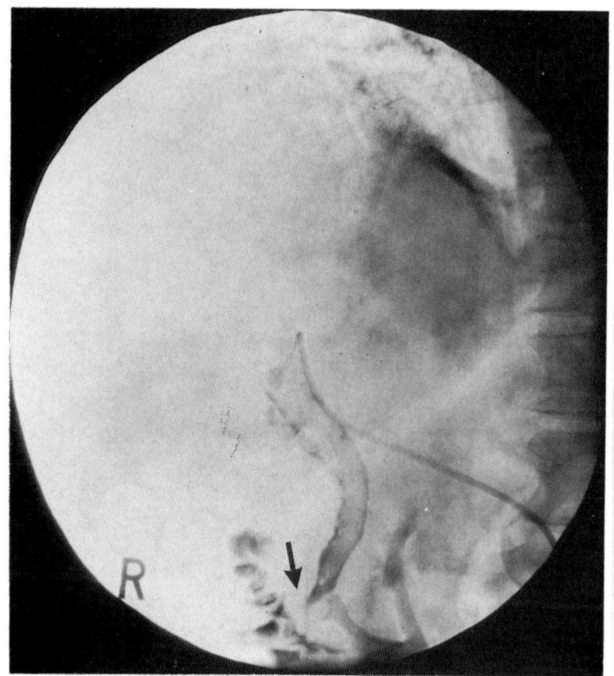

e

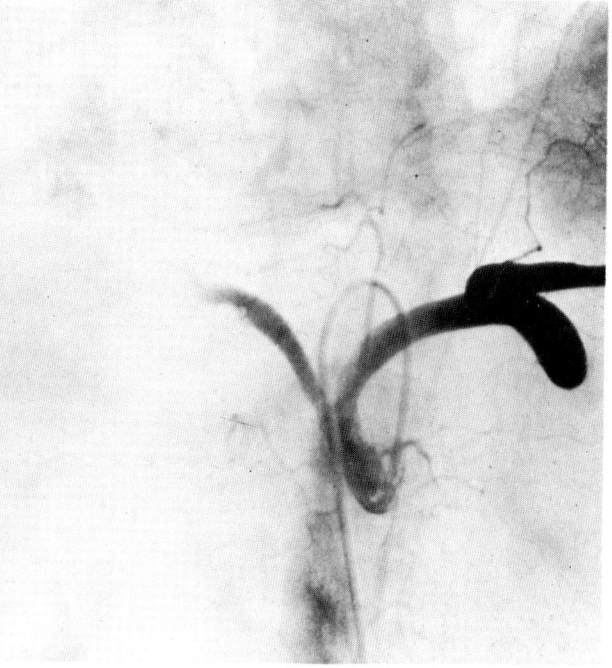
f

Fig. 21.32 *(cont'd)*

collateral routes of venous drainage may enlarge to partially decompress the system (Fig. 21.10 & 21.33). Gastric and oesophageal varices may be demonstrated by either direct or indirect venographic techniques. It is important to attempt to determine whether flow in the portal system is hepatofugal or hepatopetal, as this affects management. Careful evaluation of consecutive images may enable the angiographer to determine the direction of flow.

Transhepatic embolization of varices. This subject is covered in detail in Ch. 107.

Infection and infestation

Hepatic infection and infestation are usually diagnosed by

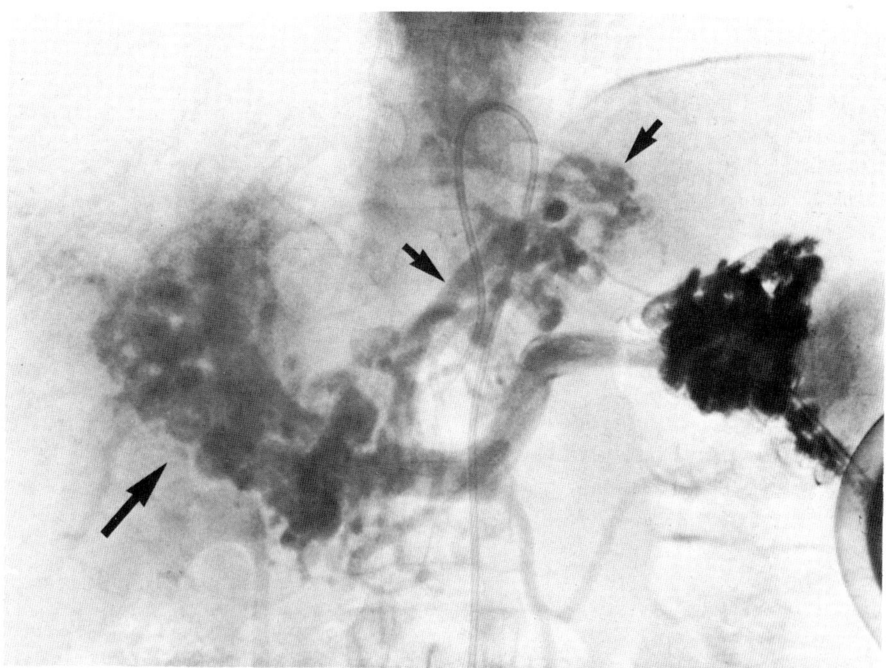

Fig. 21.33 A direct splenoportogram showing varices (short arrows) and cavernous transformation of the portal vein (long arrow)

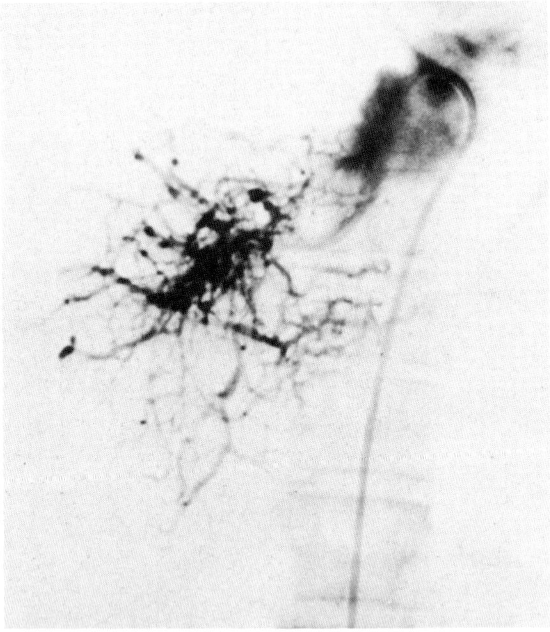

Fig. 21.34 Budd-Chiari syndrome. A catheter has been passed retrogradely into a right hepatic vein. An injection of a small volume (5 ml) of contrast medium has outlined an extensive fine network of collateral vessels. The 'spider-web' appearance is pathognomonic of the Budd-Chiari syndrome

clinical investigation and non-invasive radiological techniques, such as ultrasound and CT. Angiography may be of value in assessing the effects of abscess formation on hepatic vasculature. Displacement of both arterial and venous structures may be seen. The abscess itself is frequently avascular but may show a hypervascular ring (Nory et al 1974). Acute infection and abscess formation may produce arteriovenous shunting (Adler et al 1978) (Fig. 21.35). Multiple abscesses may be indistinguishable angiographically from metastatic disease.

A very large number of parasites may invade the liver. In certain parts of the world schistosomiasis is the most common cause of portal hypertension (Ch. 110).

Hydatid disease (Ch. 75) causes cystic change within the liver parenchyma. Angiography is not used to make the diagnosis but may be needed preoperatively to delineate anatomy. The cysts, which may reach a very large size, can cause marked displacement of arteries and displacement and compression of portal venous radicles.

Amoebic abscesses (Ch. 76) occur within the liver; as with hydatid disease angiography is infrequently indicated and then usually in preoperative assessment and not primary diagnosis.

THERAPEUTIC ANGIOGRAPHY

It is possible, with experience, to place arterial catheters into superselective positions within the hepatic arterial circulation. This capability may be employed for both infusion and embolization techniques.

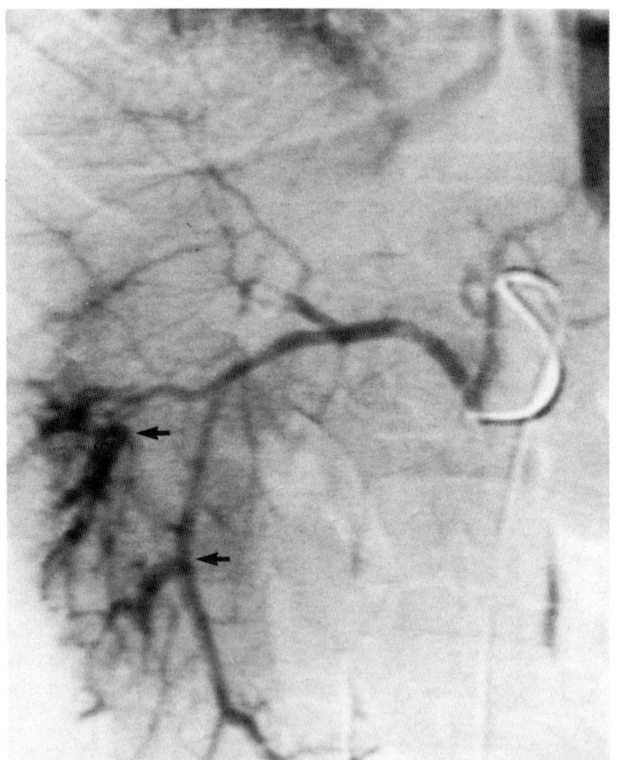

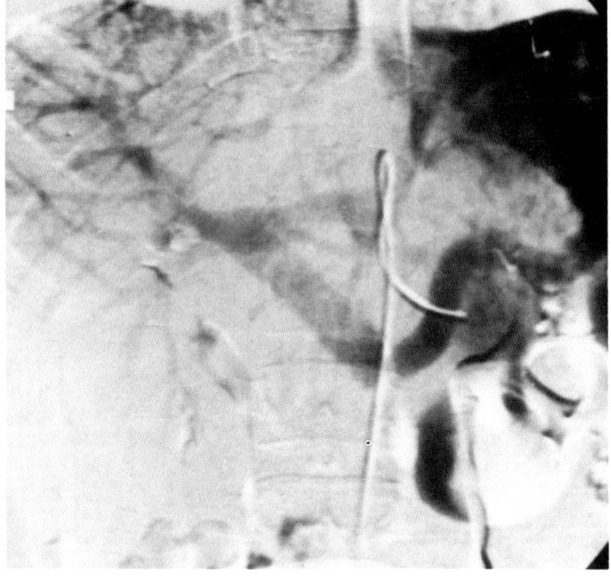

Fig. 21.35 Arteriovenous fistula—infection (abscess). a. Hepatic arteriogram shows preferential filling of vessels in the lower part of the right lobe of the liver. Multiple small arterioportal fistulae are present (arrows) b. An indirect splenoportogram shows that the portal vein segments in this area do not fill antegradely. The fistulae closed after treatment with antibiotics

Infusion techniques

The debate as to whether cytotoxic agents are more effective and cause less systemic side effects if delivered selectively to the organ of interest will not be discussed here. Arterial catheters can be inserted into the hepatic artery either percutaneously or operatively for this purpose. This technique can cause permanent arterial damage (strictures, occlusions and aneurysms have all been reported) and catheter care requires close supervision. More recently the development of labelled monoclonal antibodies has led to short-term (two to five hours) selective hepatic arterial catheterization and infusion of these antibodies to treat both primary and secondary hepatic malignancy.

Embolization techniques

Transcatheter therapeutic embolization may be used in the liver in the management of a wide variety of diseases. For further information on the types of embolic agents used and the potential hazards of the techniques the reader is referred to Ch. 94. It is worth stressing a few major guidelines at this point. Firstly, whatever the pathology, arterial embolization should not be performed in an area of the liver that does not have a portal venous supply. Secondly, it is important to observe a strict protocol with regard to patient preparation and antibiotic prophylaxis, if complications are to be avoided. Thirdly, the procedure should not be performed without the full co-operation of both an experienced surgeon and physician to manage the side effects (pain, fever) and complications (e.g. renal failure, abscess formation) that may occur. Finally, the angiographer should embolize as small an area of liver as possible, but must ensure that the desired therapeutic effect is achieved. The indications for hepatic arterial embolization are listed in Table 21.4.

Table 21.4 Indications for hepatic arterial embolization

Haemobilia	Ch. 85
Arterioportal fistula	Ch. 84
Aneurysm	Ch. 84
Liver tumour primary secondary	Ch. 94

Transhepatic embolization may be employed in the management of gastric and oesophageal varices (Ch. 107).

REFERENCES

Abeatici S, Campi L 1951 Sur les possibilities de l'angiographie hepatique — la visualisation due systeme portal (recherches experimentales). Acta Radiologica (Stockholm) 36: 83–392

Abrams R M Berenbaum E R, Santos J S, Lipson J 1969 Angiographic features of cavernous haemangioma of liver. Radiology 92: 308

Abrams R M, Meng C H, Firooznia H, Berenbaum E R, Epstein H Y 1970 Angiographic demonstration of carcinoma of the gallbladder. Radiology 94: 277–282

Abrams H L (ed) 1983 Introduction and historical notes. In: Angiography, 3rd edn. Little Brown, Boston, ch 1, p 3–13

Adler J, Goodgold M, Mity H et al 1978 Arteriovenous shunts involving the liver. Radiology 129: 315–322

Alfidi R J, Rastogitt, Buonocore E, Brown C H 1968 Hepatic arteriography. Radiology 90: 1136–1142

Allison D J 1980 Therapeutic embolization and venous sampling. In: Taylor S (ed) Recent advances in surgery 10. Churchill Livingstone, Edinburgh, p 27–64

Allison D J, Hemingway P 1983 Angiography of the gastrointestinal tract. In: Nolan D J (ed) Radiological atlas of gastrointestinal disease. John Wiley, New York, ch 9, p 281–309

Anacker H, Deveris K, Linden G 1957 Leistungsfahigkeit und Grenzen der purkutanes Splenoportographie. Fortschritte auf dem Gebiete der Rontgenstrahlen 86: 411

Baum J K, Holtz F, Bookstein J J, Klein E W 1973 Possible association between benign hepatomas and oral contraceptives. Lancet 2: 926

Baum S 1983 Hepatic Arteriography. In: Abrams H L (ed) Angiography, 3rd edn. Little Brown, Boston, Ch. 64, p 1479–1504

Bergstrand I 1983 Splenoportography. In: Abrams H L (ed) Angiography, 3rd edn. Little Brown, Boston p 1573–1604

Bierman H R, Steinbach H L, White L P, Kelley K H 1952 Portal venipuncture: percutaneous transhepatic approach. Proceedings of the Society for Experimental Biology and Medicine 79: 550

Blakemore A H, Lord J W Jr 1945 Technique of using vitallium tubes in establishing portocaval shunts for portal hypertension. Annals of Surgery 122: 476

Bron K M 1983 Arterioportography. In: Abrams H L (ed) Angiography, 3rd edn. Little Brown, Boston, p 1605–1620

Casarella W J, Knowles D M, Wolff M, Johnson P M 1978 Focal nodular hyperplasia and liver cell adenoma: Radiologic and pathologic differentiation. American Journal of Roentgenology 131: 393–402

Casteneda-Zuniga W R, Jauregui H, Rysavy J A, Formanet A, Amplatz K 1978 Complications of wedge hepatic venography. Radiology 126: 53–56

Collier N A, Carr D H, Hemingway A P, Blumgart L H 1984 Preoperative diagnosis and its effect on the treatment of carcinoma of the gallbladder. Surgery, Gynecology and Obstetrics. 159: 465–470

Dos Santos R, Lamas A, Pereira-Caldas J 1929 L'arteriographie des membres, de l'aorta et de ses branches abdominales. Bull Soc nat Chir 55: 587

Dos Santos R 1935 Phlebographie d'une veine cave inferieure suture. J Urol Med chir 39: 586

Forsberg L, Hafstorm L, Lunderquist A, Sundquist K 1978 Arterial changes during treatment with intrahepatic arterial infusion of 5 Fluorouracil. Radiology 126: 49–52

Forssmann W 1931 Ueber Kontrastdarstellung der Hohlen des levenden rechten Herzens under der Lungenschlagader. Munchen Med Mschr 78: 489–492

Goncalves A M 1982 Biography of Egas Moniz. Catalogo de exposicao itinerante da obra Egas Moniz e Reynaldo dos Santos. Publicacoes Ciencia e Vida Lda, Lisbon, p 77

Grainger R 1985 Intravascular contrast media. In: Grainger R, Allison D J (eds) Diagnostic imaging. Churchill Livingstone, Edinburgh, Ch. 7

Guida P M, Moore S W 1966 Aneurysm of the hepatic artery report of five cases with a brief review of previously reported cases. Surgery 60: 229–310

Halpern M, Turner A F, Citron B P 1968 Hereditary haemorrhagic telangiectasia. Radiology 90: 1143–1149

Hascheck E, Lindenthal O T 1896 A contribution to the practical use of the photography according to Roentgen. Wiener Klinische Wochenschrift 9:63

Kaln P C, Frates W J, Paul R E Jr 1967 The epinephrine effect in angiography of gastrointestinal tract tumours. Radiology 88: 686

Knowles D M, Wolff M M 1976 Focal nodular hyperplasia of the liver: a clinicopathologic study and review of the literature. Human Pathology 7: 533–545

Lecker G Y, Doroshaw J H, Zwelling L A, Chabrie B A 1979 The clinical features of hepatic angiosarcoma: a report of four cases and review of the English Literature. Medicine 58: 48–64

Leger L 1951 Phlebographie portale par injection splenique intraparenchymateuse. Mem Adad Chir 77:712

Lindgren E 1950 Percutaneous angiography of the vertebral artery. Acta Radiologica (Stockholm) 33: 389–404

Lunderquist A Simert G, Tylen U, Vang J 1977 Follow-up of patients with portal hypertension and oesophageal varices treated with percutaneous obliteration of gastric coronary vein. Radiology 122: 59–63

Lunderquist A, Hoevels J, Owman T 1983 Transhepatic portal venography. In: Abrams H L (ed) Angiography, 3rd edn. Little Brown, Boston, p 1505–1529

Meaney T F, Weinstein M A 1985 Digital subtraction angiography. In: Grainger R, Allison D J (eds) Diagnostic imaging. Churchill Livingstone, Edinburgh, ch. 96, p 2099–2111

Nory S B, Wallace S, Goldman A M, Ben-Menachen Y 1974 Pyogenic liver abscess. American Journal of Roentgenology 121: 388–395

Odman P 1958 Percutaneous selective angiography of the coeliac artery. Acta Radiologica (Stockholm) (Suppl 59): 1–168

Okuda K, Musha H, Yoshida T et al 1975 Demonstration of growing casts of hepatocellular carcinoma in the portal vein by celiac angiography: The thread and streak sign. Radiology 117:303

Okuda K, Obata H, Jinnovichi S et al 1977 Angiographic assessment of gross anatomy of HCC: comparison of celiac angiograms and liver pathology in 100 cases. Radiology 123: 21–29

Orrin H C 1920 The X-ray atlas of the systemic arteries of the body. Bailliere, Tindall & Cox, London

Pantoga E 1968 Angiography in liver haemangioma. American Journal of Roentgenology 104: 874–879

Peirce E C, Ramey W P 1953 Renal arteriography: a report of a percutaneous method using the femoral artery approach and disposable catheter. Journal of Urology 69: 578–585

Pliskin M 1975 Peliosis hepatitis. Radiology: 114: 29–30

Probst R, Rysavy J A, Amplatz K 1978 Improved safety of splenoportography by plugging off the needle track. American Journal of Roentgenology 131: 445–449

Rigler L G, Olfelt P C, Krumbach R W 1953 Roentgen hepatography by injection of a contrast medium into the aorta. Radiology 60:363

Ring E J 1983 Vascular disease of the liver. In: Herlinger H, Lunderquist A, Wallace S (eds) Clinical radiology of the liver. Marcel Dekker, New York, ch 29, p 953–974

Seldinger S 1953 Catheter replacement of the needle in percutaneous arteriography. Acta Radiologica (Stockholm) 39: 368–376

Shearman D J C, Finlayson N D C 1982. Diseases of the gastrointestinal tract and liver. Churchill Livingstone, Edinburgh, P 681–701

Sones P J, Oliver T W 1984 Vascular interventional techniques in liver disease. In: Bernadrino M E, Sones R J (eds) Hepatic radiology. Macmillan, New York

Soreide O Czerniak A, Blumgart L H 1985 Large hepatocellular cancers; hepatic resection or liver transplantation? British Medical Journal 291: 853–7

Sos T A 1983 Transhepatic portal venous embolization of varices: pros and cons. Radiology 148: 569–570

Travers R L, Allison D J, Brettle R P, Hughes G R V 1979 Polyarteritis nodosa: a clinical and angiographic analysis of 17 cases. Seminars in Arthritis and Rheumatism 8: 184–198

Van Breda A, Waltman A 1984 Diagnostic hepatic angiography: Mass and diffuse disease. In: Bernardino M E, Sones P J (eds) Hepatic radiography. Macmillan, New York, p 214–242

Veiga-Pires J A, Grainger R G 1982 Pioneers in angiography. M T P Press, Lancaster

Walter J F, Bookstein J J, Bouffard E V 1976 Newer angiographic observations in cholangiocarcinoma. Radiology 118: 19–23

Whelan J G, Greech J L, Tamburro C H 1976 Angiographic and radionuclide characteristics of hepatic angiosarcoma found in vinyl chloride workers. Radiology 118: 549–557

ACKNOWLEDGEMENTS

All figures except for 6c, 6d, 15, 19, 20, 22, 23, 26, 30, 31 & 35 are reproduced with permission from Grainger R, Allison D (eds) 1986 Diagnostic radiology: A textbook of organ imaging. Churchill Livingstone, Edinburgh

22

M. S. Losowsky

Liver biopsy

INTRODUCTION

Liver biopsy is a most important diagnostic tool but indications, timing and techniques must be carefully considered. All methods of liver biopsy carry their own risks and should be employed selectively and used with other diagnostic modalities. This chapter concentrates mainly on percutaneous liver biopsy. Open surgical biopsy, laparoscopically-guided needle biopsy and aspiration cytology are referred to in detail in Ch. 23, 24, 26. Techniques, indications and contraindications are discussed and the information obtained considered in perspective in relation to other diagnostic methods.

INDICATIONS

There are several clinical situations in which liver biopsy is one of the options available in order to aid in management of the patient.

The decision as to whether liver biopsy should be undertaken is necessarily complex and subjective and will be influenced by many considerations including, e.g. the information it is hoped to gain from the biopsy, whether or not it is necessary to make a precise diagnosis, the availability of alternative diagnostic methods and the presumed risks of the procedure in that particular patient.

A common reason for considering liver biopsy is the finding of *abnormal liver function tests* either when investigating an ill patient or on screening an apparently healthy person. In the first of these situations liver function tests are often non-specific, i.e. not indicating disease of the liver or biliary system; in the second abnormal liver function tests may well be due to alcohol intake.

Hepatomegaly is a frequent indication for liver biopsy. Unless the enlargement can be attributed to a known cause, such as congestive heart failure, liver biopsy is frequently necessary. The biopsy is usually preceded by an ultrasound scan of the liver to indicate whether the hepatomegaly is due to generalized or focal disease, which require different tactics in investigation.

Liver biopsy may be performed because an *abnormality has been noted at laparotomy or on a scan*, suggesting either a focal lesion or diffuse disease of the liver. It needs to be emphasized that, if there is an indication, histology is necessary even if the liver is seen by the surgeon to be macroscopically apparently clearly normal or clearly abnormal. Gross inspection can be misleading. The cirrhotic liver may be remarkably smooth and a shrunken nodular liver may be non-cirrhotic. It is, however, necessary to be cautious in the biopsy of focal lesions of the liver demonstrated by imaging techniques such as ultrasound or CAT scanning (Ch. 25). In this situation, where the question of surgery is certain to arise, and particularly as the diagnosis is indicated with some confidence by other diagnostic tests, it is probably better to defer biopsy until the time of surgery or obtain histology on the resected specimen. In particular biopsy of evidently malignant lesions, which might be susceptible to resection, or of very vascular lesions, which may bleed and precipitate early surgery, should be avoided.

Splenomegaly is a less direct, but nevertheless relatively frequent, reason for liver biopsy. The number of causes of splenomegaly is very large and not all of them can be elucidated by liver biopsy. Liver biopsy is usually preceded by some screening investigations to exclude, at least, haematological disease and certain infections.

Jaundice is a common reason for considering liver biopsy. The first information necessary is whether the jaundice is hepatic or extrahepatic and hence whether biliary decompression is required. Initial consideration of the history, physical signs and biochemistry may strongly suggest hepatocellular disease and, together with immunological investigation, may make it clear that hepatitis, alcoholic liver disease or primary biliary cirrhosis is most likely (Ch. 13). In these circumstances liver biopsy is an early investigation, but nevertheless should ideally be preceded by ultrasonic scanning of the liver to exclude dilated intrahepatic bile ducts which may add to the risk of biopsy. If initial assessment points to extrahepatic obstruction then imaging of the biliary system by trans-hepatic or endoscopic cholangiography is the preferred early investigation (Ch. 19, 20, 25). Liver biopsy, however, can be very useful in suggesting or even confirming the diagnosis of extrahepatic obstruction of the biliary system in difficult cases (Morris et al 1975).

Oesophageal varices, indicating portal hypertension, usually discovered in the investigation of haematemesis or splenomegaly, is another common indication for liver biopsy. Although portal hypertension may be caused by prehepatic obstruction within the portal venous system, either in the splenic or the portal vein, this may be a complication of chronic liver disease and thus, even if such venous obstruction is demonstrated, liver biopsy is necessary. The initial clue to posthepatic portal hypertension, due to obstruction in or just beyond the hepatic veins, is usually provided by liver biopsy.

Liver biopsy is often used in the elucidation of *prolonged pyrexia of unknown origin*. The biopsy should be cultured for relevant organisms, including tuberculosis, as well as being sent for histology.

Liver biopsy may be used in the diagnosis of a number of *conditions of obscure aetiology* (Losowsky 1966). Thus in the diagnosis of sarcoidosis, if liver function tests are abnormal and there is no clue to other tissues which might be expected to be abnormal, the biopsy is helpful in a majority of cases. In the diagnosis of collagen diseases liver biopsy may be helpful, e.g. in polyarteritis nodosa a vasculitis may be disclosed.

Liver biopsy has been suggested as a prior investigation in patients who need long-term *methotrexate therapy* for skin disease. Since methotrexate is known to produce liver damage it may be wise to exclude prior hepatic disease.

There are several *familial diseases* in which liver biopsy is an important investigation, e.g. Gaucher's disease and glycogen storage disease are conditions in which a specific diagnosis can be made by liver biopsy. Haemochromatosis and Wilson's disease are conditions in which a specific diagnosis can be made by liver biopsy and in which investigation of members of the family of the patient may reveal sub-clinical cases which will benefit from early treatment.

TECHNIQUES

Site

The standard procedure has the patient lying supine and the needle inserted horizontally and slightly cephalad, in the mid-axillary line, at the level of maximum dullness, on the right side. The sub-costal approach may be used if the right lobe is much enlarged and the needle thus kept well away from the site of the gallbladder and major bile ducts. Other approaches, with due precautions, may be used for suspected focal abnormalities in other parts of the liver. Prior sedation is not given routinely.

Aspiration biopsy

The simplest, quickest and presumed safest procedure is aspiration biopsy. A hollow needle is inserted several centimetres into the liver and suction applied, thus retaining the core of liver tissue within the needle when it is withdrawn. The Menghini needle is almost universally used (Fig. 22.1). This is a steel needle with an external bevel. There is a pin which fits in the hub of the needle to prevent the biopsy from being sucked into the syringe. Various modifications of the needle have been described and disposable commercial versions are available, allowing suction on the syringe to be maintained without further pulling on the plunger (Fig. 22.1).

Cutting biopsy

Cutting needle biopsy involves some means of cutting off the biopsy and retaining it within the needle, thus

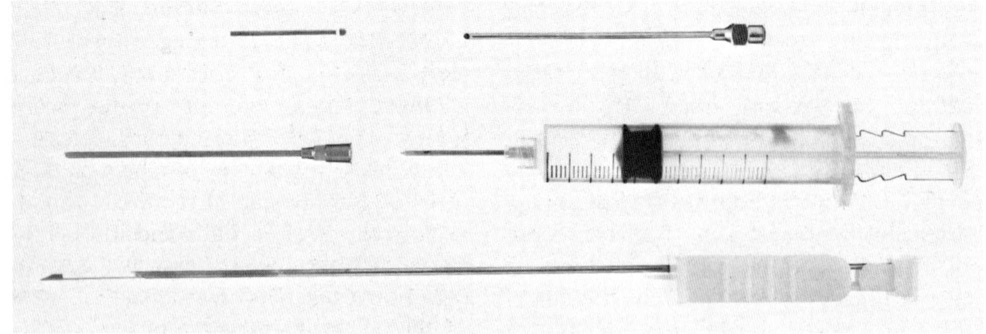

Fig. 22.1 (top) The Menghini aspiration biopsy needle. The pin, shown on the left, fits into the hub of the needle. (middle) A proprietary version of the Menghini aspiration biopsy needle. The pin is incorporated into the end of the syringe. The syringe has serrations on the plunger which can engage on a flange in the barrel thus enabling suction to be maintained without continuing to pull on the plunger. (bottom) The Tru-Cut disposable cutting biopsy needle. The internal solid trocar can be seen protruding from the end of the hollow needle. The 'bite' out of the trocar can be clearly seen

obviating the need for suction. Commonly used is the Tru-cut disposable needle (Fig. 22.1). This consists of an outer hollow needle with a plastic hub and an inner solid needle with a plastic hub. The inner needle can protrude beyond the outer needle and the protruding portion has a 'bite' removed from most of its circumference, for a length of 2 cms. The assembly is inserted into the liver with the inner needle retracted, the outer needle is then held steady and the inner needle protruded to its full extent, and the outer needle is then advanced over the inner needle cutting off the portion of liver retained within the 'bite'. The entire assembly is then withdrawn from the liver. Clearly, the number of manipulations involved means that the needle is within the liver for a longer period than with aspiration biopsy. Thus the risk of the patient breathing, coughing or moving during the procedure is greater and the risk of tearing the capsule of the liver is presumed to be greater.

Laparoscopically controlled biopsy

In some circumstances laparoscopy with direct vision of the liver can be most useful (Ch. 23). The biopsy needle may be guided directly to areas of interest and this is useful not only in obtaining biopsy of evident lesions, but also in allowing visualization and biopsy of parts of the liver thought to be normal on the basis of other investigations. Knowledge of the histological characteristics of focal lesions and of the surrounding liver tissue is often very useful in planning therapy.

Open biopsy

Laparotomy is undesirable merely as a way of obtaining biopsy material of the liver. However, where laparotomy is to be performed because of potential resectability of focal lesions, or where mini-laparotomy is indicated (Ch. 26), open biopsy may be of value and may avoid potential inaccuracies and some of the complications of closed techniques. In addition open biopsy of liver lesions encountered during operation for other conditions is mandatory, e.g. palpation of a liver nodule during surgery for excision of colorectal carcinoma demands biopsy of the nodule since simple palpation is not sufficient evidence on which to base a diagnosis of liver metastases. Liver biopsy technique is important. Surgeons should not consider it mandatory to remove a wedge of liver tissue if needle biopsy is clearly likely to be sufficient. In addition, if a wedge biopsy is taken it should not be removed from an area closely adjacent to the gallbladder bed, as a degree of fibrosis is frequently obvious in this area, but should be from some other representative site. If the liver is vascular and tends to bleed, the use of liver buffers as described by Wood et al (1976) may be helpful. If a wedge biopsy is taken it is important that a deep needle biopsy is taken also.

Other procedures

For those circumstances in which the risk of bleeding is considered too great for percutaneous needle biopsy, transvenous biopsy has been devised. The common approach is by transjugular puncture, the biopsy needle being advanced under radiological control into the vena cava and thence into the hepatic vein and into the liver parenchyma. Thus any bleeding at the puncture site will be into the vascular system.

An alternative approach to obtaining a biopsy in a patient with a bleeding diathesis is to plug the biopsy site with Gelfoam, or other haemostatic material, while withdrawing the needle (Riley et al 1984). For selected conditions, another alternative, which does not however give the same morphological information, is to use fine needle aspiration (Ch. 24).

For focal lesions within the liver, or for a liver which is shrunken and inaccessible, directed needle biopsy can be performed either under direct vision at peritoneoscopy (laparoscopy) or with scanning by ultrasound or computerized tomography (Bjork et al 1981).

Choice of technique

The Menghini procedure being simple, quick and safe is the procedure of choice for liver lesions of more or less normal consistency. An intact cylinder of good length (Fig. 22.2) can usually be obtained by an experienced operator. Aspiration biopsy of the cirrhotic liver often gives a small fragmented sample, with fibrous tissue not adequately represented (Fig. 22.3).

For a liver thought to be fibrotic or cirrhotic, cutting biopsy is preferable. By this technique the nodules, the disturbed architecture of the liver cell plates and the surrounding fibrous tissue are well represented in the specimen (Fig. 22.4).

In the diagnosis of cirrhosis of the liver, obtaining a biopsy from a selected site at peritoneoscopy, not surprisingly, improves the percentage of correct diagnoses (Pagliaro et al 1983). Comfortingly, however, blind percutaneous needle biopsy gives the correct diagnosis in over 80% of patients, avoiding the added risk, discomfort and expense of peritoneoscopy.

A comparative trial of the Tru-Cut cutting needle and the Menghini aspiration needle in a relatively small number of patients (Bateson et al 1980) disclosed no significant differences between the two for information obtained from the biopsy or for risks to the patient. The risks of either procedure are, however, sufficiently small to require a much larger series for reliable information.

Transvenous biopsy, in our experience, produces small

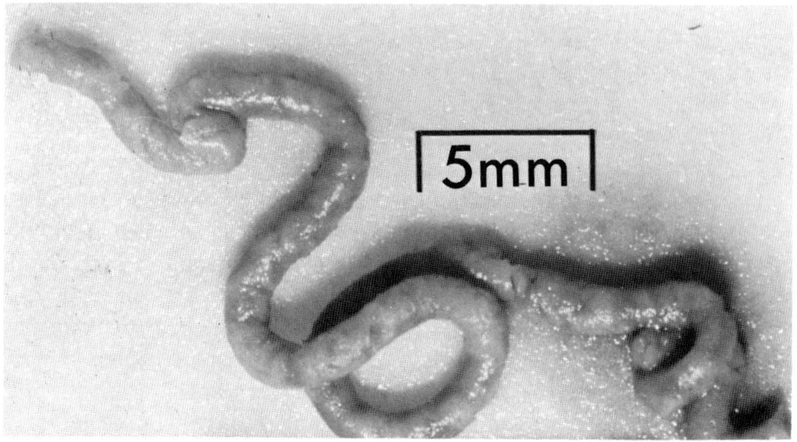

Fig. 22.2 Excellent aspiration biopsy sample obtained from a normal liver. The sample consists of a smooth cylinder, several centimetres long and unfragmented. Unfortunately the sample is mounted in a loop so that it cannot be sectioned in one plane

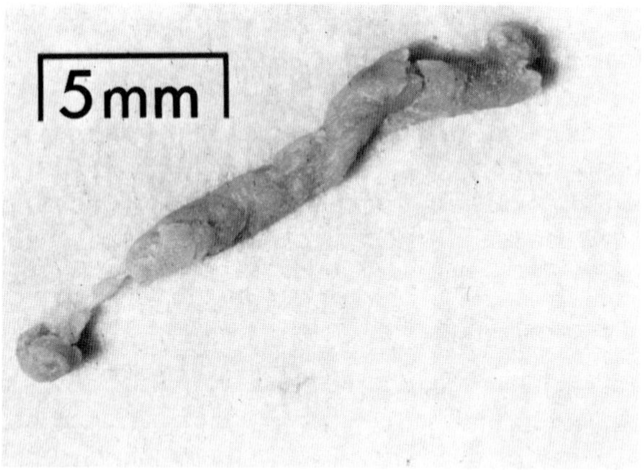

Fig. 22.3 Aspiration needle biopsy sample from a cirrhotic liver. The sample is small, irregular and fragmented. A small nodule is seen on the left and a region from which fibrous tissue has been left behind is seen just to the right of this

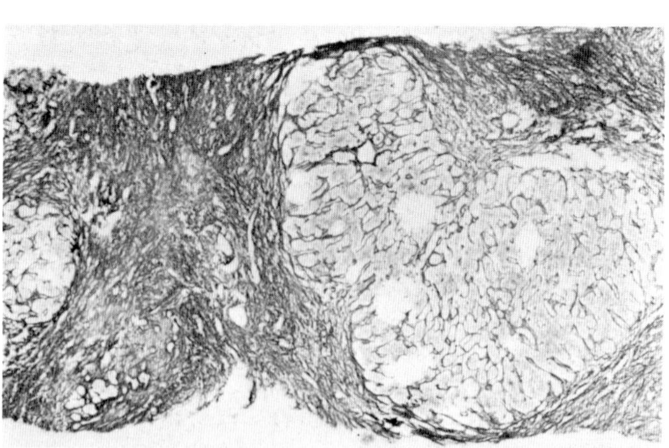

Fig. 22.4 Histological section of a cutting needle biopsy from a cirrhotic liver, stained for reticulin. Portions of nodules are clearly seen and the fibrous tissue surrounding the nodules is well represented in the section

samples often not of sufficient size for confident diagnosis. However, in almost 2000 attempts, Lebrec (1984) reported that biopsy samples large enough to allow correct evaluation of liver architecture were obtained in about two-thirds of patients with excess fibrous tissue in the liver and in virtually all those with non-fibrotic lesions. The techniques may be adapted to use a cutting needle (Bull et al 1983).

As compared with a needle biopsy, a wedge biopsy taken at operation may be more accurate in diagnosis because of the larger amount of tissue available for assessment but may also prove inaccurate in showing subcapsular artefacts and may be misleading in that there are strands of fibrous tissue which extend from the capsule and these may be misinterpreted. The surgeon should be asked to take not only a wedge biopsy but also at least one deep needle biopsy.

CONTRAINDICATIONS

Some situations pose such grave risks that they must be regarded as absolute contraindications to liver biopsy. An empyema of the pleura on the right side or an abscess in the right subphrenic space would be absolute contraindications to liver biopsy, at least by the usual route.

A most serious contraindication to needle biopsy is the likelihood that a mass within the liver is a hydatid cyst (Ch. 75). Risks of puncturing a hydatid cyst are firstly that there may be an anaphylactic reaction to the release of cyst products into the circulation and secondly that the condition may be disseminated by the procedure.

There are many other conditions which are relative contraindications to liver biopsy. For these there is, in general, little but clinical acumen and experience to guide the operator and the presumed increased risks of the procedure must be balanced against the diagnostic and therapeutic advantages. It is in some examples of this group that the alternatives of laparoscopic guided biopsy or laparotomy should be considered.

Firstly in this group a comatose, or otherwise uncooperative, patient would probably add to the risks of causing a tear in the liver capsule. The patient who is very dyspnoeic and unable to hold his breath for the two seconds which might be necessary for the procedure would be included in this category. Cholangitis is a relative contraindication to liver biopsy although sometimes in the patient with recurrent or resistant cholangitis, in whom adequate biliary drainage cannot be obtained and in whom antibiotic control has proved difficult, liver biopsy may provide a means of isolating the organisms involved and their antibiotic sensitivities.

There are a number of other conditions regarded as relative contraindications, for a variety of reasons. In the patient with gross ascites the liver will be more distant from the puncture site and may float away from the needle point. In addition any subsequent bleeding would not tamponade effectively against the parietes, would be diluted by the ascitic fluid, and would thus be more difficult to detect. In the patient with extrahepatic obstructive jaundice there is a risk of biliary peritonitis due to leakage of bile from puncture of a distended intrahepatic bile radicle under high pressure. In amyloidosis of the liver it has been suggested that the rigidity of liver substance might lead to failure of the puncture wound to seal off but, in the author's experience, this has not proved a problem. In the patient with severe anaemia, biopsy should preferably be postponed until the anaemia has been treated since the consequences of a post-biopsy bleed would be the more serious. In the congested liver, biopsy should be postponed until the congestion is relieved, if possible, since post-biopsy pain, presumably due to intrahepatic haematoma, is relatively common. One would obviously wish to avoid inserting a biopsy needle, particularly a cutting needle, into a very vascular lesion such as a haemangioma and for this reason percutaneous biopsy of mass lesions demonstrated at scanning studies must be carefully considered.

An important relative contraindication to liver biopsy is the presence of a bleeding tendency in the patient. There is, however, little evidence that this really adds to the risk of major bleeding after the procedure (Losowsky & Walker 1968, Ewe 1981). It seems likely that tearing of the liver capsule is the important cause of the very rare event of major intraperitoneal bleeding and that the risks of laboratory abnormalities of platelets or clotting factors have been over-emphasized. It is obviously prudent, nevertheless, to try to avoid liver biopsy when there is laboratory evidence of a bleeding tendency but there are occasions when it may be felt that the information to be gained outweighs the risk. It has been suggested that the source of intraperitoneal haemorrhage after liver biopsy is usually a small artery within the liver (Hegarty & Williams 1984) although it may sometimes, perhaps, be a portal vein branch.

PRECAUTIONS

The risk of infection to the operator must be borne in mind when undertaking liver biopsy in a patient with acute or chronic liver disease which may be caused by viruses. Hepatitis B is the important recognizable risk at the moment. It is possible, however, that the non-A non-B hepatitis viruses may be responsible for many cases of acute and chronic liver disease and such viruses cannot, at present, be detected by any laboratory test.

The patient should be asked if there is any known allergy to any of the agents used in performing the biopsy, e.g. the antiseptic used for skin sterilization or the local anaesthetic.

Biopsy should, of course, be undertaken only by a trained operator and only in the knowledge that there is available skilled interpretation of the histological sections.

Ideally biopsy should be undertaken only when there is easy access to blood transfusion and to skilled surgery, should these become necessary. Some operators require the patient's blood group to be known prior to biopsy. Some operators cross-match two pints of blood before the biopsy but it is not author's practice to do this.

Interference with bleeding and clotting function is very common in patients with liver disease and precautions must be taken to minimize the associated risks due to liver biopsy. For practical purposes the only pre-biopsy investigations which are usually undertaken are estimations of the prothrombin time and platelet count. A platelet count of 80 000 per mm^3 or more and a prothrombin time of 3 seconds or less above control are usually regarded as adequate. Intramuscular vitamin K may be given to attempt to improve the prothrombin time, and should be given in any case to jaundiced patients, although in severe liver disease this will usually not be of benefit. The platelet count often fluctuates from day to day and if there is no urgency to obtain the biopsy then it may be possible to wait until the platelet count is at a satisfactory level. If platelet count and/or prothrombin time remain abnormal, then other measures may be used. For example, if it is thought that the patient may have chronic active hepatitis, a short course of steroids may improve liver function without affecting the diagnostic value obtained from the biopsy. Infusions of platelets or clotting factors may be used, but there are no controlled trials to show that mortality or morbidity from liver biopsy is affected by such manoeuvres. Indeed, in view of the low mortality and morbidity, it would be extremely difficult to design a practicable trial to establish this point. Measures (transvenous biopsy, plugging of the needle track) which can be used to obtain a liver biopsy in the presence of abnormal bleeding or clotting function are referred to above. In addition to estimation of platelet count and prothrombin time it may be prudent to study platelet function if there is any reason to suspect that this will be abnormal even though the platelet count is normal. Such circumstances would include, e.g. the presence of a primary haematological disease, a dysproteinaemia or the administration of aspirin or other drugs which are known to affect platelet function.

Bacteraemia is probably quite common after liver biopsy (McCloskey et al 1973) and it would be prudent to give prophylactic antibiotics to patients with known congenital cardiac abnormalities or heart valve lesions.

If there is any question of cholangitis then it is wise to cover the procedure with broad spectrum antibiotics unless one of the objects is to obtain material for microbiological assessment. In this case antibiotics are started immediately after the procedure.

After the biopsy the patient is instructed to lie on the right side (if the biopsy was performed in the conventional manner with a lateral approach) for one hour and then to lie flat, on the back or side as preferred, until the end of twelve hours. The patient must be monitored so that any complications will be rapidly detected and can be dealt with appropriately. It is the author's practice to ask for pulse and blood pressure to be charted hourly for twelve hours, for the patient to be asked about pain, and for the medical staff to be informed if there is anything more than minor change. If there is a change in pulse or blood pressure the abdomen is examined for tenderness and guarding to detect significant leakage of blood or bile. The signs are those of peritoneal irritation, commencing in the right hypochondrium, tracking to the right iliac fossa and eventually causing generalized peritonitis. These signs develop slowly, over the space of a few hours. The key to successful management is frequent examination of the patient, the abdomen and the pulse and blood pressure charts. This should be done initially at least every half-hour once symptoms start to develop and surgical intervention should be undertaken before shock and general peritonitis supervene.

It is usual to perform needle biopsy of the liver as an inpatient and to keep the patient in bed for 24 hours after the procedure. Some recent studies, however, have shown that it is possible to perform the procedure on outpatients with safety if recommended precautions (observation for six hours, hospitalization if pain or hypotension develop) are followed and facilities for retention of the patient in hospital or urgent re-admission are available, if needed (Westaby et al 1980). Liver biopsy can be performed in patients with diseases primarily affecting clotting factors, if these can be corrected prior to the procedure. This has been well demonstrated in patients with haemophilia (Preston et al 1978).

UNTOWARD EFFECTS AND RISKS

In specialized units, complications are extremely rare after needle biopsy of the liver (Perrault et al 1978, Sherlock et al 1984). Collected experiences do, however, show a wide range of rare complications (Lindner 1966).

Death after liver biopsy is variously recorded as 1 in 600 to 1 in 7800. The incidence presumably depends upon the disease being investigated and the skill of the operator. The risks in patients with specific conditions such as extrahepatic obstructive jaundice and vascular focal lesions have been incompletely documented.

The most important risks of liver biopsy are those of significant leakage of blood or bile into the peritoneal cavity. It is presumed that the risks of major intraperitoneal bleeding are increased by impaired clotting function, an uncooperative patient or a focal vascular lesion. The risks of intraperitoneal bile leakage are increased by distended intrahepatic bile ducts secondary to extrahepatic biliary obstruction. Statistics to substantiate these beliefs, however, are not available.

Local pain is common in the first hours after needle biopsy. This presumably results from peritoneal irritation because a small amount of blood and bile leaks into the peritoneal cavity. Continuing pain, especially if spreading in the abdominal cavity and particularly if accompanied by shoulder tip pain, is of significance. Medical and nursing staff should be aware of this and be alerted to the possibility of a significant complication.

It is not unusual for there to be minor tenderness over the site of the biopsy, sometimes tracking down the paracolic gutter towards the right iliac fossa. It is rare that the pain is severe and rare that analgesics are required. Major analgesics should be avoided since they might mask the physical signs of important intraperitoneal bleeding or bile leakage. More prolonged, constant but not very severe, pain occasionally arises, particularly after biopsy of the congested liver. The pain may be due to a haematoma being located subcapsularly. Minor analgesics usually suffice and the pain subsides in a few days. Asymptomatic intrahepatic haematoma is probably not rare in apparently uncomplicated biopsy (Raines et al 1974). Delayed rupture of an intrahepatic haematoma has been reported (Reichert et al 1983).

In very rare cases the patient may show an acute hypotensive episode with bradycardia, on puncture of the peritoneum. An analogy with 'pleural shock' may be drawn. The origin is presumably vagal and, while atropine may be given, the condition recovers spontaneously within a very few minutes.

Since the conventional site for liver biopsy involves the needle traversing the pleura there is a theoretical risk of bleeding into the pleura or of pneumothorax. It must be excessively rare for either of these to be severe enough to be of clinical importance.

A further risk, largely theoretical, is the possibility of puncture of other organs with the liver biopsy needle. Organs which might be involved are the colon and the gallbladder. Presumably such an accident might occur particularly if the liver were very small or in an unusual position, if there were a loop of colon interposed between the lateral surface of the liver and the diaphragm or if there were an intrahepatic gallbladder. Such perforation may be followed by spontaneous sealing but slow leakage may be followed by peritonitis. Leakage of even large quantities of sterile bile may pass undetected with remarkably few physical signs for many hours.

Other complications described after liver biopsy include fracture of the needle (with a fragment remaining in the liver) and haemobilia, due to concurrent puncture of a vessel and bile duct (Lee et al 1977). Haemobilia can be suspected by the triad of abdominal colic, jaundice and gastrointestinal bleeding, and can be diagnosed by endoscopic observation of blood issuing from the papilla of Vater (Howdle et al 1976) or by selective hepatic angiography (Kelley et al 1983) (Ch. 21, 85). It is best treated by radiological embolization of the small vessels involved (Fagan et al 1980) but this is not always successful and operative intervention may be necessary (Fig. 22.5). Arteriovenous aneurysm within the liver is probably not uncommon but is almost always asymptomatic and probably transient (Okuda et al 1978). As a clinical problem it is an extremely rare complication of needle biopsy. If therapy is required, management here too would be by radiological embolization of the artery. Pulmonary bile embolism and septicaemia occur as exceedingly rare complications of liver biopsy.

Tumour seeding along the track of the biopsy needle is a theoretical risk but not well documented. Very large numbers of patients with primary or metastatic disease of the liver have been subjected to needle biopsy without this complication being recorded.

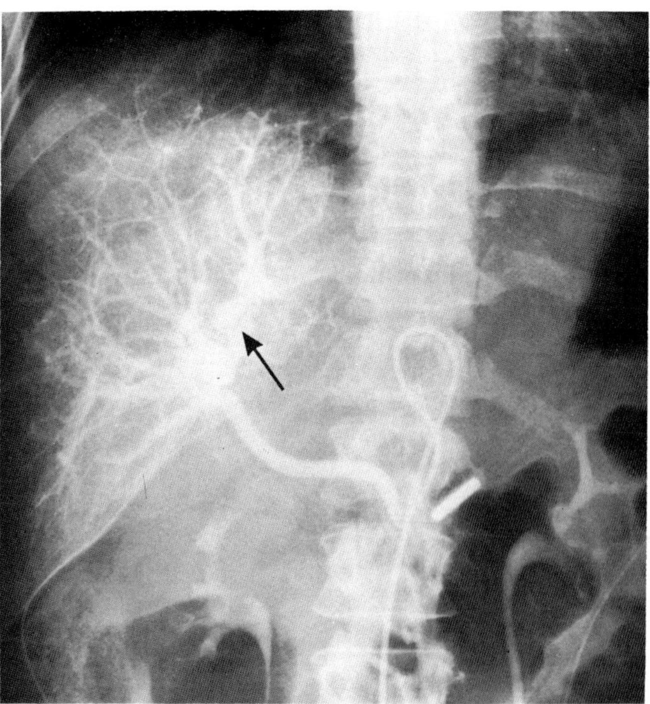

Fig. 22.5 Hepatic arteriography reveals intrahepatic arterial aneurysm (arrow) at the site of a percutaneous transhepatic liver biopsy performed two weeks previously. The patient, a 28-year-old woman who was asymptomatic, had a solitary defect demonstrated in the right lobe of the liver at CT scanning performed as part of a screening programme. The liver biopsy revealed normal liver tissue and a portion of the walls of an artery and vein. Two weeks after liver biopsy the patient presented with massive exsanguinating haematemesis as a consequence of haemobilia. The arteriogram shows a major right hepatic arterial trunk arising from the superior mesenteric artery. A previous attempt at embolization had failed to occlude the vessel and further embolization was impossible. Continued bleeding necessitated urgent operation, at which control was achieved through a right liver resection. Histology of the resected specimen revealed the original pathology to be an area of fibro-nodular hyperplasia

INFORMATION OBTAINED

The usual reason for liver biopsy is to obtain *histological information*. Macroscopic inspection may indicate particular areas of interest and these should be pointed out to the pathologist (Fig. 22.6). The fluid aspirate obtained when using the Menghini needle may be sent for cytology. A portion of the biopsy sample may be used for *metal analysis*, particularly iron and copper when there is suspicion of haemochromatosis or Wilson's disease respectively. Histology is, however, the first priority particularly in the first of these conditions and only if the sample is adequate is a portion also sent for metal analysis. A biopsy sample may be sent for *enzyme analysis* in the diagnosis of rare metabolic conditions such as glycogen storage disease or Hurler's syndrome (Lundquist & Ockerman 1970). In

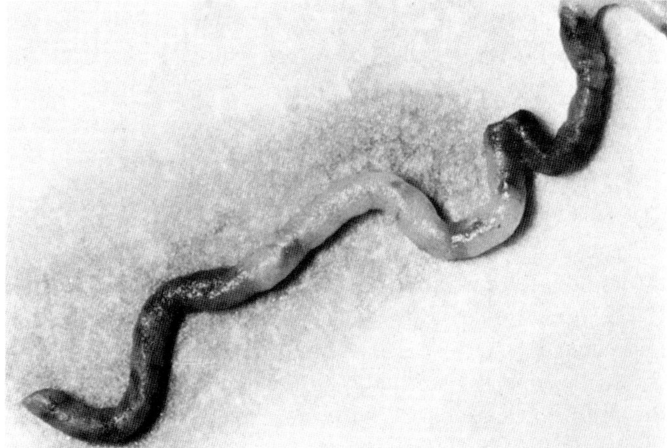

Fig. 22.6 Aspiration needle biopsy from a liver containing metastatic carcinoma. The darker portions are normal liver, the paler portions are tumour. If only a small portion of the sample looks abnormal it is important to point this out to the pathologist to ensure that it is represented in the sections reviewed

some patients with resistant cholangitis, the major reason for liver biopsy may be to obtain *microbiological information* both of the organisms concerned and of their sensitivity to antibiotics. A portion of a liver biopsy may be fixed for *electron microscopy*. Although of help in certain rare circumstances, it must be said that electron microscopy has not found a place in routine diagnosis of liver disease comparable, e.g. with its place in renal disease.

For the best results a needle biopsy must be of adequate size. Two cm is a good biopsy, 1 cm is often sufficient for diagnosis. Diagnostic information is much improved if the biopsy is not fragmented. Fragmentation may be unavoidable with a suction needle in a fibrotic liver. Fragmentation can be minimized by careful expulsion of the sample from a suction needle or gentle removal from a cutting needle. The sample should be transferred directly to a surface, such as a piece of blotting paper, to support it and avoid it breaking up. Diagnosis depends to a large extent on having adequate portal tract material within the biopsy, which, provided the sample is of adequate size, is fortuitous. Diagnostic information is much improved if multiple layers are examined and if the sample can be sectioned throughout its length and this is ensured if the sample is fixed in one plane, which is accomplished, as mentioned above, by placing it on a surface to which it adheres.

In order to obtain the maximum information to aid in the management of the patient, rather more is required than just diagnosis. In certain conditions the histologist can suggest not only the diagnosis but the aetiology, the stage of the disease, the activity of disease and the presence of certain complications. For example, with a diagnosis of cirrhosis (Scheuer 1970), histology may be expected to help to decide the aetiology as between alcohol, chronic active hepatitis, primary biliary cirrhosis, secondary biliary cirrhosis, haemochromatosis or other conditions. It should be possible for the histologist to pronounce on the activity of the cirrhosis as indicated by on-going piecemeal necrosis of liver cells and the indications of recent formation of fibrous tissue. The report may also indicate the stage of the cirrhosis, in that early cirrhosis will be manifest by relatively minor distortion of the architecture and relatively little fibrous tissue. Certain complications of the cirrhosis, such as biliary obstruction (gallstones are commoner in chronic liver disease than in the general population) or a supervening hepatocellular carcinoma, may be suspected or confidently diagnosed from the biopsy.

The limitations of diagnosis by liver biopsy must be appreciated. There are, of course, errors in interpretation, which become less with the experience of the pathologist but are never eliminated. Sampling error is additional, and the magnitude of this disputed. For example in addressing the single problem of presence or absence of cirrhosis (Scheuer 1970) different studies suggest that the error may be as small as a few per cent or as large as more than 50%. This varies with the type of cirrhosis: the missed diagnosis in macronodular cirrhosis is a well-known and not uncommon problem, while there is less of a problem in the early stages of alcoholic cirrhosis or chronic active hepatitis with cirrhosis. Sampling error is considered to be very small in viral hepatitis, particularly if severe (Soloway et al 1971). This applies to alcholic hepatitis too (Abdi et al 1979). A particular example of sampling error is the relative lack of fibrous tissue obtained using a suction needle as compared with the sample obtained by a cutting needle. Interpretation is improved by provision of all the clinical information to the pathologist so that he can then direct particular attention to, e.g. evidence of the effects of alcohol or specialized stains for rare conditions.

Certain diagnoses can only be obtained histologically. For example granulomatous hepatitis, which has a vast list of causes, is entirely a histological diagnosis pointing the way for further diagnostic efforts. It has recently been suggested that primary biliary cirrhosis, as it presents clinically, is the tip of an iceberg for a large number of asymptomatic patients who can only be diagnosed histologically.

Diagnosis is not the only point which leads to clinical benefit. Biopsies can be used to assess *prognosis* in e.g. acute hepatitis, alcoholism, lymphoma or cirrhosis. Biopsies can be used to assess *progress* in, e.g. chronic active hepatitis under treatment, haemochromatosis under treatment or acute hepatitis.

While clinical benefit to the individual patient is the only acceptable reason for undertaking liver biopsy in man, liver biopsies may also provide *epidemiological information* and may also be of use in other research avenues in aiding understanding of the *pathogenesis of diseases* or in *clinical trials* to evaluate different forms of therapy.

PERSPECTIVE

Needle biopsy is usually required in the management of 'medical' disease of the liver unless it is short-lived and self-limited.

In focal disease of the liver, in which the question of surgery must arise, needle biopsy of the liver is often required as part of the initial diagnostic process. There are, however, certain exceptions to this. Arteriography may make it clear that the lesion is malignant and there may be other indications of malignancy, e.g. a grossly elevated alpha foetoprotein level. If there is no indication of non-resectability, at angiography or computerized tomographic scanning, histology may well be postponed until the surgical specimen is available, particularly for highly vascular lesions. Haemangioma of the liver is a common, benign, focal lesion. Because it is common it is not infrequently found as a coincidental lesion in patients investigated for other conditions. Needle biopsy of haemangioma is rarely diagnostic, providing some liver tissue and some endothelial tissue which do not allow correct interpretation. Arteriography, or computerized tomography with contrast enhancement, gives much more characteristic findings but also may not be definitive.

Thus the presumed nature of the lesion in the liver, the natural history of liver disease, the alternative diagnostic facilities available and the therapeutic programme for the patient must all be taken into account in deciding whether, when and how needle biopsy of the liver should be performed.

REFERENCES

Abdi W, Millan J C, Mezey E 1979 Sampling variability on percutaneous liver biopsy. Archives of Internal Medicine 139: 667–669

Bateson M C, Hopwood D, Duguid H L D, Bouchier I A 1980 A comparative trial of liver biopsy needles. Journal of Clinical Pathology 33: 131–133

Bjork J T, Foly W D, Varma R R 1981 Percutaneous liver biopsy in difficult cases simplified by CT or ultrasonic localization. Digestive Diseases and Sciences 26: 146–148

Bull H J M, Gilmore I T, Bradley R D, Marigold J H, Thompson R P H 1983 Experience with transjugular liver biopsy. Gut 24: 1057–1060

Ewe K 1981 Bleeding after liver biopsy does not correlate with indices of peripheral coagulation. Digestive Diseases and Sciences 26: 388–393

Fagan E A, Allison D J, Chadwick V S, Hodgson H J F 1980 Treatment of haemobilia by selective arterial embolisation. Gut 21: 541–544

Hegarty J E, Williams R 1984 Liver biopsy: techniques, clinical applications, and complications. British Medical Journal 288: 1254–1256

Howdle P D, Miloszewski K J A, Glanville J N, Losowsky M S 1976 Diagnosis of biliary tract hemorrhage (hemobilia) by endoscopy. Gastrointestinal Endoscopy 23: 94–96

Kelley C J, Hemingway A, McPherson G A D, Allison D J, Blumgart L H 1983 Non-surgical management of post-cholecystectomy haemobilia. British Journal of Surgery 70: 502–504

Lebrec D 1984 Le ponction-biopsie hepatique transveineuse par voie jugulaire. Editorial. La Presse Medicale 13: 1605–1606

Lee S P, Tasman-Jones C, Wattie W J 1977 Traumatic hemobilia: A complication of percutaneous liver biopsy. Gastroenterology 72: 941–944

Lindner H 1966 Limitations and dangers in percutaneous liver biopsies with the Menghini needle. Proceedings of the First Congress of the International Society of Endoscopy: 446–448

Losowsky M S 1966 Liver biopsy in conditions other than primary liver disease. Journal of the Indian Medical Profession 13: 5707–5711

Losowsky M S, Walker B E 1968 Liver biopsy and splenoportography in patients with thrombocytopenia. Gastroenterology 54: 241–245

Lundquist A, Ockerman P A 1970 Fine-needle aspiration biopsy of human liver for enzymatic diagnosis of glycogen storage disease and gargoylism. Acta Paediatrica Scandinavica 59: 293–296

McCloskey R V, Gold M, Weser E 1973 Bacteremia after liver biopsy. Archives of Internal Medicine 132: 213–215

Morris J S, Gallo G A, Scheuer P J, Sherlock S 1975 Percutaneous liver biopsy in patients with large bile duct obstruction. Gastroenterology 68: 750–754

Okuda K et al 1978 Frequency of intrahepatic arteriovenous fistula as a sequela to percutaneous needle puncture of the liver. Gastroenterology 74: 1204–1207

Pagliaro L et al 1983 Percutaneous blind biopsy versus laparoscopy with guided biopsy in diagnosis of cirrhosis. Digestive Diseases and Sciences 28: 39–43

Perrault J, McGill D B, Ott B J, Taylor W F 1978 Liver biopsy: complications in 1000 inpatients and outpatients. Gastroenterology 74: 103–106

Preston F E et al 1978 Percutaneous liver biopsy and chronic liver disease in haemophiliacs. Lancet ii: 592–594

Raines D R, Van Heertum R L, Johnson L F 1974 Intrahepatic hematoma: a complication of percutaneous liver biopsy. Gastroenterology 67: 284–289

Reichert C M, Weisenthal L M, Klein H G 1983 Delayed haemorrhage after percutaneous liver biopsy. Journal of Clinical Gastroenterology 5:263

Riley S A, Ellis W R, Irving H C, Lintott D J, Axon A T R, Losowsky M S 1984 Percutaneous liver biopsy with plugging of needle track: A safe method for use in patients with impaired coagulation. Lancet II:436

Scheuer P J 1970 Liver biopsy in the diagnosis of cirrhosis. Gut 11: 275–278

Sherlock S, Dick R, Van Leeuwen D J 1984 The Royal Free Hospital Experience Journal of Hepatology 1: 75–85

Soloway R D, Baggenstoss A H, Schoenfield L J, Summerskill W H J 1971 Observer error and sampling variability tested.in evaluation of hepatitis and cirrhosis by liver biopsy. Digestive Diseases 16: 1082–1086

Westaby D, MacDougall B R D, Williams R 1980 Liver biopsy as a day-case procedure: selection and complications in 200 consecutive patients. British Medical Journal 281: 1331–1332

Wood C B, Capperauld I, Blumgart L H 1976 Bioplast fibrin buttons for liver biopsy and partial hepatic resection. Annals of the Royal College of Surgeons of England 58: 401–404

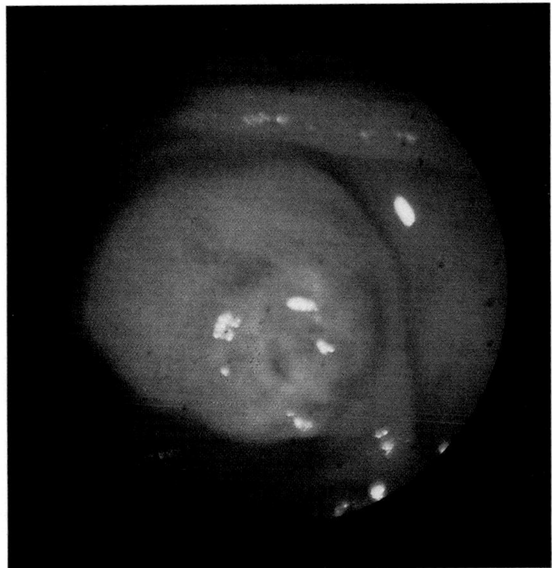

Plate 20.1 Incarcerated papillary stone causing distension of the papilla

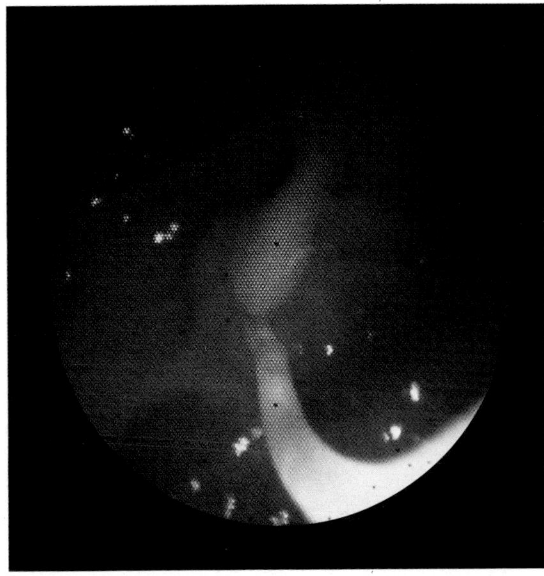

Plate 20.2 Biliodigestive anastomosis

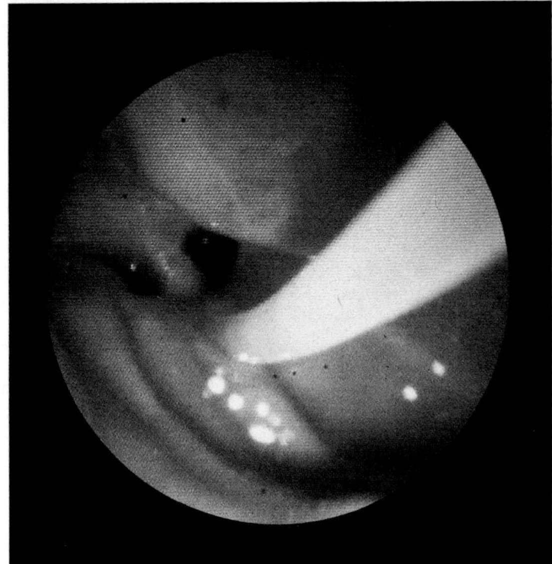

Plate 20.3 Obstruction cholangitis (choledocholithiasis) presenting with purulent outflow through the papilla

Overleaf

Plate 23.A Macronodular cirrhosis

Plate 23.B Tuberculous peritonitis. Note whitish discrete nodules on the parietal peritoneum of the anterior abdominal wall

Plate 23.C Dense adhesions with small collaterals in a patient with portal hypertension

Plate 23.D Hepatocellular carcinoma in a patient with hepatitis B viral cirrhosis. Note the macronodules and the morphology of the carcinoma on the hepatic surface adjacent to the gallbladder fossa

Plate 23.E Metastatic carcinoma from a gallbladder primary. Note the umbilication of the lesion in the foreground. Reproduced with permission from Professor A. D. Jorge

Plate 23.F Micronodular cirrhosis of alcoholic aetiology

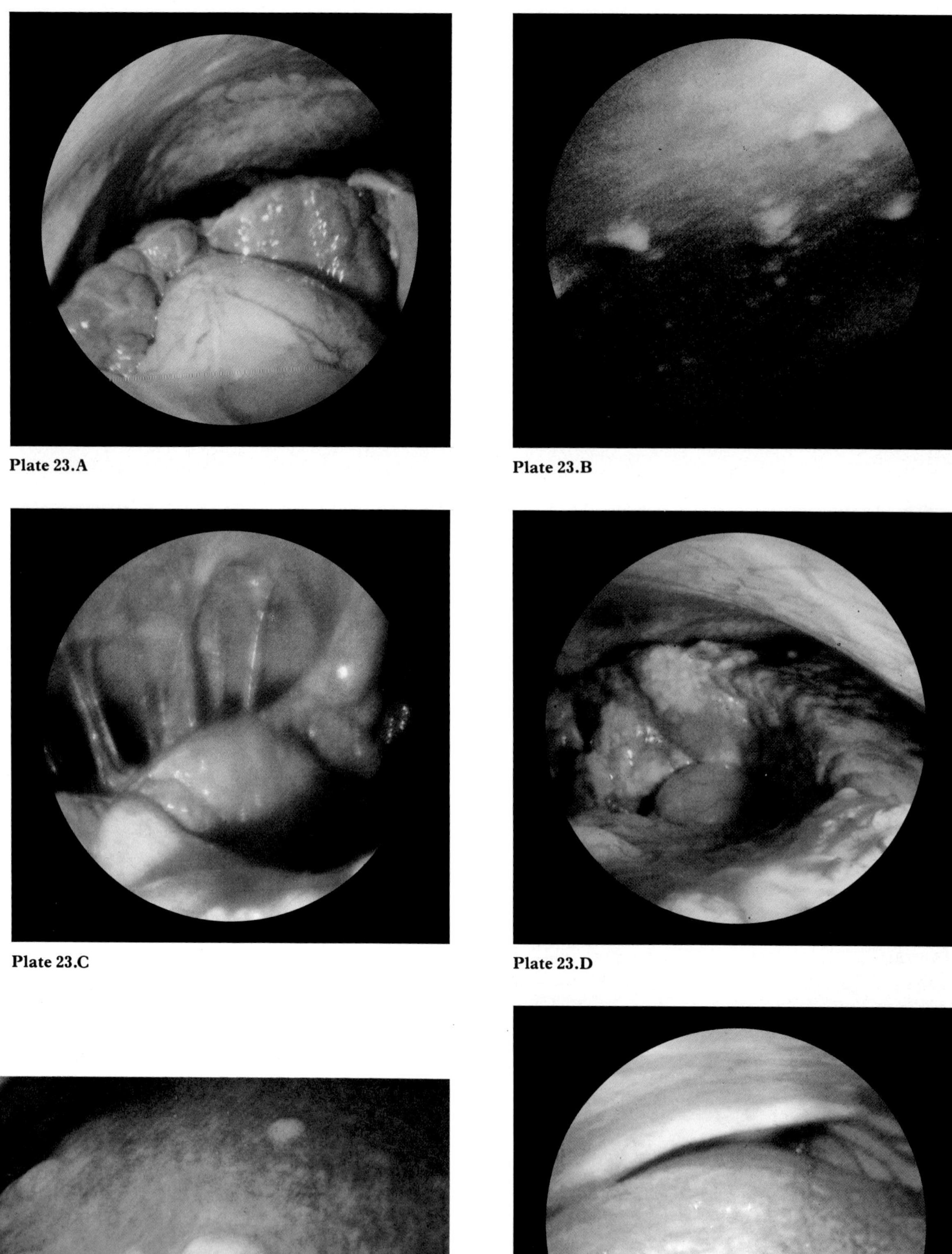

Plate 23.A

Plate 23.B

Plate 23.C

Plate 23.D

Plate 23.E

Plate 23.F

23

J. Korula, T. B. Reynolds

Laparoscopy

INTRODUCTION

Laparoscopy (or peritoneoscopy or celioscopy) refers to an examination of the peritoneal cavity and intra-abdominal organs through an endoscope. Although Ott (1901) introduced the concept when he examined the abdominal cavity through a speculum using a head mirror, Jacobaeus (1910) is credited with the pioneering examination of the peritoneal cavity in humans in 1910 using a cystoscope and with coining the term 'laparoscopy'. Interest in this procedure waxed and waned since then but was largely confined to Europe, where refinements in technique and instruments were developed during periods of enthusiasm. Kalk (1955, 1961) made significant contributions during this period, the most notable of which was the design of a laparoscope which is the basis of those used today. Though Ruddock (1934) reported on the usefulness of laparoscopy in the diagnosis of liver and peritoneal diseases at the Los Angeles General Hospital in 1934, the procedure did not gain much popularity in the United States until gynaecologists recognized its value in the diagnosis and treatment of gynaecological disorders. Having demonstrated its safety in gynaecology, they rekindled interest among hepatologists in the diagnosis of liver and peritoneal diseases. Surgeons followed, using it primarily in the preoperative evaluation of abdominal pain (Cortesi et al 1979, Sugarbaker et al 1975), following trauma (Sherwood et al 1980) or for assessment of operability (Hall et al 1980).

The evolution of non-invasive imaging techniques and the ability to obtain directed biopsies of focal lesions using this modality has resulted in a decrease in the frequency of the use of laparoscopy (Sanowski et al 1984). However, laparoscopy is still used in conditions where diagnosis depends on both visualization and biopsy of lesions.

Reviews and monographs by Kalk & Wildhirt (1961) and Wittman (1966) give an excellent detailed account of the procedure. Morphology of various disease states is effectively depicted in the colour atlases by Beck & Schaeffer (1970) and Wittman (1966); the atlas by Bruguera et al (1979) combines histopathology with the endoscopic appearances of most liver diseases.

TECHNIQUES

As with any endoscopic procedure, a thorough knowledge of the instrument and its capabilities is essential to the successful performance of laparoscopy. The instruments should be cleaned by a technician familiar with the procedure. Endoscopic transmission of hepatitis B is a rare but real problem (Birnie et al 1983) and consequently, our instruments are sterilized using ethylene oxide gas at 85°C for four hours and aerated at room temperature for 48 hours; soaking the instruments in 2% alkalinized glutaraldehyde for 10 hours, though equally effective (Bond et al 1977), may result in damage to the instruments.

Instrumentation

Veress needle. The Veress needle is an automatic needle with a spring action that combines an outer sharp point and an inner dull stylet; the former is useful for penetration of the skin, deep fascia and peritoneum. The hub of the needle contains a spring to allow the inner cannula to retract during insertion through the abdominal fascia. The blunt inner stylet springs forward with a click when the peritoneal cavity is entered. This needle was designed to reduce the possibility of perforation of a viscus and is used during development of a pneumoperitoneum.

Trocar and sleeve. These instruments are inserted into the abdomen after a succcesful pneumoperitoneum. The sleeve will ultimately house the laparoscope and is usually 1 mm greater in diameter than the trocar or laparoscope. The tip of the trocar may be conical or pyramidal; the former allows a rotary motion to aid in penetration while the latter facilitates cutting of tissue without rotary movement. Sleeves made of fibreglass are desirable in procedures where cautery is used, as electrical conductivity is reduced.

Laparoscope. The laparoscope is an indirect view type

containing optical elements that provide the operator with wide-angle view under magnification. A fibreoptic cable transmits light from an outside power source to the telescope; the latter contains fibreglass filaments which further transmit light to the distal end of the instrument. The amount of light and size of the image is directly proportional to the size of the telescope; recently, refinement in the optics has made available smaller instruments with good visibility. Telescopes are either forward viewing with an arc of 70° or forward oblique viewing with an arc of 135°. The fore-oblique gives a wider field of vision but there is greater distortion of the image at the edge of the field. Two basic types of laparoscopes are available: the diagnostic laparoscope which is used only for viewing and requires a second puncture with trocar and sleeve to facilitate passage of instruments (referred to as a two-hole or two-puncture technique); and the operative laparoscope which contains a separate channel within the scope to facilitate the passage of instruments. We frequently use the fore-oblique diagnostic laparoscope and obtain liver and peritoneal biopsies using a two-hole technique. A number of laparoscopes are available and the reader may refer to the monographs where lists of instruments and their manufacturers are available.

Light source and cables. A light source of 150 watts is required for diagnostic laparoscopy and special 1000 watt sources are available for photography.

Insufflation and type of gas

Three gases are used to achieve pneumoperitoneum. Room air was the first to be used, is readily available and simple to use. Reports of air embolism, pneumomediastinum and pneumopericardium complicating the use of room air spurred the search for an optimal gas. Both carbon dioxide (CO_2) and nitrous oxide (N_2O) need special devices that determine the rate of flow of gas and monitor the intraperitoneal pressure achieved during pneumoperitoneum. CO_2 has the advantage of being rapidly absorbed and non-combustible and would be the preferred gas if electrocautery is contemplated. However, CO_2 produces more discomfort, perhaps due to its irritant effect on the peritoneum (Sharp et al 1982, Minoli et al 1982) and the hypercarbia that predictably follows its use (El-Minawi et al 1981) may potentiate cardiac tachyarrythmias (Scott & Julian 1972); consequently, careful monitoring of cardiac activity, ventilation, acid base and blood gases is helpful and the procedure is frequently performed under general anaesthesia. Absorption of N_2O, though slower than that of CO_2, is sufficiently rapid to be well tolerated; no abnormality of cardiac rhythm, ventilation, acid base or blood gases has been observed. The combustion potential is greater than that of CO_2, and consequently it is less preferable if electrocautery is needed. The optimal rate of gas flow is one litre per minute, the volume of gas introduced is 3–4 l and the pressure achieved should range between 10–15 mmHg (Cali 1980). We use room air insufflated with a sterile sphygmomanometer bulb attached to the Veress needle. The experience at the USC Liver Unit between 1962 and 1984 using this technique demonstrates that it is a satisfactory gas for laparoscopy. We have not found post laparoscopic abdominal pain a problem probably because an attempt is made to evacuate as much of the insufflated air as possible at the conclusion of the procedure.

Technique of laparoscopy

Gynaecological laparoscopy often involves surgical manipulations through the endoscope, so it is usually performed in the operating theatre under general anaesthesia. Medical laparoscopy, on the other hand rarely causes severe pain so general anaesthesia is not required.

There is a great deal of variation in the technique of performance of laparoscopy in different centres. Some use a surgical theatre and others a procedure room or endoscopy suite. In some centres, the physicians perform a surgical scrub and wear a cap, mask and gown while in other centres sterility precautions are limited to sterile gloves and a sterile cellophane sleeve covering the laparoscope (Gips, personal communication). Some hepatologists prefer the patient to have a short acting general anaesthetic (Michel & Raynaud 1977), while others use only local anaesthesia and nitrous oxide gas without premedication (Gips, personal communication). Since the optimal technique for the performance of laparoscopy has never been established, we will simply describe our method of performing the procedure which has evolved over a 25-year period.

The procedure is performed only after obtaining informed consent which outlines the indications and the risks involved. The patient is kept fasting overnight and brought to the endoscopy room on the following morning after voiding urine to ensure an empty urinary bladder. An intravenous line is placed, preferably in the mid forearm, to allow for some movements at the wrists and elbows. The size of the intravenous needle is adequate for rapid infusion of blood or blood products in the event of a bleeding complication. Vital signs (blood pressure, heart rate and respiratory rate) are recorded at the commencement and again at the conclusion of the procedure. During the procedure the heart rate is monitored using a cardiac monitor. For premedication we use a combination of meperidine and diazepam; the former is used predominantly in patients with prior encephalopathy as its effects can be reversed with naloxone. The initial premedication dose is a small one and is titrated to achieve only a mild somnolence because patient co-operation is helpful during insertion of the Veress needle and trocar. After insertion of the trocar, further premedication may be given. Care is taken however to ensure that excessive sedation is avoided in patients with liver disease.

Procedure

The patient is placed supine on and strapped to the examining table which has capability for Trendelenburg, reverse Trendelenburg, right and left lateral tilting positions. The strapping is necessary to ensure that the patient does not slide off the table during position manoeuvres. The abdomen and right upper quadrant (if liver biopsy by a two-hole technique is required) is prepared as for an intra-abdominal surgical procedure using 10% povidone-iodine solution. The abdomen is draped in standard fashion. The operators wear surgical attire and scrub as for any surgical procedure.

Technique

An optimal site is chosen prior to infiltration of local anaesthesia; an infraumbilical midline site is frequently chosen because it avoids the peritoneal collaterals in patients with portal hypertension and because the linea alba is relatively avascular at this site (Fig. 23.1). In patients with liver disease and portal hypertension, the falciform ligament (hatched area Fig. 23.1) may contain collateral vessels or a large paraumbilical vein. Entry at this site with either the Veress needle or trocar could result in laceration of these large vessels and should be avoided. However, if the liver is impalpable, or is small as evident on scan or if a lesion near the superior aspect of the liver is suspected and cannot be reached by an infra-umbilical approach, a site 2–4 cm above the umbilicus and to the left of the midline is chosen. The skin and subcutaneous tissues are infiltrated with 1% lignocaine. A transverse incision is made that is slightly wider than the trocar sleeve. Dissection of the subcutaneous tissue is made with a curved haemostat to the linea alba or the posterior rectus sheath. Bleeding from superficial vessels usually does not require ligature since tamponade from the laparoscope trocar results in haemostasis. At this point, an attempt is made to infiltrate the parietal peritoneum with local anaesthetic. The Veress needle is then held between the thumb and forefinger of the operator's hand, about 2 cm from its distal tip (Fig. 23.2) and is inserted into the abdomen in a direction perpendicular to the skin surface with a quick thrust till a click is heard as the inner blunt cannula springs forward; this indicates that the peritoneal cavity has been entered. The patient is asked to raise the abdominal wall towards the ceiling during this insertion to prevent injury to the retroperitoneal vessels and consequently should not be too sedated at the time of insertion.

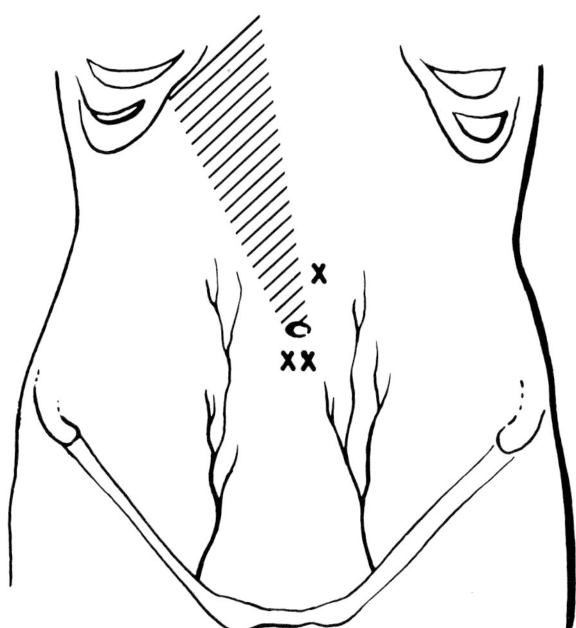

Fig. 23.1 Schematic diagram of the abdomen. Hatched area depicts location of collaterals. x indicates the optimal entry sites. Reproduced with modification from Boyce H W 1982 Diseases of the Liver, V edn. Lippincott, Pennsylvania

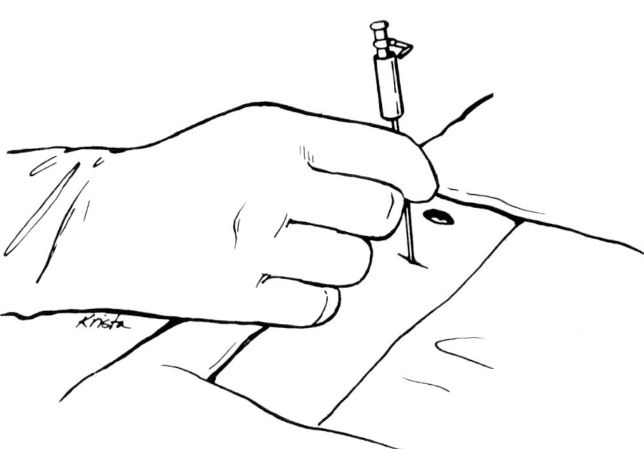

Fig. 23.2 The method of insertion of the Veress needle. Reproduced with modification from Boyce H W 1982 Diseases of the Liver, V edn. Lippincott, Pennsylvania

If ascites is present, a free flow of ascitic fluid indicates a satisfactory entry. In the absence of ascites, if the needle falls into a position parallel to the skin surface after insertion (Fig. 23.3) with easy side-to-side mobility, a satisfactory entry is likely. In obese individuals the Veress needle may not lie parallel to the skin surface after insertion. In doubtful cases, a drop of normal saline or local anaesthetic may be placed over the hub of the needle and the patient instructed to take a deep breath: if the solution disappears quickly into the needle, presumably by the negative pressure exerted, a satisfactory intraperitoneal location of

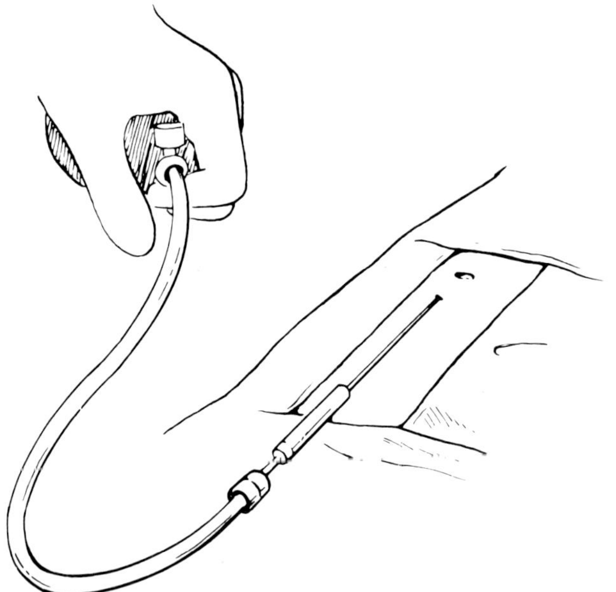

Fig. 23.3 Optimal position of the Veress needle during insufflation. Reproduced from Reynolds T B, Cowen R E 1977 Liver and Biliary Disease. W B Saunders, Pennsylvania

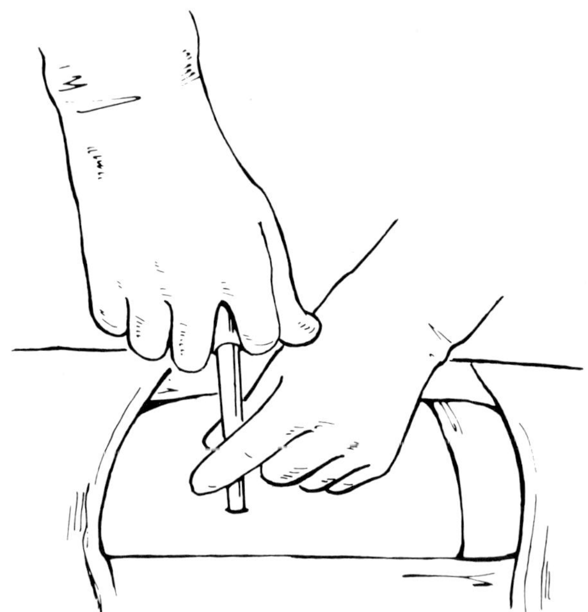

Fig. 23.4 Method of insertion of the trocar. Reproduced from Reynolds T B, Cowan R E 1977 Liver and Biliary Disease. W B Saunders, Pennsylvania

the needle is likely. If further doubt exists, the injection of saline without resistance favours a satisfactory entry. Drawing back on the syringe after the injection of saline is useful because if blood or faecal contents are aspirated, a complicated entry is likely; before insufflation of gas one must be certain of a safe and complete entry into the peritoneal cavity. Once this is achieved, room air is insufflated and should enter the peritoneal cavity without much discomfort. Tympanitic resonance over the liver confirms a satisfactory pneumoperitoneum.

If pain is experienced by the patient or if resistance to the insufflation is noted, the needle should be withdrawn and reinserted. If insufflation devices are used, a rapid rise in pressure or fall of the flow valve ball should alert one to the possibility that insufflation has occurred in an abnormal location such as subcutaneous tissues, within adhesions or into the omentum. Crepitus of subcutaneous emphysema due to the escape of gas from these planes will confirm the abnormal location of gas. The development of a satisfactory pneumoperitoneum is critical to the successful performance of laparoscopy. If ascites is obvious, the initial insertion of the Veress needle is not required and the trocar can be directly inserted.

Once gas is insufflated successfully, the end point is determined objectively by achieving a volume of 3–4 l at a pressure of 10–15 mmHg when using CO_2 or N_2O monitoring devices or by tolerable abdominal distension without pain when air is used. The Veress needle is then withdrawn, the trocar of choice is selected and the tip is inserted into the wound; the thumb and index finger of the left hand (of a right-handed operator) grips the outer sheath of the trocar about 2–3 cm from its tip to prevent the uncontrolled entry of the instrument once the peritoneum has been pierced. The right hand of the operator grips the trocar so that the hub rests against the palmar aspect of the right hand. (Fig. 23.4). The operator has better control of the thrust through the abdominal wall if the arms are somewhat extended. The patient is asked to raise the abdominal wall upwards or the assistant applies lateral compression to accomplish this as the trocar is forced into the peritoneal cavity with either a rotary movement (conical tip) or even pressure (pyramidal tip). Care must be taken not to go too deep into the peritoneal cavity during this insertion as laceration of major vessels may occur, especially in a thin individual (McDonald et al 1978). Once the trocar enters the peritoneal cavity, the hissing sound of escaping gas confirms a satisfactory entry at which time the trocar is withdrawn. Some sleeves have a trumpet valve which prevents air from escaping; a side vent is provided to insufflate air during the examination.

If ascites is present, this is removed. by siphoning following trocar insertion with the help of a cannula that has multiple perforations along its distal half; suction is rarely required. Gas is insufflated after the ascites has been removed and before the examination is begun with the laparoscope. The cable of the light source is attached to the scope and the optics and visibility are checked before inserting the endoscope into the peritoneal cavity. A few drops (0.3–0.5 ml) of a defogging solution (Ultra-Stop 'pro med' Sigma Chemie, Vienna, Austria) is placed on the distal lens of the laparoscope. Gentle warming of the instruments by placing them on an electric heating pad at low settings prior to use will also prevent the lens from fogging.

Examination

A systematic and complete method of examination is important and should be carried out even if the purpose of the examination is to identify a specific lesion of the liver or peritoneum.

The examining table is raised to a height that permits the operator to perform the examination without discomfort. As the laparoscope is advanced into the peritoneal cavity, it is important to look for evidence of blood which might alert one to a traumatic entry. The outer sheath of the trocar is advanced up to the hilt to prevent it from slipping out (Fig. 23.5) and the laparoscope is slid to and fro during the examination. The table may be tilted in the reverse Trendelenburg position while the laparoscope is directed cephalad to visualize the liver and other structures. The falciform ligament is identified; normally this has a pearly white appearance or may contain some fat. In patients with portal hypertension, tiny collateral vessels are often seen and sometimes large para-umbilical veins or a plexus of veins are present. The falciform ligament separates the anatomical right and left lobes of the liver and consequently is a useful landmark. Note is made of the location of the leading edge of both lobes of the liver in relation to the costal margin. The latter can be recognized through the laparoscope when the abdominal wall is depressed at the costal margin externally. The colour of the liver, its edge (whether sharp or rounded, the latter indicating chronic liver disease), its surface (whether smooth, irregular or undulant) the presence of nodules — micronodular (Plate 23.F), macronodular, (Plate 23.A) or a combination of both — are all important observations. The similarity or dissimilarity in the appearance of the liver lobes, the presence or absence of specific lesions sought and, if seen, the nature of the lesion whether vascular, necrotic or cystic should be recorded. Lesions in the dome of the liver are difficult to visualize.

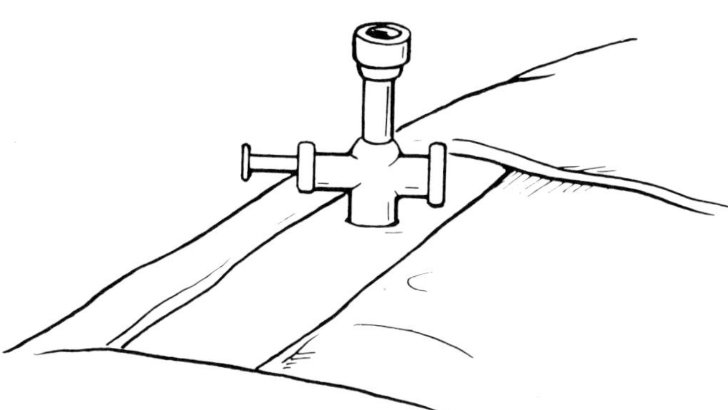

Fig. 23.5 Advancing the trocar sleeve into the abdomen prior to insertion of the laparoscope. Reproduced with modification from Boyce H W 1982 Diseases of the Liver, V edn. Lippincott, Pennsylvania

It has been suggested that a better examination is possible if two telescopes are used, the second introduced by a separate puncture further cephalad under laparoscopic view (Sugarbaker 1981). The gallbladder is identified below the leading edge of the right lobe of the liver. It may be covered by omentum in which case either a probe or the tip of the laparoscope may be used to remove this omentum. Tilting the table to either side or to a more 'head up' position may uncover the gallbladder. A normal gallbladder is robin's egg blue colour, its size varying from that of a walnut to a hen's egg. An opaque appearance to the gallbladder wall indicates chronic cholecystitis; rarely a tumour may be visible.

The peritoneum is visualized in all four quadrants if possible. The normal peritoneum has a shiny pearly appearance with tiny capillaries. In portal hypertension, peritoneal vascularity is increased and may present as a pinkish hue. In inflammatory diseases of the peritoneum, nodules or exudates are visualized; these are usually whitish, discrete, of uniform size (approximately 1–2 mm). Sometimes, there are confluent areas of nodules and exudate. 'Zuckergoose' or a sugar-coated appearance of the visceral peritoneum over the liver and/or spleen or the parietal peritoneum over the diaphragm may be seen in chronic liver disease and ascites. The genesis of this peritoneal thickening is unknown. In malignant tumours of the peritoneum, there are nodules of variable size and colour; some may even be haemorrhagic.

The spleen is not visualized unless it is enlarged and even then it is frequently covered by omentum. A change in table position may permit it to be uncovered, although if adhesions are present, visualization may not be possible. Examination of the spleen may be important in lymphoma staging. Adhesions develop following an intra-abdominal inflammatory process or after surgery; in the former, they may be of the 'violin-string type'. Adhesions may be divided through the laparoscope using cautery (Cano et al 1984) but this is not advisable in patients with portal hypertension because the collaterals that form within these adhesions (Plate 23C) could result in significant bleeding. Dense adhesions preclude adequate examination of the organs and development of pneumoperitoneum may be difficult and hazardous increasing the risk of complications.

Laparoscopic examination of the pelvis should be attempted in the female patient and this is particularly relevant when considering inflammatory or neoplastic lesions; the latter could be a cause of ascites. To achieve examination of the pelvis, the table is tilted in the Trendelenberg position to about 20–30° and the laparoscope is directed to both lower quadrants. The presence of adhesions, adherent bowel loops or omentum may preclude a complete examination.

At the conclusion of the examination, the table is

brought back to the level position and the laparoscope withdrawn. The gas is allowed to escape, enhanced by lateral compression of the flanks. When most of the gas has been removed, the trocar sleeve is removed and the abdominal incision is sutured with 3–0 silk. With the removal of the trocar one must look for bleeding since venous laceration caused at entry could have been compressed by the trocar sleeve while it was in place, only to bleed profusely later when the compression is removed. Peritoneal sutures should be attempted in patients with ascites to prevent leakage. Following the procedure, the patients's vital signs are monitored for two to three hours and normal activity and diet are resumed thereafter; if liver biopsy was performed bed rest is recommended for four hours.

Laparoscopic liver biopsy

Liver biopsies obtained at laparoscopy are frequently of adequate size (at least 2.5 cm and containing at least six portal tracts, Nord 1982) and can be obtained from specific areas of suspicious lesions. Biopsy of either right or left lobes or both can be obtained either through the operating channel or by separate puncture. For the former technique, either suction or Vim-Silverman (cutting) type needles are available. Most peritoneoscopic biopsies done at our unit utilize the separate puncture and either the Trucut needle (a cutting needle of 11.4 cm or 15.2 cm, 20 mm specimen notch* or the modified Klatskin* needle (suction needle of 1.4 mm diameter or 16 gauge). The Trucut needle is preferred in cirrhosis as fragmentation of the specimen is less likely, whereas in non-cirrhotic states either needle may be used. With the Klatskin needle, longer specimens may be obtained depending on the depth of insertion. Long specimens are useful when tissue is required for special studies such as culture, electron microscopy or quantitative heavy metal determination.

The biopsy is obtained at the end of a satisfactory laparoscopic examination. The area of the liver from which a biopsy is desired is selected and a suitable percutaneous site is chosen and infiltrated with 1% lidocaine. An attempt is made to anaesthetize the peritoneum to reduce discomfort during passage of the biopsy needle. Prominent vessels and collaterals are avoided as the biopsy needle is guided into the peritoneal cavity under laparoscopic view (Fig. 23.6). Care is taken to avoid inadvertent puncture of liver, gallbladder and other viscera. The biopsy needle is directed towards the bulk of the liver tissue, and away from the leading edge, hollow viscera and hilum. The patient is instructed to remain apnoeic if awake during insertion of the biopsy needle. Bleeding usually occurs when the needle is withdrawn but frequently stops within two to five minutes. Rarely, bleeding is excessive in amount or continues beyond five minutes. Compression of the liver surface adjacent to the bleeding site by a probe may help arrest bleeding though trauma to the biopsy site with the probe may aggravate the bleeding. Topical thrombin has been recommended by some but we have not used it.

Multiple biopsies can be obtained depending on the indication. Target biopsy or aspiration with a thin needle can be performed in the same manner. Avascular lesions such as metastatic tumour nodules can be safely biopsied; vascular lesions, on the other hand, such as hepatocellular carcinoma or angiosarcoma may bleed profusely following biopsy and aspiration cytology may be an alternative. It is hazardous to biopsy haemangiomas of the liver and when doubt exists, aspiration may be attempted. Flexible pinch biopsy forceps used in gastrointestinal endoscopy can be introduced through the operating channel of the laparoscope or through a separate trocar to obtain pinch biopsies of superficial lesions on the surface of the liver or peritoneum. Lightdale et al (1980) designed a sheathed brush for cytology to enhance the diagnostic yield from neoplastic

* Travenol laboratories, Deerfield,I L
* Becton-Dickinson, Rutherford, N J

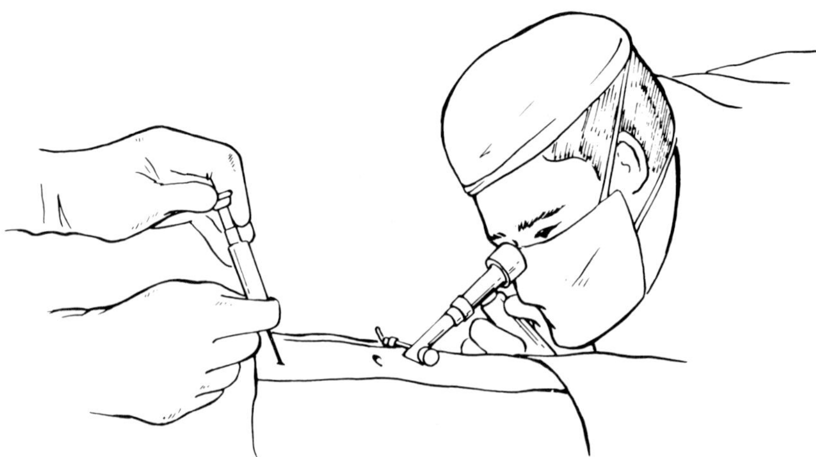

Fig. 23.6 Method of obtaining percutaneous liver biopsy (two hole technique) under laparoscopic view

lesions, and Jensen & Berci (1981) developed a 4 mm trocar used for a second puncture through which various accessories may be introduced, such as biopsy forceps, aspiration needles and quartz rod for illumination and photography.

Peritoneal biopsies are best achieved by a separate puncture using a smaller trocar. The pinch biopsy forceps is introduced through this separate puncture and guided to the desired area by the laparoscopist and the biopsies obtained. Small lesions 1 mm or less can be biopsied easily; bleeding from peritoneal lesions rarely occurs unless a blood vessel has been included in the biopsy. The flexible endoscopy forceps may also be used with the advantage of being introduced through the operating channel and obtaining biopsies beyond the reach of the standard pinch biopsy forceps.

INDICATIONS (Table 23.1)

At laparoscopy the anterior peritoneal space is exposed to view. More than two thirds of the liver surface, which includes most of the anterior surface of the left lobe, part of the right lobe and a small portion of the inferior aspects of the left lobe and rarely the right lobe may be examined. The lateral and inferior aspects of the right lobe, posterior aspects of both lobes and the hilum are inaccessible. Besides the liver, the falciform ligament, parietal peritoneum, serosal aspects of the gastrointestinal tract, spleen, gallbladder and pelvic organs can be inspected.

Evaluation of liver disease

Laparoscopy is an ideal modality for assessment of the type and severity of liver disease. The appearance of the liver surface, preferably with documentation by a colour photograph, together with a satisfactory-sized, non-fragmented liver biopsy should allow precise diagnosis and accurate staging of liver disease. In addition, the size of both liver lobes can be estimated and the amount of collateral circulation visible in the area of the falciform ligament provides an index of the portal pressure. In advanced cirrhosis, the liver surface accurately reflects the pathology and biopsy may be superfluous. Large surface nodules (5 mm in diameter) strongly suggest non-alcoholic liver disease, whereas small nodules (3 mm in diameter) are more compatible with alcoholic liver disease. With diseases characterized by portal and/or interstitial fibrosis and minimal nodular regeneration (i.e. alcoholic fibrosis or chronic active hepatitis) the surface appearance needs augmentation by needle biopsy for optimal assessment. Biopsy at laparoscopy is easily accomplished either through the biopsy channel of the instrument or by a separate puncture under direct vision. Laparoscopic biopsy is more likely to be successful than intercostal biopsy when the right lobe is small, when there is lack of dullness to percussion over the usual biopsy site on the right lower rib cage or when there is ascites. Though this has never been tested objectively, laparoscopic biopsy is probably somewhat safer than blind intercostal biopsy. The risk of biopsying bowel or gallbladder is markedly reduced. Bleeding is no less likely with laparoscopic biopsy but its severity can be assessed immediately. If multiple biopsy specimens are desirable (i.e lymphoma staging or heavy metal analysis), a decision to proceed can be based on the amount of bleeding seen after the first biopsy. Though there is objective evidence that bleeding after liver biopsy is not directly related to the prothrombin time (Ewe 1981), it is customary in most centres to avoid liver biopsy when the prothrombin time by the Quick method is prolonged by more than three seconds. Evaluation of the liver surface in such patients by laparoscopy is an alternative, since bleeding from the laparoscopic entry site in the abdominal wall is more easily controlled than bleeding from the liver.

Filling defects in the Technetium 99 m liver scan are relatively common in chronic liver disease (Boyd 1982). Differentiation between 'pseudotumour' and hepatocellular carcinoma may be uncertain with non-invasive tests such as serum alpha-fetoprotein, ultrasound, gallium scan and computerized tomography. Laparoscopic visualization of the liver surface is useful in this setting, since nodules of hepatocellular carcinoma are usually distinguishable from the surrounding cirrhotic nodules (Plate 23.D) on the basis of colour and size. Since hepatocellular carcinoma is usually multifocal when it occurs in cirrhotic livers, there is a good chance of seeing diagnosable nodules on the anterior liver surface even when the main scan defect is on the posterior or right lateral scan view. Some hepatocellular carcinomas appear highly vascular on their surface, in which case aspiration biopsy with a thin needle can be substituted for the usual needle biopsy.

Table 23.1 Indications for laparoscopy

Evaluation of liver disease:
As part of general assessment
Failure or inability to obtain percutaneous liver biopsy
1. small or no specimen on prior attempt
2. small right lobe of liver
3. Absence of hepatic dullness to percussion
4. Ascites
Prolonged prothrombin time
Evaluation of scan defect with chronic liver disease
Evaluation of focal liver lesions
Evaluation of peritoneum in exudative ascites
Determining resectability of hepatic tumour
Staging for lymphomas
Staging for metastatic disease
Miscellaneous
Surgical:
Assessment of intra-abdominal injury
Evaluation of acute abdominal pain

Evaluation of focal lesions in the liver

Focal lesions in the anterior portion of both liver lobes are easily seen at laparoscopy. Suitability for direct-vision biopsy can ordinarily be determined by the appearance of the lesion. Nodules of metastatic carcinoma are pale or white in appearance (Plate 23 E) often have a central depression or umbilication and rarely bleed when biopsied. Laparoscopy can even detect tiny lesions, much smaller than the resolution of any scanning modality (Boyd 1982).

Thin-needle guided biopsy (by ultrasound or computerized tomography) is preferred by some to direct-vision biopsy at laparoscopy (Barth et al 1981, Danielson et al 1983). Comparative studies of cost-effectiveness and frequency of complications have not been done to our knowledge. Comparisions of the frequency of diagnostic results for metastatic carcinoma with 'blind' intercostal versus laparoscopic biopsy favour the latter (Jori & Peschle 1972). However, when there are many focal lesions in the liver, then 'blind' biopsy is quite likely to be diagnostic and is simpler and less expensive than laparoscopic biopsy.

Evaluation of peritoneum in 'exudative' ascites

Laparoscopy is a very useful modality in the evaluation of ascites. In patients with chronic liver disease ascites is a transudate with a low cell count. In conditions where the ascites is exudative or haemorrhagic or where the cell count is elevated, significant peritoneal disease is likely. The not unusual combination of alcoholic liver disease and peritoneal tuberculosis may result in a 'transudative' type of ascites with a high (1000–5000/mm^3) mononuclear cell count. Laparoscopy may identify the white to yellowish nodules (Plate 23.B) with exudate of peritoneal tuberculosis (Geake et al 1981, Jorge 1984) or the variably sized, sometimes haemorrhagic lesions of tumour implants. Rarely, unusual infections such as coccidiomycosis may produce nodular lesions in the peritoneum similar to those of tuberculosis and may be identified only by culture and special histochemical stains (Ruddock & Hope 1939). When a peritoneal lesion is seen, ascites should be sent for M. tuberculosis and fungus cultures (one litre of fluid is preferred), for cytology and for carcino-embryonic antigen; fibronectin may be an additional useful measurement (Scholmerich et al 1984). Biopsy of the peritoneum should be performed for histological examination and a separate biopsy specimen should be sent for culture. Laparoscopy has been reported to be useful in the diagnosis of peritoneal mesothelioma (McCallum et al 1979) and in the Fitz-Hugh-Curtis (gonococcal perihepatitis) syndrome (Cano et al 1984).

Evaluation for surgical resectability of hepatic tumour

A less definite indication for laparoscopy is the evaluation of surgical resectability of a hepatic neoplasm. Usually, arteriography is required to determine if multicentric neoplasms or intrahepatic metastases are present. Since detection by arteriography is dependent on the vascularity of the lesions, a negative test does not exclude their presence. Laparoscopy may detect lesions on the surface of the liver and peritoneum not identified by angiography. As with angiography, failure to visualize tumours does not exclude their presence. Both modalities may be complementary to each other and there may be a place for laparoscopy prior to laparotomy for intended resection of neoplastic lesions when radiographic tests are negative or equivocal. If tumour lesions are visible on the surface of the presumed uninvolved lobe then laparotomy under general anaesthesia may be avoided. More data are needed to confirm the usefulness of this approach.

Staging of lymphomas

The use of laparoscopy in lymphoma staging, especially in Hodgkin's lymphoma, is well recognized. Tiny hepatic nodules may be seen on the liver surface and these are difficult to detect by other diagnostic modalities. The low sensitivity of the scanning modalities and the low specificity of liver test abnormalities seen in this disease are strong indications for laparotomy or laparoscopy for staging (Coleman et al 1976, Rosenberg et al 1971). Data from the National Cancer Institute and the National Tumour Institute in Milan show an 80% accuracy in detecting hepatic involvement by laparoscopy (Lightdale 1982). The diagnostic yield is directly proportional to the number of biopsies obtained and as a result at least six biopsies are considered optimal. Splenic biopsies obtained at laparoscopy did not demonstrate the same degree of accuracy (Lightdale 1982). Anderson et al (1977) state that laparoscopy may be useful in restaging hepatic involvement during clinical remission and may be preferable to percutaneous biopsy. Huberman et al (1980) increased the yield of detecting hepatic involvement in T cell lymphomas when multiple biopsies were performed at laparoscopy. The exact role of laparoscopy is not certain but it appears useful in the staging of Hodgkin's disease, in the detection of hepatic involvement of T cell lymphomas and in the restaging of non-Hodgkin's lymphoma during clinical remission.

Staging of malignancies

Laparoscopy has been advocated in the staging of metastatic disease (Sugarbaker 1984) especially with primary malignancies involving the breast (Bleiberg et al 1978, DeSouza & Shinde 1980) bronchus, (Margolis et al 1974) ovary (Ozols et al 1981, Quinn et al 1980) and pancreas (Cuschieri et al 1978). Histological diagnosis and evidence of metastasis is important to guide therapy and establish prognosis. Radionuclide scans have a 70% specificity and

80% sensitivity (Lightdale et al 1979). In an autopsy study Ozarda & Pickren (1962) showed that 90% of metastatic lesions to the liver were visible on the surface of the liver. Laparoscopy with biopsy was successful in establishing metastatic disease in 21% of 190 patients with bronchogenic carcinoma, the majority of them being small cell carcinoma (Dombernowsky et al 1978). DeSouza & Shinde (1980) evaluated the liver in 60 patients with localized breast carcinoma and detected small metastatic lesions in 8.5%. In proven hepatic metastases from breast carcinoma, laparoscopy was useful in determining response to chemotherapy objectively (Bleiberg et al 1976). In a retrospective study from the National Cancer Institute, Ozols and others (1981) reported the results of pretreatment and restaging laparoscopy in 99 patients with ovarian carcinoma who were referred for therapy following a staging laparotomy. Of the 88 pretreatment laparoscopies, new sites of disease were found in 48%; in 28% laparoscopy provided evidence of followable disease. In 32% no disease was evident. Of 28 patients with Stage I–II disease, six (21%) were upstaged to Stage III; two patients with Stage IV disease were downstaged to Stage III because hepatic capsular lesions rather than parenchymal involvement were noted at laparoscopy. 66 re-staging laparoscopies were performed while on various therapeutic regimens and in 24 patients, laparoscopy provided the only evidence of residual disease thus avoiding laparotomy in these patients. Laparoscopy documented progression in seven patients, modifying their subsequent therapy. Of the 28 patients without evidence of residual disease, 22 patients underwent exploratory laparotomy and 12 (50%) of these were found to have residual disease; the pelvis was the most common site of disease missed by laparoscopy. Laparoscopy is reported useful in the diagnosis of gallbladder carcinoma (Bhargava et al 1983) and pancreatic carcinoma (Cuschieri 1978, Ishida 1983) but more data are required to confirm its value in these latter conditions.

Miscellaneous indications

Portal hypertension can be confirmed during laparoscopy by the presence of collaterals on the falciform ligament and peritoneum. Measurement of portal pressure by cannulating a splanchnic vein in exteriorized omentum during this procedure has been reported (Yamamoto & Reynolds 1964). This may be achieved during evaluation of liver and peritoneal disease and is not a specific indication for this procedure.

Abnormalities of the biliary tree in patients presenting with jaundice can be evaluated by laparoscopy. Hilar masses may be biopsied if visualized. Cholangiography, first used by Royer et al (1950) has been performed by others (Irving 1978) where puncture of the gallbladder using a thin needle and injection of contrast delineated the obstructive lesion. To avoid bile leakage, the needle was directed transhepatically through the gallbladder bed. However, since transhepatic and endoscopic retrograde cholangiography can be performed with ease and safety and can visualize the biliary tree in almost 95% of cases, it is doubtful whether this method of biliary tract visualization would be considered a suitable alternative. Diagnosis of lesions in the pancreas have also been reported (Cuschieri et al 1978, Ishida et al 1981). Ishida (1983) reported his experience in 124 patients where supragastric pancreascopy or examination of the lesser sac (referred to as bursoscopy) was performed successfully. More data and experience are required before this procedure is considered useful in the diagnosis of pancreatic disease.

Postmortem laparoscopy may be useful in the diagnosis of intra-abdominal diseases when consent for necropsy cannot be obtained. Although this may have a certain aesthetic appeal when compared to necropsy, there are limitations to such an examination.

Surgical indications

Preoperative laparoscopy is being used by surgeons in the assessment of intra-abdominal injury in trauma cases prior to laparotomy (Diehl et al 1981, Sherwood et al 1980). Since only anterior surface of the abdominal contents is visualized, retroperitoneal injuries may be missed. Emergency laparoscopy was performed in 15 patients using a modified 5 mm (outer diameter) laparoscope (Sherwood 1980). Laparotomy was required only in two patients, both of whom had injury to the ileum, identified by sampling fluid from the left paracolic gutter for amylase content in one and by the presence of a haemorrhagic mass in the left pelvis in the other. Laparoscopy was used preoperatively in patients undergoing both routine and emergency surgery and experience in 1720 cases was reported by Cortesi et al (1979). Although Sugarbaker et al (1975) reported an improved diagnostic accuracy of preoperative laparoscopy performed for abdominal pain and in influencing decision regarding subsequent laparotomy, Jersky and others (1980) observed no advantage from such an approach. The experience resulting from the increasing use of preoperative laparoscopy might lead to its place among the definite indications in the future.

CONTRAINDICATIONS

Most contraindications are relative rather than absolute. (Table 23.2)

Laparoscopy should not be performed in an uncooperative or agitated patient unless sedation and/or general anaesthesia is considered to be safe. In obese patients with a very thick abdominal wall, satisfactory pneumoperitoneum is difficult to achieve. The trocar and telescope length may not be sufficient to perform an adequate

Table 23.2 Contraindications for laparoscopy

1. Unco-operative patient
2. Obesity
3. Large ventral hernia
4. Infected skin lesions on the abdomen
5. Previous surgery in the right upper quadrant
6. Grossly abnormal coagulation profile

examination and manoeuvrability is reduced. Infected skin lesions preclude laparoscopy because of the risk of intra-abdominal infection. Large ventral hernias may make an optimal entry site difficult to find. Adhesions from previous surgery make visualization of the intra-abdominal organs unsatisfactory, even if pneumoperitoneum is achieved. Cholecystectomy often results in adhesions that obscure the right upper quadrant from view; although excision of adhesions has been achieved through the laparoscope, this is inadvisable in patients with portal hypertension because of the risk of serious haemorrhage from collaterals within these adhesions.

Patients with significant liver disease and coagulopathy may be considered for laparoscopy without liver biopsy, as a visual assessment of morphology provides the information needed. Even though bleeding from superficial vessels is minor and easily controlled, serious bleeding from laceration of a collateral could necessitate a laparotomy. Such patients with serious liver disease tolerate surgery poorly; therefore not only must there be a strong indication to perform the procedure but every patient must be viewed as a potential surgical candidate. We have arbitrarily selected a prothrombin time of > 50% (or <4 seconds difference between patient and control if a Quick prothrombin time is used) and a platelet count of >60,000/mm^3 for laparoscopy and biopsy. Laparoscopy alone may be performed if prothrombin time is between 40–50% (or approximately less than 5 seconds difference using the Quick method). Although we recognize a lack of correlation between coagulation parameters and the risk of bleeding, the judicious selection of patients for the procedure would avoid unnecessary litigation in the event of a complication. In patients with a large right pleural effusion accompanying ascites, the presence of a small hole in the right diaphragm (Lieberman et al 1966) must be considered, since development of the pneumoperitoneum could lead to a pneumothorax. The presence of such an opening may be ascertained by injection of 500 ml of air into the peritoneal cavity followed by a chest X-ray or by the injection of radionuclide into ascites followed by scans of the chest. In patients with peritoneovenous shunts, pneumoperitoneum required for laparoscopy could result in air embolism.

Table 23.3 Complications of laparoscopy

At entry
1. bleeding from collateral vessels in peritoneum in portal hypertension
2. puncture of hollow viscus
3. puncture or laceration of major vessels

At insufflation
4. gas embolism
5. pneumomediastinum, pneumothorax
6. subcutaneous emphysema

At examination
7. rupture or tear of adhesions and bleeding
8. puncture or laceration of internal organs

At biopsy
9. bleeding
10. bile peritonitis

COMPLICATIONS

A number of complications have been reported but this procedure has a low morbidity and mortality overall. Complications frequently result when the operator is inexperienced or when patients are poorly selected. In an assessment of 63 845 procedures, Bruehl (1966) reported a mortality of 0.03% and a complication rate of 2%. A recent prospective study (Kane & Krejs 1984) showed a five- to seven-fold increase in complication rate when compared to the reported retrospective series. Although the complications in this study were frequently of a minor nature, a mortality of 0.5% was noted.

Bleeding is the most frequent complication (Table 23.3). At entry, bleeding may occur from collateral vessels in the parietal peritoneum or from adhesions; laceration of collaterals will require laparotomy. Puncture of a hollow viscus such as bowel adherent to the abdominal wall is possible. Laceration of major vessels may occur and needs prompt recognition and immediate surgical repair (MacDonald et al 1978). Bleeding can occur from laceration or puncture of intra-abdominal organs but these do not occur with a skilled operator.

Air or gas embolism is a potential and serious complication of pneumoperitoneum. It is speculated that gas enters a traumatized blood vessel which is partially collapsed due to the increase in intra-abdominal pressure. The resultant pressure gradient favours entry of gas into the circulation producing its characteristic effects (Wadhwa et al 1978, Yacoub et al 1982); in most reports of this complication it occurred when the procedure was performed under general anaesthesia. Since CO_2 and N_2O are rapidly soluble in blood, reversibility is frequent. On the other hand, room air which is least soluble is likely to be fatal. Air (or gas) can migrate to abnormal locations such as mediastinum (Ahn & Leach 1976) pleural space (Batra 1983) and pericardium (Nicholson & Berman 1979, Herrerias 1980).

Bleeding after liver biopsy occurs frequently but this usually stops within two to five minutes. Although there is little that can be done to stop the bleeding, recognition of continued bleeding can lead to prompt volume replacement and transfusion. Leakage of bile can occur from liver biopsy when there is dilatation of the ducts or from inadvertent puncture of the gallbladder. Bile peritonitis may be self-limiting or may require laparotomy and drainage but the spillage of infected bile could result in septicaemic shock (Lindner 1971, LoIudice et al 1977).

In patients with ascites, leakage of ascites may occur and may last several days. Placement of an-ostomy bag over the wound keeps the rest of the abdomen dry until the drainage ceases. Though infection of ascites is a theoretical complication, we have never recognized this event.

EXPERIENCE AT THE USC LIVER UNIT

Between 1962 and 1984, 1925 laparoscopies were performed at this unit for evaluation of liver and peritoneal diseases under the supervision of one of us (TBR). We selected 300 consecutive laparoscopies that were performed over a five year period (1979–1984) and the results of this retrospective analysis are presented. The median age of the patients was 50 years and 71% were males. The major indications for laparoscopy in these patients were as follows:

1. assessment of the type and severity of liver disease and biopsy in 33%;
2. evaluation of a focal defect on technetium 99m scan in 26%;
3. determination of the cause of exudative ascites in 16%;
4. determination of the presence of hepatocellular carcinoma in 7%;
5. laparoscopy was performed instead of a liver biopsy in 10% because of coagulopathy;
6. determination of the cause of non-exudative ascites in 4%.

Other indications included evaluation of a palpable mass, staging of lymphoma, consideration for surgical resectability of hepatocellular carcinoma in the remaining 4%.

Of the 300 laparoscopies, successful examination was carried out in 287 achieving a 96% success rate.

Morphology of the liver at laparoscopy revealed micronodular cirrhosis in 38%, micro- and macronodular cirrhosis in 13% and macronodular cirrhosis in 7%. Poorly formed nodules with interstitial fibrosis were seen in 13%. Alcoholic liver disease was the diagnosis in over 70% of the examinations.

Of the 63 patients with hepatic masses noted at laparoscopy, all of whom had focal defects on liver scan, 17 patients (27%) had metastatic carcinoma, 10 patients (16%) had hepatocellular carcinoma and four patients (6%) had haemangiomas; two patients (3%) had lymphoma. In 14 patients (22%) scar or masses with cirrhotic nodules on the surface were found and in the remaining 16 patients (26%) no lesions were visible on the surface of the liver.

The peritoneum was normal in 210 patients (73%). Adhesions with collaterals were present in 58 patients (20%). Tuberculous peritonitis was diagnosed in 11 patients (3.8%) and peritoneal metastases were diagnosed in four patients (1.4%). A white coating on the peritoneum (Zuckergoose) was seen in four patients (1.4%). In six patients (2%) with liver disease, the peritoneum contained an increased number of collateral vessels.

The falciform ligament contained collaterals in 210 patients (73%) and did not contain collaterals in 60 patients (21%). In eight patients (3%) a large single collateral vessel was present. In the remaining nine patients (3%) adhesions precluded visualization of the falciform ligament.

Both lobes of the liver were visualized in 95% of the examinations and in 88% the morphology of both lobes were similar. The right lobe was small and atrophic in 20 patients (7%) whereas left lobe atrophy was seen only in one patient (0.4%). The spleen was visualized in 60% and the gallbladder was seen only in 58%.

Laparoscopy was useful in confirming the preoperative diagnosis in 241 patients (84%) and included those patients with coagulopathy where the examination was performed instead of a biopsy, in characterizing specific lesions in 76 patients (26%) and in exclusion of preoperative diagnosis in 82 patients (28%). In 11 patients (4%), there was no benefit from the procedure. Since there was more than one indication for the procedure, the numbers exceed 100%.

Biopsies of the liver were obtained in 134 patients (43%) using a separate puncture in 80 patients (60%) and through the operating channel in 52 patients (39%). In two patients (1.5%) only aspiration of the lesions for cytology was performed. In 121 patients (90%) less than two biopsies were obtained and in eight (6%) three specimens were obtained. In three patients (2%) satisfactory biopsies were not obtained. Only six patients developed complications from the biopsy, five of whom had bleeding and one had severe pain. All complications resolved spontaneously. Peritoneal biopsies were obtained in 15 patients and in one instance the specimen was unsatisfactory. Transient pain was noted in three patients and bleeding was not encountered.

Complications of laparoscopy occurred in 19 patients (6.3%) and in 13 patients (4.3%) examination was not possible. Of these 13 patients, pneumoperitoneum was unsuccessful in two patients, severe pain during pneumoperitoneum precluded examination in four patients and in seven patients bleeding was noted at entry into the peritoneal cavity. In 10 of these patients, complications resolved spontaneously. One patient needed surgical ligation of a venous collateral that was lacerated at entry and recovered subsequently. Two patients received blood transfusions. Of the six patients who developed complications and in whom examination was completed, two patients had painful pneumoperitoneum and four patients were noted to have bleeding at the conclusion of the procedure as the trocar sleeve was removed. In two patients bleeding stopped spontaneously; one patient required surgery for repair of laceration of an abdominal venous collateral and one patient required blood transfusion. The former patient died a month later of hepatic failure despite surviving the surgery. Infection of the laparoscopy wound occurred five days after the procedure in two patients. In one Enterococcus species and in the other Pseudomonas species was grown on culture. Although both patients had ascites, neither developed infection of ascites. There were no instances of pneumothorax, pneumomediastinum, air embolism or fatalities related to the procedure. Perforation of hollow viscus or laceration of the spleen or liver were not observed in this analysis.

The apparent usefulness of this procedure in the diagnosis of liver and peritoneal diseases together with the very low complication rate evident in this analysis confirms the valuable role of laparoscopy among the investigative modalities performed in our liver unit.

REFERENCES

Ahn Y W, Leach J A 1976 A comparison of subcutaneous and periperitoneal emphysema arising from gynecological laparoscopic procedures. Journal of Reproductive Medicine 17: 335–337

Anderson T, Bender R A, Rosenoff S H, Brereton H D, Chabner R A, DeVita V T, Hubbard S P, Young R C 1977 Peritoneoscopy: a technique to evaluate therapeutic efficacy in non-Hodgkin's lymphoma patients. Cancer Treatment Reports 61: 1017–1022

Barth R A, Jeffrey R B, Moss A A, Liberman M S 1981 A comparision of computed tomography and laparoscopy in the staging of abdominal neoplasms. Digestive Diseases and Sciences 26: 253–256

Batra M S, Driscoll J J, Coburn W A, Marks W M 1983 Evanescent nitrous oxide pneumothorax after laparoscopy. Anesthesia and Analgesia 62: 1121–1123

Beck K, Schaeffer H J 1970 Colour atlas of laparoscopy. Schattauer, Stuttgart

Bhargava D K, Sarin S, Verma K, Kapur B M 1983 Laparoscopy in carcinoma of the gallbladder. Gastrointestinal Endoscopy 29: 21–22

Birnie G G, Quigley E M, Clements G B et al 1983 Endoscopic transmission of hepatitis B virus. Gut 24: 171–174

Bleiberg H, Rozencweig M, Ganji D, Heuson J C 1976 Peritoneoscopic evaluation of the effect of chemotherapeutic agents on liver metastases of breast cancer. Endoscopy 8: 217–220

Bond W N, Peterson N J, Favero M S 1977 Viral hepatitis B: Aspects of environmental control. Laboratory Health Sciences 14: 235–252

Boyd W P 1982 Relative accuracy of laparoscopy and liver scanning techniques. Gastrointestinal Endoscopy 28: 104–106

Bruehl W 1966 Zwischenfalle und Komplikationen bei der Laparoskopies und gezielten Leberpunction. Deutsche Medizinische Wochenschrift 91: 2297–2299

Bruguera M, Bordas J M, Rodes J 1979 Atlas of laparoscopy and biopsy of the liver. Translated by Galambos J T, Jinich H. Saunders, Philadelphia

Cali R W 1980 Laparoscopy. Surgical Clinics of North America 60: 407–424

Cano A, Fernandez C, Scapa M, Boixeda D, Plaza G 1984 Gonococcal perihepatitis: diagnostic and therapeutic value of laparoscopy. American Journal of Gastroenterology 79: 280–282

Coleman M, Lightdale C J, Vinciguerra V P, Degnan T J, Goldstein M, Horwitz T, Winawer S J, Silver R J 1976 Peritoneoscopy in Hodgkin's disease. Confirmation of results by laparotomy. Journal of the American Medical Association 236: 2634–2636

Cortesi N, Zambarda E, Manenti A, Gibertinin G, Gotuzzo L, Malagoli M 1979 Laparoscopy in routine and emergency surgery: experience with 1720 cases. American Journal of Surgery 137: 647–649

Cuschieri A, Hall A W, Clark J 1978 Value of laparoscopy in the diagnosis and management of pancreatic carcinoma. Gut 19: 672–677

Danielson K S, Sheedy P F, Stephens D H, Hattery R R, LaRusso N F 1983 Computed tomography and peritoneoscopy for detection of liver metastases: review of the Mayo Clinic experience. Journal of Computer Asssisted Tomography 7: 230–234

DeSouza L J, Shinde S R 1980 The value of laparoscopic liver examination in the management of breast cancer. Journal of Surgical Oncology 14: 97–103

Diehl J T, Eisenstat M S, Gillinov S, Rao D 1981 The role of peritoneoscopy in the diagnosis of acute abdominal conditions. Cleveland Clinic Quarterly 48: 325–330

Dombernowsky P, Hirsch F, Hansen H H, Hainau B 1978 Peritoneoscopy in the staging of 190 patients with small cell anaplastic carcinoma of the lung with special reference to subtyping. Cancer 41: 2008–2012

El-Minawi M F, Wahbi O, El-Bagouri I S, Sharawi M, El-Mallah S Y 1981 Physiologic changes during CO_2 and N_2O pneumoperitoneum in diagnostic laparoscopy. A comparative study. Journal of Reproductive Medicine 26: 338–346

Ewe K 1981 Bleeding after liver biopsy does not correlate with indices of peripheral coagulation. Digestive Diseases and Sciences 26: 388–393

Geake T M, Spitaels J M, Moshal M G, Simjee A E 1981 Peritoneoscopy in the diagnosis of tuberculous peritonitis. Gastrointestinal Endoscopy 27: 66–68

Gips C H 1981 A new slender laparoscope. Netherlands Journal of Medicine 24: 199–200 (abstract)

Hall T J, Donaldson D R, Brennan T G 1980 The value of laparoscopy under local anaesthesia in 250 medical and surgical patients. British Journal of Surgery 67: 751–753

Herrerias J M, Ariza A, Garrido M 1980 An unusual complication of laparoscopy: Pneumopericardium. Endoscopy 12: 254–255

Huberman M S, Bunn P A, Mathews M J, Ihde D C, Gazdar A F, Cohen M H, Minna J D 1980 Hepatic involvement in the cutaneous T cell lymphomas: results of percutaneous biopsy and peritoneoscopy. Cancer 45: 1683–1688

Irving A D, Cuschieri A 1978 Laparoscopic assessment of the jaundiced patient: a review of 53 patients. British Journal of Surgery 65: 678–680

Ishida H 1983 Peritoneoscopy and pancreas biopsy in the diagnosis of pancreatic diseases. Gastrointestinal Endoscopy 29: 211–218

Ishida H, Furukawa Y, Kuroda H, Kobayashi M, Tsuneoka K 1981 Laparoscopic observation and biopsy of the pancreas. Endoscopy 13: 68–73

Jacobaeus H C 1910 Uber die Moglichkeit die Zystoskopie bei untersuchungen seroser Hohlungen anzuwenden. Munchener. Medizinische Wochenschrift 57: 2090–2092

Jensen D, Berci G 1981 Laparoscopy: advances in biopsy and recording techniques. Gastrointestinal Endoscopy 27: 150–155

Jersky J, Hoffman J, Shapiro J, Kurgan A 1980 Laparoscopy in patients with suspected acute appendicitis. South African Journal of Surgery 18: 147–150

Jorge A D 1984 Peritoneal tuberculosis. Endoscopy 16: 10–12

Jori G P, Peschle C 1972 Combined peritoneoscopy and liver biopsy in the diagnosis of hepatic neoplasm. Gastroenterology 63: 1016–1019

Kalk H 1955 Indikationsstellung and Gefahrenmoment bei der Laparaskopie. Deutsche Medizinische Wochenshrift 61: 1831–1833

Kalk H, Wildhirt E 1961 Lehrbuch und Atlas der laparoskopie under Lieberpunction. Georg Thieme Verlag, Stuttgart p 247

Kane M, Krejs G J 1984 Complications of diagnostic laparoscopy in Dallas: a 7 year prospective study. Gastrointestinal Endoscopy 30: 237–240

Lieberman F L, Hidemura R, Peters R L, Reynolds T B 1966 Pathogenesis and treatment of hydrothorax complicating cirrhosis with ascites. Annals of Internal Medicine 64: 341–351

Lightdale C J 1982 Clinical applications of laparoscopy in patients with malignant neoplasms. Gastrointestinal Endoscopy 28: 99–102

Lightdale C J, Winawer S J, Kurtz R C, Knapper W H 1979 Laparoscopic diagnosis of suspected liver neoplasms. Value of prior liver scans. Digestive Diseases and Sciences 24: 588–593

Lightdale C J, Hajdu S I, Luisi C B 1980 Cytology of the liver, spleen and peritoneum obtained by a sheathed brush during laparoscopy. American Journal of Gastroenterology 74: 21–24

Lindner H 1971 Das Risiko der perkutanen Leberbiopsie Medizin Klin 66: 924–929

LoIudice T, Buhac I, Balint J 1977 Septicemia as a complication of percutaneous liver biopsy. Gastroenterology 72: 949–951

Margolis R, Hansen H H, Muggia F M, Kanhouwa S 1974 Diagnosis of liver metastasis in bronchogenic carcinoma. A comparative study of liver scans, function tests and peritoneoscopy with liver biopsy in 111 patients. Cancer 34: 1825–1829

McCallum R W, Maceri D R, Jensen D Berci G 1979 Laparoscopic diagnosis of peritoneal mesothelioma. Review of a case and review of the diagnostic approach. Digestive Diseases and Sciences 24: 170–174

McDonald P T, Rich N M, Collins G J, Andersen C A, Kozloff L 1978 Vascular trauma secondary to diagnostic and therapeutic procedures. American Journal of Surgery 135: 651–655

Michel H, Raynaud A 1977 Interet de laparoscopie sous anesthetisie generale. Endoscopie Digestive 2: 135–136

Minoli G, Terruzzi, Spinzi G C, Benvenuti C, Rossini A 1982 The influence of carbon dioxide and nitrous oxide on pain during laparoscopy: a double blind controlled trial. Gastrointestinal Endoscopy 28: 173–175

Nicholson R D, Berman N D 1979 Pneumopericardium following laparoscopy. Chest 1976: 605–607

Nord H J 1982 Biopsy diagnosis of cirrhosis: blind percutaneous versus guided direct vision technique — a review. Gastrointestinal Endoscopy 28: 102–104

Ott D O 1901 Ventroscopic illumination of the abdominal cavity during pregnancy. *Zeitschrift Akus. Zhensk Bolenz*

Ozarda A, Pickren J 1962 The topographic distribution of liver metastases. Its relation to surgical and isotopic diagnosis. Journal of Nuclear Medicine 3: 149–152

Ozols R F, Fisher R I, Anderson T, Makuch I, Young R C 1981 Peritoneoscopy in the management of ovarian cancer. American Journal of Obstetrics and Gynecology 140: 611–619

Quinn M A, Bishop G J, Campbell J J, Rodgerson J, Pepperell R J 1980 Laparoscopic follow up of ovarian carcinoma. British Journal of Obstetrics and Gynecology 87: 1132–1139

Rosenberg S A, Boiron M, DeVita V T Jr 1971 Report on the Committee in Hodgkin's disease staging procedure. Cancer Research 31: 1862–1863

Royer M, Mazuru P, Kohan S 1950 Biliary kinetics studied by means of peritoneoscopic cholangiography. Gastroenterology 16: 83–90

Ruddock J C 1934 Peritoneoscopy. Western Medical Journal 42: 392–405

Ruddock J C, Hope R B 1939 Coccidiodal peritonitis. Diagnosis by peritoneoscopy. Journal of the American Medical Association 113: 2054–2055

Sanowski R A, Sarles H, Bellapravulu S, Haynes W 1984 Current status and future of laparoscopy — Is it a dying procedure? Gastrointestinal Endoscopy 30: 148–149 (abstract)

Scholmerich J, Volk B A, Kottgen E, Ehlerss, Gerok W 1984 Fibronectin concentration in ascites differentiates between malignant and non malignant ascites. Gastroenterology 87: 1160–1164

Scott D B, Julian D G 1972 Observations on cardiac arrythmias during laparoscopy. British Medical Journal 1: 411–413

Sharp J R, Pierson W P, Brady C E 1982 Comparison of CO_2 and N_2O induced discomfort during peritoneoscopy under local anesthesia. Gastroenterology 82: 453–456

Sherwood R, Berci G, Austin E, Morgenstern L 1980 Minilaparoscopy for blunt abdominal trauma. Archives of Surgery 115: 672–673

Sugarbaker P H 1981 Optimizing peritoneoscopic visualisation of the liver utilizing a double telescope technique. Surgery, Gynecology and Obstetrics 152: 655–657

Sugarbaker P H 1984 Endoscopy in cancer diagnosis and management. Hospital Practice, November, 111–120

Sugarbaker P H, Sanders J H, Bloom B S, Wilson R E 1975 Preoperative laparoscopy in the diagnosis of acute abdominal pain. Lancet 1 (7904): 442–445

Wadhwa R K, Mckenzie R Wadhwa S R, Katz D L, Byers J F 1978 Gas embolism during laparoscopy. Anesthesiology 48: 74–76

Wittman I 1966 Budapest Peritoneoscopy Vols I and II. Akademiai Kiado

Yacoub O F, Cardona J, Coverler L A, Dodson M G 1982 Carbon dioxide embolism during laparoscopy. Anesthesiology 57: 533–535

Yamamoto S, Reynolds T B 1964 Portal venography and pressure measurement at peritoneoscopy. Gastroenterology 47: 602–603

O. Søreide

Percutaneous aspiration cytology

INTRODUCTION

The true nature of a mass lesion in the liver and biliary tract can only be established by microscopic examination of a specimen obtained from the lesion. Clinicians will always seek microscopic confirmation of a presumptive diagnosis as a correct diagnosis will have therapeutic and prognostic implications.

The opportunity of obtaining morphologic diagnosis safely and rapidly by use of fine needle aspiration biopsy (FNAB) is said to have been pioneered by Martin and Ellis (1930) at the Memorial Center in New York, although the first report on needle biopsy can be traced back to 1847 (Webb 1974). Frola (1935) from France also tried the fine needle aspiration technique and evaluated cytological smears, but the technique did not receive much attention and seems to have been nearly forgotten until Lopes Cordozo (1954), Söderström (1966), Wasastjerna (1969) and Lundquist (1970a) published their extensive experience. These reports have been followed by numerous others and the FNAB-technique has now been evaluated in a variety of clinical problems (Zornoza 1981, Holm & Kristensen 1985a).

The increasing popularity of the method depends largely on two factors. Firstly, the evolution of clinical cytology now allows the cytopathologist to provide a diagnosis based on the aspiration specimen which corresponds closely with that obtainable from histologic examination. Secondly, the innovations seen over the last 10–15 years with new imaging techniques such as dynamic ultrasound scanning (US) and computerized tomography (CT) provide high-resolution sectional images and allow anatomically directed aspiration techniques. In addition, despite extensive research in differences in soft tissue texture, so-called 'tissue characterization', by image analyses which might enable the examiner to suggest a specific diagnosis, it still seems necessary with an interventional method to obtain an exact, specific and tissue-confirmed diagnosis.

TECHNIQUE

Guidance

The pioneers of FNAB performed their aspirations without guidance of the needle. However, percutaneous puncture will today be performed in combination with some imaging technique such as isotopic liver scan (Johansen & Svendsen 1978), angiography (Tylén et al 1976), fluoroscopy (preferably in two planes after contrast visualization of the lesion), for instance following percutaneous transhepatic cholangiography (PTC) or endoscopic retrograde cholangio-pancreatography (ERCP) (Ho et al 1977, Goldman et al 1977) or computed tomographic scan (Whitlach et al 1984). Puncture guided by these imaging techniques is, however, cumbersome and time-consuming (Ferucci et al 1980) and has now been largely replaced by ultrasound imaging.

Ultrasound (US) has proved to be superior as a puncture guide to any other imaging modality. The development of modern high resolution scanners allows real-time visualization of the target, the surrounding tissues, the needle and the needle track. US also allows all puncture directions, it is independent of organ function and no ionizing radiation is used. US provides a dynamic image which is of importance when the target is small and moving, and the needle tip can be monitored during insertion. The method is convenient and the procedure rapid. Finally, the equipment is mobile and the patient can stay in bed during the procedure. The main disadvantages of US are related to its inability to penetrate gas and bone so that intestinal gas may interfere with imaging of the abdominal organs and the ribs may limit the accessability of certain areas.

Three different methods of ultrasonographic guiding mechanisms are available (Holm et al 1985b):

1. The freehand puncture where the needle is introduced near to the transducer and will be visualized as it enters the soundfield;

2. Puncture through a linear array puncture transducer which contains a needle canal and allows the needle to enter in the top of the soundfield;
3. A steering attachment is added to the US transducer where the needle either enters the soundfield from the side in the same plane as the soundfield, or where the needle traverses the soundfield.

Needles

A fine needle has by definition an outer diameter of 1 mm (19 gauge) or less. Needles are commercially available in different lengths, and the most commonly used diameter is 0.6–0.8 mm.

The needles are flexible and may bend when they are advanced through the abdominal wall. The fine needle can be stabilized by use of an outer guide needle of diameter 1.2 mm (10 cm long) which is first introduced through the superficial layers. This outer needle will not only ensure needle stability but will also allow multiple passes of the fine needle without inconvenience to the patient.

Needles with cutting capability have also become available and a tissue core for histological examination can be obtained (Torp-Pedersen et al 1984). This biopsy modality will not be discussed in this chapter.

Aspiration technique

The aspiration technique was pioneered by Franzén et al (1960). When the ultrasonic examination has identified a puncture target, the optimum needle route is chosen. The fine needle is fitted to a disposable syringe which will be attached to an aspiration handle (Fig. 24.1). The outer supporting needle, if needed, is introduced and the fine needle is passed through it (Fig. 24.2). When the tip of the fine needle is located within the lesion to be biopsied, the piston of the aspiration handle is retracted completely to apply full suction and the needle is moved back and forth four or five times to loosen cell clusters. With the needle still in the lesion, the negative pressure is equilibrated by slowly releasing the handle and the needle is withdrawn. The material in the needle is expelled onto glass slides. Usually several passes of the needle will be performed in slightly different directions to ensure repre-

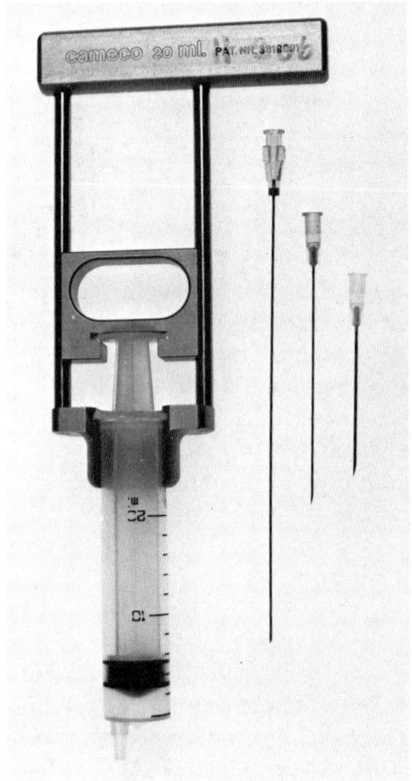

Fig. 24.1 Aspiration handle that permits a one-hand grip. The handle will fit a disposible 20 ml syringe

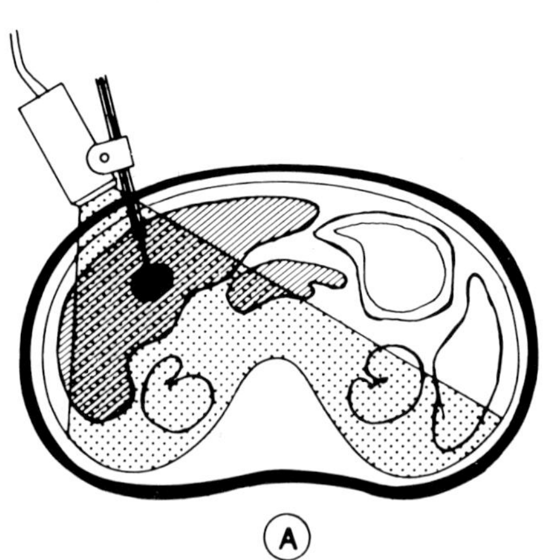

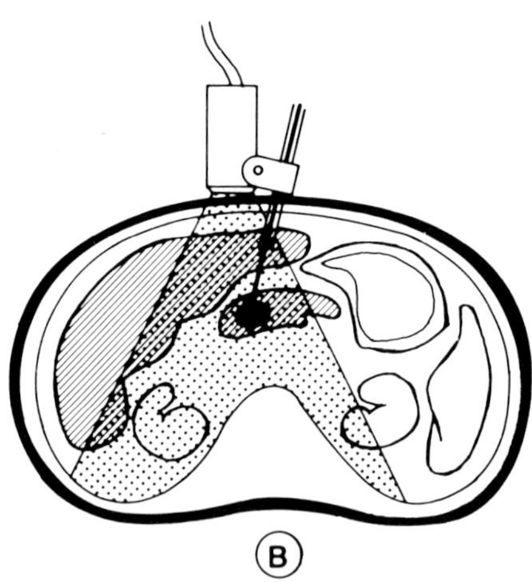

Fig. 24.2 Technique of ultrasonically guided fine needle aspiration biopsy: (A) liver lesion; (B) pancreatic mass lesion. The outer supporting needle is passed through the puncture adaptor of the sector scanner, and the fine needle for biopsy is introduced through the outer needle

sentative sampling. Expelling is facilitated by disconnecting the needle from the syringe, and filling of the syringe with air.

Experience has shown that the needle can traverse stomach, bowel and urinary bladder to reach a mass lesion. Transpleural and transpulmonal puncture should, on the other hand, be avoided, and with a puncture through the liver, the edge should be avoided as it may be lacerated if the patient moves.

FNAB can be performed on an in- and outpatient basis without preparation. The skin and subcutaneous tissues can be anaesthetized locally (rarely indicated), and diazepam might be given to an anxious patient. A small incision in the skin with a surgical blade can facilitate the entry of the needle.

Preparation of the smear

The needle content is expelled onto glass slides, and spread immediately as shown in Fig. 24.3. Fluid aspirated from cysts is spun down before being placed and spread on the slides or mixed with 50% ethanol for centrifugation later.

The biopsy material is either fixed immediately or air

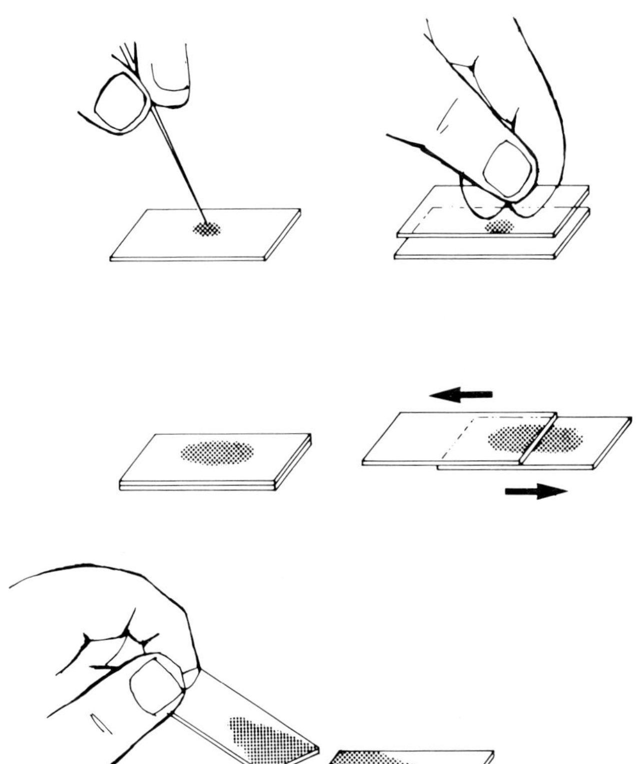

Fig. 24.3 Method of preparing aspiration biopsy smears. The needle content is expelled, and a second glass slide is put on top. The drop spreads between the slides which are then pulled in opposite directions resulting in two specimens

dried. Wet fixation is either performed in 95% ethanol or by a commercially available spray fixative (standard in our hospital) and is followed by staining before cytomorphological evaluation.

Some authors advocate that both wet and dry fixation should be done if sufficient material is obtained. Dry fixation can allow use of special stains such as immunocytochemical staining techniques.

RESULTS

It is obvious from the literature that the results will vary widely according to whether the procedure was guided by some imaging technique or was performed blindly or by palpation. The results which follow refer only to guided biopsies unless stated otherwise as this reflects the current state of the procedure.

The terminology in reported results also differs. To enable some comparison between different authors, the following terms will be used for evaluation of the results: TP = true-positive results; TN = true-negative results; FP = false-positive results; FN = false-negative results. These figures form the basis for estimation of

$$\text{Sensitivity} = \frac{TP}{TP + FN} \times 100\%$$

$$\text{Specificity} = \frac{TN}{TN + FP} \times 100\%$$

$$\text{Predictive value of a positive test } (PV_{pos}) = \frac{TP}{TP + FP} \times 100\%$$

$$\text{Predictive value of a negative test } (PV_{neg}) = \frac{TN}{TN + FN} \times 100\%$$

Not all authors report their results in this way, but the various indices can be calculated from published figures.

A general problem when reviewing the literature on FNAB is that the selection of cases may influence the results (see below). Similarly, there seems to be no consensus how to treat the non-representative or 'inconclusive' biopsies in result reporting and analysis, and the number of biopsy procedures to establish the diagnosis is rarely given. Thirdly, the verification of the final diagnosis is often a problem, especially in patients with a negative FNAB and thought to have benign disease.

Liver

FNAB of the liver is done to answer the following questions:

1. What is the nature of a lesion, i.e. is it malignant or not?
2. If malignant, can the cellular characteristics indicate the site of origin?

3. Can FNAB identify benign liver lesions and differentiate between them?

Table 24.1 gives a representative selection of recently published papers which indicate the usefulness of FNAB in diagnosing malignant liver lesions. The overall sensitivity was 93%, i.e. in those patients with malignant disease the FNAB was positive for malignancy in 93%. The specificity was 97% (or 99% if the only result not consistent with the general trend (Ho et al 1981) was excluded), i.e. patients with benign disease had a benign cytological diagnosis in 97% (99%). The predictive value of a positive (malignant) cytological test was 99%, whereas the predictive value of a negative cytology was only 77%. The interpretation of these figures is that FNAB is a highly reliable test for malignant disease when positive. However, a negative (benign) cytology is of limited value in excluding a hepatic malignancy, and further biopsies or other tests may be needed to establish the true nature of the liver lesion.

Table 24.1 may also demonstrate that FNAB has been as useful in patient series which include all types of focal liver lesion(s) (called liver mass (M) in the table) as it is in series which include only solid liver lesion(s). This is not necessarily an argument for doing FNAB of all liver lesions (see below), but simply states that if the FNAB is positive for malignancy this is highly unlikely to be false irrespective of type of lesion(s).

Many clinicians are worried about false-positive biopsies. These are exceedingly rare (Table 24.1). Analyses of the published series indicate that false-positive biopsies are due to sampling error or are based on biopsy material that often is scanty and probably should have been reported as 'not representative' (Ho et al 1981, Schwerk & Schmitz-Moormann 1981).

In contrast to other infradiaphragmatic organs, the liver may harbour a variety of malignant tumours. Secondary liver tumours, especially in the Western hemisphere, are more common than liver primaries. The cytological characteristics of aspirates from several liver lesions have been clearly established (Eklund & Wasastjerna 1971, Wasastjerna 1979, Tao et al 1984). The trained cytologist is able to give a cytological diagnosis which corresponds closely to the histology of the tumour (Jacobsen et al 1983, Droese et al 1984). By establishing the histogenetic origin, the clinician can then direct further investigations to organ systems, for instance to the gastrointestinal tract in the case of an adenocarcinoma. Bile duct carcinomas which make up 15–25% of primary carcinoma of the liver are said to be often misdiagnosed as metastatic (Wasastjerna 1979), but data in the literature is difficult to evaluate. Of 20 patients with a focal lesion of bile duct origin 16 (80%) had a positive diagnosis of malignancy, but the histogenetic nature of the lesions was not given (Montali et al 1982, Tatsuta et al 1984, Whitlach et al 1984, Haubek 1985).

The value of FNAB in the diagnosis of benign focal liver lesion(s) is difficult to establish. It is clear from numerous papers that the cytological diagnoses in these patients have been non-specific, i.e. that of 'no malignant tumour cells found'. The fact that differentiation between lesions even within the benign group is essential for the type of treatment advocated, combined with the unreliability of a negative cytology, suggest that the general picture of the usefulness of FNAB is less positive than that outlined for malignant tumours.

Simple liver cysts are a frequent finding in clinical practice. If the lesion exhibits the typical ultrasonographic or tomographic characteristics of a simple cyst, it is a general opinion that FNAB probably is unnecessary and unhelpful (Haubek 1985).

The literature on FNAB of benign solid focal liver lesions is sparse. Solbiati et al (1985) performed FNAB in

Table 24.1 Results of percutaneous FNAB in the diagnosis of malignant liver lesions

Author(s)	No. of patients	Type of lesions(s)	Sensitivity	Specificity	PVpos	PVneg
Ho et al 1981	40	M	93%	80%	93%	80%
Montali et al 1982	108	M	92%	100%	100%	70%
Rosenblatt et al 1982	59	M	94%	100%	100%	80%
Jacobsen et al 1983	55	S	100%	100%	100%	100%
Pagini et al 1983	100	S	95%	100%	100%	56%
Schwerk et al 1983	130	S	92%	93%	98%	77%
Droese et al 1984	100	S	94%	100%	100%	89%
Whitlach et al 1984	86	M	87%	100%	100%	76%
Tatsuta et al 1984	41	M	94%	96%	94%	96%
Haubek 1985	380	S	91%	100%	100%	65%
Holm et al 1985b	247	S	92%	100%	100%	60%
overall	1346		93%	97%	99%	77%

S = solid liver lesion(s): M = liver mass(es) of any type

33 patients with a liver haemangioma. The cytological diagnosis was based on the absence of malignant cells and the presence of capillary vessels in addition to blood and endothelial cells. A confident cytologic diagnosis was made in four (12%), and a probable diagnosis in another four (12%), indicating that FNAB is highly unreliable in the diagnosis of haemangiomas.

This author has been unable to find any report on FNAB of hepatic adenoma, focal nodular hyperplasia and fatty focal infiltration. The hepatocytes of FNH are cytologically normal and are indistinguishable from those of normal liver although they may contain excess glycogen (Knowles & Wolff 1976).

Table 24.2 Results of percutaneous FNAB in the diagnosis of extrahepatic bile duct tumours

Author(s)	No. of patients	% Positive cytological diagnosis
Evander et al 1978	19	53%
McLoughlin et al 1978	2	100%
Evander et al 1980	33	42%
Chitwood et al 1982	12	67%
Blumgart et al 1984	22	59%*
Dalton-Clark et al 1986	6	67%
Overall	94	54%

*both pre- and intraoperatively

Extrahepatic bile ducts

The literature on percutaneous FNAB of the extrahepatic bile duct is sparse, which may reflect the view taken by Longmire et al (1973) that a tissue confirmed diagnosis is not required when dealing with bile duct obstruction.

Table 24.2 gives the results in six reports, although the paper published by Evander et al (1980) may contain some or all of the patients reported by the same group in a previous publication (Evander et al 1978). There is no specific information concerning the guidance used by these authors although the reports indicate that PTC (percutaneous transhepatic cholangiography) and US were most commonly used.

Of the FNAB performed in 94 patients, 51 (54%) proved to be positive for malignancy. There is no information regarding the site of the tumours (proximal, mid-duct, distal or retro-duodenal) in relationship to diagnostic accuracy, nor concerning the number of biopsies obtained. None of the authors have described false-positive biopsies.

Pancreas

FNAB of the pancreas was pioneered by Christoffersen & Poll (1970), and percutaneous biopsies were first obtained by Oscarson et al in 1972.

Several series of percutaneous FNAB of pancreatic mass lesions have been published, however, many with only a limited number of patients. Table 24.3 gives a representative selection of the major series with a total number of patients of 863. A positive cytology for malignancy (i.e. the sensitivity) has been obtained in an average of 71% of patients with verified cancer ranging from 58% to 86%. The implication of the figures is that the frequency of false negatives (or not representative biopsies (see below)) is

Table 24.3 Results of percutaneous FNAB in the diagnosis of pancreatic cancer

Author(s)	No. of patients	Type of lesion	Positive cytology in patients with cancer	False-positive(s)
Tylén et al 1976	29	M	76%	–
Goldstein et al 1977	18	M + B	57%	0/4
Evander et al 1978	52	M	60%	–
Yamanaka & Kimura 1979	28	M + B	86%	0/6
Hancke 1981	72	M + B	60%	72
Mitty et al 1981	53	M + B	86%	0/10
Hovdenak et al 1982	55	M + B	76%	0/9
Schwerk et al 1983	70	M + B	69%	0/18
Hancke et al 1984	203	M + B	71%	2/77 (2.6%)
Bree et al 1984	32	M + B	86%	0/11
Holm et al 1985b	190	M + B	72%	2/73 (2.7%)
Søreide et al 1985	61	M + B	58%	0/24
Overall	863		71%	4/304 (1.3%)

M = malignant tumours of the pancreas

M + B = malignant and benign pancreatic mass lesions

fairly high, and that a negative biopsy does not exclude malignancy.

The accuracy of FNAB of the pancreas seems to be independent of type of lesion, i.e. whether the biopsies were performed in patients with a malignant tumour only, or whether the biopsies were taken from any benign and malignant pancreatic mass lesion. This means that when malignant cells are demonstrated cancer is accurately diagnosed.

The problem of false-positive biopsies is also outlined in Table 24.3. Out of 304 patients with benign disease, four (1.3%) biopsies were reported as showing malignant cells. However, in two of these (Holm et al 1985b), the false-positives were due to misinterpretation of the specimen by the cytopathologist. Thus, false-positive biopsies occur in less than 1% of patients with benign pancreatic disease. The remaining two false-positives were obtained from patients with chronic pancreatitis (Hancke et al 1984). We have also reported two false-positive intraoperative FNAB in a patient with chronic pancreatitis (Søreide et al 1985). In chronic pancreatitis both architectural and cytological changes may mimic carcinoma. We believe that most of these false-positives can be avoided by applying strict criteria for what constitutes a representative biopsy.

A specific problem for pancreatic FNAB seems to be the relatively high frequency of non-representative specimens, by some authors also called 'insufficient material' or 'inconclusive' cytology. The figures range from 3.2% (Hancke 1981) to 44% (Søreide et al 1985). The high figure in the latter series may reflect the strict criteria formulated by the cytologists for a representative biopsy (Søreide et al 1985). The high frequency of non representative biopsies may probably also reflect the relative inaccessability of the pancreas, and imaging problems especially experienced with US.

Lastly, it must be emphasized that recognition of cells from an adenocarcinoma in FNAB of the pancreas does not necessarily mean that the tumour originates in this gland. Cytological examination alone cannot exclude origin in other or adjacent structures, e.g. intestines, stomach and distal bile duct. Similarly, experience seems to be insufficient to permit description of all variants of islet cell tumours, and cytologists state that extreme care is necessary in judging the biological behaviour of these tumours on the basis of the cytological picture (Stormby 1979).

COMPLICATIONS AND RISKS

The relative safety of FNAB of intra-abdominal organs has recently been studied by two independent groups. Livraghi et al (1983) reviewed the literature and tabulated the results of 11700 FNAB of the abdomen including 552 patients of their own. Smith (1985) did a hospital survey with 214 responders. The report comprises a total of 15 777 abdominal aspiration biopsies carried out for the year in question, and with an estimated number of FNAB for the period when the procedure had been employed of 63108. These two reports will form the basis of the review of FNAB-related complications and deaths.

The overall complication rate of FNAB in Smith's study was 0.16%. Livraghi reported an incidence of major complications of 0.05%, and an incidence of minor problems (mostly pain) of 0.5% (58/11700). In comparison, Holm et al (1985b) reported two complications following 2000 fine needle punctures of the abdomen giving a complication rate of 0.1%, and Lundquist (1970b) had one complication in 2611 fine needle liver biopsies (0.04%).

The potential hazards in percutaneous biopsy are bleeding, bile leak, infection and tumour seeding or implantation in the needle tract. Table 24.4 gives the frequency of these complications. Bleeding is most common, and may ultimately lead to death (Smith 1985). Of 27 patients in Smith's series with bleeding (defined as patients requiring blood transfusion), three died. No information is given concerning the type of lesion biopsied.

As pointed out by Smith (1985) the frequency of bile leak (bile leak is not defined in either study) is probably overinflated by inclusion of leaks following transhepatic cholangiography. If we look for the entity of 'bile peritonitis', only five cases have been reported (incidence of 0.007%).

The infection group includes patients with generalized peritonitis after abscess puncturing, bacteraemia, and patients will so-called generalized infections. The risk is small. It is apparent from the literature that both bacterial and parasitic abscesses can be punctured without any significant risk (Smith 1985, Grønvall 1985), and even hydatid cysts, often regarded as an absolute contraindication to biopsy, have been punctured without hazard to the patient.

The risk of needle tract tumour seeding following biopsy of a malignant lesion has been used as an argument against FNAB. However, experimental work (Ryd et al 1983) as well as clinical experience (Table 24.4) have indicated that the risk is very small indeed.

Table 24.4 Complication rates in abdominal FNAB

Complication	Frequency of complication Livraghi et al 1983 (n = 11700 biopsies)	 Smith 1985 (n = 63108 biopsies)
Bleeding	7 (0.06%)	27 (0.04%)
Bile leak	2 (0.02%)	51 (0.08%)**
Infection	3 (0.03%)*	16 (0.02%)
Needle tract seeding	2 (0.02%)	3 (0.005%)
Deaths	1 (0.008%)	4 (0.006%)

* 12 patients with fever not included

** Probably inflated by inclusion of transhepatic cholangiography

Others have reported complications such as pancreatitis (one fatal), haematuria, GI-tract bleeding, and chylous ascites.

The risk of dying following FNAB was in these two series 0.006%–0.008% respectively. Of the five deaths reported, three were caused by bleeding and the remaining two by pancreatitis.

In conclusion, the hazards of FNAB are small indeed, and can compare favourably with any invasive diagnostic modality used in clinical practice.

THE ROLE OF PERCUTANEOUS FNAB IN PATIENTS WITH HEPATOBILIARY SURGICAL DISEASES — A PERSONAL VIEW

The results presented in this chapter may indicate that FNAB is a highly valuable diagnostic tool which can be performed safely in any patient. The problem with any collected review is that it provides general figures taken out of a clinical context, often in highly selected patients, where the authors naturally will give as good results as possible (i.e. the problem related to the number of biopsy procedures needed to establish the cytological diagnosis), and where the information obtained from the FNAB may only add marginal additional information or just confirm what the clinician knows (or should know) from the history or other clinical and laboratory results.

The author's view is that FNAB should not be done indiscriminately in any or all patients just because it is simple and safe. On the other hand, if FNAB is included in a plan for management of specific problems (see below), FNAB can be accepted as an integrated and valuable investigation which will prove to be highly cost effective. The following personal recommendations for percutaneous FNAB are briefly outlined.

Liver

Simple cysts

These are frequent incidental findings, but infrequently symptomatic. If a typical appearance is found on imaging (US or CT), no fine needle aspiration is required as FNAB is generally unhelpful (usually the cytological material is too sparse or completely missing to allow any diagnosis) and recurrence of the cyst(s) is a rule after emptying.

'Atypical' cysts

A cyst with irregular linings or margins and with an inhomogeneous content in an afebrile patient should be investigated and evaluated as a solid focal liver lesion (see below). If the patient is septicaemic or presents with signs of an ongoing infection, immediate needling of the lesion is advocated to obtain material for culture. In an area where hydatid disease is endemic, serologic tests should be done and FNAB deferred.

Multiple solid liver lesions

The typical patient is one with primary extrahepatic malignant lesion previously treated. FNAB should be performed in these patients early to establish the true nature of the disease and to avoid overinvestigation, but in some patients the diagnosis of advanced malignant disease will be so obvious that FNAB will be of only academic interest and will add to the discomfort of the patient. In patients with no known primary tumour, FNAB is indicated early in the diagnostic process as the cytology may establish the histogenetic type of tumour and thus be helpful in identifying the very few for whom treatment is worthwhile (lymphomas, germ cell tumours, etc.).

A solid focal lesion

In the symptomatic patient with a solid, potentially resectable focal liver lesion, percutaneous FNAB should only be considered after the patient has been fully investigated, e.g. according to the algorithm outlined by Thompson et al (1985). The reasons for this attitude are: the fact that a negative FNAB is unreliable and further investigations are often required: the fact that FNAB cannot identify the benign liver lesions and differentiate between them: and the obvious fact that a primary malignant liver lesion should be resected whenever possible. Thus, most patients in this group will eventually come to laparotomy irrespective of the cytological findings. For the benign lesions where surgery is not indicated (i.e. haemangiomas) the diagnosis will be established by CT and angiography and not by FNAB.

In patients with a solid, focal liver lesion and with a history of a previous or synchronous malignancy, FNAB should, however, be performed early in the diagnostic process.

Extrahepatic bile ducts and pancreas

The clinical problem related to tumours of the extrahepatic bile ducts and pancreas is that of investigation of a jaundiced patient. The first step in the diagnostic strategy for such patients is abdominal ultrasound (Benjamin 1983).

If US shows extrahepatic bile duct dilatation, and a pancreatic tumour or mass, FNAB during the initial US examination is advocated. A positive cytology for malignancy early in the diagnostic process will obviate the need for more sophisticated and invasive tests in patients unfit for major pancreatic surgery, or enable the surgeon to plan further investigations with the view to evaluating resectability.

For patients with extrahepatic bile duct obstruction not caused by a pancreatic mass, a full and comprehensive investigation including PTC (and/or ERCP) and angiography should be undertaken (Ch. 25). For patients with a resectable lesion, surgery should be undertaken. Percutaneous FNAB should be reserved for those with an irresectable lesion, and should be guided by US if the lesion can be identified ultrasonographically, or by fluoroscopy following PTC or ERCP (for discussion of criteria of irresectability in patients with a cholangiocarcinoma, see Ch. 65).

FNAB OR COARSE NEEDLE BIOPSY?

It is a generally accepted fact that the complication rate increases with increasing diameter of the needle (Menghini 1970). As shown in Table 24.4, the complication rate of FNAB is extremely low, and favourable when compared with that of 5.9% following coarse liver biopsy (Perrault et al 1978).

Percutaneous coarse needle biopsy is, in the author's opinion, contraindicated in pancreatic and bile duct lesions. Whether FNAB is as accurate as coarse needle biopsy in diagnosing malignant liver disease is still under discussion and comparative studies are not conclusive (Jacobsen et al 1983, Pagani 1983, Haaga et al 1983). However, the difference in morbidity rates and the fact that an inconclusive FNAB can be repeated without adding any significant risk to the patient, lead to the conclusion that FNAB is probably superior to conventional liver biopsy techniques in the evaluation of focal liver lesions. Coarse liver biopsy should probably only be performed in patients where the structural information is decisive, e.g. a biopsy of the non-tumourous liver in a patient with hepatocellular carcinoma to exclude underlying cirrhosis.

The technique of obtaining histological material using a fine, cutting needle is new, and it is too early to draw any firm conclusion and to determine its role versus traditional FNAB (Torp-Pedersen et al 1985).

REFERENCES

Benjamin I S 1983 Biliary tract obstruction. Surgical Gastroenterology 2: 105–120

Blumgart L H, Benjamin I S, Hadjis N S, Beazley R 1984 Surgical approaches to cholangiocarcinoma at confluence of hepatic ducts. Lancet i: 66–69

Bree R L, Jafri S Z H, Schwab R E, Farah J, Bernacki E G, Ellwood R A 1984 Abdominal fine needle aspiration biopsies with CT and ultrasound guidance: techniques, results and clinical implications. Computerized Radiology 8: 9–15

Chitwood W R, Meyers W C, Heaston D K, Herskovic A M, McLeod M E, Jones R S 1982 Diagnosis and treatment of primary extrahepatic bile duct tumours. American Journal of Surgery 143: 99–105

Christoffersen P, Poll P 1970 Peroperative pancreas aspiration biopsies. Acta Pathologica Microbiologica et Immunologica Scandinavica, Supplement 112: 28–32

Dalton-Clarke H J, Pearse E, Krause T, McPherson G A D, Benjamin I S, Blumgart L H 1986 Fine needle aspiration cytology and exfoliative biliary cytology in the diagnosis of hilar cholangiocarcinoma. European Journal of Surgical Oncology 12: 143–145

Droese M, Altmannsberger M, Kehl A, Lankish P G, Weiss R, Weber K, Osborn M 1984 Ultrasound-guided percutaneous fine needle aspiration biopsy of abdominal and retroperitoneal masses. Accuracy of cytology in the diagnosis of malignancy, cytologic tumour typing and use of antibodies to intermediate filaments in selected cases. Acta Cytologica 28: 368–384

Eklund P, Wasastjerna C 1971 Cytological identification of primary hepatic carcinoma cells. Acta Medica Scandinavica 189: 373–375

Evander A, Ihse I, Lunderquist A, Tylén U, Åkerman M 1978 Percutaneous cytodiagnosis of carcinoma of the pancreas and bile duct. Annals of Surgery 188: 90–92

Evander A, Fredlund P, Hoevels J, Ihse I, Bengmark S 1980 Evaluation of aggressive surgery for carcinoma of the extrahepatic bile ducts. Annals of Surgery 191: 23–29

Ferucci J T Jr, Wittenberg J, Mueller P R, Simeone J F, Harbin W P, Kirkpatrick R H, Taft P D 1980 Diagnosis of abdominal malignancy by radiologic fine needle aspiration. American Journal of Roentgenology 134: 323–330

Frola E 1935 Etude clinique l'etat functionnel du foie par la ponction hepatique. Presse Medicale 43: 1198–1202

Franzen S, Giertz G, Zajicek I 1960 Cytological diagnosis of prostatic tumours by transrectal aspiration biopsy — a preliminary report. British Journal of Urology 32: 193–196

Goldman M L, Naib Z M, Galambos J T, Rude J C, Oen K-T, Bradley E L, Salam A, Gonzales A C 1977 Preoperative diagnosis of pancreatic carcinoma by percutaneous aspiration biopsy. Digestive Diseases and Sciences 22: 1076–1082

Goldstein H M, Zornoza J 1978 Percutaneous transperitoneal aspiration biopsy of pancreatic masses. Digestive Diseases and Sciences 23: 840–843

Grønvall S 1985 Diagnostic and therapeutic puncture of intraabdominal fluid collections. In: Holm H H, Kristensen J K (eds) Interventional ultrasound. Munksgaard, Copenhagen, p 154–159

Haaga J R, LiPuma J P, Bryan P J, Balsara V J, Cohen A M 1983 Clinical comparison of small- and large-caliber cutting needles for biopsy. Radiology 146: 665–667

Hancke S 1981 Ultrasound in the diagnosis of pancreatic cancer. Scanning and percutaneous fine needle biopsy. Almquist and Wiksell, Stockholm

Hancke S, Holm H H, Koch F 1984 Ultrasonically guided puncture of solid pancreatic mass lesions. Ultrasound in Medicine and Biology 19: 613–615

Haubek A 1985 Puncture of focal liver lesions. In: Holm H H, Kristensen J K (eds) 1985 Interventional ultrasound. Munksgaard, Copenhagen, p 43–53

Ho C-S, McLaughlin M J, McHattie J D, Tao L-C 1977 Percutaneous fine needle aspiration biopsy of the pancreas following endoscopic retrograde cholangio-pancreatography. Radiology 125: 351–353

Ho C S, McLoughlin M J, Tao L C, Blendis L, Evans W K 1981 Guided percutaneous fine needle aspiration biopsy of the liver. Cancer 47: 1781–1785

Holm H H, Kristensen J K (eds) 1985a Interventional ultrasound. Munksgaard, Copenhagen

Holm H H, Torp-Pedersen S, Larsen T, Juul N 1985b Percutaneous fine needle biopsy. Clinics in Gastroenterology 14: 423–449

Hovdenak N, Lees W R, Pereira J, Beilby J O W, Cotton P B 1982 Ultrasound-guided percutaneous fine-needle aspiration cytology in pancreatic cancer. British Medical Journal 285: 1183–1184

Jacobsen G K, Gammelgaard J, Fuglø M 1983 Coarse needle biopsy versus fine needle aspiration biopsy in the diagnosis of focal lesions of the liver. Ultrasonically guided needle biopsy in suspected hepatic malignancy. Acta Cytologica 27: 152–156

Johansen P, Svendsen K 1978 Scan-guided fine-needle aspiration

biopsy in malignant hepatic disease. Acta Cytologica 22: 292–296
Knowles D M II, Wolff M 1976 Focal nodular hyperplasia of the liver: a clinicopathologic study and review of the literature. Human Pathology 7:533
Livraghi T, Damascelli B, Lombardi C, Spagoli I 1983 Risk in fine needle abdominal biopsy. Journal of Clinical Ultrasound 11: 77–79
Lopes Cordozo P 1954 Clinical cytology. Stafleu, Leiden
Longmire W P, McArthur M, Basounis E, Hiatt J 1973 Carcinoma of the extrahepatic biliary tract. Annals of Surgery 178: 333–345
Lundquist A 1970a Fine needle aspiration biopsy for cytodiagnosis of malignant tumour of the liver. Acta Medica Scandinavica 188: 465–470
Lundquist A 1970b Liver biopsy with a needle of 0.7 mm outer diameter. Acta Medica Scandinavica 188: 471–474
Martin H E, Ellis E B 1930 Biopsy by needle puncture and aspiration. Annals of Surgery 92: 169–181
McLoughlin M J, Ho C S, Langer B, McHattie J, Tao L C 1978 Fine needle aspiration biopsy of malignant lesions in and around the pancreas. Cancer 41: 2413–2419
Menghini G 1970 One-second biopsy of the liver — problems of its clinical application. New England Journal of Medicine 283: 582–584
Mitty H A, Efremidis S C, Yeh H C 1981 Impact of fine-needle biopsy on management of patients with carcinoma of the pancreas. American Journal of Roentgenology 137: 1119–1121
Montali G, Solbiati L, Croce F, Ierace T, Ravetto C 1982 Fine-needle aspiration biopsy of liver focal lesions ultrasonically guided with a real-time probe. Report of 126 cases. British Journal of Radiology 55: 717–723
Oscarson J, Stormby N, Sundgren R 1972 Selective angiography in fine-needle aspiration cytodiagnosis of gastric and pancreatic tumours. Acta Radiologica 12: 737–749
Pagani J J 1983 Biopsy of focal hepatic lesions. Comparison of 18 and 22 Gauge needles. Radiology 147: 673–675
Perrault J, McGill D B, Ott B J, Taylor W F 1978 Liver biopsy: complications in 1000 patients. Gastroenterology 74: 102–106
Rosenblatt R, Kutcher R, Moussouris H F, Schrieber K, Koss L G 1982 Sonographically guided fine-needle aspiration of liver lesions. Journal of the American Medical Association 248: 1639–1641
Ryd W, Hagmar B, Eriksson O 1983 Local tumour cell seeding by fine-needle aspiration biopsy: a semiquantitative study. Acta Pathologica Microbiologica et Immunologica Scandinavica 91(A): 17–21
Schwerk W B, Schmitz-Moormann P 1981 Ultrasonically guided fine-needle biopsies in neoplastic liver disease: cytohistologic diagnosis and echo pattern of lesions. Cancer 48: 1469–1477
Schwerk W B, Dürr H K, Schmitz-Moormann P 1983 Ultrasound guided fine-needle biopsies in pancreatic and hepatic neoplasms. Gastrointestinal Radiology 8: 219–225
Smith E H 1985 Fine needle aspiration biopsy: are there any risks? In: Holm H H, Kristensen J K (eds) Interventional ultrasound. Munksgaard Copenhagen, p 169–177
Solbiati L, Livraghi T, De Pia L, Ierace T, Masciadri N, Ravetto C 1985 Fine-needle biopsy of hepatic hemangioma with sonographic guidance. American Journal of Roentgenology 144: 471–474
Stormby N 1979 Pancreas. Monographs in Clinical Cytology 7: 194–211
Söderström N 1966 Fine needle aspiration biopsy. Grune and Stratton, New York
Søreide O, Skaarland E, Pedersen O M, Larssen T B, Arnesjö B 1985 Fine needle biopsy of the pancreas. Results of 204 biopsies in 190 patients. World Journal of Surgery 9: 960–965
Tao L C, Ho C S, McLaughlin M J, Evans W K, Donat E E 1984 Cytologic diagnosis of hepatocellular carcinoma by fine-needle aspiration biopsy. Cancer 53: 547–552
Tatsuta M, Yamamoto R, Kasugai H, Okano Y, Noguchi S, Okuda S, Wada A, Tamuta H 1984 Cytohistologic diagnosis of neoplasms of the liver by ultrasonically guided fine-needle aspiration biopsy. Cancer 54: 1682–1686
Thompson J N, Gibson R, Czerniak A, Blumgart L H 1985 Focal liver lesions: a plan for management. British Medical Journal 290: 1643–1645
Torp-Pedersen S, Juul N, Vyberg M 1984 Histological sampling with a 23 gauge modified Menghini-needle. British Journal of Radiology 57: 151–154
Tylen U, Arnesjö B, Lindberg L G, Lunderquist A, Åkerman M 1976 Percutaneous biopsy of carcinoma of the pancreas guided by angiography. Surgery, Gynecology and Obstetrics 142: 737–739
Wasastjerna C 1969 A cytochemical method for the study of bile canaliculi in fine needle aspirates of the liver. Acta Pathologica Microbiologica et Immunologica Scandinavica 77: 399–404
Wasastjerna C 1979 6. Liver. In: Zajicek J Aspiration biopsy cytology. Part 2: Cytology of infradiaphragmatic organs. S Karger, Basel, p 167–192
Webb A J 1974 Through a glass darkly. (The development of needle aspiration biopsy). Bristol Medico-Chirurgical Journal 89: 59–68
Whitlach S, Nuñez C, Pitlik D A 1984 Fine needle aspiration biopsy of the liver. A study of 102 consecutive cases. Acta Cytologica 28: 719–725
Yamanaka T, Kimura K 1979 Differential diagnosis of pancreatic mass lesions with percutaneous fine-needle aspiration biopsy under ultrasonic guidance. Digestive Disease and Sciences 24: 694–699
Zornoza J 1981 Percutaneous needle biopsy. Williams and Williams Baltimore

25

I. S. Benjamin, L. H. Blumgart

Assessment of diagnostic techniques for biliary obstruction and liver masses

INTRODUCTION

Much of this work has been devoted to diagnostic techniques used in the investigation of liver and biliary tract disorders. Advances in both the understanding of disease processes and of radiological and other techniques have made available to the clinician a rich selection of investigative procedures. Choice of the appropriate procedure for each case will depend to a large extent on the availability of individual investigative modalities in each centre. However, it is important that a systematic approach be developed, particularly for the commonly occurring clinical syndromes, in order to optimize the use of diagnostic facilities and to strike a balance between the goal of accurate preoperative diagnosis and overuse of investigations which are often invasive and expensive. The object of this chapter is to outline, for a number of clinical situations, an approach which has proved valuable to the authors in practice. For more detailed consideration of the use of individual diagnostic techniques the reader is referred to the appropriate chapters.

It is perhaps important at the outset to justify the use of extensive investigation in patients who are likely ultimately to require operative management. Firstly, even in the most straightforward case there are exceptions to a clinically obvious diagnosis. In some cases this may be of little consequence, since confirmation of the diagnosis will be sought and readily obtained at laparotomy, e.g. in a patient with cholelithiasis it is not usually necessary to determine preoperatively whether there are or are not stones in the common bile duct. However, there may be cases in which laparotomy may be positively contraindicated, as in the case of the elderly patient who presents with jaundice and who has cholelithiasis based on ultrasound evidence, but whose jaundice is not obstructive in nature and is due to active hepatitis. In such a case, operation may be injurious to the patient, and such management would amount to a return to the procedure of 'diagnostic laparotomy' for jaundice which was widespread practice less than two decades ago. Furthermore, establishment of the cause of biliary tract obstruction is by no means always straightforward at laparotomy, and this is especially so when the problem is an incomplete stricture in the upper parts of the biliary tree. While standard textbook descriptions suggest that diagnosis in such cases can be established by ductal exploration with choledochoscopy and biopsy, this is by no means always easy or successful, and it is not uncommon to receive cases for evaluation in whom no satisfactory diagnosis has been reached following surgical exploration even by experienced surgeons. Finally, preoperative diagnosis is valuable in permitting planning of a treatment strategy which takes account of such factors as the patient's general condition, the presence of benign or malignant disease, the extent of the disease process, its amenability to operative correction, and the availability of alternative non-operative methods of management. Such full preoperative diagnosis will also facilitate informed discussion with the patient and his relatives, and allow a reasonable assessment of the prognosis, operative risks and therapeutic alternatives. Using these approaches it is now rare in our practice to undertake treatment without full preoperative information regarding the presence or absence of malignant disease and the likelihood of resectability: e.g. in 94 cases of hilar cholangiocarcinoma, it was established preoperatively that there was an irresectable tumour in 64 cases, and at laparotomy in the remaining 30 patients, it was possible to proceed with resection in 18 cases (Blumgart et al 1984).

It is important to state that not only the nature of the disease, particularly in the case of biliary tract obstruction, but also its extent, the condition of the liver, the presence or absence of cirrhosis or the atrophy/hyperplasia complex (Ch. 6), and the patient's general condition with regard to nutritional status, sepsis and other potential risk factors must each form a part of the complete diagnosis before surgery in the liver and biliary tract is undertaken, and this should be the objective in every case of major biliary and hepatic pathology.

In this chapter two categories of diagnostic problems will be considered: biliary tract obstruction and the intrahepatic mass.

BILIARY OBSTRUCTION

Introduction

Approaches to diagnosis must consider the concepts of incomplete biliary obstruction in addition to the more straightforward case of obstructive jaundice (Ch. 10). The majority of approaches to biliary obstruction now rely heavily upon radiological imaging techniques. However, non-imaging methods remain important in initial assessment of these patients. A careful and thorough *history* and examination may suggest the diagnosis in a proportion of patients with biliary tract obstruction, and may direct the sequence of radiological investigations. In the case of patients presenting with jaundice *de novo*, it is well established that progressive painless jaundice is frequently associated with malignant biliary obstruction, although in our experience pain is common both with pancreatic cancer and with hilar biliary tumours, pain being a feature in 27 of 94 patients with hilar cholangiocarcinoma in our series (Blumgart et al 1984). Pain was also a feature in more than half of the patients with carcinoma of the gallbladder seen at Hammersmith Hospital. Similarly, obstruction due to previously undetected gallstones may be painless. Nevertheless, a long history of symptoms consistent with biliary tract pain prior to the onset of obstructive jaundice is still strongly suggestive of benign biliary tract disease. In the *postcholecystectomy patient*, a history of the previous surgery is particularly important. Examination of previous hospital records is valuable but not always possible, and it is important to question the patient specifically as to the use of external drainage tubes after the operation, the presence of prolonged or high volume external biliary drainage, and the presence of major infective episodes after surgery. A history of gastrointestinal bleeding in this situation may also suggest the complication of portal hypertension, and may dictate the use of endoscopy and angiography (Ch. 58).

Examination is important, and should be repeated when appropriate to elicit valuable transient or intermittent signs, such as an intermittently palpable gallbladder associated with periampullary tumours (Blumgart & Kennedy 1973). It is also important to seek the stigmata of chronic hepatocellular failure (such as palmar erythema or spider naevi): such signs may suggest the secondary effects of prolonged and severe biliary tract obstruction, but should also raise the suspicion of unrelated intrinsic parenchymal liver disease (Ch. 7).

Standard *biochemical testing* is performed as a routine in all cases of suspected biliary disease. It has been noted elsewhere in this book that such tests are inevitably non-specific, and may be of more value in following the course of a disease after treatment than in providing diagnostic information. However, minor changes in the liver enzymes, and in particular alkaline phosphatase, should not be ignored as they may on occasion be the only clue to continuing biliary tract pathology in the absence of jaundice or other biochemical abnormalities. It is not usually necessary to perform the more complex serological tests, such as auto-antibody estimations, unless there is a strong suspicion of intrinsic liver pathology. It may thus be possible to avoid the time and expense associated with such tests in the majority of cases. However, it is the authors' practice to carry out Hepatitis B antigen screening routinely for all new referrals: this is particularly important in patients from overseas, especially from areas where Hepatitis B is endemic. The use of clearance studies to assess liver function may be valuable in assessing the difficult case. Conventional dye clearances (using substances such as BSP or indocyanine green) are not indicated as a routine, but the use of antipyrine clearance as an index of hepatocellular oxidative capacity may be a potentially valuable prognostic indicator in patients undergoing major liver and biliary surgery (Ch. 10).

In the initial biochemical assessment of patients with biliary obstruction, assessment of the patient's general condition must include evaluation of *renal function* by means of creatinine clearance and of *nutritional status*. This can be crudely assessed by use of haemoglobin and albumin values, but if these are abnormal then a more sophisticated assessment of nutritional status may be indicated (Ch. 32).

It is important whenever possible to gain some initial assessment of the presence of *infection* in each patient. If there is external drainage from a tube or fistula this should be cultured immediately for both aerobic and anaerobic organisms. Patients who are febrile should also have culture of the blood before undertaking any investigation or treatment, and at every episode of invasive radiology involving entry to the biliary system, bile should be aspirated and cultured. The importance of having bacteriological information in advance of any septic episodes which may complicate the patient's course cannot be too strongly emphasized. This will both allow an informed choice of prophylactic antibiotics when indicated, and direct the clinician to appropriate therapy for infective complications (Ch. 11).

If the possibility of malignant disease is entertained but unproven then any aspirated bile should also be sent for cytological examination. We have found this valuable preoperatively in a number of patients with hilar cholangiocarcinoma (Dalton-Clarke et al 1986). The place of direct fine needle aspiration cytology is considered in relation to individual clinical problems below.

The nature and sequence of biliary imaging techniques and the decision to use angiography will depend upon the nature of the presentation and the presumed site of the problem within the biliary tract. These procedures will therefore be considered separately.

The jaundiced patient

In the majority of patients presenting initially with jaundice, a combination of clinical history and physical examination may reveal the diagnosis. The distinction between 'medical' and 'surgical' jaundice may be obvious in the majority of cases, but it is in the difficult case that a carefully ordered approach to diagnosis is important. Numerous algorithmic schemes have been described (e.g. Benjamin et al 1978, Karran et al 1985), and most now rely on ultrasound to detect the existence of dilated intra- or extrahepatic bile ducts. While the classical sign of 'surgical' jaundice has long been dilatation of the intrahepatic ducts, it is important to emphasize the exceptions to this finding. Biliary obstruction without ductal dilatation may be found in a significant proportion of cases — 16% in one series (Beinart et al 1981). Thus in the presence of a history and physical findings strongly suggestive of one of the variants of biliary obstruction, the finding of non-dilated intrahepatic ducts on ultrasound should not be taken to exclude extrahepatic biliary obstruction. It should on the other hand alert the clinician to the possibility of severe secondary biliary fibrosis or concomitant hepatic pathology. Conversely, ductal dilatation of a gross degree may occur in the presence of intermittent gallstone obstruction (Ch. 46). However, ductal dilatation should not be accepted as a normal finding, and a subtle or intermittent form of obstruction should always be sought in such cases.

As a means of determining the obstructive nature of jaundice *ultrasound* has held pride of place for several years, and an accuracy of greater than 90% may be achieved (Koenigsberg et al 1979, Ferrucci et al 1983). However, with advances in ultrasound equipment definition of the *level of obstruction* is also possible in the majority of patients. In a recent prospective study in our own hospital ultrasound was able to define the level of obstruction correctly in 95% of 65 patients with biliary obstruction (Gibson et al 1985). This was at least as good and possibly superior to the performance of CT in this prospective series, with a prediction level of 90%. Moreover, ultrasound produced valuable diagnostic information in the majority of cases, and was able to distinguish with 88% accuracy between benign and malignant aetiology, again somewhat better than the performance of CT scanning (63%). Detection of cholelithiasis is of course very reliable with ultrasound examination, although small bile duct stones, particularly lying in the distal biliary tree, still pose difficulties. All of these advances have raised the possibility that surgeons might be prepared to operate on the evidence of ultrasound alone in the presence of obstructive jaundice. Eyre-Brook and his colleagues (1983) showed a 95% correct interpretation of ultrasound scanning in 132 patients who underwent laparotomy for jaundice. These authors concluded that it was safe to proceed directly to surgery only when an experienced ultrasonographer has demonstrated findings 'typical' of distal common bile duct obstruction due to gallstones or tumour. We would concur with this view, although we advocate duodenoscopy prior to operation in order to detect unsuspected periampullary tumours, and we would further emphasize the importance of full biliary imaging, particularly for cases of proximal obstruction. It is also important not to assume that in the presence of ultrasonographically demonstrated biliary calculi, obstruction is due to this cause. There is of course a strong association between cholelithiasis and gallbladder carcinoma, and a less definite but noteworthy association with ductal cholangiocarcinoma in our experience (33 of 84 cases for whom clear data were available). Notwithstanding this rather guarded approach, it must be stated that advances in both the technology and the operator's skill in diagnostic ultrasound have been dramatic and are continuing. In our own prospective series ultrasound was in fact as accurate in predicting the cause of obstruction as direct cholangiography (88% and 89% respectively), so that there are certainly cases in which percutaneous or retrograde cholangiography may be omitted, thus avoiding a small but significant complication rate (Ch. 19).

If ultrasonography is not satisfactory or incompletely diagnostic, the choice lies between retrograde (ERC) and percutaneous (PTC) *cholangiography* as the next diagnostic test. We have generally preferred percutaneous cholangiography for cases of proximal bile duct obstruction and ERC/ERCP for cases with suspected distal obstruction. There have been published controlled studies comparing the value of these two modalities (Elias et al 1976, Matzen et al 1982). Such comparisons however are not particularly helpful in clinical practice. The tests are complementary and the order in which they are performed will usually be defined by the experience and expertise of the institution. Either technique will have a success rate of 70–90% and each has its specific advantages and contraindications. PTC is contraindicated in patients with severely deranged coagulation, although in our experience this has not been a major problem, and can usually be overcome by the use of fresh frozen plasma and platelet infusion at the time of the investigation. The only recent case of haemorrhage following PTC in our practice was in a patient with normal coagulation. Gross ascites is a more important contraindication, particularly in the presence of gross biliary obstruction, because of the risk of diffuse biliary peritonitis. ERCP on the other hand may fail to obtain full visualization of the proximal intrahepatic biliary tree, particularly when there is asymmetrical stricturing at the hilus. Some operators have used balloon catheters to overcome this problem, but we prefer the percutaneous route to obtain complete evaluation of the intrahepatic biliary tree in this situation. The chief advantage of ERCP is that it allows visualization of the periampullary region and also pancreatography in a majority of cases. This is particularly helpful when periampullary tumours or iatrogenic choledochoduodenal fistulae are suspected, and also when obstruction may be due to adenocarcinoma of the pancreas or to chronic pancreatitis. Advantages claimed for either technique on the basis of availability of interventional methods are probably irrelevant, since the choice of the route of biliary intubation will usually depend upon local practice and experience. The exception to this is the availability of endoscopic papillotomy as an option for patients with choledocholithiasis, and for this reason ERCP is preferred when necessary in cases of gallstone obstruction (Ch. 35).

Angiography is of value in the patient with biliary obstruction due to tumour. Its use in assessment of resectability for tumours of the extrahepatic biliary tree is considered in Chapters 64 & 65. Until recently we have used angiography in all potentially resectable cases in order to define the arterial anatomy and particularly to assess tumour involvement, especially of the portal vein. However, more recently the advances in ultrasonography referred to above have allowed us to avoid angiography in some patients. Our results have suggested that good quality ultrasound is at least as accurate as indirect portography in predicting tumour involvement of the portal vein and its main branches. However, if ultrasound visualization of the portal vein is not technically adequate then angiography with indirect portography is indicated (Gibson et al 1985). In the case of distally placed tumours, particularly those of the pancreatic head, irresectability may be inferred from the existence of arterial encasement as well as venous involvement. Ultrasound is less reliable in our experience at demonstrating tumour involvement of arteries than of large veins, so that in such cases arteriography may still be indicated. The specific cases of hilar and of distal obstruction are further considered below.

Thus, in summary, in our approach to the jaundiced patient detailed ultrasonography is the key to accurate diagnosis. In cases where distal bile duct obstruction due to a clearly demonstrated pancreatic tumour or to uncomplicated cholelithiasis and choledocholithiasis has been demonstrated, ultrasound may be the only preoperative imaging required. However, in our practice this constitutes a minority of cases, and usually direct biliary imaging is undertaken. The choice of ERCP or PTC depends upon the probable site of the lesion, and on any contraindications present. Occasionally both modalities are required (Benjamin et al 1978). If ultrasound shows no evidence of biliary obstruction or any other suspicious pathology, and if the clinical history, physical examination and biochemical investigations are consistent with the possibility of a non-obstructive cause of the jaundice, we would then proceed to percutaneous liver biopsy, if indicated. We regard the use of needle biopsy of the liver without prior demonstration of non-dilated ducts on ultrasonography as a potentially hazardous procedure, and do not recommend its use in this manner in the jaundiced patient (Benjamin et al 1977, Conn 1975).

Hilar obstruction

Obstruction of the confluence of the hepatic ducts in the absence of previous surgery is commonly due to tumour, arising in the bile ducts or gallbladder or secondary to tumour elsewhere within or outside the liver. Thus, when biliary obstruction at this level has been identified by ultrasonography, the direction of investigation should be towards elucidating the nature and extent of a potentially malignant process. It has been noted that ultrasonography may define adequately the level of the lesion and suggest its malignant nature in the majority of cases. Ultrasound is not so effective in our experience in defining intrahepatic extension of tumour. Involvement of second order hepatic ducts in the intrahepatic biliary tree (an important indicator of irresectability, Ch. 65) was underestimated in almost 50% of cases in our recent prospective study (Gibson et al 1985). Thus, biliary contrast imaging is almost always required in hilar obstruction, and PTC is the preferred approach. When the obstruction is complete it may be necessary to use ERC to define the lower end of the stricture, although in cases where ultrasonography has been adequate this may not be an essential step. It is important to allow time to elapse and to carry out delayed films with the patient tilted head up before accepting that there is a complete obstruction at the confluence of the hepatic ducts. When there is separation of the right and left hepatic ductal systems, separate punctures may be necessary in order to obtain complete imaging, which is mandatory in assessment of these cases (Ch. 19). It is important to note the significant sub-group of patients with hilar cholangiocarcinoma who present without jaundice, and in whom PTC demonstrates unilateral segmental hepatic duct obstruction (Hadjis et al 1986).

Carcinoma of the gallbladder causing hilar obstruction may produce specific subtle cholangiographic signs, particularly distortion of the intrahepatic bile ducts of segment V (Collier et al 1984a). Metastatic tumour or filling defects due to primary hepatocellular carcinoma have specific features which are discussed in Chapter 19. Ultrasound may also be valuable in demonstrating the features of an extraductal hilar mass or loose tumour within the biliary system, while PTC may identify the rare cases of polypoid tumours within the hilar ductal system. This distinction may be important because of the possibility of local excision or curettage with a relatively good prognosis (Gouma et al 1984).

At the time of PTC, bile should be aspirated both for bacteriological and cytological examination. In our experience in a small number of such cases exfoliative cytology was positive in 73%, with no false positive results. This was somewhat inferior to fine needle aspiration cytology which was positive in 95% of cases (including both preoperative and operative specimens). Thus it may be valuable to obtain fine needle aspiration cytology using PTC for guidance, or at the time of ultrasonography in cases where a hilar mass is demonstrated (Dalton-Clarke et al 1986 (Ch. 24, 65).

As noted above, it has been our practice in the past to carry out angiography in all cases of cholangiocarcinoma thought at initial ultrasound and PTC to be potentially resectable (Voyles et al 1983). A combination of cholangiography and angiography gives a high degree of definition of irresectability of hilar tumours (Ch. 65). However, it may now be possible to rely more upon high quality ultrasound and avoid angiography in certain cases.

The role of CT scanning in assessment of hilar cholangiocarcinoma remains undetermined. Importantly it is valuable for demonstrating lobar or segmental atrophy of the liver, although this is often suggested on cholangiography. CT was inferior in our experience in demonstrating the cause and level of biliary obstruction, and indeed in defining the malignant nature of the lesion. Contrast enhanced CT was inferior to ultrasound in defining portal venous involvement by tumour, a situation in which paradoxically ultrasound proved more accurate than indirect portography in a number of cases (Gibson et al 1985). Involvement by tumour of the caudate lobe (segment I) has been an area of considerable difficulty in assessing resectability of hilar tumours. CT scanning in theory might be valuable for defining this area preoperatively, but this has rarely proved to be the case in our experience and this remains a 'blind spot' in preoperative evaluation.

It is extremely important to note the incidence of cases in which there is an apparent tumour at the hilus of the liver which proves to be due to a benign cause. Cholangiography and ultrasonography may define patients with the Mirizzi syndrome (Koehler et al 1979) preoperatively, and should be suspected when gallstones are seen in a shrunken gallbladder in association with a hilar obstruction. However, we have now seen a number of cases of localized sclerosing cholangitis (Smadja et al 1983) and other benign strictures not associated with gallstones (Hadjis et al 1985) 'masquerading' as hilar cholangiocarcinomas. It is critically important to define such cases, particularly when non-surgical methods of treatment such as biliary endoprosthesis are proposed, since it may often be impossible to define the benign nature of these lesions without surgical resection (Ch. 65).

In summary, when dealing with a hilar obstruction we would recommend fine needle PTC in the majority of cases as the investigation to follow ultrasonography. Complete cholangiography is essential, and this may require several passes and occasionally subsequent ERC. Bile must be obtained for culture and cytology, and in selected cases fine needle aspiration cytology of the hilar region is also valuable. In potentially resectable cases of hilar malignancy the presence or absence of vascular involvement should be established, and if this cannot be achieved by high quality ultrasound then angiography is indicated. It is important to be wary of the benign stricture presenting as a possible hilar malignancy. The specific case of benign postcholecystectomy strictures is considered below.

Distal obstruction

Ultrasonography will usually define the level of obstruction, although duodenal gas may make precise definition of obstructions of the distal bile duct difficult. ERCP should be performed unless contraindicated on anatomical grounds or because of recent incompletely resolved pancreatitis or pancreatic cyst formation. Careful attention should be paid during endoscopy to the first and second parts of the duodenum as evidence of choledochoduodenal fistulation may be found. The papilla should be inspected carefully, and biopsies and both brush and aspiration cytology should be carried out if there is any suspicion at all of periampullary or pancreatic malignancy. Cholangiography should be as complete as possible, if necessary by use of a balloon catheter if the obstruction is higher than originally suspected. Pancreatography should also be obtained wherever possible. The option of endoscopic papillotomy has already been mentioned.

A combination of ultrasound and ERCP may adequately define a malignant obstruction of the distal bile duct or may demonstrate a clearly benign cause such as cholelithiasis. Further investigation is indicated in two situations: firstly, when the presence of malignancy cannot be confirmed or excluded, and secondly when a malignant lesion has been shown which is potentially resectable. In the first instance, cytology may prove helpful. The difficult situation is that in which an obstruction is shown in the intrapancreatic portion of the distal bile duct in association with pancreatic ductal changes which may be due to chronic pancreatitis or pancreatic cancer. The appearances of distal bile duct strictures due to pancreatitis have been well described (Scott et al 1977), the classical feature being a long smooth stricture through the pancreatic head. Obstruction due to a pancreatic cyst may also occur and should normally have been defined by ultrasonography and ERCP avoided. In cases where the dilemma persists, particularly when ultrasonography has demonstrated a mass in the pancreatic head, then further definition by means of CT scanning may be valuable. Fine needle aspiration of a pancreatic head mass should be performed (Ch. 24). Angiography may be valuable both in demonstrating portal venous occlusion (which is non-specific and may occur with chronic pancreatitis) and regional arterial encasement (which rarely occurs in benign disease). It is not always possible positively to exclude malignancy, but if the history is consistent with obstruction due to chronic pancreatitis then a period of observation may be warranted provided jaundice (if present) is resolving. There remains a small and difficult group of patients in whom laparotomy and possibly 'blind' resection may be the final arbiter of the diagnosis. In one large series from a centre in which operative biopsy of the pancreas is avoided whenever possible, a radical resection was often performed based on clinical judgement alone, and in this series 8% of resections performed proved to be for chronic pancreatitis (Lee 1982).

When malignancy has been demonstrated, assessment of resectability will depend on evidence of spread beyond the limits of normal resection margins or on the invasion of local structures, particularly the portal vein. A combination of ultrasonography, CT scanning and angiography will define the majority of such cases. In cases of periampullary carcinoma we do not normally perform angiography since portal venous involvement is very rare. It had been our practice in the past to carry out angiography in order to define those patients in whom a hepatic artery accessory to or replacing the right hepatic artery arises from the superior mesenteric artery passing behind the head of the pancreas (Ch. 3). However, this can be avoided when ultrasound is of sufficient quality to demonstrate the presence of such a vessel.

In summary, ERCP is preferred for patients with distal obstruction, and the objective is to define the presence of malignancy, preferably with cytological or biopsy diagnosis. Angiography may be required in selected cases, to help define resectability, although this can often be achieved by ultrasound alone.

Postcholecystectomy patients

It is important at the outset to say that while some 10–40% of patients suffer symptoms following cholecystectomy, many of these are unrelated to the biliary tract, and only a minority of patients have symptoms related to biliary tract obstruction. However, unless a positive diagnosis is achieved implicating factors outwith the biliary tract, the possibility of retained common bile duct stones, benign stricture formation, a biliary-enteric fistula, one of the variety of periampullary problems, or an undisclosed biliary or periampullary tumour must be sought (Ch. 55).

As with several other types of biliary problem, the use of ultrasound as an intial non-invasive and extremely versatile diagnostic technique may be recommended. If fistulae or indwelling biliary tubes are present then these should be used to obtain fistulograms or tubograms, although often in such cases direct cholangiography may be required because of incomplete imaging. Endoscopy is mandatory in investigation of the postcholecystectomy patient, since a high proportion of patients may have a lesion identified by endoscopy alone. It may be valuable to perform both end-viewing and side-viewing endoscopy to ensure a complete examination, but if this is to be combined with ERCP then two separate sessions may be necessary. ERCP remains the lynchpin of diagnosis in this group of patients. Care must be taken to exclude iatrogenic biliary-enteric fistula, which may be responsible for persistent late symptoms (Blumgart et al 1977, Hunt & Blumgart 1980). Others have recognized these choledochoduodenal fistulae but have questioned their importance as a clinical problem (Martin & Tweedle 1984).

If a benign iatrogenic bile duct stricture is encountered at ERCP, it may be necessary also to undertake PTC to obtain full cholangiography. Stenosis of the papilla of Vater secondary to surgical interference or instrumentation may be difficult to diagnose, and failed cannulation at ERCP may suggest this: in such cases also PTC may be necessary. We have abandoned the use of intravenous cholangiography entirely for investigation of these patients. The findings are rarely diagnostic and a negative investigation may be seriously misleading.

Cholangitis

The classic case of acute cholangitis, with fever, rigors and jaundice, may require little investigation. Blood cultures are mandatory, preferably before commencing antibiotic therapy, but biliary imaging is not necessarily indicated in the emergency situation. Ultrasonography may again be of value in defining the state of dilatation of the biliary tree. In the absence of any preceding history, surgery or other known biliary lesion, primary cholangitis is usually associated with choledocholithiasis, and this may be demonstrated by ultrasound. If biliary imaging is undertaken, this should be done under full antibiotic cover and with a readiness to undertake a drainage procedure if necessary. Bile should be aspirated either at ERCP or at PTC before any volume of contrast is injected into the already distended and inflamed biliary tree. There have been recent reports of improved mortality and morbidity by means of endoscopic papillotomy for gallstone related suppurative cholangitis (Costamagna et al 1985), though the debate as to whether endoscopic or surgical methods are indicated is beyond the scope of this chapter. For the present purpose however it must be stated that, in cases with suppurative cholangitis and unrelieved obstruction, minimal diagnostic intervention should be used and urgent biliary drainage following adequate resuscitation is the only effective approach (Ch. 72).

Intermittent attacks of cholangitis of a less clamant nature may be associated with the follow-up of patients with known incomplete biliary obstruction or may occur in the course of follow-up in patients following biliary-enteric reconstruction for malignant or benign disease. It is known that the biliary tree may take months to years to return to normal structure and function, following biliary bypass of a long-standing stricture. Episodes of recurrent cholangitis should be carefully investigated since progressive intrahepatic changes may have serious consequences (Ch. 58). In this context we have found HIDA scanning particularly valuable, especially in patients with a persistently elevated alkaline phosphatase. If HIDA scans show normal curves of hepatic uptake and biliary-enteric excretion then invasive cholangiography may be avoided. If symptoms persist, even in the face of a normal HIDA scan, then direct cholangiography is essential. It has already been noted that intravenous contrast agents invariably produce insufficient biliary definition to be of value in this context. When the biliary bypass is in the form of a choledochoduodenostomy or sphincteroplasty then endoscopic cholangiography may be applicable. However, when there is an hepaticojejunostomy then fine needle PTC cannot be avoided. It may be difficult to distinguish in these cases small filling defects due to debris or intrahepatic stones from air bubbles, and this investigation requires a careful technique and an experienced radiologist. The investigation may also take considerable time with re-positioning of the patient in order to elucidate these features fully. Full cholangiography is important since segmental obstructions may give rise to cholangitis in the absence of jaundice or HIDA scanning abnormalities.

In *sclerosing cholangitis* ERCP and PTC may be required several times during the course of the disease to monitor its progress. Repeated investigation is not necessary in the relatively asymptomatic patient, but may be important in the patient with progressive symptoms since in some cases a dominant stricture in the extrahepatic biliary tract may be the principal cause of obstruction and bypass above this level may allow a long symptom-free period before advancement of intrahepatic disease causes further relapse. Most other imaging modalities are useless in this situation.

Benign iatrogenic biliary stricture (Ch. 58)

Many of these patients present as postcholecystectomy problems, so that ERCP may be performed early in the diagnosis of chronic strictures. The high stricture is usually not delineated by ERCP since most strictures are a result of disruption of the common bile duct. PTC is usually the only means of obtaining cholangiography. All separately obstructed segments should be identified at PTC. There is no difficulty in the decision to investigate such patients by direct cholangiography. The use of angiography in patients with benign hilar strictures is, however, less widespread. There is an incidence of portal hypertension in benign iatrogenic biliary stricture of up to 20%, due in part to secondary hepatic fibrotic changes and in part to direct trauma to the hilar vessels. We have restricted the use of angiography in this situation to selected groups of patients: 1. those with a history of major bleeding at the time of initial operation, suggestive of vascular damage; 2. those with a history of gastrointestinal haemorrhage suggestive of portal hypertension with oesophageal varices; 3. patients with splenomegaly detected clinically or on scanning, or those with oesophagogastric varices seen on routine endoscopy; 4. those with established lobar atrophy on cholangiography or on ultrasound or CT scanning. The previous comments on ultrasonography as a means of vascular assessment also apply in this situation, although local postoperative fibrotic changes make interpretation more difficult. If there is any doubt, and particularly if there is evidence of the atrophy/hypertrophy complex with rotation of the liver, then angiography may be essential both for full diagnosis and as a guide to the best surgical approach. These cases are at the extreme of the range of successful treatment by any surgeon, and this is a situation which should be treated in a specialist centre.

Some patients with chronic incomplete bile duct strictures may merit needle biopsy of the liver to define the degree of hepatic damage before undertaking surgery.

THE LIVER MASS

Patients may present with a mass in the epigastrium or in the right upper quadrant thought to be arising from the liver, either initially, or quite commonly as part of the investigation of known or suspected malignant disease elswhere, and particularly in the gastrointestinal tract. As with the investigation of biliary tract obstruction discussed above, in the majority of cases the diagnosis may be evident at an early stage, but there are numerous pitfalls and exceptions, so that an ordered approach to investigation is advised. It is important to state at the outset that we do not recommend immediate percutaneous needle biopsy of a liver mass at an early stage of investigation. This point will be justified and emphasized below, but it is an essential point of departure in discussing the approach to investigation of the liver mass, since in many non-specialist units biopsy may be considered to be the most direct route to complete diagnosis. For the present it must be stated that we believe that biopsy of focal liver lesions is not only often unhelpful to the management of these patients, but does carry the risk of serious and sometimes life-threatening complications and may also jeopardize subsequent curative treatment.

Clinical assessment

Abdominal palpation will normally have revealed already the presence of a suspected liver mass. It is not necessary to detail the steps required for a full clinical examination of the patient, but the clinician should direct his attention to the following points in particular: jaundice, signs of hepatocellular insufficiency and of collateral circulation, nutritional impairment, lymphadenopathy, abnormal chest signs, cutaneous or ano-rectal malignancies or mucocutaneous angiomata. In the abdomen attention should be paid to the mass itself, whether it is regular or irregular, whether there is a palpable or ballottable gallbladder, separate masses within the abdomen, splenomegaly, or ascites. A bruit may be audible in some cases of haemangioma, arterio-venous malformation or malignant liver tumour. It must be remembered that not all masses suspected of being intrahepatic on presentation and even on initial investigation prove to arise from the liver (Collier et al 1984b): we have seen duodenal, renal, and adrenal tumours as well as retroperitoneal sarcomas and a leiomyosarcoma of the inferior vena cava present in this manner. While it may not always be possible to identify these clinically, one may sometimes palpate a plane of cleavage between the mass and the liver which moves with respiration. However, some masses which appear separate are in fact pedunculated liver tumours, e.g. arising from the lower margin of the quadrate lobe (segment IV).

Biochemistry

Full initial screening of haematological and biochemical parameters will normally be performed. Hepatitis B antigen screening is carried out as a routine, particularly in view of the association between primary hepatocellular carcinoma and hepatitis B. More specialized tests will naturally reflect the previous experience and referral pattern of an individual unit. However, we perform as a routine alpha-fetoprotein and carcino-embryonic antigen estimation, and in appropriate cases blood samples are also taken for hydatid serology, and fasting bloods for hormone levels in case the lesion is a primary or secondary endocrine tumour. In addition, we estimate plasma neurotensin and serum vitamin B12 binding capacity because these are useful tumour markers for the fibrolamellar variant of hepatocellular carcinoma (Paradinas et al 1982, Collier et al 1984c). It is not of course necessary to await the results of these specialized investigations before proceeding with further diagnostic evaluation.

Radiological imaging

Further investigation of the liver mass may most usefully follow an algorithmic approach. The procedures adopted will be different depending on whether hepatic lesions are thought to be focal or multicentric, and whether they are cystic or solid. Thus, the first investigation will normally be ultrasonography which will permit early separation into cystic or solid lesions and will also exclude large bile duct obstruction. In the majority of cases it will also exclude multiple hepatic lesions. In the very obese patient or where overlying bowel gas obscures ultrasonography then CT scanning may be necessary at an early stage. We have recently published an algorithmic approach to investigation of the focal liver lesion, and the diagrammatic representation of these procedures is shown in Fig. 25.1 and 25.2 (Thompson et al 1985). While these diagrams are largely self-explanatory certain points deserve special emphasis.

Most haemangiomata are diagnosed with confidence on CT scanning, particularly with the use of rapid sequence scanning after intravenous contrast. However, not all haemangiomas produce the typical appearances of enhancement commencing peripherally, and in particular small and involuting haemangiomas may have atypical appearances both on CT and ultrasound. Indeed, not all enhancing lesions are haemangiomata and primary malignant liver tumours may have a very similar appearance. In this situation percutaneous biopsy may result in life-threatening haemorrhage and we have been forced to operate four times in the last year following such a biopsy at a referring hospital. When there is doubt, angiography may resolve the difficulty, but on occasions direct visualization at laparoscopy or mini-laparotomy (Ch. 23, 26) may be necessary finally to confirm the diagnosis.

Patients must be routinely assessed for evidence of extrahepatic secondary tumour by clinical findings (as noted above), chest X-ray, and where appropriate a radionucleide bone scan. Upper and lower gastrointestinal endoscopy or barium studies and mammography in female patients may be valuable in the patient with a single liver secondary. Our major indication for angiography is a proven solitary solid lesion with no evidence of primary tumour elsewhere and no other sites of secondary spread. However, this is only necessary if the patient's general condition suggests that he will be a candidate for hepatic resection. We now rarely use hepatic isotope scanning because the level of resolution with CT scanning is greater. We have a growing experience with Nuclear Magnetic Resonance, but the place of this investigation is not yet well defined. Moreover, with the present technology it remains a very time-consuming procedure with the possiblity of scanning only limited regions of interest. However, it has been useful in differentiating between tumour and fatty infiltration in some cases (Ch. 17). In patients who proceed to angiography multiple tumours not detected on ultrasound or CT scanning may occasionally be found, or a mass may give the characteristic appearances of a haemangioma. In patients with lesions close to the inferior vena cava we also perform inferior vena cavography at the time of angiography, since compression or invasion of the cava may be found. This information is of value at operation (Ch. 97).

Biopsy (Ch. 22, 23, 26)

A combination of the investigations outlined will normally determine whether a solitary liver lesion requires and is

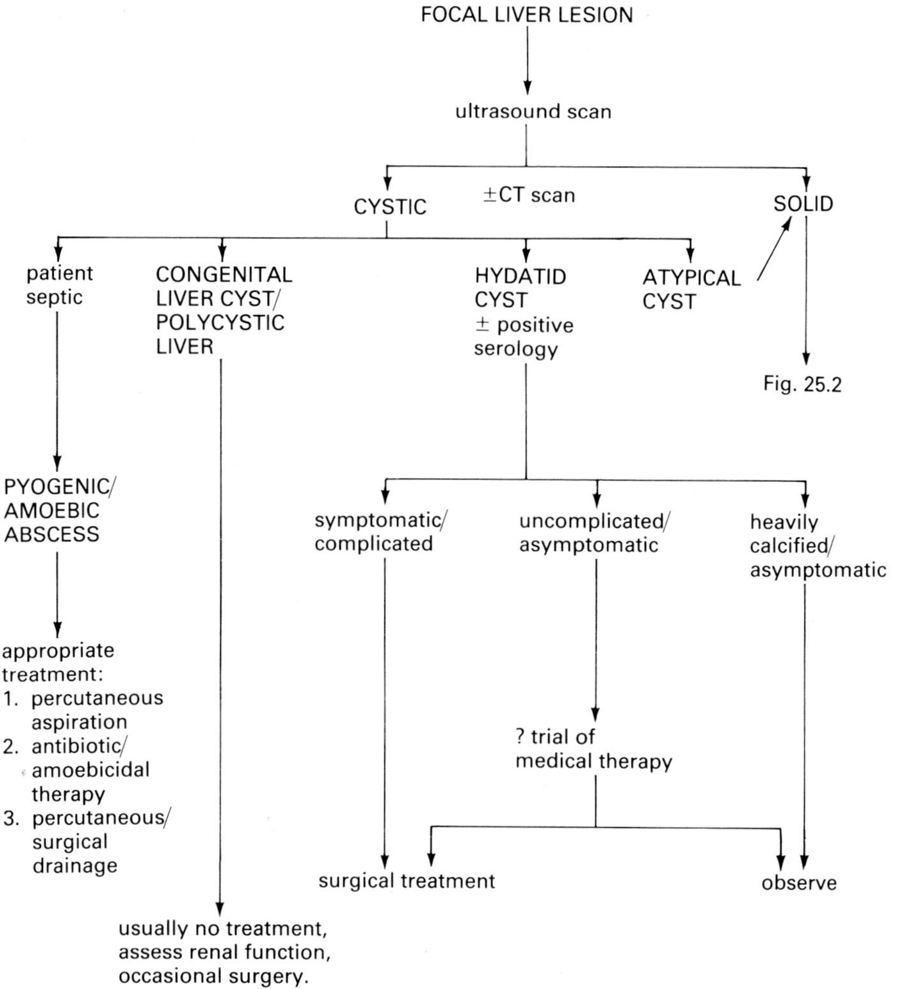

Fig. 25.1 An algorithm for investigation of the suspected focal liver lesion: management of lesions found to be cystic on ultrasound.

amenable to surgical resection in an eligible patient. In this case it is not normally necessary to obtain the formal tissue diagnosis until the time of laparotomy. However, in certain circumstances for resectable lesions and in cases where pathological confirmation is necessary in patients with a contraindication to resection, then the choice lies between percutaneous fine needle aspiration cytology (under ultrasound or CT guidance unless the tumour is readily palpable) or needle biopsy using the Tru-cut needle. If needle biopsy is to be undertaken, we prefer to use visual control by means of laparoscopy. This allows accurate localization of the biopsy into tumour tissue, which is best approached through uninvolved liver. Occasionally, needle biopsy may be performed under ultrasound guidance. In patients with primary hepatocellular carcinoma, it may be valuable to perform biopsy of the *uninvolved* liver in order to determine the possibility of cirrhosis, as this is a relative contraindication to major hepatic resection. There may be some advantages to biopsy during angiography, since immediate embolization is then possible should major haemorrhage occur. It is also now possible to perform direct embolization of a needle biopsy track (D J Allison, personal communication).

It has already been stated that we avoid early biopsy of focal hepatic lesions until their nature and extent has been adequately defined. The complication rate of percutaneous liver biopsy clearly varies from one centre to another, and will reflect the type of patients undergoing investigation. A complication rate of some 6% has been reported in a series of 1000 liver biopsies recently (Perrault et al 1978). Complications are likely to be higher in biopsies done for focal lesions than those done predominantly for elucidation of cirrhosis or hepatocellular disorders, though it is difficult to acquire evidence from the reported literature to support such an assumption. Biopsy is obviously contraindicated in those with an audible bruit and those who have highly vascular tumours on investigation, and in suspected hydatid disease. The risk of tumour dissemination by liver biopsy must be small but finite. Fine needle aspiration cytology appears to carry less risk than needle biopsy (Ferrucci et al 1980), but we have seen one case of primary hepatocellular carcinoma in which tumour seeding

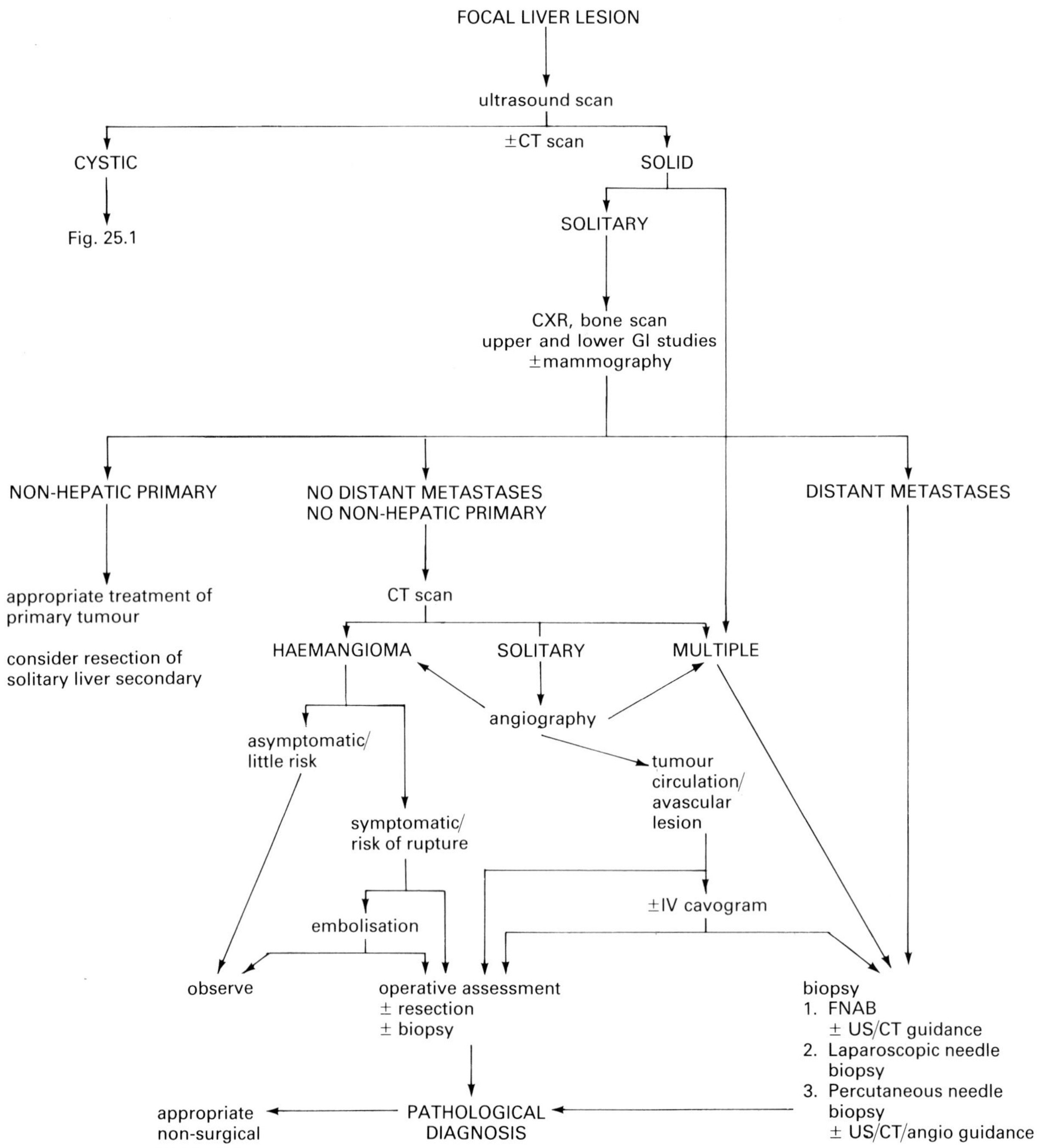

Fig. 25.2 As Fig. 25.1, but for lesions found to be solid on ultrasound.

occurred and progressed rapidly at the site of an aspiration cytology needle track. False-negatives may occur in up to one-third of cases of fine needle aspiration for focal liver lesions (Zornoza et al 1980), and an experienced cytologist is required. There are some potential benefits to pre-operative cytological and histological biopsy. On occasion laparotomy may be avoided because of a firm diagnosis of a benign lesion, such as focal nodular hyperplasia or liver cell adenoma, although even for these benign tumours direct inspection is often indicated and resection may sometimes be required.

The relative place of laparoscopy and mini-laparotomy is discussed in Chapters 23 and 26.

Assessment of resectability

It is important to note that the criteria for resectability of solid hepatic tumours must be very carefully defined. Size alone, especially as seen at CT scanning, is rarely a contraindication to attempted resection of a solitary primary hepatocellular tumour (Ch. 97). Moreover, multiple colonic secondary deposits confined to one hepatic lobe do not contraindicate resection, and the criteria for potentially curative surgery have to be considered carefully in this light (Ch. 92).

The management plan outlined in these algorithms has proved a useful guide in the management of focal liver lesions in a Unit where the principal referral practice is of potentially resectable tumours. Any such algorithm must be viewed in the context of the individual surgical practice, and must be modified in that light. However, as with other areas of hepatic, biliary and pancreatic surgery, and tumours in particular, complete and accurate preoperative diagnosis is the key to rational and successful management.

REFERENCES

Beinart C, Efremedis S, Cohen B, Mitty H A 1981 Obstruction without dilation. Importance in evaluating jaundice. Journal of the American Medical Association 245: 353–356

Benjamin I S, Imrie C W, Blumgart L H 1977 Liver biopsy in 'difficult' jaundice. British Medical Journal (ii): 578

Benjamin I S, Allison M E M, Moule B, Blumgart L H 1978 The early use of fine needle percutaneous transhepatic cholangiography in an approach to the diagnosis of jaundice in a surgical unit. British Journal of Surgery 65: 92–98

Blumgart L H, Kennedy A 1973 Carcinoma of the ampulla of Vater and duodenum. British Journal of Surgery 60: 33–40

Blumgart L H, Carachi R, Imrie C W, Benjamin I S, Duncan J G 1977 Diagnosis and management of postcholecystectomy symptoms — the place of endoscopy and retrograde choledochopancreatography (ERCP). British Journal of Surgery 64: 809–816

Blumgart L H, Benjamin I S, Hadjis N S, Beazley R M 1984 Surgical approaches to cholangiocarcinoma at the confluence of hepatic ducts. Lancet i: 66–70

Collier N A, Bloom S R, Hodgson H J F, Weinbren K, Lee Y C, Blumgart L H 1984a Neurotensin secretion by fibrolamellar carcinoma of the liver. Lancet i: 538–540

Collier N A, Carr D, Hemingway A, Blumgart L H 1984b Preoperative diagnosis and its effect on the treatment of carcinoma of the gallbladder. Surgery, Gynecology and Obstetrics 159: 465–470

Collier N A, Allison D J, Vermess M, Blumgart L H 1984c Right upper quadrant abdominal masses mimicking hepatic tumours: an approach to management. Australian and New Zealand Journal of Surgery 54: 113–118

Conn H 0 1975 Liver biopsies in extrahepatic biliary obstruction and other 'contraindicated' disorders. Gastroenterology 68: 817–821

Costamagna G, Nuzzo G, Coppola R, Colosimo C Jnr, Luna R, Colagrande C, Puglionisi A 1985 Urgent endoscopic decompression of the bile ducts for acute cholangitis. Chirurgia Epatobiliare 4: 25–31

Dalton-Clarke H J, McPherson G A D, Pearse E, Krause T, Benjamin I S, Blumgart L H 1986 Fine-needle aspiration cytology and exfoliative biliary cytology in the diagnosis of hilar cholangiocarcinoma. European Journal of Surgical Oncology 12: 143–145

Elias E, Hamlyn A N, Jain S et al 1976 A randomized trial of percutaneous transhepatic cholangiography with the Chiba needle versus endoscopic retrograde cholangiography for bile duct visualisation in jaundice. Gastroenterology 71: 439–443

Eyre-Brook I A, Ross B, Johnson A G 1983 Should surgeons operate on the evidence of ultrasound alone in jaundiced patients? British Journal of Surgery 70: 587–589

Ferrucci J T, Wittenberg J, Mueller P R et al 1980 Diagnosis of abdominal malignancy by radiologic fine-needle aspiration biopsy. American Journal of Radiology 134: 323–330

Ferrucci J T, Adson M A, Mueller P R, Stanley R J, Stewart E T 1983 Advances in the radiology of jaundice: a symposium and review. American Journal of Radiology 141: 1–20

Gibson R N, Yeung E, Thompson J N, Carr D H, Hemingway A P, Bradpiece H A, Benjamin I S, Blumgart L H, Allison D J 1986 Bile duct obstruction: radiologic evaluation of level, cause and tumour resectability. Radiology 160: 43–47

Gouma D J, Mutum S S, Benjamin I S, Blumgart L H 1984 Intrahepatic biliary papillomatosis. British Journal of Surgery 71: 72–74

Hadjis N S, Collier N A, Blumgart L H 1985 Malignant masquerade at the hilum of the liver. British Journal of Surgery 72: 659–661

Hadjis N S, Benjamin I S, Blenkharn J I, Blumgart L H 1987 Anicteric presentation of hilar cholangiocarcinoma: anatomical and pathological considerations. Digestive Surgery (submitted for publication)

Hunt D R, Blumgart L H 1980 Iatrogenic choledochoduodenal fistula: an unsuspected cause of postcholecystectomy symptoms. British Journal of Surgery 67: 10–13

Karran S, Dewbury K C, Wright R 1985 Investigation of the jaundiced patient. In: Wright R, Alberti K G M M, Karran S, Millward-Sadler G D T (eds) Liver and biliary disease: Pathophysiology, diagnosis, management 2nd edn. Saunders, London, Ch. 27, p 647–658

Koehler R E, Melson G L, Lee J K T, Long L 1979 Common hepatic duct obstruction by cystic duct stone: Mirizzi syndrome American Journal of Roentgenology 132: 1007

Koenigsberg M, Wiener S N, Walzer A 1979 The accuracy of sonography in the differential diagnosis of obstructive jaundice: a comparison with cholangiography. Radiology 133: 157–165

Lee Y T N 1982 Tissue diagnosis for carcinoma of the pancreas and periampullary structures. Cancer 49: 1035–1039

Martin D F, Tweedle D E F 1984 The aetiology and significance of distal choledochoduodenal fistula. British Journal of Surgery 71: 632–634

Matzen P, Malchow-Moller A, Lejerstofte J, Stage P, Juhl E 1982 Endoscopic retrograde cholangiopancreatography and transhepatic cholangiography in patients with suspected obstructive jaundice. A randomized study. Scandinavian Journal of Gastroenterology 17: 731–735

Paradinas F J, Melia W M, Wilkinson M L et al 1982 High serum vitamin B12 binding capacity as a marker of the fibrolamellar variant of hepatocellular carcinoma. British Medical Journal 285: 840–842

Perrault J, McGill D B, Ott B J, Taylor W F 1978 Liver biopsy: complications in 1000 inpatients and outpatients. Gastroenterology 74: 103–106

Scott J, Summerfield J A, Elias E, Dick R, Sherlock S 1977 Chronic pancreatitis: a cause of cholestasis. Gut 18: 196–201

Smadja C, Bowley N B, Benjamin I S, Blumgart L H 1983 Idiopathic localized bile duct strictures: relationship to primary sclerosing cholangitis. American Journal of Surgery 146: 404–408

Thompson J N, Gibson R N, Czerniak A, Blumgart L H 1985 Focal liver lesions: a plan for management. British Medical Journal 290: 1643–1645

Voyles C R, Bowley N B, Allison D J, Benjamin I S, Blumgart L H 1983 Carcinoma of the proximal extrahepatic biliary tree. Radiological assessment and therapeutic alternatives. Annals of Surgery 197: 188–194

Zornoza J, Wallace S, Ordonez N, Lukeman J 1980 Fine-needle aspiration biopsy of the liver. American Journal of Radiology 134: 331–334

Operative diagnostic techniques

N. A. Collier, L. H. Blumgart

Laparotomy and mini-laparotomy

INTRODUCTION

Over the past decade there has been a rapid development of new radiological and endoscopic techniques in the diagnosis of hepatobiliary and pancreatic disease. These techniques usually lead to an accurate diagnosis preoperatively without the need to resort to exploratory laparotomy. This has resulted in a change in emphasis in the diagnostic approach to liver and biliary disease which has been particularly marked in the investigation of obstructive jaundice (Ch. 25).

The range of techniques developed by the interventional radiologist and endoscopist has not only led to improved diagnosis, but also to a variety of non-operative therapeutic options in the management of hepatobiliary diseases. However, there remain significant problems with interventional radiological techniques, partly related to inappropriate selection and partly to the intrinsic dangers such as bleeding, bile leakage and tumour dissemination which may follow percutaneous needling of the liver. Variation in individual technical skills and the availability of equipment will to a large degree determine the preoperative investigations used and the choice of non-operative approaches to therapy.

Clinicians in peripheral hospitals often face the difficult decision of whether to deal with a potentially complex problem with limited investigation or to refer a patient to a specialist centre. It is in this situation that the experience and judgement of the clinician is of major importance. A well-timed exploratory laparotomy may resolve diagnostic uncertainty and save the patient the anxiety of a possibly unnecessary referral to another hospital. Clinicians must also consider cost factors when determining patient management. The expense of sophisticated tests must be balanced against the likely benefit to the patient. Routinely used multiple imaging modalities will prolong hospital stay without necessarily obtaining additional diagnostic information. In selected patients, short-circuiting of the investigation process and early laparotomy may not only produce rapid diagnosis and a shortened hospital stay but also avoid some of the more invasive and potentially dangerous investigations.

There is little doubt that the indications for exploratory laparotomy and mini-laparotomy have contracted with the recent advances in radiological and endoscopic techniques. This chapter attempts to define the place of laparotomy and mini-laparotomy and discusses both indications and techniques. The intraoperative investigations which may be carried out are also described with particular reference to the use of aspiration cytology in the diagnosis of malignant disease of the liver and biliary tract.

INDICATIONS

Obstructive jaundice

There is no longer any place for diagnostic laparotomy in differentiating intrahepatic from extrahepatic cholestasis and operation in these circumstances may not only fail to yield a diagnosis but also carry a significant risk (Blumgart 1978). By assessment of the clinical features, liver biochemical tests and abdominal ultrasonography, accurate differentiation between extrahepatic and intrahepatic cholestasis should be achieved in nearly 100% of cases (Benjamin & Blumgart 1979) (Ch. 25).

Once mechanical obstruction to the biliary tree is confirmed, further investigation should be directed at determining the level, degree and nature of the biliary obstruction. Before the introduction of fine needle percutaneous cholangiography (Okuda et al 1974) and endoscopic retrograde cholangiography (McCune et al 1968, Oi 1970), contrast studies performed to outline the biliary tree were inaccurate and often dangerous. Intravenous cholangiography rarely gave diagnostic information and now should no longer be used.

Before the introduction of the fine needle technique, and because of the risk of biliary peritonitis after percutaneous cholangiography, mini-laparotomy combined with open transhepatic cholangiography became popular in the early 1970s (Strack et al 1971, Stein 1975). This method provided a high diagnostic yield with low morbidity as the needle puncture site on the liver surface could be controlled. Stein et al (1977) reported successful cholangiography in 134 of 148 patients (91%) and, in 95 patients with dilated ducts, the biliary system was demonstrated in all but one. The procedure was combined with finger exploration of the surface of the liver, gallbladder and porta hepatis and with needle liver biopsy. Postoperative bile leakage occurred in only one patient and a correct diagnosis was achieved in 92% of patients. Further operation was avoided in 24 patients because of the finding of non-operable disease.

The reported advantages of this technique were rapid diagnosis with shortened hospital stay, using a procedure which could be performed under local anaesthetic and in the presence of abnormal clotting studies. In practice, fine needle percutaneous transhepatic cholangiography (PTC) has virtually replaced open cholangiography. In most patients in whom PTC is unsuccessful either because of technical factors such as non-dilated ducts or cirrhosis, or where the risk is too high because of grossly deranged clotting or marked ascites, endoscopic retrograde cholangiopancreatography (ERCP) will yield diagnostic information. Mini-laparotomy and cholangiography should be reserved for those few patients in whom ERCP fails or is impossible or for the rare instances when the risks of percutaneous liver biopsy and cholangiography are considered too high.

Another method by which the bile ducts may be outlined is by insertion of a needle through the right lobe of the liver and into the hepatic surface of the gallbladder, guided under vision by laparoscopy (Berci et al 1973). This approach, although reported to carry a low morbidity, has been largely superseded by percutaneous 'blind' techniques. The major drawback of transhepatic cholecystography is that unless there is obstruction of the common bile duct below the level of the cystic duct, filling of the intrahepatic biliary tree is often inadequate.

In some instances of obstructive jaundice, preliminary laparotomy may be used to assess resectability of a malignant obstructing lesion and to combine the procedure with preliminary biliary decompression. This approach has been used particularly for malignant obstruction of the distal common bile duct due to carcinoma of the pancreas, ampulla or duodenum. Whipple, when describing his original pancreatico-duodenectomy (Whipple et al 1935), recognized the dangers of undertaking major resective surgery in the presence of obstructive jaundice. He described an initial assessment of the tumour at laparotomy combined with a cholecysto-gastrostomy to relieve jaundice before proceeding to definitive resection. The disadvantage of this approach is that the initial laparotomy carries a significant morbidity and mortality related to the effects of obstructive jaundice. Benjamin (1981) reported a pooled mortality rate of 21.9% for eight series reported between 1970 and 1979 in which simple biliary bypass had been carried out for irresectable pancreatic and periampullary cancers. The morbidity and mortality result largely from the effects of renal impairment, clotting abnormalities, increased susceptibility to infection and hypoalbuminaemia. Braasch & Gray (1977) showed that the incidence of postoperative haemorrhage, renal failure and death were related to the depth of jaundice at the time of surgery.

Hopes that the use of non-operative biliary decompression, as a precursor to surgery in obstructive jaundice, would reduce the complication and death rate related to the definitive procedure have yet to be borne out by controlled clinical trials of percutaneous transhepatic intubation (McPherson et al 1984, Hatfield et al 1982), although endoscopic intubation especially for low bile duct obstruction may well prove valuable (Ch. 69). Nevertheless a two-stage approach to malignant obstruction of the distal bile duct still has a place in selected patients. In the younger patient with a potentially resectable lesion of the

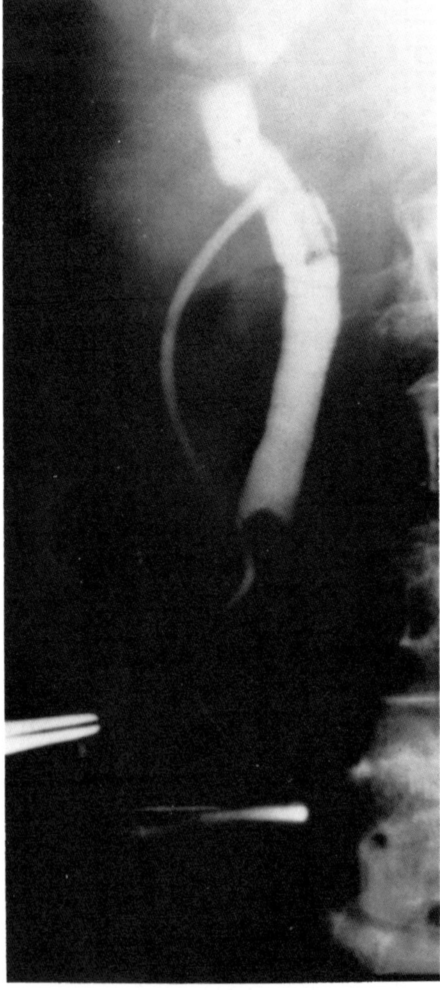

Fig. 26.1 T-tube inserted in the common bile duct above an obstructing ampullary carcinoma. The tumour was excised transduodenally at a second procedure

pancreas or ampulla, every effort should be made to achieve complete tumour clearance as this appears to be the only possible way of prolonging survival. If any adverse factors such as malnutrition, infection or renal dysfunction are present then preliminary laparotomy with tumour assessment and either T–tube biliary drainage (Fig. 26.1) or simple biliary-enteric bypass should be considered as an initial procedure. If this can be performed safely, resection can be delayed for several weeks to months until the patient's condition has improved to a point where resection can be carried out.

Primary liver tumours

Though primary liver cancer is rare in Western patients, thorough assessment of such patients is essential as successful resection can be followed by excellent long term survival. Adson & Weiland (1981) have reported three, five and ten year survival rates of patients surviving resection of primary malignant liver lesions of 65%, 36%, and 33% respectively. The preoperative investigation of such patients may include the use of laparoscopy, mini-laparotomy or laparotomy to confirm the histological diagnosis and to assess resectability (Blumgart & Benjamin 1983).

A clinical situation which has become increasingly common is the finding of an unsuspected mass lesion during investigation for unrelated upper abdominal pathology, usually gallstones. The improved imaging obtained with grey-scale ultrasonography has been the major factor behind the increased rate of detection of liver lesions, as has the increased use of abdominal CT scan. The majority of such lesions will be of a benign nature, but once detected, they must be thoroughly investigated to rule out malignancy. A combination of ultrasound, CT scan and angiography may clarify the nature of the lesion, but in most cases will not differentiate a benign from a malignant condition (Fig. 26.2).

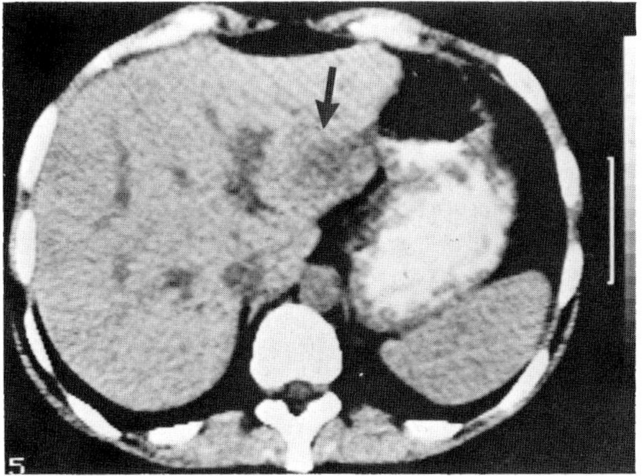

Fig. 26.2 Abdominal CT scan demonstrating a tumour in the left lobe of the liver (arrow). Left lobectomy was performed for an hepatic adenoma

Simple cysts, haematomas and echinococcal cysts can usually be defined by ultrasound alone. Capillary and cavernous haemangiomas, which are relatively common, may also show characteristic features on investigation. The larger lesions will show evidence of contrast pooling within venous lakes on angiography and on CT scanning intravenous contrast enhancement may demonstrate peripheral followed by central contrast pooling within the lesion. These changes, although characteristic, are not invariable and it is not uncommon for doubts to persist as to the nature of the lesion, even after thorough investigation. (Bernadino & Lewis 1982).

Other benign tumours such as areas of focal nodular hyperplasia and liver cell adenomas, although rare, may have a potential for malignant transformation and the adenomatous lesion particularly may be complicated by haemorrhage or necrosis (Foster 1982). Histological diagnosis is eventually required for most liver lesions whether symptomatic or discovered incidentally. This may be achieved by a number of methods. Percutaneous needle biopsy may be carried out blindly or guided by radiological imaging or laparoscopy. Alternatively, fine needle aspiration of the lesion may be carried out for cytological studies. Finally, open biopsy using either mini-laparotomy or laparotomy may be carried out; each of these approaches has relative merits and disadvantages.

Guided biopsy has the obvious advantage over blind needle puncture of accurate needle placement with a higher chance of a positive result. Using laparoscopy to perform guided biopsy has the added advantage over radiological techniques that areas of obvious surface vascularity may be avoided and the diathermy attachment of the laparoscope may be used to control minor haemorrhage. Also, further information may be obtained regarding the presence of tumour peritoneal seeding, retroperitoneal node enlargement and the extent of the primary tumour, thus assisting in the assessment of tumour resectability. The liver tissue not involved with tumour should be visualized and biopsied to rule out coincidental parenchymal liver disease.

The reported complication rate associated with fine needle liver aspiration is very low (Lundquist 1970, Ferrucci et al 1980). In contrast, the risks associated with the commonly used wider bore biopsy needles appear significant, particularly in the biopsy of vascular liver lesions (Ch. 22). Severe abdominal haemorrhage had occurred following percutaneous biopsy in four patients with liver tumours who were referred to the Hepatobiliary Unit, Hammersmith Hospital, in the past 12 months. If there is clinical evidence of hypervascularity of the lesion with an abdominal bruit, or where angiography indicates a vascular lesion, percutaneous biopsy should be avoided. The presence of ascites should also be considered a relative contraindication as abdominal wall tamponade of the puncture site will not occur. If percutaneous biopsy of a vascular lesion is imperative, biopsy at the time of angiography can be carried out and combined with arterial embolisation to reduce the risk of haemorrhage.

Another potential risk of biopsy is seeding of tumour along the biopsy track. This risk has been frequently reported following standard needle biopsy of a variety of organs including the lung, salivary glands, pancreas and prostate (Clarke et al 1953, Wolinsky & Lischner 1969, Berg & Robbins 1962). More recently, this complication has been reported after biopsy of a liver tumour (Sakurai et al 1983) and may also occur at the exit sites of percutaneous drains. Although reported after fine needle aspiration biopsy (Ferrucci et al 1979), malignant seeding appears to be a very small risk. Needle puncture of hydatid cysts carries a high risk of peritoneal seeding and anaphylaxis and these complications are avoidable by performing the relevant serological tests when hydatid disease is suspected.

We would therefore recommend the use of laparoscopy (Ch.23) as a useful addition to the investigations of malignant liver lesions. It is able to detect and accurately biopsy lesions only a few millimetres in size on the liver surface (Lightdale 1982). Up to 80% of the liver surface can be inspected and a good indication of the extent of any liver tumour can be obtained as well as detection of the presence of cirrhosis. There are, however, limitations to the use and effectiveness of laparoscopy where mini-laparotomy and laparotomy may provide substantially more information. When previous upper abdominal surgery has been performed, laparoscopy is rarely possible because of the presence of adhesions. Also deeply placed lesions or tumours originating from the caudate lobe will generally not be seen laparoscopically and if scanning and angiography have provided inadequate information, mini-laparotomy may be a useful means of obtaining additional evidence of resectability. Another clinical situation where mini-laparotomy is superior to laparotomy is in the differentiation between large retroperitoneal infra-hepatic masses and tumours arising from the liver. Large right hypochondrial lesions can produce pressure atrophy of the right or left lobe of the liver and give a scan appearance identical with that of a primary tumour (Collier et al 1984) (Fig. 26.3). Lesions such as renal, adrenal and other retroperitoneal tumours may obtain their blood supply partly from the hepatic artery and thus not be easily differentiated from liver tumours on angiographic studies. In this situation, mini-laparotomy will generally clarify the origin of the tumour.

The specific techniques involved in performing mini-laparotomy are discussed in the section below. With reference to the assessment of liver tumours, particular points of importance are the palpation of the coeliac and portal node areas, as thorough an exploration of the liver as can be obtained and wedge or needle biopsy of any liver lesion. A biopsy of the liver not involved with tumour is also mandatory so that cirrhosis may be ruled out.

The relative accuracy of laparotomy compared with other methods used in the diagnosis of hepatic tumours is difficult to assess. Before CT scanning became available, angiography and radioisotope scanning were the most accurate methods of non-operative diagnosis. Almersjo et al (1974) compared the accuracy of serum tests, angiography and scintigraphy with laparotomy in the diagnosis of hepatic tumours. They concluded that these preoperative diagnostic methods were considerably less accurate than laparotomy, and that laparotomy was superior in detecting small tumours and in determining resectability. More recently, Harbin et al (1980) have pointed out that the accuracy of CT scanning may exceed that of laparotomy, particularly in the diagnosis of deep-seated hepatic and retroperitoneal lesions. A balanced approach, making use of the advantages of new radiological techniques combined with prudent use of laparotomy, is likely to yield the highest rate of diagnosis with the maximum benefit to the patient (Williamson et al 1980).

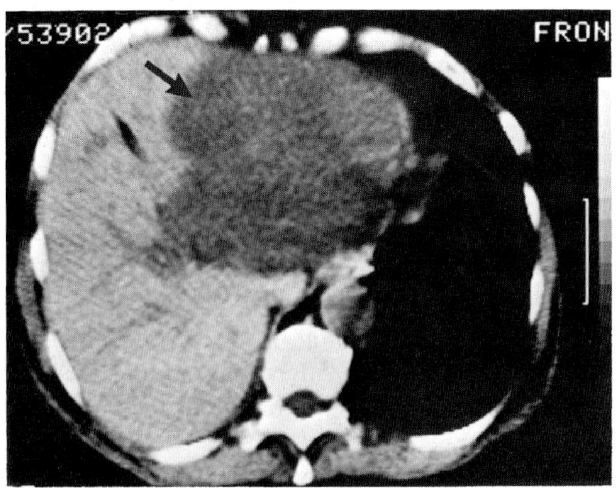

Fig. 26.3 Abdominal CT scan. The large circumscribed mass (arrow) was a leiomyosarcoma of the retroperitoneum with no liver invasion

Metastatic liver tumours

Laparotomy and mini-laparotomy have only limited use in the assessment of the resectability of metastatic liver tumours. There is rarely any need to obtain histological proof of the nature of the liver lesion, particularly for colorectal metastases when a previous abdominal exploration will have been performed. Thorough laparotomy is of course undertaken at the time of any definitive attempt at liver resection and occasionally, despite thorough investigation, it will be revealed that the tumour is not resectable because of bilateral liver metastases or extrahepatic tumour deposits.

The place of the so called 'second look' laparotomy following previous curative resection of a colorectal carcinoma is becoming increasingly recognized. Early detection of local tumour recurrence or solitary or localized liver metastases may increase the possibility of complete tumour clearance with possible prolongation of survival (Attiyeh & Stearns 1981). Frequent monitoring of the serum carcino-embryonic antigen (CEA) levels appears to be the best guide to the presence of tumour recurrence. Wood et al (1980) recognized two patterns of CEA elevation associated with recurrent colorectal cancer. They noted a 'fast' rise in serum concentrations of CEA in those patients with metastatic disease and more commonly a 'slow' rise in those with local recurrence alone. By monitoring CEA levels, Attiyeh & Stearns (1981) achieved a 43% resectability rate at second look laparotomy for recurrent colorectal cancer. This included seven 'curative' resections in the 18 patients found to have metastatic liver disease. Encouraging results in terms of prolongation of patient survival following liver resection for colorectal metastases (Ch. 92) suggest that a second look laparotomy, based on clinical or biochemical evidence of tumour recurrence, is a worthwhile proposition (Bengmark et al 1982).

The laparotomy assessment of the liver for metastatic disease does have limitations. To detect small metastases, palpation of the liver must be carried out meticulously using a bimanual technique with a hand above and below the liver gently compressing the liver substance in a systematic manner. Gray (1980) in a retrospective study showed that an incorrect negative assessment of the liver occurred in 6% of 116 patients with gastrointestinal cancer and in 8% the liver was incorrectly assessed as containing tumour. This and other studies (Pejchl & Chaloupka 1981) highlight the importance of operative biopsy of any suspected metastatic lesion and may explain the unexpected longevity of some patients with supposed liver metastases.

Portal hypertension

Visualization of portal venous anatomy is essential if portal-systemic shunting is being considered in cases of portal hypertension. The earliest portography was obtained by the open cannulation of a major intra-abdominal portal venous radicle (Moore & Bridenbaugh 1950). Strack et al (1971) described the use of omentoportography and portal pressure measurement at the time of mini-laparotomy investigation of portal hypertension. They were able not only to measure portal pressure but also to demonstrate patency of splenic and portal veins, assisting in the selection of patients suitable for portal-systemic shunting and the selection of the appropriate form of shunt. Omentoportography was also used to provide evidence of encroachment of the portal vein by periampullary cancer indicating tumour irresectability.

The advantage of open splenoportography was that direct splenic pulp injection could be avoided: this was particularly relevant in those patients with clotting abnormalities. The method used involved delivery of a segment of the greater curvature of the stomach through the mini-laparotomy wound and insertion of a catheter into a gastro-epiploic vein. Contrast material was then injected at a rate of 10 to 15 ml per sec and rapid interval X-rays obtained.

This method of assessment of portal venous anatomy has now been almost entirely superceded by newer angiographic techniques. Selective cannulation of the splenic artery and late venous phase films of the splenic arterial contrast injection will usually adequately demonstrate portal anatomy. If splenectomy has been performed then similar studies of the superior mesenteric artery will usually prove adequate. An alternative approach to indirect splenoportography is direct splenoportography by percutaneous puncture of the spleen and bolus contrast injection.

The newer methods of digital vascular imaging seem likely to further refine the non-operative methods of obtaining portal venography (Mistretta et al 1981). Only very rarely, when non-operative techniques have failed to visualize the portal system adequately, will open omentoportography be necessary. Also, when laparotomy or mini-laparotomy is being carried out for diagnostic purposes without prior angiographic studies, omentoportography may still have an occasional place.

Other indications

Chronic abdominal pain for which no cause can be found is a common and frustrating clinical problem. The use of exploratory laparotomy for undiagnosed upper abdominal pain remains a controversial subject. Laparotomy for pain in the presence of normal extensive investigations is usually futile and may lead to complications which cloud further assessment of the patient (Piedrahita & Butterfield 1976, Devor & Knauft 1968). If, on the other hand, objective clinical findings such as an abdominal mass or jaundice are present, then positive laparotomy findings are likely. With the use of newer imaging techniques such as CT scanning and ERCP, laparotomy except in the emergency situation should rarely be necessary without a clear picture of the probable diagnosis and the possible procedures which may need to be performed.

One circumstance where diagnosis can often be elusive is abdominal pain following a previous cholecystectomy, the so called 'post-cholecystectomy syndrome'. Although mini-laparotomy employing open transhepatic cholangiography, liver biopsy and omentoportography has been strongly recommended for the investigation of this syndrome in the past (Mehta & Del Guercio 1974), ERCP is now the investigation of first choice and combined with thorough gastrointestinal endoscopy is likely to produce a diagnosis in a large percentage of patients (Blumgart et al 1977) (Ch. 55). Diagnoses such as retained common bile

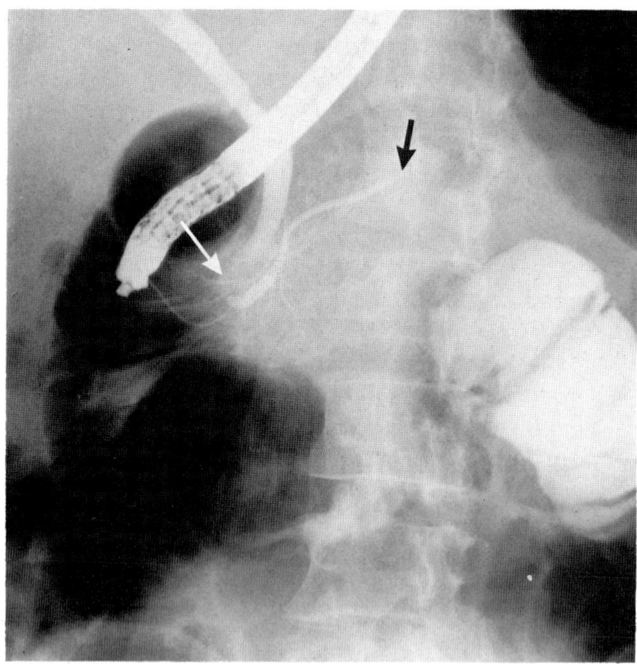

Fig. 26.4 ERCP in a patient with post-cholecystectomy pain. There is a choledocho-duodenal fistula (white arrow) and pancreatic duct obstruction (black arrow) due to a chronic pancreatitis

duct calculi, bile duct strictures, choledochoduodenal fistulae and pancreatic disease are now readily identified by ERCP (Fig. 26.4) which is now routinely available in most major centres (Ch. 20).

TECHNIQUE

Mini-laparotomy

A standard method of mini-laparotomy used to diagnose liver disease has been described by Strack et al (1971) and Stein (1975). Patients are fasted for six hours before the procedure and receive a standard premedication. A 4 to 5 cm midline sub-xyphoid incision is made using local anaesthesia. If the liver edge is palpable below this point, the incision is made at the liver edge. A short subcostal incision may be more appropriate for assessment of right lobe liver lesions.

If ascitic fluid is encountered, specimens are taken for cytological examination and for microbiology. The surface of the liver, gallbladder, and porta hepatis are examined as completely as is possible through the limited incision. Finger examination of the retroperitoneal node areas may also be possible as may palpation of the pancreas. A mediastinoscope can also be used to visualize the peritoneal cavity.

A wide range of intraoperative procedures are then possible, depending on the condition under investigation. Needle and wedge biopsies of any liver lesion can be obtained; biopsy of apparently normal liver may also give useful information. If open transhepatic cholangiography is being performed, a 20 gauge Teflon catheter with internal stilette is inserted through the surface of the liver aiming at the confluence of the bile ducts. This catheter is inserted for about 15 cm and then withdrawn progressively under fluoroscopic control while injecting 30% Urografin. If a bile duct is successfully entered, the biliary system is completely filled with contrast material while the fluoroscopic screening is continued. Plain radiographs are then taken concentrating on areas of interest or abnormality. The catheter is then withdrawn and the surface puncture site sutured with fine catgut.

Omentoportography, when required, can be performed by isolating a segment of the greater curvature of the stomach which can be delivered into the wound with a Babcock clamp. A suitable gastro-epiploic vein is cannulated using a fine umbilical catheter. Portal pressure is measured and contrast material is then injected under fluoroscopic control. A series of radiographs may be taken to display the relevant anatomical details with care being taken not to exceed the safe dosage of intravenous contrast. Any history of a contrast allergy will of course be a contraindication to this form of investigation.

A limited number of other intraoperative procedures may be possible. Aspiration biopsy of a pancreatic or bile duct mass may be performed as described below. Readily accessible lymph nodes can be biopsied although it is unwise to attempt any extensive dissection through the limited exposure afforded by the mini-laparotomy incision. More extensive procedures such as hepatic arterial ligation or cannulation are better performed through a formal laparotomy under general anaesthetic. If an inoperable tumour is encountered, metal clips may be placed to guide postoperative radiotherapy.

After the procedure the abdominal wall is closed with a non-absorbable mass suture technique. A layered closure may be preferred if ascites is present. Postoperatively the patient is usually able to eat on the same day and no special instructions are necessary. Using this technique Stein et al (1977) during the investigation of 168 patients were able to make a definitive diagnosis in 92%. Further operation was avoided in 24 patients because of the demonstration of non-operable disease. Two deaths occurred which may have been related to mini-laparotomy. One followed a biliary leak and another patient died of renal failure probably contributed to by the contrast load during cholangiography. Nineteen patients in the series had elevated prothrombin times but bleeding occurred in only two patients, neither serious, both of whom had normal prothrombin times. Strack et al (1971) in a series of 100 patients achieved a 100% rate of diagnosis. Complications included one case of bile leakage and one case of intra-abdominal bleeding. Two minor wound infections also occurred.

Finally should a situation be encountered which allows safe immediate definitive operation, the incision can be extended and the relevant surgery performed.

Laparotomy

The technical aspects of exploratory laparotomy in the investigation of hepatobiliary disease are in keeping with standard general surgical principles. Preoperatively, particular attention must be paid to abnormalities of blood coagulation, renal function, nutrition and hypoproteinaemia and awareness of the increased susceptibility to infection, of jaundiced patients in particular, should make the use of prophylactic antibiotics mandatory.

General anaesthesia in the presence of jaundice carries a significant risk of renal failure and the maintenance of a normal circulating blood volume combined with induced osmotic diuresis using mannitol will usually prevent this complication. Jaundiced patients will therefore require a urinary catheter at the commencement of the procedure. The abdominal incision will depend to some extent on the site and type of pathology under investigation. In general a right sub-costal or midline incision will provide adequate exposure. Particular attention to haemostasis must again be taken to avoid late wound complications.

Thorough abdominal exploration is then carried out. If it is apparent that another operative procedure will be necessary, perhaps at a referral centre, then excessive mobilization of organs such as the liver or pancreas should be avoided as this may compromise dissection at a later date. The liver is carefully assessed using bimanual palpation by systematically compressing the liver substance between a hand over the diaphragmatic surface and one placed beneath the liver. For this method to be complete and reliable it may be necessary to mobilize the triangular ligament of the liver, particularly on the right side (Ch. 97). In addition a full assessment of the liver demands that the lesser sac be opened and the caudate lobe digitally explored. This method when performed meticulously can detect small unsuspected lesions deep within the liver substance. Relevant biopsies are then taken using a needle or wedge technique. Thorough examination of all other organs is then carried out with particular reference to the porta hepatis, retroperitoneal lymph nodes and pancreas, which may involve widely opening the gastro-colic omentum for complete examination. Biopsy or aspiration cytology of suspected abnormalities is then taken and the abdominal wound is closed without drainage.

Complications such as wound and chest infection occur in all recorded series of laparotomies and are particularly common in high risk patients. Death from cardiovascular disease, pulmonary embolus, or renal failure provide a not insubstantial risk. Pollock (1981) prospectively recorded the incidence of complications and death following 1207 laparotomies: 122 deaths occurred following operation, 42 of which were due to preventable complications and 13 due to myocardial infarction or stroke. The dangers in jaundiced patients, as previously noted, are considerably higher. The risks of exploratory laparotomy must be viewed in perspective, taking into account the likely diagnostic yield and the relative danger to the patient.

Intraoperative cytology

Fine needle aspiration cytology is now used widely in the histological diagnosis of carcinoma of the breast. It has also been used in the investigation of prostatic, bone, renal, thyroid, skin and lymph node tumours (Melcher et al 1981).

Percutaneous fine needle aspiration is now also being widely practised in the investigation of hepatobiliary disease (Gompels & Pike 1979) (Ch. 24). Accurate placement of the aspiration needle using ultrasound guidance can achieve cytological diagnosis in a large percentage of cases of liver and pancreatic tumour. The intra operative use of fine needle aspiration biopsy has been less widely practised. Biopsy under vision can be obtained from most organs using either wedge or core cut techniques. The authors have used operative fine needle aspiration commonly in two circumstances. The first is in the investigation of pancreatic masses where core cut or wedge biopsy may be dangerous because of the complication of pancreatic fistula and haemorrhage. The second is in the investigation of suspected bile duct tumours where the tumour is either too small to allow incisional biopsy or is so placed that needle or incisional biopsy could lead to a high risk of bleeding or biliary fistula.

Technique is all important if adequate specimens are to be obtained which can be correctly interpreted by the cytologist. A disposable 10 or 20 ml syringe with a 21 gauge venepuncture needle is used. The cytology technician is present in the theatre at the time of specimen collection so that fresh cells can be immediately fixed for maximum preservation. The needle is inserted into the centre of the lump under investigation. The syringe plunger is withdrawn to create a negative pressure and without removing the needle from the lump, it is moved carefully through the tissues of the lump while the negative pressure on the syringe sucks cells into the lumen of the needle. The syringe plunger is released *before* the needle is withdrawn from the tissue. The syringe and needle are then handed to the cytologist who expels the contents of the needle on to a microscope slide for fixation and immediate examination.

This procedure may be repeated several times until an adequate specimen is obtained. Heavily blood stained specimens are technically unsatisfactory. If a large amount of fluid is aspirated either from the pancreatic duct or biliary system, this may be examined cytologically but is less likely to provide diagnostic material. Care should be taken to avoid puncturing a major blood vessel, in particular the portal vein behind the head of the pancreas or adjacent to a bile duct tumour. This cannot always be avoided and if portal puncture occurs, pressure should be applied until haemostasis ensues. Only one significant complication has occurred using this technique at the Hammersmith Hospital resulting in a temporary pancreatic fistula following direct needle aspiration of the pancreatic head. The pancreas may also be punctured through the medial wall of the second part of the duodenum decreasing the risk of fistula but for fine needle aspiration this measure is not usually necessary.

With careful attention to technique and with the back-up of a good cytologist, a high diagnostic yield may be achieved. In a study of 18 patients with suspected tumours in the hilus of the liver we were able to obtain positive aspiration cytological diagnosis in 13 out of 15. In the same group of patients the bile was examined in 17 and positive cytology was achieved in only eight (Dalton-Clark et al 1983). This technique is particularly applicable to hilar cholangiocarcinoma as the tumour is often inaccessible to normal biopsy methods and lies adjacent to major vascular structures making core cut or wedge biopsy dangerous.

CONCLUSIONS

Because of new radiological imaging techniques, there has been a change in the approach to the investigation of hepatobiliary disease. Mini-laparotomy and laparotomy, which in the past have been used to make up for the inadequacies of radiology, have now been displaced from their position of importance by sophisticated imaging techniques.

However, indications for laparotomy techniques still exist in selected cases. Where the necessary radiology is not available, where there are difficulties in analysis of films, if radiographs are of poor quality, or where adverse factors such as obesity or ascites are present, mini-laparotomy and laparotomy may provide additional useful information. A severe bleeding diathesis or dense upper abdominal adhesions will limit the use of percutaneous techniques and laparoscopy and an open method of investigation may be a necessary alternative.

A carefully timed laparotomy in a well selected patient may lead to rapid diagnosis with shortening of hospital stay and curtailment of prolonged and expensive investigation. The selection and timing of such an intervention invariably will depend on the experience and judgement of the surgeon, who must be aware of limitations and be prepared to act upon information obtained at an exploratory operation.

REFERENCES

Adson M A, Weiland L H 1981 Resection of primary solid hepatic tumors. American Journal of Surgery 141: 18–20

Almersjö O, Bengmark S, Hafstrom L O, Rosengren K 1974 Accuracy of diagnostic tools in malignant hepatic lesions. A comparative study using serum tests, angiography, scintiscanning and laparotomy. American Journal of Surgery 127: 663–668

Attiyeh F F, Stearns M W 1981 Second-look laparotomy based on CEA elevations in colorectal cancer. Cancer 47: 2119–2125

Bengmark S, Hafstrom L, Jeppsson B, Jonssoon P E, Ryden S, Sundqvist K 1982 Metastatic disease in the liver from colorectal cancer: an appraisal of liver surgery. World Journal of Surgery 6: 61–65

Benjamin I S 1981 Tumour and host: aims and decisions in pancreatic cancer. In: Cohn I Jr, Hastings P R (eds) Pancreatic cancer. U.I.C.C., Geneva

Benjamin I S, Blumgart L H 1979 Biliary bypass and reconstructive surgery. In: Wright R, Alberti K G M M, Karran S, Millward-Sadler G H (eds). Liver and biliary disease: Pathophysiology, diagnosis, management. W. B. Saunders, London, p 1219–1246

Berci G, Morgenstern L, Short J M, Shapiro S 1973 A direct approach to the differential diagnosis of jaundice. Laparoscopy with transhepatic cholecystocholangiography. American Journal of Surgery 126: 372–378

Berg J W, Robbins G F 1962 A late look at the safety of aspiration biopsy. Cancer 15: 826–827

Bernadino M E, Lewis E 1982 Imaging hepatic neoplasms. Cancer 50: 2666–2671

Blumgart L H 1978 Biliary tract obstruction : new approaches to old problems. American Journal of Surgery 135: 19–31

Blumgart L H, Benjamin I S 1983 Surgical aspects of liver and biliary cancer. In: Hodgson HJF, Bloom SR (eds) Gastrointestinal and hepatobiliary cancer. Advances in Gastroenterology series. Chapman and Hall, London, Ch. 10

Blumgart L H, Carachi R, Imrie C W, Benjamin I S, Duncan J G 1977 Diagnosis and management of post-cholecystectomy symptoms : the place of endoscopy and retrograde choledochopancreatography. British Journal of Surgery 64: 809–816

Braasch J W, Gray B N 1977 Considerations that lower pancreatoduodenectomy mortality. American Journal of Surgery 133: 480–484

Clarke B G, Leadbetter W F, Campbell J S 1953 Implantation of cancer of the prostate in site of perineal needle biopsy: report of a case. Journal of Urology 70: 937–939

Collier N A, Allison D J, Vermess M, and Blumgart L H 1984 Right upper quadrant abdominal masses mimicking hepatic tumours: an approach to management. Australian & New Zealand Journal of Surgery 54: 113–118

Dalton-Clark H, McPherson G A D, Ruston M, Krause T, Pearse E, Blumgart L H 1983 Fine needle aspiration versus exfoliative cytology in the diagnosis of hilar cholangiocarcinoma. Clinical Oncology 10 (1):88

Devor D, Knauft R D 1968 Exploratory laparotomy for abdominal pain of unknown etiology. Archives of Surgery 96: 836–839

Ferrucci J T, Wittenberg J, Margolies M N, Carey R W 1979 Malignant seeding of the tract after thin-needle aspiration biopsy. Radiology 1340: 345–346

Ferrucci J T, Wittenberg J, Mueller P R, Simeone J F, Harbin W P, Kirkpatrick R H, Taft P D 1980 Diagnosis of abdominal malignancy by radiological fine-needle aspiration biopsy. American Journal of Radiology 134: 323–330

Foster J H 1982 Benign liver tumours. World Journal of Surgery 6: 25–31

Gompels B M, Pike C P 1979 Fine needle aspiration cytology. Lancet ii: 424

Gray B N 1980 Surgeon accuracy in the diagnosis of liver metastases at laparotomy. Australian & New Zealand Journal of Surgery 50: 524–526

Harbin W P, Wittenberg J, Ferrucci J T, Mueler P R, Ottinger L W

1980 Fallibility of exploratory laparotomy in detection of hepatic and retroperitoneal masses. American Journal of Radiology 135: 115–121
Hatfield A R W, Tobias R, Terblanche J, et al 1982 Preoperative external biliary drainage in obstructive jaundice. A prospective controlled clinical trial. Lancet ii: 896–899
Lightdale C J 1982 Laparoscopy and biopsy in malignant liver disease. Cancer 50: 2672–2675
Lundquist A 1970 Fine-needle aspiration biopsy for cytodiagnosis of malignant tumour in the liver. Acta Medica Scandinavica 188: 465–470
McCune W S, Shorb P E, Moscovitz H 1968 Endoscopic cannulation of the ampulla of Vater : a preliminary report. Annals of Surgery 167: 752–756
McPherson G A D, Benjamin I S, Hodgson H J F, Bowley N B, Allison D J, Blumgart L H 1984 Preoperative percutaneous transhepatic biliary drainage: the results of a controlled trial. British Journal of Surgery 71: 371–375
Mehta M, Del Guercio L R M 1974 Minilaparotomy: an integrated procedure for rapid diagnosis in post-cholecystectomy biliary tract symptoms. Annals of the Royal College of Surgeons of England 54: 301–305
Melcher D H, Linehan J J, Smith R S 1981 Fine needle aspiration cytology. In : Anthony P P, MacSween R N M (eds). Recent advances in histopathology. Churchill Livingstone, Edinburgh, Ch. 17
Mistretta C A, Crummy A B, Strother C M 1981 Digital angiography : a perpective. Radiology 139: 273–276
Moore G E, Bridenbaugh R B 1950 Portal venography. Surgery 28: 827–831
Oi I 1970 Fiberduodenoscopy and endoscopic pancreato-cholangiography. Gastrointestinal Endoscopy 17: 59–62
Okuda K, Tanikawa K, Emura T et al 1974 Non surgical, percutaneous transhepatic cholangiography — diagnostic significance in medical problems of the liver. American Journal of Digestive Diseases 19: 21–36
Pejchl S, Chaloupka F 1981 Possibilities of laparotomy in the diagnosis of hepatic metastases of malignant tumours. Ceskoslovenska Gastroenterologie A Vyziva 35: 210–215
Piedrahita P, Butterfield W C 1976 Abdominal exploration as a diagnostic procedure. American Journal of Surgery 131: 181–184
Pollock A V 1981 Laparotomy. Journal of the Royal Society of Medicine 74: 480
Sakurai M, Seki K, Okamura J, Kuroda C 1983 Needle tract implantation of hepatocellular carcinoma after percutaneous liver biopsy. American Journal of Surgical Pathology 7: 191–195
Stein H D 1975 The diagnosis of jaundice by the mini laparotomy open transhepatic cholangiogram. Annals of Surgery 181: 386–389
Stein H D, Saalfrank V, Meng C H 1977 Mini laparotomy as an aid to diagnosing liver disease. Surgery, Gynecology and Obstetrics 145: 49–54
Strack P R, Newman H K, Lerner A G et al 1971 An integrated procedure for the rapid diagnosis of biliary obstruction, portal hypertension and liver disease of uncertain etiology. New England Journal of Medicine 285: 1225–1231
Whipple A O, Parsons W B, Mullins C R 1935 Treatment of carcinoma of the ampulla of Vater. Annals of Surgery 102: 763–779
Williamson B W A, Blumgart L H, McKellar N J 1980 Management of tumours of the liver. American Journal of Surgery 139: 210–215
Wolinsky H, Lischner M W 1969 Needle track implantation of tumour after percutaneous lung biopsy. Annals of Internal Medicine 71: 359–162
Wood C B, Ratcliffe J G, Burt R W, Malcolm J H, Blumgart L H 1980 The clinical significance of the pattern of elevated serum carcinoembryonic antigen (CEA) levels in recurrent colorectal cancer. British Journal of Surgery 67: 46–48

27

R. E. Hermann, T. A. Broughan

Intraoperative radiology

INTRODUCTION

The use of intraoperative radiology during operations on the biliary system provides a valuable adjunct to the completeness of the operative procedure. During cholecystectomy or common bile duct exploration, operative cholangiography provides visualization of the entire biliary system, from the intrahepatic bile ducts to the distal common bile duct, and demonstrates patency by the passage of contrast material into the duodenum. The principal advantages of intraoperative cholangiography are that it shows the anatomy of the biliary system including anatomical variations and that it identifies pathology which might otherwise be missed by the surgeon, such as stones, strictures, inflammatory changes, or tumours. Finally, it provides a permanent radiographic record of the biliary system at that particular time, which can be referred to by other physicians and which can be compared with changes which might develop in later years.

Operative cholangiography was introduced by Mirizzi (1937) in Argentina and was subsequently recognized by many surgeons as an important addition to biliary surgery. Although there has been little disagreement as to the value of operative cholangiography for difficult or complicated biliary operations, there has been disagreement through the years as to whether it should be used routinely or selectively (Hermann & Hoerr 1965, Jolly et al 1968, Stark & Loughry 1980).

Advocates of its routine use, since its inception, have recognized its value in identifying the entire biliary system at operation so that unsuspected pathological findings are not missed. Of most frequent importance is that an unsuspected bile duct stone is not left in the biliary system after operation. The routine use of operative cholangiography has identified an incidence of unsuspected stones or other pathology in the range of 6–8% (Pagana & Stahlgren, 1980, Levine et al 1983) (Fig. 27.1 and 27.2). Additionally, routine use of intraoperative cholangiography improves the speed and efficiency as well as the skill, accuracy, and effectiveness of the procedure.

The principal argument against routine operative cholangiography, and the argument for using it selectively, is whether it is cost-effective (Stark & Loughry 1980, Skillings et al 1979). Stark & Loughry (1980) believe that the cost of the procedure does not justify its benefit when used routinely, but that it should be used selectively. A comparison of routine versus selective operative cholangiography was performed using a cost-benefit analysis by Barnes & Barnes (1977). In this study, despite a high incidence of false-positive cholangiograms and an estimated conservative figure for the cost of death ($200,000), an overall saving of approximately 11% per patient was calculated if operative cholangiography was used routinely.

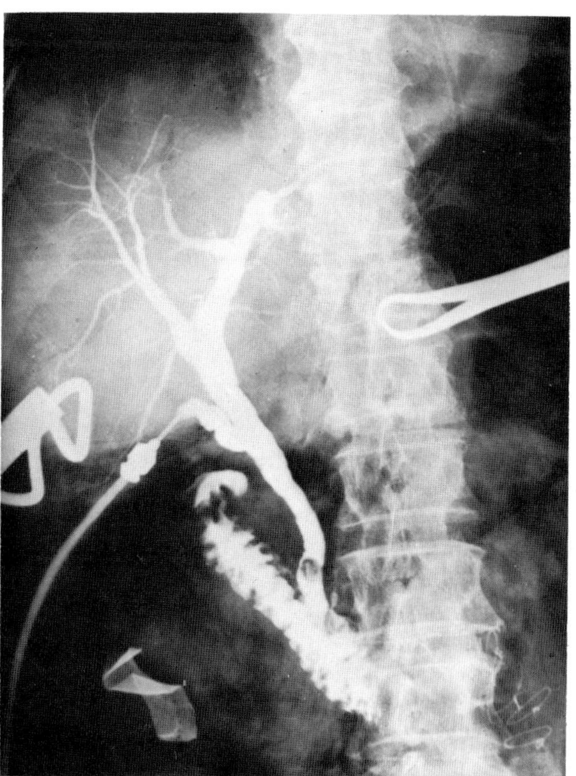

Fig. 27.1 Operative cholangiogram shows a small stone in the distal, intrapancreatic bile duct, unsuspected by the surgeon

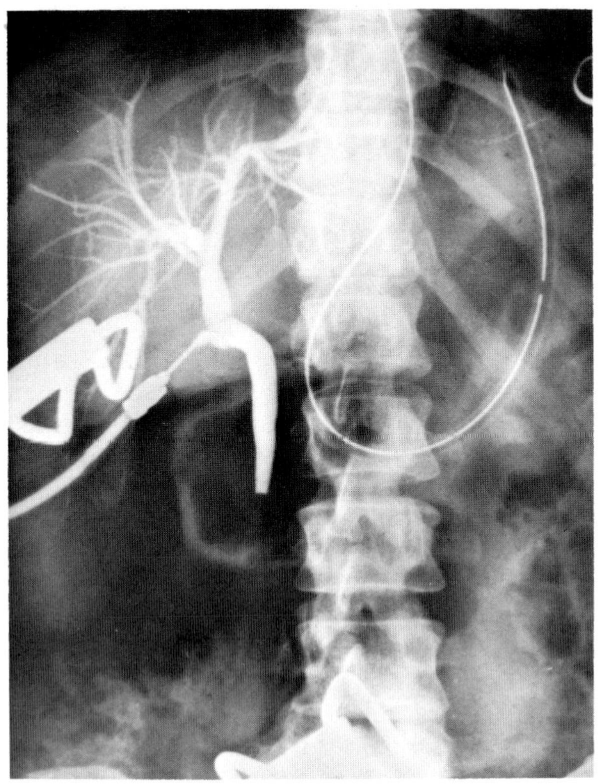

Fig. 27.2 Operative cholangiogram shows an unsuspected distal bile duct obstruction due to a small stone. The patient had no prior history of jaundice or pancreatitis

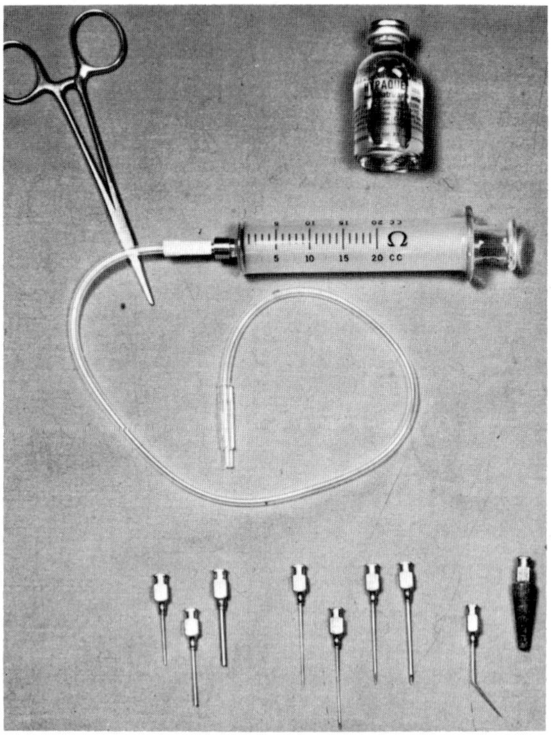

Fig. 27.3 Instruments used for operative cholangiography include a selection of blunt-tip needles, some sharp needles, polyethylene tubing, a 20 ml syringe and a vial of contrast material, Renograffin-60

TECHNIQUES OF OPERATIVE CHOLANGIOGRAPHY

We have used operative cholangiography routinely during all biliary procedures at the Cleveland Clinic for the past 35 years. The instruments we use are shown in Fig. 27.3. Five techniques are used: 1. cystic duct cholangiography when the gallbladder is present and will be removed; 2. cholecystocholangiography when the gallbladder is present and may be preserved; 3. common duct cholangiography when the gallbladder is absent or when the common bile duct is dilated and appears to be the major site of disease; 4. transhepatic cholangiography when the anatomy of the extrahepatic bile duct is unclear or distorted from multiple previous operations on the bile ducts; and 5. post-exploration T-tube cholangiography performed after exploration of the common bile duct prior to terminating the operative procedure. The techniques, indications, and advantages of these methods will be discussed individually.

Cystic duct cholangiography

After the gallbladder is dissected from the liver bed, the cystic duct is identified. Any stones in the cystic duct are milked back into the gallbladder, and the neck of the gallbladder is ligated. Another ligature is placed around the distal cystic duct and left untied. The instruments used in cholangiography are prepared by the surgical nurse; 15 ml of Renograffin-60 (iodine concentration of 29%) is drawn into a 20 ml syringe attached to a short length of polyethylene tubing and a blunt 18 gauge needle. Care is taken to remove all air bubbles from the system. The contrast material should be warmed to body temperature. The cystic duct is then partially divided and the blunt 18 gauge needle attached to the syringe and tubing is inserted into the duct (Fig. 27.4). The distal ligature is tied around the duct and needle to secure them in place. Bile is gently aspirated into the tubing to confirm the position of the needle in the bile duct and to aspirate any air from the system back into the tubing and the syringe. The radiographic field is cleared of radiopaque material and equipment but the retractors and drapes are not removed (retractors used during operations on the biliary system are purposely placed in such a way that they do not obstruct the radiographic visualization of the biliary system).

15 ml of Renograffin-60 is used for the operative cholangiogram. Approximately 3.0 ml are used for the initial injection and a roentgenogram is taken. An additional 10–12 ml is used for the second injection and a second roentgenogram is taken. While awaiting development of the films, which takes approximately 10

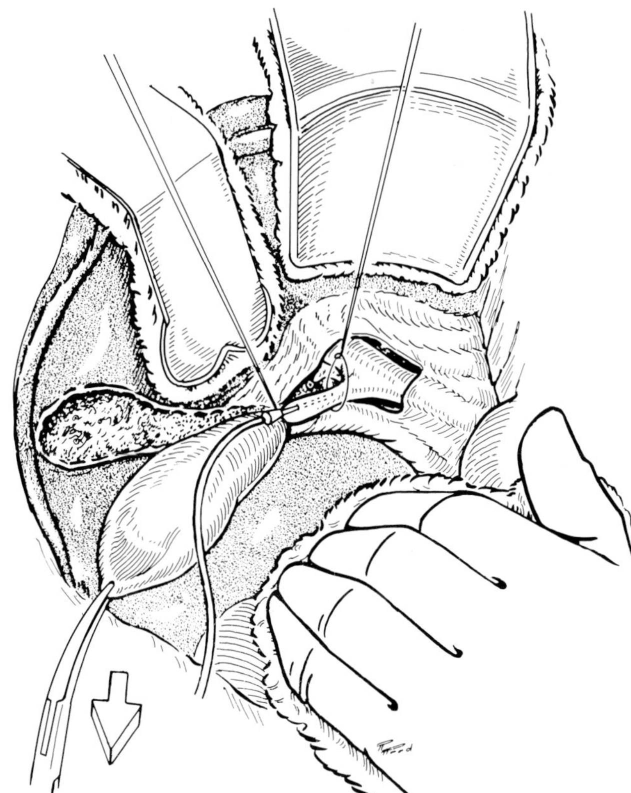

Fig. 27.4 Technique of cystic duct cholangiography

minutes, the needle and tubing are removed from the cystic duct, the duct is ligated close to its junction with the common bile duct, and the duct is divided and the gallbladder removed.

The indications for a cystic duct cholangiogram performed during cholecystectomy are that it is performed routinely in all cases. This includes patients with acute and chronic cholecystitis as well as those with jaundice or palpable stones in the common bile duct in whom a bile duct exploration will be performed.

The advantages of routine intraoperative cholangiography have previously been enunciated. We find it to be the most accurate indication for common bile duct exploration. Before the advent of operative cholangiography, various preoperative and perioperative criteria were followed to determine the need for bile duct exploration (Glenn 1952, Bartlett & Waddell 1958, Saypol 1961). These included:

1. a palpable stone in the common bile duct;
2. a history of jaundice or cholangitis;
3. a thickened or dilated bile duct;
4. multiple small stones in the gallbladder or a single faceted stone;
5. a cystic duct larger than the stones in the gallbladder;
6. a past history of pancreatitis;
7. a patient over 60 with a long history of biliary disease (because of the greater incidence of common bile duct stones in elderly patients).

The use of these clinical criteria alone led to a number of unnecessary common bile duct explorations. Saypol (1961) and Appleman et al (1964) reported that when clinical indications alone were used as a guide, biliary pathology was found in only 30–50% of the common bile ducts explored. In these early studies, more than half the patients having common bile duct exploration were treated unnecessarily (Leichtling et al 1959, Appleman et al 1964, Saypol 1961).

When cystic duct cholangiography is performed routinely and is used as the principal guide to the need for common bile duct exploration, pathology is found in the common bile duct in 90–95% of patients (Pagana & Stahlgren 1980). An error of 5–10% of false-positive operative cholangiograms is still found or an error in interpretation is made, leading to an unnecessary duct exploration (Isaacs & Daves 1960, Havard 1970, Holmin et al 1980). The major benefit of operative cholangiography, however, is the demonstration of unsuspected pathology in the bile ducts. Predominantly, the pathology found is an unsuspected stone; no good data on the incidence of unsuspected neoplasms or strictures are available. The clinical significance of an unsuspected stone has been questioned (Glenn 1974, Stark & Loughry 1980) with one estimate (Stark & Loughry 1980) that only one in 10 unsuspected stone becomes clinically important. The incidence of anatomical anomalies of the biliary system noted during routine operative cholangiography has been identified in up to 47% of patients (Hayes et al 1985). The incidence of a significant biliary anomaly where a surgical injury might occur if it

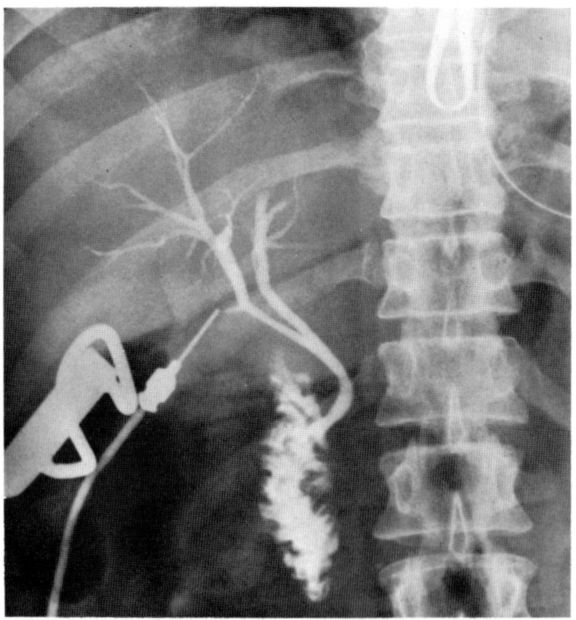

Fig. 27.5 Operative cholangiogram shows a significant anomaly of the biliary system; the cystic duct inserts into the main right hepatic duct

was not identified, was noted by Isaacs & Daves (1960) to be 3.4% (Fig. 27.5 and 27.6).

We believe the aim of an operative procedure on the biliary system is to identify or remove all pathology, leaving the patient's bile ducts unobstructed postoperatively, while avoiding an unnecessary bile duct exploration (Ch. 46). Unrecognized or untreated pathology of the biliary system leads to continuing ill health, possible secondary operative procedures or further complications, such as jaundice, cholangitis, or pancreatitis. Since the clinical criteria for exploration of the common bile duct, used alone, lead to a high percentage of unnecessary bile duct explorations, these should be supplemented or refined by more exact criteria. Operative cholangiography, used routinely, provides these criteria.

Unnecessary common bile duct explorations are potentially dangerous. McSherry & Glenn (1980) reported a 0.5% mortality for cholecystectomy alone as compared to a 2.1% mortality for cholecystectomy with common bile duct exploration. Glenn (1952) further related the mortality for common bile duct exploration to the age of the patient: 1.5% for patients under 50 and 9.6% for patients over 50. We have found in our studies that older patients have a higher incidence of common bile duct stones (Table 27.1) (Hermann 1983). Thus, it is increasingly important to use operative cholangiography routinely when operating on older patients.

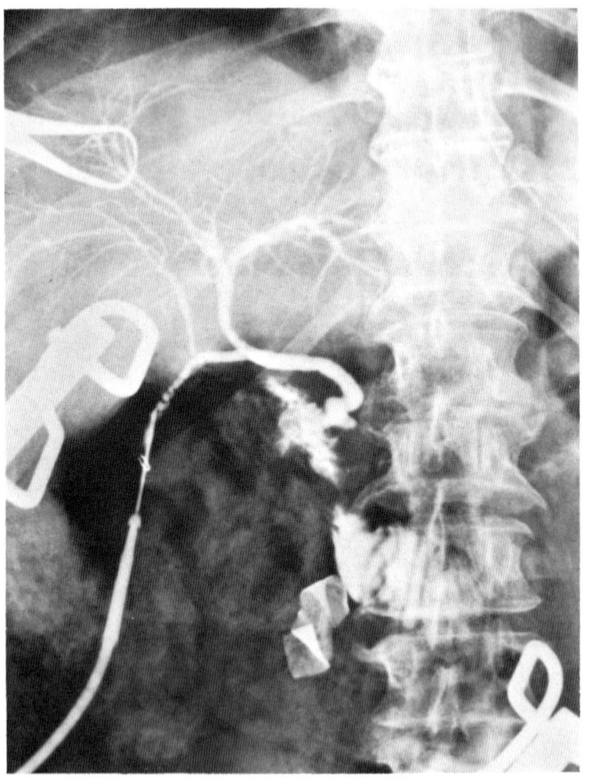

Fig. 27.6 Operative cholangiogram shows the cystic duct joining a sectoral right hepatic duct

Table 27.1 Incidence of bile duct stones at cholecystectomy

Age (years)	All patients/ patients with bile duct stones	Percent
10–20	25/4	16
21–30	92/11	12
31–40	226/21	9
41–50	325/28	9
51–60	473/67	14
61–70	275/85	31
71–80	116/56	48
81–90	11/10	96
Total	1543/282	18

The risk of cystic duct cholangiography performed routinely has never been an issue. Its risk is minimal and no morbidity or mortality can be attributed to its use. However, in spite of this lack of risk, many surgeons have been slow to use it routinely or frequently. Early advocates of its routine use have included Partington & Sachs (1948), Nienhuis (1961), Hicken & McAllister (1964), Hermann & Hoerr (1965), Jolly et al (1968) and others. Jolly et al in 1968 surveyed the membership of the American Surgical Association and found that only 18% of surgeons at that time used operative cholangiography routinely. A survey of the Ohio Chapter of the American College of Surgeons (1970) showed that operative cholangiography was used in only 25% of cholecystectomies performed in Ohio in the 1960s. Studies from Sweden in 1980 show that it is now used in 96% of biliary operations in Sweden (Holmin et al 1980). An informal survey taken at the Clinical Congress of the American College of Surgeons in 1984 indicate that it is now used routinely by about 80% of American surgeons.

Cholecystocholangiography

Cholecystocholangiography is a technique of operative cholangiography performed through the gallbladder when the cystic duct is patent and the surgeon may wish to preserve the gallbladder. Indications for this technique include the adult patient with obstructive jaundice due to an unresectable carcinoma of the head of the pancreas, when visualization of the biliary system is desired but the gallbladder may be used for a biliary bypass procedure. Another example is the patient with unexplained jaundice in whom a preoperative cholangiogram has not been possible and, at operation, a collapsed biliary system is found. In such a patient, it may be desirable to have a picture of the gallbladder, extrahepatic and intrahepatic bile ducts to determine whether bile duct obstruction is present. A final example is the baby with neonatal jaundice explored for the possibility of biliary atresia. A cholecystocholangiogram gives access to the biliary system for visualization of the system to look for the presence of bile ducts.

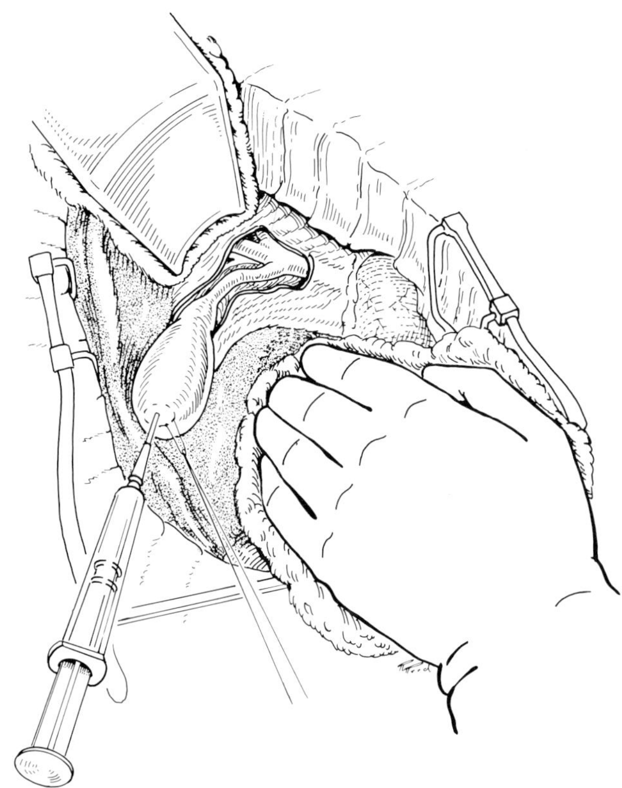

Fig. 27.7 Technique of cholecystocholangiography

Our technique includes the placement of a purse-string suture in the fundus of the gallbladder. A 15 or 18 gauge needle is used to puncture the gallbladder through the purse-string suture and the gallbladder is emptied of bile (Fig. 27.7). Approximately 15–30 ml of Renograffin-60 is then instilled into the gallbladder, the needle and syringe are withdrawn, and the purse-string suture is tied. With traction on the purse-string suture, the surgeon then squeezes the contrast material out of the gallbladder into the biliary system and two cholangiograms are obtained.

This technique of operative cholangiography provides visualization of the biliary system and demonstrates anatomy, but is less accurate than cystic duct cholangiography in the identification of small stones or other subtle pathology. It is important to express as much of the contrast medium out of the gallbladder as possible prior to obtaining the cholangiogram, since retention of a large amount of contrast material in the gallbladder may tend to obscure detail if it overlies any segment of the biliary system.

Common duct cholangiography

An operative cholangiogram may be obtained directly through the wall of the common bile duct if the gallbladder has been removed previously or if the common bile duct is dilated and appears to be the primary site of disease, even though the gallbladder may be present. A small, 21 or 23 gauge needle, such as a scalp vein needle used in children, attached to a segment of tubing and a 20 ml syringe, is inserted into the common bile duct. Occasionally, bending the needle into a right-angle aids in the insertion into the duct (Fig. 27.8). Bile is aspirated to be certain of needle placement and to remove any air in the system. After removal of air bubbles, 10–15 ml of contrast material is gently introduced into the bile duct and two X-rays are again taken, one after the instillation of approximately 3–4 ml and the second after the instillation of the remainder of the contrast material.

We obtain common duct cholangiograms prior to exploration of the common bile duct whenever we explore the bile duct for stones. This pre-exploration cholangiogram helps to define the location and number of stones in the bile ducts and is a valuable guide to the surgeon (Fig. 27.9 and 27.10). Occasionally, when a satisfactory preoperative percutaneous transhepatic cholangiogram or endoscopic retrograde cholangiogram has been performed, we will omit the pre-exploration cholangiogram at the operating table and proceed directly to a common bile duct exploration.

Transhepatic cholangiography

In the patient who has had multiple previous operations on the biliary system, especially when the anatomy or

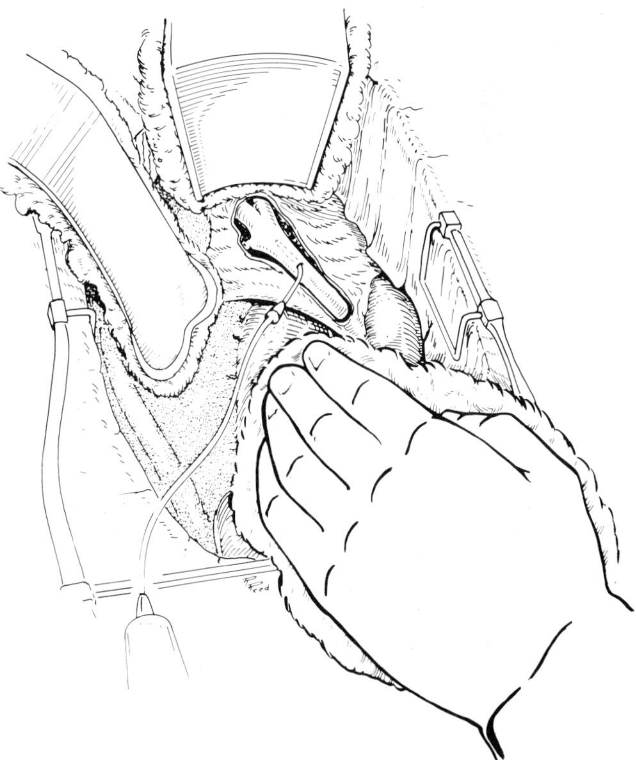

Fig. 27.8 Technique of common duct cholangiography

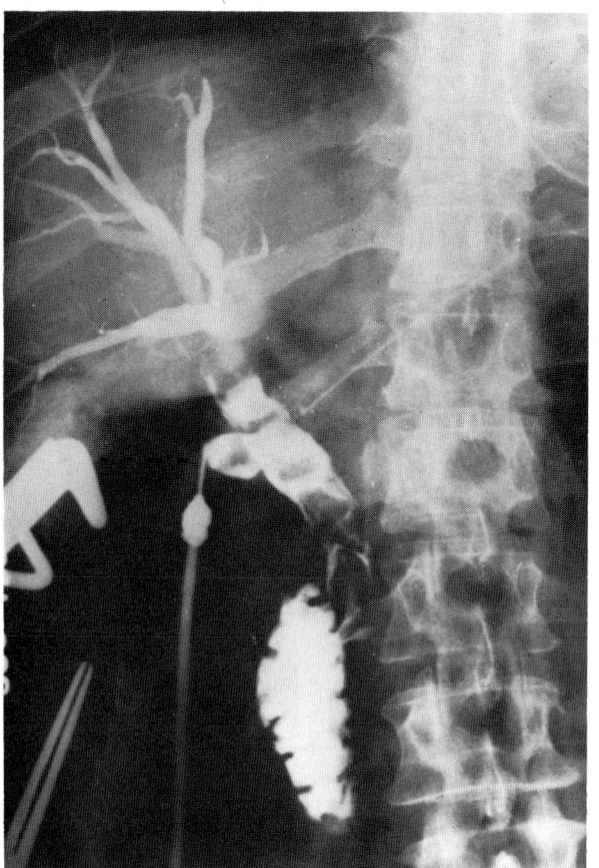

Fig. 27.9 A common duct cholangiogram shows multiple stones in the common bile duct

location of the bile duct is unclear to the surgeon, a direct needle puncture of the intrahepatic bile ducts is essential to identify the location of the biliary system and to instill contrast material to identify the anatomy and the location of a biliary obstruction (Fig. 27.11). An example is the patient with a recurrent stricture of the bile duct who has had multiple previous operations. Ideally, a preoperative percutaneous transhepatic cholangiogram will have been performed to identify the stricture and dilated bile ducts. In spite of this information, however, at operation it may be difficult to identify the biliary system. At this time, after dissection of the porta hepatis and identification of the common hepatic artery, a direct needle puncture of the liver may be performed to identify the intrahepatic bile ducts to aid in location of the biliary system.

A 21 gauge needle directly attached to a 20 ml syringe is used and, after aspiration of bile, approximately 10 ml of contrast material is injected. The major value of this cholangiogram is the identification of the biliary system and demonstration of its anatomy to visualize the point of obstruction (Fig. 27.12 and 27.13).

Post-exploration T-tube cholangiography

After exploration of the common bile duct, we always place a T-tube in the bile duct to provide access to the biliary system and for post-exploration cholangiograms.

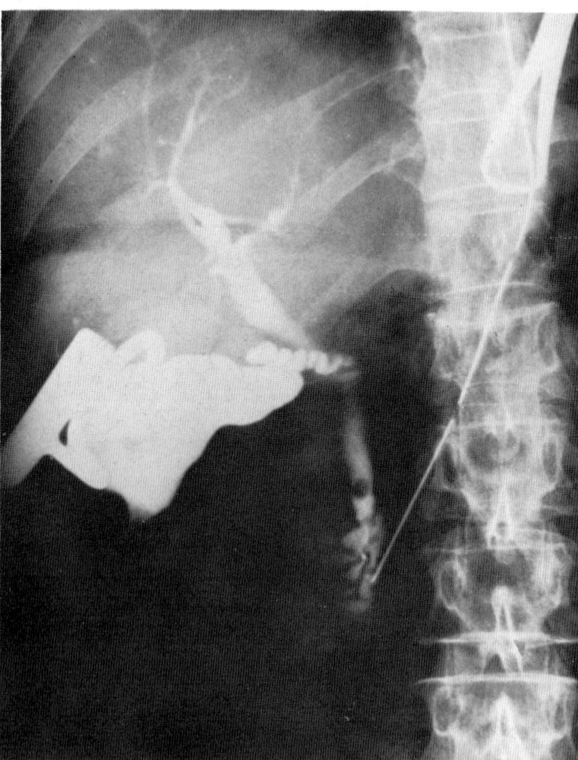

Fig. 27.10 A cholecystocholangiogram shows a solitary stone in the common bile duct

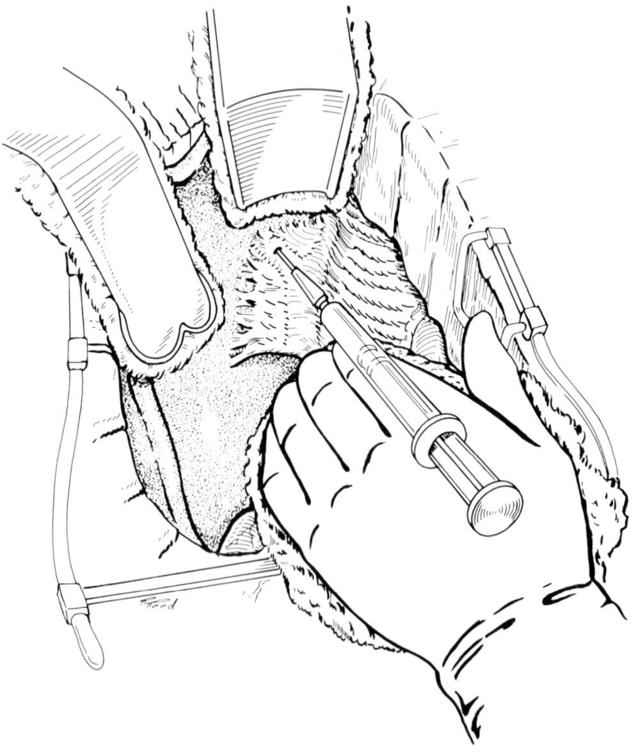

Fig. 27.11 Artist's drawing of a transhepatic cholangiogram into the hilar area of the liver. The extrahepatic anatomy is scarred from multiple previous operations to correct bile duct strictures

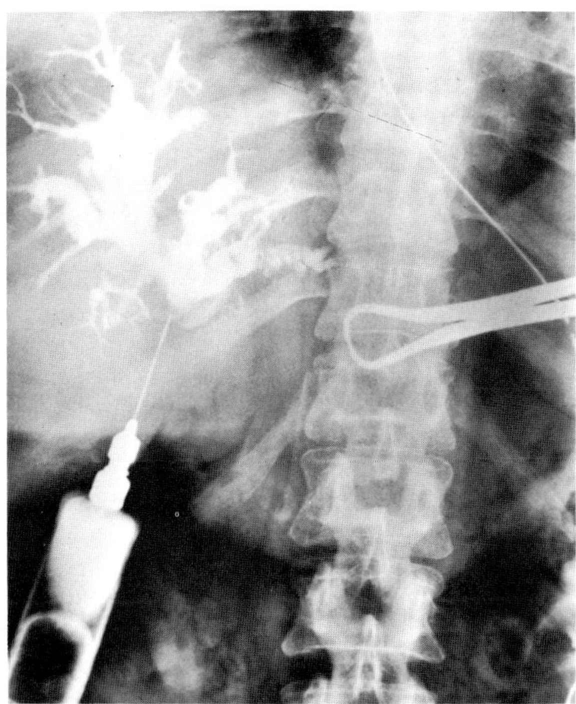

Fig. 27.12 Transhepatic cholangiogram performed to identify and locate an obstructed bile duct (stricture)

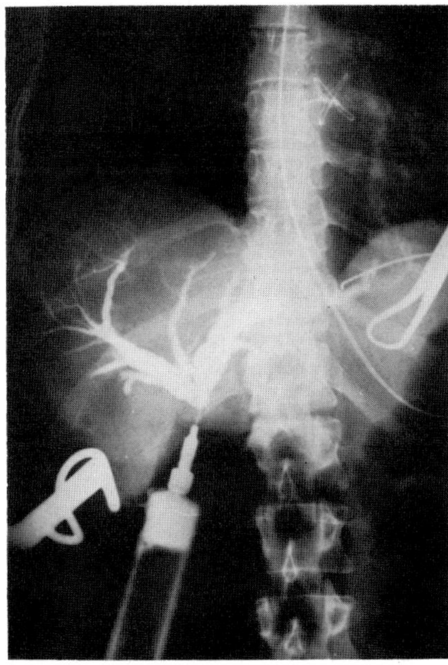

Fig. 27.13 Another transhepatic cholangiogram shows a stricture of the bile duct

We use a T-tube size 14F–18F in most patients, a purposefully large tube so that post-exploration extraction of any retained stones through the matured T-tube tract is possible.

A completion, post-exploration cholangiogram should be obtained intraoperatively while the patient is under anaesthesia before the abdominal incision is closed, so that if any stones or other pathology have been overlooked or remain in the biliary system, these can be corrected before the operative procedure is terminated. We perform a completion T-tube cholangiogram in all patients immediately following common bile duct exploration when stones have been removed or other pathology corrected. (Ch. 46). We now, ocassionally, omit this completion cholangiogram when a questionable defect has appeared on intraoperative cholangiography and a negative common bile duct exploration has been performed, especially if operative choledochoscopy has been a part of the bile duct exploration. The omission of this post-exploration T-tube cholangiogram is debatable and one might argue its value in all cases. In any case, we always obtain a final T-tube cholangiogram on the 8th to 10th postoperative day, prior to removing the T-tube if this study is normal.

It has been shown in a number of surgical studies that T-tube cholangiography is more accurate than common bile duct exploration alone (Hicken & McAllister 1964, McCormick et al 1974, Mullen et al 1971, Way et al 1972). That is, stones have been identified on the post-exploration T-tube cholangiogram that were not seen by the surgeon during open common bile duct exploration (Fig. 27.14). Way et al (1972) demonstrated that completion T-tube cholangiography reduced the likelihood of finding a residual stone on a later, postoperative T-tube cholangio-

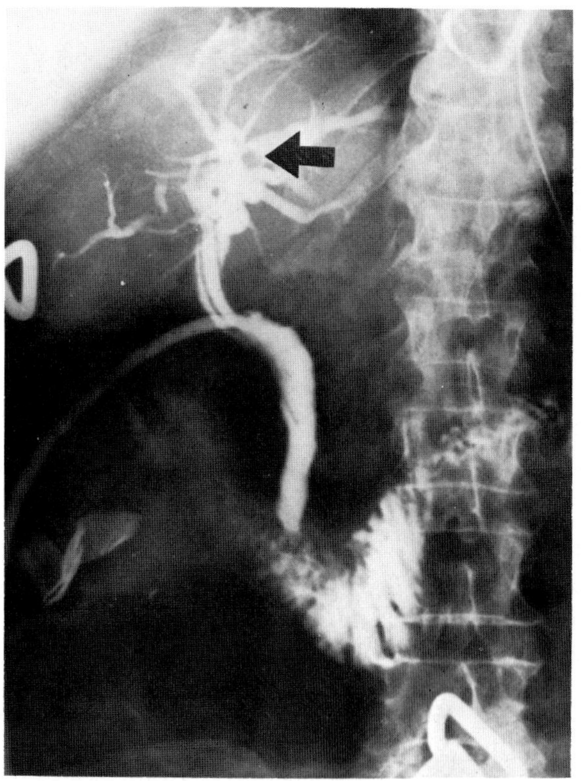

Fig. 27.14 A post-exploration T-tube cholangiogram identifies a residual stone in the intrahepatic bile ducts, missed during operative exploration of the bile duct

gram, from 30% to 7%. Hicken & McAllister (1964) similarly showed that completion T-tube cholangiograms reduced the incidence of residual bile duct stone from 11% to 4%. Similar excellent results have been reported by LeQuesne & Bolton (1980).

Our technique of completion T-tube cholangiography is to fill the right upper quadrant with saline solution, placing the biliary system underwater. Saline is then used to irrigate and remove all air from the biliary system. A 20 ml syringe is attached directly to the T-tube and two cholangiograms are obtained, one after the instillation of approximately 5 ml of contrast medium and the second after the instillation of an additional 10 ml. The most common abnormal finding on this completion cholangiogram is sphincter spasm with no contrast material entering the duodenum. If the distal bile duct tapers smoothly and no stone deformity is seen and the patient has had normal exploration of the distal bile duct with passage of Bakes' dilators into the duodenum, we disregard this spasm. If, however, there is any concern that this represents an organic obstruction, 5 ml of 20% magnesium sulphate solution may be injected through the wall of the duodenum onto the mucosa of the papilla of Vater. This will relax the sphincter, permitting a second injection study which will demonstrate patency.

Other techniques of postexploratory cholangiography using a balloon catheter prior to insertion of the T-tube have been shown extremely effective (Myat et al 1973) (Ch. 52).

INTERPRETATION OF CHOLANGIOGRAMS

Interpretation of intraoperative cholangiograms is extremely important and is usually performed by the surgeon. For this reason, high quality films must be obtained. It is important to position the patient in such a way that the common bile duct is to the right of and does not overlie the lumbar spine. This means that the patient must be tilted slightly on the operative table so that the left side is elevated or the radiological projection used must be slightly oblique. The contrast material should not be too concentrated and the quantity should not be so great as to obscure small stones in the duct. The contrast material must be warm and gently instilled into the biliary system so that sphincter spasm does not occur. The entire biliary system should be identified including both intrahepatic and extrahepatic bile ducts and flow of contrast into the duodenum. The total time involved in obtaining the cholangiogram should be less than 10 minutes.

LeQuesne (1960) presented guidelines for the interpretation of cholangiograms. The normal duct should be no larger than 12 mm in size; contrast media must flow freely into the duodenum in all films; at least one film should show the junction of the distal bile duct with its characteristic notch and the wider proximal duct; no filling defects should be present; and the hepatic ducts should be seen, but not overfilled. Visualization of the pancreatic duct is of no significance or harm, although we note that, in a review of our own operative cholangiograms, the pancreatic duct is visualized more frequently in patients who have had a history of pancreatitis.

If high quality cholangiograms are not being obtained, this negates the value of the procedure. Air bubbles, leakage of dye from the needle or ducts, over-penetration or under-penetration, or other problems of technique lessen the whole value of intraoperative cholangiography (Hall et al 1973). These considerations imply that the surgeon, the nurse who prepares the equipment, and the radiology team all require frequent practice in obtaining intraoperative cholangiograms. When operative cholangiography is performed routinely, optimal conditions for excellent cholangiograms are obtained. When it is performed infrequently or selectively, there is a greater chance for poor quality studies.

In some centres, intraoperative cholangiography and intraoperative manometric studies (Ch. 28) of the biliary system are combined (Mallet-Guy 1952, McCarthy 1977, White & Bordley 1978). We do not perform manometric studies at the Cleveland Clinic, as we do not believe that they provide sufficient information in the anaesthetized patient to justify the additional time and cost involved.

Intraoperative choledochoscopy (Ch. 29) is a valuable adjunct to both intraoperative cholangiography and common bile duct exploration (Berci 1978, Escat 1984, Keighley & Kappas 1980, King & String 1983, Sohein et al, 1963). We use it frequently to aid in the identification of bile duct changes seen on intraoperative cholangiography.

OPERATIVE FLUOROSCOPY AND CHOLANGIOGRAPHY

Berci et al (1978) have been strong advocates of operative fluoroscopy and cholangiography for several years. They report that the addition of fluoroscopy has reduced the incidence of retained stones to 1%. A permanently installed unit with the capacity to take operative cholangiograms is necessary; six to 12 films are taken in addition to fluoroscopy. Multiple views and flow rates are possible. The average time for a study is no longer than five minutes in their experience. The rate and amount of contrast material injected can be optimized. Fluoroscopy is also a valuable tool for analysing and observing sphincter function (Mallet-Guy 1957). The sphincter may relax sporadically and fluoroscopy is more likely to detect emptying into the duodenum.

Feeley & Peel (1982) have demonstrated a wide variation in biliary system volumes and emphasize the importance of observing early filling of the bile duct. The importance of early filling decreased as duct size increased. In 34 out of 41 patients whose bile ducts were filled by 2.0 ml or less of contrast material, the first film was the most important diagnostically. Of 66 patients having ductal volumes greater than 10 ml, the first film was diagnostic in only seven.

The cost of installation of an intraoperative fluoroscopy and cholangiogram unit is (now) greater than $150,000. Berci et al (1978) believe that the cost of the unit is defrayed in three years if it is shared with other operative services, such as orthopaedics, in the hospital.

RESULTS

We have now performed intraoperative cholangiography in more than 8000 patients at the Cleveland Clinic during the past 35 years. Our experience continues to be favourable. Used routinely, operative cholangiography is a standard part of biliary surgery. All patients are placed on an operating table equipped for intraoperative radiology, radiology technicians are stationed in the operating room, the nurses are prepared with instruments ready, and the surgeon and his team gain daily experience with the use and interpretation of operative cholangiograms.

Our complication rate for operative cholangiography is nil. In the experience of the senior author (R.E.H) over the past 22 years, a single problem cannot be remembered which could be attributed to operative cholangiography. More specifically, no instances of pancreatitis, cholangitis, or sepsis can be related to the procedure. In patients with a known allergy to iodine dyes, operative cholangiography has been safe and no allergic reactions have been seen.

We have reviewed our own operative cholangiograms and find an overall incidence of unsuspected pathology, predominantly unsuspected stones in the bile duct, to be 7% (unpublished data). Pathology encountered, other than stones, includes unsuspected strictures of the duct (Fig. 27.15), inflammatory changes such as sclerosing

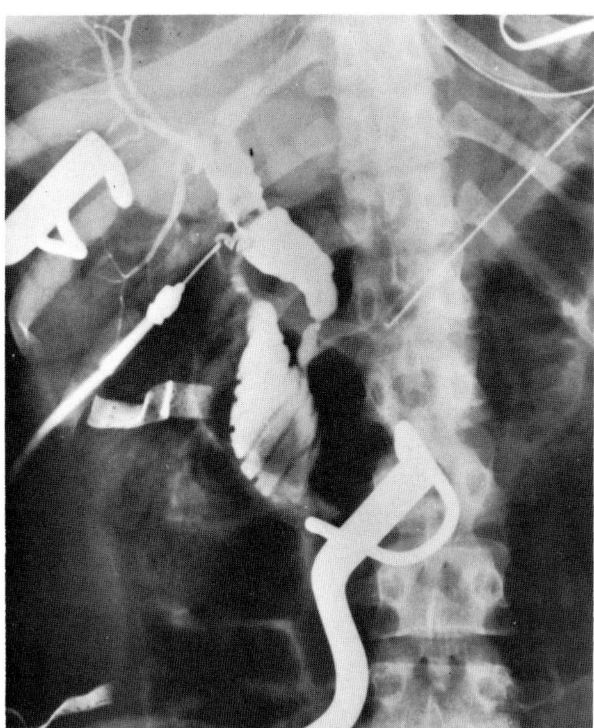

Fig. 27.15 Operative cholangiogram shows a congenital stricture of the distal bile duct. There are stones in the bile duct

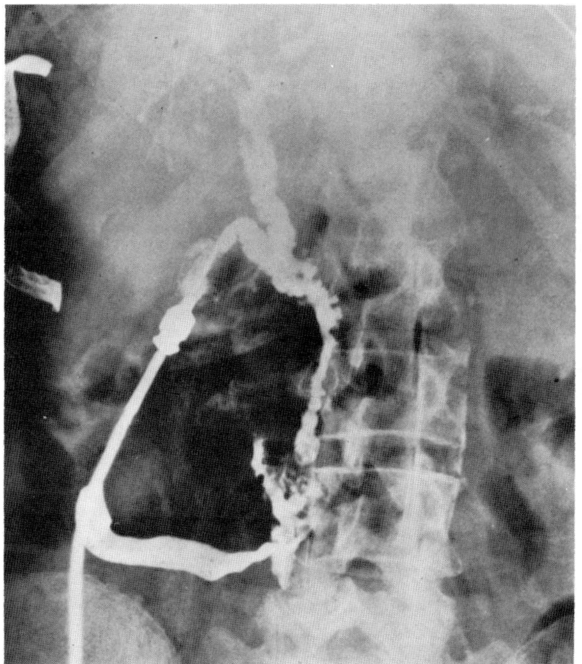

Fig. 27.16 Operative cholangiogram shows sclerosing cholangitis of the biliary system, unsuspected preoperatively or by the surgeon.

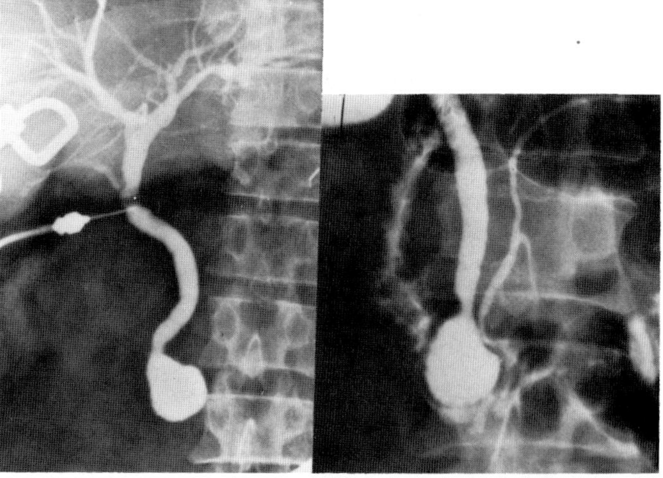

Fig. 27.17 Cystic duct cholangiogram shows a choledochal cyst (choledochocele) of the distal bile duct, unsuspected by the surgeon

cholangitis (Fig. 27.16), congenital anomalies (Fig. 27.17), and tumours of the biliary system (Fig. 27.18). We have found intraoperative cholangiography to be our most valuable indication for exploration of the biliary system. Our incidence of false-positive cholangiograms with resultant unnecessary bile duct exploration, has been approximately 10%. Our incidence of false-negative cholangiograms (difficult to ascertain) is in the range of 2%. We believe the routine use of this procedure has reduced our incidence of retained bile duct stones to less than 2% (Broughan et al 1985).

We use operative cholangiography to provide evidence for stenosis of the sphincter of Oddi and, along with bile duct exploration and inability to pass Bakes' dilators through the sphincter, use it as an indication for sphincteroplasty. Operative cholangiography also identifies distal bile duct stenosis in patients with recurrent bile duct stones (Fig. 27.19) and contributes information which we use as an indication for biliary-intestinal bypass (choledochoduodenostomy or choledochojejunostomy). Finally, in patients with intrahepatic duct changes or intrahepatic bile duct stones (Fig. 27.20), operative cholangiography has led us to perform the occasional transhepatic bile duct exploration or resection of a portion of the liver to remove a diseased area of intrahepatic cystic dilatation with stones and sepsis.

We believe intraoperative cholangiography should be a routine part of all operative procedures on the biliary system.

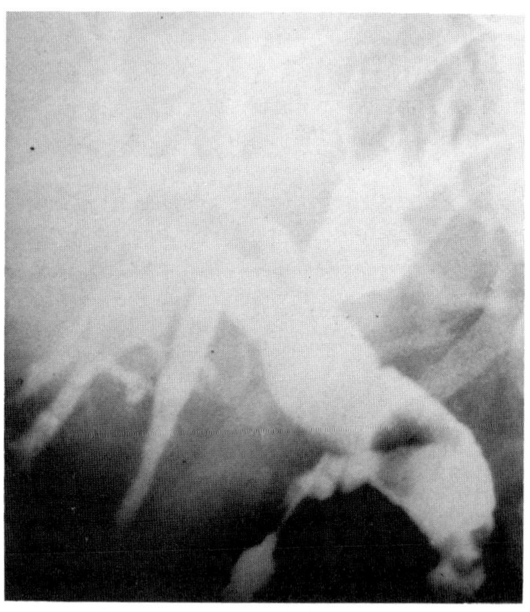

Fig. 27.19 Cystic duct cholangiogram shows a dilated bile duct with multiple stones and moderate stenosis of the distal bile duct. Because of the distal duct stenosis, a choledochoduodenostomy was performed after common bile duct exploration

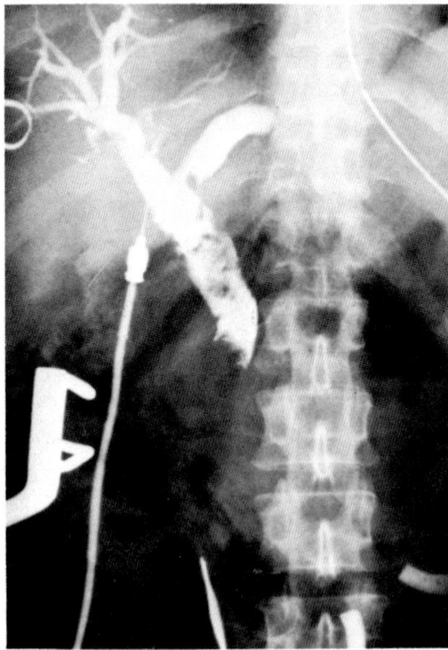

Fig. 27.18 Operative cholangiogram shows an abrupt obstruction of the distal bile duct. A soft, villous tumour of the distal bile duct was found

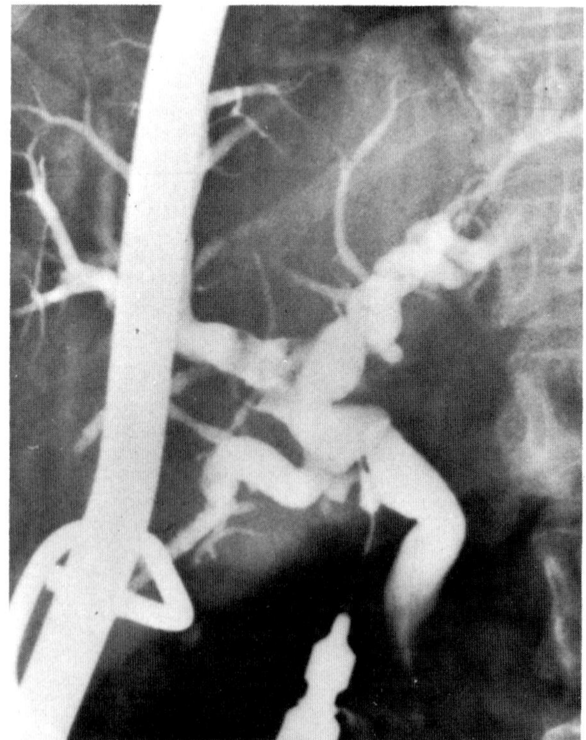

Fig. 27.20 Operative cholangiogram shows several stones in the intrahepatic bile ducts

REFERENCES

Appleman R M, Priestley J T, Gage R P 1964 Cholelithiasis and choledocholithiasis: factors that influence relative incidence. Mayo Clinic Proceedings 39: 473–478

Barnes B A, Barnes A B 1977 Evaluation of surgical therapy by cost-benefit analysis. Surgery 82: 21–33

Bartlett M K, Waddell W R 1958 Indications for common duct exploration: evaluation in 1000 cases. New England Journal of Medicine 258: 164–167

Berci G, Hamlin J A, Morgenstern L, Fisher D L 1978a Modern operative fluorocholangiography: utopia or overlooked entity? Gastrointestinal Radiology 3: 401–406

Berci G, Shore J M, Morgenstern L, Hamlin J A 1978b Choledochoscopy and fluorocholangiography in the prevention of retained bile duct stones. World Journal of Surgery 2: 411–427

Broughan T A, Sivak M V, Hermann R E 1985 The management of retained and recurrent bile duct stones. Surgery 98: 746–750

Daniel O 1972 The value of radiomanometry in bile duct surgery. Annals of the Royal College of Surgeons of England 51: 357–372

Deitch E A, Voci V E 1982 Operative cholangiography: the case for selective instead of routine operative cholangiography. American Surgeon 48: 297–301

Escat J, Glucksman D L, Maigne C, Fourtanier G, Fournier D, Vaislic C 1984 Choledochoscopy in surgery for choledocholithiasis: six-year experience in three hundred eighty consecutive patients. American Journal of Surgery 147: 670–671

Feeley M, Peel A L 1982 A critical assessment of fluoroscopy in per-operative cholangiography. Annals of the Royal College of Surgeons of England 64: 180–182

Glenn F 1952 Common duct exploration for stones. Surgery, Gynecology and Obstetrics 95: 431–438

Glenn F 1974 Retained calculi within the biliary ductal system. Annals of Surgery 179: 528–539

Hall R C, Sakiyalak P, Kim S K, Rogers L S, Webb W R 1973 Failure of operative cholangiography to prevent retained common duct stones. American Journal of Surgery 125: 51–63

Havard C 1970 Operative cholangiography. British Journal of Surgery 57: 797–807

Hayes M A, Goldenberg I S, Bishop C C 1958 The developmental basis for bile duct anomalies. Surgery, Gynecology and Obstetrics 107: 447–456

Hermann R E 1983 Common bile duct stones. In: Moody F G (ed) Advances in diagnosis and surgical treatment of biliary tract disease. Masson, New York, p 69–78

Hermann R E, Hoerr S O 1965 The value of the routine use of operative cholangiography. Surgery, Gynecology and Obstetrics 121: 1015–1020

Hicken N F, McAllister A J 1964 Operative cholangiography as an aid in reducing the incidence of 'overlooked' common bile duct stones: a study of 1293 choledocholithotomies. Surgery 55: 753–758

Holmin T, Jonsson B, Lingren B et al 1980 Selective or routine intraoperative cholangiography: a cost-effectiveness analysis. World Journal of Surgery 4: 315–322

Isaacs J P, Daves M L 1960 Technique and evaluation of operative cholangiography. Surgery, Gynecology and Obstetrics 111: 103–112

Jolly P C, Baker J W, Schmidt H M, Walker J H, Holm J C 1968 Operative cholangiography: a case for its routine use. Annals of Surgery 168: 551–565

Keighley M R, Kappas A 1980 Evaluation of operative choledoscopy. Surgery, Gynecology and Obstetrics 150: 357–359

King M L, String S T 1983 Extent of choledochoscopic utilization in common bile duct exploration. American Journal of Surgery 146: 322–324

Leichtling J J, Rubin S, Breidenbach L 1959 The significance of in vivo measurement of the common bile duct. Surgery, Gynecology and Obstetrics 109: 773–777

Le Quesne L P 1960 Cholangiography. Proceedings of the Royal Society of Medicine 53: 852–855

Le Quesne L P, Bolton J P 1980 Choledocholithiasis: incidence, diagnosis, and operative procedures. In: Maingot R (ed) Abdominal operations VIIth ed. vol I, Appleton-Century-Crofts, New York, p 1055–1102

Levine S B, Lerner H J, Leifer E D, Lindheim S R 1983 Intraoperative cholangiography: a review of indications and analysis of age-sex groups. Annals of Surgery 198: 692–697

Mallet-Guy P 1952 Value of peroperative manometric and roentgenographic examination in the diagnosis of pathologic changes and functional disturbances of the biliary tract. Surgery, Gynecology and Obstetrics 94: 385–393

Mallet-Guy P 1957 Television radioscopy during operations on the biliary passages. Surgery, Gynecology and Obstetrics 106: 747–748

McCarthy J D 1977 Radiomanometric guides to common bile duct exploration. American Journal of Surgery 134: 697–701

McCormick J S, Bremner D N, Thomson J W, McNair T J, Philp T 1974 The operative cholangiogram: its interpretation, accuracy and value in association with cholecystectomy. Annals of Surgery 180: 902–906

McSherry C K, Glenn F 1980 The incidence and causes of death following surgery for nonmalignant biliary tract disease. Annals of Surgery 191: 271–275

Mehn W H 1954 Operating room cholangiography. Surgical Clinics of North America 34: 151–158

Mirizzi P L 1937 Operative cholangiography. Surgery, Gynecology and Obstetrics 65: 702–710

Mullen J L, Rosato F E, Rosato E F, Miller W T, Sullivan M 1971 The diagnosis of choledocholithiasis. Surgery, Gynecology and Obstetrics 133: 774–778

Myat Thu Ya, Robinson D, Gunn A A 1973 Peroperative cholangiography. British Journal of Surgery 60: 711–712

Nienhuis L I 1961 Routine operative cholangiography: an evaluation. Annals of Surgery 154: 192–202

Ohio Chapter, American College of Surgeons 1970 28,621 cholecystectomies in Ohio. American Journal of Surgery 119: 714–717

Orloff M J 1978 Importance of surgical technique in prevention of retained and recurrent bile duct stones. World Journal of Surgery 2: 403–410

Pagana T J, Stahlgren L H 1980 Indications and accuracy of operative cholangiography. Archives of Surgery 115: 1214–1215

Partington P F, Sachs M D 1948 Routine use of operative cholangiography. Surgery, Gynecology and Obstetrics 87: 299–307

Reasbeck P G 1981 The results of cholecystectomy at a district general hospital: a reappraisal of operative cholangiography. Annals of the Royal College of Surgeons of England 63: 359–362

Saypol G M 1961 Indications for choledochostomy in operations for cholelithiasis: analysis of 525 cases. Annals of Surgery 153: 567–574

Schein C J, Stern W Z, Hurwitt E S, Jacobson H G 1963 Cholangiography and biliary endoscopy as complementary methods of evaluating the bile ducts. American Journal of Radiology 89: 864–875

Seif R M 1977 Routine operative cholangiography: a critical appraisal. American Journal of Surgery 134: 566–568

Skillings J C, Williams J S, Hinshaw J R 1979 Cost-effectiveness of operative cholangiography. American Journal of Surgery 137: 26–31

Stark M E, Loughry C W 1980 Routine operative cholangiography with cholecystectomy. Surgery, Gynecology and Obstetrics 151: 657–658

Taylor T V, Torrance B, Rimmer S, Hillier V, Lucas S B 1983 Operative cholangiography: is there a statistical alternative? American Journal of Surgery 145: 640–643

Way L W 1973 Retained common duct stones. Surgical Clinics of North America 53: 1139–1147

Way L W, Admirand W H, Dunphy J E 1972 Management of choledocholithiasis. Annals of Surgery 176: 347–359

White T T, Bordley J IV 1978 One per cent incidence of recurrent gallstones six to eight years after manometric cholangiography. Annals of Surgery 188: 562–569

J. Perissat

Intraoperative manometry in biliary surgery

Biliary manometry consists in measuring pressure in the biliary tract. The method was initiated in France (Caroli 1945, 1946). Originally introduced as complementary to operative cholangiography (Ch. 27) it soon became common practice initially in France and then in Europe (Mortola et al 1977, Naveau 1979) but was adopted only very slowly and partially in the Anglo-Saxon world (Beneventano et al 1967, White & Bordley 1978, Cuschieri, Hughes & Cohen 1972, Daniel 1972, McCarthy 1970, 1977, Mieny et al 1974).

The technique is used almost exclusively as an intraoperative investigation in cases of biliary lithiasis and has two main aims: 1. The detection of stones not previously demonstrated at operative cholangiography; 2. The demonstration of abnormality of the sphincter of Oddi (in most cases an organic or functional stenosis responsible for poor duct drainage, recurrent calculi, chronic cholestasis and residual pain after cholecystectomy).

Intraoperative manometry demands appropriate equipment, time and patience. It adds significantly to the duration of surgery and consequently to the period of general anaesthesia and moreover sometimes yields false positive results.

Since the 1970s investigation of the biliary tree has become more efficient. The development of endoscopic retrograde cholangiography, ultrasonography and computerized tomography have added new dimensions (Ch. 25). In addition new techniques for the intraoperative exploration of the duct have been developed including refinements in choledochoscopy (Ch. 29). Furthermore the advent of endoscopic papillotomy makes it possible to remove retained stones without the need for laparotomy or anaesthesia (Ch. 35).

With the advent of all these new techniques should intraoperative manometry still be considered useful in the investigation of the common bile duct during surgery for gallstones? No biliary surgeon can afford to ignore this question which this chapter attempts to answer.

TECHNIQUES

There are three techniques for intraoperative biliary manometry.

1. Simple radio-manometry. This assists in the assessment of the elevation of pressure levels in an open circuit with a varying flow and pressure of injection. It is perfectly adequate for routine surgical practice.
2. Radio-mano-flowmetry. This consists of measurement of the changes in flow rate under a constant injection pressure.
3. Radio-kinesimetry. This consists of the measurement of pressure variation at a constant flow rate.

The latter two methods, which are more difficult to practise, are usually reserved for cases when more thorough investigation is required.

Whichever of these techniques is used correct practice is subject to a number of important considerations.

Radiological Good image intensification is required. In some systems images can be stored and examined at a later date. In others a video recorder is included making it possible to store the most interesting dynamic sequences. A very efficient system of radiologically guided surgical exploration has been developed by Rives et al (1981) which combines television techniques with high intensity radiography yielding very high quality X-rays.

Anaesthetic participation Both premedication and the early stages of anaesthesia must be totally without morphinomimetic substances (which produce spasm of the sphincter of Oddi) and para-sympatheticolytic substances (which relax it). During manometry such drugs should be injected at the surgeon's request in order to assess the functional potential of the sphincteric mechanism.

A faultless hydraulic circuit The probe must be placed within the lumen of the common bile duct without touching its sides. Introduction is via the cystic duct. The tip of the probe is olive-shaped, to ensure good position within the duct (Fig. 28.1).

Simple radio-manometry

The common bile duct is cannulated by means of a catheter introduced into the cystic duct and connected via a three–way tap system to a manometer and a perfusion bottle open to atmospheric pressure (Fig. 28.1). The following readings can then be taken: Basal pressure (BP) in the common bile duct measured by opening the connection from the duct to the manometer, the perfusion bottle being excluded from the circuit (position no.1) (Fig. 28.2). The pressure required to open the papilla, opening pressure, (OP). This is measured by perfusion of the common bile duct at increasingly higher pressures starting from the basal pressure (BP). The first moment of flow into the duodenum is visualized on the display screen and the pressure carefully noted (position no. 2) (Fig. 28.3).

X-ray of the whole biliary system with perfusion pressures two or three times above BP is carried out so that the biliary tree is allowed to fill. This allows for thorough radiological examination with a view to detecting any congenital or pathological abnormality.

The resting pressure (RP) is taken after the high pressure phase. The reservoir is again clamped from the circuit. The time needed for resting pressure (RP) to return to the basal level (BP) is an indication of the functional status of the sphincter of Oddi (position no. 1).

Apparatus

The early versions of the apparatus used for simple radiomanometry were developed by Caroli (1945, 1946). The perfusion reservoir was a bottle which slides up and down a vertical scale. The zero mark was adjusted to the level of the common bile duct. A glass tube alongside the vertical scale served as the water manometer. Both the manometer and the reservoir were connected to the main bile duct by means of a Y-connection attached to a cannula which passed through the cystic duct. It was possible to sterilize the whole system. Nevertheless there were definite drawbacks; the apparatus took a long time to set up, did not record pressure curves and broke easily. The device was therefore modified by successive users and in particular more recent versions (White & Bordley 1978, Tondelli & Allgower 1980) should be mentioned, although all aim at a concomitant study of the flow rate and pressure levels.

No complex tailor-made equipment is needed nowadays: it would be difficult to come by and to maintain in

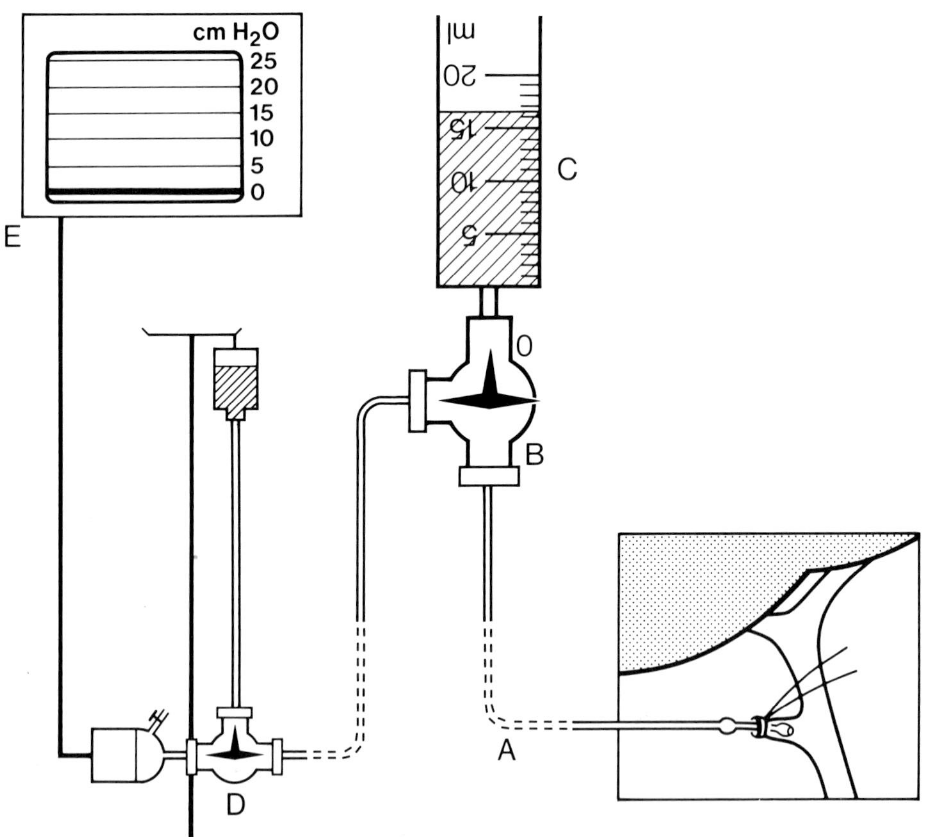

Fig. 28.1 Hydraulic circuit for simple radiomanometry. The common bile duct has been cannulated and the cannula (A) is connected via a 3-way tap (B) to a manometer and display screen (D/E) and a perfusion bottle (C) open to atmospheric pressure

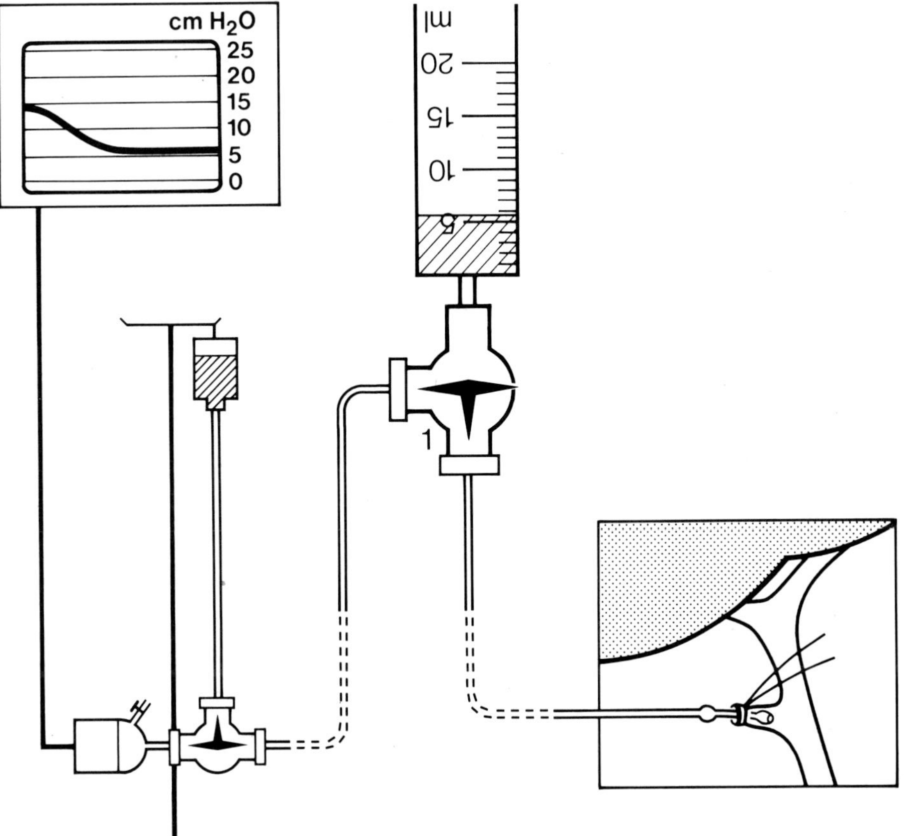

Fig. 28.2 Basal pressure (BP) is measured with the tap in position no. 1 as shown here. The perfusion bottle is excluded from the circuit

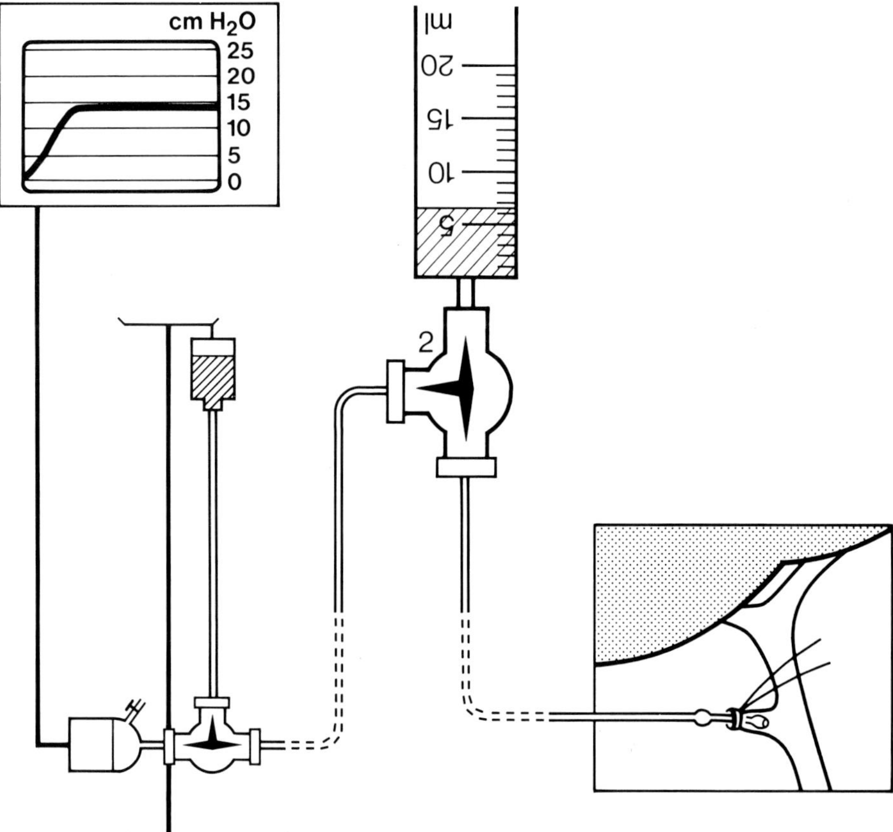

Fig. 28.3 Measurement of opening pressure (OP). The tap is in position no. 2. The common bile duct is perfused at increasing pressure starting from a basal pressure (BP). The first moment of flow into the duodenum is visualized on the display screen and the pressure clearly noted.

good working order. A simple system of intraoperative radio-manometry can be quickly improvised in any non-specialized modern operating theatre. The author's personal solution is a trans-cystic intubation cannula equipped with a three-way tap system connected to a membrane pressure sensor. The reservoir for injection is a simple disposable 20 ml syringe. The contrast medium used is a 30% solution of Uroselectan® diluted in equal parts of isotonic saline previously heated to 37°C. All measurements are taken using television control and video recording (Fig. 28.1).

All modern operating theatres should now be equipped with at least a radio television with image intensifier and video recording system and a system for constant reading and recording of pressure levels. Once these are installed the additional costs for intraoperative biliary manometry relate only to the disposable materials used on each occasion.

Simple radio-manometry is thus an easily implemented, intraoperative investigative method of reasonable cost.

Results (Fig. 28.4)

Basal pressure (BP) is usually recorded at 8 to 12 cm of water. The pressure required to open the sphincter of Oddi (OP) lies between 12 and 15 cm of water. The most important phase during X-ray investigation is precisely the point at which the opening pressure is assessed. Indeed the biliary system fills only very slowly at low pressure during which time a whole series of X-rays and a television recording should be taken. Such gradual filling of the biliary tract ensures that even very small stones are not obscured.

Once OP has been obtained injection pressure is raised to about 30 cm of water thus filling the whole of the main biliary channel, the confluence of the right and left hepatic ducts and the intrahepatic ducts. Complete radiological study of the whole biliary tract is then possible. After perfusion is stopped the resting pressure (RP) is measured. This should return to the basic pressure (BP) within one or two minutes.

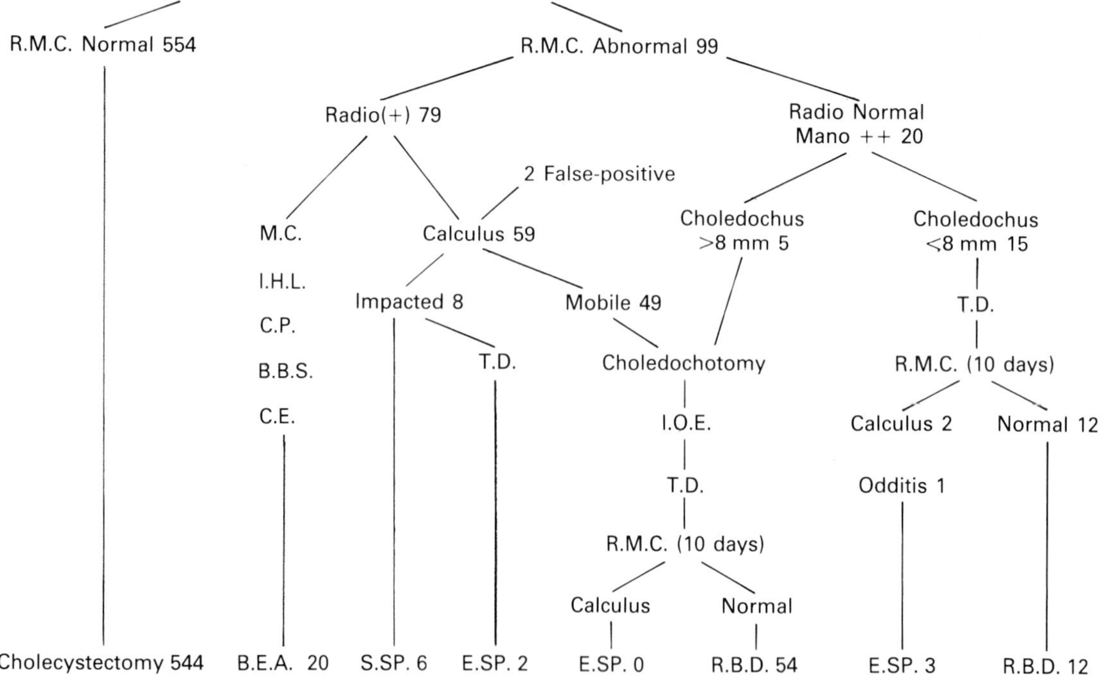

Fig. 28.4
Key

M.C.:	Multiple calculi
I.H.L.:	Intrahepatic lithiasis
C.P.:	Chronic pancreatitis
B.B.S.:	Benign biliary stricture
C.E.:	Congenital enlargement
B.E.A.:	Biliary enteric anastomosis
T.D.:	Trancystic drainage
S.SP.:	Surgical sphincterotomy
E.SP.:	Endoscopic sphincterotomy
I.O.E.:	Intraoperative endoscopy
R.B.D.:	Removal of biliary drainage

There are four possible findings:

1. Both X-ray and manometry results are normal (Fig. 28.5). If this is the case no further investigation of the main biliary duct is necessary. The catheter is removed from the cystic duct which is ligatured. Simple cholecystectomy is performed. In the author's personal records, 544 such cases were investigated and no residual calculi have been demonstrated in any of these patients.

2. Stones within the common bile duct are radiologically demonstrated. Manometric investigation is then of no use at all. The stones are removed surgically. Intraoperative choledochoscopy is employed to ensure that no residual stones are left. A trans-cystic catheter is left in situ after choledochotomy and is employed ten days later for a radiomanometric postoperative check. This may show either the presence of a residual calculus, which is then removed if necessary by means of endoscopic papillotomy (no such case has appeared in our statistics) or there is a persistance of high pressure levels even after the pharmaco-dynamic tests. This is a sign of residual, so-called, Odditis which again may be treated by means of endoscopic papillotomy (the authors have had no such case).

3. No stones are shown to be present in the duct on X-ray but manometry reveals high basal and opening pressures and a resting pressure that remains high or only subsides very slowly, these findings being in a common bile duct over 8 mm in diameter (Fig. 28.6). This combination of findings makes it advisable to perform choledochotomy together with intraoperative choledochoscopy. This will show either the presence of small stones (microstones) that have escaped X-ray observation (in which case the therapeutic procedure is the same as in 2. above) or a common duct free of stones, in which case the choledochotomy opening should be closed leaving the trans-cystic drain in place. This is then used ten days later for further radio-manometric studies to assess any residual organic lesion. If a positive finding is then obtained endoscopic papillotomy should be performed. In the author's personal series of 20 patients with a common bile duct over 8 mm in diameter and with a high pressure reading, microstones were found in five cases and had not been observed in previous X-ray study (Fig. 28.4).

4. The common bile duct is found to be radiologically stone free but manometry reveals basal and opening pressures to be high and resting pressure to remain high even after pharmaco-dynamic tests (we use Hymecromone iv). The common duct is under 8 mm in diameter. In this instance an external temporary trans-cystic drain should be left in place for further radiomanometric observation ten days later. If pressures are still abnormally high, endoscopic sphincterotomy should be carried out. In the author's series there were two cases of microlithiasis and one of probable sclerosing Odditis. These three cases came from a total of 15 with normal X-rays results and a persistently high manometric level associated with a common bile duct under 8 mm diameter as described above. In most cases the radio-manometric findings are within normal limits within 10 days and transcystic drainage can then be stopped without any need for further investigation or treatment. This was the case in the remaining 12 patients all of whom were seen again for a check-up one year later and none of whom showed any biliary disorder.

To summarize, simple radio-manometry enables the surgeon to make sure that the main bile duct is normal (544 cases of simple cholecystectomy) with no residual calculi, to detect any microstones not spotted on X-ray examination (seven out of 20 cases) and to decide in favour

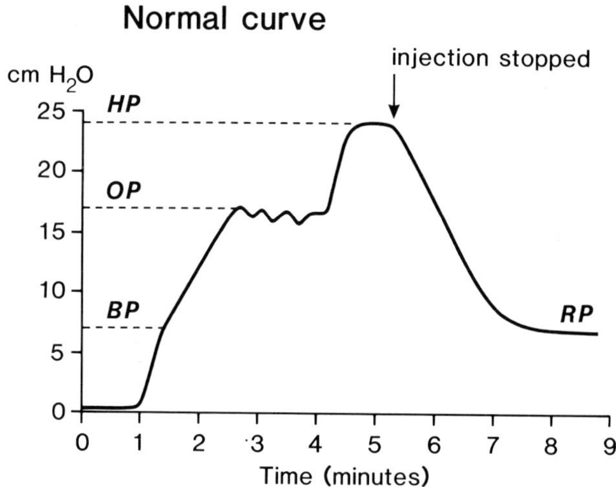

Fig. 28.5 Simple radiomanometric curve. BP = basal pressure, OP = opening pressure, HP = hyper pressure, RP = residual pressure. Normal findings

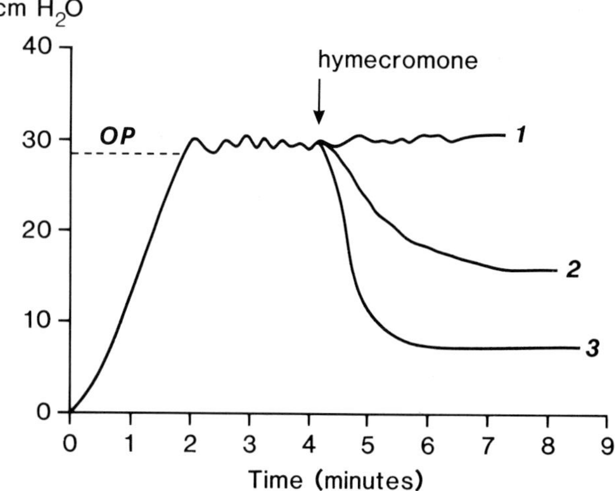

Fig. 28.6 Simple radiomanometry. Abnormal curves. 1. Curve obtained with obstructive disease (calculi or papillary stenosis)
2. Odditis (there is a high residual pressure)
3. Spasm of the sphincter of Oddi (there is a normal residual pressure after hymecromone injection.

of either intraoperative choledochoscopy, when the common duct is over 8 mm in diameter, or to leave an external temporary biliary drain, when it is under 8 mm in diameter, thus allowing a postoperative check 10 days later. The results of the latter examination may lead to endoscopic sphincterotomy if necessary (three cases in the author's records, of which two were performed for lithiasis and one for Odditis) (Fig. 28.4).

While manometry is of no value when X-ray results show calculi to be present it should always be used as a complementary examination when the X-ray results are normal. In the author's experience of 643 cases of radiomanometric investigation, 20 were normal at X-ray and positive manometry led to the discovery of eight organic lesions, either immediately managed or treated at an interval by means of endoscopic papillotomy.

Thus it may be said that in 1987 radio-manometry enables the surgeon to decide: on choledochotomy in order to allow intraoperative choledochoscopy; whether it is necessary to place a temporary external biliary drain or not; and whether postoperative sphincterotomy should be performed within the next 10 days or not.

For these reasons the technique is still extremely useful as an intraoperative investigative method. However simple radio-manometry gives no precise indication as to the functional state of the sphincter of Oddi. The main criticism is that it does not take into account the flow rate of the bile into the duodenum. This is why, since no other therapeutic possibilities were available before the 1970s, the radio-manometric method was improved and perfected.

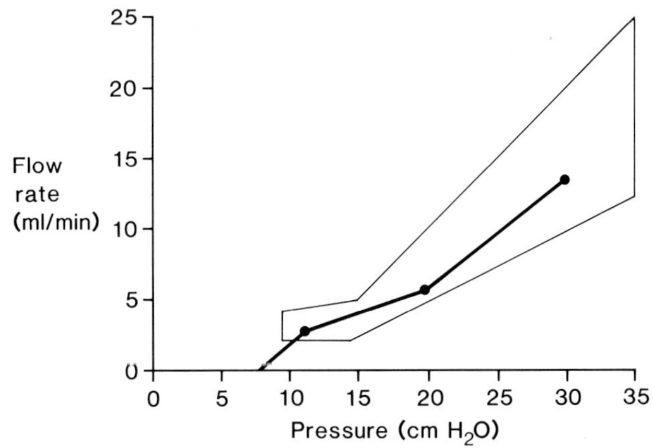

Fig. 28.7 Radio-mano-flowmetry (radiomanodebimetry). Pressure levels and flow rates from a large series are used to obtain a nomogram; the findings for each patient under investigation can be plotted

Radio-mano-flowmetry

As in simple manometry the basal pressures in the biliary tract (BP) and the pressure required to open the sphincter of Oddi (OP) are first assessed. A new element consists in measuring the flow rate of the liquid in the bile duct and on into the duodenum under various constant pressures: OP to start with, then BP × 2 and 3. By plotting pressure levels as abscissae and the flow rates as the ordinates, a graph is obtained which shows the functioning of the sphincter of Oddi for each patient under investigation. The method has been widely used in France and large series have allowed a nomogram to be plotted, which enables any biliary surgeon while operating on a patient to place him into one of three possible categories according to the hydrodynamic quality of the sphincter of Oddi (Fig. 28.7) (Vayre & Jost 1981). The categories are: a normal biliary duct, a hypotonic bile duct with high flow rate and hypertonic bile duct with low flow rate.

In the latter case it is essential to determine whether the hypertonicity is due to an organic obstacle or simply to spasm of the sphincter of Oddi. This is done by means of the same pharmaco-dynamic tests as above. Hypertonicity curves resulting from an organic lesion are in the high pressure area right from the start. Increasing the pressure does not make the flow rate any higher and the gradient of the curve remains moderate. Sphincter relaxants do not increase the flow rate. Spasm is characterized by normal flow rate under low pressure which does not rise in proportion to the pressure increase. This then constitutes a case of low flow rate under high pressure. In such circumstances a high flow rate will suddenly be restored by sphincter relaxants, the television image then demonstrating the sudden opening of the sphincter of Oddi followed by a massive flow of contrast fluid into the duodenum confirming that the spasm has been relieved.

Apparatus

The apparatus is not significantly different from that used in simple manometry. The only modification is a scale which is added to the perfusion bottle to allow for direct readings of flow rate within a given time. Diameters must be constant throughout the tubing system. More particularly the trans-cystic intubation cannula must have an inside diameter of 1 mm, in order to simplify calculations. As in simple manometry the hydraulic manometer can be replaced by a membrane manometer with electronic recording of pressure levels and flow variation. The most sophisticated apparatus is that developed by Stalport (1964), the system allowing flow rate to be read directly on a meter which works basically on the same principle as the differential pressure recorder.

Results

In a total series of 1400 direct observations at initial operation Vayre & Jost (1981) reported a 0.64% rate of residual stones or of organic stenosis of the sphincter of Oddi. Similar results are reported by White & Bordley

(1978), Tondelli & Allgower (1980), Arianoff (1976, 1979) and Yvergneaux et al (1974, 1977a, 1977b). Using his highly sophisticated apparatus Stalport (1964) obtained some even more impressive results and worked out a format for assessing 'dilatability' for the main duct and sphincter, assessing resistance of the sphincter (resistivity) and for assessing systolic activity of the common bile duct. Such refinements are exceptional and indeed Stalport remarks that 'sphincterotomy should never be based on hydro-dynamic results only'.

Radio-kinesimetry

While radio-mano-flowmetry has reached a stage of near perfection as a technique it is sometimes criticized for not allowing direct readings of the opening and closing movements of the sphincter of Oddi, or for possible interference in this mechanism as a result of contraction of the duodenal muscular wall. For this reason some authors have chosen to use a third method of manometric investigation of the biliary system, namely radio-kinesimetry.

Radio-kinesimetry consists of recording pressure variation in the main bile duct with the perfusion flow being constant. Average bile flow rate through the sphincter of Oddi is considered to be 1 ml per minute.

First, the basal pressure (BP) is measured. The bile duct is then infused regularly increasing flow rates from 1 ml/min to 6 ml/min. For each of these different constant flow rates pressure is recorded for three to five minutes, which thus demonstrates a series of oscillations on the graph. Wide oscillations correspond with the patient's breathing movements. More moderate oscillations (5 cm of water once or twice a minute) correspond with variations in pressure because of muscular contraction of the duodenum, as shown in studies based on simultaneous recordings of duodenal and common bile duct pressure. The third type of oscillation (1 to 3 cm of water up to five times a minute) corresponds with the opening and closing movements of the sphincter of Oddi. Experimental studies using electromyographic recording in conjunction with pressure measurements have shown a correlation to exist between rapid oscillation and the electrical activity of the sphincter of Oddi, irrespective of electrical activity and pressure increase due to duodenal contraction.

Perfusion is stopped after three to five minutes recording, the evolution of the curve to resting pressure being documented.

Apparatus

Perfusion is obtained simply by gravity, the reservoir being connected directly to the biliary tract. A water manometer records pressure variations. Modifications of the apparatus (Kapandji 1972) allowed automatic recording of pressure variations (Fig. 28.8).

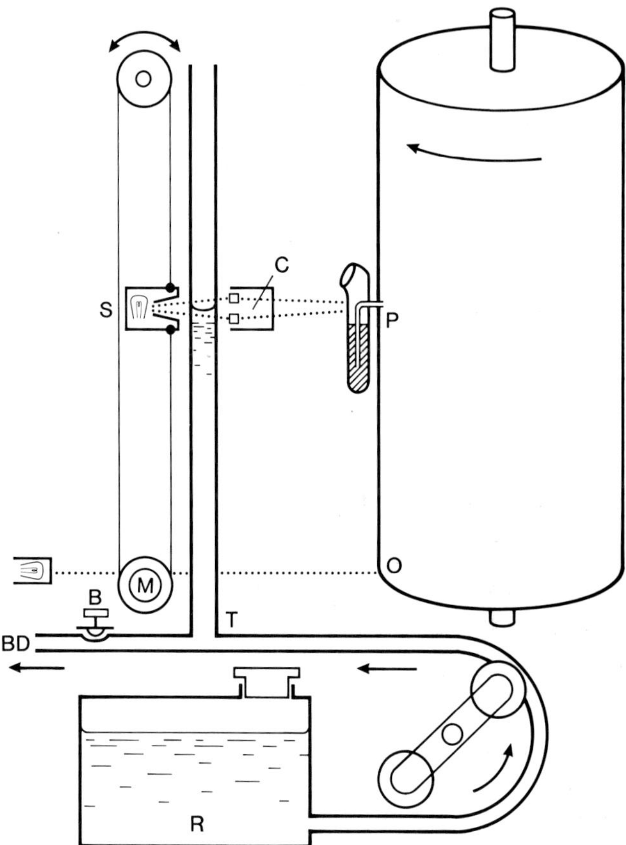

Fig. 28.8 Radiokinesimetry. The apparatus illustrated allows biliary study during surgery by measuring the flow rate and pressure of a continuous perfusion of a radio-opaque fluid. Variations in the level of liquid in the tube (T) are registered by an electronic follower (S) composed of a lamp which shines on two cells (C). As the level rises or falls the difference in light intensity received by the cells induces a motor (M) to move the follower unit to restore the level equally between the two cells. This is accomplished with the help of a logic circuit. A pen fixed to the follower unit (P) traces the curve on a cylinder (30 cm in height and 40 cm in diameter) which holds calibrated paper and makes a complete revolution every 13 minutes. The curve is easily zeroed with the help of a guide at a spot (O) sending a light beam horizontally to the lower edge of the cylinder. The height of the operating table can be adjusted so that the spot of light is projected level with the patient's sphincter of Oddi. A peristaltic pump perfuses the liquid from the tank (R) to tube (T) and to the biliary ducts of the patient (BD). The rate of flow can be adjusted to 40, 80, 120 or 200 drops per minute. A push button (B) closes the circuit and allows the establishment of a standard slope. The entire hydraulic system can be dismantled and sterilized in an autoclave. The system is compact and easy to transport.

A photo-amplifier attached to the ceiling of the operating theatre, with a C-shaped arm enabling movement in all directions is used. The generator is a 150 Kw/800 mAmp X-ray model. X-rays taken in rapid succession make it possible to compare morphological aspects of the functioning of the sphincter of Oddi. In addition, many authors cannulate the duodenum with a probe bearing a pressure sensor (Cushieri et al 1972, Cushieri 1981, Larrieu & Benoit 1978) thus making it possible to distinguish between the muscular activity of the sphincter of Oddi and the duodenum. The use of pharmaco-dynamic testing helps further with interpretation. Hyperkinesis of the second part of the duodenum may be induced and then stopped by intravenous injection of glucagon, the sphincter of Oddi recovering its autonomous rhythm of contraction.

Results

Radio-kinesimetry makes it possible to assess basal pressure (BP) in the biliary system. Infusing this in a succession of predetermined increasing flow rates, from 1 ml/min to 6 ml/min, makes it possible to assess the functional condition of the sphincter of Oddi when no organic obstacle is present, e.g. a stone obstructing the lower common bile duct immediately above the sphincter.

There are broadly speaking three possible types of curves:

Normo-tonic (Fig. 28.9) The curve rises steadily from basal to opening pressure at 15 cm of water. At this point the curve suddenly falls 2 to 3 cm thus indicating that the sphincter has opened. It then starts to rise slowly again as the sphincter closes. This oscillating movement occurs two to three times per minute, clearly representing the morphological aspect of bile evacuation, which takes the form, not of a steadily passive flow, but of a succession of spurts. The general configuration of the curve shows a progressive decrease towards a mean pressure of about 10 cm of water. Perfusion is then stopped and the ensuing fall of the curve records the evolution of the resting pressure. This should have a falling configuration returning to basal figures.

Hyper tonic In the case of an organic lesion (microstone or stenosis of the sphincter of Oddi) the curve shows a steady rise in pressure from BP. Under very high pressure the curve stabilizes as a plateau with no signs of oscillation corresponding to the opening and closing of the sphincter. Stopping perfusion does not lower the resting pressure, which remains high. If the case is one of functional stenosis of the sphincter, the initial portion of the curve is the same as above but, for a pressure considerably greater than the normal opening pressure of the sphincter, one notes a sudden fall in oscillation compared with those in the normal curve. This demonstrates that the sphincter has started functioning again, but only under a much higher pressure than normal. Once perfusion is stopped, the resting pressure decreases slowly in a succession of plateaux, often stabilizing at a level higher than the basic pressure. Injecting a sphincter relaxant at this point ensures that normal resting pressure is restored within three to five minutes.

Hypo-tonic The pressure required to open the sphincter is under 15 cm of water, immediately followed by a sudden return to an average evacuation pressure in the common bile duct very near basal pressure. The oscillation shows that the closing and opening movements of the sphincter are often of very low amplitude and frequency, a sign of sphincteric akinesia or hypokinesia. Cessation of perfusion soon brings the resting pressure back down to the level of basal pressure. Sometimes there is a new rise in the resting pressure (ascending RP), which can be a sign that the liquid has refluxed from the duodenum through a gaping sphincter. This back flow is visible radiologically. Such curves thus show both the tonicity or pressure in the common bile duct and of the sphincter of Oddi's kinesia or ability to move.

The different types of results can therefore be classified as follows:

A hypertonic curve with akinesia of the sphincter is a sign either of obstructing stone above the sphincter (ascertained by X-ray) or of irreversible stenosis of the sphincter.

A hypertonic curve with normo-kinetic or hyperkinetic curve is a sign of a functional obstacle in the region of the sphincter of Oddi. This can be corrected using a pharmacodynamic test.

A normo-tonic, normo-kinetic curve.

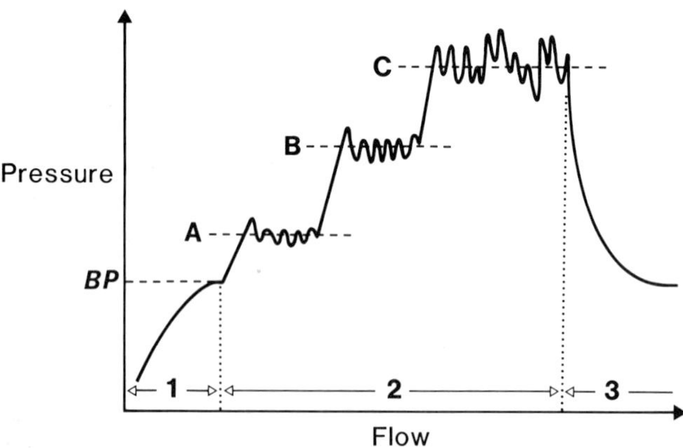

Fig. 28.9 Radiokinesimetry. The procedure can be performed in three steps.

Step 1. Initial intracavity pressure. The previously emptied tube (T) (Fig. 28.8) is connected to the biliary tract and the level goes up to a certain height. This is the initial intracavity basal pressure (BP) which is usually 8–10 cm of water.

Step 2. Kinesimetry. Perfusion at a rate of 40 drops per minute for which a standard flow is established. The level reaches a new height (A), at which pressure the sphincter opens and flow through the sphincter of Oddi is equal to the flow rate of the perfusion. At that level some contraction waves can be seen corresponding to the opening and closing of the sphincter of Oddi. Occasionally the curve rises immediately to the top during the standardization stage. This indicates an organic block (calculus or tumour).

An increase in flow rate results in a further rise in the curve which stabilizes at a fresh level (B) and (C). Note that these levels may be affected by duodenal waves which are longer and more spread out than the Oddian undulations.

Step 3. Residual pressure. The end of the perfusion is followed by a drop in the pressure (residual curve). Should the residual curve begin to rise again or remain high a pharmacodynamic test using amylnitrite or hymercromone permits the distinction of spasm from an organic obstacle.

Kinesimetry is the only biliary exploration carried out during surgery which gives functional information on the sphincteric mechanism and the duodenum.

A hypo-tonic curve with a normokinetic, hypokinetic or akinetic curve is a sign that the sphincter of Oddi is gaping.

One should refrain from interpreting curves in excessive detail but nevertheless the method seems to constitute the only way of assessing with precision the functional condition of the sphincter of Oddi. Indeed, Larrieu & Benóit (1978) found this the only method by which mobility of the sphincter could be demonstrated and, according to these authors, irreversible Odditis is diagnosed when there occurs the association of an enlarged common bile duct visualized radiologically, a high pressure level during flow into the duodenum and an absence of sphincteric movement. In such a case sphincterotomy is definitely advocated.

WHICH OF THE ABOVE TECHNIQUES IS APPLICABLE TODAY?

40 years after the inception of the method, should intraoperative manometric investigation still be used in biliary surgery? The two-fold aims of the method are important, namely the detection of stones not visualized radiologically (because of their small size) and the assessment of the functional potential of the sphincter of Oddi (with a view to diagnosing stenosing papillitis) and thus the avoidance of post-cholecystectomy morbidity. Of course, intraoperative manometry is entirely pointless if stones have been diagnosed and demonstrated radiologically or when the main bile duct has already been opened and endoluminal instruments have been used. These cause severe spasm of the sphincter and invalidate all results.

Locating calculi

Manometry enhances the quality of X-ray investigations. The main bile duct is filled in a paraphysiological fashion making it possible to inject small amounts of contrast fluid and thus ensuring that no small stones are obscured and that interference with the opening and closing of the sphincter of Oddi and with contraction of the duodenal wall is kept to a minimum.

When no stones are visualized on X-ray in a main bile duct smaller than 8 mm in diameter, normal manometric results:

avoid choledochotomy to allow intraoperative choledochoscopy

avoid temporary external biliary drainage

give a 99% assurance of trouble-free recovery after cholecystectomy

give a 99% assurance against post-cholecystectomy symptoms.

When no stone is visible radiologically and high pressure is shown to persist, manometry leads to:

either choledochotomy and choledochoscopy if the common bile duct is over 8 mm in diameter;

or trans-cystic external bile drainage if the common bile duct is under 8 mm in diameter. Radio-manometric investigation is repeated 10 days later and if the results are normal the drain is removed. If on the other hand the results point to disorders owing to microlithiasis or organic stenosis of the sphincter of Oddi, treatment should probably be through endoscopic papillotomy.

Analysing the functional potential of the sphincter of Oddi

Analysis of the functioning of the sphincter of Oddi was one of the main objectives when the methodology was developed and the results were used to justify adjuvant surgical sphincterotomy during the course of operation. With the development of more precise investigative techniques diagnosis of organic stenosis of the sphincter of Oddi has been made less often. Kinesimetry shows the incidence of true organic stenosis of the papillary region requiring sphincterotomy to be under one per cent. Since 1973 it has been possible to perform endoscopic papillotomy. This eliminates the need to decide whether to operate on the sphincter of Oddi at the time of initial surgery. The surgeon may decide to wait, using a temporary external trans-cystic biliary drain and perform radiomanometry 10 days later. Should this confirm the presence of organic stenosis in the lower part of the biliary system, endoscopic sphincterotomy would usually provide simple treatment. So it can be said that in 1987 a sophisticated analysis of the functioning of the sphincter of Oddi is no longer essential. In ordinary surgical routine simple radiomanometry is desirable.

In conclusion it is the author's opinion that, until new techniques (such as intraoperative ultrasonography) (Ch. 30) are proved more efficient, biliary manometry will remain a valid method of intraoperative investigation during operations for common bile duct stones. The technique is easy, requires little specific equipment and is low in cost. It allows for high quality and reliability of X-ray study, enables the surgeon to dispense with choledochoscopy and unnecessary external biliary drains and guarantees a speedy recovery after cholecystectomy with a low incidence of post-cholecystectomy symptoms.

REFERENCES

Arianoff A A 1976 Evaluation de l'apport des techniques radiologiques a la pathologie chirurgicale biliare, Acta Gastroenterologica Belgica vol XXXIX, p. 7–20

Arianoff A A 1979 Biligraphie pre-operatoire versus radiodebitmanometrie per-operatoire. J Chir Paris 116, no. 6–7: 451–452

Beneventano T, Jacobson H G, Hurwitt E S, Schein C J 1967 Cine-cholangiomanometry: physiologic observations. American Journal of Roentgenology, Radium Therapy and Nuclear Medicine 100: 673–679

Caroli J 1945 La radio-manometrie biliaire. Etudes techniques. Semaine des Hopitaux de Paris 21: 1278–1282

Caroli J 1946 La radiomanometrie biliaire. Sem Hop Paris 43: 1085–2000

Cuschieri A 1981 Cholangiomanometry. British Journal of Surgery 68: 369–370

Cuschieri A, Hughes J H, Cohen M 1972 Biliary-pressure studies during cholecystectomy. British Journal of Surgery 59: 267–273

Daniel O 1972 The value of radiomanometry in bile duct surgery. Annals of the Royal College of Surgeons of England 51: 357–372

Kapandji I A 1972 Le kinesigraphe en chirurgie biliaire. La Nouvelle Presse Medicale 1: 417–418

Larrieu H, Benoit G 1978 Kinesimetrie et oddite — A propos de 500 observations. Chirurgie 104: 178–183

McCarthy J D 1970 Radiomanometry during biliary operations. Archives of Surgery 100: 424–429

McCarthy J D 1977 Radiomanometric guides to common bile duct exploration. American Journal of Surgery 134: 697–701

Mieny C J, Mendelow D, Cooke P 1974 Radiomanometry in the diagnosis of common bile duct disease. South African Journal of Surgery 12: 189–191

Mortola G P, Rivara A, De Salvo L Cafiero F, Parodi E, Berti Riboli E 1977 La cholangiomanometria intraoperatoria — Revisione critica e proposta di una metodica originale. Minerva Chirurgica 32: 279–290

Naveau S, Vauzelle D, Larrieu H 1979 Radiokinesimetrie couplee biliaire et duodenale—Premiers resultats. Médecine et Chirurgie Digestives 8 no. : 615–618

Rives J, Falment J B, Palot J P, Delattre J F 1981 La radiologie moderne per-operatoire en chirurgie biliaire — Resultats obtenus dans une serie continue de 341 observations. Journal de Chirurgie (Paris) 118, no. 1: 19–24

Stalport J 1964 Etude, par debitmetrie de la physiopathologie oddienne. Journal de Chirurgie T. 88, no. 1: 11–32

Tondelli P, Allgower M 1980 Gallenwegschirurgie. Indikationen und operative verfahren bei gutartigen gallenwegserkrankungen. Springer-Verlag:

Vayre P, Jost J L 1981 La radiomanodebitmetrie per-operatoire — Incidences sur la chirurgie des voies biliaires extra-hepatiques pour 1600 operes depuis plus de 5 ans. Journal de Chirurgie (Paris) 11: 625–635

White T T, Bordley J 1978 One per cent incidence of recurrent gallstones six to eight years after manometric cholangiography. Annals of Surgery 188: 562–569

Yvergneaux J P, Bauwens E, Van Outryve L, Yvergneaux E 1977a Benign stenosis of the papilla of Vater — Diagnosis of 119 cases with conventional and selective low radiomanometry. Acta Chirurgica Belgica 76: 523–532

Yvergneaux J P, Bauwens E, Van Outryve L, Yvergneaux E 1977b Etude de la papillo-infundibulotomie mesuree avec suture, a l'aide de la radiomanometrie et de la debitmetrie electronique — Etude preliminaire. Acta Gastroenterologica Belgica 11: 413–428

Yvergneaux J P, Bauwens E, Yvergneaux E 1974 Analyse de 58 reinterventions biliaires et d'une statistique personnelle de 1,604 interventions biliaires avec radiomanometrie. Acta Gastroenterologica Belgica 37: 58–74

FURTHER READING

Bismuth H, Lazorthes F 1981 Les traumatismes operatoires de la voie biliaire principale. Monographies de l'Association Francaise de Chirurgie. Masson Paris.

Caroli J, Porcher P, Pekinio G, Delattre M 1965 Contributions of cine-radiography to study the function of human biliary tract. American Journal of Digestive Diseases 677–696

Champault G, Patel J C 1980 Exploration radiologique per-operatoire de la voie biliaire principale — Interet des modificateurs du tonus oddien. Médecine et Chirurgie Degestives 9 no. 5: 445–447

Escat J, Fourtanier G, Lacroix A, Anduze-Achez Y 1979 L'endoscopie biliaire per-operatoire dans le traitement de la lithiase. Chirurgie 105: 221–224

Faris I, Thompson J P S, Grundy D J, Le Quesne L P 1975 Operative cholangiography: a reappraisal based on a review of 400 cholangiograms. British Journal of Surgery 62: 966–972

Ferri O, Cagliani P, Arienti E, Maestri L 1980 Elettrofisiologia — Ruolo della elettromanometria nello studio intra-e postoperatorio delle vie biliari. Min Diet e Gastr 26: 271–286

Gordon F, Cassie, Kapadia C R 1981 Short notes and case reports — Operative cholangiography or extraductal palpation: an analysis of 418 cholecystectomies. British Journal of Surgery 68: 516–517

Hagenmuller F, Ossenberg F, Classen M 1977 Duodenoscopic manometry of the common bile duct. In: Delmont J (ed) The sphincter of Oddi. Karger, Basle, 72.76

Havard C 1970 Operative cholangiography. British Journal of Surgery 57: 797–807

Hepp J 1974 Reflexions sur la radiomanometrie per-operatoire. Cahiers de Medecine 15 (12): 791–794

Hess W 1954 Die primare stenosierente Papillitis. Helvetica Chirurgica Acta 21: 433–437

Hollender L F, Meyer C H, Goldschmidt P, Vouge M, Marrie A 1981 A propos de la fiabilite des explorations radiographiques de la voie biliaire principale pour lithiase. Journal de Chirurgie (Paris) 118, no. 8–9: 463–365

Kapandji I A 1947 La kinesimetrie et la kinesigraphie en chirurgie biliaire. Annales de Chirurgie 3: 293–297

Kavlie H, White T T 1972 Flow rates and manometry in the assessment of the common bile duct. Acta Chirurgica Scandinavica 138, no. 8: 817–826

Keighley M R B, Kappas A 1980 Evaluation of operative choledochoscopy. Surgery, Gynecology and Obstetrics 150: 357–359

Kock J P, Jensen S K 1982 Operative pressure profile at Oddi's sphincter and in the choledochus duct through the cystic duct (development of a normal curve). Acta Chirurgica Scandinavica 148, no. 2: 159–161

Larrieu H 1975 Abord de la kinesimetrie dans l'exploration des voies biliaires. J. de Radiologie et d'Electrologie 56:633

Lataste J, Albou J C 1977 Le reflux dans le canal de Wirsung au cours de la radiomanometrie biliaire per-operatoire — A propos de 200 cas. Journal de Chirurgie (Paris) 113, no. 1: 3–14

Mallet-Guy B 1952 Value of peroperative manometric and roentgenographic examination in the diagnosis of pathologic changes and functional disturbances of the biliary tract. Surgery, Gynecology and Obstetrics 94:385

Mallet-Guy P, Rose D F 1956 Preoperative manometry and radiology in biliary tract disorders. British Journal of Surgery 44–55

Michon H 1961 L'exploration per et post-operatoire de la fonction oddienne per la kinesimetrie. These de Paris

Mirizzi P L 1932 La cholangiographia durante las operaciones de las vias biliares. Bol. Y. Trob. Soc. de Cirugia, Buenos-Aires 16, no. 24: 25, 30, 31

Moody F G 1981 Surgical applications of sphincteroplasty and choledochoduodenostomy. Surgical Clinics of North America 61, no. 4: 909–921

de Nunno R, Ballabio R 1979 Nuovo colangioflussimanometro elettronico per la chirurgia biliare. Minerva Chirurgica 34: 1335–1337

Ordner C, Bloch P, Hollender L F, Meyer C 1979 Cholangiographie per-operatoire et calculs oublies. Medecine et Chirurgie Digestives 8, no. 7: 625–627

Oster M J, Csendes A, Funch-Jensen P, Skjoldborg H 1980 Intraoperative pressure measurements of the choledochoduodenal junction, common bile duct, cysticocholedochal junction and gallbladder in humans. Surgery, Gynecology and Obstetrics 150: 385–389

Poilleux F, Goidin E, Tricarita A 1958 Notes sur une nouvelle methode d'exploration des voies biliaires: la kinesimetrie. Arch. Mal. App. Dig. date 47, no. 3: 153–164

Poilleux F, Michon H Controle de la fonction oddienne par la kinesimetrie per et post-operatoire — Incidences therapeutiques. per-operatoire. Memoire de l'Academie de Chirurgie 79: 304–312
Rattner D W, Warshaw A L 1981 Impact of choledochoscopy on the management of choledocholithiasis — Experience with 499 common duct explorations at the Massachusetts General Hospital. Annals of Surgery 194, no. 1: 76–79
Ribeiro B F, Williams J T, Lees W R, Roberts M, Le Quesne L P 1980 An evaluation of cholangiomanometry with synchronous cholangiography. British Journal of Surgery 67: 863–868
Rosch W, Koch H, Demlang L 1976 Manometric studies during ERCP and endoscopic papillotomy. Endoscopy 8: 30–33
Ross H 1980 An aid to the complete visualisation of the bile duct with the Storz choledochoscope. Surgery, Gynecology and Obstetrics 150, 4: 574–575
Roux M, Debray C H, Le Canuet R 1953 Reflexion a propos de 260 observations de chirurgie biliaire sous controle radio-manometrique per-operatoire. Memoire de l'Academie de Chirurgie 79: 304–312
Seiyo Ikeda, Masao Tanaka, Hideo Yioshimoto, Hideaki Itoh, Fumio Nakayama 1981 Improved visualisation of intrahepatic bile ducts by endoscopic retrograde balloon catheter cholangiography. Annals of Surgery 194: 171–175
Sigel B, Machi J, Beitler J C, Donahue P E, Bombeck T, Baker R J, Duarte B 1983 Comparative accuracy of operative ultra sonography and cholangiography in detecting common duct calculi. Surgery 94: 715–720
Stalport J, Nicolas E, Demelenne A, Horeckzki G 1963 A propos d'une nouvelle methode d'enregistrement debitmetrique. Acta Chirurgica Belgica 2: 220–223
Van Sonnenberg E, Ferrucci J T, Neff C C, Mueller P R, Simeone J F, Wittenberg J 1983 Biliary pressure: manometric and perfusion studies at percutaneous transhepatic cholangiography and percutaneous biliary drainage. Radiology 148: 41–50

Choledochoscopy

Bakes (1923) was the first to draw attention to the fact that manipulation within a tubular organ, without direct vision, is difficult and accompanied by a high failure rate. He recommended an ear funnel with a mirror and a small electrical globe to allow inspection of the distal common bile duct. McIver (1941) suggested using a cystoscope telescope system in right-angled configuration with an electrical light source; but he was unable to generate interest. In Europe Wildegans popularized choledochoscopy by advertising an endoscope with a 60° angulation and interchangeable sheath (Wildegans 1953, 1960). The author started using this instrument but with limited success (Berci 1961). One of the main problems was the configuration of this instrument since manipulation was difficult in patients in whom the rib cage was near to the incision. In addition, the optical image was not satisfactory.

With the introduction of the Hopkins rod lens system the author was able to design a small instrument with a better image quality and illumination and published the first results 14 years ago (Shore & Berci 1971, Griffin 1976). Since then, this instrument has been widely accepted. With the advent of the flexible endoscope, flexible choledochoscopes were soon available (Yamakawa & Mieno 1975). Choledochoscopy has introduced an important new parameter into biliary surgery, especially in the management of common bile duct stones, in assessment and biopsy of tumours of the bile ducts and in allowing choledochoscopic approaches, not only intraoperatively but in the postoperative period.

Gallstones in the common bile duct, however, remain the major problem. Ever since Kehr (1913), published his unique textbook of biliary surgery, the problem of the retained common bile duct stone has plagued patients and surgeons alike. The real incidence of this complication is not known but is reported as between five and 28% (Schein et al 1966, Smith et al 1957, Hicken et al 1959, Corlette et al 1978, Gartell & McGinn 1984, Berci & Cuschieri 1984, Berci & Hamlin 1984). The results depend on the accuracy of follow-up. It is essential that all postoperative T-tube cholangiograms should be recorded in a hospital for a period of five years, so as to allow an accurate reflection of the problem since the incidence may fluctuate from year to year. The number of common bile duct explorations is relatively small and accounts for only 15–20% of patients submitted to cholecystectomy. If the common bile duct is primarily closed after exploration, or a biliary-enteric bypass is performed, then these patients should be excluded from the evaluation. The rapid rise of endoscopic papillotomy for common bile duct stones in the cholecystectomized patient also indicates that more stones are missed than surgeons are willing to believe. In the overwhelming majority of such cases, common bile duct stones were overlooked at first or second operation.

Gallstone disease is one of the most frequent reasons for surgical operation, 750 000 cholecystectomies and approximately 120 000 common bile duct explorations per annum being carried out in the United States alone (Wood 1979). The socio-economic aspects are also of importance since if a patient has to accommodate an indwelling T-tube for a period of six weeks, he or she cannot continue normal physical activities. Even the simplest, safest and most successful second procedure, stone removal through the T-tube tract, needs one or more sessions (Berci & Hamlin 1981a). Endoscopic papillotomy usually requires a stay of one to three days in hospital. A second surgical exploration means a minimum of eight to ten days' institutional care. On a national scale the retained common duct stone adds significantly to the ever-increasing cost of health delivery.

The author, having been personally involved in the development of choledochoscopy over 23 years, must ask the question: Does intraoperative choledochoscopy really decrease the incidence of retained stones? Some authors find the technique of great value and claim only 0–3% of missed stones with the routine use of choledochoscopy (Griffin 1976, Finnis & Towntree 1977, Lennert 1980, Reitsma 1981, Yap et al 1980); whereas others do not support these claims (Feliciano et al 1980, Rattner & Warshaw 1981). All agree, however, that, if choledochoscopy is employed after the standard attempts at stone extraction, further stones are recovered in 10–15% of cases (Berci & Cuschieri 1984).

What are the factors which contribute to the great variation in reported results, and which is the best method of learning choledochoscopy? The author has recently conducted a survey of 184 large Californian hospitals (total population of California 20 million). 87% of these institutions had purchased a rigid or flexible choledochoscope. However, surgeons used it routinely in only 8% of cases (Shulman & Berci 1985). Thus, even though the instruments are available, surgeons are reluctant to use them (King & String 1983). What are the reasons for this?

In California the average surgeon may perform 30–40 cholecystectomies per year. However, this means that the experience of common bile duct exploration is limited to three to five cases per surgeon per year. Thus, although during the last 14 years the concept of intraoperative biliary endoscopy has been theoretically accepted, it is possible to conclude that it has not been on a large scale.

The advantages of choledochoscopy and definition of unsuspected lesions of the biliary tract, in the biopsy and diagnosis of liver tumours and its use postoperatively or following percutaneous transhepatic drainage utilizing the track of drainage tubes have been even less fully appreciated.

This chapter outlines a practice of choledochoscopy, learning techniques, operative methods and an assessment of relevance to other diagnostic modalities.

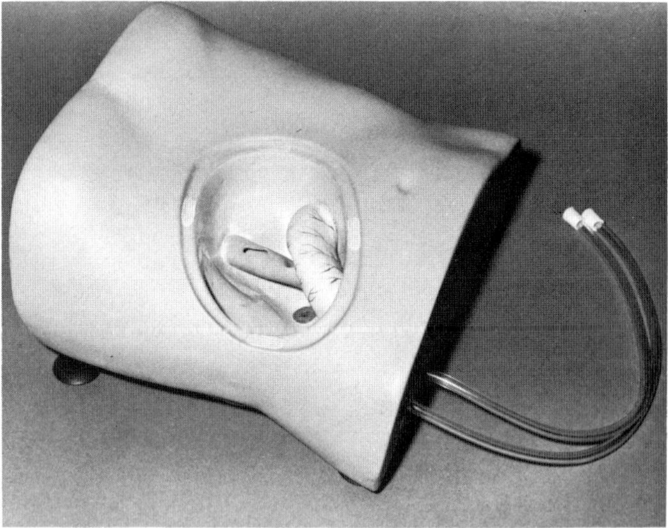

Fig. 29.1 Biliary model. The common bile duct and the duodenum are pliable and simulate physiological conditions. During practice irrigation can be used

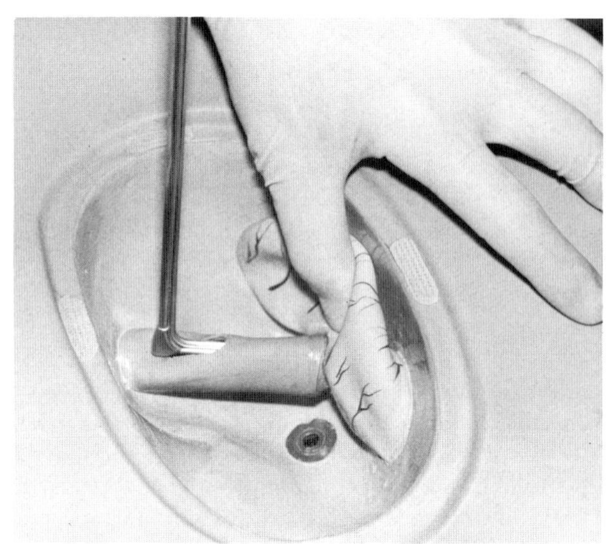

Fig. 29.2 The duodenum has to be kept on a traction to allow improved vision of the sphincter area

TRAINING

Adequate training in choledochoscopy can be acquired by practice under supervision in the operating room and particularly if television choledochoscopy (see below) is practised. On the other hand, learning basic techniques using models of the biliary system is of value.

Animal model

A satisfactory model of the dilated common bile duct can be created from the inferior vena cava of mongrel dogs. The vena cava is ligated immediately below the renal veins. The lumbar veins are also dissected and ligated and a tie is placed below the bifurcation, creating a closed tubular system. Incising the isolated cava, a dilated 'common bile duct' is created. Choledochoscopy and various stone-removal manoeuvres can then be practised. This is a time-consuming, expensive dissection but is a not-unreasonable approach in those hospitals with appropriate animal laboratory facilities.

Biliary model

Early models displaying the shape or size of the extrahepatic biliary system were not ideal since they were rigid and did not simulate anatomical conditions. A plastic biliary phantom has been designed* in which the 'duodenum' has to be kept under tension in order to keep the distal duct on the stretch so as to improve visualization of the sphincter region. The Kocher manoeuvre is essential and overlooked by many surgeons employing choledochoscopy. This important step, which should never be omitted, can be practised on the model. Furthermore,

* Gaumard Scientific Co. 7030, SW 46th Str. Miami, Fla. 33155. USA

during choledochoscopy, continuous irrigation of the duct with fluid is required. In the model described this can be employed, allowing the surgeon familiarity with the difficulties of working underwater (Fig. 29.1 & 29.2).

Team effort

During choledochoscopy a good assistant is essential since four hands are required to keep the duodenum on the stretch and to introduce and manipulate instruments. Should a stone come into vision, accessory instruments are introduced and the stone is withdrawn. The old concept of introducing the choledochoscope and, if a stone is discovered, withdrawing and subsequently using standard instruments reintroduced semi-blindly, is erroneous (see below). As soon as the surgeon is in a good position, no further time should be wasted. The assistant should advance the most suitable accessory stone-grasping instrument and deliver the stone. During choledochoscopy, the first opportunity is the best one and in an oedematous, inflamed duct, unnecessary prolonged manipulation should be avoided.

Television choledochoscopy

Choledochoscopy is greatly facilitated if the enlarged image of the intraluminal duct can be seen from a convenient distance and discussed together with the entire surgical team. Orthopaedic surgeons have long appreciated that delicate procedures can be performed through an arthroscope coupled to a TV camera, the surgeon and assistant both participating. These approaches are also useful in teaching and practice of choledochoscopy (Berci et al 1985).** There is no reason why the cost of the television camera cannot be spread by allowing its use between orthopaedic surgeons, general surgeons, and those in other disciplines (Fig. 29.3 & 29.4).

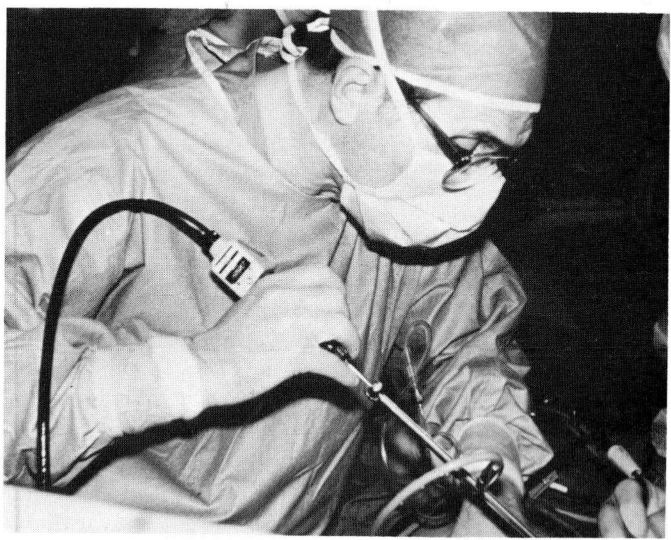

Fig. 29.3 Choledochoscopy and stone removal under visual control is a team effort. Four hands and co-ordinated movements are required. A miniature TV camera — which can be sterilized — is attached to the instrument

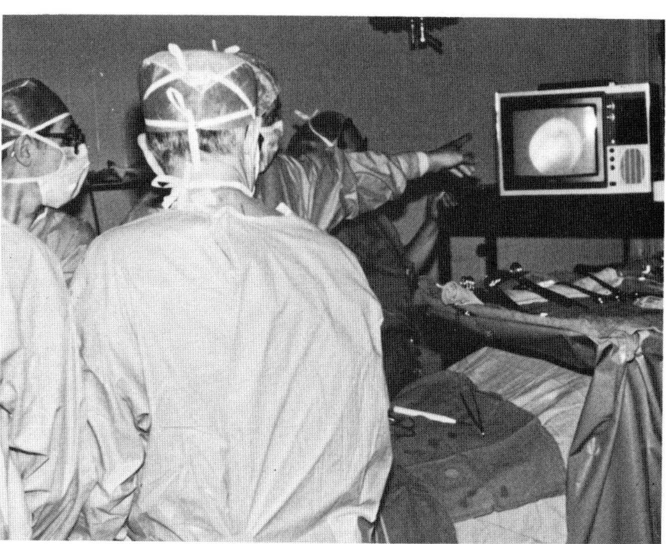

Fig. 29.4 The entire surgical team can follow the procedure. It is easy for the assistant to introduce stone retrieving instrument(s) and observe manipulations with the operator

TECHNIQUE

Surgical approach

Several incisions may be used to afford access to the biliary tree (subcostal, transverse, right paramedian, midline). The most important fact, however, is that an adequate approach to the anatomy should allow exposure of the gallbladder, liver, extrahepatic biliary system, duodenum and head of the pancreas. Choledochoscopy, as with any other manipulation involving the extrahepatic biliary system, needs an incision that allows good access and good illumination.

Operative cholangiography (see Ch. 27)

Choledochoscopy does not exclude cholangiography. Both are complementary and should be employed. The author routinely uses operative cholangiography with exceedingly good results (Berci & Hamlin 1981). Although this important intraoperative modality has been available for decades, surgeons continue to be sceptical and some claim it is too time-consuming, its technical failure rate is unacceptably high, as is the false-positive and false-negative rate and, furthermore, that it is not cost-effective. When operative cholangiography falls short of expectations,

** Circon Corp. 749 Ward Drive Santa Barbara, Ca. 93111. USA

surgeons point to the radiologist, blaming equipment failure, poor exposure techniques, time delay and interpretative errors. The surgeon feels frustrated by the lack of understanding and control of radiological factors. Radiologists consider the examination as substandard because they lack direct control, blaming the surgeons for not understanding the basic techniques such as the necessity of good scout films, the importance of patient positioning, careful injection of contrast material and the removal of opaque clamps and instruments from the field. If progress is to be achieved, a co-operative effort must be made by both disciplines.

An initial cystic duct or initial choledocho-cholangiogram is preferred because under these conditions there is still a closed system without the introduction of possible artefacts caused by manipulation. The films provide a valuable baseline of information to the surgeon *early in the course of the operation.*

The timely display of ductal anatomy aids in subsequent dissection. Attention is drawn to important ductal anomalies of surgical interest and the number and location of stones will usually be displayed. With a well-performed negative cholangiogram, unnecessary exploration of the common bile duct which is accompanied by an increased morbidity can be avoided (Berci & Hamlin 1981).

Technique of choledochoscopy

Choledochoscopy should be carried out under strictly sterile conditions. Sometimes the surgeon has worked for an hour or so in an extremely well-illuminated field and then must suddenly change to a small monocular eyepiece. These changes can make perception difficult. The requirements for sterilizing the instrument and the limited vision have perhaps inhibited successful wide application of choledochoscopy but recent developments in optical technology have made a major advance. In particular, the development of miniature, sterilizable, attachable television cameras have made a contribution to significant recent changes in endoscopic technique.

There are basically two types of choledochoscope, the rigid and the flexible. It does not matter which instrument is employed as long as the operator is familiar with it. The authors prefer the rigid choledochoscope since it is simple to manipulate, easy to learn, and less expensive (Berci & Shore 1981, Berci & Cuschieri 1984, Iseli & Marshall 1978).

Instrumentation

Before the procedure is started, the surgeon should check with the nurse that the endoscope and accessory instruments are available and in good condition. It is advisable to keep the choledochoscope on a separate sterile table.

The rigid choledochoscope consists of a right-angled telescope with a built-in irrigation channel and a fibre-optic light carrier. The outside diameter is 5 × 3 mm and allows its insertion even into a non-dilated duct. The standard 40 mm horizontal limb usually suffices but on occasion the distal duct can be long and a second 60 mm instrument is needed to visualize the ampulla (Fig. 29.5–29.9).† It is of the utmost importance to obtain an initial cholangiogram so as to visualize the site of drainage and the configuration of the distal duct, since this will determine which instrument will be employed (the short or the long one) and what difficulties can be anticipated because of a long or tortuous duct.

The attachable instrument channel is one of the most important accessories. In case of choledocholithiasis it should be attached immediately and introduced with the scope. Instead of blind manipulation, the Dormia stone basket is applied. Calculi can be entrapped with precision under visual control. The same instrument channel can be used for the advancement of a balloon catheter. In case of manipulations an assistant is required and therefore a teaching attachment (Fig. 29.5) or television camera is ideal. This provides the possibility of simultaneous observation and co-ordinated manipulation in extracting calculi.

With the employment of orthodox techniques, the biliary balloon catheter is introduced blindly into the duodenum, inflated and palpated. During withdrawal the balloon has to be deflated to be able to pass the sphincter. During this manoeuvre the balloon may suddenly 'jump'

† Karl Storz Endoscopy, 7200 Tuttlingen, P O Box 4752 W. Germany

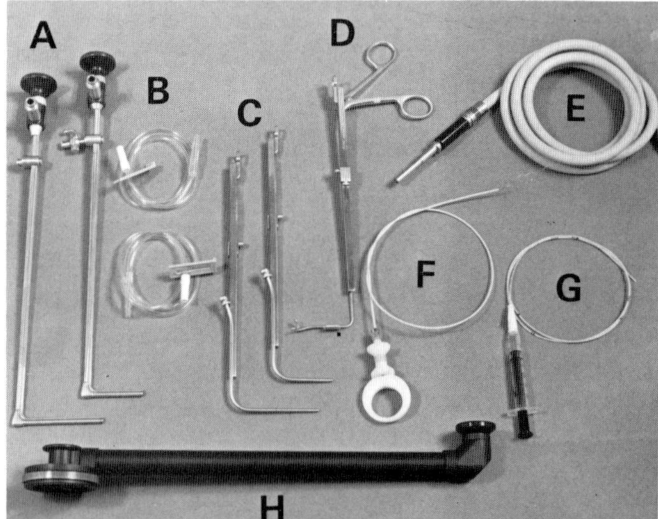

Fig. 29.5 A. A shorter and a longer rigid choledochoscope. Shorter: horizontal length 40 mm, longer limb: 60 mm. B. Two venous extension tubes. C. Instrument guide channel. D. Biopsy forceps. E. Fibre-optic light guide. F. Dormia stone basket to be introduced through the instrument guide channel which is attached to the telescope. G. Fr. 4 balloon catheter to be introduced to the same (C) instrument guide channel. H. A teaching attachment which can be gas sterilized

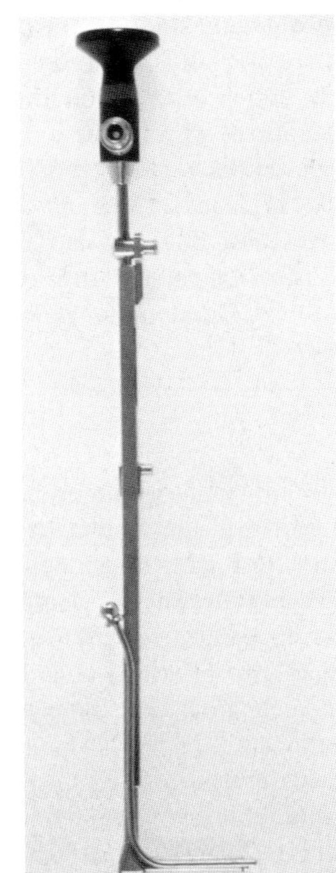

Fig. 29.6 Instrument guide channel attached to the choledochoscope

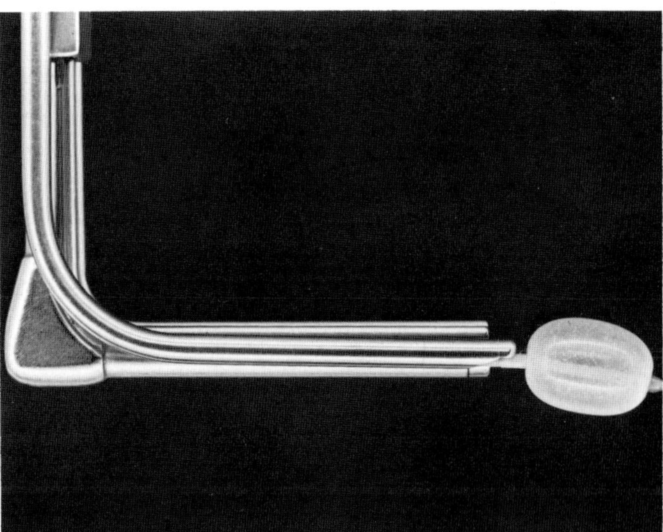

Fig. 29.8 Fr. 4 balloon catheter. The balloon is passed beyond the stone. The endoscope with the stone is withdrawn (together) into the incision

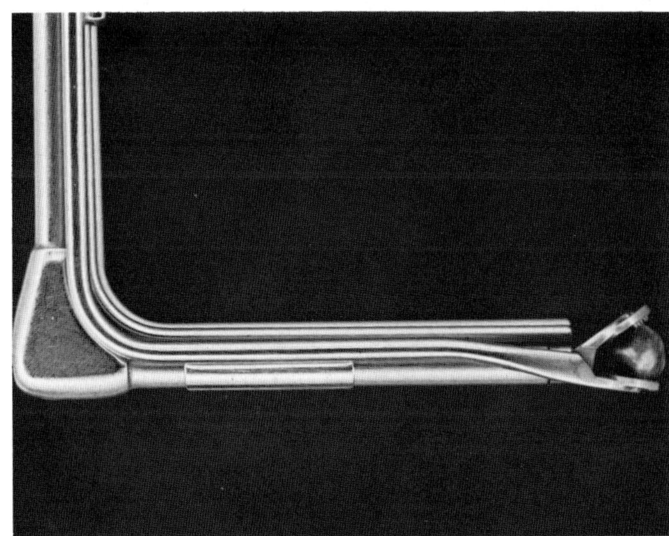

Fig. 29.9 For removal of impacted stones (distal duct) this attachable stone forceps can be of great help

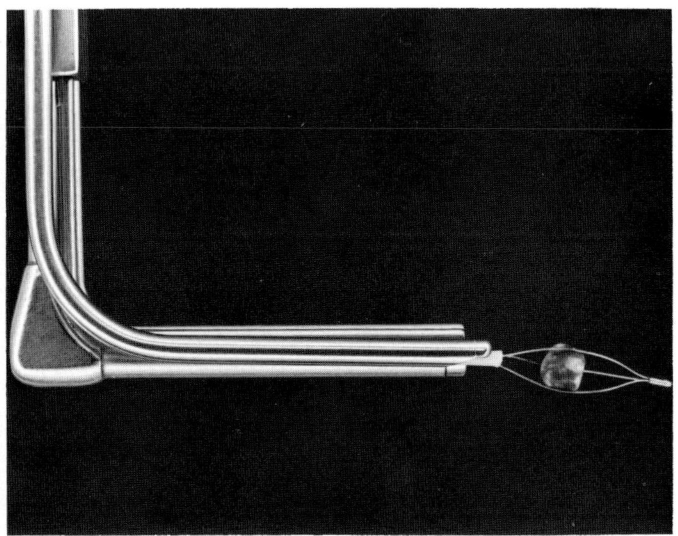

Fig. 29.7 Dormia stone basket. The position of the basket and stone can be easily observed and necessary movements carried out to entrap the calculus

and despite immediate re-inflation a calculus in the sphincteric area can be bypassed. The same manoeuvre can be performed under endoscopic control which allows the position of the balloon in relation to the sphincter to be observed. Impacted stones can be removed with stone forceps but the Dormia basket and balloon catheter (size Fr. 4) are the major tools for stone extraction.

To provide adequate irrigation for the proper distension and clearing of the ducts a Fenwal pressure irrigation system, available in every operating theatre, is used. A cuff pressure of 150 mmHg, monitored by a manometer ensures proper visualization. The saline is delivered to the bile duct under low pressure because there is high resistance created by the narrow irrigation channel. A saline drip, under hydrostatic pressure only, does not suffice. Illumination is provided from an external light source via a flexible fibre-optic cable. An attachable biopsy forceps is provided to obtain tissue samples of suspicious areas.

The flexible fibre-optic choledochoscope (Fig. 29.10)

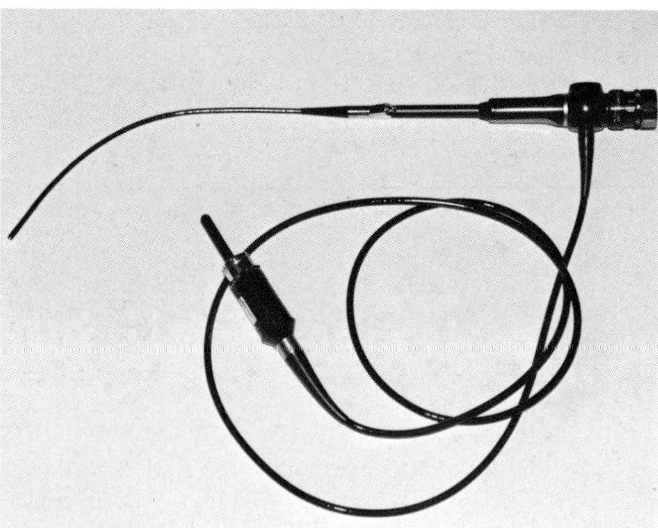

Fig. 29.10 Flexible choledochoscope with instrument channel O.D: 5 mm. This instrument is used mainly in the postoperative period for extraction of retained stones through the T-tube tract

should not exceed an outside diameter of 5 mm.* The tip movements (up and down) can be controlled at the eyepiece by the thumb. Due to the fact that the tip can be moved only in one plane, it is sometimes necessary for the assistant to apply a rotational force. For stone removal, a stone basket or the same Fr 4 balloon catheter mentioned above, can be advanced through the instrument channel. The irrigation conditions are the same as described above. The assistant has to advance the basket or balloon catheter. New versions of the totally immersible flexible endoscopes have made sterilization easier. This instrument needs extreme care in handling, maintenance and operation because it is extremely fragile and expensive.

Exploration of the bile duct and choledochoscopic procedures

Stay sutures are placed and a small standard choledochotomy incision, not exceeding 10 mm, is made in the common bile duct. A suction tube should be placed beside the common bile duct to remove overflow of irrigation fluids. The sutures are held by haemostats and crossed after the insertion of the endoscope, thus decreasing leakage.

The most important step, often overlooked and probably the main factor in unsuccessful endoscopic procedures of the distal ducts, is the omission or insufficient mobilization of the duodenum. It is not enough to divide the peritoneal reflection of the anti-mesenteric border of the second part of the duodenum. The duodenum must be widely mobilized since only if this is done can it be kept on an adequate stretch allowing one to straighten a tortuous or curved distal duct and thus facilitate adequate visualization. During the endoscopic examination, one hand must always be placed on the mobilized duodenum. The endoscope can then be felt as a probe and the wall of the duct can be stretched in front of the advancing instrument, keeping it straight and allowing better vision. It is not necessary to pass the instrument through the sphincter of Oddi and on into the duodenum, provided the sphincter is well observed.

Endoscopic appearances

Immediately after introducing the endoscope, a yellowish or red disc will be seen. This indicates that the tip of the endoscope is in contact with the ductal wall. This can be corrected by slow withdrawal or tilting of the endoscope until the tubular appearance of the duct or the sphincter is seen. In case of the proximal duct system, the bifurcation is easily recognized. The best views are generally obtained on withdrawal of the instrument, followed by slow advancement under direct visual control.

After the distal duct is examined, the endoscope is withdrawn, rotated 180° and re-introduced towards the hepatic ducts. Once the bifurcation is identified, the endoscope is rotated to bring the right main hepatic ductal orifice into view. It is then advanced along the tributaries as far as possible. The variations of the normal anatomy (proximal duct) are numerous but after a little experience it is possible to examine each orifice systematically. Upon slow withdrawal and slight rotation to the right, the orifice of the left main hepatic duct can be seen and this in turn is followed peripherally. It is not unusual to be able to examine even tertiary bifurcations of the bile ducts. An important further technical point is worthy of mention. The cystic duct *stump*, which may be quite long (Berci & Hamlin 1981), should be independently checked. This is important since a small calculus can easily remain hidden in such a long and possibly tortuous stump. This is particularly so in cases with multiple stones in a dilated duct. The cystic duct stump is checked by introducing a flexible probe or catheter and passing it on into the common bile duct. This will deliver any calculi into the duct where they can be visualized at (repeated) choledochoscopy and removed.

The normal mucous membrane of the common bile duct is pale pink in appearance with a faint yellow tinge. There are usually several longitudinal folds present which are flattened by the pressure of the irrigating liquid. A delicate, submucosal vascular reticulum is usually visible. Approaching the ampulla, the duct narrows, becoming funnel-shaped and curves towards the right posteriorly. The sphincter area itself has a characteristic appearance which must be identified to ensure complete distal examination. The orifice is seen as outlined against the darker

* Olympus Co. Tokyo.

background of the adjacent duodenal lumen. It usually appears stellate but may look somewhat fish-mouthed, be pinpoint or patulous in nature. The mucosa in the papillary area is coarser and raised into folds, covered sometimes by a fibrinous exudate. Failure to visualize the sphincter area precludes any diagnostic conclusions regarding the state of the distal duct. The orifice of the pancreatic duct is hardly ever seen. Bifurcation of the common hepatic duct is similar to the appearance of the main bifurcation of the bronchial tree seen at bronchoscopy. The right hepatic duct soon divides into its main sectoral branches, whereas the left duct usually has no major visible tributary. The mucosa of the hepatic duct is paler than that of the distal duct. Variations in the hepatic ductal anatomy or orifices are very common (Ch. 2). In particular, a sectoral tributary of the right hepatic duct may join the left hepatic duct and give the appearance of a trifurcation. The ducts may be dilated, allowing examination of segmental (tertiary) hepatic ducts. The identification of the major bifurcation is mandatory in order to achieve hepatic duct visualization.

Cholangitis is a very common finding in patients with choledocholithiasis and can be of varying degree, ranging from mucosal congestion and oedema to marked ulcerative cholangitis with fibrinous exudation. These inflammatory changes become more marked in the papillary regions. At times, the examination of the sphincter area is obscured by an inflammatory exudate which has accumulated in this region. Removal of this debris by irrigation or stone forceps, after temporary withdrawal of the endoscope, usually improves visualization. The changes are far less conspicuous in the proximal duct and in the hepatic ducts.

Gallstones are easily identified and may be free-floating. Indeed, they sometimes evacuate spontaneously on withdrawal of the endoscope. At times a stone can be found impacted in the orifice of an hepatic duct or at the ampulla, partially embedded in the ductal wall or in a diverticulum of the distal duct. Multiple stones and biliary mud are frequently found behind a larger calculus. Repeated endoscopic examinations are necessary to make sure that a complete stone-free duct is left behind after exploration. Multiple small calculi in the hepatic ductal branches associated with biliary mud in a dilated duct and in an elderly patient should cause the surgeon to consider biliary-enteric bypass (Ch. 46). In the case of impacted intrahepatic stones it is important to manipulate with precision under endoscopic control (careful basket or balloon movements beyond the stone) to avoid perforation or haemobilia, which can be induced by perforating the wall of the bile duct and damaging adjacent vessels (Ch. 85).

In general terms, in the case of floating stones, the basket or balloon should be positioned beyond the stone. The basket is then carefully opened and the position of the stone observed. The endoscope is tilted or moved, together with the basket, and these manipulations allow the stone to be entrapped. The endoscope and the basket are then withdrawn together.

There are several important points worthy of emphasis. The best opportunity to remove stones in a difficult situation is the first one; therefore, if the endoscope is in a good position, it should not be withdrawn or moved. The position should be maintained and the assistant advance the basket, balloon catheter, or stone-grasper. The stone is then entrapped and the instrument removed together with the stone. To enable this teamwork, a teaching attachment for the endoscope or an attached television camera is necessary.

The *normal ampullary area* is soft and pliable. If the area is observed for a minute or so, the opening and closing phases of the sphincter can be seen. *Sphincter stenosis* presents as a pinpoint opening which does not change in configuration but the appearance is unfortunately not diagnostic since a similar change can be caused by prolonged spasm due to frequent manipulation.

Neoplasms of the biliary system can be visualized and biopsied, and specimens can also be obtained for cytological examination. Papillary tumours in particular protrude into the lumen of the biliary tract and are readily seen and biopsied. Even though the biopsy specimens obtained are small, they are usually adequate for diagnosis. Extrinsic ductal obstruction due to a neoplasm of extraductal origin (e.g. pancreatic carcinoma, metastatic disease, lymphoma) create an appearance of complete occlusion of the ductal system through which the instrument cannot be advanced. There may or may not be breaching of the mucosal integrity. Extrinsic compression of the distal common bile duct by an inflammatory mass is indistinguishable from a malignant lesion. Choledochoscopic examination in cases of papillary bile duct tumour, particularly low bile duct tumours, is important and the whole biliary tree should be examined since multicentric tumours may be found in up to 7% of cases (Ch. 65).

Bile duct tumours may be unexpectedly encountered on exploration of the common bile duct for stone and it is important to remember this possibility.

COMPLICATIONS

The author is not aware of any major complications which have followed choledochoscopy. 500 patients submitted to choledochoscopy have been observed and no case of perforation of the common bile duct or haemobilia noted (Berci & Cuschieri 1984). The incidence of wound infection and subphrenic abscess is not known to be increased in cases in which choledochoscopy has been employed intraoperatively.

CONCLUSIONS

The general surgeon should become familiar with the use of a choledochoscope at operation. Such familiarity will allow developing skills in the use of flexible choledochoscopes employed in the postoperative period through the T-tube tract and their use following dilatation of previously-placed transhepatic percutaneous drains.

Familiarity and expertise with choledochoscopic techniques would reduce the incidence of retained common bile duct stones very considerably and improve the diagnosis of bile duct tumours. Removal of stones and biopsy of tumours under direct vision is much more precise than the employment of blind techniques and complete removal of stones without damage to the ducts is much more likely using direct visual control.

While intraoperative cholangiography remains mandatory, especially for the early demonstration of anatomical abnormalities and as an index for duct exploration (Ch. 27, 46), choledochoscopy is probably the best method for exploring the duct and for ensuring a complete clearance of stones. Post-exploratory cholangiography (Ch. 46, 52) is also very effective if used in an expert manner but in the author's opinion is less satisfactory and probably less accurate than the employment of choledochoscopic techniques.

Taken together, the appropriate use of intraoperative diagnostic tests, including operative cholangiography and intraoperative choledochoscopy will greatly improve the standard of biliary tract surgery and reduce the retained stone rate to acceptable levels. The techniques are safe and should be appropriately taught in all institutions. The expense of acquiring adequate instrumentation will be more than offset by the saving to the health care services engendered as a result of a reduction in the number of retained common bile duct stones.

REFERENCES

Bakes J 1923 Die Choledochopapilloskopie. Archiv fuer Klinische Chirurgie 126: 473–483

Berci G 1961 Choledochoscopy. Medical Journal of Australia 2:861

Berci G, Shore J M, Morgenstern L 1971 An improved rigid choledochoscope. American Journal of Surgery 122: 567–568

Berci G, Hamlin J A 1981a Retrieval of retained stones. In: Operative biliary radiology. Williams & Wilkins, Baltimore, p 147–159

Berci G, Hamlin J A 1981b The fluorocholangiogram. In: Operative biliary radiology. Williams & Wilkins, Baltimore, p 63–109

Berci G, Shore J M 1981 Operative biliary endoscopy. In: Berci G, Hamlin J A (eds) Operative biliary radiology. Williams & Wilkins, Baltimore, p 169–187

Berci G, Cuschieri A 1984 In: Common bile duct exploration. Martinus-Nijhoff, Boston-Lancaster, p 54–61

Berci G, Hamlin J A 1984 Postoperative removal of retained stones through the T-tube tract. In: Cuschieri A, Berci G (eds) Common bile duct exploration. Martinus Nijoff, Boston-Lancaster, p 89–99

Berci G, Cuschieri A, Morgenstern L, Shulman A 1985 Television-choledochoscopy. Surgery, Gynecology and Obstetrics 160: 177–78

Corlette M B, Achatzky S, Ackroyd F 1978 Operative cholangiography and overlooked stones. Archives of Surgery 113: 729–733

Feliciano D V, Mattox K L, Jordan G L 1980 The value of choledochoscopy in exploration of the CBD. Annals of Surgery 191: 649–652

Finnis D, Towntree T 1977 Choledochoscopy in the exploration of the common bile duct. British Journal of Surgery 64: 661–664

Gartell P C, McGinn F P 1984 Choledochoscopy: are stones missed? A controlled study. British Journal of Surgery 71: 767–7770

Griffin W T 1976 Choledochoscopy. American Journal of Surgery 132: 697–698

Hicken N F, McAllister J A, Walker G 1959 The problems of retained common duct stones. American Journal of Surgery 97: 173–183

Iseli A, Marshall V C 1978 Choledochoscopy: A comparison of a rigid and a flexible instrument. Medical Journal of Australia 1: 131–132

Kehr H 1913 Praxis der Gallenwege Chirurgie. Lehman, Munich

King M, String J 1983 Extent of choledochoscopic utilization in CBD explorations. American Journal of Surgery 146: 322–324

Lennert K 1980 Choledochoskopie. Springer, Heidelberg

McIver M A 1941 An instrument for visualization of the interior of the common bile duct at operation. Surgery 9: 112–114

Rattner D W, Warshaw A L 1981 Impact of choledochoscopy on the management of choledocholithiasis. Annals of Surgery 194: 76–79

Reitsma B J 1981 Common duct stones (thesis). University of Limburg, Maastricht

Schein C J, Stern W Z, Jacobson H G 1966 Residual stones. In: Schein C J (ed) The common bile duct. Thomas, Springfield, p 266–271

Shore J M, Morgenstern L, Berci G 1971 An improved rigid choledochoscope. American Journal of Surgery 122: 567–568

Shulman G, Berci G 1985 The use of the choledochoscope: A survey of California hospitals. American Journal of Surgery 149: 703–704

Smith S, Engel C, Averbook B, Longmire W P 1957 Problems of retained and recurrent common bile duct stones. Journal of the American Medical Association 164: 231–236

Wildegans J 1953 Grenzen der Cholangiography und Aussichten der Endoskopie der tiefen Gallenwege. Medizinische Klinik 48: 1270–1273

Wildegans H 1960 Die operative Gallengang Endoskopie. Urban & Schwartzenberg, Munich

Wood M 1979 Eponyms in biliary tract surgery (presidential address). American Journal of Surgery 138: 746–749

Yamakawa T, Mieno K 1975 An improved choledochofiberscope. Gastrointestinal Endoscopy 17: 459–462

Yap P C, Atacador M, Yap A G,Yap R G 1980 Choledochoscopy as a complimentary procedure to operative cholangiography in biliary surgery. American Journal of Surgery 140: 648–650

30

J. J. Jakimowicz

Intraoperative ultrasound — biliary disease

INTRODUCTION

Before cholecystectomy is performed, a decision has to be made as to whether or not to explore the common bile duct. This decision is based upon the clinical indications, on findings at the preoperative diagnostic work-up, on peroperative findings and on the results of a peroperative diagnostic procedure, if one is used. Despite improvements in diagnostic methods it remains difficult to obtain reliable preoperative information on the condition of the common bile duct.

To improve the results of surgery on the gallbladder and biliary tract, a variety of peroperative diagnostic procedures are available.

Peroperative cholangiography (Ch. 27) alone or combined with biliary manometry (Ch. 28) has been frequently advocated as a screening procedure to detect asymptomatic common bile duct pathology. However with the exception of a few countries in the world, it has not gained general popularity (Puglionesi 1978). Similarly, peroperative cholangiography in the Netherlands is not universally applied (Hessling 1983). On the other hand, the percentage of unexpected, unpredictable common bile duct stones, which later may induce morbidity and necessitate therapy and even reoperation, ranges from 3% to 7% of cholecystectomized patients.

If peroperative cholangiography is performed, unexpected pathology may be detected. However, in up to 30% of cases there is a false positive cholangiogram (Skillings et al 1979, Saltzstein et al 1973, Start & Loughry 1980) and a relatively high score of negative, unnecessary common bile duct explorations which have made the value of this method as a screening procedure open to debate.

Thus there are reasons to search for a simple, safe, rapid and reliable peroperative screening procedure. If a peroperative screening procedure is expected to gain general popularity, it has to fulfil most of the following criteria:

be easy to perform and interpret
confirm or exclude the presence of anticipated pathology
detect unexpected pathology
demonstrate the location and extent of pathology
provide anatomical information
be generally applicable
be if possible non-invasive
show positive results in a cost benefit analysis

In a prospective study results of peroperative cholangiography, ultrasonography and manometry were evaluated in the light of the above criteria (See also Table 30.6).

The idea of the peroperative use of ultrasound imaging is almost 20 years old. The first reports on the use of ultrasound for diagnostic purposes were published in the early 1960s (Hayaski et al 1962, Knight & Newell 1963). Eiseman et al (1965) published their experience on the intraoperative use of ultrasound A-scan for detection of common bile duct stones during operation, showing a high degree of accuracy when compared with operative cholangiography. Technical limitations of the A-scanners related to the one-dimensional image (as only the analog signal was available for interpretation) were the main drawbacks which prevented this method from gaining popularity. Important developments in medical ultrasound which have taken place in the last 24 years have resulted in the production of a new generation of mobile, high resolution ultrasound scanners. High quality, two-dimensional images in real-time are provided and are much easier to interpret. Very encouraging reports on the use of real-time, B-mode ultrasound imaging in biliary and pancreatic surgery appeared in the late 1970s (Sigel et al 1979, Lane & Crocker 1979).

EQUIPMENT

A detailed and comprehensive review of the principles of medical ultrasonography may be found in books dealing with diagnostic ultrasound (White 1976, Wells 1977) and a brief review of basic information and practical hints regarding the use of intraoperative ultrasonography has been recently published (Sigel 1982).

In practical terms the ultrasonography equipment

consists of two main components: a dedicated digital electronic system, a so-called scanner, and a transducer probe. These two components are connected by a cable. The scanner provides an adequate electric signal which is used to stimulate the crystal within the transducer probe. The crystal then emits a series of ultrasonic pulses, part of which are reflected within the structure scanned, detected by the transducer crystal and converted into electrical signals. These electrical signals are transmitted along the cable back to the scanner and are amplified, processed and finally displayed in a two-dimensional image on the video screen of the scanner.

After two-and-a-half years' experience of peroperative ultrasonography, in particular of the biliary tract, the author opines that intraoperative ultrasound equipment should fulfil the following basic criteria:

The scanner should be a compact, mobile, real-time B-mode system providing a high quality image. It should be easy to operate so that the presence of a technician is not necessary.

The scanner should have two options, enabling the use of a mechanical sector or a linear array transducer. Current experience recommends that for the purpose of biliary tract screening the mechanical sector transducers should be used and for the purpose of liver and pancreas examination the linear array transducer is more suitable.

The scanner should be provided with equipment for documentation of the findings, allowing a hard copy of the image or a videotape record. The latter is very useful, particularly for teaching purposes.

As this equipment is used in the operating theatre it has to satisfy the safety conditions for electrical devices in order to avoid potential electrical hazards during the procedure.

The main limitations of ultrasound equipment are related to the transducer probe. Most of the existing commercially available transducer probes were developed for external transcutaneous use, and are thus relatively large in size. The limited space in the operative field and its specific topography for operations upon the biliary tract is one of the main drawbacks to adapting existing equipment for peroperative use. It is obvious that the transducer has to be small in size and its shape must enable easy and comfortable manipulation within the limited space available.

The cable connecting the transducer with the scanner has to be long enough to keep the scanner far enough away from the operative field to maintain sterility and to enable positioning of the scanner for easy observation of the image on the videoscreen.

Although the transducer can usually be sterilized by ethylene oxide gas, it is desirable that a sterile plastic sleeve be used to cover it during use. This makes it possible to use the same transducer for several procedures on the same day. Peroperative ultrasound examination is almost always either contact screening of the examined structures (organ) or close range screening. The technical specifications of the transducer for contact screening are essentially different from those necessary for transcutaneous use. The specifications for a transducer probe for screening of the biliary tract should be as follows:

mechanical sector
trapezoidal field of view
sector angle from 60 ° up to 100 °
ultrasound frequency 5 to 10 MHz
depth of view 4 to 6 cm with a focus of 1.5 to 2 cm
lateral resolution of at least 1 mm
small in physical size

The trapezoidal configuration of the field is one of the crucial requirements. This allows observation of a long (5–8 cm) segment of the common bile duct in one section and this is not only of importance for the reliability of the examination, as the whole duct may be seen in a few sections, but also significantly simplifies the examination as the image resembles the cholangiographic pictures to which surgeons are accustomed. This may shorten the period necessary for learning the technique. Such trapezoidal configuration of the field is achieved by mounting an adaptor on the front of the transducer. A contact area of approximately 4–6 cm should be possible between the transducer and the screened structure (Fig. 30.1). In the author's experience a frequency of 7.5 MHz is the most appropriate. The use of frequencies higher than 10 MHz may result in information of no clinical importance and lead to unnecessary exploration of the common bile duct.

In Eindhoven a mechanical sector transducer, manufactured by Philips and commercially available, is used for screening of the biliary tract and also for examination of the pancreas and liver. Initially, the Sonor Diagnost 2000

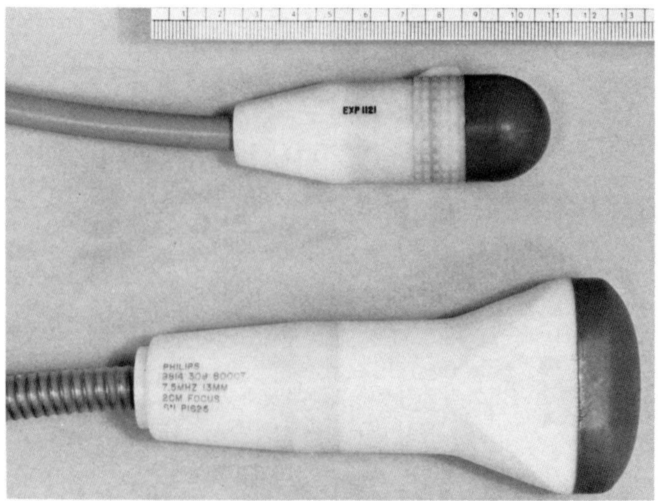

Fig. 30.1 Ultrasound transducers: the so called 'miniature' (top) and the 'small parts' transducer (bottom)

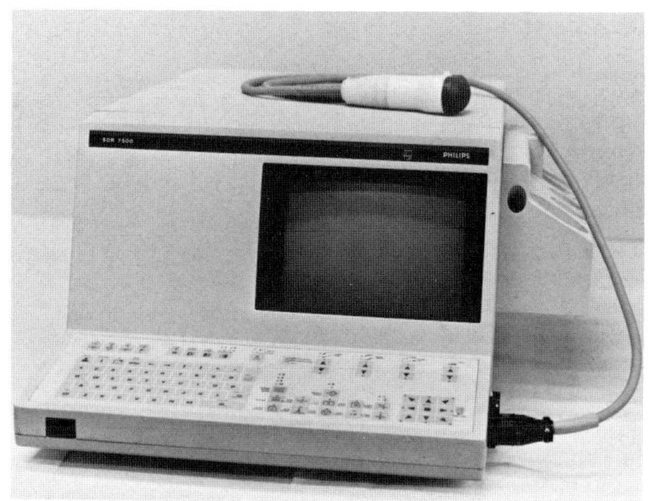

Fig. 30.2 The Philips SDR 1500 mobile, real-time B-mode ultrasound scanner

was used, later the 3000 SDR, and recently the new SDR 1500 compact mobile, real-time B-mode scanner (Fig. 30.2). This scanner offers both a mechanical sector and a linear array option.

For bile duct and pancreas examination a so-called small parts transducer is used which fulfils most of the requirements previously listed (Fig. 30.1).

Technical data of the transducers used by different investigators and in the current series are presented in Table 30.1.

TECHNIQUE

The technique of intraoperative ultrasound examination of the biliary tract has been previously documented (Sigel 1982, Carol et al 1983, Jakimowicz 1985). Ultrasonography of the biliary tract is performed after removal of the gall-bladder and ligation of the cystic duct. The duodenum is mobilized by means of Kocher's manoeuvre and usually held displaced slightly upwards and medially. The clean and non-sterile transducer is placed within a disposable, sterile plastic cover, its tip covered with methylcellulose gel. The plastic cover must fit the rubber membrane of the transducer very closely with the layer of gel between the two, so as to assure acoustic contact. The transducer is then placed in the operative field and positioned under visual control directly on the antero-lateral aspect of the common bile duct. The space between the transducer and the surface of the duct is filled with warm saline solution, avoiding the creation of air bubbles which may disturb the image.

Table 30.1 Specifications of the ultrasound transducers used by different investigators

Author	Sigel B et al 1983	Sigel B 1984	Own series	
Manufacturer of equipment	High stoy	Diasonics	Philips	
Transducer type	Mechanical sector	Mechanical sector	Mechanical sector 'small parts'	Mechanical sector 'miniature'
Frequency	7.5 MHz/ 10 MHz	10 MHz	5 MHz/ 7.5 MHz	3.5 MHz/ 5 MHz
Sector	18 °	30 °	30 ° and 60 °	50 ° and 100 °
Focus field	20 mm/ 15 mm	0–40 mm	0–40 mm	0–50 mm
Depth of view	60 mm	40 mm	40 mm	110 mm
Peroperative application	biliary tract pancreas	biliary tract pancreas	biliary tract pancreas	liver

Peroperative ultrasonography is a contact screening method. To achieve reliable results the technique of examination should be rigorously standardized. This also results in performance of the examination without unnecessary interference and without prolongation of the operation. The transducer is kept in direct contact with, or at a very close range to, the structure under examination. The hand holding the transducer probe should rest over the costal margin or on the chest of the patient. In this way disturbance of the image caused by respiratory movements is eliminated. The transducer must not exert any pressure on the pliable, hollow structure of the common bile duct, otherwise it will disturb the image and make accurate examination impossible. The scanning manoeuvres involve longitudinal scanning along the antero-lateral aspect of the duct, but turning in the distal part towards the lateral aspect. The common bile duct image should be continuously visible on the video screen. To achieve this, slight angulation and rotation of the transducer during the screening may be necessary.

When examining the common bile duct move the transducer very slowly along the duct first in the direction of the liver, until the liver tissue and intrahepatic ducts are seen. Then the probe is moved in the direction of the papilla, until the pancreatic tissue comes in view. The retroduodenal part of the duct and the papilla are examined from the anterolateral to the lateral aspect of the duct, holding the duodenum anteriorly. This is the crucial and most difficult part of the examination because this part of the duct is usually narrow and it may often be difficult to distinguish the ductal and the duodenal walls. If, on thorough observation, an echogenic zone or acoustic shadow is found, it is important that on repeated examination it is constant and really intraluminal, since a 'partial volume effect' caused by kinking of the duct or by the adjacent wall of the duodenum may be mistaken for a stone. For examination of the retroduodenal part of the common bile duct, Sigel (1984) advocates a transduodenal approach, using the duodenum as an acoustic window. With this approach great care is necessary because the air in the duodenum may disturb the image considerably. The normal common bile duct is an echolucent structure and the portal vein is often seen behind it as a broad echolucent element (Figs. 30.3, 30.8, and 30.9). Bile duct stones may be easily recognized as an echogenic element within the echolucent duct producing, in most instances, an acoustic shadow (Fig. 30.4 and 30.5). Thus sonography enables not only detection of the stone but also its localization and estimation of the number of calculi (Fig. 30.4). Not only a large stone but also bile sludge and gravel and multiple small stones, with a diameter of one mm or less, may be seen usually as an echogenic element at the bottom of the duct sometimes accompanied by a narrow acoustic shadow or, in the case of a massive gravel layer, a broad acoustic shadow (Fig. 30.6). The ultrasound features of the stones are strongly dependent on their nature (hard or soft), their size and location. It is important to note that soft primary bile duct stones are only moderately echogenic and usually do not produce an acoustic shadow. An acoustic shadow may sometimes become lost within an echolucent, markedly dilated duct or in the underlying portal vein.

Ultrasonography also enables measurement of the internal diameter of the common bile duct. However,

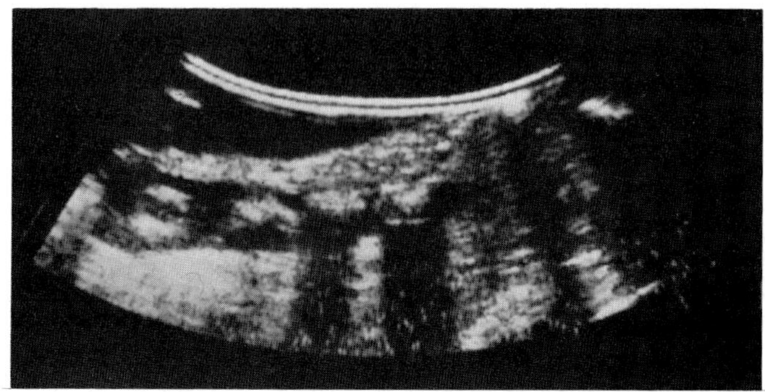

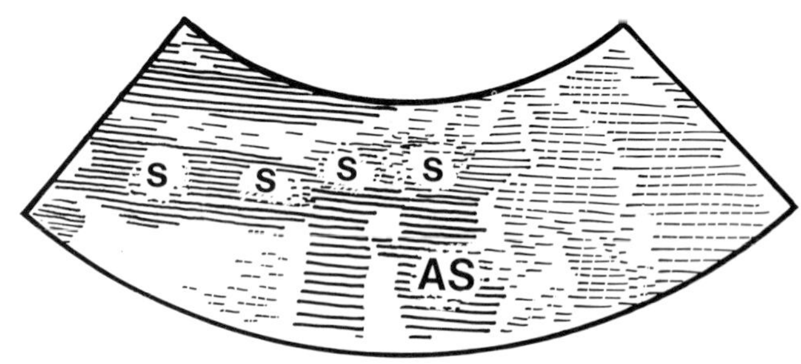

Fig. 30.4 Four stones (S) in the distal common bile duct: one to the right close to the papilla. Two of these stones produce an obvious acoustic shadow (AS)

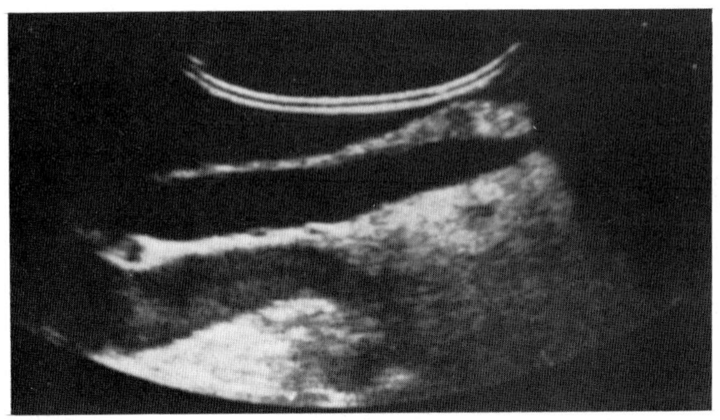

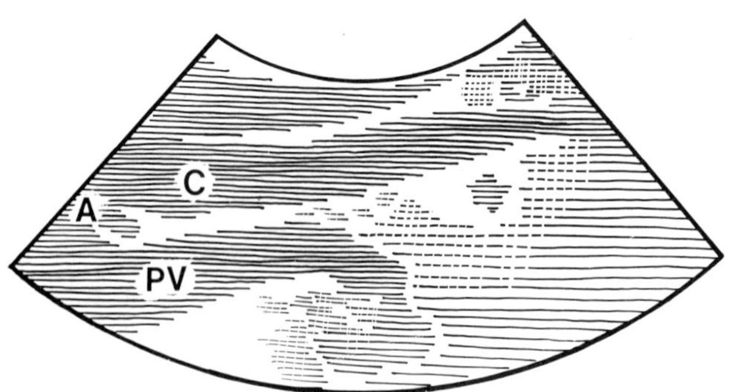

Fig. 30.3 A common bile duct (C) of 8 mm internal diameter with the portal vein in the background (PV). Notice the length of the duct in view (7.5 cm) and the right hepatic artery (A)

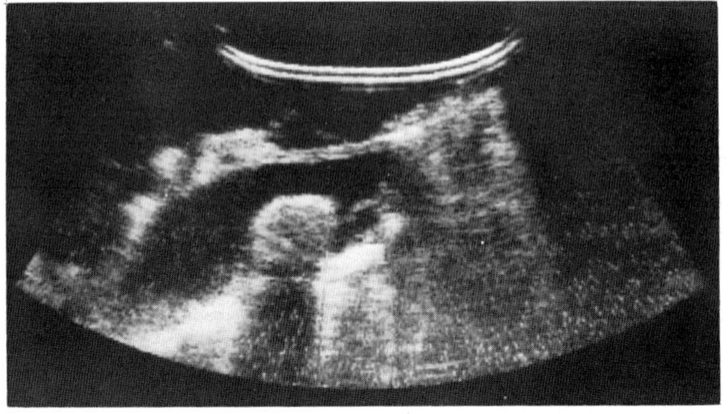

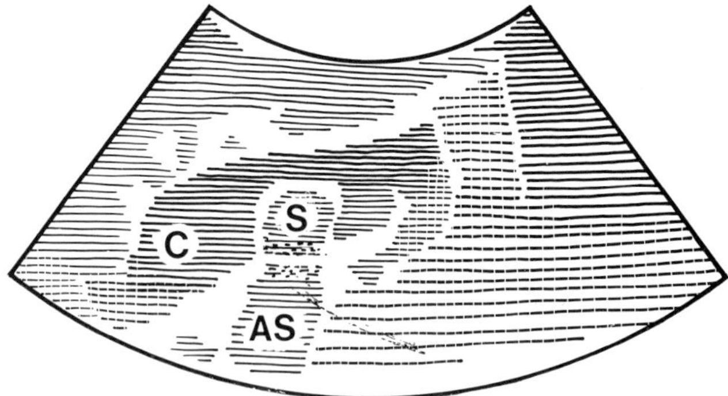

Fig. 30.5 A common bile duct (C) of 1.3 cm internal diameter with two stones (S) of which the largest is causing a massive acoustic shadow (AS)

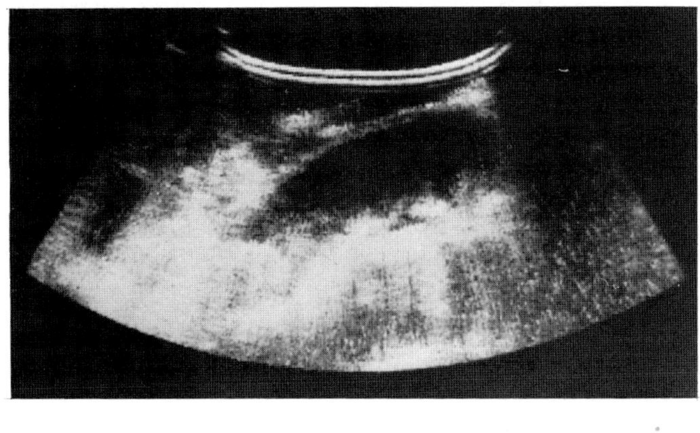

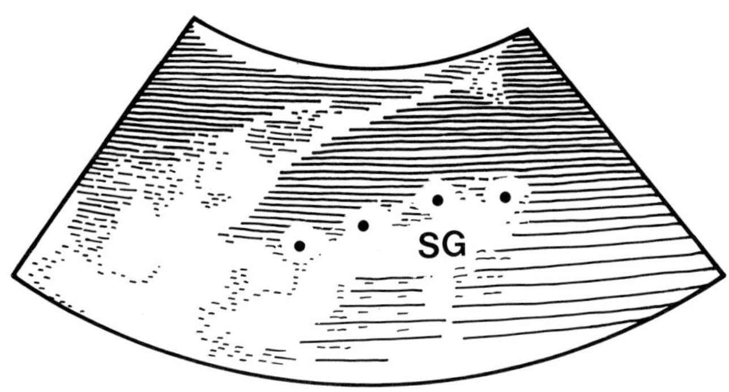

Fig. 30.6 A dilated common bile duct with sludge and gravel at the bottom (SG)

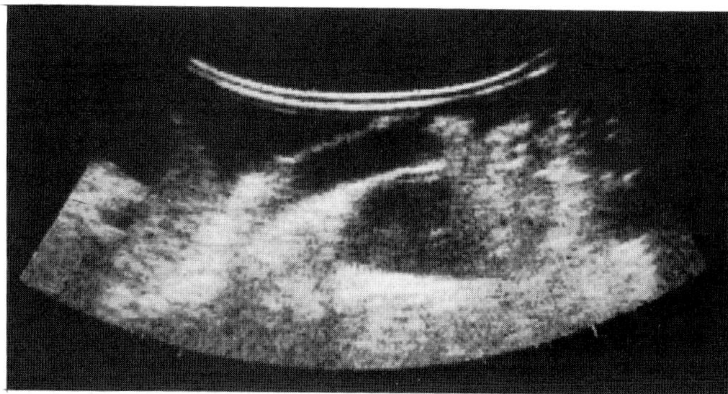

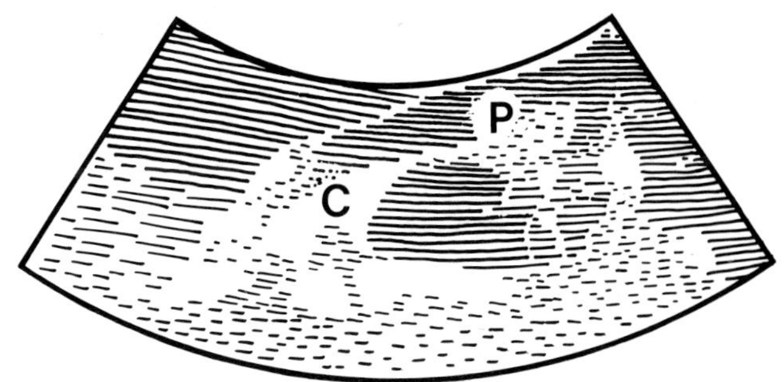

Fig. 30.7 A common bile duct (C) with a polyp (P) of 5 mm diameter in the distal part of the duct

current experience has shown that even a bile duct with an internal diameter of only 5 mm may contain stones.

Not only stones but also other pathology of the duct may be detected by ultrasonography. In the current series a polyp, tumours in the distal and proximal (Fig. 30.7) part of the duct, strictures and narrowing of the duct caused by compression of the duct due to a cyst in the pancreatic head or to a tumour of the pancreas were demonstrated. In the case of tumour of the common bile duct, ultrasonography enables not only its detection but also determination of the depth of tumour involvement of the surrounding structures, such as the portal vein (Figs. 30.8 and 30.9). If the pancreatic duct is dilated, it too can be seen at ultrasound examination.

EVALUATION

In the course of a prospective study at Eindhoven, the value of peroperative ultrasonography has been evaluated and compared with peroperative cholangiography and peroperative biliary manometry using a new manometry technique. In an attempt to reduce, as far as possible, the incidence of retained biliary stones, post-exploratory choledochoscopy was used routinely. In a period of 34 months, 321 patients entered this comparative study. All underwent both peroperative ultrasonography and cholan-

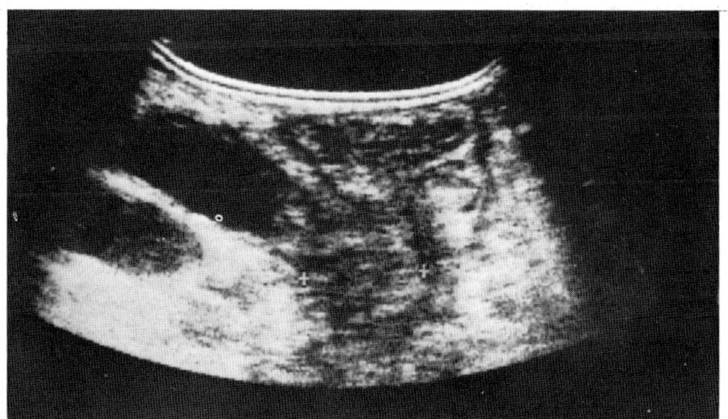

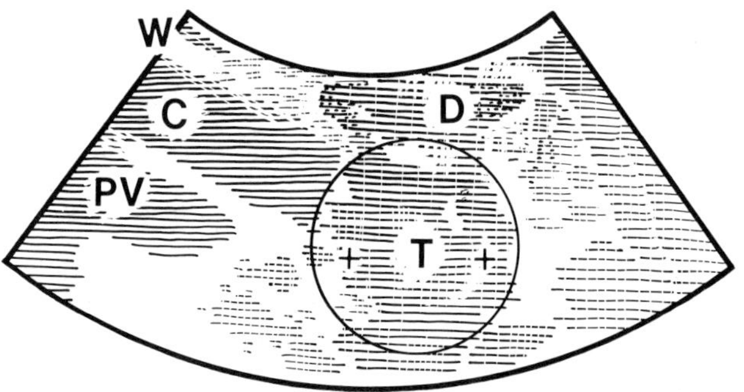

Fig. 30.8 A papillary tumour (T) of 1.7 cm diameter obstructing the distal common bile duct (C). The duodenum (D) is seen in the right upper part of the field. Notice the thickened wall of the bile duct (W)

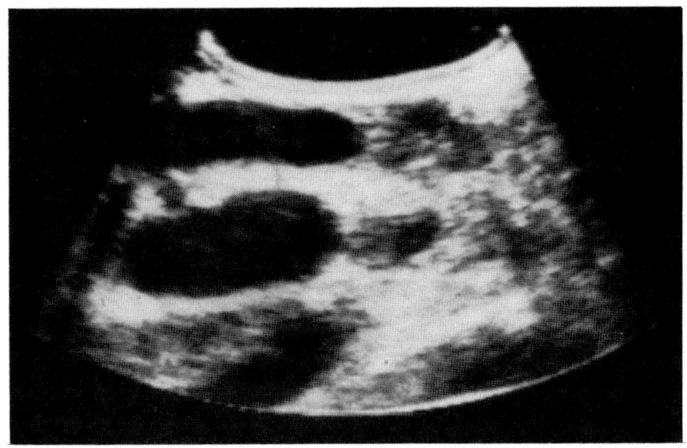

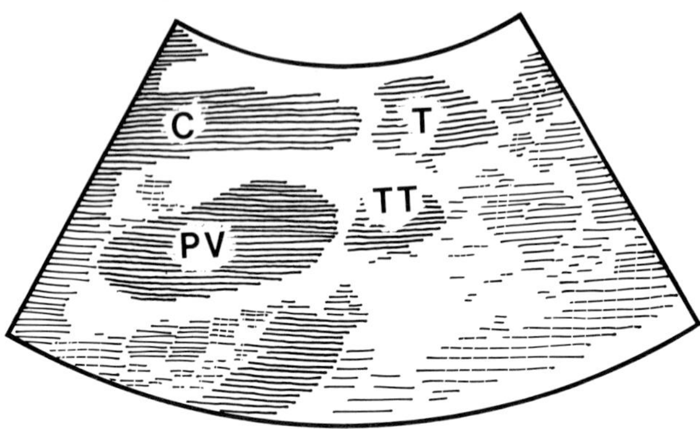

Fig. 30.9 A tumour (T) of the distal common bile duct (C). Ultrasonography also demonstrates the presence of tumour infiltration in the portal vein (PV) and the presence of a tumour thrombus (TT)

giography. In 181 patients biliary manometry was also performed.

Ultrasonography was carried out using the previously described equipment and techniques. Intraoperative cholangiography was performed using X-ray fluoroscopy equipment providing both a screen image and X-ray pictures. Biliary manometry was carried out using a micro-transducer catheter technique. The equipment used and the technique have been previously reported (Carol & Jakimowicz 1984). The method enables a reliable measurement of the exact intraductal pressure and provides permanent records of measured pressures eliminating the possibility of observer related error. Preliminary results (Carol & Jakimowicz 1984) show that the so-called pMax (maximum ductal pressure), measured during a constant infusion of contrast medium with a flow of 1.5 cc per minute, has the best discriminative capacity. To enable a comparison of different examinations, pressure values measured were plotted on graph paper in order to find a clear pressure value differentiating patients having common bile duct pathology from those having no pathology (Fig. 30.10). A significant overlap of measured values was found if a line was arbitrarily placed at 15 mmHg, the optimal position (Fig. 30.10) (Tables 30.3 and 30.4). It has to be stressed that in the case of biliary manometry this distribution was solely related to the ratio of cholecystectomy to common bile duct exploration (respectively 2.1 to 1).

For the purpose of peroperative choledochoscopy, which is used as a final procedure after routine instrumental common bile duct exploration, a flexible choledochoscope (Olympus) was used.

The data is presented in Table 30.2. It is worth emphasizing that the use of a peroperative diagnostic procedure led to the detection of clinically unsuspected stones in 12 (5.6%) of the 218 patients in whom no indication for exploring the common bile duct was present.

The results of operative ultrasonography, cholangiography and biliary manometry for the whole group of patients are presented in Table 30.3 and separately for the group of patients who underwent common bile duct exploration in Table 30.4. In 103 patients undergoing common bile duct exploration the results of peroperative diagnostic procedures were verified by choledochoscopy and finally

Table 30.2 A comparison of peroperative ultrasonography and peroperative cholangiography in the assessment of the bile ducts at biliary surgery: patient data

Total no. of patients: 321	Male: 73 Female: 248
Cholecystectomy	219
Cholecystectomy + choledochotomy	99
Choledochotomy	4
Choledocho-duodenostomy	7
Papillotomy	4
Roux-Y	1
Whipple	1
Positive duct exploration	74 (71.8%)
Negative duct exploration	29 (28.2%)
Unpredicted stones found	12
Retained stones	0
Overall morbidity	(9.8%)
Overall mortality	1 (0.3%)

Table 30.3 A comparison of peroperative diagnostic procedures for common bile duct pathology in 321 patients

	Ultrasonography n = 321	Cholangiography n = 321	Manometry n = 181
True negative	245	225	120
True positive	66	61	22
False negative	6	8	19
False positive	3	13	20
Technically unsatisfactory	1	14	--
Sensitivity	91.6%	88.4%	53.6%
Specificity	98.8%	94.5%	86.6%
Accuracy	97.1%	93.1%	78.4%
Predictive value of a negative test	97.6%	96.5%	86.3%
Predictive value of a positive test	95.6%	82.4%	55.0%
Prevalence	22.5%	22.6%	

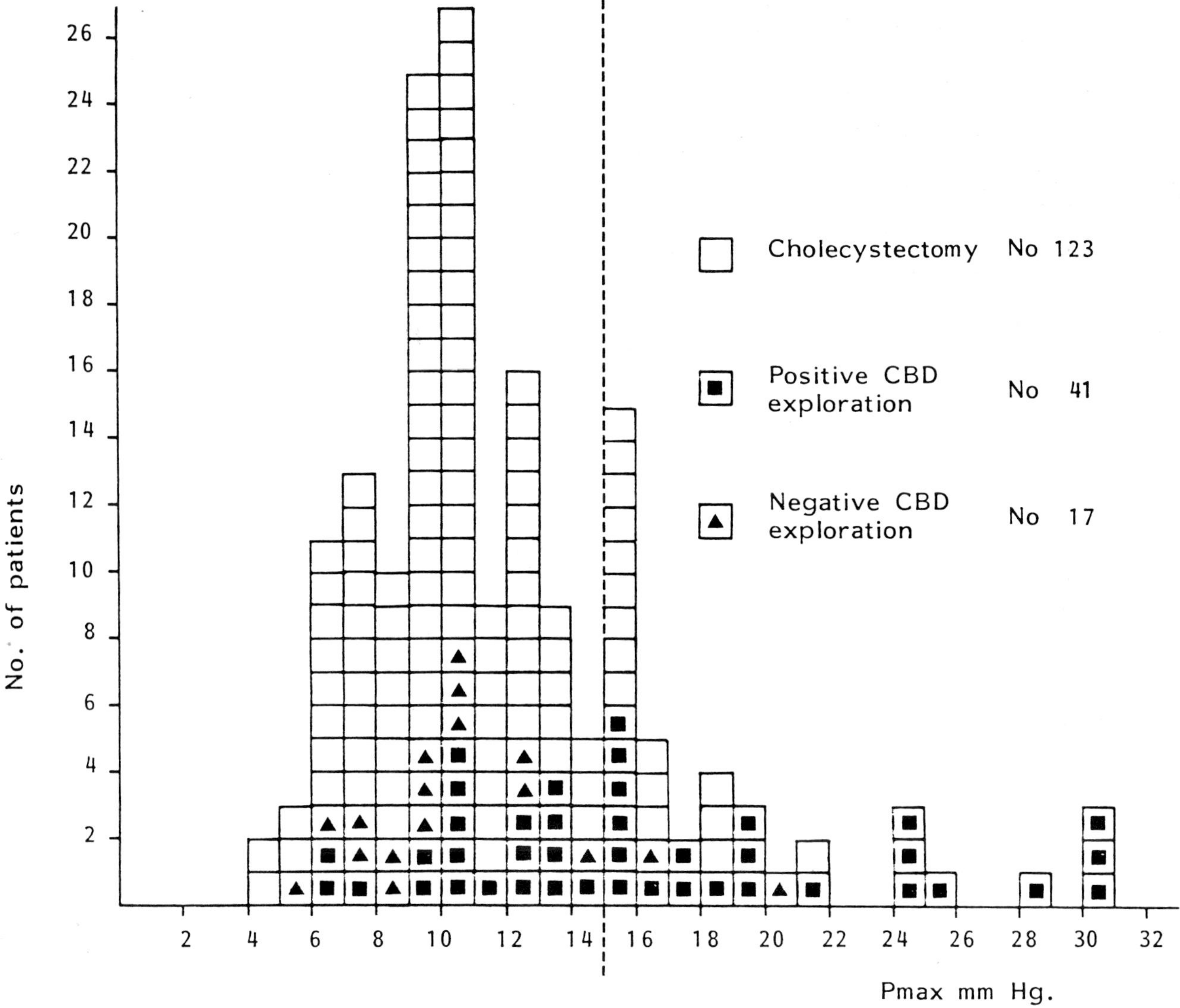

Fig. 30.10 Results of biliary manometry in 129 patients: distribution of 'positives' and 'negatives' by borderline pressure value at 15 mmHg

Table 30.4 A comparison of peroperative diagnostic procedures in patients who underwent common bile duct exploration

	Ultrasonography n = 103	Cholangiography n = 103	Manometry n = 58
True negative	27	17	15
True positive	66	61	22
False negative	6	8	19
False postive	3	13	2
Technically unsatisfactory	1	4	--
Sensitivity	91.6%	88.4%	53.6%
Specificity	90.0%	56.6%	90.4%
Accuracy	91.2%	78.8%	63.7%
Predictive value of a negative test	81.8%	68.0%	44.1%
Predictive value of a positive test	95.6%	82.4%	91.6%
Prevalence	70.6%	69.7%	70.6%

postoperatively by T-tube cholangiogram (Table 30.4). For patients in whom duct exploration was not performed (218) the presumption of true negativity of the examination was based upon the assumption that if both peroperative ultrasonography and cholangiography were negative and other clinical signs of pathology were absent, then no pathology was present. Although this does not give absolute certainty of the absence of pathology, it allows a reasonable comparison of accuracy of both procedures.

To enable comparison between different diagnostic procedures and with previously reported series, we used the same indices to assess results as have others. The predictive value of a positive test indicates how often a test outcome was correct, that is, how often common bile duct exploration proved the presence of the expected pathology. The prevalence was definite, being a % figure of how often pathology was found in the total population examined. The accuracy of peroperative ultrasonography versus cholangiography and biliary manometry is shown in Tables 30.3 and 30.4. Comparison with manometry is possible since even though not all 321 patients underwent this examination, the prevalence of stones was similar to that for both other tests. It is clear that peroperative ultrasonography and cholangiography have a similar accuracy with the exception of the predictive value of a positive test. In addition, when we look separately at the patients who underwent common duct exploration, the accuracy of ultrasonography was 91.2% versus 78.8% for cholangiography (Table 30.4).

Biliary manometry proved to be less reliable due to the limited discriminative capacity of the pressure measurement as a diagnostic procedure. In no patient was the common bile duct explored solely on the basis of biliary manometry. Manometry thus gave only supplementary information supporting the results of peroperative ultrasonography or peroperative cholangiography or both. Peroperative ultrasonography in this series revealed not only the presence of stones, but also enabled detection of other pathology. In two patients a tumour of the common bile duct could be demonstrated and in another two compression of the duct by pancreatic cyst or tumour was shown. Benign stenosis of the distal common bile duct was seen in one patient. A tumour of the papilla of Vater was detected in two patients. In one patient a benign polypoid lesion of the distal common bile duct was detected solely by peroperative ultrasonography and this finding was subsequently confirmed by choledochoscopy.

The results of choledochoscopy were as follows:

All 103 patients underwent completion choledochoscopy after exploration of the common bile duct, using a flexible choledochoscope.

In 6 patients, stones, missed by exploration, were found at choledochoscopy, thus preventing retained stones in 6% of the patients.

In all patients, including those with choledochoduodenostomy, a T-tube cholangiogram was performed and no retained biliary stones were encountered.

Peroperative ultrasonography appears to be an important diagnostic test in liver biliary and pancreatic surgery. Peroperative examination of the gallbladder is indicated only when performing emergency operations or in a patient with morbid obesity and then only if no adequate preoperative examinations are available and when at palpation no stones are felt (Herbst et al 1984).

For examination of the biliary tract, ultrasonography can be used not only as a diagnostic procedure but also for operating in difficult circumstances such as the presence of an inflammatory mass or tumour or at reoperation. The method often enables the recognition of vital structures such as the common bile duct and large vessels in otherwise difficult situations.

The use of peroperative ultrasonography of the pancreas has also been studied (Lane & Glazer 1980, Sigel 1982, Sigel et al 1982 a & b, Klotter et al 1983). Valuable additional information is often gained relative to peroperative decision making. The exact location of pancreatic lesions is possible and recognition of important anatomical structures and their relation to the lesion may be displayed. Time-consuming and sometimes risky dissection of tissue can be avoided and, in the case of malignancy, operability can be determined. Finally, ultrasonographically guided biopsies may enable an exact diagnosis.

A representative series of patients operated upon for pancreatic pathology has been reported recently by Sigel et al (1983a). In this series, during operations for complications of pancreatitis, peroperative ultrasonography was found to be useful in 60% of the patients. It enabled an accurate localization of pseudocysts and dilated sections of the pancreatic duct, the pinpointing of lesions and their relationship to the vessels and the biliary tract. When operating upon a pancreatic tumour, the surgeon was aided by peroperative ultrasonography in 62% of the cases. Experience reported recently by other investigators confirms the statement of Sigel (1984) that ultrasound not only contributes to the diagnosis, but helps in operative decision making. Differences in ultrasonic patterns of the pancreatic tissue and changed appearance of the pancreatic duct may be useful in differentiating between a benign and a malignant lesion (Klotter et al 1983). Ultrasound guided fine-needle biopsies of the suspect regions improve diagnostic accuracy.

Peroperative ultrasonography has also been found useful in locating insulinoma of the pancreas (Sigel et al 1983b, Klotter et al 1983). Unnecessary dissection and blind resection of pancreatic tissue are thus avoided. For the purpose of examination of the pancreas both mechanical sector as well as array ultrasound transducers can be used.

As biliary lithiasis is a common disease and a leading cause of hospitalization and surgical therapy in many countries, one can expect that the use of peroperative ultrasonography during biliary surgery will become the main peroperative application of this method. First reports on the assessment of B-mode, real-time ultrasonography as a peroperative diagnostic procedure were made by Sigel et al (1979) and Lane & Crocker (1979). These preliminary reports underlined the usefulness of this non-invasive diagnostic tool in the detection of biliary stones. Results of a prospective study comparing ultrasonography and cholangiography in 100 patients showed that both examinations have a similar accuracy (Lane et al 1982). In this study the sensitivity of peroperative ultrasonography was 96% and specificity 93%, while peroperative cholangiography had both a specificity and sensitivity of 96%. It can be concluded from these studies that peroperative ultrasonography is a rapid and reliable method for the detection of common bile duct stones and a reliable alternative to routine peroperative cholangiography. From their experience with a large group of patients, Sigel et al (1983c) suggest that peroperative ultrasonography has the potential of being not only safe and reliable, but also the simplest and most cost-effective diagnostic procedure for detecting common bile duct stones.

Comparison of results of the two biggest series of patients, that of Sigel et al (1983c) and the current series, is possible since the same indices for assessment were used by both groups (Table 30.5). On the other hand, this comparison has to be considered with some caution since the prevalence of ductal stones in the two series is significantly different. Such a comparison of different series may easily lead to erroneous conclusions if the patient populations are not comparable. Nevertheless, it is evident that in both series peroperative ultrasonography and peroperative cholangiography have a similar screening accuracy with the exception of the predictive value of a positive test. This is significantly higher for peroperative ultrasonography. In practical terms, both series suggest that if exploration of the common bile duct were to be undertaken solely on the grounds of positive ultrasound examination, fewer unnecessary, negative common bile duct explorations would be performed. For the current series (Tables 30.3 & 30.4) the rate of negative explorations would be

Table 30.5 Accuracy of peroperative ultrasonography and peroperative cholangiography in different series

	Ultrasonography		Cholangiography	
	Sigel et al	Present series	Sigel et al	Present series
	n = 350	n = 321	n = 350	n = 321
Sensitivity	93.8%	91.6%	90.9%	88.4%
Specificity	98.6%	98.8%	95.4%	94.5%
Accuracy	98%	96.1%	94.8%	93.1%
Predictive value of negative test	99%	97.6%	98.7%	96.5%
Predictive value of positive test	91%	95.6%	73.2%	81.4%
Prevalence	13.9%	22.5%	12.1%	22.4%

significantly lower (3% versus 13%). However, neither peroperative cholangiography nor ultrasonography is perfect (Table 30.6). The advantages and disadvantages of both have been recently reviewed (Sigel et al 1983c, Lane et al 1982, Jakimowicz et al 1984).

The main advantage of ultrasonography is that it is completely non-invasive, so that the use of contrast material and ionizing radiation can be avoided. It is easily repeated and the ability to produce multiple images in real-time shortens the time necessary for adequate examination (Table 30.7). The cost of a single examination is relatively low, being somewhat less than a half of the cost of cholangiography. Finally, in experienced hands, it seems to be more reliable than peroperative cholangiography.

The main disadvantage of the method should be stressed. In comparison with cholangiography, ultrasonography cannot provide the same degree of anatomical detail of the biliary tract, and examination of the intrahepatic ducts is not easy. The passage of bile into the duodenum cannot, as yet, be demonstrated by peroperative ultrasonography. There are some other aspects of the method which create problems. These are solely related to the technique itself and the images produced. These are more complex than the cholangiographic pictures surgeons are accustomed to and result in a longer learning period before accurate interpretation is possible. Specifically designed ultrasound equipment for peroperative use has only recently become available so that surgeons' experience is limited. There is a need to develop ultrasound systems specifically for peroperative use. Well-organized teaching programmes are also required.

Peroperative ultrasonography has a great potential for further development which implies the need for further prospective studies to evaluate the merits and limitations of this new intraoperative technique.

CONCLUSIONS

Peroperative ultrasonography meets most of the criteria that a peroperative diagnostic procedure should fulfil. It

Table 30.6 Comparison of peroperative ultrasonography, cholangiography, biliary manometry and choledochoscopy in view of different criteria

	Peroperative ultrasonography	Peroperative cholangiography	Billiary manometry	Peroperative choledochoscopy
be easy to perform and interpret	+	+	–	+
confirm or exclude the presence of anticipated pathology	+	+	–	+
detect unexpected pathology	+	+	–	+
demonstrate the location and extent of pathology	+	+	(+) –	+ (–)
provide anatomical information	+	+	–	+ (–)
be generally applicable	+	+	–	+
be, if possible, non-invasive	+	–	–	(+) –
show positive results in a cost and benefit analysis	+	(+) –	–	+

Table 30.7 Comparison of peroperative ultrasonography, peroperative cholangiography, biliary manometry and choledochoscopy

	Ultrasonography	Cholangiography	Manometry	Choledochoscopy
Repeatability	good	limited	limited	good
Time required	5–7 min.	10–15 min.	10 min.	5–10 min.
Learning period	long	short	long	short
Cost of single examination	low	high	limited	low
Visualization of bile flow	not possible	possible	possible	possible
Detection of intrahepatic stones	limited	good	not possible	limited
Potential for further improvement	high	low	low	limited
Detection of pathology of the papilla	good	good	good	possible

is reliable in the detection of pathology, demonstrates its location and extent, provides information on anatomy and is generally applicable. The costs of a single examination are acceptably low and, when correctly learned, the procedure is reliable and easy to perform and interpret. Peroperative ultrasonography may become, in the future, the alternative to, if not a substitute for peroperative cholangiography as a screening procedure. It is indicated instead of cholangiography in juvenile patients and in pregnant women, to avoid exposure to X-rays. The current experience proves the importance of the use of peroperative diagnostic procedures during biliary surgery since it leads to detection of unexpected pathology in more than 6% of patients. The use of peroperative ultrasonography in combination with choledochoscopy in patients undergoing common bile duct exploration in this large series resulted in no retained stones.

Biliary manometry appears to have an inferior role and supplies only supplementary diagnostic information. It has a limited ability to indicate the necessity for exploration of the common bile duct.

Peroperative ultrasonography or peroperative cholangiography is recommended as a screening procedure during cholecystectomy or surgery on the biliary tract. If common bile duct exploration is undertaken, it should be supplemented by completion choledochoscopy.

REFERENCES

Carol E J, Jakimowicz J J 1984 A peroperative pressure measurement in the biliary tract using the microtransducer catheter. Digestive Surgery 1: 217–221

Carol E J, Jakimowicz J J, Jürgens Ph J 1983 Intraoperative ultrasonography of the bile ducts. Medicamundi 28 (2): 114–117

Eiseman B, Greenlaw R H, Gallagher J G 1965 Localization of common duct stones by ultrasound. Archives of Surgery 91: 195–198

Hayaski S, Wagai T, Miyazawa R 1962 Ultrasonic diagnosis of breast tumour and cholelithiasis. Western Journal of Surgery 70: 34–40

Herbst C A, Mittelstaedt C A, Staab E V, Buckwalter J A 1984 Intraoperative ultrasonography evaluation of the gallbladder in morbidly obese patients. Annals of Surgery 200: 691–692

Hessling E J 1984 Pre- and postoperative manometry of the biliary tract: an assessment of its diagnostic value, using an improved technique. Thesis, University of Groningen

Jakimowicz J J 1985 Operative ultrasonography in biliary and pancreatic surgery. In: Hess W, Cireni A, Rohner A, Akowbiantz A (eds) Bilio-pankreatische Chirurgie. PICCIN, Padova

Jakimowicz J J, Carol E J, Jürgens Ph J 1984 The peroperative use of real-time B-mode ultrasound imaging in biliary and pancreatic surgery. Digestive Surgery 1: 55–60

Klotter H J, Kuhn F P, Rückert K, Hinkel E, Kümmerle F 1983 Intraoperative Ultraschalluntersuchungen bei Pankreaseingriffen. Deutsche Medizinische Wochenschrift 108: 1463–1468

Knight P R, Newell J A 1963 Operative use of ultrasonics in cholelithiasis. Lancet i: 1023–1025

Lane R J, Crocker E F 1979 Operative ultrasonic bile duct scanning. Australian and New Zealand Journal of Surgery 49 (4): 454–458

Lane R J, Glazer G 1980 Intraoperative B-mode ultrasound scanning of the extrahepatic biliary system and pancreas. Lancet ii: 334–337

Lane R J, Graham A, Coupland G A E 1982 Ultrasonic indications to explore the common bile duct. Surgery: 268–274

Puglionesi A 1978 Risultati di un'inchiesta conoscitiva presso 163 centri chirurgici e valutazione dei principali aspetti dell' indagine diagnostica. Atti Societa' Italiana Chirurgia 1: 383–397

Saltzstein E C, Subbarao V E, Mann R W 1973 Routine operative cholangiography. Archives of Surgery 107: 289–291

Sigel B (ed) 1982 Operative ultrasonography. Lea & Febiger, Philadelphia

Sigel B 1984 Personal communication

Sigel B, Spigos D G, Donahue Ph E, Pearl R, Popky G L, Nyhus L M 1979 Intraoperative ultrasonic visualization of biliary calculi. Current Surgery 36: 158–159

Sigel B, Coelho J C U, Machi J, Flanigan D P, Donahue Ph E, Schuler J J et al 1983a The application of real-time ultrasound imaging during surgical procedures. Surgery, Gynecology and Obstetrics 157: 33–37

Sigel B, Duarte B, Coelho J C U, Nyhus L M, Baker R J, Machi J 1983b Localization of insulinomas of the pancreas at operation by real-time ultrasound scanning. Surgery, Gynecology and Obstetrics 156 (2): 145–147

Sigel B, Machi J, Beitler C, Donahue Ph E, Bombeck C Th, Baker R J et al 1983c Comparative accuracy of operative ultrasonography and cholangiography in detecting common bile duct calculi. Surgery 94 (4): 715–720

Sigel B, Coelho J C U, Donahue Ph E, Nyhus L M, Spigos D G, Baker R J et al 1982a Ultrasonic assistance during surgery for pancreatic inflammatory disease. Archives of Surgery 117: 712–716

Sigel B, Coelho J C U, Nyhus L M, Velasco J M, Donahue Ph E, Wood D K et al 1982b Detection of pancreatic tumours by ultrasound during surgery. Archives of Surgery 117: 1058–1061

Skillings J C, Williams J S, Hinshaw J R 1979 Cost-effectiveness of operative cholangiography. American Journal of Surgery 137: 26–31

Stark M E, Loughry C W 1980 Routine operative cholangiography with cholecystectomy. Surgery, Gynecology and Obstetrics 151: 657–658

Wells P N T 1977 Biomedical ultrasonics. Academic Press, London.

White D N 1976 Ultrasound in medical diagnosis. Ultramedison, Kingston, Ontario

SECTION 3

Pre- and postoperative care and anaesthesia

M. E. M. Allison

The kidney and the liver. Pre- and postoperative factors

'Operations on patients with obstructive jaundice offer three avenues of danger, aside from the so-called accidents of surgery: (1) Haemorrhage, (2) Uraemia, and (3) Hepatic Insufficiency.'

Walters & Parham 1922

HISTORICAL PERSPECTIVE

For almost one hundred years surgeons have approached their jaundiced patients with justifiable trepidation. Liver disease per se, and in particular obstructive jaundice, apparently predisposed the sufferer to inumerable postoperative complications, not least of which was death from uraemia. The first clear description of this was from two German surgeons, Clairmont and von Haberer, in 1911, who described five previously healthy young women who died with renal failure shortly after cholecystectomy.

By 1938 the correlation had become so well recognized that Ayer could write 'fatal anuria has been observed frequently following operations on the biliary passages'. The cause of this problem exercised the minds of many investigators during the 1920s and 1930s. Definite abnormalities in renal structure and function were documented in clinical and experimental biliary tract obstruction (Wilbur 1934, Stewart & Cantarow 1935, Elsom 1937, Ayer 1938). Bile salts or other potential nephrotoxins originating in the obstructed liver were generally held responsible. Ravdin (1929) and later Shorr et al (1948) believed that specific vasodepressor substances were released from the obstructed liver which could result in profound postoperative shock. This is interesting today in the light of our understanding of endotoxaemia and the vasodepressor effect of cholaemia.

Lassen & Thomson expressed a different view in 1958 when they reported on 30 consecutive patients with obstructive jaundice and renal failure. Most were critically ill with pyrexia and hypotension before the onset of acute renal failure (ARF). It was unnecessary to evoke the presence of 'a mysterious nephrotoxic substance'; their patients had ARF due to shock.

The classic observations of Dawson (1964, 1968) on patients undergoing surgery for obstructive jaundice and on experimental animals reconciled these views. Postoperative ARF occurred more frequently in patients with obstructive jaundice than in non-jaundiced control patients undergoing surgery of comparable magnitude. He suggested that the presence of obstructive jaundice might 'render the kidney more sensitive to decreased blood flow — that is anoxia'.

The terms 'hepatorenal failure' and 'hepatorenal syndrome' are often used to describe any patient with jaundice and renal failure. Unfortunately, these expressions mean 'many things to many people' (Conn 1973) and their use can obscure proper consideration of underlying pathophysiological processes. Initially Helwig & Schutz (1932) used the expression 'hepatorenal failure' to refer to patients who were not necessarily jaundiced but who died with uraemia after biliary tract surgery or acute liver injury. Today the phrase should only be used to describe patients with cirrhosis, salt and water retention and terminal renal failure, in whom there is no evidence of pre-renal oliguria or established acute tubular necrosis (ATN) (Papper 1983).

Two aspects of liver and kidney function of relevance to the surgeon are considered in this chapter:

1. Obstructive jaundice and renal failure.
2. Chronic cirrhosis of the liver with ascites, sodium retention and renal failure, including the 'hepatorenal syndrome' (HRS).

OBSTRUCTIVE JAUNDICE AND RENAL FAILURE

It is difficult to find up-to-date well matched figures for the incidence of postoperative ARF in obstructive jaundice but it continues to affect 6–18% of such patients. In 1960 Williams et al reported that uraemia occurred in 6% of 350 patients with obstructive jaundice after surgery and was the commonest cause of postoperative death. In Glasgow Royal Infirmary Renal Unit, an analysis of 251 patients treated for established ARF between 1959 and 1970 showed that in 12% renal failure was preceded by biliary tract surgery. 69% of these patients died (Kennedy et al 1973).

Today, despite improvements in anaesthesia and perioperative care ARF after biliary tract surgery continues to be a significant problem, involving 6–18% of patients and associated with a high mortality rate (Pitt et al 1981, Blamey et al 1983, Armstrong et al 1984). Table 31.1 shows the fate of 114 patients after surgery on their liver, biliary tract or pancreas, in a specialized unit in Glasgow Royal Infirmary during 1976. Before surgery 36 were jaundiced and one had renal failure; 78 were non-jaundiced and none had renal failure. All were very ill, half of them having been referred from other hospitals because of complex hepatobiliary problems. Many of them had previously had biliary tract surgery and they were often infected and malnourished. Postoperative shock and ARF was significantly more common in the patients who were jaundiced before surgery and all of the patients who developed ARF died. The combination of liver disease, biliary tract surgery and renal failure is particularly sinister.

The pathophysiology of acute renal failure

At a clinical level, the definition of ARF is reasonably clear. *Potential* acute renal failure is often seen in the critically ill patient in association with hypotension, hypovolaemia and infection. These patients develop pre-renal oliguria, which is a normal physiological response to acute haemorrhage, a fall in cardiac output, anaesthesia or surgery itself. Glomerular filtration rate (GFR) falls. There is a marked rise in the secretion of antidiuretic hormone (arginine vasopressin, AVP) and aldosterone, resulting in increased tubular reabsorption of salt and water. The patient with acute circulatory failure and pre-renal oliguria thus produces a small volume of concentrated urine, with urine/plasma osmolality ratio greater than 1.05. Tubular reabsorption of urea also increases significantly and hence the plasma urea/creatinine ratio rises. Potential ARF is often reversible if appreciated and dealt with expeditiously (Luke et al 1970).

Table 31.1 Fate of 114 Patients after surgery on liver/biliary tract/pancreas

Preoperative	Number	Postoperative Shock/Septicaemia	Postoperative Acute Renal* Failure
Jaundiced	36	13/36 = 36%	6/36 = 17%**
Non-jaundiced	78	15/78 = 19%	1/78 = 1%

*Mortality Rate 100%
**Only 1 had preoperative renal impairment

Established acute renal failure, however, may rapidly ensue. This should be defined simply as a rise in endogenous serum creatinine above normal in a patient with previously good renal function and which persists despite absence or correction of adverse haemodynamic or obstructive factors. Most patients are oliguric. A small number of non-oliguric or high output ARF problems also occur, probably more commonly than is generally recognized. In a recent prospective study, Anderson et al (1977) observed that 54 out of 92 patients with progressive azotaemia had urine volumes in excess of 600 ml per day. In 80% the urine volume exceeded 1 litre per day. The morbidity and mortality in this group was lower than in the oliguric patients.

This relatively simple clinical definition of ARF covers a multitude of complex pathophysiological events (Fig. 31.1). A wide variety of animal models have been studied, some of which have little obvious relevance to clinical practice. Two situations of particular interest for those involved with patients who have obstructive jaundice and renal failure are the effects of ischaemia and of endotoxaemia. Both models have been studied at four levels: whole animal, whole kidney, single nephron and single cell function. Both involve four mechanisms within the kidney itself: renal vasoconstriction, tubular obstruction, a fall in glomerular ultrafiltration co-efficient and back leakage of filtrate across damaged tubular cells (Figs. 31.1(B), 31.6). The relative importance of each depends on the precise precipitating cause and changes as the situation evolves.

Ischaemic acute renal failure

Two mechanisms have been used to produce acute renal ischaemia in experimental animals. Most commonly, the left renal artery is clamped for a varying period of time and then released. Less frequently the effect of systemic hypovolaemia, produced by a period of haemorrhage followed by retransfusion, is studied.

As an example of the first situation a severe and reproducible (from rat to rat) model of ischaemic ARF can be produced in the rat by cross clamping the left renal artery for one hour. The presence of the contra-lateral kidney ensures the survival of the animal and allows sequential observations during recovery. In this model the course of renal failure can be divided into three phases: an initial phase, a maintenance phase and an early and late recovery phase. During the initial 24 hours after release of the clamp there is a profound fall in urine flow rate, a reduction in GFR to less than 2% of control values and a fall in renal blood flow (RBF) to 20–50%. The decrease in GFR, however, is due at this stage not to a fall in glomerular capillary hydrostatic pressure, which is within the normal range, but to tubular obstruction. Restoration of RBF to normal by volume expansion with isotonic sodium chloride does not improve the GFR.

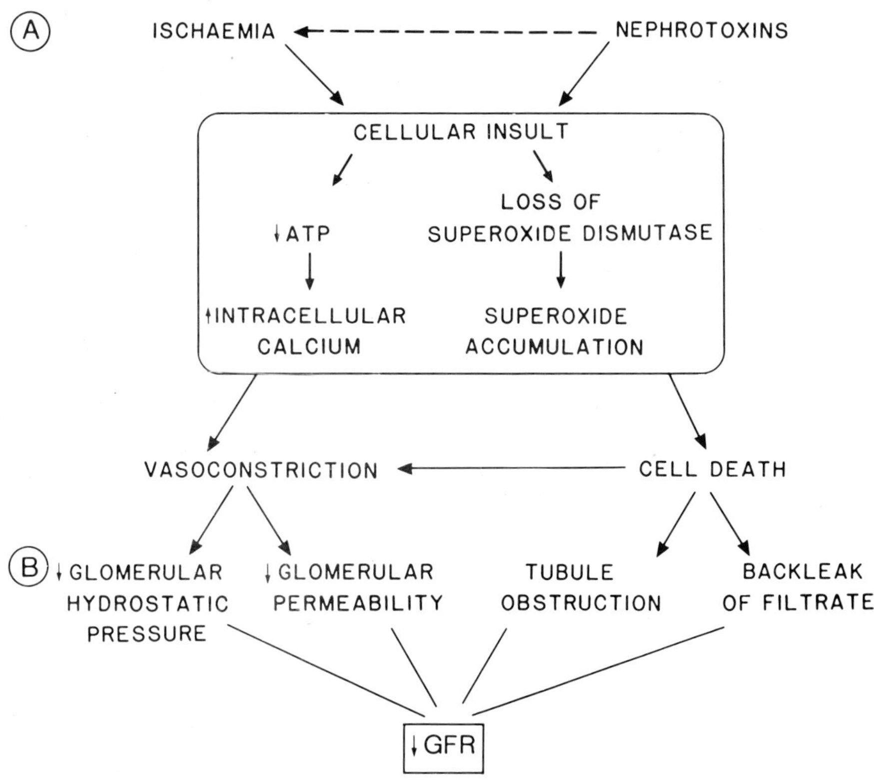

Fig. 31.1 Acute renal failure. (A) The onset is due to cellular insult resulting in intrarenal vasoconstriction and cell death. (B) Four mechanisms maintain the fall in GFR

Twenty-four hours later the renal failure is maintained because of a marked fall in glomerular capillary hydrostatic pressure and hence in single nephron filtration rate. This fall in glomerular capillary hydrostatic pressure is due to a marked increase in pre-glomerular vascular resistance. In addition, there is evidence of back leakage of glomerular filtrate across the damaged tubular epithelium.

Over the following one to four weeks recovery occurs in a bi-phasic manner. First there is regeneration and repair of tubular epithelium with a decrease in transtubular leakage and a loss of intratubular casts. Later there is progressive vasodilatation, a rise in glomerular hydrostatic pressure and a return of GFR towards normal.

The duration of ischaemia and the presence or absence of an untouched contra-lateral kidney is critical to the severity of renal failure. Prolonged ischaemia, two hours or more, leads to irreversible injury while 25 minutes or less results in only a mild form of renal failure. The degree of recovery of renal function is enhanced in a solitary ischaemic kidney as compared to a kidney subjected to a similar episode in the presence of a normally functioning contra-lateral organ.

Renal ischaemia produced by transient hypovolaemia is of more relevance to those interested in clinical shock. This is usually produced by bleeding the animal to some pre-determined blood pressure for a set period of time and then re-transfusing the shed blood. During severe haemorrhagic hypotension there is patchy hypoperfusion of the renal cortex with a fall in RBF and a rise in renal vascular resistance. About 20% of the animals die during this period.

Re-transfusion of shed blood in the survivors is followed by a 24-hour period of diuresis with loss of urinary concentrating ability. Micropuncture studies have shown this to be due to a fall in reabsorption beyond the proximal convoluted tubule (Tanner & Selkurt 1970).

Very interesting changes take place in cell structure and function during and after ischaemia. Studies of cell biology show that, on exposure to anoxia, all cells die in a similar fashion, be they renal tubular cells, cardiac myocytes or hepatocytes. Leaf et al (1983) have reviewed these in detail (Fig. 31.1(A)).

Early morphological changes involve the mitochondria which first lose their matrix granules, then become condensed and finally appear swollen. Blebs appear on the cell surface and the whole cell appears swollen. Up to this point recovery is still possible if the ischaemic insult is removed. Continued anoxia, however, results in disruption of cellular membrane structures and death is inevitable. These structural abnormalities are associated with loss of calcium from the mitochondria into the cell cytoplasm and a significant rise in cytosolic ionized calcium. Membrane pumps are inhibited by the lack of ATP, since oxidative phosphorylation is quickly inhibited in the mitochondria by anoxia. Ion gradients are changed and the cell gains solute and water and hence appears swollen. Restoration of oxygen delivery brings another insult, namely the production of superoxide radicals (Paller et al 1984).

These changes have been described in some detail for two reasons. Firstly, it has been reported that bilirubin and bile salts also impair cellular metabolism and a number of membrane transport systems. Bilirubin can uncouple oxidative phosphorylation in isolated mitochondria. Changes in ultrastructure of glomerular endothelial cells have been described in rats with obstructive jaundice similar to those seen in anoxia (Figs 31.2, 31.3) (Allison et al 1978). An increased 'sensitivity' of these cells to anoxia, therefore, might not be too surprising.

Secondly, an understanding of the cellular effects of anoxia has led to the rational use of measures designed to attenuate these changes. Thus, the use of intravenous mannitol, a solute which penetrates cell membranes poorly and hence exerts an osmotic effect, has been shown to be of use clinically when given early during a period of anoxic insult. More recently calcium channel blocking drugs, such as verapamil, have been effective experimentally in animal models of ARF. Free radical scavengers such as superoxide dismutase and dimethylthiourea protect against renal failure during reflow after a 60-minute period of warm ischaemia in the rat (Paller et al 1984). As yet these substances await clinical trial but their use would be based on the results of careful studies of cell biology.

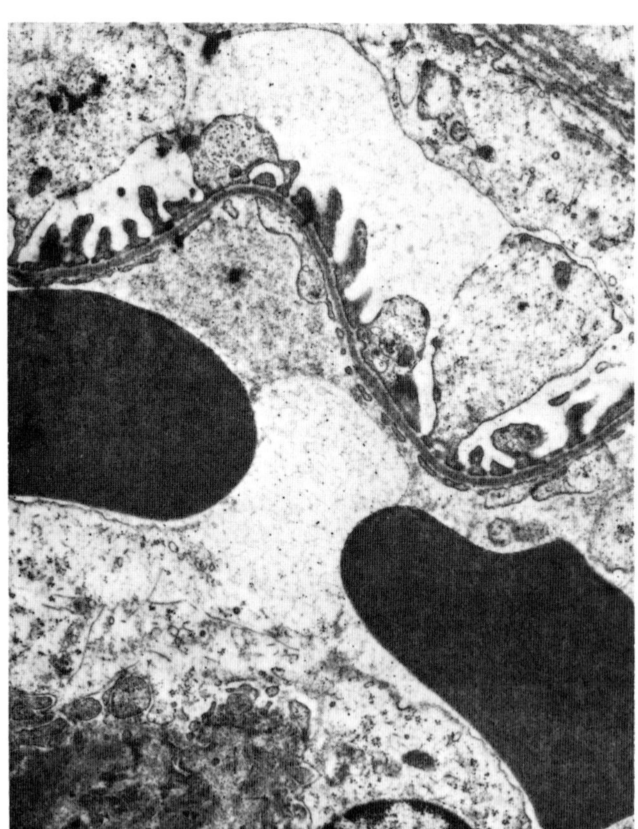

Fig. 31.2 Electron micrograph (original × 17,500) of glomerulus from sham operated control rat. The three layers of the basement membrane are clearly delineated and the epithelial and endothelial cells appear quite normal with no evidence of increased cytoplasmic activity. The normal fenestrated endothelial configuration is clearly visible, as are the epithelial foot processes. From Allison et al 1978.

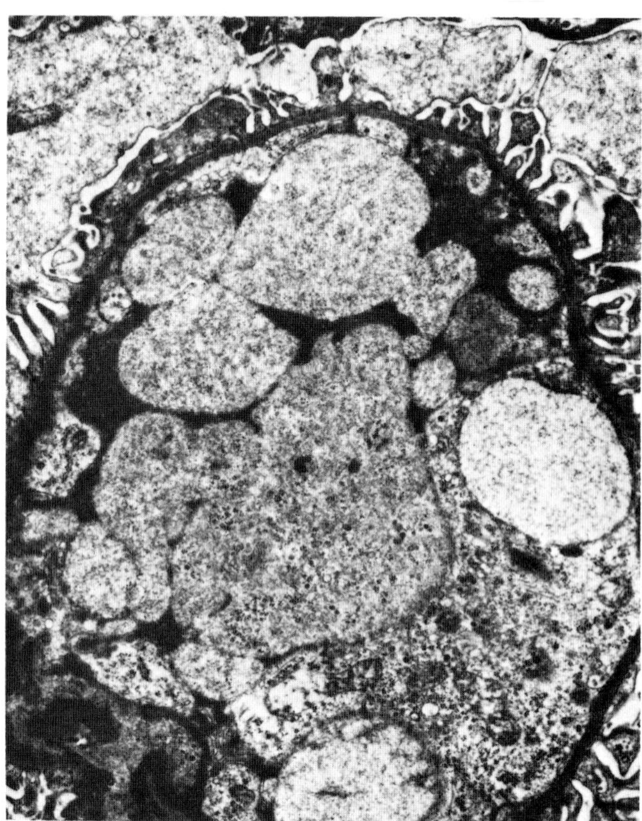

Fig. 31.3 Electron micrograph (original × 17,500) of a glomerulus from a rat with obstructive jaundice. There is an increase in activity of both epithelial and endothelial cells with marked endothelial cell swelling. The basement membrane appears muddy and the three layers are not clearly delineated. From Allison et al 1978

Endotoxin and acute renal failure

> 'Few, if any, biological substances have such varied effects on so many systems as does endotoxin'.
>
> Nolan 1981

Endotoxins are lipopolysaccharide components of the outer cell membrane of gram negative bacteria which are normally present in the gut. They are released on the death of the cell and if able to reach the circulation have profound and disastrous effects on cell and organ function (Ch. 12).

The renal effects are summarized in Figure 31.4 (Wardle 1980).

Intense renal vasoconstriction occurs with profound damage to the endothelium with loss of its normal protective role in preventing thrombosis. This may be due to a

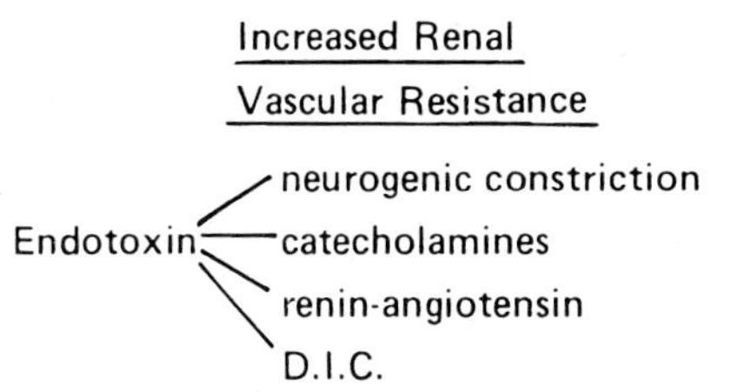

Fig. 31.4 Endotoxin and acute renal failure. From Wardle 1980

change in the balance between the production by the endothelial cells of prostacycline, a potent vasodilator and anti-platelet agent, and thromboxane, a most potent platelet aggregator and vasoconstrictor released by platelets. Administration of prostacycline or indomethacin, a prostaglandin synthatase inhibitor, can protect the rat with obstructive jaundice from renal fibrin deposition and death after intravenous endotoxin (Fletcher et al 1982).

In healthy subjects endotoxin is virtually absent from the peripheral circulation. In obstructive jaundice, however, endotoxaemia, as detected by the limulus lysate assay, is found in 50–75% of patients in the peroperative period (Wardle 1975, Bailey 1976). Absence of bile salts, gut anoxia and decreased liver perfusion all contribute to the escape of endotoxin into the circulation. Patients with endotoxaemia appear to be at particular risk of ARF. In rat studies Wardle & Wright (1970) showed that a single dose of intravenous endotoxin to an animal with obstructive jaundice produced ARF with intense intrarenal fibrin deposition. Increased endotoxin release in obstructive jaundice may thus lead to low grade disseminated intravascular coagulation. In particular, patients with increased fibrin degradation product levels (FDP) before operation have a poor prognosis (Allison et al 1979). 44% of patients with raised FDP levels died after operation compared with no deaths in those with normal levels of FDP. Renal failure was confined to those with increased levels of FDP.

Why is the patient with obstructive jaundice particularly susceptible to acute renal failure?

Cholaemia and liver damage per se are associated with adverse effects on renal structure and function, on circulatory homeostasis and on the integrity of the gastrointestinal barrier. It is scarcely surprising, therefore, that patients with obstructive jaundice have an increased risk of postoperative ARF.

Renal structure

There are well documented abnormalities in renal structure which 50 years ago investigators called 'cholemic nephrosis'. Light microscopy showed dilated tubules, lined by degenerating cells. Pigment casts were present in the distal convoluted tubule and collecting duct. The patients had albuminuria and there were cellular casts containing bile pigments in the urine.

Electron microscopic studies have confirmed that 'toxic' cellular degenerative changes occur, particularly in the middle segment of the proximal convoluted tubule. Within 12 hours of bile duct obstruction in the rat there is an increase in pinocytotic organelles in the sub-apical cytoplasm of the proximal convoluted tubule cells, presumably due to increased active transport of bile acids. Rats fed a bile acid rich diet show similar changes. Significant changes in glomerular morphology are found in experimental animals with obstructive jaundice, similar to those seen in the human glomerulus in cirrhosis of the liver. Black granules appear in the basement membrane and subendothelial space, together with epithelial foot process fusion and considerable thickening of the basement membrane. We observed marked endothelial cell swelling with loss of the normal fenestrated appearance, a 'muddy' basement membrane and epithelial cell swelling with the presence of inclusion bodies in rats with obstructive jaundice (Fig. 31.2, 31.3) (Allison et al 1978).

The mechanism of these changes in cell structure remains unknown despite extensive studies of the noxious effects of bilirubin and bile salts on the integrity of cells in vitro and in vivo. The constituents of bile are potentially nephrotoxic in a number of ways. Bilirubin can uncouple oxidative phosphorylation in mitochondria and decrease cell respiratory rate. Unfortunately, the relative toxicity of conjugated as compared to unconjugated bilirubin remains unclear. Bile acids can inhibit ATPase activity, disrupt lysosomes, cause haemolysis and disrupt membranes. It should be noted that these changes in intracellular structure and function in cholaemia resemble the effects of anoxia on cellular activities. Presumably these cells would be especially sensitive to a small fall in oxygen delivery.

Renal function

> 'The disturbance in renal function incident to jaundice may . . . . . . become a matter which greatly influences the practical management of patients with biliary obstruction; hence its degree and course should be carefully assessed.'
>
> Elsom 1937

There are numerous descriptions of impaired kidney function in association with obstructive jaundice per se, in the absence of any surgical insult. As many as 30% of patients with obstructive jaundice have been found to have a significant decrease in creatinine clearance before surgery (McPherson et al 1982a). Preoperative acute renal failure has been found especially in the presence of cholangitis and sepsis (Sorenson et al 1971, Bismuth et al 1975).

We found an impairment in urinary concentrating ability in 24 patients with obstructive jaundice before surgery (Allison et al 1979). The mean GFR for the group as a whole was not different from controls. However, there was a small subgroup (5/24) in whom GFR was significantly reduced. After surgery, three of these five subjects had significant renal failure. More precise studies of renal function have been made in rats, dogs, rabbits and baboons. Unfortunately there is great variability in the effects of chronic bile duct ligation in different species making direct comparison difficult.

The general consensus of opinion can be summarized as follows (Better 1983): Firstly, most investigators have found a fall in total RBF, particularly outer cortical blood flow. Indeed, medullary flow has been shown to rise and this has been used as an explanation for the fall in renal concentrating ability found in obstructive jaundice. This decrease in RBF could be due to an increased sensitivity of the renal vasculature to catecholamines, as shown both in vivo and in vitro (Bomzon & Kew 1983). As yet the factor or factors responsible for this remain speculative, but it would appear to involve stimulation of α adrenergic receptors and seems to be associated with the rise in the β lipoprotein fraction found in obstructive jaundice.

Secondly, in contrast to the significant decrease seen in RBF, whole kidney and superficial single nephron GFR are normal.

Thirdly, urinary concentrating ability is significantly decreased.

Finally, salt retention is rare in obstructive jaundice. Indeed, Alon et al (1982) have shown that the intrarenal infusion of diluted bile or bile acids, but not bilirubin, produces a diuresis and natriuresis in animals. Hence patients with obstructive jaundice may be especially vulnerable to salt and water depletion.

Circulatory homeostasis

Patients with obstructive jaundice seem more likely to develop haemorrhagic hypotension during surgery than non-jaundiced subjects. This decreased tolerance to even small volumes of blood loss can be demonstrated in the experimental animal. Thus a large and sometimes fatal fall in arterial blood pressure in the jaundiced rat could be precipitated by loss of only 10% of blood volume (Aarseth et al 1979). We found that 40% of rats with obstructive jaundice became hypotensive and died during routine surgery in preparation for kidney micropuncture studies (Allison et al 1978). The vasodepressor effects of cholaemia per se have been extensively examined and are summarized in Fig. 31.5 (Green et al 1984).

Theoretically, hypotension could result from a change in one or more of four primary factors: cardiac output, left ventricular performance, total plasma volume and its

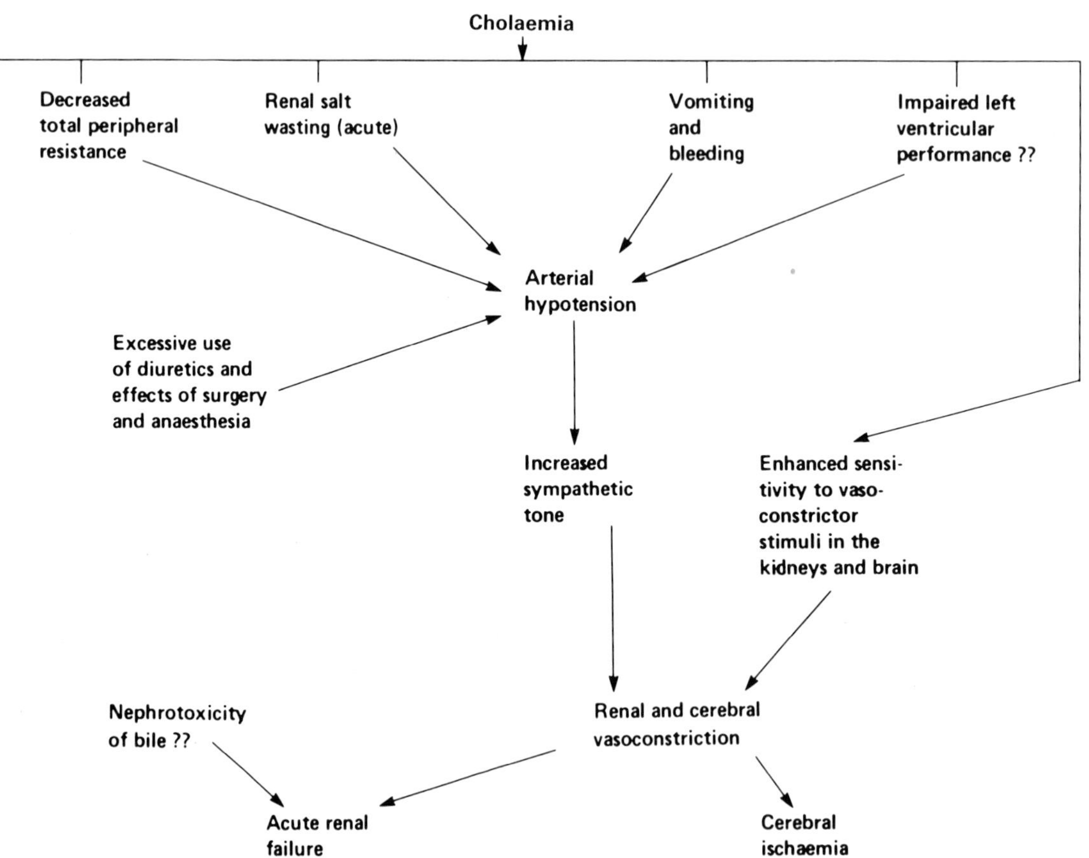

Fig. 31.5 Pathogenesis of arterial hypotension and renal failure in cholaemia. From Green et al 1984

distribution between the splanchnic and systemic vascular beds and peripheral resistance. A significant fall in peripheral resistance and hence in arterial blood pressure is found when cholaemia is produced either by ligation of the common bile duct or by diversion of the bile duct to the inferior vena cava. In addition, there is a redistribution of the total blood volume with trapping of blood in the splanchnic circulation in obstructive jaundice. Effective blood volume is thus reduced.

Cardiac output appears to be relatively unchanged in obstructive jaundice. Acute blood loss, however, results in a more marked fall in cardiac output with delayed recovery than that seen in control animals. The constituents of bile, in particular bile acids, have a cardiodepressor activity on left ventricular function. The precise factor or factors responsible for this remain speculative.

Integrity of the gastrointestinal barrier

The normal intestine and hepatobiliary system form a very efficient barrier against enteric pathogens, including endotoxins. Obstructive jaundice greatly reduces the efficacy of this barrier, putting the sufferer at increased risk of perioperative renal failure.

Bile salts, sodium taurocholate and deoxycholate act as surfactants and disrupt endotoxin, both in vitro and in vivo. In obstructive jaundice this important action of bile salts is lost, resulting in excessive endotoxin being absorbed into the portal blood system. This observation was first made in 1966 (Rudbach et al 1966) but only recently has its practical potential been appreciated and investigated (Bailey 1976, Evans et al 1982). Oral bile salts may prove to be an effective protection against endotoxaemia and hence renal failure in patients with obstructive jaundice.

It is well recognized that liver disease is associated with a progressive decrease in the reticulo-endothelial phagocytic capacity of the Kupffer cell system. Approximately 50% of patients with obstructive jaundice can be shown to have a decrease in the clearance of micro-aggregated iodinated human albumin (Drivas et al 1976) or of Tc labelled sulphur colloid (Ingoldby 1983) indicating impaired reticulo-endothelial activity. These patients are especially at risk of developing postoperative endotoxaemia. Tragically, endotoxins can themselves further suppress reticulo-endothelial cell activity and the function of hepatocytes, thus prolonging their active life. These changes have been attributed to a combination of the noxious metabolic effects of conjugated bilirubin, the detergent action of bile acids retained in the liver and to poor liver perfusion. Maintenance of normal liver blood flow therefore forms the third factor in the defence mechanisms of the gut and hepatobiliary tree.

In all forms of surgery good liver perfusion and freedom from hepatocellular anoxia is a well recognized prerequisite for health. In 1946 it was shown that death from haemorrhagic shock in dogs could be prevented only if liver blood flow, and hence oxygen delivery, to the liver cells was maintained during bleeding (Frank et al 1946). Unfortunately, the effect of obstructive jaundice per se on liver blood flow in the human is unknown but in experimental animals liver blood flow has been shown to decrease at least in the early stages of biliary tract obstruction (Ch 7). What is most important is that surgery and anaesthesia can be associated with a significant fall in liver perfusion in the human (Gelman 1976).

There are two reasons why this might be especially important in patients with obstructive jaundice. The first is that liver anoxia could result in a further decrease in the clearance of endotoxin from portal blood. Secondly, the liver normally plays a crucial role in the removal of lactate from the extracellular fluid. Lactic acid, formed from pyruvate as the end product of anaerobic glycolysis in skeletal muscle, gut, brain, skin and red blood cells, is removed via gluconeogenesis in the liver (approximately 60%) and kidney (approximately 30%) (Park & Arieff 1983). Decreased lactate clearance is found in some types of liver disease and surgery or anaesthesia will presumably further decrease clearance, resulting in profound metabolic acidosis.

Which patients are particularly at risk?

Rapid identification of high risk patients with obstructive jaundice is an essential prerequisite for good surgical management. Uncontrolled observations on small numbers of patients have suggested that the general risk factors for surgery such as advancing age, hypoalbuminaemia, poor renal function, infection and weight loss are important (Allison et al 1979).

Statistical evaluation of risk factors measured in large numbers of patients undergoing biliary tract surgery have now been reported. Dixon et al (1983) studied 373 patients with obstructive jaundice and reported that a high plasma bilirubin (> 200 μmols/litre), a low haematocrit and malignant disease were important independent risk factors for postoperative mortality. Both Pitt et al (1981) and Blamey et al (1983) found eight clinical and laboratory factors preoperatively which correlated significantly with postoperative mortality. Seven of the eight factors were common to both studies: malignant disease, age over 60 years, haematocrit less than 30%, albumin less than 30 g/litre, white blood count greater than 10 000 per mm^3, hyperbilirubinaemia and a raised serum alkaline phosphatase. A major difference between the two was in the statistical significance of a raised preoperative serum creatinine, which in the study of Pitt et al did not reach statistical significance. Blamey et al found it to be a factor of major prognostic importance. This is especially curious since renal failure was the commonest postoperative complication observed by Pitt et al, accounting for 18.1% of total morbidity.

Linear discriminant analysis by Blamey et al further showed that serum creatinine and serum albumin in the week before surgery had independent significance in predicting mortality. Postoperative ARF occurred as a complication in 8% of their patients, especially when there was pre-existing renal impairment but also in association with hyperbilirubinaemia, hypoalbuminaemia, diabetes mellitus or malignancy.

McPherson et al (1982b) have suggested that measurement of antipyrine half-life might help in selecting high risk patients with obstructive jaundice. This may well prove to be a useful measure of the hepatic deficit accompanying obstructive jaundice and of the rate of recovery, but further substantiation is required.

Prevention/amelioration of acute postoperative renal failure

Table 31.2 outlines the methods currently advised for the peroperative management of patients with obstructive jaundice.

Avoid delay

An impressive array of laboratory tests (Ch. 25) are available which enable prompt and precise diagnosis. Delay in investigation should not occur since it is recognized that the prognosis deteriorates as the depth and duration of the jaundice increases. Attention should be focused on sepsis and pre-existing renal impairment as the two most important associated problems, especially in the high risk group with raised serum creatinine concentration and a low serum albumin concentration.

Assess renal function

Renal function is best assessed simply by the measurement of serum creatinine concentration on two or three consecutive days. Hyperbilirubinaemia and obstructive jaundice per se do not interfere with the measurement of creatinine by the Jaffe reaction (M Smith, personal communication). Measurement of creatinine clearance, involving 24-hour urine collections, is unnecessary and in any case usually notoriously inaccurate in clinical practice. Serum creatinine concentration should accurately reflect GFR in the absence of significant muscle breakdown. On the other hand, blood urea will not accurately reflect kidney function, since urea production is altered by liver disease and infection.

Table 31.2 Peroperative management of patients with obstructive jaundice

General	Avoid prolonged hyperbilirubinaemia Treat known infection, especially cholangitis Use aminoglycosides carefully Avoid pre-renal failure Correct anaemia, coagulation defects, hypoalbuminaemia Avoid all NSAID*
Specific	IV saline and mannitol pre- and postoperatively Maintain good liver perfusion at surgery
No conclusive evidence for: Preoperative percutaneous biliary drainage Gut sterilization Polymyxin B Oral bile salts	

* Non steroid anti-inflammatory drugs

Treat infection

Infection of the biliary tree usually occurs in association with cholelithiasis or after previous biliary tract surgery. About 10% of these patients develop ARF (Bismuth et al 1975). Our practice is to give all patients an aminoglycoside (e.g. netilimicin, 100 mg i.v.) just before any invasive procedure, together with metronidazole 1 g rectally. If the patient is pyrexial this is continued postoperatively. Peak and trough aminoglycoside levels should be monitored daily and the dose adjusted to keep peak levels between 5 and 10 mg per litre and trough levels between 2 and 3 mg per litre. In renal impairment aminoglycoside dosages must be greatly reduced and in those patients with a severe deficit in renal function who are dialysis dependent as little as 40 mg i.v. after each dialysis may be sufficient.

Correct pre-renal deficits

Patients with obstructive jaundice are often elderly and malnourished. They tolerate anoxia, hypovolaemia and hypotension poorly. Careful assessment of fluid balance should be made with attention to skin turgor, presence or absence of oedema and cardiac failure. A serum albumin concentration less than 30 g per litre in association with diminished skin turgor generally denotes significant volume depletion. Before any invasive procedure patients should have their volume defects corrected by the use of appropriate intravenous fluids. Plasma protein solution is useful to correct protein and salt deficiency. Concentrated albumin is available to increase albumin concentration to greater than 30 g/litre when there is a danger of fluid overload. Haemoglobin should be 10 g/dl or greater.

All patients are empirically given vitamin K before surgery but routine coagulation screen may detect other defects. The finding of diffuse intravascular coagulation carries an especially bad prognosis since it is generally associated with bacteraemia and endotoxaemia.

Avoid dangerous drugs

All non-steroidal anti-inflammatory drugs (NSAID) should be stopped. They impair renal prostaglandin synthesis and can precipitate ARF especially in the elderly, hypovolaemic and anoxic patient. Prostaglandins are required for the maintenance of intrarenal blood flow when this is threatened by hypovolaemia and its associated increase in AVP (Yared et al 1985). In addition, NSAID can themselves produce acute interstitial nephritis and renal failure.

Mannitol and saline

Mannitol is a simple sugar, molecular weight 182. When given intravenously it is not metabolized but is freely filtered by the glomeruli into the tubular fluid where it acts as an osmotic diuretic. Intravenous mannitol in healthy individuals results in a profound diuresis and natriuresis.

The protective effect of mannitol in the ischaemic kidney was first noted by Selkurt in 1945 and studied in more depth by Barry & Malloy in 1962 and by Eliahou in 1964. To date it remains the best substance available for the prophylaxis of ischaemic ARF.

In the 1960s Dawson reasoned that since renal ischaemia seemed particularly dangerous to patients with obstructive jaundice mannitol should be especially useful. He went on to demonstrate that this was indeed so. Patients with obstructive jaundice were given a constant infusion of 10% mannitol, equivalent to 50 g for two hours before surgery. After surgery 10% mannitol infusion was continued to maintain a urine flow rate greater than 60 ml per hour. He was thus able to prevent a postoperative fall in GFR.

There are four good theoretical reasons why mannitol is effective. Firstly, it is an osmotic diuretic and by increasing tubule flow rate should flush out tubular casts and debris. Secondly, and the more important, it increases RBF even during hypotension. This is shown by the rise in partial pressure of oxygen found in the urine during mannitol infusion. Thirdly, it appears to prevent the endothelial cell swelling which occurs during ischaemia, thus stopping the 'no reflow phenomenon' (Flores et al 1972). Finally, mannitol appears to be an effective hydroxyl radical scavenger. This is a fascinating observation in view of the recent recognition of the damaging effects of free radicals on cell function (Paller et al 1984).

Twenty years of clinical experience have established that renal function can be well maintained in patients with obstructive jaundice provided that adequate intravenous fluids and mannitol are given. Our practice is to give a bolus of 20 g (100 ml of 20% mannitol) two hours before surgery and again during anaesthesia. All jaundiced patients are catheterized so that hourly urine volumes can be monitored. After surgery 20 g mannitol is repeated if the urine flow rate falls to less than 50 ml per hour on two successive occasions. Adequate intravenous saline must also be given because a marked natriuresis is seen during the two or three immediate postoperative days when mannitol is being used (Allison et al 1979).

Injudicious overindulgence in mannitol might result in excessive intravascular volume expansion, hyponatraemia and intracellular dehydration. During anuria 200 g mannitol given intravenously could theoretically expand the extracellular space by 2 litres. One anuric patient given a total of 300 g mannitol over 24 hours did become semicomatose with a serum sodium of only 96 mmol/litre (Feldman et al 1971). However, 20 g mannitol repeated up to five times over a 24-hour period in a patient with some renal function is innocuous and should be used as the drug of first choice.

Anxiety over mannitol led to the use of the diuretics frusemide and ethacrynic acid to improve renal function in potential ARF. These drugs increase solute excretion and hence urine flow rate, primarily by poisoning the chloride pump in the thick ascending limb of Henle's loop and there is no evidence that they have a beneficial effect on cell function during hypoxia. They should not be used as prophylactic drugs during or after surgery on patients with obstructive jaundice unless the patient is in cardiac failure. Otherwise the use of frusemide treats the doctor, who sees an increase in urine flow rate, rather than the patient, whose kidney cells continue to deteriorate.

There is evidence in favour of low dose dopamine infusion, 1–2 μg/kg body weight per minute in the early stages of incipient ARF (Henderson et al 1980). At this dose dopamine produces a rise in RBF and should be given when hourly urine volumes are less than 50 ml per hour on two successive occasions. Large inotropic doses of dopamine or dobutamine sometimes have to be used to sustain blood pressure but will have little beneficial effect on RBF.

Preoperative percutaneous biliary drainage

It might seem logical to suppose that preoperative biliary decompression (Molnar & Stockum 1974) should improve the prospects for later definitive surgery especially in high risk patients (Ch. 37).

Initial results seemed favourable. The technique was described as being relatively safe, simple and, for the high risk patient, resulted in improved kidney function and better nutritional status.

Well controlled clinical trials of external biliary drainage have failed to substantiate these claims (Hatfield et al 1982, McPherson et al 1984, Pitt et al 1985). Sepsis has proved to be a major problem when using external drainage although this can be overcome by careful attention to technique. The only objective improvement seems to be a significant fall in bilirubin. Although overall renal function in terms of creatinine clearance improved this was also seen in the control group treated by simple rehydration alone prior to definitive surgery. All these studies failed to demonstrate a decrease in mortality by the use of this technique. It is possible that preoperative internal biliary drainage may be more effective in preventing renal failure

(Smith et al 1985) but this remains to be proven in a large trial.

Oral bile salts

Despite apparently adequate peroperative intravenous fluids, albumin, mannitol and antibiotics, patients with obstructive jaundice still succumb to postoperative renal failure (Evans et al 1982, Ingoldby 1983). The clue may lie in the presence of endotoxaemia (Ch. 12), the incidence of which after surgery in obstructive jaundice ranges from 50–81% (Wardle 1975, Bailey 1976, Ingoldby 1983).

Attempts to reduce peroperative endotoxaemia in obstructive jaundice by means of gut sterilization with antibiotics (Hunt et al 1982) or by administration of an anti-toxin such as polymixin B (Ingoldby 1980) have been unsuccessful.

Evidence is accumulating, however, that preoperative oral bile salts can significantly reduce the incidence of endotoxaemia in obstructive jaundice in rats (Bailey 1976) and man (Cahill 1983). Bile salts can reduce the anaerobic gut pool as well as having a direct surfactant effect on endotoxins. This may prove to be an innocuous but effective method not only of reducing endotoxaemia but of preventing the ARF which might follow (Cahill 1983). A final verdict awaits the outcome of controlled clinical trials in adequate numbers of patients undergoing surgery for obstructive jaundice.

The management of established acute renal failure

Preoperative ARF

A small number of patients with cholangitis, sepsis and obstructive jaundice will develop acute renal insufficiency (Bismuth et al 1975). The management of these patients is especially critical. They should be resuscitated with fluid replacement, correct antibiotics and, if necessary, dialysis before definitive surgery. The timing of the operation is determined by the evolution of the sepsis. Death from renal insufficiency may be prevented by adequate dialysis until postoperative recovery occurs.

Postoperative ARF

This is more difficult to manage since the patient has been the subject of a surgical insult and often has multi-organ failure. In general, such patients are best managed by a team of experts in an intensive care environment. Established ARF should always be considered to be potentially reversible since, should the patient survive the other problems, renal function will usually recover. The principles of management are quite simple: control of fluid balance, control of electrolytes, especially potassium, provision of adequate calories and amino acids and careful scrutiny for developing complications. No patient should be allowed to die of uraemia, electrolyte imbalance or starvation. Dialysis can be carried out either by the use of an external semi-permeable membrane (haemodialysis) or across the peritoneal membrane. Peritoneal dialysis is often neither feasible nor desirable in a patient recovering from surgery for obstructive jaundice and will not be considered further.

Haemodialysis is generally carried out by the use of cellulosic based membranes such as cupraphane. In classic haemodialysis substances of a molecular weight less than 1000 daltons will pass across such a semi-permeable membrane quite freely, diffusing from an area of high concentration to an area of low concentration. Thus urea and creatinine, present in the blood in high concentration in uraemia, will diffuse down a concentration gradient into the dialysate which bathes the membrane. The passage of water occurs by convection, necessitating a relatively high transmembrane hydrostatic pressure gradient. Water removal by cellulosic based membranes is thus limited and pressure dependent.

Recently exciting advances have been made in membrane technology. Highly permeable membranes, chiefly polysulphone and polyacrilonitrile membranes have appeared. They allow the free passage of substances up to a molecular weight of approximately 5000 daltons. Considerable passage still occurs up to a molecular weight of 50 000 daltons. They are very permeable to water and only a small transmembrane pressure gradient will result in a large flux of water. The permeability characteristics of these membranes are therefore similar to those of the glomerular basement membrane complex and they have been termed the 'artificial glomerulus'. Such membranes can be used to produce a pure ultrafiltrate of plasma simply by the hydrostatic pressure of the arterial blood. This is known as haemofiltration. Up to 20 litres of ultrafiltrate can be removed from the plasma in the course of 24 hours, thus keeping the concentration of blood urea etc. relatively constant. Replacement fluids must be given simultaneously to prevent loss of essential plasma electrolytes.

By combining simple ultrafiltration with dialysis (haemodiafiltration) one can use these membranes continuously to give smooth control of extracellular fluid composition over three to six weeks in patients with ARF (Simpson et al 1985). In addition these membranes enable removal of substances of molecular weight 1000–5000 daltons, an attribute of considerable theoretical interest to those involved in managing patients with hepatic failure (Ch. 102).

RENAL FUNCTION IN CIRRHOSIS OF THE LIVER

> 'It is not the purpose of this article to review in its entirety the abundant literature ..... but rather to attempt an

appraisal and interpretation of some of the available information pertinent to Laennec's Cirrhosis of the Liver.'

Papper 1958

A vast multitude of clinical and experimental studies on the role of the kidney in cirrhosis of the liver have appeared over the past 100 years. Interested readers are referred to six excellent reviews (Papper 1958, Epstein 1983a and b, Vaamonde 1983, Papper 1983, Levensen et al 1983, Levinsky 1983). The treatment of these conditions has recently been well reviewed by Epstein 1984.
Three aspects will be considered:

1. The nature of the renal problem in cirrhosis.
2. Renal failure in advanced cirrhosis.
3. Management of renal failure in cirrhosis.

1. Renal structure and function in cirrhosis

Renal structure

'The morbid alteration of the kidney, known to the name of Bright's disease, frequently accompanies cirrhosis, having been met with 15 times in 42 cases.'

Becquerel 1840

Despite this bold statement made over 100 years ago, attempts to correlate glomerular structure and function in cirrhosis of the liver have, until recently, been notoriously disappointing. For decades light microscopists examined autopsy material and considered degeneration of tubule cells to be the outstanding renal lesion. The recent introduction of electron microscopy and immunofluorescent techniques to examine renal biopsy material has yielded fascinating information. Significant glomerular abnormalities are present in over 95% of 116 renal biopsies examined by various authors (Eknoyan 1983). There is an increase in mesangial matrix, irregular thickening of the capillary basement membrane and occasionally pronounced glomerulosclerosis. Sakaguchi et al (1965) coined the term 'hepatic glomerulosclerosis' to describe these changes, since they were seen in a wide variety of liver diseases irrespective of the nature, duration or severity of the condition. Two distinct forms can be described. The first, a non-proliferative form, is associated with mesangial deposits of IgA. Patients usually do not have proteinuria. The second and more severe proliferative form shows both endothelial and epithelial cellular proliferation and intramembranous deposits of IgA. Patients often have pronounced proteinuria and haematuria. Hypocomplimentaemia and cryoglobulinaemia have been described in patients with cirrhosis.

Unfortunately, few studies have attempted to correlate these abnormalities in structure with functional changes. Indeed, Eknoyan in a recent review states that 'the glomerular lesions are accompanied by neither clinical manifestations nor biochemical abnormalities indicating renal dysfunction'. Detailed sequential studies correlating renal structure and function in cirrhosis of the liver are needed.

One recent interesting observation concerning the pathogenesis of renal failure in patients with liver disease has recently been made by histopathologists. Lecithin:cholesterol acyltransferase (LCAT) is an enzyme, made in the liver, which is responsible for the esterification of plasma cholesterol. Familial deficiency of the enzyme is associated with the appearance of unesterified cholesterol-rich lipoprotein in the plasma. A major problem for these sufferers is renal failure. Their glomeruli show deposition of cholesterol and phospholipids in the glomerular basement membrane, in the mesangium and significantly in the subendothelial space. These changes will develop within five to six months of the transplantation of a healthy kidney into a sufferer.

In 1978 Hovig et al found low plasma LCAT activity in patients with cirrhosis of the liver and renal failure. Theoretically, endothelial cell swelling and damage due to these substances could result in a decreased ability of the cells to produce prostacycline or other cytoprotective vasoactive polypeptides in response to stress. It should be remembered that endothelial cell swelling and damage is also a histological feature in animals with experimental biliary tract obstruction (Fig. 31.2, 31.3).

Renal function

It is well established that cirrhosis of the liver is associated with a profound but variable degree of salt and water retention. Indeed, at times these patients can excrete urine which is almost free of sodium. Since this can occur when the glomerular filtration rate, and hence the filtered load of sodium, is within normal or only slightly decreased, these patients must have a very significant rise in the tubular reabsorption of sodium. In 1977 Lopez-Novoa et al were able to confirm significant increased proximal reabsorption in the nephrons of rats with chronic cirrhosis by the use of kidney micropuncture techniques. The normal circadian rhythm for sodium excretion is changed, nocturnal sodium loss being increased in comparison to the reverse in normal subjects. In some patients the ability to excrete a water load is diminished, those with ascites and oedema being particularly affected.

Recent studies (Naccarato et al 1981) have shown that increased tubular reabsorption of sodium can be found very early in the evolution of cirrhosis and pre-date the development of ascites. Levy and colleagues have described two phases in fluid retention. In the early or first phase (Unikowsky et al 1983) sodium retention may be the result of stimulation of a stretch receptor or a low pressure baroreceptor within the liver. Early intrahepatic hypertension would cause reflex stimulation of sympathetic nerves and increased tubular sodium reabsorption. This early first phase occurs before ascites formation and is associated with expansion of plasma volume.

Later ascites develops, effective arterial blood volume decreases and plasma renin, aldosterone and oestrogen concentrations rise. Increased tubular reabsorption of sodium continues and such patients are often unable to excrete a water load. They have dilutional hyponatraemia.

The precise pathophysiological mechanisms in ascites are still the subject of considerable research and have been discussed elsewhere (Ch. 103).

2. Renal failure in advanced cirrhosis

Renal failure is distressingly common in cirrhosis of the liver, being found at some time in 50–75% of sufferers (Wilkinson et al 1975). Uraemia has been described as the commonest extrahepatic cause of death in these patients (Clermont et al 1967). In many instances renal failure is due to pre-renal deficits and/or ATN. In some, however, there is no obvious cause for renal failure and these patients are described as having 'the hepatorenal syndrome'. This has been defined by Papper (1983) as 'incompletely explained renal failure in patients with liver disease in the absence of clinical, laboratory or other known cause of renal failure'. Patients with HRS are often in the terminal stages of liver failure and the mortality rate is extremely high, although spontaneous recovery has been reported.

Table 31.3 contrasts the clinical and laboratory features of the three forms of renal failure which are found in cirrhosis of the liver. In both pre-renal oliguria and in established ATN a clear precipitating event is usually obvious, with acute circulatory failure, infection or exposure to nephrotoxins. The patients need not necessarily have ascites. Pre-renal oliguria is further characterized by a high urine/plasma osmolality ratio and a low urinary sodium excretion, indicating relatively intact tubular function. Replacement of measured deficits with or without the addition of dopamine or mannitol is generally successful in correcting the oliguria, provided the initiating events are under control. In established ATN, tubular function is lost, with a fall in the urine/plasma osmolality ratio to 1 or less and a high urinary sodium loss. Once tubular cell death has occurred volume expansion will not improve oliguria. These points have been covered in the first section of this chapter.

Table 31.3 Differential diagnosis of oliguria in cirrhosis

	Pre-renal	ATN (established)	HRS
Clinical features	Associated with acute hypotension, hypovolaemia infection	Follows pre-renal or nephrotoxins	Minor degree of salt/H_2O depletion or hypotension slow to develop
Urine sodium mmol/L	< 10	> 50	< 10 initially
Urine: Plasma osmolality (no diuretics)	> 1.05	1 or less	> 1.05 initially
Response to volume expansion ± dopamine, mannitol	yes	no	no

The HRS is therefore a clinical diagnosis of exclusion. Those at risk are generally in hospital, suffering from alcoholic cirrhosis with portal hypertension, are usually jaundiced and have moderate to severe ascites. They may be relatively hypotensive but not clinically shocked. Almost all have dilutional hypoatraemia and the majority have hypoalbuminaemia. Interestingly, a sense of false security may be given from observation of a normal serum creatinine concentration in these patients. Measurement of GFR by inulin clearance has shown this to be significantly reduced in many patients with advanced cirrhosis and ascites (Papadakis and Arieff, 1984). They conclude that HRS may represent only a slight deterioration in function in an already compromised kidney. Initially, tubular function is well maintained with a high urine/plasma osmolality ratio and a low urine sodium concentration. Unlike pre-renal oliguria, however, volume expansion, whilst it may produce a very small and temporary improvement in renal function, has no long lasting beneficial effects.

Pathophysiology of HRS

Many factors present in cirrhosis of the liver may predispose the sufferer to both pre-renal oliguria and HRS. Some of these, such as the noxious effects of cholaemia and endotoxaemia have already been discussed in the section on obstructive jaundice and will not be considered again.

The hallmark of renal function in cirrhosis of the liver is vascular instability, with active cortical vasoconstriction. This was beautifully demonstrated in 1970 by Epstein et al using ^{133}xenon washout technique and selective renal arteriography to study renal blood flow and its distribution in 15 patients with cirrhosis of the liver and differing renal function. In cirrhotic patients with renal failure there was marked variability and irregularity of xenon washout, in contrast to other patients without liver disease but with renal failure. Blood flow through the outer cortical compartment decreased in approximate proportion to the decrease in creatinine clearance.

The dynamics of forces normally governing glomerular ultrafiltration are now the subject of intense scrutiny. Each nephron's glomerular filtration rate is determined by the balance of hydrostatic and oncotic forces acting across the capillary bed together with the permeability and surface area of the capillary available for filtration, Kf (Fig. 31.6). High affinity glomerular receptors for vasoactive agents, such as angiotensin II, norepinephrine, AVP, PGE_2, PGI_2,

$$\text{sngfr} = K_f(\bar{P}_{GC} - P_T) - (\bar{\Pi}_{GC} - \Pi_T)$$

Fig. 31.6 The factors determining the rate of ultrafiltration in a single glomerulus.
Sngfr: Single nephron glomerular filtration rate.
Kf: Glomerular capillary permeability, determined by local effective hydraulic permeability and the surface area available for filtration. Reduced by contraction of mesangial cells.
$\bar{P}_{GC}$: Mean hydraulic pressure within glomerular capillary, determined by efferent/afferent arteriolar constriction and systemic blood pressure.
P_T: Mean hydraulic pressure in Bowman's Space.
π_{GC}: Mean oncotic pressure within glomerular capillary, determined by plasma albumin concentration and glomerular filtration rate. Oncotic pressure rises exponentially with filtration.
π_T: Oncotic pressure within Bowman's Space (negligible)

thromboxane A_2, acetylcholine, bradykinin, histamine, dopamine and serotonin have been described (Dworkin et al 1985). It is likely that a nice balance normally exists between intrinsic renal vascular tone, determined by AVP, prostaglandins and angiotensin II, and extra-renal vascular tone dependent on sympathetic nerves and cardiac output.

In cirrhosis of the liver, however, there may be a grave imbalance between renal vasoconstrictive mechanisms (e.g. AVP, angiotensin II, sympathetic nerve activity) and vasodilatory mechanisms (e.g. PGE_2, PGI_2, bradykinin). This is outlined in Fig. 31.7. As a result there is variable renal cortical ischaemia and loss of the protective mechanisms normally at work to maintain GFR in the face of systemic hypotension and hypovolaemia. The evidence for this can be summarized as follows:

Firstly, immunoreactive circulating AVP is high in cirrhosis. This is due partly to an increased half-life but also to increased secretion due to a re-setting of normal osmoreceptor control. Exogenous AVP is a potent renal and systemic vasoconstrictor agent. Most important, AVP can also decrease GFR by decreasing glomerular capillary hydraulic permeability, Kf.

Secondly, renal PGE_2 production is increased in cirrhosis of the liver. This can be considered to be a compensatory adaptation to balance the renal vasoconstrictor effects of AVP. In advanced cirrhosis, however, or after administration of NSAID, renal PGE_2 release decreases. These drugs can cause a significant fall in GFR and renal plasma flow in patients with alcoholic liver disease. There is also evidence that glomerular thromboxane release may be increased in HRS, causing a fall in Kf.

Thirdly, the renin-angiotensin system is activated in patients with cirrhosis and ascites, with a marked rise in plasma renin levels. Indeed, these patients may be dependent on angiotensin II to maintain systemic blood pressure, administration of converting enzyme inhibitors resulting in profound hypotension. Unfortunately, angiotensin II can also cause renal afferent arteriolar vasoconstriction and a decrease in Kf, resulting in a fall in GFR.

Finally, activation of the sympathetic nervous system may play an important role (Gottschalk et al 1985). Raised plasma norepinephrine levels are found in patients with decompensated cirrhosis and correlate significantly with

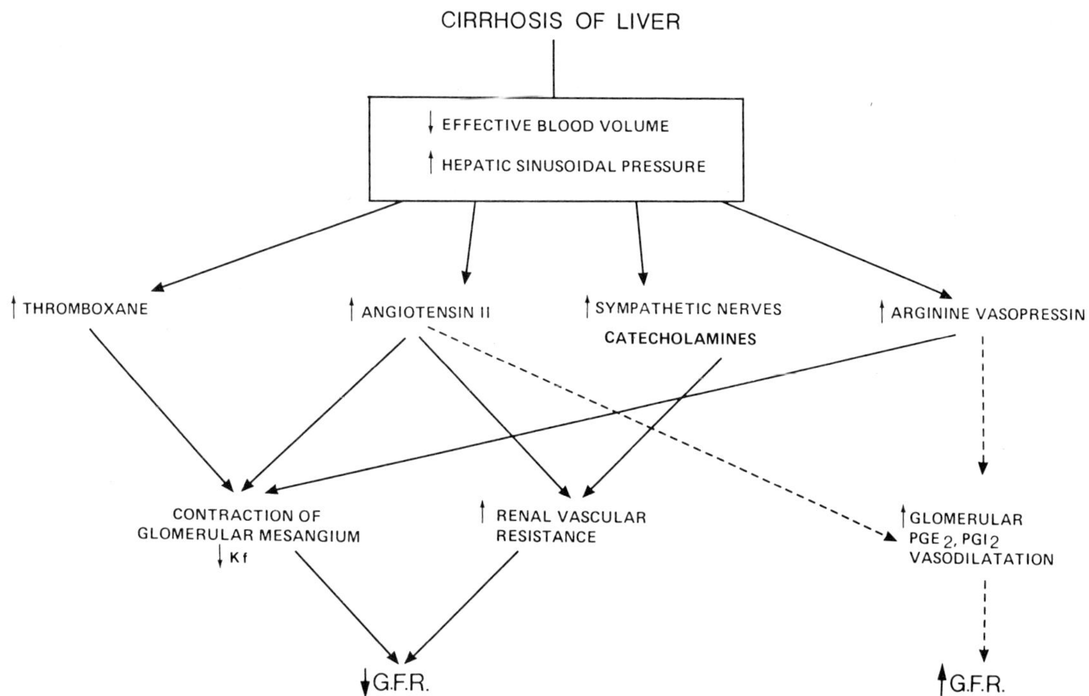

Fig. 31.7 Schematic representation of the possible intrarenal action of vasoactive hormones which might predispose to renal failure in cirrhosis of the liver. Endothelial cell damage (e.g. due to LCAT) may reduce ability to produce 'protective' vasodilatory PGE_2, and PGI_2

the decrease in RBF and the extent of sodium retention. Increased sympathetic nerve activity is thus believed to produce both renal vasoconstriction and an increase in sodium reabsorption from the proximal tubule. The precise mechanisms for activation remain speculative, but could involve baroreceptors in the liver and portal vein. Animal studies have shown the existence of both a hepato-renal reflex and a splanchno-renal reflex.

3. Management of renal failure in cirrhosis of the liver

> 'The hepatorenal syndrome is one of the most frustrating diseases in medicine'.
>
> Conn 1973

For those without access to liver transplantation the old addage that 'prevention is better than cure' certainly applies to renal failure in liver disease. All patients in hospital with cirrhosis of the liver should have renal function carefully monitored, especially when salt and water restriction or diuretics are in use, when gastrointestinal bleeding is likely or if surgery is proposed. Table 31.4 lists the basic requirements.

Renal failure in cirrhosis may often be iatrogenic (Epstein 1984). For example, NSAID will prevent the intrarenal production of PGE_2 and PGI_2, vasoactive substances which play an essential protective role in normal glomerular haemodynamics and which are especially essential in cirrhosis of the liver. These drugs can cause renal impairment in liver disease (Boyer et al 1979, Zipser et al 1979). The hepatorenal syndrome begins insidiously and the surgeon cannot be too obsessional in carefully examining the patient daily in terms of weight loss, presence or absence of oedema, sodium balance and serum creatinine concentration. 'Therapeutic' paracentesis in patients with ascites is best avoided. If required urgently to relieve symptoms, it should always be accompanied by the simultaneous intravenous infusion of concentrated albumin to maintain or increase plasma volume and improve plasma albumin concentration. Re-infusion of concentrated ascitic fluid is also possible, although much less practical (See below).

Table 31.4 Prevention of renal failure in cirrhosis

Examine daily	weight tissue turgor ascites/oedema blood pressure temperature
Measure	Urine volume and osmolality sodium balance serum: creatinine, urea, sodium, potassium and albumin concentration Haemoglobin/haematocrit Liver function
Avoid	NSAIDs* Nephrotoxins Excessive weight loss (> 0.5 kg/day) due to diuretics, paracentesis or lactulose Hypoalbuminaemia Infection

*Non steroid anti inflammatory drugs

In the first instance all patients with cirrhosis who develop oliguria should be considered to have either pre-renal oliguria or established ATN (Table 31.3). Reversible volume depletion will respond to volume expansion with colloid, if albumin is low, or with saline. Patients with HRS given colloid will also respond favourably in the first instance but this is not sustained. A history of nephrotoxic drugs, severe infection or urinary obstruction would suggest ATN. Theoretically, these patients should recover once the aggravating factors have been corrected or removed. Haemodialysis support may be needed for three to six weeks while this occurs and should best be done using the more permeable polysulphone or polyacrilonitrile membranes and haemodiafiltration.

The outlook for patients with true HRS, however, is grim indeed; 'very few cases survive' (Conn 1973). Essentially, improvement in renal function appears to be almost totally dependent on recovery of the liver and, indeed, kidney function in patients treated by liver transplantation returns to normal (Iwatsuki et al 1973). The advent of charcoal haemoperfusion, plasma exchange and the new permeable membranes for haemodiafiltration have led to reports of improvement in liver function in the short term with associated renal recovery. Such manoeuvres may buy time to enable liver repair to occur and may occasionally be of benefit in the long term.

Somewhat in desperation an impressive array of 'specific medications' have been tried (Levenson et al 1983). While some are based on sound theoretical grounds, none have as yet been shown to be really effective in the long term. Two manoeuvres of particular interest to the surgeon are peritoneovenous shunting of ascitic fluid (Le Veen et al 1974) (PVS) (Ch. 103) and portacaval shunting. Both have been claimed to improve renal function in advanced cirrhosis and the HRS (Schroeder et al 1970, Wapnick et al 1977).

Role of peritoneovenous or portacaval shunting in improving renal function

Hypovolaemic shock and renal failure often follow rapid and injudicious paracentesis. It is an old clinical observation that this can be prevented by simultaneous intravenous re-infusion of the ascitic fluid. This manoeuvre was early shown to produce a significant, but unfortunately transient, improvement in GFR and effective renal plasma flow with a diuresis and a natriuresis. Kaiser et al (1962) claimed this technique to be of great value in the per-operative management of cirrhotic patients with ascites, conserving protein and maintaining renal function. It was quickly recognized that intravenous infusion of albumin, preferably as a 25% solution with a normal sodium concentration, would produce similar results, although the cost of the procedure was increased. Recently the development of a polyacrilonitrile membrane has enabled successful ultrafiltration of the ascitic fluid with the removal of salt and water before re-infusion (Parbhoo et al 1974).

While the short-term beneficial effects of this technique have been clearly demonstrated, it is doubtful if it provides more than a little palliation or perhaps a useful adjunct in the management of patients with ascites being prepared for surgery. Long-term observations of renal function and survival in cirrhotic patients subjected to either daily or weekly re-infusion treatments or managed by conventional diuretics and salt restriction have shown no difference in the frequency of ultimate renal failure or survival (Clermont et al 1967).

The development by LeVeen et al in 1974 of a satisfactory valve first made possible long term PVS of ascitic fluid. Subsequent modifications were made to prevent shunt occlusion (Denver shunt, Cordis-Hakim valve). Despite significant morbidity due to fever, diffuse intravascular coagulation and infection many thousands of these devices have now been implanted in ascitic patients. Significant improvement in nutritional and immunological well-being with reduction in ascitic fluid accumulation seems to occur in a significant proportion (Ch. 103).

The technique has also been widely advocated as an effective treatment for the HRS. Epstein (1982) has critically reviewed the evidence for this claim and found it lacking. There is good evidence that pre-renal oliguria can be prevented or even reversed by successful PVS. Improvement in renal function with a diuresis and natriuresis is found for up to two weeks after shunt insertion. Simultaneously cardiac output increases, calculated peripheral resistance falls and both plasma renin activity and aldosterone concentration decrease (Schroeder et al 1979, Blendis et al 1979). In some patients these improvements have been noted for as long as up to six months after implanting the shunt (Greig et al 1981).

The evidence for improvement of renal function in HRS itself, however, is not good. Most investigators have claimed improvement in patients who undoubtedly had pre-renal oliguria. Only the study of Schroeder et al (1979) is considered by Epstein to fulfil all the correct criteria for the diagnosis of HRS. They compared two techniques, either creation of a side-to-side portacaval shunt or a mesocaval shunt or insertion of a LeVeen shunt in 10 cachectic patients with massive ascites and oliguric renal failure. Interestingly renal function improved and plasma renin activity fell to normal in seven of the 10 patients after either a portacaval shunt or a successful PVS. However, three of the five patients given á portacaval anastomosis died of liver failure postoperatively. The authors conclude 'that the efficacy of these procedures in prolonging the survival of patients with hepatorenal syndrome remains to be proven by controlled prospective study'.

REFERENCES

Aarseth S, Bergen A, Aarseth P 1979 Circulatory homeostasis in rats after bile duct ligation. Scandinavian Journal of Clinical Laboratory Investigation 39: 93–97

Allison M E M, Moss N G, Fraser M M, Dobbie J W, Ryan C J, Kennedy A C et al 1978 Renal function in obstructive jaundice: a micropuncture study in rats. Clinical Science and Molecular Medicine 54: 649–659

Allison M E M, Prentice C R M, Kennedy A C, Blumgart L H 1979 Renal function and other factors in obstructive jaundice. British Journal of Surgery 66: 392–397

Alon U, Berant M, Mordechovitz D, Hashmonai M, Better O S 1982 Effect of isolated cholemia on systemic haemodynamics and kidney function in conscious dogs. Clinical Science 63: 59–64

Anderson R J, Linas S L, Berns A S 1977 Non-oliguric acute renal failure. New England Journal of Medicine 296: 1134–1138

Armstrong C P, Dixon J M, Taylor T V, Davies G C 1984 Surgical experience of deeply jaundiced patients with bile duct obstruction. British Journal of Surgery 71: 234–238

Ayer D 1938 Renal lesions associated with deep jaundice. Archives of Pathology 22: 26–41

Bailey M E 1976 Endotoxin, bile salts and renal function in obstructive jaundice. British Journal of Surgery 63: 774–778

Barry K G, Malloy J P 1962 Oliguric renal failure. Evaluation and therapy by the intravenous infusion of mannitol. Journal of the American Medical Association 179: 510–513

Becquerel A 1840 Recherches anatomico-pathologiques sur la cirrhose du foie. Archives Generoles de Médécine 3rd series, 8: 40–79

Better O S 1983 Bile duct ligation: an experimental model of renal dysfunction secondary to liver disease. In: Epstein M (ed) The kidney in liver disease. Elsevier Science Publishers, p 295–311

Bismuth H, Kuntziger H, Corlette M B 1975 Cholangitis with acute renal failure. Annals of Surgery 181: 881–887

Blamey S L, Fearon K C H, Gilmour W H, Osborne D H, Carter D C 1983 Prediction of risk in biliary surgery. British Journal of Surgery 70: 535–538

Blendis L M, Greig P D, Langer B, Baigrie R S, Ruse J, Taylor B R 1979 The renal and haemodynamic effects of peritoneovenous shunt for intractable hepatic ascites. Gastroenterology 77: 250–257

Bomzon L, Kew M C 1983 Renal blood flow in experimental obstructive jaundice. In: Epstein M (ed) The kidney in liver disease. Elsevier Science Publishing, p 313–326

Boyer T D, Zia P, Reynolds T B 1979 Effect of Indomethacin and Prostaglandin A_1 on renal function and plasma renin activity in alcoholic liver disease. Gastroenterology 77: 215–222

Cahill C J 1983 Prevention of post-operative renal failure in patients with obstructive jaundice — the role of bile salts. British Journal of Surgery 70: 590–595

Clairmont P, von Haberer H 1911 Ueber Aurie nach Gallensteinoperationen. Mitteilunger aus den Grenzgebieten der Medizen und Chirurgie 22: 159–172

Clermont R J, Vlahoevic Z R, Chalmers T C, Adham N F, Curtis G W, Morrison R S 1967 Intravenous therapy of massive ascites in patients with cirrhosis. II Long term effects on survival and frequency of renal failure. Gastroenterology 53: 220–228

Conn H O 1973 A rational approach to the hepatorenal syndrome. Gastroenterology 65: 321–340

Dawson J L 1964 Jaundice and anoxic renal damage: the protective effect of mannitol. British Medical Journal 1: 810–811

Dawson J L 1968 Acute post-operative renal failure in obstructive jaundice. Annals of the Royal College of Surgeons of England 42: 163–181

Dixon J M, Armstrong C P, Duffy S W, Davies G C 1983 Factors affecting morbidity and mortality after surgery for obstructive jaundice: a review of 373 patients. Gut 24: 845–852

Drivas G, James O, Wardle N 1976 Study of reticuloendothelial phagocytic capacity in patients with cholestases. British Medical Journal 1: 1568–1569

Dworkin L D, Brenner B M 1985 Biophysical bases of glomerular filtration. In: Seldin D W, Giebisch G (eds) The kidney: physiology and pathophysiology. Raven Press, New York, p 397–426

Eknoyan G 1983 Glomerular abnormalities in liver disease. In: Epstein M (ed) The kidney in liver disease. Elsevier Science Publishing, New York, p 199

Eliahou H E 1964 Mannitol therapy in oliguria of acute onset. British Medical Journal 1: 807–809

Elsom K A 1937 Renal function in obstructive jaundice. Archives of Internal Medicine 60: 1028–1033

Epstein M, Berk D P, Hollenberg N K, Adams D G, Chalmers T C, Abrams H L et al 1970 Renal failure in the patient with cirrhosis. The role of active vasoconstriction. The American Journal of Medicine 49: 175–185

Epstein M 1982 Peritoneovenous shunt in the management of ascites and the hepatorenal syndrome. Gastroenterology 82: 790–799

Epstein M 1983a Renal sodium handling in cirrhosis. Seminars in Nephrology 3: 225–240

Epstein M 1983b The renin-angiotensin system in liver disease. In: Epstein M (ed) The Kidney in liver disease. Elsevier Science Publishers, New York, p 353–346

Epstein M 1984 Therapy of renal disorder in liver disease. In: Suki W N, Massry S G (eds) Therapy of renal diseases and related disorders. Martinus Nijhoff, Dordrecht p 335–346

Evans H J R, Torrealba V, Hudd C, Knight M, 1982 The effect of pre-operative bile salt administration on post-operative renal function in patients with obstructive jaundice. British Journal of Surgery 69: 706–708

Feldman B H, Kjellstrand C M, Fralby E E 1971 Mannitol intoxication. Journal of Urology 106: 622–623

Fletcher M S, Westwick J, Kakkar V V 1982 Endotoxin, prostaglandins and renal fibrin deposition in obstructive jaundice. British Journal of Surgery 69: 625–629

Flores J, Dibona D R, Beck C H, Leaf A 1972 The role of cell swelling in ischaemic renal damage and the protective effect of hypertonic solute. Journal of Clinical Investigation 51: 118–126

Frank H A, Seligman A M, Fine J 1946 Traumatic Shock XIII. The prevention of irreversibility in haemorrhagic shock by the viviperfusion of the liver. Journal of Clinical Investigation 25: 22–29

Gelman S I 1976 Disturbances in hepatic blood flow during anaesthesia and surgery. Archives of Surgery 111: 881–883

Gottschalk C W, Moss N G, Colindres R E 1985 Neural control of renal function in health and disease. In: Seldin D W, Giebisch G (eds) The kidney: physiology and pathophysiology. Raven Press, New York, p 599–600

Green J, Beyar R, Bomzon L, Finberg J P M, Better O S 1984 Jaundice, the circulation and the kidney. Nephron 37: 145–152

Greig P D, Blendis L M, Langer B, Taylor B R, Colapinto R F 1981 Renal and haemodynamic effects of peritoneovenous shunt. II Long term effects. Gastroenterology 80: 119–125

Hatfield A R W, Terblanche J, Sataar S, Kernoff L, Tobias R, Girdwood A H et al 1982 Pre-operative external biliary drainage in obstructive jaundice. Lancet ii: 896–899

Helwig F C, Schutz C B 1932 A liver, kidney syndrome. Surgery, Gynecology and Obstetrics 55: 570–580

Henderson I S, Beattie T J, Kennedy A C 1980 Dopamine hydrochloride in oliguric states. Lancet ii: 827–828

Hovig T, Blomhoff J P, Holme R, Faltmark A, Gjone E 1978 Plasma lipoprotein alterations and morphological changes with lipid deposition on the kidneys of patients with hepatorenal syndrome. Laboratory Investigation 38: 540–549

Hunt D R, Allison M E M, Prentice C R M, Blumgart L H 1982 Endotoxaemia, disturbance of coagulation and obstructive jaundice. American Journal of Surgery 144: 325–329

Ingoldby C 1980 The value of Polymixin B in endotoxaemia due to experimental obstructive jaundice and mesenteric ischaemia. British Journal of Surgery 67: 565–567

Ingoldby C 1983 Endotoxaemia and renal failure in obstructive jaundice. Thesis submitted for Master of Surgery of the University of Cambridge

Iwatsuki S, Popoutzer M M, Corman J L, Ishikawa M, Putnam C W, Katz F H et al 1973 Recovery from 'hepatorenal syndrome' after orthotopic liver transplantation. New England Journal of Medicine 289: 1155–1159

Kaiser G C, Lempke R E, King R D, King H 1962 Intravenous infusion of ascitic fluid. Archives of Surgery 85: 83–91

Kennedy A C, Burton J A, Luke R G, Briggs J D, Lindsay R M, Allison M E M et al 1973 Factors affecting prognosis in acute renal failure. Quarterly Journal of Medicine 42: 73–86

Lassen N A, Thomsen A C 1958 The pathogenesis of the hepatorenal syndrome. Acta Medica Scandinavica CLX: 165–171

Leaf A, Cheung J Y, Mills J W, Bonventre J V 1983 Nature of the cellular insult. In: Brenner B M, Lazarus J M (eds) Acute renal failure, W B Saunders, Philadelphia, p 2–20

LeVeen H H, Christoudias G, Ip M, Luft R, Falk G, Grosberg S 1974 Peritoneovenous shunting for ascites. Annals of Surgery 180: 580–591

Levenson D J, Skorecki K L, Narins R G 1983 Acute renal failure associated with hepatobiliary disease. In: Brenner B M, Lazarus J M (eds) Acute renal failure. W B Saunders, Philadelphia, p 467–498

Levinsky N G 1983 The hepatorenal syndrome. Medical Grand Rounds 2: 160–169

Lopez-Novoa J, Rengel M A, Rodicio J L, Hernando L 1977 A micropuncture study of salt and water retention in chronic experimental cirrhosis. American Journal of Physiology 232: 315–318

Luke R G, Briggs J D, Allison M E M, Kennedy A C 1970 Factors determining the response to mannitol in acute renal failure. American Journal of Medical Science 259: 168–174

McPherson G A D, Benjamin I S, Habib N A, Bowley N B, Blumgart L H 1982a Percutaneous transhepatic drainage in obstructive jaundice. British Journal of Surgery 69: 261–264

McPherson G A D, Benjamin I S, Boobis A R, Brodie M J, Hampden C, Blumgart L H 1982b Antipyrine elimination as a dynamic test of hepatic functional integrity in obstructive jaundice. Gut 23: 734–738

McPherson G A D, Benjamin I S, Hodgson H J F, Bowley N B, Allison D J, Blumgart L H 1984 Pre-operative percutaneous transhepatic biliary drainage: the results of a controlled trial. British Journal of Surgery 71: 371–375

Molnar W, Stockum A E 1974 Relief of obstructive jaundice through a transhepatic catheter — a new therapeutic method. American Journal of Roentgenology 122: 356–367

Naccarato R, Messa P, D'Angelo A, Fabris A, Messa M, Chiaramonte M et al 1981 Renal handling of sodium and water in early chronic liver disease. Gastroenterology 81: 205–210

Nolan J P 1981 Endotoxin, reticuloendothelial function and liver injury. Hepatology 1: 458–465

Paller M S, Hoidal J R, Ferris T F 1984 Oxygen free radicals in ischaemic acute renal failure in the rat. Journal of Clinical Investigation 74: 1156–1164

Papadakis M A, Arieff A T 1984 Hepatorenal syndrome: an expanded definition. Kidney International 25: 173

Papper S 1958 The role of the kidney in Laennec's cirrhosis of the liver. Medicine (Baltimore) 37: 299–316

Papper S 1983 Hepatorenal syndrome. In: Epstein M (ed) The kidney in liver disease. Elsevier Science Publishers, New York, p 87–106

Parbhoo S P, Ajdukiewicz A, Sherlock S 1974 Treatment of ascites by continuous ultrafiltration and reinfusion of protein concentrate. Lancet 12: 949–952

Park R, Arieff A I 1983 Lactic acidosis: Current concepts. In: Schade P S (ed) Clinics in endocrinology and metabolism. W B Saunders, Philadelphia, Vol 12, No. 2, p 339

Pitt H A, Cameron J L, Postier R G, Gadacz 1981 Factors affecting mortality in biliary tract surgery. American Journal of Surgery 141: 66–72

Pitt H A, Gomes A S, Lois J F, Mann L L, Deutsch L S, Longmire W P 1985 Does pre-operative percutaneous biliary drainage reduce operative risk or increase hospital costs. Annals of Surgery 201: 545–553

Ravdin I S 1929 Vasodepressor substances in the liver after obstruction of the common duct. Archives of Surgery 18: 2191–2201

Rudbach J A, Anacker R L, Haskins W T, Johnson A G, Milner K C, Ribi E 1966 Physical aspects of reversible inactivation of endotoxin. Annals of New York Academy of Sciences 133: 629–643

Sakaguchi H, Dachs S, Grisham E, Paronetto F, Salomon M, Churg J 1965 Hepatic glomerulosclerosis. An electron microscopic study of renal biopsies in liver disease. Laboratory Investigation 14: 535–545

Schroeder E T, Numann P J, Chamberlain B E 1970 Functional renal failure in cirrhosis. Recovery after portacaval shunt. Annals of Internal Medicine 72: 923–928

Schroeder E T, Anderson G H, Smulyan H 1979 Effects of portacaval or peritoneovenous shunt on renin in the hepatorenal syndrome. Kidney International 15: 54–61

Selkurt E E 1945 Changes in renal clearance following complete ischaemia of the kidney. American Journal of Physiology 144: 395–404

Shorr E, Zweifach B W, Furchgott F 1948 Hepatorenal factors in circulatory homeostasis: III The influence of hormonal factors of hepatorenal origin on the vascular reaction to haemorrhage. Annals of The New York Academy of Science 49: 571–592

Simpson H K, Allison M E M, Telfer ABM 1986 Improving the prognosis in acute renal and respiratory failure. Renal Failure (in press)

Smith R C, Pooley M, George C R P, Faithful G R 1985 Pre-operative percutaneous transhepatic internal drainage in obstructive jaundice: a randomised, controlled trial examining renal function. Surgery 97: 641–647

Sorensen F H, Anderson J B, Ornsholt J, Skjoldborg H 1971 Acute renal failure complicating biliary tract disorders. Acta Chirurgica Scandinavica 137: 87–91

Stewart H L, Cantarow A, 1935 Renal lesions following injection of sodium dehydrocholate in animals with and without biliary stasis. Archives of Pathology 20: 866–881

Tanner G A, Selkurt E E 1970 Kidney function in the squirrel monkey before and after haemorrhagic hypotension. American Journal of Physiology 219: 597–603

Unikowsky B, Wexler M J, Levy M 1983 Dogs with experimental cirrhosis of the liver but without intrahepatic hypertension do not retain sodium or form ascites. Journal of Clinical Investigation 72: 1594–1604

Vaamonde C A 1983 Renal water handling in liver disease. In: Epstein M (ed) The kidney in liver disease. Elsevier Science Publishers, New York, p 55–86

Walters W, Parham D 1922 Renal and hepatic insufficiency in obstructive jaundice. Surgery, Gynecology and Obstetrics 35: 605–609

Wapnick S, Grosberg S, Kinney M, LeVeen H H 1977 LeVeen continuous peritoneal-jugular shunt: Improvement in renal function in ascitic patients. Journal of The American Medical Association 237: 131–133

Wardle E N, Wright N A 1970 Endotoxin and acute renal failure associated with obstructive jaundice. British Medical Journal 4: 472–474

Wardle E N 1975 Endotoxaemia and the pathogenesis of acute renal failure. Quarterly Journal of Medicine 44: 389–398

Wardle E N 1980 Endotoxin shock. In: Karran S (ed) Controversies in surgical sepsis. Praeger, New York, p 199–206

Wilbur O L 1934 The renal glomerulus in various forms of nephrosis. Archives of Pathology 18: 157–185

Wilkinson S P, Hirst D, Portman B, Williams R 1975 Pathogenesis of renal failure in cirrhosis and fulminant hepatic failure. Postgraduate Medical Journal 51: 503–505

Williams R D, Elliot D W, Zollinger R W 1960 The effect of hypotension in obstructive jaundice. Archives of Surgery 81: 335–340

Yared A, Kon V, Ichikawa I 1985 Mechanism of preservation of glomerular perfusion and filtration during acute extracellular volume depletion. Journal of Clinical Investigation 75: 1477–1487

Zipser R D, Hoefs J C, Speckart P F, Zia P K, Horton R 1979 Prostaglandins: modulation of renal function and pressor resistance in chronic liver disease. Journal of Clinical Endocrinology and Metabolism 48: 895–900

A. W. Halliday, G. M. Flannigan

Pre- and postoperative nutrition in hepatobiliary surgery

'Life, like the flicker of a candle, is dependent on nutrition.'
Leonardo da Vinci

INTRODUCTION

Central role of the liver and biliary system in metabolism

Five hundred years ago Leonardo da Vinci wrote of the importance of the liver in metabolism and nutrition, 'The liver is the distributor and dispensor of vital nourishment to man. The bile is the familiar or servant of the liver which sweeps away and cleans up all the dirt and superfluities left after the food has been distributed to members by the liver.'

In the nineteenth century Claude Bernard first demonstrated the ability of the liver to synthesize glycogen from food substances. Later work showed that the liver was central to the control of carbohydrate, protein and fat metabolism, as well as vitamin storage, plasma protein and coagulation factor production.

Amino acid, fat and protein metabolism

During starvation the body's store of glycogen is depleted within 24 hours. The body's glucose needs are met by gluconeogenesis from glycogenic amino acids, lactase, pyruvate and glycerol. Muscle and fat stores are mobilized to make the precursor substances available. During starvation, sepsis and injury, fatty acid mobilization leads to ketone body production. The biochemical and metabolic pathways involved in ketosis have been well summarized by Cahill (1981).

Bile salt production and exocrine pancreatic secretion control the normal digestion and absorption of fat. Glycolysis, lipogenesis and fat deposition are promoted by the action of insulin, using energy from the tricarboxylic acid cycle. When insulin levels fall during ketosis the beta-oxidation of fatty acids leads to ketogenesis, gluconeogenesis and lipolysis. Half of the body's deposit of fat is stored in the subcutaneous tissues and the rest is found mainly around the kidneys, in the omentum and the gut mesentery. The presence of cirrhosis may alter the normal metabolism of fat.

After protein digestion, amino acids are absorbed into the splanchnic circulation. Glutamate, aspartate and glutamine are utilized by the intestine after absorption and the other amino acids pass to the liver. In the liver they may be absorbed by hepatocytes, or pass into the general circulation. Leucine, isoleucine and valine, known as the branched-chain amino acids, are metabolized preferentially by muscle tissue. The muscle itself produces alanine and glutamate which undergo gluconeogenesis in the liver and kidneys.

The synthesis of plasma proteins is an important function of the liver. Albumin is essential to maintain oncotic pressure, and to carry unconjugated bilirubin and other poorly soluble substances. Transferrin and caeruloplasmin control the carriage of iron and copper, and prealbumin and retinol binding protein are the carriers for thyroxine and vitamin A. The immunoglobulins, with the exception of gammaglobulin, are also produced by the liver and have an important role to play in the maintenance of the immune response.

SPECIFIC NUTRITIONAL PROBLEMS IN HEPATOBILIARY DISEASE

Malnutrition may develop in association with or as a result of any of the conditions shown in Table 32.1.

Obstructive jaundice

The development of obstructive jaundice leads to malabsorption of fat and offensive steatorrhoea. The patient may feel nauseated by fatty foods but this symptom is not invariably present. At first the clinician often prescribes a low fat diet, regardless of the cause of obstructive jaun-

Table 32.1 Specific nutritional problems in hepatobiliary disease

Problem	Nutritional defects	Solutions
Obstructive jaundice	Anorexia Malabsorption of fats and fat-soluble vitamins	Oral/enteral bile salts Intravenous fat/vitamins Intramuscular vitamin K Relief of obstruction
Cirrhosis/Hepatocellular failure	Glucose intolerance/insulin resistance Branched-chain amino acid deficiency Vitamins A, C, E, Folate, Zinc deficiency	Oral/enteral vegetable protein Branched chain supplements Intravenous feeding with fat supplements and vitamins
Traumatic/Elective liver resection	Hypoglycaemia Hypoalbuminaemia Abnormal lipid metabolism	Intravenous dextrose Albumin supplements Medium-chain triglycerides
Infection/Inflammation	Increased metabolic rate V/Q imbalance with ↑ CO_2 production Glucose intolerance/insulin resistance	Intravenous/enteral feeding with ↑ fat and ↓ dextrose Antibiotics/abscess drainage
Cancer	Anorexia ↑ lactic acid, glucose uptake ↑ albumin/protein catabolism Weight loss, hypoalbuminaemia, oedema	Oral/enteral supplements Intravenous feeding ± albumin Tumour resection

dice. Attempts to prevent weight loss, with a high carbohydrate, high protein diet, are usually unsuccessful. Dietary alterations become even more complicated in the presence of diabetes. When jaundice has been present for some time, malnutrition may result in hypoalbuminaemia and the presence of clinical oedema and ascites. Low protein diets, which may be prescribed in these circumstances, will exacerbate this problem.

Many patients with obstructive jaundice may tolerate dietary fat well and if they are able to absorb even small amounts of fat, a low fat diet should not be prescribed. Carbohydrate tolerance is normal in the presence of obstructive jaundice, except when pancreatic damage is also present. In a recent study at Hammersmith Hospital, Flannigan et al (1985) measured the ability of patients with biliary obstruction to clear intravenous alanine and glucose. Glucose clearance and hepatic gluconeogenesis were unaltered in the presence of severe obstructive jaundice (Figs 32.1, 32.2). Where the patient is unable to eat and intravenous feeding is indicated, a normal balanced regimen should be used, there being little evidence to support the idea that jaundiced patients have a limited tolerance of intravenous fat solutions.

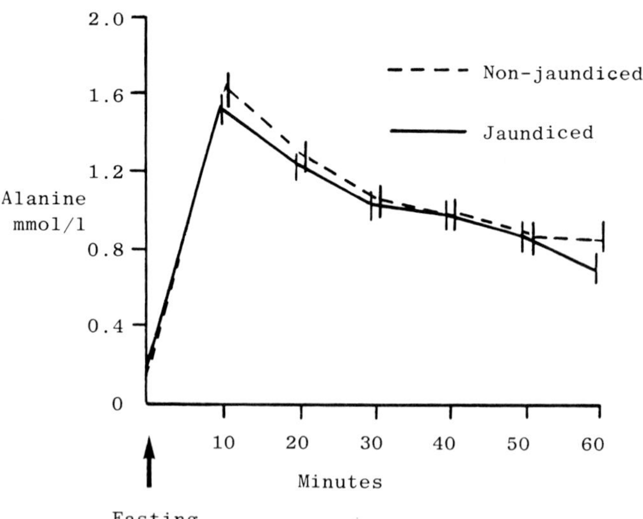

Fig. 32.1 The clearance of intravenous L-alanine (12 g) in jaundiced and non-jaundiced patients

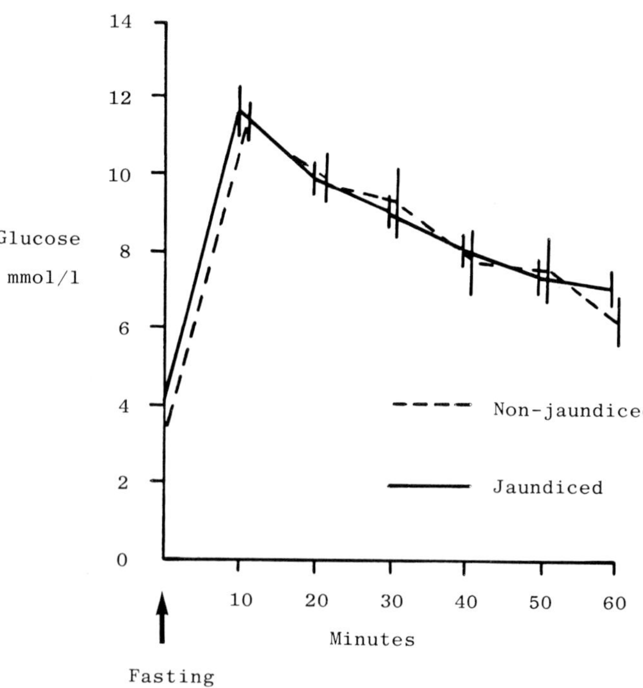

Fig. 32.2 The clearance of intravenous glucose (25 g) in jaundiced and non-jaundiced patients

Cirrhosis and hepatocellular failure

The presence of cirrhosis alters normal fat and carbohydrate metabolism and Mezey (1978) noted that glucose intolerance due to insulin resistance is present in 50–80% of cirrhotics. Patients who develop liver failure because of cirrhosis require special management. Lean body mass is often reduced although they may gain weight because of ascites. Deficiencies of vitamins A, C & E and folate leave them at risk of postoperative complications such as wound infection and dehiscence. Zinc deficiency can result from low levels of retinol alcohol dehydrogenase (Smith & Goodman 1971). A characteristic abnormal amino acid pattern is associated with cirrhosis and hepatocellular failure, with low levels of the branched-chain amino acids (BCAA). There is also evidence that normal immune defence mechanisms are compromised. Munro and his colleagues (1975) postulated that insulin resistance, a characteristic of cirrhotic patients, causes a decrease in BCAA levels and an increase in peripheral metabolism, leading to muscle breakdown. Promotion of anabolism by specially formulated diets using vegetable protein, or branched-chain biased amino acid components, has been found helpful. Fischer et al (1976) showed that, using a specially formulated 23% dextrose, BCAA-enriched solution, which was low in other amino acids, encephalopathy could be reversed. Although other studies have suggested that these solutions may be capable of improving the patient's nutritional status, a multicentre trial (Wahren et al 1983) showed no evidence of improved survival using branched-chain biased solutions.

Trauma and elective liver resection

The ability of the liver to function normally after a resection depends on the proportion of normal hepatic parenchymal tissue remaining, and on the presence or development of septic complications. Albumin synthesis is reduced for one to three weeks in patients having 70% of the liver resected (Almersjö & Bengmark 1969, Augustine & Swick 1980). Lipid metabolism is significantly altered following hepatic resection, leading to increases in free fatty acid and blood ketone levels. Glucose and/or insulin administration may be required during the first few postoperative days. Glucose administration is usually indicated to avoid hypoglycaemia immediately after operation. Energy production from glucose is usually restored to normal within 3–4 days of operation.

Infection and inflammation

Hepatobiliary and pancreatic disease may present as infection or inflammation. Viral or alcohol-induced hepatitis can result in a serious reduction in normal dietary intake. For the surgeon, pancreatitis and cholangitis are more common problems. Cholangitis may be a feature of gallstone disease, bile duct stricture or sclerosing cholangitis. The combination of obstructive jaundice, fever and rigors results in anorexia, malabsorption of fat and an increase in the metabolic rate leading to a loss of lean body mass. If recurrent attacks of cholangitis or pancreatitis occur, then malnutrition may become evident, but, in patients with benign biliary stricture or early sclerosing cholangitis, malnutrition is not a common problem.

Cancer

The development of malnutrition in cancer patients is due both to the changes in metabolism caused by the tumour itself and to the effects of the tumour on other organs. De Wys (1979) has reviewed the problems of anorexia in cancer patients and noted that taste changes occur and that appetite is often better earlier in the day. Small intestinal atrophy and hyposecretion have been observed in cancer patients. Burt et al (1983) showed that lactic acid output and glucose uptake are increased in cancer patients, leading to increased protein metabolism and a lowering of plasma insulin levels. Theologides (1979) noted that fat mobilization and albumin metabolism are increased in cancer while protein synthesis is reduced.

Hepatobiliary and pancreatic cancer are associated with pain, anorexia, weight loss, fever and jaundice (Adson & Weiland 1981). Pain causes a decrease in appetite, fever increases metabolic rate and jaundice impairs fat absorption. Malnutrition in the preoperative period has been reported by several workers (Collure et al 1974, Blumgart et al 1984).

IDENTIFICATION OF MALNUTRITION BY NUTRITIONAL ASSESSMENT

The goals of nutritional assessment were defined by Bistrian (1976) to be a 'model to accurately identify the subset of surgical patients that are at increased risk of developing nutritionally-based complications, in whom

Table 32.2 Measuring malnutrition

Dietary intake	
Height/Weight index	
Weight loss	
Muscle function:	dynamometry
	adductor pollicis function
Body composition:	fat
	body cell mass
	total body potassium
	total body nitrogen
Protein turnover studies	
Urinary urea, creatinine, 3-methyl histidine	
Serum albumin, prealbumin, retinol-binding protein	
Delayed hypersensitivity skin testing	

preoperative nutritional support will reduce the incidence of postoperative morbidity and mortality'. The guidelines for measuring malnutrition are shown in Table 32.2.

History

Dietary history and physical examination form the basis of sound nutritional assessment. In each institution and for each particular problem, special investigations can be selected according to their availability and the appropriateness of their use.

Dietary history has been shown by Mueller & Thomas (1975) to be valuable in revealing areas of deficient intake. Fat intolerance and low protein intake can be defined and objectively measured.

Anthropometry

Weight and height measurements may be used to calculate the severity of nutritional depletion. The type of tissue involved in weight loss may be difficult to determine and the time course of this loss is also important. Simple measurements, such as weight or weight/height ratio do not take account of body build. A more accurate estimate requires a weight/height/frame table such as that suggested by Grant et al (1981).

Recent weight loss exceeding 10% of the original healthy weight is a valuable indicator of malnutrition, and is of significance in predicting surgical mortality in patients with malignant hepatobiliary disease (Halliday et al, 1985a). However, its use is subject to accuracy of patient recall and it may therefore be imprecise when used for assessing progress during nutritional supplementation.

Body fat stores are measured using skinfold thickness. This should be done by a single operator and four sites (suprailiac, subscapular, biceps and triceps) should be used. Single site (triceps) measurement is inaccurate and standard normal values vary with different populations and with time. The same problems apply to mid-arm muscle circumference measurement, with the additional observation that the humeral diameter is not accurately measured and the arm is not a true cylinder. Hypoalbuminaemia may cause tissue oedema leading to inaccurate skinfold thickness measurement and a falsely optimistic evaluation.

Muscle function can be measured by a simple hand grip dynamometer (Klidjian et al 1982), or by assessment of adductor pollicis function by electrical stimulation (Lopes et al 1982). These are the only dynamic tests of nutritional status available but there have been criticisms of dynamometry, one being that it may alter with learning.

Body composition analysis

Body cell mass may be estimated by indirect measurement, using skinfold thickness to determine the percentage body weight as fat (Durnin & Womersley 1974) and thereby calculating fat-free mass. One disadvantage of this method is that it depends on serum albumin and packed-cell volume being within the normal limits and this estimation may not therefore be of value in severely malnourished patients.

Total body potassium has been used as an index of body cell mass. Since 98% of body potassium is intracellular, a low value is indicative of muscle cell loss. Shizgal & Spanier (1977), using an isotope dilution method, estimated total exchangeable potassium and showed that, in critically ill patients, body cell mass could only be maintained by supplying a minimum of 46 kcal/kg per day. Total exchangeable potassium has been shown to underestimate true total body potassium by about 12%, and recently more accurate estimations have been made by direct measurement, using a whole body counter. The subject lies in the whole body counter for a half-hour period. Gamma radiation, produced from native ^{40}K, is detected by sodium iodide crystals. This isotope represents a constant (0.012%) proportion of total body potassium. Measurement of total body potassium can therefore be expressed as a percentage of the expected normal for a patient of the same sex, weight, height and age, using previously calibrated measurements. One advantage of this method is that potassium measurement is unaffected by the administration of diuretics and by the presence of oedema. Casey et al (1965) noted that the normal liver only contained 90mEq of potassium, and that cirrhotic patients often had a low total body potassium. However when Soler et al (1976) gave potassium supplements to cirrhotic patients for six months, they failed to improve total body potassium. The deficiency in potassium was therefore a lack of cell mass rather than an abnormality in potassium metabolism.

The use of this measurement of malnutrition was further demonstrated in 1979 by Walesby et al who studied patients undergoing cardiac surgery and found that a low total body potassium was associated with postoperative sepsis and death. Moreover, these patients could not be selected preoperatively by observation alone, and this method provided an effective screening test for malnutrition.

Total body nitrogen analysis was described by Hill and his co-workers in 1978, using prompt gamma ray analysis. It is thought by some workers to be a more accurate method of analysis of protein-containing tissue than total body potassium. However, after a period of successful intravenous nutrition, total body nitrogen may not alter significantly whereas total body potassium may increase (McNeill et al 1982). In 1965, Garrow et al predicted that the 'nature, distribution and concentration of protein, rather than its absolute amount' was probably of more importance in determining clinical outcome.

Protein/nitrogen turnover studies

Urinary 3-methylhistidine, urea and creatinine have been used to measure protein loss. 24-hour urinary nitrogen is useful as a monitor of changes during nutritional therapy, and may indicate the presence of sepsis. However, inaccurate results may be obtained if urine collections are incomplete, and the value of 3-methylhistidine is limited by rapid alterations in protein turnover resulting from operative or septic stress.

Visceral protein status is usually assessed by serum albumin ($t\frac{1}{2}$ = 12 days), transferrin ($t\frac{1}{2}$ = 8 days) or a shorter half-life transport protein such as thyroxine-binding prealbumin ($t\frac{1}{2}$ = 2 days). Bozzetti et al in 1975 showed poor wound healing to be associated with protein deficiency. Seltzer et al (1979), Pitt et al (1981), Blamey et al (1983), and Armstrong et al (1984) all support the value of hypoalbuminaemia as a predictor of poor surgical outcome, particularly in hepatobiliary surgery. Transferrin and thyroxine-binding prealbumin (TBPA) have also been suggested as good indicators of protein synthesis and nutritional status. Unlike albumin they have a shorter half-life and reflect changes in nutritional status more rapidly. Transferrin has been criticized by Rowlands et al (1982) because levels are altered by iron deficiency and by blood transfusion. Shetty et al (1979) have recommended pre-albumin and retinol-binding protein (both short half-life proteins) as sensitive indicators of subclinical malnutrition, their estimations being independent of renal function. Following liver resection they will not be affected by exogenous albumin infusion (Vanlandingham et al 1982). Halliday et al (1985b) found thyroxine-binding prealbumin to be of value as an indicator of serious malnutrition in jaundiced patients. Prediction of operative mortality was possible using this measurement preoperatively (Fig. 32.3).

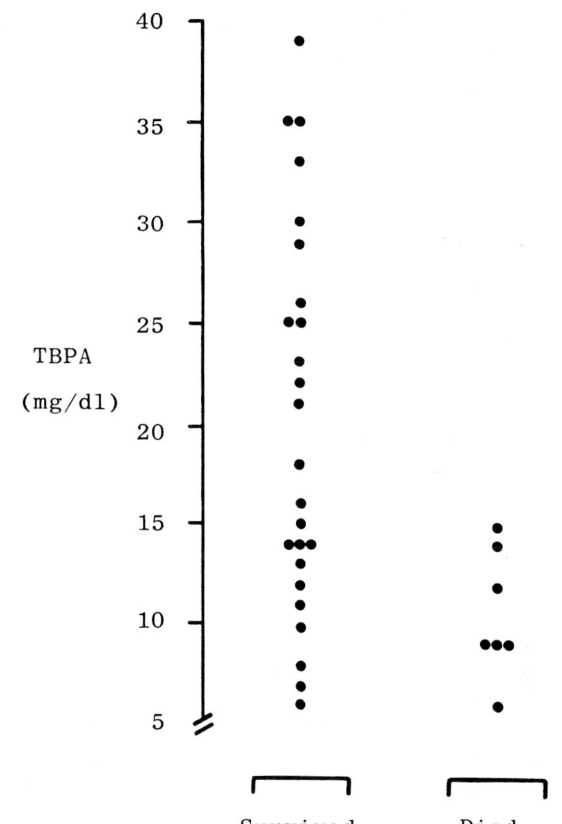

Fig. 32.3 Preoperative TBPA and survival following surgery for malignant hepatobiliary disease

Immune status

The measurements used to determine immune status in patients before surgery include total lymphocyte count, mixed leucocyte response, antibody production, complement levels, lymphokine production and delayed hypersensitivity skin testing. The last of these has been in wide use and many workers have claimed that it is a valuable prognostic test. Caution in the interpretation of these tests was expressed by Bates, Suen & Tranum (1979) who, in reviewing the literature, found that there was no uniform method of either administering or interpreting skin tests. They made recommendations for the uniform dilutions, measurement, interpretation and types of antigens. Twomey, Ziegler & Rombeau (1982) reviewed 500 papers dealing with nutrition and the immune response and concluded that the rationale for the use of skin testing was not clear. In a study of patients with cirrhosis of the liver, anergy was found to be common, but this was not correlated with poor nutritional status (Mills et al 1983). Anergy and relative anergy are associated with mortality following hepatobiliary surgery for cancer (Fig. 32.4) but it has not been possible to effect changes in skin test results by the use of intravenous nutrition (Halliday et al 1985a).

IDENTIFICATION OF NUTRITIONAL RISK FACTORS

General surgical risk factors

In 1936, Studley showed that patients who died following surgery for peptic ulcer had lost significantly more weight than those who survived. Since then, other studies have identified nutritional 'risk factors': those nutritional measurements which are associated with a greater postoperative morbidity and mortality. Buzby et al (1980) developed a prognostic nutritional index for gastrointestinal surgery. This was a linear predictive model based on values of albumin, skinfold thickness, transferrin and skin test results:

PNI % (percent chance of developing complications) = 158 − 16.6 × (albumin) − 0.78 × (triceps skinfold thick-

	Survived	Died
Reactive	14	1
Rel. Anergic Anergic	1	6

Fig. 32.4 Preoperative skin test reactivity and survival following surgery for malignant hepatobiliary disease

ness) $-0.20 \times$ (transferrin) $-5.8 \times$ (delayed hypersensitivity response)

The formula was complicated and, although these workers validated it for their patients, others did not always find it of use. Its value lies in the objectivity of their approach to nutritional status and operative risks. Unfortunately Buzby et al were unable to demonstrate improvements in the prognostic nutritional index following 7–10 days feeding. They attributed this to the fact that the parameters they used were unlikely to change in such a short period of time and suggested that the values of shorter half-life proteins such as prealbumin and retinol binding protein might provide a more accurate method of assessing improving nutritional status.

Hepatobiliary surgical risk factors

In patients undergoing hepatobiliary surgery, serum albumin <3.0 g/dl, haematocrit <30%, and a weight loss of >10% of the original weight have been shown to help in the identification of patients at risk (Pitt et al 1981, Dixon et al 1983).

The authors have studied 32 patients with malignant hepatobiliary disease and measured weight loss, calorie intake, arm circumference, total body potassium, body fat, skin test reactivity and serum albumin and thyroxine-binding prealbumin. Weight loss and total body potassium were the most useful measurements for predicting the development of serious life-threatening complications after operation. The prediction of death could be accurately assessed using weight loss, arm circumference, total body potassium, skin testing and prealbumin (Fig. 32.5) (Halliday et al 1985c).

Improvement in total body potassium from a high risk to a lower risk level can be achieved using preoperative feeding (Fig. 32.6) and predicted postoperative complications can be significantly reduced (Halliday et al 1985c).

PREOPERATIVE AND POSTOPERATIVE SUPPLEMENTAL NUTRITION — INDICATIONS FOR USE

Preoperative nutrition

Several controlled trials have now been undertaken to evaluate the use of preoperative nutrition. Trials which have shown that morbidity and mortality can be reduced (Moghissi et al 1977, Dietel et al 1978, Heatley et al 1979,

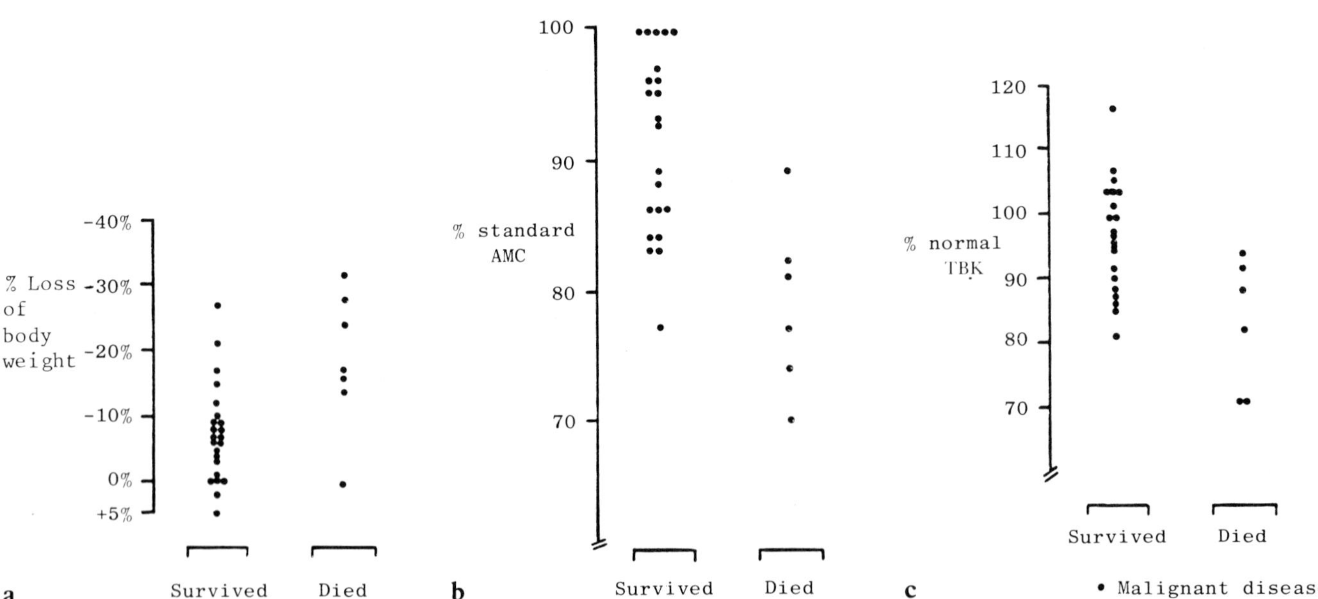

Fig. 32.5 Preoperative (a) weight loss, (b) arm circumference and (c) total body potassium, and survival following surgery for malignant hepatobiliary disease

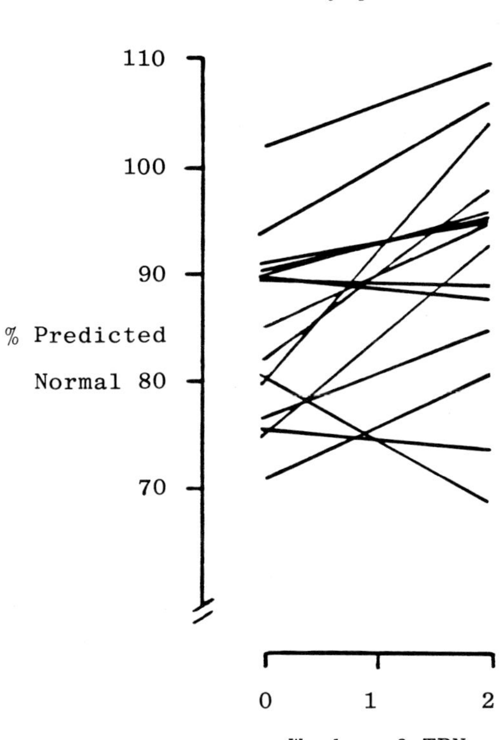

Fig. 32.6 Changes in total body potassium during two weeks of parenteral nutrition

Muller et al 1982) suggest that maximum benefit can probably be obtained following a minimum of 10–14 days preoperative parenteral nutrition. Heatley et al (1979), studying patients with oesophageal or gastric cancer, found that the incidence of postoperative wound sepsis was reduced by 7–10 days preoperative intravenous feeding. Dietel et al (1978) had found, retrospectively, that fewer deaths occurred in nutritionally-depleted cancer patients when fed pre- and postoperatively but their study contained many sub-groups of patients and wide variations in duration of support. Since then, the decision to withhold nutritional support as part of a randomized trial has proved difficult to justify ethically, and few controlled trials have been reported. Improvements of nutritionally-related changes in immune function and anthropometry have been demonstrated, following preoperative nutritional support, but it has not been possible to link these changes with improved outcome.

In the Hepatobiliary Unit at Hammersmith Hospital, patients undergo initial screening for malnutrition. Where the patient has a weight loss of greater than 10% of original weight or a subnormal serum albumin (<30 g/l) then total body potassium is measured and intensive feeding is instituted. Success in restoring TBK is usually apparent within two weeks. During this time diagnostic evaluation can take place and investigations requiring periods of starvation (ultrasound, angiography, percutaneous cholangiography) will not therefore worsen the patient's nutritional state. The temptation to perform a 'simple, quick' operation, such as biliary bypass, should be avoided in the presence of malnutrition as there is evidence that this can be extremely hazardous. Collure et al (1974) reported oedema in 20%, and hypoalbuminaemia in 40% of a series of patients with carcinoma of the pancreas or ampulla of Vater. Although 60% of their patients had palliative bypass procedures, and only 2% had radical operation, the overall mortality was 20%, and over 50% of patients had major postoperative complications. In a recent review by Blumgart et al (1984) of 94 cases of hilar cholangiocarcinoma, jaundice was noted in 94%, weight loss in 85%, anaemia in 25% and hypoalbuminaemia in 20% of cases, indicating that malnutrition is a serious problem in this condition.

The high 30 day mortality (20%–53%) following percutaneous or endoscopic decompression of malignant biliary obstruction (Ch. 37) may be related to similar nutritional problems. Preoperative transhepatic biliary drainage (PTBD) has been used to relieve jaundice due to obstructing bile duct carcinoma and to allow time for improvement of nutritional status. This procedure may be hazardous (McPherson et al 1982) and can cause biliary and hepatic parenchymal sepsis. In a study at Hammersmith Hospital it has been shown that, if sepsis can be avoided, vigorous nutritional therapy can improve nutritional status. During drainage, 12 patients were given at least 3000 calories per day by oral, enteral or parenteral routes. Drainage was carried out for a mean of 26 days (range 10–45 days). Six of 12 patients developed biliary sepsis during drainage. Those patients without sepsis improved their hepatic protein synthesis, as shown by increases in prealbumin levels during drainage (Fig. 32.7) and they developed fewer postoperative complications. These results suggest that during PTBD nutritional status can be improved, providing the bile remains sterile (Halliday et al 1985b).

Postoperative nutritional supplementation

The major postoperative complications of hepatobiliary and pancreatic surgery are jaundice, intra-abdominal sepsis, wound infection, respiratory infection, biliary and pancreatic fistula, gastrointestinal haemorrhage and renal failure (Armstrong et al 1984).

Following liver resection liver function tests, clotting factors, glucose and albumin production may be temporarily deranged (Iwatsuki et al 1983, Stone 1975, Thompson et al 1983). Patients should begin to drink within days of resection and recommence diet by the end of the first postoperative week. Should any major complications occur the early institution of nutritional support is vital. Knowledge of the factors influencing the regenerative response is of great importance. Liver resection in the presence of cirrhosis is particularly hazardous and liver

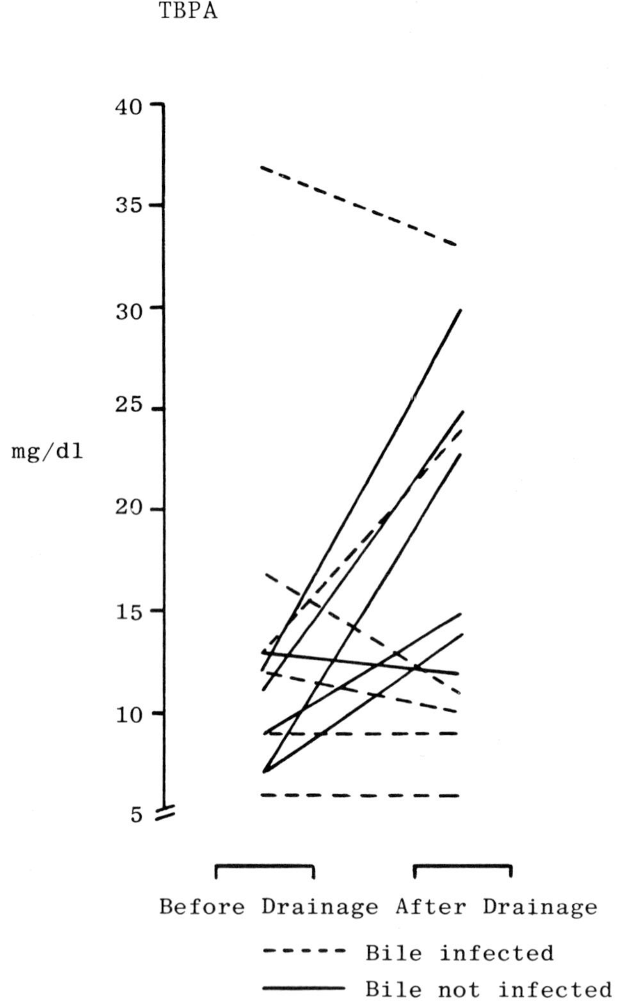

Fig. 32.7 Changes in TBPA during percutaneous transhepatic biliary drainage

failure may result from relatively conservative procedures. When possible, preoperative anticipation of this by an estimation of residual normal functioning liver tissue should be made. There is some evidence to suggest that BCAA solutions may be of special value after liver resection (Saint-Aubert et al 1983).

Renal failure is a well recognized postoperative complication in the patient with preoperative hepatic dysfunction. It is of serious prognostic significance and should be treated aggressively. Haemodialysis or haemofiltration are often required and full volumes of normal parenteral nutrition solutions can be used, because dialysis will remove excess fluid. In the more common situation, where mild renal dysfunction is seen, careful fluid management, alteration in diet or the use of special renal failure enteral solutions may be indicated.

Patients undergoing major liver surgery frequently encounter postoperative respiratory problems. If ventilatory support is necessary and sepsis develops, then special nutritional requirements have to be met. Amino acid infusions increase ventilatory drive but glucose infusions can cause detrimental effects. Glucose-based parenteral nutrition regimens are now regarded as harmful (Elwyn et al 1981). Fat is the main oxidative substrate during sepsis, as glucose oxidation is reduced in the presence of normal insulin concentrations. When insulin resistance develops, control of glucose metabolism by the addition of exogenous insulin becomes difficult. Excessive glucose in the infusion regimen leads to overproduction of CO_2 and worsens respiratory distress. The septic patient can clear and oxidize fat (Stoner et al 1983) and a suggested regimen for this clinical situation includes 20% dextrose (1 litre), 12–18 g nitrogen and 500–1000 ml 20% fat solution daily. Branched-chain amino acid solutions may be substituted when liver function is inadequate. The calorie to nitrogen ratio may safely and effectively be reduced to 50–70:1 under septic conditions.

Biliary fistulae may occur after hepatic resection or bile duct surgery. Conservative therapy is generally employed until the patient's condition is satisfactory for surgery. A policy of waiting and restricting the bile flow stimulation by parenteral nutritional supplementation frequently leads to spontaneous closure of the fistula. Loss of sodium bicarbonate, chloride and potassium from biliary fistulae can be significant, and these should be replaced either in the intravenous solution or by oral electrolyte administration.

Pancreatic fistulae also respond well to conservative therapy based on restriction of oral intake and support with parenteral nutrition. It has recently been observed that lipid infusions increase exocrine pancreatic secretion (Matsuno et al 1981) and this should be borne in mind when formulating the parenteral mixture. The administration of histamine H_2 receptor antagonists and pancreatic enzymes helps decrease fistula output (Ihse et al 1977).

GUIDELINES FOR PRACTICAL NUTRITIONAL MANAGEMENT

There are three routes for nutritional supplementation: oral, enteral and parenteral. The choice is based on the severity of the malnutrition, the presence of anorexia or sepsis, and the time available before operation or definitive treatment.

Oral

Ideally a well balanced hospital diet offers the least expensive and simplest nutritional support. Since anorexia is a common problem the patient may not be able to take full advantage of this method. To succeed, daily intake should be recorded by the patient, recommended targets should be set, and daily weighing is essential to monitor progress. However, the patient should understand that daily weight variation is to be expected, and that the target is an upward trend. Additional dietary supplements should be provided by the hospital dietician, or by the patient's relatives, and these can, if appetizing, improve the patient's motivation.

Enteral feeding

The costs of enteral feeding are comparable to that of a special diet (i.e. 4–5 times the basic hospital diet cost). It may be well tolerated in some anorectic patients because they do not have to look at or taste the diet. Feelings of being bloated, diarrhoea or tube displacement may cause problems. Daily intakes of 3000 calories and 70–80 g of protein a day can be achieved by this method. The problem of diarrhoea has been investigated by Keohane et al (1983) who found that it was not caused by high osmolarity or rapid infusions of solutions, but that the most significant factor was the concurrent administration of antibiotics. In patients with cancer, preoperative negative nitrogen balance is well documented (Moghissi & Teasdale 1980) and the calculated energy required to reverse this balance is 40–45 kcal/kg/day and 0.2–0.25 g N/kg/day. Thus, a 60 kg man would require a minimum of 2.5 litres/day of standard enteral feeding (1 cal/ml) to reach this target.

Standard enteral nutrition of 2.5–3 litres/day is usually well tolerated in patients with obstructive jaundice. Special formula enteral nutrition has been developed for use in patients with chronic liver disease who may require dietary supplementation. This formula contains a BCAA-biased protein source, as well as carbohydrate and fat. Patients with cirrhosis require a minimum oral intake of 50 gm protein/day, and can tolerate up to 80 g/day without psychomotor impairment. Protein synthesis is relatively normal in cirrhotic patients without encephalopathy but protein catabolism is increased. There is some evidence to suggest that BCAA solutions may help suppress increased catabolism in these patients (O'Keefe et al 1980). Another use of BCAA-enriched enteral solutions is in the treatment of sepsis where this may be present preoperatively. During severe catabolism, glucose resistance and diminished fatty acid utilization create a deficit of muscle protein as fuel. This deficit can be met by BCAA-enriched solutions.

Care should be taken in inserting enteral feeding tubes. Although the risks of this method are less than those of parenteral nutrition, unusual complications such as pneumothorax or oesophageal perforation have been reported.

Simple small bore silicone tubes with an internal stylet are now widely available. These are usually well tolerated and their position can be checked by aspiration of gastric juice, auscultation over the epigastrium while injecting air, or by plain abdominal X-ray. Isosmolar enteral feeds may be commenced at full strength, and the delivery rate increased to the maximum required over a two to three day period. Some patients prefer bolus feeding and the freedom of tube disconnection during the day. Most patients manage a total daily intake of 2.5–3 litres without difficulty. Feelings of fullness or vomiting may result from inaccurate gravity drip-feeding. New pumps and side-screw clips are now available to control flow rate more accurately. Diarrhoea may be controlled by the cessation of antibiotic therapy, use of antispasmodic agents or reduction in the delivery rate of enteral solutions. Hyperosmolar solutions may cause unpleasant abdominal cramps and are not often required. The formulation of enteral feeding in preparation for and following hepatic surgery should take account of the patient's clinical condition. Low fat, high carbohydrate and high protein mixtures are usually well tolerated by patients with cirrhosis or obstructive jaundice who may be fat intolerant. Balanced formula enteral feeds provide adequate nutrition under most circumstances. Each hospital stocks a selected range of enteral feeds. These cover many different clinical situations and their contents may be discussed with pharmacists and dieticians.

Parenteral

Although parenteral feeding is considerably more expensive than other methods, once started it provides an easily measurable, usually adequate amount of daily nutrition. Methods of insertion of feeding lines are well summarized by Grant et al (1981). Subclavian approaches to line insertion may cause pneumothorax, subclavian or carotid artery puncture as well as inappropriate line positioning, e.g. in the jugular vein or right atrium.

Catheters may be placed in the superior vena cava via the basilic vein, or by direct puncture of the subclavian or internal jugular vein. Other methods of insertion include cephalic vein cutdown (Ellis & Fielding 1977) and subclavian vein cutdown (Oosterlee & Dudley 1980). Chest X-ray should be performed immediately after insertion to check line position and to detect pneumothorax. In experienced units, catheter complications are rarely serious, but subclavian artery, carotid artery, phrenic and major nerve trunk injury have all been reported. Catheter tip embolisation, catheter migration and air embolism are rare but potentially fatal complications of central venous line placement (Fielding & Ellis 1981). Blocked catheters can be cleared using heparin saline flush in a 1 ml syringe. A scrupulous sterile technique is required during insertion and after care. The lines should be secured by Luer lock as accidental disconnection may cause fatal air embolism. Provided that a careful antiseptic technique is used during insertion and after care, the indicence of catheter sepsis should be less than 5%. Lines should be inserted in the operating theatre and no additional solutions (e.g. blood, plasma or drugs) should be introduced through the nutrition catheter and no blood samples withdrawn through it. Careful instructions should be given to nursing staff about its care. Tunnelling the line under the skin may reduce the likelihood of sepsis but this has not been conclusively shown.

A persistent pyrexia may be caused by catheter sepsis, and a period of 24–48 hours should be allowed for this pyrexia to resolve after removing the line. Peripheral intravenous feeding may also be useful, avoiding the dangers of central line insertion and sepsis, but the peripheral cannula should be changed every 24–36 hours.

Patients with deranged liver function tests are often denied intravenous feeding because of the fear of causing further deterioration. In patients with established cirrhosis, portal hypertension or hepatic failure, the plasma amino acid pattern may be abnormal and caution is advocated when choosing the type and amount of protein infusate. BCAA solutions are suitable for these patients as they are mainly metabolized in muscle and fatty tissue. The first solution of this type, F080, developed by Fischer, provided only small amounts of methionine, phenylalanine and tryptophan, but large quantities of BCAA (valine, leucine and isoleucine). There is evidence to suggest that nutritional improvement can be achieved in patients who are cirrhotic (Leweling & Kanuff 1979, Fisher & Freund 1981). The aims of treatment are to normalize the plasma amino acid profile and to achieve positive nitrogen balance.

Glucose intolerance is commonly encountered in patients with severe parenchymal liver disease. In patients with obstructive jaundice without cirrhosis, glucose solutions of 20%, 40% or even 50% are usually well tolerated. Only minimal amounts of insulin are required unless sepsis supervenes. Where glucose intolerance develops, the calorie source should be based on a dual lipid-glucose mixture. Messing et al (1977) in France showed that the massive fatty infiltration of the liver caused by prolonged parenteral nutrition was due to the sole use of glucose as the non-protein calorie source. In the United States, lipid is usually administered twice weekly, rather than daily. Stein et al (1980), from Pennsylvania, reported that after 7–10 days of preoperative intravenous feeding which included twice weekly lipid, peroperative liver biopsies showed fatty infiltration. This suggested that essential fatty acid deficiency may occur despite apparently adequate lipid administration. Recent work has shown that an amino acid and glucose–lipid mixture administered daily promotes nitrogen retention more effectively than an infusion of amino acids and glucose only (McFie & Smith 1981).

Hyperlipaemia may occur during lipid infusion in patients with liver disease. The administration of small amounts of heparin during lipid infusion reduces the levels of circulating triglycerides to lower values. However, accurate measurement of oxidation of lipid after infusion requires the use of radioactive tracer techniques and the usual test of plasma examination 12 hours after lipid infusion indicates clearance but not oxidation of lipids.

MONITORING NUTRITIONAL SUPPLEMENTATION

Careful recording of daily calorie and nitrogen intake is essential in normal patients and in patients with abnormal liver function. A baseline nutritional assessment, including urea and electrolytes and liver function tests, is essential. It is important to set nutritional goals: e.g., improvement of total body potassium to within an acceptable 'risk' range. Achievement of these goals will depend on the clinical condition and the metabolic demands following operation.

Oral nutrition

Intake (calories and nitrogen) and output (nitrogen) measurements are essential. If the patient has obstructive jaundice then levels of bilirubin, alkaline phosphatase and aspartate transaminase should be checked twice weekly to detect any deterioration. Anthropometric (skin fold thickness) measurement is useful when checked at one to two weekly intervals, but should be interpreted with caution in the presence of hypoalbuminaemia. Serum albumin is unlikely to improve significantly in less than two weeks but measurement of short half-life proteins such as TBPA or retinol binding protein should show an improvement within two days if nutrition is adequate.

Enteral nutrition

The same measurements apply when monitoring enteral nutrition. Because of the large quantity of liquid which may be given, patients with heart failure should be monitored particularly carefully.

Parenteral nutrition

Certain special hazards may be encountered during parenteral nutrition. Measurements of pulse, temperature and blood pressure and urine testing for glycosuria should be performed three to four times daily when starting parenteral nutrition. Daily serum urea, electrolytes, blood glucose and weight should be recorded. A weight gain of greater than 0.5 kg/day is undesirable and indicates water retention. Serum calcium, phosphate and liver function tests should be checked twice weekly. Hypophosphataemia may occur within days of starting feeding and should be promptly corrected. Weekly estimations of magnesium and zinc may also be of help. Zinc deficiency is not uncommon in patients with chronic liver disease.

Vitamin and trace metal requirements

Vitamin and trace metal deficiencies are well recognized in patients with chronic alcoholic liver disease (Morgan

1982). Many of the patients have deficiencies of thiamine, folic acid, pyridoxine, nicotinic acid, ascorbic acid and zinc. Other vitamin and trace metal deficiencies have been described but in liver disease, liver surgery and hepatobiliary cancer the daily requirements are not well understood. Tables of minimum daily requirements refer usually to healthy individuals. A policy which will help patients with liver disease must be based on the measurement of baseline values for those vitamins and trace metals most likely to be affected by the disease process. Morgan (1982) has summarized the methods available for measuring these nutrients. Not all of these methods will give a true value of the body store.

Zinc is largely bound to albumin. It is also in equilibrium with cysteine and histidine-bound zinc and some is complexed with alpha-2 macroglobulin. Erythrocyte zinc levels do not accurately reflect even severe zinc deficiency and, under conditions of sepsis and stress, leucocyte endogenous mediator (LEM) can cause wide fluctuations in plasma zinc levels. Deficiency of zinc in cirrhotic patients may cause night blindness. This is because of reduced action of retinol alcohol dehydrogenase, a zinc-containing enzyme. Appetite and taste, cell-mediated immunity and wound healing are also adversely affected by chronic zinc deficiency. Acute zinc deficiency can occur in patients on parenteral nutrition (Kay & Tasman-Jones 1975) and causes skin lesions resembling acrodermatitis, diarrhoea, alopecia and mood disturbances. Zinc supplementation is often inadequate and levels of 1.3–3.0 μmol/kg per day may be required for severely catabolic patients.

Copper is carried by caeruloplasmin, an alpha-2 macroglobulin formed in the liver. It is essential for normal iron metabolism and patients on long-term parenteral nutrition are at risk of developing copper deficiency. The plasma levels of copper are also affected by sepsis and the release of LEM. The administration of iron, in the presence of inadequate copper stores, may lead to the deposition of iron in Kupffer cells and hepatocytes. Adequate copper levels during intravenous feeding are usually achieved by the administration of 2–4 mg of copper sulphate/day.

Folate and vitamin B_{12} uptake are reduced in patients with cirrhosis (Glass & Mersheimer 1960) and they may be released from storage more rapidly than normal. Cancer patients require regular folate and bolus doses may be given either weekly or in daily infusions. Tetrahydrofolate metabolism is regulated by *vitamin C* intake. Leucocyte ascorbic acid (LAA) concentration is reduced following surgical operations (Irvin 1978) and drugs such as tetracycline will also reduce LAA levels. Anaemia associated with scurvy is rare in liver disease, but LAA levels are often reduced in cirrhosis. Bed sores developing in malnourished, septic patients may respond to the addition of 500 mg of vitamin C to their daily diet.

Vitamins A, D, E and K are all fat soluble and vitamin A is carried by retinol binding protein (RBP). Zinc is necessary for the hepatic synthesis of RBP. Adequate levels of vitamins A, D and K are therefore necessary for patients with severe liver disease. Although they may be supplied as an injectable preparation added to fat emulsion the intravenous vitamin requirement is higher than the oral one (BMJ editorial 1978). Over-enthusiastic vitamin supplementation can cause exfoliative dermatitis (hypervitaminosis A) and hypercalcaemia (hypervitaminosis D). Weekly administration of 5000 units vitamin A, 500 units vitamin D, and 17.5 units of vitamin E has been recommended (Ota et al 1978). The use of vitamin K in patients with liver disease is important before and after surgery. Daily injections of 10 mg are given to jaundiced patients on our unit. B and C vitamins may also be administered orally or as high dose injectable preparations. Thiamine deficiency is associated with postoperative confusion in the elderly.

SUMMARY

The liver is central to the well being and nourishment of man. The elucidation of its role in fat, protein and carbohydrate metabolism has helped in the recognition of malnutrition in hepatobiliary surgery. Manipulation of this central role to treat malnutrition in hepatobiliary disease has meant that oral, enteral and parenteral support can now be tailored to patients' needs. The aims and objectives of reduction of morbidity and mortality in hepatobiliary and pancreatic surgery depend on careful assessment of the patient's nutritional state. In the future, early correction of malnutrition in the jaundiced and cirrhotic patient should be possible before major surgery. Important early indices of the risks of postoperative complications include weight loss of more than 10% of healthy body weight, hypoalbuminaemia, and a reduction in total body potassium. Postoperatively the problems of sepsis and deteriorating liver and renal function may be effectively treated by appropriate antibiotic therapy, surgical drainage of infected collections and aggressive nutritional support.

REFERENCES

Adson M A, Weiland L H 1981 Resection of primary solid hepatic tumours. American Journal of Surgery 141: 18–21

Almersjö O, Bengmark S 1969 Changes in serum protein fractions after 20–80 percent liver resections in man — especially albumin changes. Acta Chirurgica Scandinavica 135: 311–319

Anon 1978 Deficiencies in parenteral nutrition. British Medical Journal Editorial 2: 913

Armstrong C P, Dixon J M, Taylor T V, Davies G C 1984 Surgical experience of deeply jaundiced patients with bile duct obstruction. British Journal of Surgery 71: 234–238

Augustine S L, Swick R W 1980 Turnover of total proteins and ornithine amino-transferase during liver regeneration in rats. American Journal of Physiology 238: E46–E52

Bates S E, Suen J Y, Tranum B L 1979 Immunological skin testing: a plea for uniformity. Cancer 43: 2306–2314

Bistrian B R, Blackburn G L, Vitale J 1976 Prevalence of malnutrition in general medical patients. Journal of the American Medical Association 235: 1567–1570

Blamey S L, Fearon K C H, Gilmour W H, Osborne D H, Carter D C 1983 Prediction of risk in biliary surgery. British Journal of Surgery 70: 535–538

Blumgart L H, Hadjis N S, Benjamin I S, Beazley R 1984 Surgical approaches to cholangiocarcinoma at confluence of hepatic ducts. Lancet i: 66–69

Bozzetti F, Terno G, Longoni C 1975 Parenteral hyperalimentation and wound healing. Surgery, Gynecology and Obstetrics 141: 712–714

Burt M E, Aoki T T, Gorschboth C M, Brennan M F 1983 Peripheral tissue metabolism in cancer-bearing man. Annals of Surgery 198: 685–689

Buzby G P, Mullen J L, Matthews D C, Hobbs C L, Rosato E F 1980 Prognostic nutritional index in gastrointestinal surgery. American Journal of Surgery 139: 160–167

Casey T H, Summerskill W H J, Orvis A L 1965 Body and serum potassium in liver disease. Gastroenterology 48: 198–215

Cahill G F 1981 Ketosis. Journal of Parenteral and Enteral Nutrition 5: 281–287

Collure D W D, Burns G P, Schenk W G 1974 Clinical, pathological and therapeutic aspects of carcinoma of the pancreas. American Journal of Surgery 128: 683–689

De Wys W D 1979 Anorexia as a general effect of cancer. Cancer 43: 2013–2019

Dietel M, Vasic V, Alexander M A 1978 Specialised nutritional support in the cancer patient — is it worthwhile? Cancer 41: 2359–2363

Dixon J M, Armstrong C P, Duffy S W, Davies G C 1983 Factors affecting morbidity and mortality after surgery for obstructive jaundice: A review of 373 patients. Gut 24: 845–893

Durnin J V G, Womersley J 1974 Body fat assessed from total density and its estimation from skin fold thickness. British Journal of Nutrition 32: 77–79

Ellis B W, Fielding L P 1977 Advanced techniques of intravenous therapy. In: Rob, Smith (eds) Operative surgery — General Principles, 3rd edn. Butterworth, Sevenoaks, p 26–34

Elwyn D H, Askanazi J, Kinney J M 1981 Kinetics of energy substrates. Acta Chirurgica Scandinavica Suppl. 507: 209–219

Fielding L P, Ellis B W 1981 Intravenous nutrition — technical aspects. In: Nutrition and the surgical patient. Churchill Livingstone, Edinburgh

Fischer J E, Rosen H M, Ebeid A M, James J H, Keane J M, Soeters P B 1976 The effect of normalisation of plasma amino-acids on hepatic encephalopathy in man. Surgery 80: 77–91

Fischer J E, Freund H R 1981 Hepatic failure. In: Nutrition and the surgical patient. Churchill Livingstone, Edinburgh

Flannigan G M, Peterson J L, Sapsed S M, Hall G, Blumgart L H 1985 Glucose and alanine metabolism in obstructive jaundice. Clinical Nutrition (Supp.) 4: 26

Garrow J S, Fletcher K, Halliday D 1965 Body composition in severe infantile malnutrition. Journal of Clinical Investigation 44: 417–425

Glass G B J, Mersheimer W L 1960 Metabolic turnover of Vitamin B12 in the normal and diseased liver. American Journal of Clinical Nutrition 8: 285–292

Grant J P, Custa P B, Thinlow J 1981 Current techniques in nutritional assessment. Surgical Clinics of North America 61: 437–463

Halliday A W, Benjamin I S, Blumgart L H 1985a Nutritional risk factors in hepatobiliary surgery. Clinical Nutrition (Supp.) 4: 21

Halliday A W, McPherson G A D, Benjamin I S, Blumgart L H 1985b Does preoperative biliary drainage allow an improvement of nutritional status in the jaundiced patient? Clinical Gastroenterology

Halliday A W, Benjamin I S, Blumgart L H 1985c Nutritional risk factors in malignant hepatobiliary and pancreatic disease: a prognostic index. Clinical Nutrition (Supp.) 4:

Heatley R V, Williams R H P, Lewis M H 1979 Preoperative intravenous feeding — a controlled trial. Postgraduate Medical Journal 55: 541–545

Hill G L, McCarthy I D, Collins J P, Smith A H 1978 A new method for the rapid measurement of body composition in critically ill surgical patients. British Journal of Surgery 65: 732–735

Ihse I, Lilja P, Lundquist I 1977 Feedback regulation of pancreatic enzyme secretion by intestinal trypsin in man. Digestion 15: 303–308

Irvin T T 1978 Effects of malnutrition and hyperalimentation on wound healing. Surgery, Gynecology and Obstetrics 146: 33–37

Iwatsuki S, Shaw B W, Starzl T E 1983 Experience with 150 liver resections. Annals of Surgery 197: 247–253

Kay R M, Tasman-Jones C 1975 Zinc deficiency and intravenous feeding. Lancet ii: 605

Keohane P P, Atrill H, Love M, Frost P, Silk D B A 1983 Double blind controlled trial of 'starter regimes' in enteral nutrition. Gut 24: A495

Klidjian A M, Archer T J, Karran S J 1982 Detection of dangerous malnutrition. Journal of Parenteral and Enteral Nutrition 6: 19–121

Leweling H, Kanuff H G 1979 Amino acid imbalance in patients with liver failure: effect of amino acid infusions. Journal of Parenteral and Enteral Nutrition 3: 290

Lopes J M, Russel D M, Whitwell J, Jeejeebhoy K N 1982 Skeletal muscle function in malnutrition. American Journal of Clinical Nutrition 36: 602–610

McFie J, Smith R C 1981 Glucose or fat as a non protein energy source? Gastroenterology 80: 103–107

McNeill K G, Harrison J E, Mernagh J R, Stewart S, Jeejeebhoy K N 1982 Changes in body protein, body potassium and lean body mass during TPN. Journal of Parenteral and Enteral Nutrition 6: 106–108

McPherson G A D, Benjamin I S, Habib N A, Bowley N A, Blumgart L H 1982 Percutaneous transhepatic drainage in obstructive jaundice: Advantages and problems. British Journal of Surgery 69: 261–264

Matsuno S, Miyashira E, Sadaki K, Sato T 1981 Effects of intravenous fat emulsion on exocrine and endocrine pancreatic function. Japanese Journal of Surgery 11: 323–329

Messing B, Bitoun A, Galion A, Mary J Y, Goll A, Bernier J J 1977 La steatose hepatique au cours de la nutrition parenterale depend-elle de l'apport calorique lipidique? Gastroenterology Clinical Biology 1: 1015–1025

Mezey E 1978 Liver disease and nutrition. Gastroenterology 74: 770–783

Mills P R, Shenkin A, Anthony R S, McLellan A S, Main A N H, MacSween R N M, Russell R 1983 Assessment of nutritional status and in vivo immune response in alcoholic liver diseases. American Journal of Clinical Nutrition 38: 849–859

Moghissi K, Hornshaw J, Teasdale P R, Dawes E A 1977 Parenteral nutrition in carcinoma of the oesophagus treated by surgery: nitrogen balance and clinical studies. British Journal of Surgery 64: 125–128

Moghissi K, Teasdale P R 1980 Parenteral feeding in patients with carcinoma of the oesophagus treated by surgery: energy and nitrogen requirements. Journal of Parenteral and Enteral Nutrition 4: 371–375

Morgan M Y 1982 Alcohol and nutrition. British Medical Bulletin 38: 21–29

Mueller C B, Thomas E J 1975 Nutritional needs of the normal adult. In: Manual of surgical nutrition. W B Saunders, Philadelphia

Muller J M, Brennan U, Dienst C, Pichlmaier H 1982 Preoperative parenteral feeding in patients with gastrointestinal carcinoma. Lancet i: 68–71

Munro H N, Fernstrom J D, Wurtman R J 1975 Insulin, plasma amino-acid imbalance and hepatic coma. Lancet i: 722–724

O'Keefe S J D, Abraham R R, Davis M, Williams R 1980 Protein turnover in acute and chronic liver disease. Acta Chirurgia Scandinavica Suppl 507: 91–101

Oosterlee J, Dudley H A F 1980 Central catheter placement by puncture of the exposed subclavian vein. Lancet i: 19–20

Ota D M, Imbembo A L, Zuidema G D 1978 Total parenteral nutrition. Surgery 83: 503–520

Pitt H A, Cameron J L, Postier R G, Gadacz T R 1981 Factors affecting mortality in biliary tract surgery. American Journal of Surgery 141: 66–72

Rowlands B J, Jensen T, Dudrick S J 1979 Comparison of two methods of measurement of serum transferrin. Journal of Parenteral and Enteral Nutrition 3: 504 (abstract)

Saint-Aubert B, Astre C, Andriguetto P C, Yakoun M, Joyeux H 1983 Influence of nutrition on liver regeneration. In: New aspects of clinical nutrition. Karger, Basel, p 548–557

Seltzer M H, Bastidas J A, Cooper D M, Engler P, Slocum B, Fletcher H S 1979 Instant nutritional assessment. Journal of Parenteral and Enteral Nutrition 3: 157–159

Shetty P S, Jung R T, Wastrasiewicz K E, James W P T 1979 Rapid turnover transport proteins: an index of subclinical protein-energy malnutrition. Lancet ii: 230–232

Shizgal H M, Spanier A H 1977 Caloric requirements of the critically ill patient receiving intravenous hyperalimentation. American Journal of Surgery 133: 99–104

Smith F R, Goodman D S 1971 The effects of diseases of the liver, thyroid and kidneys on the transport of Vitamin A in human plasma. Journal of Clinical Investigation 50: 2426–2436

Soler N G, Jain S, James H, Paton A 1976 Potassium status of patients with cirrhosis. Gut 17: 152–157

Stein T P, Buzby G P, Hargrove W C III, Leskiw M J, Mullen J L 1980 Essential fatty acid deficiency in patients receiving simultaneous parenteral and oral nutrition. Journal of Parenteral and Enteral Nutrition 4: 343–345

Stone H H 1975 Major hepatic resections in children. Journal of Paediatric Surgery 10: 127–134

Stoner H B, Little R A, Frayn K N, Elibute A R, Tresadern J, Gross E 1983 The effect of sepsis on the oxidation of carbohydrate and fat. British Journal of Surgery 70: 32–35

Studley H O 1936 Percentage of weight loss. A basic indicator of surgical risk in patients with chronic peptic ulcer. Journal of the American Medical Association 106: 458–460

Theologides A 1979 Cancer cachexia. Cancer 43: 2004–2012

Thompson H H, Tompkins R K, Longmire W P Jr 1983 Major hepatic resection: A 25 year experience. Annals of Surgery 197: 375–388

Twomey P, Ziegler D, Rombeau J 1982 Utility of skin testing in nutritional assessment: a critical review. Journal of Parenteral and Enteral Nutrition 6: 50–58

Vanlandingham S, Spiekerman A M, Newmark S R 1982 Prealbumin: a parameter of visceral protein levels during albumin infusion. Journal of Parenteral and Enteral Nutrition 6: 230–231

Wahren J, Denis J, Desurmont P, Eriksson L S, Escoffier J M, Gauthier A P et al 1983 Is intravenous administration of branched chain amino acids effective in the treatment of hepatic encephalopathy? A multicenter study. Hepatology 3: 475–480

Walesby R K, Goode A W, Spinks T J, Herring A, Ranicar A S O, Bentall H H 1979 Nutritional status of patients requiring cardiac surgery. Journal of Thoracic and Cardiovascular Surgery 77: 570–576

33

J. G. Whitwam and M. Morgan

Anaesthesia for major hepatobiliary surgery

This section is concerned with the provision of anaesthesia for major surgery of the hepatobiliary system and thus will include hepatic resection; biliary reconstruction and restoration of biliary drainage by the anastomosis of the bowel to the intrahepatic biliary system; surgery for portal hypertension; surgery for closed and penetrating injuries of the liver; pancreatic lesions, which may include tumours that secrete hormones and peptides; cholecystectomy. The general principles of managing such patients will be discussed together with specific problems presented by certian types of tumours.

Patients with hepatobiliary disease requiring operation, although frequently jaundiced, are not usually suffering from severe primary hepatocellular failure, which is discussed elsewhere (Ch. 102)

The special problems that they may present are:

1. Massive blood loss
2. Reduction of body temperature during prolonged surgery with consequent changes in peripheral vascular resistance
3. Coagulation defects
4. Severe postoperative pain
5. Severely reduced liver function postoperatively due to extensive hepatic resection, compromise of its blood supply either intra-operatively or postoperatively, or due to the effect of drugs, episodes of systemic hypotension and associated hypoxia during the procedure
6. In many patients, infection at the start of surgery
7. Compromised renal function in patients with hepatobiliary disease; hepato- and pseudohepatorenal renal syndromes (Hishon 1981) (Ch. 31)
8. Air or tumour embolism
9. A possible need for extensive access to the inferior vena cava requiring a high exposure above the diaphragm and possibly within the pericardium via a sternotomy. It may be necessary to place a conduit in the inferior vena cava to maintain venous drainage (Ch. 84, 97). Rarely it may be neccessary to use bypass techniques to protect the arterial supply to the brain and other organs while problems associated with venous drainage are being resolved.

At the outset it should be said that currently, in most centres, conventional anaesthetic techniques suitable for any form of abdominal surgery are used. This comprises: preoperative medication, usually with an opioid and an anticholinergic; induction of anaesthesia with thiopentone followed by a neuromuscular blocking drug and tracheal intubation; maintenance with nitrous oxide in oxygen and an opioid such as morphine, papaveretum or fentanyl with the addition of small concentrations of any one of the three major inhalational agents, halothane, enflurane or isoflurane. The lungs are mechanically ventilated and a positive end-expiratory pressure is applied when required to minimize the risk of air embolism. .

Good venous access is essential and monitoring will include the electrocardiogram, central venous and arterial pressures, blood gas tensions, haemotocrit, electrolytes, glucose, a coagulation screen when necessary and temperature. Provision will be made for maintenance of body temperature.

Thus, as in other areas of anaesthesia, attention to basics and a common sense approach provide the important ingredients of good practice rather than over indulgence in irrelevant theoretical considerations and the mindless application of expensive, often distracting and sometimes potentially dangerous technology merely because it is available. However, such an approach could imply complacency and developments during the past decade make this a particularly opportune time to review the anaesthetic management of these patients.

GENERAL CONSIDERATIONS

The following broad issues must be considered by any group setting up protocols and policy for the management of these patients:

1. In most published reports, surgery for obstructive jaundice still carries a relatively high mortality rate, which is at least in part due to infection and the development of renal failure (Hishon 1981).

2. Previous surgery may make access slow and tedious and the principal surgery may take several hours. However, some patients may be inoperable and may not justify admission to an intensive care unit so that at the start the anaesthetic technique has to be sufficiently flexible to allow relatively rapid recovery and the return of spontaneous respiration.

3. Nitrous oxide is not completely inert as has been previously thought. It has metabolic effects so that a policy is required for its continued use.

4. All the inhalational agents which are metobolized in significant amounts are capable of producing hepatocellular damage, and a policy is required for their use.

5. Periods of hypotension and/or hypoxia may compromise liver function and may lead to renal failure more readily than in other patients.

6. There may be derangements of carbohydrate and protein metabolism with associated disorders of blood coagulation.

7. There may be a need for the rapid transfusion of substantial amounts of blood and blood products and a policy is required for the use, or otherwise, of blood filters.

8. Patients who have had previous surgery, biliary obstruction or cholangitis are potentially infected, even if they are afebrile, and a policy is required for the use of antibiotics.

9. Postoperative pain may make the use of drugs in the epidural space desirable and there must be a clear policy on the use of epidural catheters in patients who may develop coagulation defects during and after surgery and who are potentially infected and may develop bacteraemia.

10. Liver dysfunction, biliary obstruction or renal failure may modify the pharmacokinetics and dynamics of anaesthetic agents.

PHYSIOLOGICAL AND PHARMACOLOGICAL CONSIDERATIONS

Practically all anaesthetic techniques for major procedures, whether local or general, cause a reduction in splanchnic and liver blood flow.

The interaction of patients with liver disease and anaesthetic agents can be discussed under three broad headings. The effect of anaesthetic agents on liver function and their ability to cause hepatocellular damage in patients whose reserve of liver function may either already be impaired or become so as a consequence of hepatic resection, is the most important aspect of the subject. The effect of impaired liver function on the pharmacokinetics and pharmacodynamics of anaesthetic drugs is the second heading; and third is metabolic interactions of anaesthetic agents with non-anaesthetic drugs due to the effects of the former.

Effects of anaesthesia on liver function

Minor reversible adverse changes in liver function follow most surgical procedures and can be related to the extent of the surgery (Clarke, Doggart & Lavery 1976). Discounting the effects of removal of the liver and physical trauma due to retraction or damage to its blood supply, hepatic injury associated with surgery is almost always caused either by tissue hypoxia or the anaesthetic agent used (Aldrete 1969, Gelman 1976).

Hepatic toxicity of anaesthetic agents

Halothane, enflurane, isoflurane Some halogenated hydrocarbons, such as chloroform and carbon tetrachloride, are intrinsically hepatotoxic and can cause a dose dependent acute hepatic injury which is due to the production of free radicals and often fatal (Zimmerman 1978). Halothane, the first of the modern fluorinated alkane anaesthetics, represented a major advance in that this problem did not occur. However, after its introduction in 1956, a number of cases of hepatic injury were reported, nearly half of which have been fatal, in which fever developed within 72 hours and jaundice after an average period of seven days (range 4–15 days). The lesion is associated with cellular necrosis, abnormal liver function tests and eosinophilia in a number of patients. However, this is a rare unpredictable occurrence, probably with an incidence of 1 in 100 000 on first exposure, which increases to between 1 in 7000 to 1 in 20 000 with repeat exposures within a short period of time. The incidence of halothane toxicity on the liver is increased dramatically by previous enzyme induction with other drugs.

Various causes have been put forward to explain 'halothane hepatitis' (Brown 1985) and include hypoxia, hypersensitivity and metabolic degradation to a toxic metabolite via a specific reductive pathway, instead of the normal oxidation and the formation of a metabolite-hapten complex with hepatocellular toxicity. Those at greatest risk are obese women over the age of 40 years who have been exposed to halothane several times in a short period of time (e.g. within 28 days). The possibility of a genetic susceptibility factor has been suggested and this is supported by recent in vitro work (Farrell, Prendergast & Murray 1985). Using a test that detects cell damage from electrophilic drug intermediates, Farrell et al found that lymphocytes from patients with halothane hepatitis exhibited an increase in cytotoxicity that was eight times greater than the increase in healthy controls. Patients with other liver disease and those recently exposed to halothane without adverse effects did not differ from healthy controls. Family studies revealed a high incidence of abnormal results and these workers concluded that there is a familial, constitutional susceptibility factor that predisposes to halothane hepatitis.

While there is no contraindication to the use of halothane in the majority of jaundiced patients, simple prudence suggests that it should be avoided in patients undergoing hepatobiliary surgery if only to remove one preventable, albeit rare, addition to the list of potential causes of postoperative jaundice.

The recently introduced agent enflurane can cause a similar type of jaundice, but the incidence is much lower and the subject has been reviewed by Lewis et al (1983). The most recently introduced agent, isoflurane, which is an isomer of enflurane, does not appear to cause liver injury even when given for prolonged periods, or under conditions in which the other anaesthetics induce liver injury, namely enzyme induction plus hypoxia. Isoflurane anaesthesia does not cause glutathione depletion in mice (Zumbiel et al 1978) suggesting that it does not produce reactive metabolites. The physical stability of isoflurane and its resistance to biodegradation suggest that it should be free from hepatotoxic effects. So far there have been no reports in medical journals of 'halothane like' hepatitis in response to isoflurane. However, compared to the other agents it has only been used extensively for a relatively short period of time.

Unlike halothane, isoflurane and enflurane do not appear to cause bromsulphthalein (BSP) retention (Stevens et al 1973), and halothane may impair this aspect of liver function for up to seven days following anaesthesia in volunteers (Stevens et al 1973). In contrast, in these volunteers no change in serum LDH or SGOT were seen in response to enflurane or isoflurane. In general, serum levels of liver enzymes (SGOT, SGDT, LDH) increase slightly following surgery using isoflurane anaesthesia but these changes are relatively transient and are more marked with halothane.

The properties of isoflurane were reviewed by Eger (1981) and the properties, potency and relative toxicity of all three agents are summarized in tables 33.1, 33.2, 33.3 and 33.4.

On the evidence so far available, in terms of hepatotoxicity, isoflurane is the volatile anaesthetic agent of choice if such an agent is to be used in patients with potential hepatic dysfunction.

Nitrous oxide The prolonged use of nitrous oxide in animals and man causes a reduction of methionine synthe-

Table 33.1 Properties of the three principal volatile anaesthetic agents currently in use

Property	Isoflurane	Enflurane	Halothane
Formula	F H F F-C-C-O-C-H F Cl F	Cl F F H-C-C-O-C-H F F F	Br F H-C-C-F Cl F
Molecular weight	184.5	184.5	197.4
Specific gravity (25 °C)	1.50	1.52	1.86
Boiling point (C)	48.5	56.5	50.2
Vapour pressure (mmHg)			
18 °C	218.7	156.3	224.1
20 °C	239.5	171.8	244.1
22 °C	261.8	188.6	265.5
24 °C	285.8	206.6	288.3
26 °C	311.5	226.1	312.7
Odour	ethereal	ethereal	organic solvent
Pungency	mild	mild	none
Preservative	not needed	not needed	required
Stability in			
soda lime	stable	stable	decomposes
UV light	stable	stable	decomposes
Reacts with metal	no	no	yes
Minimum flammable concentration (%) in 70% N_2O/30% O_2	7.0	5.8	4.8

Table 33.2 Relative potencies of commonly used inhalational anaesthetic agents. MAC-Minimal alveolar concentration required to prevent reflex movement in response to nociceptive stimulation of the skin in 50% of subjects (Modified from Eger)

MAC in middle-aged human subjects

	MAC (% atm) In O_2	In N_2O
Halothane	0.75	0.29
Isoflurane	1.15	0.50
Enflurane	1.68	0.57
Nitrous oxide	110	—

MAC values are listed in order of decreasing potency. Sources: halothane, Saidman & Eger 1964; isoflurane, Stevens et al 1975; enflurane, Gion & Saidman 1971, Torri et al 1974; nitrous oxide, Winter et al 1972.

Table 33.3 Comparison of hepatotoxic potential of halothane, ethrane and isoflurane

	halothane	enflurane	isoflurane
Likelihood of injury enhanced by multiple exposure	+	+	−
Hepatic enzyme induction	+	±	−
Type of hepatic necrosis	centrilobular	centrilobular	−
% agent metabolized	15–25	<3	0.2
BSP retention	+	+	−
Hepatic enzyme elevation during surgery	++	+	+

Table 33.4 Liver function after halothane or isoflurane anaesthesia in patients (Modified from Eger)

Postoperative day	Bilirubin (mg %)		SGOT (IU/ml)	
	halothane	isoflurane	halothane	isoflurane
Preoperative	0.71 ± 0.03	0.61 ± 0.02	29.6 ± 2.7	34.1 ± 2.1
Day 2	0.87 ± 0.06*	0.68 ± 0.04*	37.8 ± 3.5	40.2 ± 2.8
Day 4	0.69 ± 0.04	0.59 ± 0.04	40.3 ± 3.7*	36.2 ± 3.1
Day 7	0.54 ± 0.03*		35.2 ± 2.5	35.6 ± 3.7

* Significantly different from the preoperative level ($p < 0.05$)

tase (Koblin et al 1982) leading to vitamin B_{12} deficiency and megaloblastic anaemia. It has been confirmed from liver biopsies in this unit that anaesthesia with nitrous oxide and either enflurane or isoflurane causes complete depletion of this enzyme within four to six hours. In one study, nitrous oxide was incriminated in the relatively higher mortality rate in patients undergoing intensive care (Amos et al 1982). The whole subject of nitrous oxide toxicity and the controversies surrounding its continued use have been reviewed in a recent monograph edited by Eger (1985). Currently this agent is used routinely as a background agent during general anaesthesia and is not generally perceived as a harmful drug. While this may be true in otherwise healthy patients, whether it should be used for prolonged anaesthesia in critically ill patients is now open to question. However, there are so many factors involved in the successful outcome of major surgery that it is extremely difficult to implicate a single anaesthetic agent as having critically harmful effects.

Until the availability of isoflurane, the authors have used nitrous oxide as a background to general anaesthetic techniques, enflurane being added in situations where the use of large doses of intravenous supplements (e.g. opioids or benzodiazepines) and a prolonged recovery were undesirable. In the current state of the procedure, isoflurane would appear to be the most suitable inhalational agent in these patients although arguably inhalational anaesthesia should be avoided and there is a potential problem in relation to prolonged use of nitrous oxide. Unfortunately, a move to wholly intravenous anaesthesia could lead to problems in recovery, particularly where hepatocellular function is compromised. Awareness is also a problem with a total intravenous technique, particularly in view of the potential 'resistance' of some of these patients to intravenous anaesthesia due to altered pharmacokinetics. However, in general, intravenous agents such as the barbiturates, opioids and benzodiazepines have only a minimal, if any, effect on hepatic function and hence any general anaesthetic technique can be based, to a large extent, on these three groups of drugs.

The whole subject of drugs and liver damage has been the subject of a recent review (Stricker & Stoelstra 1985).

Effect of impaired liver function and blood flow on the kinetics and dynamics of anaesthetic drugs

Available information on the effect of hepatic and renal disease on drug distribution, excretion and effect has been reviewed by Stanski & Watkins (1982). Hepatic disease can affect hepatic drug clearance by several mechanisms.

1. Hepatic blood flow may be altered, either by a change in total flow or by altered intrahepatic shunting of blood. Liver blood flow plays a significant role in the clearance of drugs and also affects the activity of drug metabolizing enzymes. Normally at rest approximately one-quarter of the cardiac output goes to the liver, one-quarter to one-third of which is supplied by the hepatic artery and the remainder by the portal vein. The age related reduction in cardiac output causes a reduction in hepatic blood flow and drug clearance.

2. Drug clearance can be altered due to reduction of hepatocellular function, either due to an altered number of hepatic cells or to an alteration in the function of the cells.

3. Plasma protein concentrations and composition can be altered which affects drug binding. It is only the unbound, unionized portion of drug which is pharmacologically active and alterations in the level of plasma proteins can markedly alter the response to drugs that are highly protein bound e.g. diazepam.

Such changes in liver function can have a marked effect on many of the drugs used in anaesthesia.

Thiopentone

In patients with chronic hepatic dysfunction, Shideman et al (1949) observed a decreased dose requirement of thiopentone and a longer duration of effect of this drug. The precise causes in the change in thiopentone kinetics and dynamics in hepatic dysfunction remains unknown; however, an increased free thiopentone fraction has been demonstrated due to decreased protein binding. Clinically this is of little importance, as the drug is given slowly until consciousness is lost, so that the minimum amount is used, and repeated doses are not normally used.

Neuromuscular blocking drugs

Dundee & Gray (1953) reported that there was an abnormal 'resistance' to curare in patients with liver disease, which was attributed to abnormal protein binding. However, subsequent studies have shown that the protein binding of curare is unaffected by liver disease. Much more work has been performed on the use of pancuronium in patients with hepatocellular and obstructive biliary disease.

Westra et al (1981) found that in patients with obstructive jaundice, pancuronium clearance was reduced while the volume of distribution was increased and its terminal half-life prolonged. In contrast, Duvaldestin et al (1978) found a different pharmacokinetic profile for pancuronium in patients with hepatic cirrhosis undergoing portocaval anastomosis, and who did not have oedema or ascites at the time of surgery. The elimination half-life was significantly increased due to an increased volume of distribution. However, clearance was only slightly decreased. They observed a significant delay in the onset of paralysis and the peak effect of the drug occurred up to 10 minutes after its administration compared with the normal time of two to three minutes.

These studies indicate that different types of liver disease have different effects on pancuronium pharmacokinetics. In obstruction of the biliary tract and obstructive jaundice, total clearance of pancuronium is decreased, presumably due to decreased elimination of pancuronium and its metabolites into the bile, or alternatively, by decreased pancuronium metabolism. The resulting prolonged elimination half-life causes a slower rate of recovery from paralysis. Thus in obstructive jaundice, large doses of pancuronium result in a significantly longer duration of paralysis. In cirrhosis, the altered volume of distribution of pancuronium has a profound effect on paralysis. Lower initial plasma concentrations and a slower rate of distribution to tissues, including the neuromuscular junction, result in a slow onset of paralysis and the need for an increase in the dose to obtain the required degree of paralysis. Once peak paralysis is achieved in a patient with cirrhosis, the rate of recovery will be delayed because of the prolonged terminal elimination half-life.

Little information is available on the pharmacokinetics of the other competitive neuromuscular blocking drugs in patients with liver disease. Alcuronium has been used in this unit with no untoward effect. The newer and relatively short-acting steroid relaxant, vecuronium, is mainly eliminated via the biliary system and hence its effects can be expected to be prolonged in liver disease and biliary obstruction. Its short duration of action, however, means that during prolonged surgery it has to be given by continuous infusion with monitoring of neuromuscular transmission. Of more interest is the drug atracurium, whose action is terminated by Hofmann elimination (non-enzymatic alkaline hydrolysis, accelerated by an increase in temperature) and is therefore independent of hepatic and renal function. Again, this agent is relatively short-acting and to date there are no reports of its use by continuous infusion in patients with hepatobiliary disease.

Benzodiazepines

Diazepam The liver is the primary site of diazepam metabolism. The hepatic extraction ratio is low, resulting in a low clearance which is sensitive to changes in plasma protein binding and to the degree of hepatic enzyme activity (Branch et al 1976). Several investigators have found that hepatic cirrhosis doubles the terminal elimination half-life of diazepam due to a reduction in clearance and also to an increase in the volume of distribution at a steady state. The increased free fraction in cirrhosis may explain the greater volume of distribution. The decreased clearance is a direct effect of hepatic dysfunction on the ability of the liver to metabolize diazepam. The elimination half-life is also increased significantly in acute viral hepatitis as a result of reduced hepatic clearance; immediately after recovery, the half-life returns almost to normal. Because of the uncertain relationship between plasma levels of diazepam and its effects on the central nervous system, it is difficult to determine how hepatic disease should alter the use of diazepam. Theoretically, however, either the dose should be reduced or a different benzodiazepine should be used which does not undergo extensive metabolism, such as oxazepam, lorazepam, or temazepam. However, all these drugs depend on biliary excretion for their elimination which could be prolonged in the presence of biliary obstruction.

Lorazepam In subjects with hepatic cirrhosis, the volume of distribution of lorazepam is significantly increased, but the total clearance is unchanged and the terminal elimination half-life is prolonged. These alterations might be due to an increase in the free plasma fraction which increases from 6.8 to 11.4%. This increase in free, unbound drug results in more extensive tissue distribution as measured by the volume of distribution.

Midazolam Data on the effects of hepatic disease on the pharmacokinetics and pharmacodynamics of midazolam have not as yet been published. Midazolam, which is water soluble, has a much higher clearance than diazepam and this might be related to its slightly lower protein binding and the consequent higher free concentration of the drug so that its rate of metabolism by the liver is greater. One could predict that a decrease in liver function would cause a marked increase in the duration of action of midazolam.

Narcotic analgesics

Narcotic analgesics given in small doses intravenously form part of the standard balanced anaesthetic technique and supplement the analgesia provided by nitrous oxide. The drugs most commonly used are morphine, or its derivatives, e.g. papaveretum or diamorphine, and drugs derived from pethidine e.g. fentanyl, sufentanil, alfentanil. Fentanyl has become increasingly popular in recent years. It is 50 to 100 times more potent than morphine, and has a more rapid onset and shorter duration of action after a single injection than either morphine or pethidine.

The clearance of morphine, pethidine and fentanyl from the body is mainly due to hepatic metabolism. All three drugs have a high hepatic extraction ratio and their elimination is dependent on hepatic blood flow. Reduction of liver blood flow during the course of surgery and anaesthesia will reduce the clearance of the narcotics, but this will be of little clinical importance in patients with normal liver function. In patients with hepatocellular disease, however, the action of narcotics is markedly extended and prolonged coma can follow the use of normal doses. Very few pharmacokinetic measurements have been made in such patients, although the elimination half-life of pethidine is more than twice the normal in patients with acute viral hepatitis and cirrhosis (Klotz et al 1974, McHorse et al 1975). Great caution must be exercised in the use of narcotic analgesics in patients with advanced liver disease.

Metabolic interactions of anaesthetic agents with other drugs

Reilly et al (1985) have shown that halothane can cause a 60% reduction in the clearance of propranolol, which they related more to a change in the metabolizing capacity of the liver rather than a reduction in its blood supply. This is yet another example of a general principle that inhalational agents, which cause an acute reduction of hepatocellular function, whether this be mediated directly or indirectly through a reduction in the hepatic blood flow, will reduce the clearance of all drugs which are metabolized in the liver, including intravenous anaesthetic agents such as the barbiturates and benzodiazepines.

Hepatic blood flow

The maintenance of the blood flow and delivery of oxygen to the liver should as far as possible be maintained during anaesthesia. All anaesthetic techniques, whether general or local, will cause a reduction in liver blood flow, though the mechanisms vary. Whatever may be the direct effect of the inhalational agents on the intrahepatic blood vessels, the principal effects on blood flow appear to be due to a general depression of the circulation either through effects on cardiac output or peripheral vascular resistance.

Hughes, Campbell & Fitch (1980) compared the effects of halothane and enflurane on hepatic blood flow in dogs, and found a dose dependent effect. At equipotent concentrations, enflurane caused a greater reduction in systemic vascular resistance and mean arterial pressure than halothane. However, hepatic arterial resistance was decreased with enflurane but not halothane, so that the effects on liver blood flow were not dissimilar. Neither agent significantly affected hepatic oxygen consumption when administered in concentrations up to 2.0% and 3.0% for halothane and enflurane respectively.

Isoflurane has very little effect on the myocardium and its principal effect on the circulation is to reduce systemic vascular resistance. As yet there appears to be no published data on its effect on liver blood flow, but there is no reason to suppose that its effect at low concentrations will be dramatically different from enflurane and halothane.

Other factors may effect hepatic blood flow. In general it will be reduced by hypoxia, hyperventilation with a reduction in $PaCO_2$, increased sympathetic activity which is mediated by α-adrenoceptors and drugs which block peripheral β_2-adrenoceptors. β_2-agonists increase hepatic blood flow.

Survival of liver tissue is critically dependent on its blood supply. Episodes of severe hypotension and hypoxia should be avoided. In general the aortic pressure should be maintained at a level commensurate with the age of the patient.

Blood coagulation (Ch. 12)

A full discussion of the clotting system is beyond the scope of this short chapter and for further information reference should be made to Bayer (ed) Clinics in Haematology (1984). The following general points can be made for guidance.

Problems with the clotting system may arise for three principal reasons :

1. Hepatocellular dysfunction. All the proteins involved in blood coagulation appear to be synthesized in the liver, with the exception of factor VIII which is probably produced in the reticulo-endothelial system. The liver is also necessary for the de-activation of activated clotting factors and clotting inhibitors (e.g. plasmin). The production of both of these may be increased in patients undergoing major surgery particularly in the presence of infection. Hence this aspect of liver dysfunction may lead to coagulation defects by several mechanisms.
2. Vitamin K deficiency will lead to deficiencies of factors II, VII, IX and X, of which factor VII is probably the best marker. The prothrombin time is prolonged.
3. Acute peroperative loss of platelets and clotting factors due to the replacement of blood with materials deficient in these factors.

The assessment of clotting will include: a full blood count, including platelets and a coagulation screen; partial thromboplastin time (APTT — intrinsic system); prothrombin time (PT extrinsic system); thrombin time (TT). If required it should include an assessment of fibrinolytic activity, e.g. the presence of fibrin degradation products and clot lysis time.

Measurement of factors V, VII and VIII together with a platelet count offers a quick discriminatory appraisal of the likely major cause of the coagulation defect, since factor VIII is not produced in the liver and factor V is not dependent on vitamin K for its synthesis.

During the management of major surgery the thrombin time in the form of the accelerated clotting time (ACT-

Haemocron) provides a rapid easy assessment of the final stage of the production of fibrin. The ACT is in effect a slow thrombin time (approximately 100 sec) which allows the introduction of blood into the test system without incurring unacceptable errors in time. It is a sensitive index of either a reduction in fibrinogen or, e.g. the presence of anticoagulants such as heparin, and its principal use is in cardiac surgery. An increase in the ACT could indicate: a reduction in fibrinogen; activation of the clotting system (DIC syndrome) or failure of the liver to deactivate either activated clotting factors or inhibitors of coagulation. An increase in the ACT from baseline readings alerts the anaesthetist to the presence of a problem; he then needs either to transfuse clotting factors or to investigate the development of a more serious underlying problem. For example, simple observation of pink serum during the measurement of the haematocrit could indicate a blood transfusion reaction.

PREOPERATIVE ASSESSMENT

The preoperative visit is an essential part of the anaesthetic management of any patient about to undergo surgery. A general examination of the cardiovascular and respiratory systems is made. Inspection of the face and neck allows an assessment to be made of the ease or otherwise of tracheal intubation and note is taken of the state of the teeth and any previous dental work. The veins of the arms are examined for ease of access and an Allan's test performed to assess the adequacy of the arterial circulation to the hand if radial artery cannulation is contemplated.

The extent and nature of the surgical problem should be known because of its anaesthetic implications. The presence of jaundice could imply a prolonged prothrombin time due to non-absorption of vitamin K from the gut due to lack of bile salts. There is an increased incidence of postoperative renal failure in patients with obstructive jaundice (Dawson 1965) (Ch. 31), which might be due to endotoxins from the patients own bowel flora caused by the reduction in bile salts (Bailey 1976). As this postoperative renal failure can be prevented by a preoperative diuresis, consideration should be given to the use of mannitol pre-, per- and postoperatively. The use of diuretics demands repeated measurement of serum potassium levels with appropriate therapy if these are below 4.0 mmol/litre. Most of these patients have a modest hypokalaemia when they are presented to the anaesthetist. The presence of sepsis requires antibiotic therapy and it should be borne in mind that high blood levels of the aminoglycoside antibiotics, such as occurs following topical application of these drugs, will potentiate competitive neuromuscular blocking agents.

Many of these patients are elderly and hypertensive. Anti-hypertensive therapy must be continued up to the time of surgery and every effort must be made to reduce the blood pressure to levels commensurate with the patient's age. In untreated hypertensives, marked falls in blood pressure can occur on induction of anaesthesia and the consequent reduction in coronary blood flow can result in myocardial ischaemia and even infarction. Conversely, in these patients tracheal intubation can be associated with very large rises in arterial blood pressure and heart rate, with a great increase in myocardial work, which again is undesirable since this also can lead to myocardial infarction.

Patients with chest disease will require preoperative physiotherapy, with or without the use of bronchodilators. The sputum should be cultured and antibiotic therapy instituted if necessary. These patients will often receive postoperative analgesia via the epidural route. Enquiries should be made into the alcohol intake of the patient, which may not only cause resistance to anaesthetic drugs, but also the presence of an alcoholic neuropathy will preclude the use of regional anaesthesia. The nutritional state of the patient should be noted, as if this is poor a more difficult postoperative course can be anticipated.

Insulin dependent diabetics will require the intravenous administration of insulin and glucose peroperatively, which are best given by continuous infusion and repeated and regular estimations of blood glucose levels will be necessary. In those diabetics controlled by oral therapy, stopping the drug is all that is necessary preoperatively, but these and those controlled by diet alone might become insulin dependent during the peroperative period. Also, oral drugs can cause hypoglycaemia up to two to three days after their withdrawal if the patient undergoes even a limited period of starvation e.g. on the day of the operation.

Preoperatively the presence of any other hormone secreting tumour and the appropriate work up will be noted, e.g. carcinoid, vipomas, insulinomas.

The possibility of an anaphylactic reaction must be borne in mind in patients with hydatid disease and all necessary drugs should be immediately available to deal with this event.

Preoperative investigations

Essential

Certain investigations are mandatory before embarking on major hepatobiliary surgery.

1. Liver function tests, including plasma protein levels, should be measured and will form the baseline for subsequent management.

2. A clotting profile should be performed and efforts made to ensure that this is as normal as possible. Jaundiced patients will frequently have a prolonged prothrombin time due to the inability to absorb vitamin K from the gut,

but hepatocellular damage may be a contributory factor. Vitamin K should be given intramuscularly for several days preoperatively, and failure to restore the prothrombin time to normal values after this treatment indicates the presence of hepatocellular disease. Fresh frozen plasma and or preparations of clotting factors should be available under these circumstances.

3. The haemoglobin and haematocrit. Most anaesthetists will accept patients for major surgery with haemoglobin levels above 9 g/dlitre, but levels lower than this will require preoperative transfusion and the cause of the low haemoglobin must be sought.
4. Electrocardiogram
5. Chest X-ray
6. Urea, creatinine as a rapid assessment of renal function, and also electrolytes. Preoperative hypokalaemia will require treatment.

When indicated

1. Lung function test and blood gas analysis are necessary in patients with significant preoperative lung disease. These can be repeated to assess the outcome of preoperative physiotherapy and bronchodilator therapy and will serve as a baseline for intraoperative and postoperative measurements. Lung function tests may also be indicated prior to operation for very large liver lesions, which by abdominal distension and infradiaphragmatic pressure limit respiratory excursion.
2. In patients with large vascular intrahepatic tumours, measurements of the blood volume and a baseline cardiac output are desirable. (The baseline cardiac output will usually be measured immediately before the induction of anaesthesia when the patient is sedated after premedication.)
3. Hormone secreting tumours will be fully investigated by the time of surgery.

Blood grouping

An adequate amount of blood should be available and a sample of blood should be kept in the blood transfusion laboratory for urgent cross-matching should more be required. As far as possible the blood transfusion laboratory should be warned in advance when a patient might require large amounts of blood. It is assumed that large quantities of fresh frozen plasma, plasma protein fraction, and plasma substitutes are always readily available. Platelets in large amounts may be required and will usually be ordered 24–28 hours in advance.

During massive transfusion, after the blood volume has been replaced 2–3 times, it is the antibodies in the circulating blood which are more important in receiving further red cells rather than those endogenous to the patient at the outset. Because of the need to administer not only further red cells but also ABO compatible platelets and fresh frozen plasma, it is desirable to check compatibility with the patient from time to time and the use of one blood group throughout is desirable. It is the policy at Hammersmith Hospital that during continued rapid transfusion, after 10 units of blood have been administered, only ABO compatibility is checked if further blood is required. If the transfusion is stopped, then a full reappraisal of compatibility is performed before a second transfusion (e.g. during the postoperative period). The introduction of red cell transfusion which are virtually plasma free (SAGM), together with purified protein fraction, will make the situation potentially safer.

PROPOSED SCHEME OF ANAESTHETIC MANAGEMENT

Premedication

These patients are usually very anxious, may be hypertensive and some have coronary artery disease. Hence heavy premedication resulting in a well sedated patient is desirable. Overnight sedation provided with lorazepam 1–5 mg administered orally, and papaveretum and hyoscine (10–20 mg and 0.2–0.4 mg respectively) administered intramuscularly with 5 mg of droperidol approximately 1.5 hours prior to surgery provides a situation which permits initial cannulation of vessels with minimal distress. It also provides amnesia for events on the day of surgery. However, in patients with severe hepatocellular disease who are in a poor nutritional state or the elderly, these doses are reduced.

Anaesthesia

Upon the patient's arrival in the anaesthetic room, the ECG is monitored and the arterial blood pressure is recorded. One large bore (13 gauge) peripheral venous cannula is introduced into an arm vein through which an infusion of Hartmann's solution is commenced. A radial artery cannula (20–22 G Abbocath) is also introduced under local analgesia and the arterial pressure is then continuously recorded and displayed. Anaesthesia is induced with thiopentone (3–4 mg/kg) intravenously, or midazolam (0.2–0.3 mg/kg) followed by a long-acting neuromuscular blocking drug such as pancuronium, alcuronium or d-tubocurarine. Suxamethonium is only used, together with cricoid pressure, when rapid intubation is required in emergency cases or in those likely to have a full stomach. This is followed by an opioid such as diamorphine 0.1 mg/kg or fentanyl 10μg/kg. The lungs are manually ventilated with 100% oxygen until muscle relaxation is sufficient to allow passage of a disposable, non-irritant plastic tracheal tube. A nasogastric tube is also inserted at this time. Ventilation is then continued either with approximately 70% nitrous oxide in oxygen or oxygen enriched air* and the end-tidal carbon concentration is maintained around 5%. If the clotting profile is normal and there is no evidence of septicaemia, a mid-thoracic epidural catheter is introduced and diamorphine 0.1 mg/kg (in a concentration of 1 mg/ml in water) is injected via this catheter instead of the intravenous route as this provides relatively prolonged analgesia (e.g. 6–12 hours). In patients managed with an epidural opioid further intravenous narcotics are not required and hypnosis is maintained either with inhalational agents or midazolam administered intravenously.

During surgery, isoflurane 0.5–2.0% is added to the inspired gas and the concentration will be increased to the upper part of this range when there are signs of inadequate anaesthesia such as lacrimation, sweating, increased blood pressure and heart rate. Alternatively, anaesthesia can be maintained entirely with drugs administered intravenously. Incremental doses of the neuromuscular blocking drug are given to maintain muscle relaxation and large doses are often required. A typical case lasts between four and six hours and, as the patients are transferred to the intensive care unit and artificial ventilation continued, then reversal of the relaxant is not required. Similarly, narcotics can be used in generous doses, intravenously if necessary, e.g. up to 50 μg/kg of fentanyl or equivalent doses of other narcotics. Such doses will only be used in patients where an epidural catheter is not being used for the administration of the opioid. In such patients hypnosis is maintained with the inhalational agent isoflurane or midazolam administered intravenously.

Infusions and cardiovascular monitoring

A minimum of two large (13 gauge) peripheral cannulae for infusions are established. If major bleeding is anticipated two additional peripheral infusions may also be included. Two cannulae (16 gauge) are inserted percutaneously into the right internal jugular vein, unless this vein is needed for surgical purposes (e.g. to establish perfusion of the patient). In this case, either the left internal jugular or subclavian veins will be used. These cannulae permit measurement of central venous pressure and drug administration and can be used for infusions if necessary. In the presence of very large tumours or if a vena caval conduit is to be used, a catheter is passed into the inferior vena cava (i.v.c.) via a femoral vein to measure i.v.c. pressure. When measurements of portal venous pressure are required these are related to the i.v.c. rather than the superior vena caval pressures.

Throughout, heart rate, central venous pressure and arterial pressure are continuously displayed.

Pulmonary artery catheters Monitoring of left atrial pressure and measurement of cardiac output are desirable when major haemorrhage may be anticipated as may occur in the presence of large vascular tumours such as haemangiomata or if the patient has severe pulmonary or myocardial disease. In these patients a thermodilution, balloon-tipped flow directed catheter of the Swan–Ganz type is inserted via the right internal jugular vein.

Haemodynamic data at the start of operation from 16 patients is shown in Table 33.5. However, in two other patients with large haemangiomas, cardiac outputs of over 12 litres/minute have been recorded at the start of the procedure. Even after removal of the tumour, a high cardiac output may persist for many hours into the postoperative period in this particular type of patient and hence rational blood volume replacement requires a wide haemodynamic profile. In addition to the usual measurements of heart rate and arterial and venous pressure, the measurement of cardiac output allows observations of systemic vascular resistance and cardiac index. This is extremely valuable in patients with known coronary or other myocardial disease.

If a pulmonary artery catheter is used, the pulmonary artery pressure is continuously displayed. The wedging procedure should only be carried out for the briefest possible time necessary to record left atrial pressure, since this procedure is always a potential cause of damage to or rupture of the relevant pulmonary artery.

Respiratory monitoring and acid base balance

During the procedure, the inspired oxygen concentration is monitored with an in-line oxygen monitor. The end-tidal carbon dioxide concentration is measured, together with continuous monitoring of the expired minute volume and

*Footnote — Some anaesthetists including one of the authors (J.G.W.) have ceased to use nitrous oxide in these patients because of its effects on methionine synthetase described above.

Table 33.5 Haemodynamic data before induction of anaesthesia of 16 patients (10 male 6 female) undergoing major hepatobiliary surgery

	Age (yrs)	Weight (kg)	Height (cm)	Blood pressure (mmHg) Systolic	Diastolic	Mean (bpm)	Heart rate	CVP (mmHg)	Cardiac output (l/min)	PaO_2 (kPa)	$PaCo_2$ (kPa)	pH
Mean	57.1	63.8	172.8	134.1	64.9	88.4	74.8	4.6	5.66	12.7	4.8	7.41
SEM	2.64	2.23	2.35	4.58	3.57	3.65	2.68	0.55	0.30	0.33	0.15	0.003

inflation pressure. Arterial oxygen, carbon dioxide and acid-base status are measured hourly, or more frequently if indicated, and the ventilation adjusted accordingly. The $PaCO_2$ is maintained around 5.3 kPa (40 mmHg) and the PaO_2 above 16 kPa (120 mmHg) to minimize the potential effects of ventilation on hepatic blood flow (Liponati et al 1973).

Following catheterization of the right internal jugular vein, the rare possibility of a pneumothorax must be borne in mind; this would be indicated by a low PaO_2, increasing inflation pressure and a falling arterial pressure without any immediately obvious cause.

Temperature

Core temperature is measured via a thermistor thermometer placed either in the nasopharynx or lower quarter of the oesophagus and is maintained above 35 °C. This is achieved by the use of a heated mattress under the patient, a high capacity cascade humidifier in the ventilator circuit set to maintain a temperature of 38 °C at the tracheal tube (Linko et al 1984) and the use of blood warmers in the major infusion lines. The skin temperature of one toe may also be recorded to follow the core-peripheral temperature gradient. Normally the temperature of the skin of the big toe will be in the range 28–32 °C.

Urine flow

After induction of anaesthesia, the bladder is catheterized and a urine production of at least 1 ml/min is maintained by the infusion of mannitol. It is unusual to exceed a total dose of 0.5 g/kg. If there is no response to mannitol, frusemide in repeated doses of 5 mg intravenously is administered.

Plasma potassium This is measured regularly at the time of arterial blood gas sampling. These patients often start with relatively low values, e.g. around 4 mmol/litre and they remain so during massive blood transfusion. Usually an infusion of 10–30 mmol KCI will return the values to the normal range (4.5–5.5 mmol/litre). However, if urine production is low, or if there is any doubt about renal function, then it is prudent to leave the plasma potassium concentration below normal at this stage.

Fluid and blood replacement

Blood loss is assessed by the simple conventional method of measuring suction volumes and weighing swabs. Five principal factors may interact to produce alterations in systemic arterial pressure: blood loss, inferior vena caval occlusion, effects of anaesthetic agents, myocardial depression and peripheral cooling with vasoconstriction. Hence it is essential to measure blood loss and relate these to the measured haemodynamic variables and also the possibility of distortion of the inferior vena cava during manipulation of the liver.

In the past, with the general availability of whole blood, there was no requirement to measure the plasma albumin or oncotic pressure. With the introduction of concentrated red cells suspended in a protein free solution (e.g. SAGM blood), in addition to the haematocrit, it is desirable to measure the plasma oncotic pressure in procedures requiring large blood transfusions.

In order to conserve plasma and blood, during the initial stages of transfusion a maximum of four units of a starch solution are used (Hespan) to prevent adverse effects on the clotting system (Mishler 1984). After this, plasma protein fraction (PPF) is used and when the haemocrit has fallen to 30–32%, red cells are introduced and further volume replacement consists either of plasma protein fraction (PPF), fresh frozen plasma (FFP) or blood so that the haemocrit remains around this level. The oncotic pressure is maintained above 16–18 mmHg (2.13–2.4 kPa) by the administration of concentrated albumin solutions. Towards the end of the procedure, when surgical bleeding is under control, FFP is introduced and platelets are administered as indicated. A full clotting screen is performed and if required specific factors such as factor VIII can be administered. However, in view of the hepatitis risk and other infective disorders with such concentrates, the policy whenever possible is to use only FFP, platelets, red cells and albumin.

Autotransfusion A cell separator is desirable so as to use as much of the patient's own red cells as possible. This has the added advantage of reducing the risk of transfusion transmitted disease.

When the arterial supply to a large haemangioma is occluded, the patient may receive a substantial autotransfusion from the tumour. This has on one occasion required the removal of over 2 litres of blood from a patient to prevent massive overtransfusion and to restore a satisfactory haemodynamic state. Such blood can be taken into suitable packs and retransfused when this becomes necessary at a later stage.

All intravenous fluids are warmed during infusion. Calcium is not administered routinely. If during an episode of rapid blood loss and replacement the arterial pressure is lower than would be expected, if there is inferior vena caval occlusion, the superior vena caval pressure is above starting values and isoflurane has been withdrawn, then 2.5–5.0 ml of 10% calcium chloride is usually effective. Ideally plasma calcium level should be measured.

Very rarely in patients with heart disease, inotropic myocardial support is desirable. Dopamine is the preferred drug (4–10 μg/kg/min) by intravenous infusion, since it may also improve renal blood flow.

In addition to blood loss, there is a background fluid replacement during long procedures of Hartmann's solution at a rate of 5 ml/kg/hour.

Blood filtration This is a controversial subject which has recently been reviewed by Derrington (1985).

There is little doubt that microaggregates do form in stored blood. They consist principally of fibrin, leucocytes and platelets. Their sizes range from 10–300μ and there may be over a million in one unit of whole blood which has been stored for more than a few days. Since the pulmonary arteriolar and capillary diameters are in the range 5μ–150μ these microaggregates can cause micro-emboli in the lung and pulmonary damage. However, microaggregates can form in the circulation normally, and are then phagocytosed in the reticulo-endothelial system (R.E.S) by opsonins. Antibodies and complement are associated with this type of activity. The alpha-2-surface binding glycoprotein, fibronectin, has also been shown to assist this process and appears to be important in the phagocytosis of microaggregates by the R.E.S. (Saba & Jaffe 1980). Fibronectin survives well in stored blood and is concentrated in cryoprecipitate (Snyder, Ferri & Mosher 1984).

Blood is not infrequently transfused rapidly under pressure and this may result in rupture of cells trapped in the filter so that potentially dangerous mediators are released. Mean plasma histamine levels of 5.3 ng/ml have been found in blood downstream of the filter, and levels can be reached which are found in life threatening reactions (Roger et al 1982). Other problems which may be associated with the use of filters are haemolysis with depth filters under pressure, complement-activation (nylon filters), release of debris into the blood, channelling and unloading of microaggregates (depth filters), and removal of viable platelets. Hence fresh blood and platelets should not be passed through filters. Studies of changes in pulmonary function with and without filters are not conclusive concerning the role of microaggregates in the deterioration of pulmonary function. The logistical aspects of the use of filters make them cumbersome to use and they slow down maximum transfusion rates which may be the dominant issue. For all these reasons filters are not used routinely during blood transfusion, and perhaps increased use of cryoprecipitate, and hence the administration of fibronectin, is a more rational approach.

Air embolism

This may become a potential problem during dissection of major hepatic veins or the vena cava and at these times a positive end-expiratory pressure (PEEP) is applied and the patient is put in a head down position (20°–30°). A PEEP of 10–15 cmH_2O (0.1–1.5 kPa) is used provided this does not cause a fall in arterial blood pressure due to reduction of venous return to the heart and consequent fall in cardiac output. Except in a crisis the PEEP is introduced progressively but rapidly in steps of 2.5 cmH_2O (0.25 kPa).

High frequency ventilation

A system has been developed which allows the administration of conventional inhalational anaesthesia from an anaesthetic machine via a cascade humidifier at both normal and high frequencies of ventilation (Chakrabarti & Whitwam 1983, Whitwam et al 1983). This provides a reduction of airway pressures and a smaller diaphragmatic excursion during inflation of the lungs. The optimum frequency of ventilation appears to be 30–80 breaths per minute. It can be useful in the presence of very large liver tumours where there is a high diaphragm and a gross reduction of lung volume. Other indications include patients with severe cardiopulmonary disease. Also, during the application of PEEP, excessively high peak inflation pressures can be avoided.

Special procedures

Inferior Vena Cava On occasion it may be necessary to use a veno-venous bypass which diverts blood from the retro-hepatic inferior vena cava and the region of the hepatic veins. Systemic heparinization can be avoided by use of heparin impregnated tubes and the use of an appropriate pump (Ch. 121). To provide platelet protection and prevent thrombus formation, prostacyclin (PGI_2) is administered as an infusion starting at 4 ng/kg/min increasing to a range of 20–40 ng/kg/min. This causes a reduction in both systemic and pulmonary vascular resistance. After an initial fall in systemic arterial pressure, compensation occurs and it returns to acceptable levels. However, there is a large continuing reduction in pulmonary vascular resistance and it is currently the best drug for reducing pulmonary artery pressure. It is important that the pressure in the inferior vena cava below the conduit is measured and compared with the pressure in the superior vena cava. As mentioned above, portal venous pressure should be related to the pressure in the I.V.C.

Non-anaesthetic drugs

Antibiotics are administered routinely at the start of the procedure. Currently the preferred drugs are piperacillin (4.0 g) and tobramycin (120 mg) intravenously. Vitamin K may be required and it should be remembered that cremophor is present in its formulation and this has been implicated in anaphylactoid reactions (Morgan & Whitwam 1984).

The above remarks on anaesthetic management apply to the requirements for extensive surgical procedures. Most biliary bypass procedures, e.g. hepaticojejunostomy, require only good venous access, and the direct recording of systemic arterial pressure. Intraoperative blood loss only rarely exceeds three to four units and the procedure lasts less than four hours. Accordingly, a more conventional anaesthetic technique is used e.g. thiopentone 4 mg/kg, pancuronium 0.1 mg/kg, diamorphine 0.1–0.15 mg/kg or fentanyl 10–15 μg/kg, all given intravenously and the patients' lungs are ventilated either with oxygen enriched air or nitrous oxide-oxygen with isoflurane 0.5–2%. After closure of the abdomen, the muscle relaxant is reversed with neostigmine 2.5–3.5 mg mixed with either atropine 1.2 mg or glycopyrronium 0.6 mg. The patients rapidly become rousable and breathe spontaneously and are extubated on the operating table or in the recovery ward. They are retained in a recovery area three to four hours and then are either transferred to a high dependency unit or occasionally to the intensive care unit if there is a significant ongoing blood loss or a requirement for the administration of analgesic drugs via an epidural catheter.

Oxygen therapy is used at all times during recovery to supply an inspired concentration of 40–50%. Postoperative analgesia is provided either with epidural diamorphine (0.1 mg/kg of a solution containing 10 mg in 10 ml of dextrose), or an intravenous infusion of diamorphine (1–3 ml/ hour of a solution containing 60 mg in 60 ml 5% dextrose). On return to the normal ward, the patient is given further analgesia by intramuscular papaveretum 10–20 mg intra-muscularly on an on-demand basis.

For operations such as cholecystectomy lasting approximately one hour, and where blood loss is minimal, a conventional thiopentone (4 mg/kg) pancuronium (0.1 mg/kg) fentanyl (5 μg/kg) N_2O/O_2 isoflurane (0.5–2%) sequence is used with reversal of the muscle relaxant at the end of the procedure. The trachea is extubated on the operating table and the patients are transferred via the recovery area to the postoperative surgical ward.

SPECIFIC PROBLEMS

Portocaval anastomosis

Any procedure to relieve portal hypertension can be extensive and prolonged, and the basic principles outlined above apply. Great care must be taken with the use of narcotic analgesics and other central nervous system depressant drugs in patients with cirrhosis who have compromised hepatocellular function.

The Budd-Chiari syndrome is a specific problem involving thrombosis of the hepatic veins, and there is still a high peroperative mortality (Maddry 1984, McDermott et al 1984). The syndrome can occur in patients with paroxysmal nocturnal haemoglobinuria, and in these patients acute cardiac arrest has been described during the induction of anaesthesia (Sugimore et al 1983). These patients have abnormal bone marrow stem cells, and may not deal adequately with active complement fragments. Careful preoperative preparation is therefore essential (Braren, Jenkins & Python 1981). Anaesthesia should be based on drugs which are least likely to cause complement activation, e.g. benzodiazepines and opioids.

Hydatid disease

Very rarely in these patients anaphylactic shock may occur during operation with profound hypotension and bronchospasm. Steroids are indicated as part of the premedication. Should anaphylactic shock occur the usual resuscitative measures should be applied, which include adrenaline (0.2 μg/kg intravenously, repeated as necessary), bronchodilators (salbutamol 8 mg in 200 ml 5% dextrose infused rapidly) and antihistamines, including both an H_1 and H_2 receptor antagonist (chlorpheniramine and ranitidine respectively). The circulating volume should be maintained with a colloid solution. These drugs must therefore be immediately available during surgery for hydatid disease. The haematocrit should be measured repeatedly to allow assessment of fluid replacement. Late complications e.g. after 12–24 hours, can include full disseminated intravascular coagulation and adult respiratory distress syndromes, although disseminated intravascular coagulation has been known to occur in the immediate postoperative period.

Pancreatic resection

These patients are managed like any other major surgical procedure. However, one important feature is the degree of postoperative pain, and unless it is contraindicated an epidural catheter should be placed and postoperative pain managed with epidural opioids (e.g. diamorphine) or local analgesics (e.g. bupivacaine).

Endocrine secreting tumours

The three major types of tumour are carcinoid, with metastases in the liver, insulinoma and tumours secreting vasoactive intestinal peptide (Verner-Morrison Syndrome, WDHA syndrome). The principal features of the APUD cell series of tumours and their anaesthetic implications have been reviewed by Whitwam (1977).

Carcinoid

Carcinoid tumours are rare, but produce a variety of active substances such as serotonin, bradykinin and prostaglandins which are responsible for the flushing, diarrhoea, headache, palpitations and bronchospasm which are the features of the carcinoid syndrome. As a result, complications such as hyper- or hypotension, severe tachycardia and bronchospasm have been reported in more than 50% of patients during anaesthesia, and may be precipitated by manipulation of the tumour (Mason & Steane 1976).

Dery (1971) has classified the disturbances occurring

during anaesthesia as either serotoninergic or bradykininergic in origin. Serotonin has positive inotropic and chronotropic effects on the myocardium and raises the arterial blood pressure. It is responsible for the diarrhoea that is seen in patients with the carcinoid syndrome and also by its effects on carbohydrate metabolism for the hyperglycaemia which is seen in a number of patients. Bradykinin is a polypeptide which is formed by the action of kallikreins, a number of proteolytic enzymes, on an inactive precursor kallikreinogen. Bradykinin has been shown to be released from hepatic venous blood during a flushing attack (Oates, Pettinger & Doctor 1966). It is a potent vasodilator, and causes hypotension, increased capillary permeability and bronchospasm.

Because of the paucity of reports of patients with the carcinoid syndrome, definitive statements on anaesthetic management cannot be made. Mason & Steane (1976) reported that most of the life-threatening events seen during anaesthesia, such as hypotension and brochospasm, were caused by bradykinin. They therefore suggested the use of the kallikrein-bradykinin inhibitor aprotonin (Trasylol®) pre- and peroperatively. If symptoms are mainly serotoninergic in origin, then it would be logical to use anti-serotonin drugs preoperatively. Until recently, a specific serotonin blocker has not been available. However, Tornebrandt et al (1983) reported no major significant cardiovascular changes in 11 patients with carcinoid syndrome who received no pretreatment with anti-serotonin drugs, but significant changes in heart rate, pulmonary artery pressure, cardiac index and left and right ventricular stroke work in patients who received the non-specific antagonist levopromazine. These changes did not correlate with changes in plasma serotonin levels. The new serotonin antagonist, ketanserin, is now being used in these patients, particularly to control the gastro-intestinal symptoms.

Insulinomas

These are found principally in the pancreas, and the main problem is to avoid hypoglycaemia. The patients will receive a glucose infusion sufficient to prevent this until the tumour or hyperplastic region is removed. It is advisable to maintain blood glucose levels above normal, e.g. 6.0–8.0 mmol/litre. Manipulation of the tumour does not cause acute release of insulin. The blood level of insulin will fall to normal on satisfactory removal of the tumour. Blood glucose and insulin levels should be measured for several days postoperatively to ensure that all the lesion has been removed.

V.I.P. secreting tumours

These are found in the pancreas and the gut. Patients present with watery diarrhoea, achlorhydria and hypokalaemia. The reduction in serum potassium may be severe, e.g. to below 2.0 mmol/litre and they may present with related disorders of the central nervous system. Vasoactive intestinal peptide when injected intravenously stimulates respiration via the peripheral chemoreceptors and it also causes hypotension and hyperglycaemia. Preparation of these patients for surgery must include measures to restore the serum potassium to acceptable levels e.g. >3.5 mmol/litre. Tumour manipulation causes release of the hormone, with an increase in its blood level which can be associated with severe hypotension (Taylor et al 1977). At Hammersmith Hospital infusions of angiotensin II have been used to prevent severe hypotension and the value of this substance is clearly illustrated in fig. 33.1. Angiotensin II is prepared by dissolving 2.5 mg in 50 ml of 5% dextrose. It is infused at rates varying between 1 and 20 μg/kg/min and its effects are like an inverted 'mirror image' of sodium nitroprusside, which is used to lower blood pressure.

PAEDIATRIC HEPATOBILIARY SURGERY

Managing children is a question of scale, and their different physiological parameters, e.g. in relation to temperature control, renal function, blood volume,

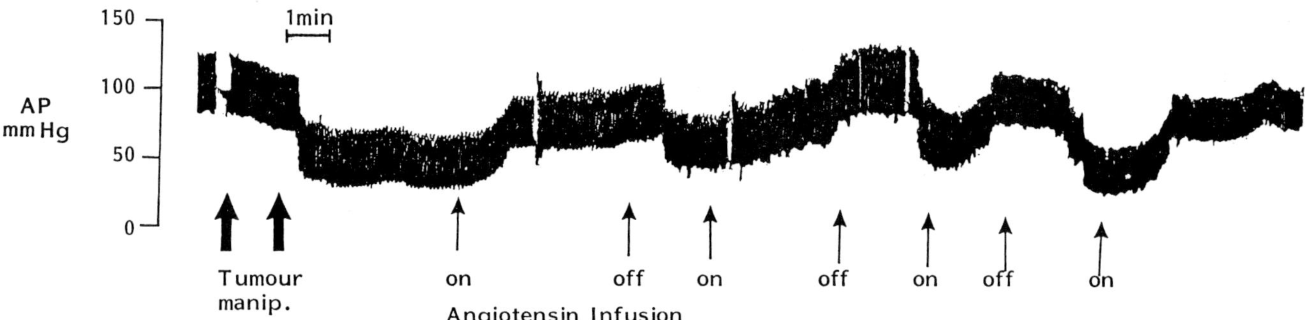

Fig. 33.1 Systemic arterial pressure recorded via a radial artery cannula during manipulation of a pancreatic tumour secreting vasoactive intestinal peptide illustrating the effect of starting and stopping an infusion of angiotensin II. Within 5–10 min of removing the tumour cardiovascular stability returned and the angiotensin II infusion was discontinued

haemoglobin and haematocrit, cardiac index, lung mechanics and function, and their poor ability to cope with extreme changes brought about by the infusion of blood and fluids. Blood volume replacement must be handled with extreme care and fresh blood should always be available. Temperature control is critical. Sodium overload must be avoided and a background fluid regimen of 5% dextrose is to be preferred to sodium-containing solutions. Measurements of the plasma electrolytes and the acid base status should be made regularly. Children are also more likely to become hypoglycaemic and frequent measurements of blood glucose concentration should be made.

CONCLUSION

In conclusion, anaesthesia for major hepatobiliary surgery provides one of the most interesting and stimulating areas of clinical practice. It encompasses virtually all the techniques, skills and fundamental physiological and pharmacological considerations relevant to the speciality and provides major opportunities for research. It is to be hoped that this chapter, apart from providing a current overview of the subject, will encourage interest and research into the problems presented by these patients.

REFERENCES

Aldrete J A 1969 Anesthesia and intraoperative care. In: Starzl T E, Putman C W (eds) Experience in hepatic transplantation. W B Saunders, Philadelphia, p 83–92

Amos R J, Amess J A L, Hinds C J, Mollin D L 1982 Incidence and pathogenesis of acute megaloblastic bone marrow changes in patients receiving intensive care. Lancet ii: 835–839

Bailey M E 1976 Endotoxin, bile salts and renal function in obstructive jaundice. British Journal of Surgery 63: 774–778

Bayer W L (ed) 1984 Clinics in haematology. Blood transfusion and blood banking W B Saunders, London

Branch R A, Morgan M H, James J, Read A E 1976 Intravenous administration of diazepam in patients with chronic liver disease. Gut 17: 975–983

Braren V, Jenkins D E, Python J M 1981 Peroperative management of patients with paroxysmal nocturnal hemoglobinuria. Surgery, Gynecology and Obstetrics 133: 151–520

Brown B R 1985 Halothane hepatitis revisited. New England Journal of Medicine 313: 1347–1348

Chakrabarti M K, Whitwam J G 1983 A new valveless all-purpose ventilator. Description and laboratory evaluation. British Journal of Anaesthesia 55: 1005–1015

Clarke R S J, Doggart J R, Lavery T 1976 Changes in liver function after different types of surgery. British Journal of Anaesthesia 48: 119–128

Dawson J L 1965 Postoperative renal function in obstructive jaundice: effect of mannitol diuresis. British Medical Journal I, 82–86

Derrington M C 1985 The present status of blood filtration. Anaesthesia 40: 334–347

Dery R 1971 Theoretical and clinical considerations in anaesthesia for secreting carcinoid tumours. Canadian Anaesthetist's Society Journal 18: 245

Dundee J W, Gray T C 1953 Resistance to d-tubocurarine chloride in the presence of liver disease. Lancet ii: 16–17

Duvaldestin P, Agoston S, Henzel, Kersten U W, Desmonts J M 1978 Pancuronium pharmacokinetics in patients with liver cirrhosis. British Journal of Anaesthesia 50: 1131–1136

Eger EI 1981 Isoflurane. A review. Anesthesiology 55: 559–576

Eger E I 1985 Nitrous oxide. E J Arnold, London

Farrell G, Prendergast D, Murray M 1985 Halothane hepatitis. Detection of a constitutional susceptibility factor. New England Journal of Medicine 313: 1310–1314

Gelman S I 1976 Disturbances in hepatic blood flow during anesthesia and surgery. Archives of Surgery (Chicago), III: 881–883

Gion H, Saidman L J 1971 The minimum alveolar concentration of enflurane in man. Anesthesiology 35: 361–364

Hishon S 1981 The hepatorenal syndrome. Hospital Update: 1027–1035

Hughes R L, Campbell D, Fitch W 1980 Effect of enflurane and halothane on liver blood flow and oxygen consumption in the greyhound. British Journal of Anaesthesia 52: 1079–1086

Klotz V, McHorse T S, Wilkinson G R, Schenker S 1974 The effects of cirrhosis on the disposition and elimination of meperidine in man. Clinical Pharmacology and Therapeutics 16: 667–675

Koblin D D, Waskell L, Watson J E, Stokstead, ELR, Eger E I 1982 Nitrous oxide inactivates methionine synthetase in human liver. Anesthesia and Analgesia 61: 75–78

Lewis J H, Zimmerman H J, Ishak K G, Mullick F G, (1983) Enflurane hepatotoxicity. A clinicopathologic study of 24 cases. American Journal of Internal Medicine 98: 984–992

Linko K, Honkavaara P, Nieminemm T 1984 Heated humidification in major abdominal surgery. European Journal of Anaesthesiology i: 285–291

Liponati M, Malsch E, Price H L, Coperman L H, Baum S, Harp J 1973 Splanchnic circulation during methoxyflurane anesthesia. Anesthesiology 38: 466–472

Maddry W C 1984 Hepatic vein thrombosis. Hepatology 4: 1445–1446

Mason R A, Steane P A 1976 Carcinoid syndrome: its relevance to the anaesthetist. Anaesthesia 31: 228–242

McDermott W V, Stone M D, Both A, St Trey C 1984 Budd-Chiari syndrome. Historical and clinical review and analysis of surgical corrective procedures. American Journal of Surgery 147: 463–467

McHorse T S, Wilkinson, G R, Johnson R F, Schenker S 1975 Effects of acute viral hepatitis in man on the disposition and elimination of meperidine. Gastroenterology 68: 775–780

Mishler J M 1984. Synthetic plasma volume expanders. Their pharmacology, safety and clinical efficacy In: Bayer W L (ed) Clinics in haematology. W B Saunders, London, P 15–92

Morgan M, Whitwam J G 1984 Althesin. Anaesthesia 40: 121–123

Oates J A, Pettinger W A, Doctor R B 1966 Evidence for release of bradykinin in carcinoid syndrome. Journal of Clinical Investigation 45: 173

Reilly C S, Wood A J J, Koshakji R P, Wood M 1985 The effect of halothane on drug disposition: contribution to changes in intrinsic drug metabolising capacity and hepatic blood flow. Anesthesiology 62: 70–76

Roger H D. Lorenz W, Lennartz H, Kusch J, Dietz W, Gerdes B, Parkin J V 1982 Plasma histamine levels in patients in the course of several standard operations. Influence of anaesthesia, surgical trauma and blood transfusion. Klinische Wochenschrift 60: 926–934

Saba T M, Jaffe E 1980 Plasma fibronectin (apsonic glycoprotein): its synthesis by vascular endothelial cells and role in cardiopulmonary integrity after trauma as related to ventricular-endothelial function. American Journal of Medicine 68: 577–594

Saidman L J, Eger E I II 1964 Effects of nitrous oxide and narcotic premedication on the aveolar concentration of halothane required for anesthesia. Anesthesiology 25: 302–306

Shideman F E, Kelley A R, Lee L E et al 1949 The role of the liver in the detoxication of thiopental (Pentothal) by man. Anesthesiology 10: 421–428

Snyder E L, Ferri P M, Mosher D F 1984 Fibronectin in liquid and frozen stored blood components. Transfusion 24: 53–56

Stanski D R, Watkins W D 1982 Drug disposition in anesthesia. Grune & Stratton, New York

Stevens W C, Eger E I, Joas T A, Cromwell T H, White A, Dolan W M 1973 Comparative toxicity of isoflurane, halothane, fluroxane

and diethyl ether in human volunteers. Canadian Anaesthetists' Society Journal 20: 357–368
Stevens W C, Dolan W M, Gibbons R T, White A, Eger E I, Miller R D et al 1975 Minimum alveolar concentrations (MAC) of isoflurane with and without nitrous oxide in patients of various ages. Anesthesiology 42: 197–200
Stricker B H, Stoelstra P 1985 Drug induced hepatic injury. Drug induced disorders 1: Elsevier, Amsterdam
Sugimori T, Nakawishi T, Kuse S, Hokuriku 1983. Cardiac arrest and haemolytic episode in paroxysmal nocturnal haemoglubinuria after induction of anaesthesia. Hokuriku Journal of Anesthesiology 17: 83–92
Taylor A R, Chulajata D, Jones D M, Whitwam J G 1977 Adrenal tumour secreting vasoactive intestinal peptide and nor-adrenaline. Anaesthesia 32: 1012–1016
Tornebrandt K, Nobin A, Ericsson M, Thomson D 1983 Circulation, respiration and serotonin levels in carcinoid patients during neurolept anaesthesia. Anaesthesia 38: 957–967
Torri G, Damia G, Fabiani M L 1974 Effect of nitrous oxide on the anaesthetic requirement of enflurane. British Journal of Anaesthesia 46: 468–472
Westra P, Vormeer G A, de Lange A R, Scaf A H J, Meijer D K F, Wessling H 1981 Hepatic and renal disposition of pancuronium and gallamine in patients with extrahepatic cholestasis. British Journal of Anaesthesia 53: 331–338
Whitwam J G 1977 APUD cells and the apudomas. A concept relevent to anaesthesia. Anaesthesia 32: 879–888
Whitwam J G, Chakrabarti M K, Konarzewski W H Askitopoulou H G 1983 A new valveless all purpose ventilator. Clinical evaluation. British Journal of Anaesthesia 55: 1017–1023
Winter P M, Hornbe T F, Smith G et al 1972 Hyperbaric nitrous oxide anesthesia in man: determination of anesthetic potency (MAC) and cardiorespiratory effects. Abstracts of scientific papers. Annual Meeting of the American Soceity of Anesthesiologists, p 102–104
Zimmerman H J 1978 Hepatoxocity. The B adverse effects of drugs and other chemicals on the liver. Appleton Century-Crofts, New York, P 370–394
Zumbiel M A, Fiserova-Bergerova V, Malinin T I, Holaday D A 1978 Glutathione depletion following inhalational anesthesia. Anesthesiology 49: 102–108

Postoperative intensive care

Postoperative intensive care is a relatively new concept and probably arose out of two main developments: firstly, the use of muscle relaxant drugs during surgery and the evolution of efficient machines for artificial ventilation of the lungs; and secondly the surgeon's desire and ability to operate upon increasingly sick patients (Stoddart 1980). It was recognized that an intensive care unit was an 'economic arrangement for the treatment of grave illness' and improved the chances of survival of desperately ill patients (B M A Planning Unit Report 1967). The components of patient management in such a unit are resuscitation, diagnosis, monitoring, specific therapy and systems support (Dobb 1984), to which must be added all the requirements of general patient care.

INDICATIONS FOR INTENSIVE CARE

There can be no hard and fast rules governing admission of patients to the intensive care unit after major surgery. Clinical judgement will be the principal basis for admission, but must take into account a number of factors such as the nature of the disease process, operability, age, likely short-term outcome and the availability of beds. Patients who require artifical ventilation of the lungs or monitoring of intravascular pressures, and those in hepatic or renal failure will require admission to an intensive care unit in the postoperative period.

GENERAL CARE

Nursing care

With the amount of high technology that exists in an intensive care unit, it is easy to forget the application of basic nursing principles. This particularly applies to heavily sedated or unconscious patients attached to ventilators whose general condition can rapidly deteriorate with lack of basic care. It is essential that the eyes are protected to prevent corneal drying and entry of foreign bodies. The eyelids should be kept closed and methylcellulose drops instilled at regular intervals. Particular care must be taken of the skin to prevent decubitus ulceration, which will rapidly develop in immobile patients who may have a low cardiac output. Patients should be turned two hourly and pressure areas inspected for signs of redness, and any further pressure on such areas avoided. Padded rings should not be used as they concentrate pressure on specific points. Air beds, ripple mattresses etc. are useful but not essential. Attention to oral hygiene is still important and often overlooked.

Nasogastric tubes should routinely be inserted in unconscious and ventilated patients. Their position in the stomach must be checked as they can be passed into a bronchus even in the presence of a tracheal tube (Sweatman et al 1978). The tube should be fixed away from the nares to prevent ulceration.

Intra-arterial lines should be constantly flushed with heparinized saline and a check regularly made on the circulation of the hand. Proper care will ensure a very low incidence of complications (Mandel & Danchot 1977). Intravenous lines also require meticulous care to prevent dislodgement and infection. They should be securely fixed, preferably by suturing, and the entry site sprayed twice daily with antiseptic solution.

Wounds and dressings must be cared for in the usual fashion according to local protocol.

Physiotherapy

This is essential in the prevention and treatment of chest infections, and will include chest vibration, percussion and postural drainage. Particularly at risk are patients with depressed conscious levels and those attached to ventilators. In the latter, a simulated cough is used by 'bag squeezing' (Clement & Hubsch 1968), followed by tracheal suction. Damage can occur to the tracheobronchial mucosa during this manoeuvre (Sackner et al 1973), which may also be associated with hypoxaemia, a reduction in cardiac output (Barrell & Abbas 1978) and the development of arrythmias. In patients who are critically ill and who need extensive chest physiotherapy it is desirable to attach some form of continuous monitoring of oxygenation such as an oximeter or transcutaneous oxygen electrode, to avoid inadvertent falls in oxygen content to potentially dangerous levels (Rithalia et al 1979). If mixed venous oxygen tension ($P\bar{v}O_2$) is being monitored continuously e.g. by a pulmonary artery catheter, then this will provide similar information regarding the transient effects of physiotherapy on oxygenation of the patient.

Physiotherapy is also necessary to encourage active limb movement where appropriate to reduce the possibility of deep vein thrombosis and to decrease muscle wasting, while passive movement will help to prevent contractures and stiffening of joints.

Prophylactic therapy

Antibiotics

The use of prophylactic antibiotic therapy as a routine in patients admitted to the intensive care unit is controversial, but most authorities seem to agree that it has little place (Dobb 1984). However, many of the patients undergoing hepatobiliary surgery may have had several previous operations and may already be undergoing therapy for cholangitis and a variety of other infections. Clearly such therapy must be continued in these patients into the postoperative period and the currently preferred regimen at Hammersmith Hospital is based on piperacillin and tobramycin.

Anticoagulants

Low dose subcutaneous heparin is effective in reducing the incidence of deep vein thrombosis and fatal pulmonary embolism in surgical patients (Sagar et al 1975). However, in patients who have undergone massive transfusion and have the potential for continued bleeding postoperatively, efforts are usually directed towards restoring a normal coagulation system. The use of heparin under these circumstances would require critical judgement, e.g. in the presence of a disseminated intravascular coagulation syndrome.

Antacids

A number of critically ill patients develop gastrointestinal haemorrhage as a result of stress ulceration (Croker 1979). It has therefore been suggested that the pH of the gastric contents be maintained above 3.5 with antacid therapy or with H_2-receptor blockade in order to prevent this complication (Menguy 1980). However, it is not the authors' practice to use such therapy routinely.

Radiology

Regular chest X-rays are mandatory in these patients to help in the diagnosis and monitoring of the progress of pulmonary infections, pulmonary oedema, pneumothoraces and other postoperative complications. Radiology is also extremely valuable in locating the position of tracheal tubes, central venous catheters and nasogastric tubes. Consultation with a radiologist concerning interpretation of X-rays is essential.

Psychological support

Intensive care units can be intimidating places for some patients. Instead of the quiet environment to be expected for someone recovering from major surgery, noise levels approaching that of a busy street corner (70–80 dB) have been recorded at times during 24 hours in an intensive care unit (Bentley et al 1977). Hale et al (1977) reported that 7% of patients admitted to an intensive care unit required psychiatric consultation for depression, anxiety, psychosis or organic brain syndrome.

Sleep deprivation is a problem and patients become disorientated as they are unable to distinguish between night and day. Mean sleep times of less than two hours per night have been reported by Aurell & Elmquist (1985), and they noted that nursing staff grossly misjudged the amount of sleep. These authors concluded that pain and environmental disturbance played only a minor role in this sleep deprivation and suggested that the grossly abnormal sleep patterns may be due to some fundamental derangement of the 'sleep-wake' regulating mechanisms. The simple provision of a clock can do much to help these patients and arguments have been made for the provision of large picture windows to provide relief from monotony and as an aid to general patient well-being (Keep 1977).

Nutrition

The majority of patients admitted to the intensive care unit after major hepatobiliary surgery only spend 24–48 hours in the unit and in this relatively short period, nutritional problems rarely arise. At particular risk are those patients who require further surgery and are re-admitted to the unit after spending some time on a general ward, where, in spite of the efforts of the staff, the high nutritional requirements of these patients have not been met. Enteral feeding may not be possible and a parenteral regime is necessary which will require a high calorie and glucose content and is discussed elsewhere (Ch. 32).

Analgesia

In 1980, Spence stated 'It is the scandal of modern surgery that a large proportion of patients suffer severe pain in the postoperative period.' This statement is supported by the published views of eminent members of the medical profession who have undergone major surgery (Donald 1976, Rhodes 1983) and by the general public, one of whom was moved to comment after major surgery, '. . . the grave defect in English public hospital treatment . . . which is a cruel and callous disgrace' and condemned the 'nonchalant attitude of the medical profession to quite unnecessary suffering' (MacInnes 1976). Patients in intensive care units and particularly those attached to ventilators are very likely to have their needs for analgesia ignored by staff who are paying much more attention to monitoring systems. One of the main problems in this respect is the great difficulty in actually measuring pain and its relief.

Postoperative pain is most severe following upper abdominal surgery (Parkhouse et al 1961, Loan and Dundee 1967) and this is especially true for the large subcostal incisions commonly used for hepatobiliary surgery and which may be associated with sternotomy. Pain is also more severe following long operations (Banister 1974) which again applies to these patients. It must also be remembered that coughing induced by tracheal suction in patients attached to ventilators can cause excruciating pain.

There are two points of paramount importance to be remembered concerning postoperative pain and its treatment. Firstly, apart from purely humanitarian considerations, relief of pain helps to restore normal physiological functions. Thus respiratory function is improved following adequate analgesia with a consequent increase in oxygenation (Spence & Smith 1971) and also increased mobility mitigates against deep vein thrombosis. Complete pain relief will also result in a reduction in circulating catecholamines and hence the incidence of hypertensive episodes and of arrhythmias will be reduced (Ruthberg et al 1984). Secondly, analgesia must not be confused with sedation. All the narcotic analgesics in current use for postoperative pain are excellent sedatives, but the converse is not true. Not only may sedatives not have analgesic properties, but some, notably the barbiturates and phenothiazines, actually increase sensitivity to somatic pain (Whitwam 1984).

Nor must it be forgotten that pain and discomfort arise not only from the operative incision, but also from the sites of intravenous infusions, intra-arterial lines, badly positioned drains and nasogastric tubes.

Care must also be taken to ensure that the bladder is draining correctly since a patient with a full bladder may not only be in pain but is likely to be extremely restless.

Opioid analgesics

These drugs remain the main method of treatment of pain in the intensive care unit as in the general ward. With regard to the degree of analgesia produced, there is nothing to choose between any of these drugs, whether they be pure agonists or partial agonists, provided that adequate doses are administered. The differences between them lie only in the speed of onset, duration of action and incidence and severity of side effects. However, a feature of the partial agonists (e.g. pentazocine) which may not be generally appreciated and which is not found with the pure agonists (e.g. morphine, pethidine) is the production of psychic phenomena such as hallucinations, anxiety and agitation. But the most serious complication of all opioid drugs, whether pure or partial agonists, is respiratory depression. Cardiovascular depression should not be a problem in the doses used. The only advantage of the partial agonists is that drug dependence (addiction) does not occur, although the authors know of no reports of the use of pure agonist drugs, such as morphine, in the intensive care unit leading to this problem. Choice of drug therefore often reflects individual preference.

The duration and efficiency of analgesia is markedly influenced by the route of administration. It must also be remembered that there is a very wide individual susceptibility to opioid drugs and that optimum analgesia can only be achieved by titrating the dose against each individual patient's needs.

Intramuscular Intermittent intramuscular opioids given on an 'as required' basis, with a limit on the number of doses and given at the discretion of a nurse, is an extremely inefficient method of analgesia (Utting & Smith 1979), and has no place in an intensive care unit. The staffing levels in such units allow each dose of the drug to be given immediately when they are needed.

Intravenous The administration of small doses of opioids intravenously at frequent intervals is a much more efficient method of analgesia and the dose can be titrated against the patients's needs. However, this method is practical only if a member of staff is always present to assess the effect of the drug and the need for further doses. Therefore, continuous intravenous infusions of opioids are being used more frequently, and provide a background of analgesia against which further bolus doses can be given if necessary (Church 1979). The continuous infusion of diamorphine (60 mg in 60 ml) at a rate of 1–3 ml/hour in the average adult, depending on the patients' response to pain and respiratory side effects, provides a pain-free tranquil state in spontaneously breathing patients and is probably the best available technique other than the use of the epidural route. However, some units use patient controlled analgesia (Chakravarty et al 1979, Tamsen et al 1979) where the patient activates a mechanism which delivers a preset dose intravenously. Limits must be set on the dose and frequency of administration to avoid complications. This method demands relatively expensive apparatus and also requires patient co-operation, so that unlike the continuous infusion of opioids it is not practical for the majority of patients requiring artificial ventilation.

Sedation produced by opioids may tend to render the

patient unable to co-operate with physiotherapists, and these drugs also depress the cough reflex. Although nausea and vomiting is also extremely distressing, the most serious complication with these drugs is respiratory depression. During continuous infusions, periods of apnoea can occur with marked arterial desaturation (Catley et al 1982), with the potential development of arrhythmias. These patients therefore need constant observation and preferably some form of respiratory monitor (e.g. end-tidal CO_2, external magnetometer or some other electronic device). Although muscle rigidity has been described following the administration of highly potent opioids (e.g. alfentanil and fentanyl) (Muldenhauer & Hug 1984) this does not seem to occur in intensive care situations.

Local analgesia

Intercostal block Intercostal blockade with bupivacaine, which must be bilateral for paramedian and bilateral subcostal incisions, will provide complete somatic analgesia for periods up to 10 hours (Moore 1975). However, repeating the block at intervals thereafter is not a feasible proposition in patients in an intensive care unit.

Epidural block There is no doubt that thoracic epidural analgesia is the best method of pain relief following upper abdominal surgery. With the use of bupivacaine, pain is completely abolished with all the consequent beneficial effects on lung function and the patient remains fully alert and co-operative. However, the price paid for this complete analgesia is high in terms of complications (Conacher et al 1983). The most serious is hypotension due to sympathetic blockade, and it is essential that this technique is not used in the presence of hypovolaemia. A vasopressor might be needed to restore arterial pressure and must always be to hand. Retention of urine is frequent in uncatheterized patients and tachyphylaxis to the local anaesthetic agent is also a problem.

Following the discovery of opiate receptors in the spinal cord (Pert & Snyder 1973) these drugs were soon given epidurally and intrathecally to relieve postoperative pain. There are now a large number of reports attesting to their efficacy when administered in this way (Cousins & Mather 1984), and although analgesia is long lasting, it is not complete analgesia as produced by the local anaesthetics. Epidural opioids have the distinct advantage of having no cardiovascular effects, but common complications include nausea and vomiting, pruritus and retention of urine. Again, respiratory depression is the most serious problem, but is even more sinister than when given by other routes because it can be delayed for up to 12 hours after administration of the drug (Morgan 1982). Thus a patient given a top-up epidural dose in the intensive care unit may not develop respiratory depression until much later, by which time he may have been returned to a general ward. The drug particularly involved in this complication is morphine, which is one of the least fat soluble of the currently used opioids. It should therefore not be used epidurally since this complication is much rarer following use of the more fat soluble drugs, such as diamorphine or fentanyl.

Epidural block is contraindicated in the presence of septicaemia because of the possibility of abscess formation, and also in the presence of a coagulation defect. A normal clotting profile is therefore necessary in patients with obstructive jaundice prior to performing the block. Also, the epidural catheter should be inserted prior to surgery, as massive blood transfusion during the procedure may result in a deranged clotting mechanism. Nevertheless, Odoom & Sih (1983) have performed 1000 epidural blocks on 950 patients with a coagulation defect with no adverse effects. Epidural analgesia is the most usual method of pain relief in the authors' unit. The preferred method is epidural diamorphine in a dose of 0.1 mg/kg given through an epidural catheter inserted in the mid-thoracic region prior to the start of surgery. If an epidural is contraindicated, the drug is given by continuous intravenous infusion as described above.

All opioid drugs cause an increase in common bile duct pressure due to spasm of the sphincter of Oddi. This increase in pressure can result in epigastric distress or even biliary colic (Radnay et al 1980), but is of no consequence when the bile duct is being surgically drained. Interestingly, recent experimental work has shown that whereas intravenous morphine or fentanyl caused significant increases in bile duct pressure for some two or three hours, there were no such increases following administration of the same doses by the epidural route (Vatashky et al 1984).

Inhalational analgesia Some procedures performed in the intensive care unit, such as removal of drains or tracheal suction, are extremely painful for a short time. For these, inhalation of 50% nitrous oxide in oxygen (Entonox) can provide marked analgesia for this very short time, and it can also be administered to patients attached to ventilators. Alternatively, small doses of ketamine (e.g. 0.3 mg/kg intravenously) combined with a benzodiazepine (e.g. diazepam 5–10 mg or midazolam 2–4 mg intravenously) provide excellent short term analgesia for these painful manoeuvres.

It must be remembered when considering pain relief in the intensive care unit, that it is the requirements of patients attached to artificial ventilators which are likely to be ignored. They are unable to communicate verbally and are usually sedated so that they appear to be asleep and are assumed to be pain free. Assessment of their analgesic needs is very difficult. Only changes in autonomic function e.g. in heart rate, blood pressure, pallor, sweating may indicate that they are in pain (Campbell 1974), but there are many other reasons for the appearance of such signs.

PATIENTS REQUIRING ARTIFICIAL VENTILATION

INDICATIONS FOR ARTIFICIAL VENTILATION

The main reason for admission to an intensive care unit is a continuing need for artificial ventilation, which might be indicated for a number of reasons.

1. Persisting effects of large doses of anaesthetic and neuromuscular blocking drugs, used during prolonged surgery, into the postoperative period.

2. Massive intraoperative blood loss and replacement. Continuing artificial ventilation will ensure optimum oxygenation, although care must be taken to avoid a reduction in cardiac output by the application of a positive end-expiratory pressure in hypovolaemic patients.

3. Anticipation of further bleeding, when the potentially serious haemodynamic consequences of re-induction of anaesthesia to allow artificial ventilation will be avoided.

4. Any episode of cardiac arrest during surgery.

5. Significant pre-existing lung disease. In these patients, the temporary depression of lung function with resultant hypoxaemia in the first few postoperative days (Hewlett & Branthwaite 1975, Craig 1981) is accentuated, and artificial ventilation will be required to maintain oxygenation.

6. Failure to maintain adequate arterial oxygenation, e.g. an arterial oxygen tension (PaO_2) of less than 70 mmHg (9.3 kPa) with an inspired oxygen concentration of 50–60% and/or an alveolar-arterial oxygen tension difference ($A\text{-}aDO_2$) of greater than 450 mmHg (47 kPa) following the administration of 100% inspired oxygen for 10 minutes. Some degree of pulmonary collapse might result if the chest has been opened or from prolonged traction on the diaphragm. It is important to exclude a pneumothorax as a cause of arterial hypoxaemia, which might result from trauma to the apex of the lung during attempts to cannulate the internal jugular vein. Other causes would include aspiration of gastric contents during induction of anaesthesia, or at a later stage when re-admission to the unit might be necessary for chest infections, septicaemia or adult respiratory distress syndrome.

7. Any case where sternotomy has been performed and/or total cardiopulmonary or left heart bypass has been used.

MODERN ASPECTS OF ARTIFICIAL VENTILATION

Practically all the patients undergoing hepatobiliary surgery have relatively normal cardiorespiratory function and can be managed with conventional ventilation techniques. However, in those few patients who have serious pre-existing lung disease or who develop adult respiratory distress syndrome, e.g. as the result of septicaemia or adverse reactions to drugs, blood products or other infusions, the following considerations apply:

1. Positive end expiratory pressure (PEEP) should be used to reduce the intrapulmonary vascular shunt from say 30–50% to a more manageable 15–20%. This can be achieved by arbitrarily applying 5–15 cmH_2O of PEEP and observing the PaO_2 or more systematically by the simultaneous measurement of PaO_2, mixed venous oxygen tension ($P\bar{v}O_2$) and cardiac output, which will require the insertion of a pulmonary artery catheter. PEEP should always be applied in incremental steps of 2–5 cmH_2O since the cardiovascular tolerance of hypovolaemic patients is limited and it may cause falls in arterial pressure.

2. If the peak inflation pressures are high, these should be reduced by using smaller tidal volumes and higher frequencies of ventilation; that is, high frequency ventilation (HFV). Equipment is now available for this purpose and minimum inflation pressures are achieved at ventilation frequencies below 100 breaths per minute, since above this frequency the advantage of a low tidal volume in relation to a low pulmonary compliance is offset by the high gas flows required due to the short inspiratory times which have to be driven through the airways resistance.

The setting up procedure is: 1.ventilate the patient with 100% oxygen; 2. find the ventilation frequency at which the airway pressure is minimal while maintaining a normal $PaCO_2$; 3. apply PEEP to reduce the shunt fraction and increase the PaO_2; 4. reduce the inspired oxygen concentration to the lowest level compatible with maintaining a PaO_2 which is either normal or at least above 70 mmHg (9.3 kPa). If necessary the patient should continue to be ventilated with 100% oxygen since there is little evidence that patients with severe lung disease and a low PaO_2 who are ventilated with 100% oxygen to ensure short term survival suffer any long term effects which can be related to oxygen toxicity.

It should always be remembered that increasing the oxygen content of arterial blood need not necessarily cause an increase in oxygenation of the tissues, if accompanied by a fall in cardiac output (Askitopoulou et al 1984). This is why a rational approach to the artificial ventilation of patients with severe adult respiratory distress syndrome requires the measurement of cardiac output and both mixed venous and arterial blood gas values. A diminished arterio-venous oxygen content difference and a low cardiac output also indicates severe derangement of tissue metabolism and a potentially terminal state, e.g. in septic shock.

Care of patients attached to ventilators

Communication

Patients attached to ventilators are not always unconscious and can be fully aware of the environment, including conversation between staff. It is imperative that nursing and medical staff talk to these patients, even though they may give no indication that they can hear what is being said. Under no circumstances should the patients's condition, further treatment or prognosis be discussed by groups of medical staff within hearing distance. Any changes in management should be communicated to the patient. Similarly, the patients should be told of any manoeuvres that are to be performed such as turning, suctioning, removal of drains or intramuscular injections. Facilities should be available for the patients to be able to write their requests, remembering that they might normally wear spectacles. A list of common requirements should be written in large letters so that the patient can point to the appropriate item. These should be available in the patients' own language if an interpreter is not available.

Sedation

Synchronization with the ventilator is mandatory to achieve optimum gaseous exchange. Similarly, a distressed patient is likely to be hypertensive and in conjunction with hypoxaemia, arrhythmias are very likely to occur. Some drug or combination of drugs is therefore necessary to allow control of ventilation and tolerance of the tracheal tube. Opioid drugs, such as papaveretum, besides producing analgesia, are excellent sedatives and also decrease the sensitivity of the respiratory centre to carbon dioxide, thereby facilitating control of ventilation.

Large doses of opioids, however, will result in a high incidence of nausea and vomiting and also respiratory depression which will make weaning from the ventilator difficult. Most centres therefore use a combination of an opioid and a tranquilliser, such as one of the benzodiazepines. Diazepam has the disadvantage of having a long half-life, (<30 hr) and active metabolites, (e.g. the desmethyl derivative with a half-life >100 hr) and hence accumulates and has a prolonged effect. Midazolam has a much shorter half-life (<2 hr) but nonetheless cumulative effects have been reported in patients requiring artificial ventilation (Byatt et al 1984). It is important to realize that the neuromuscular blocking drugs have no central action and their use should be restricted to facilitating synchronization with the ventilator when this cannot be achieved by any other means.

However, the combination of opioids and benzodiazepines is undesirable in patients who require regular neurological assessment. Here, rapid drug clearance is required so that the assessment can be made without the influence of central depressant drugs. The intravenous anaesthetic agents Althesin and etomidate were ideal in this respect when given by continuous infusion. However, the former has been withdrawn because of an unacceptable incidence of anaphylactoid reactions and the latter because of the suppression of cortisol production (Ledingham & Watt 1983, Owen & Spence 1984). It remains to be seen whether the new agent di-isopropylpherol (Diprivan) will be useful in this respect since recovery following infusion is extremely rapid (O'Callaghan et al 1982, Fragen et al 1983).

Humidification of inspired gases

Water in the airways is essential for: 1. alveolar gas exchange, as solubility in the aqueous layer is a prerequisite for diffusion into and out of the blood; 2. ciliary activity; and 3. to maintain the mobility of secretions. Humidification of the inspired gas is therefore necessary whenever the nose is bypassed by a tracheal tube or tracheostomy.

Experimentally it has been shown that the airway mucosa remains intact as long as inspired gases are 100% saturated between temperatures of 25 and 30°C (Tsuda et al 1977), while Forbes (1973) has shown that good clearance of mucus requires a relative humidity in the inspired gases of 75% at 37°C. The commonest humidifiers contain heated water and with these temperature of the inspired gas near the patient should be kept around 35°C. Ultrasonic nebulisers are efficient, but increase airway resistance and can cause water intoxication (Hulands 1980). In recent years the use of disposable condenser humidifiers (artificial noses) have become more popular, but only those with large volumes (e.g. 60–100 ml) are efficient.

Disconnections

Patients can become accidentally detached from a ventilator at any time, even in the best run units. This is particularly dangerous in those who have received neuromuscular blocking drugs as no respiratory efforts can be made and death or permanent neurological damage rapidly ensues. Various devices are therefore available which give audible alarms following such an event. There is a tendency at the present time for a large number of alarms to be used on many items of equipment, e.g. ventilators, infusion pumps, pressure monitors, gas analysers. The bedlam caused by such alarm systems in an average intensive care unit is such that they are frequently misinterpreted or ignored, and there is no substitute for frequent observation of visual displays.

Indications for cessation of artificial ventilation (Weaning)

The classical criteria for weaning require satisfactory results from three tests of respiratory function.

1. Tests of mechanical capability
   a. resting minute volume of less than 10 litres which can be doubled with maximum voluntary ventilation
   b. peak inspiratory force of greater than 20–30 cmH_2O

   c. vital capacity greater than 10–15 ml/kg body weight
   d. forced expiratory volume in one second (FEV_1) greater than 10 ml/kg body weight.
2. Tests of oxygenation
   a. A-aDO_2 less than 300 mmHg (40 kPa) when breathing 100% oxygen
   b. shunt fraction less than 10–20% of the cardiac output
   c. PaO_2 greater than 70–80 mmHg (9.3–10.6 kPa) with an inspired oxygen of 50–60%.
3. Tests of ventilation
   a. normal arterial carbon dioxide tension in the absence of severe chronic respiratory disease
   b. a physiological deadspace — tidal volume ratio of less than 50%.

However, weaning is rarely a problem after major hepatobiliary surgery as the patients usually have relatively normal lung function preoperatively. Problems might arise in patients who have been re-admitted to the intensive care unit with adult respiratory distress syndrome or septicaemia. Very occasionally a patient may be resistant to attempts to discontinue mechanical ventilation and become hypoxaemic when the inspired oxygen concentration is reduced. In these patients, a period of intermittent mandatory ventilation, followed by spontaneous breathing with a continuous positive airway pressure to raise the functional residual capacity, may be necessary before spontaneous ventilation is adequate to maintain normal gaseous homeostasis (Downs 1983).

MONITORING

Many aspects of vital function are constantly monitored in intensive care units. A continuous display of relevant information allows rapid detection of changes and releases nursing time for other tasks. However, such monitoring requires invasive techniques with all the attendant complications such as infection, infarction and electrocution. In addition there may be problems with calibration and hence the misinterpretation of data.

The introduction of computers to correlate data provides two major advantages. Firstly, it allows staff to be alerted to deviations from normal responses and trends. Secondly, it assists teaching and training of staff. Long term storage of data from many patients allows retrieval of information and correlation of related events can be obtained which may not be obvious without such facilities.

Cardiovascular monitoring

Electrocardiogram

This should be displayed continuously, together with the heart rate, for immediate recognition and treatment of arrhythmias.

Arterial blood pressure

This is usually measured directly from a percutaneously catheterized radial artery. It is essential that the catheter be continuously flushed and that no air bubbles are present in manometer tubing connecting it to the transducer. Automatic blood pressure devices involving intermittent cuff inflation are not satisfactory in the intensive care unit as the frequent cuff inflations disturb the patient.

Central venous pressure

This is monitored by a catheter whose tip lies in the superior vena cava. Such catheters are usually inserted via the right internal jugular vein, a subclavian vein or a vein in the antecubital fossa. Great care must be taken during their introduction to prevent infection and air embolism. The latter is most likely to occur when the subclavian or neck veins are used and when central venous pressure is low. Normally the latter is an excellent guide to changes in the effective circulating volume, and reductions during blood loss may occur before there are any significant changes in heart rate or arterial pressure.

Flow directed catheters

Insertion of a balloon-tipped, flow-directed catheter into the pulmonary artery is being increasingly used in seriously ill patients. Patients undergoing hepatobiliary surgery usually have normal cardiorespiratory function and it is not therefore the authors' practice to insert such catheters routinely. Their use is associated with a number of potentially serious complications such as trauma to the tricuspid valve, damage to the endocardium, arrhythmias, perforation of the heart, pulmonary infarction, rupture of the pulmonary artery, knotting, infection and electrocution. They are used by the authors in those patients who are seriously ill with low output states, particularly with septic shock, pre-existing cardiac disease or pulmonary hypertension.

All these catheters allow the measurement of central venous pressure (right atrial pressure), pulmonary artery pressure, pulmonary artery wedge pressure (which reflects left atrial pressure) and also intermittent blood sampling for measurement of mixed venous oxygen tension. Catheters incorporating a thermistor allow measurement of core temperature and cardiac output by the thermodilution technique, and hence calculation of total peripheral resistance. More sophisticated devices (and hence potentially prohibitively expensive for routine use) would include facilities for continuous measurement of mixed venous oxygen tension, pH and potassium.

Probably the most valuable information provided by these catheters relates to decisions on volume replacement, drug therapy and the management of oncotic pressure. The normal pulmonary artery wedge pressure is

8–10 mmHg, and pressures above 11 mmHg may indicate a deterioration of left heart function.

$$\text{TPR} = \frac{(\text{Cardiac output}) \times 80 \text{ dynes/sec/cm}^{-5}}{(\text{mean arterial blood pressure})}$$

Normal range 800–1600

A raised total peripheral resistance is an indication for arterial vasodilation (e.g. with sodium nitroprusside or α-adrenoceptor blockade), and if the pulmonary artery wedge pressure remains high after restoration of the peripheral resistance to normal, then the use of inotropic agents should be considered (e.g dopamine, dobutamine). A high pulmonary artery pressure together with a raised central venous pressure may be an indication for the reduction of right ventricular and pulmonary artery pressure preload with nitroglycerine. When very high pulmonary artery pressures occur, use of prostacyclins should be considered. If all pressures and the cardiac output are low, then the blood volume is reduced.

A serious reduction in tissue oxygen consumption will be indicated by a reduction in the arterial to mixed venous oxygen tension difference and may be of grave prognostic significance in, e.g. septic shock. In units where facilities are available, terminal tissue metabolic failure is confirmed by measurement of substrate metabolism and the amino-acid profile ('footprint') of the blood; this is beyond the scope of this chapter.

Respiratory monitoring

Spontaneous ventilation

In these patients, clinical observation of colour, respiratory rate and the effort of breathing are the most useful observations, while signs of carbon dioxide retention will be indicated by an increasing heart rate and blood pressure, sweating and cutaneous vasodilatation. These observations can be supplemented when indicated by spirometry and measurement of blood gas tensions.

Artificial ventilation

Constant monitoring is necessary in patients whose lungs are being artificially ventilated. The following measurements should be made: 1. inspired oxygen concentration; 2. airway pressures; 3. expired minute volume; 4. end-tidal carbon dioxide concentration; 5. arterial blood gas tensions. More recently transcutaneous methods of measurement of oxygen saturation and oxygen tension have become available (Rithalia et al 1979).

Temperature

Core temperature of the body should be constantly displayed and may be measured in the lower quarter of the oesophagus, nasopharynx, external auditory meatus or the pulmonary artery. Skin temperature, e.g. of the big toe, can be a useful measurement in patients who have just returned from the operating theatre or who are shocked. The core-peripheral temperature gradient gives an indication of the state of the peripheral circulation, an improvement being indicated by a rise in skin temperature and a reduction in the gradient. It can therefore be used as a simple monitor of the efficacy of treatment in shocked patients. The normal core and toe temperatures are 37°C and 28–32° respectively.

Haematological monitoring

1. Blood loss and blood volume. The haemoglobin and haematocrit should be measured routinely. In addition to the observation of external losses of blood, the simple measurement of abdominal girth usually indicates the internal accumulation of blood or fluid. This is performed routinely on all patients who have undergone extensive liver resection. Although in the postoperative period a falling haemoglobin is usually indicative of continued blood loss or haemolysis, it should not be forgotten that folic acid and vitamin B12 deficiency can occur in patients who have been seriously ill for prolonged periods. Drug induced bone marrow depression may occur and can be associated with the use of Intralipid (Gibson et al 1978).

2. Oncotic pressure should be measured routinely in these patients. Normal values are 20 mmHg or above and albumin should be administered if it falls below this value. This is particularly necessary in patients with high pulmonary artery and wedge pressures to reduce the tendency to pulmonary oedema.

3. Coagulation. In the immediate postoperative period, where there has been massive intraoperative blood loss and transfusion, the measurement of platelets and a simple coagulation screen should be performed, the frequency being indicated by the state of the patient, previous results and intervening therapy with platelets and clotting factors, usually in the form of fresh frozen plasma.

Bacteriological monitoring

Patients in an intensive care unit are very vulnerable to the acquisition of infection from the environment. Routine specimens from such patients may show that potential sites of infection have been colonized with certain organisms, which might lead to infection (Sanderson 1980). Thus antibiotic sensitivities can be discovered at an early stage. Sanderson (1980) has suggested the following routine bacteriological monitoring of patients in an intensive care unit: tracheal aspirate and pharyngeal swab daily; culture of urine from catheterized patients every 48 hours; peritoneal dialysis fluid daily; intravenous catheters on removal. Faeces, wounds (including tracheostomy) and drain sites should be swabbed when clinically indicated.

It is essential in these patients who are particularly at risk that all staff, medical and nursing, are meticulous in their application of procedures to prevent cross infection.

It is well known that 10% of central venous cannulae introduced percutaneously, albeit with sterile precautions, will show bacterial contamination on their tips within four days of insertion and this may well be associated with a bacteraemia. Although great care may be taken with the introduction of these cannulae, subsequent injections and infusions through taps and entry ports attached to them are performed in a much less disciplined way. For crystalloid solutions the use of bacterial filters is recommended. Prolonged intravenous therapy should be performed through intravenous lines in which skin and venous entry points are separated by a subcutaneous tunnel and which are introduced with full sterile precautions. Thereafter, ideally, handling of connections should be performed under sterile conditions.

Proper understanding of the therapeutic value and dangers of antibiotics is essential for all clinicians working in an intensive care unit and close co-operation with a microbiologist is mandatory. Choice of the appropriate drug will be made in the light of the organisms grown and their sensitivities. Renal and hepatic function must also be taken into account according to the drug used, and in some cases (e.g. gentamicin) blood levels should be measured to avoid toxicity. The intravenous route of administration is the most appropriate for such drugs.

Biochemical monitoring

Routine biochemical measurements will include electrolytes, urea, creatinine, tests of liver function, glucose and acid-base balance. The frequency of these tests will depend on the patient's illness and its severity.

Blood glucose levels must be closely followed after extensive hepatic resection. The rapidity of onset and magnitude of the fall in blood glucose is related to the preoperative liver glycogen stores, to preoperative and peroperative liver perfusion and the amount of normal liver resected (Stone 1977). Glucose should be administered intravenously when necessary to maintain blood glucose. Maintenance of blood glucose levels and concern about glucose administration is usually only important for some 48 hrs (Vajrabukka et al 1975) but in some cases may be required for up to three weeks postoperatively (Stone 1977).

Similarly, hypo-albuminaemia may result from extensive hepatic resections and plasma albumin levels must be monitored either directly or by the measurement of oncotic pressure. A significant reduction in albumin does not usually occur until the third or fourth postoperative day, at which time such patients have normally returned to the general ward (Stone et al 1969). Albumin levels must be maintained in order to prevent fluid shifts and pulmonary oedema. The need for such replacement therapy diminishes as liver regeneration occurs (Blumgart & Vajrabukka 1972, Vajrabukka et al 1975.)

Liver failure

This is a rare occurrence following major hepatobiliary surgery, but will be seen more frequently as an end-stage of hepatic cirrhosis following operations for portal hypertension and very occasionally after liver resection. The patient passes through a stage of hepatic encephalopathy into coma, with clinical and biochemical signs of hepatic decompensation.

In chronic liver disease, a number of factors may precipitate encephalopathy. These include azotaemia, sedative, anxiolytic or narcotic analgesic drugs, gastrointestinal haemorrhage, hypokalaemia, alkalosis, infection or protein intoxication. There are increases in the blood levels of ammonia (which only poorly correlates with the degree of hepatic encephalopathy), pyruvate, lactate, citrate and α-ketoglutarate. Short chain fatty acids and amino-acids also accumulate, and the latter probably play an important role in the production of encephalopathy, possibly by adversely affecting the synthesis of neurotransmitters. There will be water retention, potassium depletion and sodium retention due to secondary hyperaldosteronism. Cerebral oedema is common. Bleeding may occur due to diminished synthesis of clotting factors. The serum bilirubin and particularly serum aspartate transaminase (formerly SGOT) and alanine amino transferase (formerly SGPT), which are markers of liver cell damage, will be elevated. In these circumstances, a falling blood urea is a particularly grave sign as it indicates lack of production by the liver.

Briefly, treatment will consist of the maintenance of fluid and electrolyte balance, feeding with a high carbohydrate, protein-free diet, vitamin supplementation and correction of clotting abnormalities. Measures should be taken to prevent renal failure. Newer methods of treatment would include dialysis, exchange transfusion and plasmapheresis, isolated liver perfusion, adsorbent haemoperfusion with coated charcoal and ultimately liver transplantation.

Renal failure

Renal failure is far more likely to be seen following major surgery on the liver and bile ducts than is liver failure (Ch 31). The term hepatorenal syndrome has been used to describe the renal failure that sometimes follow surgery for obstructive jaundice, but hepatologists now restrict its use to the unexplained renal failure that sometimes complicates hepatic cirrhosis (Hishon 1981).

In these patients, urine output must be monitored with daily plasma and urinary urea estimations. In the presence of oliguria, a urinary urea of less than 300 mmol/litre or a specific gravity of less than 1014 is suggestive of renal failure, whereas a higher urea and a specific gravity of more than 1018 is indicative of dehydration (Gilbertson & Goldsmith 1980).

Dialysis is now the main form of treatment of renal failure persisting after correction of potential causes, and after abdominal surgery will usually consist of haemodialysis. Gilbertson & Goldsmith (1980) have summarized the criteria for dialysis, either alone or in combination as: marked overhydration, especially in conjunction with hyponatraemia and pulmonary oedema; rising plasma urea above 30 mmol/l; rising plasma potassium above 5.0 mmol/l; falling standard bicarbonate of less than 18 mmol/l. Further reasons for early dialysis include old age, cardiac disorders and anticipation of gastrointestinal haemorrhage. While preparing for haemodialysis in the presence of severe hyperkalaemia, a glucose-insulin regimen may be considered appropriate.

This chapter has summarized the basic care and monitoring required by a patient admitted to an intensive therapy unit following major surgery. Following major operations on the liver and bile ducts, it is very rare for patients to require intensive care for more than 24–48 hours, and adherence to the basic principles of management outlined above will ensure a safe passage through the unit. Re-admission may be occasioned for such reasons as massive haemorrhage, overwhelming sepsis, renal or hepatic failure.

The peroperative mortality in patients undergoing major hepatobiliary surgery at Hammersmith Hospital is virtually zero. Their problems usually occur at a later stage and are most frequently related directly or indirectly to infection.

REFERENCES

Askitopoulou H, Chakrabarti M K, Morgan M, Sykes M K 1984 Failure of large tidal volumes to improve oxygen availability during anaesthesia. Acta Anesthesiologica Scandinavica 28: 348–350

Aurell J, Elmquist D 1985 Sleep in the surgical intensive care unit: continuous polygraphic recording of sleep in nine patients receiving postoperative care. British Medical Journal 290: 1029–1032

Banister E H D'A 1974 Six potent analgesic drugs. A double blind study in post-operative pain. Anaesthesia 29: 158–162

Barrell S E, Abbas H M 1978 Monitoring during physiotherapy after open heart surgery. Physiotherapy 64: 272–275

Bentley S, Murphy F, Dudley H 1977 Perceived noise in surgical wards and an intensive care area — an objective analysis. British Medical Journal 2: 1503–1506

Blumgart L H, Vajrabukka T 1972 Injuries to the liver: analysis of 20 cases. British Medical Journal 1: 158–164

B M A Planning Unit Report 1967 Intensive Care British Medical Association, London

Byatt C M, Lewis L D, Dawling S, Cochrane G M 1984 Accumulation of midazolam after repeated dosage in patients receiving mechanical ventilation in an intensive care unit. British Medical Journal 289: 199–200

Campbell D 1967 Pain relief in patients on ventilators. British Journal of Anaesthesia 39: 736–742

Catley D M, Thornton C, Jordan C, Royston D, Lehane J R, Jones J G 1982 Postoperative respiratory depression associated with continuous morphine infusion. British Journal of Anaesthesia 54: 235P

Chakravarty T, Tucker W, Rosen M, Vickers M D 1979 Comparison of buprenorphine and pethidine given intravenously on demand to relieve post-operative pain. British Medical Journal 2: 895–897

Church J J 1979 Continuous narcotic infusion for relief of post-operative pain. British Medical Journal 1: 977–978

Clement A J, Hubsch 1968 Chest physiotherapy by the 'bag squeezing' method: a guide to technique. Physiotherapy 54:355

Conacher I D, Paes M L, Jacobson L, Phillips P D, Heaviside D W 1983 Epidural analgesia following thoracic surgery. A review of two years' experience. Anaesthesia 38: 546–551

Cousins M J, Mather L E 1984 Intrathecal and epidural administration of opioids. Anesthesiology 61: 276–310

Donald I 1976 At the receiving end: a doctor's personal recollection of second-time valve replacement. Scottish Medical Journal 21: 49–57

Downs J B 1983 Weaning from ventilatory support. Annual Refresher Course Lectures. American Society of Anesthesiologists p 203

Forbes A R 1973 Humidification and mucus flow in the intubated trachea. British Journal of Anaesthesia 45: 874–878

Fragen R J, Hanssen E N J H, Denissen P A F, Booij L H D J, Crul J F 1983 Disoprofol (ICI 35868) for total intravenous anaesthesia. Acta Anaesthesiologica Scandinavica 27: 113–116

Gilbertson A A, Goldsmith J J 1980 Renal failure in the general intensive therapy unit. In: Gray T C, Nunn J F, Utting J E (eds) General anaesthesia 4th edn. Butterworths, London, 1687–1696

Hale M, Koss N, Kerstein M, Camp K, Barash P 1977 Psychiatric complications in a surgical I C U. Critical Care Medicine 5: 199–202

Hewlett A M, Branthwaite M A 1975 Postoperative pulmonary function. British Journal of Anaesthesia 47: 102–107

Hishon S 1981 The hepatorenal syndrome. Hospital Update: 1027–1035

Hulands G H 1980 General care of patients in the intensive therapy unit. In: Gray T C, Nunn J F, Utting J E (eds) General anaesthesia 4th edn. Butterworths, London, p 1573–1589

Keep P J 1977 Stimulus deprivation in windowless rooms. Anaesthesia 32: 598–600

Ledingham I A, Watt I 1983 Influence of sedation on mortality in critically ill multiple trauma patients. Lancet i:1270

Loan W B Dundee J W 1967 The clinical assessment of pain. Practitioner 198: 759–768

MacInnes C 1976 Cancer ward. New Society 36: 232–234

Mandel M, Danchot P J 1977 Radial artery cannulation in 1000 patients: precautions and complications. Journal of Hand Surgery 2: 482–485

Menguy R 1980 The prophylaxis of stress ulceration. New England Journal of Medicine. 302:461

Moldenhauer C C, Hug C C 1984 Use of narcotic analgesics as anaesthetics. Clinics in Anaesthesiology. Intravenous anaesthesiology 2: 107–138

Moore D C 1975 Intercostal nerve block for postoperative somatic pain following surgery of thorax and upper abdomen. British Journal of Anaesthesia 47: 284–286

Morgan M 1982 An assessment of epidural and intrathecal opiates in the management of postoperative pain. Anaesthesia 37: 527–529

O'Callaghan A C, Normandale J P, Grundy E M, Lumley J, Morgan M 1982 Continuous intravenous infusion of disporofol (ICI 35868, Diprivan). Comparison with Althesin to cover surgery under local analgesia. Anaesthesia 37: 295–300

Odoom J A, Sih I L 1983 Epidural analgesia in anticoagulant therapy. Experience with one thousand cases of continuous epidurals. Anaesthesia 38: 254–259

Owen H, Spence A A 1984 Etomidate. British Journal of Anaesthesia 56: 555–557

Parkhouse J, Lambrechts W, Simpson B R 1961 The incidence of postoperative pain. British Journal of Anaesthesia 33: 345–353

Pert C B, Snyder S H 1973 Opiate receptor: demonstration in nervous tissue. Science 179: 1011–014

Radnay P A, Brodman E, Markiher D, Duncalf D 1980 The effect of equi-analgesic doses of fentanyl, morphine, meperidine and pentazocine on common bile duct pressure. Anaesthetist 29:26

Rhodes P 1983 Getting a new hip joint. British Medical Journal 127: 747–748

Rithalia S V S, Rozkovec A, Tinker J 1979 Characteristics of transcutaneous oxygen tension monitoring in normal adults and critically ill patients. Intensive Care Medicine 5:147

Rutberg H, Hakanson E, Anderberg B, Jorfeldt L, Martensson J, Schuldt B 1984 Effects of extradural administration of morphine, or bupivacaine, on the endocrine response to upper abdominal surgery. British Journal of Anaesthesia 56: 233–238

Sackner M A, Landa J F, Greeneltch N, Robinson M J 1973 Pathogenesis and prevention of tracheobronchial damage with suction procedures. Chest 64:284

Sagar S, Massey J, Sanderson J M 1975 Low-dose heparin prophylaxis against fatal pulmonary embolism. British Medical Journal 4: 257

Sanderson P J 1980 Control of infection in the intensive therapy unit. In: Gray T C, Nunn J F, Utting J E (eds) General anaesthesia 4th edn. Butterworths, London, p 1611–1625

Spence A A 1980 Uses of anaesthesia. Postoperative care. British Medical Journal 281: 367–368

Spence A A, Smith G 1971 Postoperative analgesia and lung function: a comparison of morphine with extradural block. British Journal of Anaesthesia 43: 144–148

Stoddart J C 1980 Intensive therapy. In: Gray T C, Nunn J F, Utting J E (eds)) General anaesthesia 4th edn. Butterworths, London, p 1543–1556

Stone H H 1977 Preoperative and postoperative care. In: Madding G F, Kennedy P A (eds) The Surgical Clinics of North America. Symposium on hepatic surgery 57: 409–419

Stone H H, Long W D, Smitth R B III, Haynes C D 1969 Physiologic considerations in major hepatic resections. American Journal of Surgery 117: 78–84

Sweatman A J, Tomasello P A, Longhead M G, Orr M, Datta T 1978 Misplacement of nasogastric tubes and oesophageal monitoring devices. British Journal of Anaesthesia 50: 389–392

Tamsen A, Hartif P, Dahlstrom B, Lindstrom B, Hison-Holmdahl M 1979 Patient controlled analgesia therapy in the postoperative period. Acta Anaesthesiologica Scandinavica 23: 462–470

Tsuda T, Noguchi H, Takumi Y, Aochi O 1977 Optimum humidification of air administered to a tracheostomy in dogs. Scanning electron microscopy and surfactant studies. British Journal of Anaesthesia. 49: 965–977

Utting J E, Smith J M 1979 Postoperative analgesia. Anaesthesia 34: 320–332

Vajrabukka T, Bloom A L, Sussman M, Wood C B, Blumgart L H 1975 Postoperative problems in management after hapatic resection for blunt injury to the liver. British Journal of Surgery 62: 189–200

Vatashky J E, Haskel Y, Beilin B 1984 Common bile duct pressure in dogs after opiate injection — epidural versus intravenous route. Canadian Anesthetists' Society Journal 31: 650–653

Whitwam J G 1984 Intravenous induction agents. Clinics in Anaesthesiology. Intravenous anaesthesiology 2: 515–535

SECTION 4

Interventional radiological and endoscopic techniques

35

P. R. Salmon

Interventional endoscopy

INTRODUCTION

Whilst the role of the flexible fibre-optic endoscope in the diagnosis of biliary tract disorders was rapidly established by the introduction of endoscopic retrograde cholangio-pancreatography (ERCP) (Oi et al, 1970, Salmon et al 1971) and the ability to obtain a tissue diagnosis in some cases, interventional (therapeutic) endoscopy, whereby the endoscope is used as a delivery system for various therapeutic devices, developed much later.

At present a growing number of interventional procedures are available (Table 35.1) for the biliary tract and liver but the precise place of some of these procedures has not yet been defined by randomized clinical trials. It is already clear, however, that endoscopic sphincterotomy is a major advance in the treatment of the elderly and of high risk patients with duct stones, and in many cases may be preferable to surgery and common duct exploration (Ch. 47, 50). This chapter aims at giving an overview of the currently available procedures whilst details of specific aspects are covered in other chapters.

Table 35.1 Interventional endoscopy in biliary tract disease

Endoscopic sphincterotomy
Endoscopic biliary drainage
Endoscopic balloon dilatation of biliary strictures
Endoscopic lithotripsy
Iridium wire placement

ENDOSCOPIC SPHINCTEROTOMY

Endoscopic sphincterotomy, first described by Classen & Demling (1974) and Kawai et al (1974), has proven to be a major advance in the management of common bile duct stones. The technique has been fully detailed in the literature (Cotton 1980, Cremer et al 1977) and is covered in Chapter 47.

Endoscopic sphincterotomy may be performed in a number of different clinical situations (Table 35.2 and 35.3) each of which is reviewed in this chapter.

Table 35.2 Current indications for endoscopic sphincterotomy

Choledocholithiasis
Post-cholecystectomy patients
Gallbladder in situ
Acute gall stone pancreatitis
Papillary stenosis
Endoscopic placement of biliary endoprosthesis
Patients with periampullary malignant disease
'Sump' syndrome
Accessory sphincterotomy
Trans-ampullary extraction of pancreatic calculi

Table 35.3 Indication for endoscopic sphincterotomy (USA experience 21 centres)

Indications	No	%
Common duct stones	1106	88.5
Post-cholecystectomy	(1013)	
Gallbladder in situ	(93)	
Papillary stenosis	126	10.0
Ampullary tumour	8	0.7
Miscellaneous	10	0.8
Total	1250	100.0

(After Geenen et al 1981)

Choledocholithiasis

The overall success rate for sphincterotomy and for stone removal (extraction or spontaneous passage) is about 95% and 85% respectively (Safrany 1981, Reiter et al 1984, Nakajima et al 1979, Cotton & Vallon 1981, Geenen et al 1981). Sphincterotomy may be difficult to achieve in the presence of a periampullary diverticulum, previous Billroth II partial gastrectomy or impacted gallstones but these conditions are not contraindications. Endoscopic sphincterotomy may also be performed in cases of acute cholangitis with stones or in acute gallstone pancreatitis (Ch. 47). Even in the more difficult situations cited, experienced operators can achieve relatively high success rates (Safrany et al 1980).

Not all published series give data allowing calculation of true success which can only be judged following radiological confirmation of a clear biliary system. In practice this usually means endoscopic stone extraction at the time of sphincterotomy.

In cases of large stones (>2 cm) a double pigtailed endoprosthesis may be positioned across the stone endoscopically (Huibregtse & Tytgat 1982) or a nasobiliary tube may be inserted (Wurbs & Classen 1977, Cotton et al 1979). This latter technique allows further per-nasal cholangiography to monitor progress and the tube may also be used for chemical dissolution therapy with bile salt–EDTA solution or glyceryl-mono-octanoin. These techniques give effective bile duct decompression and should be considered as an alternative to surgery in acute obstructive suppurative cholangitis.

There is clearly a case for endoscopic sphincterotomy in some patients with the gallbladder in situ and this will include the elderly high risk patient with common bile duct stones (Ch. 47). Table 35.4 shows the results in several series of such cases and the subsequent need for surgery. Follow-up after endoscopic sphincterotomy for up to eight years (Table 35.5) demonstrates the low rate of subsequent cholecystectomy or repeat endoscopic stone removal necessary.

Table 35.4 Endoscopic sphincterotomy with gallbladder in situ

Series	No	Successful sphincterotomy	Clear duct	Failure	Surgery acute GB	Elective
Viceconte et al 1981	41	28	28	0	4	9
Yin et al 1984	159	158	142	15	3	19
Neoptolemos et al 1984	100	98	91	3	2	37
Escourrou et al 1984	255	234	222	8?	0	—

Table 35.5 Follow-up after endoscopic sphincterotomy with gallbladder in situ

Series	No	Follow-up Months	Cholecystectomy	Repeat endoscopic treatment
Yin et al 1984	109	12–96	7	1
Neoptolemos et al 1984	56	16–34	1	0
Escourrou et al 1984	130	6–66	10	2

Acute gallstone pancreatitis

Acute gallstone induced pancreatitis (Ch. 43) may be approached by a policy of urgent endoscopic sphincterotomy. There is limited evidence that such an approach is successful (Safrany & Cotton 1981) (Ch. 47) but on theoretical grounds alone a facility to remove an obstructive ampullary lesion should be employed where available. Further results are required but the mortality currently cited (6.3%) of acute gallstone pancreatitis may be lower following endoscopic stone removal.

Papillary stenosis (see also Ch. 56)

This much discussed and misunderstood condition is defined as benign disease of the papilla of Vater (sclerosis or adenomyomatosis) which impedes the passage of bile and/or pancreatic juice and produces symptoms as a result. Whilst diagnosis has formerly been largely the domaine of the surgeon following transpapillary flow-metry, manometry and pressure controlled cholangiography at surgery (Ch. 28, 56), endoscopic diagnosis is now possible (Ch. 9). ERCP demonstrates a dilated bile duct, absence of stones and no flow of contrast into the duodenum (Geenen et al 1981). Whilst surgical transduodenal sphincteroplasty can produce excellent results in cases diagnosed by these strict criteria, several recent publications (Table 35.6) document the efficacy of endoscopic sphincterotomy in post-cholecystectomy papillary stenosis.

Table 35.6 Endoscopic sphincterotomy in post-cholecystectomy papillary stenosis

Series	No of patients	Symptomatic relief	
Seefeld et al (1981)	14	11/14	79%
Viceconte et al (1981)	49	41/49	84%
Seiffert (1981)	813	111/127	87%

Objective diagnosis of papillary stenosis by endoscopic manometry of the sphincter of Oddi is not a routine procedure but it is a desirable objective where the equipment is available (Ch. 9). Further studies are required to establish the normal range of sphincteric pressure and to establish the range consistent with the diagnosis of papillary stenosis (Geenen et al 1984, Tanaka et al 1983, Schupisser & Tondelli 1984).

Endoscopic placement of biliary endoprosthesis (see also Ch. 37, 69)

Biliary drainage may be affected following endoscopic sphincterotomy (Table 35.1) by placing a biliary endoprosthesis. This may be employed in patients with malignant bile duct obstruction for temporary preoperative decompression, or as a definitive palliative procedure in inoperable malignancy. It may also be employed in patients with primary sclerosing cholangitis, post-traumatic surgical strictures, biliary trauma, in patients with very large (>2 cm) common duct stones and in chronic pancreatitis.

The development of endoscopic techniques of biliary drainage has followed logically from the technique of percutaneous drainage which, however, carries appreciable

Table 35.7 Results of endoscopic insertion of large-bore endoprosthesis in malignant biliary disease (Huibregtse and Tytgat 1984)

	Papillary tumour	Distal common duct	Mid common duct	Hilum
Male	9	80	25	28
Female	15	71	30	39
Age (yr)	71 (43–84)	69 (41–91)	71 (35–91)	66 (33–85)
Surgical bypass	2	13	2	0
30 day mortality	0	18 (11.9%)	12 (21.8%)	16 (23.8%)
Died (No)	8	80	30	30
Median survival (days)	104	128	116	96
Range (days)	57–414	34–394	31–266	31–782
Alive (No)	14	40	11	21
Median interval (days)	213	144	223	168
Range (days)	61–535	60–530	62–601	55–810
Early cholangitis	0	12 (7.9%)	8 (14.5%)	28 (41.8%)
Reduction in jaundice	24 (100%)	143 (94.7%)	39 (71%)	48 (71.6%)
No reduction in jaundice	0	8 (5.2%)	16 (29%)	19 (28.3%)

hazards (Ch. 36) (Ferrucci & Meuller 1981, Burcharth et al 1981, Meuller et al 1982), but which has suggested a reduction of operative mortality in cases of surgical jaundice (Nakayama et al 1978, Denning et al 1981). Currently used endoscopic endoprostheses are between 8 to 11.5 Fr diameter and are either straight (Amsterdam Endoprosthesis) or double pigtail in design. Other shapes are commercially available.

Endoscopic biliary large-bore endoprosthesis is an advance in the management of malignant mid and distal common duct strictures (Table 35.7). A combination of percutaneous and endoscopic insertion of endoprosthesis may be an effective palliative treatment of bifurcation tumours but evaluation of these techniques is still in progress (Ch. 37).

Complications of endoscopic insertion of a biliary endoprosthesis (Table 35.8) developed in 100 out of 380 patients compiled by international enquiry (Hagenmüller 1984). Cholangitis, usually occurring early after endoprosthesis insertion, is seen in 15 to 20% of patients, and for this reason prophylactic antibiotics are recommended. Cholangitis following this procedure has a number of causes. It may be due to early clogging of the endoprosthesis by blood clots or more likely is due to cholangitis developing in an undrained part of the biliary tree. This complication may occur in spite of gas sterilization of all

Table 35.8 Complications of endoscopic insertion of biliary endoprosthesis

Cholangitis
Perforation
Endoprosthesis blocked
Early clogging
Late clogging
Dislodgement
Cystic duct occlusion with acute cholecystitis
Occlusion by tumour growth
Duodenal erosion or ulceration

ancillary equipment and conscientious disinfection of the endoscope with aqueous glutaraldehyde.

Perforation is a rare complication. Blocking of the endoprosthesis usually occurs after two to seven months following insertion. The nature of the occluding material is not certain and is not solely due to the rate of bile flow which itself is a function of the endoprosthesis diameter. Ultrasonography and HIDA scintiscanning can be used to detect tube blockage but re-development of cholestasis and cholangitis usually mark its occurrence. A rise of alkaline phosphatase usually heralds clogging and ultrasonography is recommended.

In some cases two or three large-bore endoprostheses have been inserted and all have blocked suggesting that increasing the diameter of the endoprosthesis is not in itself sufficient. Further research into tubing material, choleretic drugs, antibiotics, stone dissolution agents and correlation with liver function and bile flow are needed. A blocked endoprosthesis can be simply exchanged by the endoscopist. Some endoscopists routinely change the endoprosthesis after three to four months.

Patients with periampullary malignant disease

Two approaches have been made with ampullary tumours.

Endoscopic sphincterotomy has been performed in order to relieve jaundice prior to pancreaticoduodenectomy (Alderson et al 1981) or to provide long-term relief of obstruction by insertion of a biliary endoprosthesis (Huibregtse & Tytgat 1984). In this series 24 patients (9 male, 15 female) were treated with a biliary endoprosthesis and two with a pancreatic endoprosthesis in addition because of marked dilatation of the pancreatic duct. In 22 patients the endoprosthesis was the definitive treatment. Fourteen patients remained alive after a median time interval of 213 days (mean 254 days, range 61–535 days) and eight patients died after a median survival of 204 days (mean 160 days, range 57–414 days). In all cases the bilirubin level returned to normal.

'Sump' syndrome

Baker et al (1985) found that five out of eight patients with the 'sump' syndrome improved following endoscopic sphincterotomy. This condition is not often associated with acute cholangitis or steatorrhoea and plain radiographs showing air in the biliary tree are not sufficient evidence that the stoma (choledochoduodenostomy) or the papilla is functioning properly.

Accessory sphincterotomy

Endoscopic pancreatography has refocussed attention on congenital anomalies of the pancreatic duct system. The most common of these, pancreas divisum, described by Opie (1903, 1910), occurs when the ventral pancreatic duct (duct of Wirsung) fails to fuse with the dorsal anlage so that drainage of the dorsal pancreas (body and tail) occurs solely through the dorsal duct (duct of Santorini) and the accessory papilla. When papillary stenosis of the accessory papilla occurs a clinical syndrome of abdominal pain may result in which endoscopic or surgical attempts to improve drainage may provide effective treatment.

The frequency of pancreas divisum is probably about 5 to 6% of all cases coming to post-mortem (Millbourn 1950, Hand 1963). ERCP series are usually heavily biased due to case selection and cannot be relied on to provide an accurate indication of the prevalence of pancreas divisum. Nevertheless, a survey of 17 series of ERCP (102–6003) cases totalling 22 224 cases gave an overall incidence of 4.6% (1.3–6.9%) which correlates well with autopsy studies and Kruse (1981) in a survey of 40 000 European ERCPs showed an incidence of pancreas divisum in idiopathic pancreatitis of 10% (4–40%) compared with 4% in patients with biliary tract disease.

Several groups have reported encouraging results following accessory sphincterotomy, whether endoscopic or surgical (Sahel et al 1982, Keith et al 1982, Warshaw et al 1983, Gregg et al 1983, Traverso et al 1982, Cooperman et al 1982) but only long-term follow-up will resolve the existing problem of correlating symptoms with the anatomical anomaly and show that true improvement follows dorsal duct drainage.

Endoscopic balloon dilatation of bile duct strictures

Dilatation of the ampulla and biliary tree is not a new procedure (Bakes 1928). Biliary strictures have been successfully dilated down T-tube tracts (Burhenne & Morris 1980) but endoscopic dilatation of a bile duct stricture was not attempted until 1977 when a Fogarty balloon catheter was employed to dilate a biliary stricture through a choledochoduodenostomy (Lee & Kato 1977).

Currently Gruntzig type balloons are used (Gruntzig & Bollinger 1973) and large channel (2.8, 3.7, 4.2 mm) side viewing endoscopes are employed, allowing 5 to 8 Fr Gruntzig type balloon catheters to be passed (balloons 4–8 mm diameter). Pressures of up to five atmospheres (75 psi) can be generated in these balloons. Balloon dilatation was successful in 18 out of 27 patients (Table 35.9), largely for postoperative bile duct strictures. Follow-up is required for long-term confirmation of these results and care should be exercised in selecting suitable cases (Ch. 58).

Table 35.9 Endoscopic balloon dilatation of biliary strictures

Type	Attempts	Early success
Inflammatory		
(Idiopathic)	4	2
Postoperative	10	9
Sclerosing cholangitis	4	2
Choledochoduodenostomy	2	2
Malignant	7	3
	27	18

After Geenen 1984

Table 35.10 Complications following endoscopic balloon dilatation of biliary strictures

Complication	No
Sepsis	1
Bleeding	0
Perforation	0
Pancreatitis	5
	6

Geenen 1984

Experience is currently developing with balloon dilatation of pancreatic duct strictures. The complication rate appears to be low (9.2%) (Table 35.10) but long-term results are not yet available and prospective multicentre trials are now being performed in order to evaluate this potentially valuable procedure.

Endoscopic lithotripsy

Nearly all (about 90%) bile duct stones can be removed at the time of endoscopic sphincterotomy, by either basket or balloon extraction (Ch. 48). Large stones (>2 cm diameter), however, may require mechanical lithotripsy. The original report of a suitable device (Demling & Riemann 1982) has not been followed by entirely satisfactory new devices but the original group have subsequently quoted successful mechanical lithotripsy in 86.9% of 145 patients.

Table 35.11 Long-term follow-up following endoscopic sphincterotomy. International survey 1982 (6 centres)

Indication	Total	Symptom free	Improved	Unchanged	Worse
Post cholecystectomy choledocholithiasis	654	568 (89.9%)	41 (6.3%)	38 (5.8%)	7 (1.0%)
Choledocholithiasis (gallbladder in situ)	109	91 (83.5%)	14 (12.8%)	3 (2.7%)	1 (1.0%)
Papillary stenosis	159	113 (71.1%)	14 (8.8%)	30 (18.9%)	2 (1.2%)
Riemann et al	922	782 (84.8%)	59 (6.4%)	71 (7.7%)	10 (1.1%)

New designs based on the original mechanical lithotripter are currently being produced. Other techniques such as electrohydraulic lithotripsy based on a high voltage spark (Koch et al 1977) have been employed and in vitro studies of giant pulsed (Q-switched) laser impulses for stone fragmentation have been initiated.

Iridium wire placement

Iridium wire implants have recently been employed in cases of pancreatic carcinoma and cholangiocarcinoma and further experience is currently awaited.

COMPLICATIONS OF ENDOSCOPIC SPHINCTEROTOMY

The complication rate for endoscopic sphincterotomy is now well documented at about 8 to 9% with a mortality of less than 1% (Geenen et al 1981). Sepsis, haemorrhage, perforation and pancreatitis account for the great majority of complications which nearly always become apparent within 24 to 48 hours of the procedure.

Sepsis is an especially important hazard since the bile in obstructing choledocholithiasis is usually infected and tends to spread intravascularly during pressure changes (Hultborn et al 1962), especially via the lymphatics (Huang et al 1969). Prophylactic antibiotics are essential when there is bile duct obstruction and manipulation of the bile duct is planned as there is good evidence that the use of appropriate antibiotics will reduce thc incidence of septicaemia even though the obstructed bile may not be sterilized (Keighley et al 1976).

Long-term follow-up studies are as yet few (Ch. 47) but some (Riemann et al 1983) have shown most patients symptom-free (Table 35.11). If the symptom-free and improved patients from these series are aggregated, 93.2% of patients have benefited from endoscopic sphincterotomy. If the causes of death in patients who have since died following endoscopic sphincterotomy are analyzed (Table 35.12) it is found that 75% of patients died of causes unassociated with biliary disease. Nine deaths (1.6%), including four patients who died following cholecystectomy, were due to disease of the biliary system. Two occurred following stone extraction and two following septic cholangitis.

Table 35.12 Long-term follow-up endoscopic sphincterotomy

549 patients. Follow up of 2–9 years (mean = 3 years)		
Biliary tract surgery		61
Cholecystectomy	39	
CBD exploration	17	
Sphincteroplasty	5	
Deaths		66
Biliary	9	
Non-biliary	45	
Unknown	12	

Riemann et al 1983

REFERENCES

Alderson D, Lavelle M I, Venables C W 1981 Endoscopic sphincterotomy before pancreaticoduodenectomy for ampullary carcinoma. British Medical Journal 282: 1109–1111

Baker A R, Neoptolemos J P, Carr-Locke D L, Fossard D P 1985 Sump syndrome following choledochoduodenostomy and its endoscopic treatment. British Journal of Surgery 72: 433–435

Bakes J 1928 On the drainage-less surgery of the bile passages and on the methodical dilatation of the papilla. Zentralblatt für Chirurgie 55: 1858

Burcharth F, Efsen F, Christiansen L A 1981 Non surgical internal biliary drainage by endoprosthesis. Surgery, Gynecology and Obstetrics 153: 857–860

Burhenne H J, Morris D C 1980 Biliary stricture dilatation: use of the Gruntzig balloon catheter. Journal of the Canadian Association of Radiologists 31: 196–197

Classen M, Demling L 1974 Endoscopische sphincterotomie der Papilla Vater, und steinextraktion aus Ductus Choledochus. Deutsche Medizinische Wochenschrift 99: 496–497

Cooperman M, Ferrara J J, Fromkes J J, Carey L C 1982 Surgical management of pancreas divisum. American Journal of Surgery 143: 107–112

Cotton P B 1980 Non operative removal of bile duct stones by duodenoscopic sphincterotomy. British Journal of Surgery 67: 1–5

Cotton P B, Vallon A G 1981 British experience with duodenoscopic sphincterotomy for removal of bile duct stones. British Journal of Surgery 68: 373–375

Cotton P B, Barney P G J, Mason R R 1979 Transnasal bile duct catheterization after endoscopic sphincterotomy. Gut 20: 285–287

Cremer M, Gulbis A, Toussaint J, De Teouf J, Van Laethem A, Hermanus A 1977 La sphincterotomie endoscopique. Contribution belge a l'experience mondiale. Acta Gastroenterologica Belgica 40: 41–54

Demling L, Riemann J F 1982 Mechanischer Lithotriptor. Deutsche Medizinische Wochenschrift 107: 555

Denning D A, Ellison E C, Carey L C 1981 Pre-operative percutaneous transhepatic biliary compression lowers operative mortality in patients with obstructive jaundice. American Journal of Surgery 141: 61–64

Escourrou J, Cordova J A, Lazorthes F, Frexinos J, Ribet A 1984 Early and late complications after endoscopic sphincterotomy for biliary lithiasis with and without the gall bladder 'in situ'. Gut 25: 598–602

Ferrucci J J, Meuller P R 1981 Interventional radiology of the biliary tract. Gastroenterology 82: 974–985

Geenen J E 1984 Balloon dilatation of bile duct strictures. In: Classen M, Geenen J E, Kawai K (eds) Non-surgical Biliary Drainage. Springer-Verlag, Heidelberg, p 105–108

Geenen J E, Vennes J A, Silvis S E 1981 Resume of seminar on endoscopic retrograde sphincterotomy (ERS). Gastrointestinal Endoscopy 27: 31–38

Geenen J E, Hogan W, Toouli J, Dodds W, Venu R 1984 A prospective randomized study of the efficiency of endoscopic sphincterotomy for patients with presumptive sphincter of Oddi dysfunction. Gastroenterology 86: A105

Gregg J A, Monaco A P, McDermott W V 1983 Pancreas divisum: results of surgical intervention. American Journal of Surgery 145: 488–493

Gruntzig A, Bollinger A 1973 Perkutane Rekanalisation chronischer arterieller Verschlüsse nack Dotter — eine nicht operative Kathetertechnik. Schweizer Medizinische Wochenschrift 103: 825–831

Hagenmüller F 1984 Bilioduodenal drainage in malignant bile duct stenosis. In: Classen M, Geenen J E, Kawai K (eds) Non-surgical biliary drainage. Springer-Verlag, Heidelberg, p 94–104

Hand B H 1963 An anatomic study of the choledochoduodenal area. British Journal of Surgery 50: 486–494

Huang T, Bass J A, Williams R D 1969 The significance of biliary pressure in cholangitis. Archives of Surgery 98: 629–632

Huibregtse K, Tytgat G N J 1982 Palliative treatment of obstructive jaundice by transpapillary introduction of a large-bore bile duct endoprosthesis. Gut 23: 371–375

Huibregtse K, Tytgat G N J 1984 Endoscopic placement of biliary prosthesis. In: Salmon P R (ed) Gastrointestinal endoscopy: Advances in diagnosis and therapy Vol.1 p 219–231

Hultborn A, Jacobsson B, Rosengren B 1962 Cholangiovenous reflux during cholangiography. An experimental and clinical study. Acta Chirurgica Scandinavica 123: 111–124

Kawai K, Akasata Y, Murakami K, Tada M, Nakajima M 1974 Endoscopic sphincterotomy of the ampulla of Vater. Gastrointestinal Endoscopy 20: 148–151

Keighley M R B, Drysdale R B, Quoraishi A H 1976 Antibiotics in biliary disease — the relative importance of antibiotic concentrations in the bile and serum. Gut 17: 495–500

Keith R G, Shapero T G, Saibil F G 1982 Treatment of pancreatitis associated with pancreas divisum by dorsal duct sphincterotomy alone. Canadian Journal of Surgery 25: 622–626

Koch H, Stolte M, Walz V 1977 Endoscopic lithotripsy in the common bile duct. Endoscopy 9: 95

Kruse A 1981 Pancreas divisum. Praxis 70(46): 2064–2067

Lee T G, Kato 1977 Endoscopic retrograde cholangiodilatation: a preliminary report. Gastrointestinal Endoscopy 23: 171–172

Meuller P R, Van Sonnenberg E, Ferrucci J T 1982 Percutaneous biliary drainage: technical and catheter related problems in 200 procedures. American Journal of Radiology 138: 17–23

Millbourn E 1950 On excretory ducts of pancreas in man with special reference to their relation to each, to common bile duct and to duodenum. Radiologic and anatomic study. Acta Anatomica 9: 1–34

Nakajima M, Kizu M, Akasaka Y, Kawai K 1979 Five years experience of endoscopic sphincterotomy in Japan. A collective study of 25 centres. Endoscopy 2 138–141

Nakayama T, Ikeda A, Okuda K 1978 Percutaneous transhepatic drainage of the biliary tract. Technique and results in 104 cases. Gastroenterology 74: 554–559

Neoptolemos J P, Carr-Locke D L, Fraser I, Fossard D P 1984 The management of common bile duct calculi by endoscopic sphincterotomy in patients with gall bladders in situ. British Journal of Surgery 71: 69–71

Oi I, Kobayashi S, Kondo T 1970 Endoscopic pancreaticocholangiography. Endoscopy 2:103

Opie E 1903 The anatomy of the pancreas. Johns Hopkins Hospital Bulletin 150: 229–232

Opie E 1910 Disease of the pancreas. J B Lippincott, Philadelphia

Reiter J J, Bayer H B, Mennicken C, Manegold P C 1984 Results of endoscopic papillotomy; a collective experience from 9 endoscopic centres in West Germany. World Journal of Surgery 2: 505–507

Riemann J F, Lux G, Forster P, Altendorf A 1983 Long term results after endoscopic papillotomy 15: 165–168

Safrany L 1981 Endoscopic papillotomy in the treatment of biliary tract disease; 258 procedures and results. Digestive Diseases and Sciences 26: 1057–1064

Safrany L, Cotton P B 1981 A preliminary report. Urgent duodenoscopic sphincterotomy for acute gallstone pancreatitis. Surgery 89: 424–428

Safrany L, Neuhaus B, Porto-Carrero G, Krause S 1980 Endoscopic sphincterotomy in patients with Billroth II gastrectomy. Endoscopy 12: 16–22

Sahel J, Cros R C, Bourry J, Sarles H 1982 Clinico-pathologic conditions associated with pancreas divisum. Digestion 23: 1–8

Salmon P R, Brown P, Htut T, Burwood R, Read A E 1971 Duodenoscopy. Lancet i: 1298–1299

Schupisser J P, Tondelli P 1984 Papillary stenosis. In: Salmon P R (ed) Gastrointestinal endoscopy: Advances in diagnosis and therapy, Vol.1 p 181–192

Seefeld U, Buhler H, Woodtli W, Deyhle P 1981 Endoskopische papillotomie bei narbiger papillenstenose nach Cholecystektomie. Zeitschrift für Gastroenterologie 19:505

Seiffert 1981 (cited by Schupisser & Tondelli 1984)

Tanaka M, Ikeda S, Nakayama F 1983 Continuous measurement of common bile duct pressure with an indwelling microtransducer catheter introduced by duodenoscopy: new diagnostic and for postcholecystectomy dyskinesia — preliminary report. Gastrointestinal Endoscopy 29: 83–88

Traverso L W, Perry W W, Musser G, Frey C F 1982 Pancreas divisum: the role of pancreatic duct drainage. Surgical Gastroenterology 1: 11–16

Viceconte G, Viceconte G W, Pietropaelo V, Montori A 1981 Endoscopic sphincterotomy: indications and results. British Journal of Surgery 68: 376–380

Warshaw A L, Richter J M, Schapiro R H 1983 The cause and treatment of pancreatitis associated with pancreas divisum. Annals of Surgery 198: 443–452

Wurbs D, Classen M 1977 Transpapillary longstanding tube for hepatobiliary drainage. Endoscopy 9: 192–193

Yin T P, Leung J W C, Vallon A G, Cotton P B 1984 Sphincterotomy with gall bladder in situ; one to eight year follow up. Gut 25:A1186

Interventional radiological techniques in the liver and biliary tract

Interventional radiology has rapidly become an alternative to surgical procedures in many fields. New methods are developed, tested, continuously refined and compared with surgery in terms of success rate, discomfort to the patients, complications, hospitalization time, and general costs.

When the first excitement which attends almost all new methods has subsided, a more objective evaluation takes place which finally provides the guide lines for their use.

During the last 15 years diagnostic angiography has become less and less important. Presently angiography is almost never performed to initially diagnose abnormalities within the liver, bile ducts or pancreas. The diagnosis is made with the aid of ultrasound, computerized tomography or endoscopy. On the other hand, when the diagnosis has been made, the technical skill gained from angiographic procedures can be used in the treatment of patients if surgery is not possible.

In the following a review will be made of interventional radiology of the liver and the bile ducts today, and suggestions for future development made.

THE LIVER

Liver cysts

Indications

Benign non-parasitic cysts (Ch. 80, 81) occur in the liver in 0.1–0.2% of cases reported from autopsy materials. If the cysts are large symptoms may occur with upper abdominal discomfort. In spite of extensive hepatomegaly from these cysts, liver insufficiency or portal hypertension is rare. Treatment therefore aims to reduce the discomfort from the pressure of the cyst.

Technique

Under local anaesthesia and guided by ultrasound or CT the cyst is punctured with a sheathed needle. The sheath is coiled up in the cyst with the aid of a guide wire and the content of the cyst is evacuated. 10 to 40 ml of absolute alcohol is injected into the cyst in order to sclerose its wall. After 5–10 minutes the alcohol is aspirated, the catheter is removed and the patient sent back to the ward for observation until the following day.

We have treated seven patients with large liver cysts in this way (Fig. 36.1). Three patients became totally free of symptoms after one to seven treatments. Another three patients were markedly improved after two to seven treatments. In one patient with multiple medium sized cysts there was no discernible effect.

Complications

Ethanol sclerosing of liver cysts has been shown to be a useful technique to reduce the volume of large hepatic cysts. Complications are few. Slight elevation of serum ethanol may be seen and in rare cases up to 8 mmol/l has been found. Leak of ethanol through the puncture hole to the peritoneum may occur resulting in abdominal pain. Severe side reactions have, however, not been encountered.

Drainage of liver abscesses

Indications

Ultrasonography (US) and computerized tomography (CT) are very effective techniques to localize subphrenic, intrahepatic and subhepatic abscesses. US is somewhat more precise in the localization of subphrenic abscess since with CT it is often difficult to separate a pleural lesion from a subphrenic collection. US also gives better information about the content of the abscess: if it is mature; if there is a fluid content and if the cavity is divided by septa. CT, on the other hand, often gives better information regarding the topography of adjacent organs when a safe route for percutaneous drainage is to be selected.

There is an indication for percutaneous drainage of many major subphrenic, intra- and subhepatic abscesses, where US and/or CT show that they can be approached

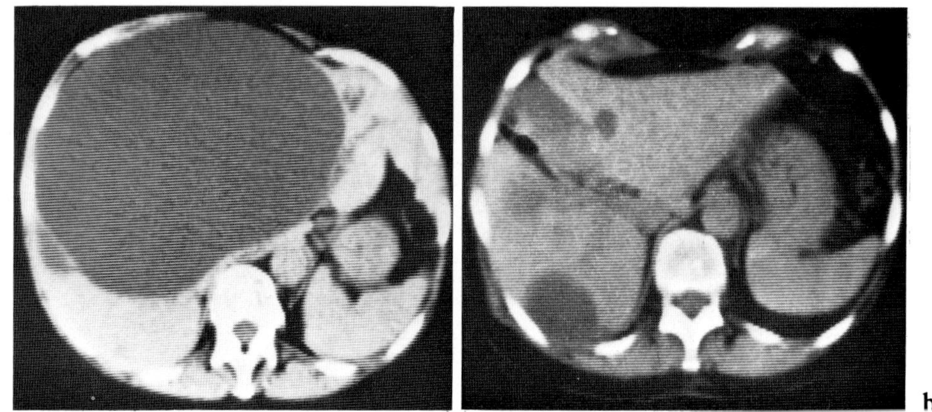

Fig. 36.1 Patient with large benign hepatic cyst in the liver. CT a. before and b. after percutaneous sclerosing with absolute alcohol

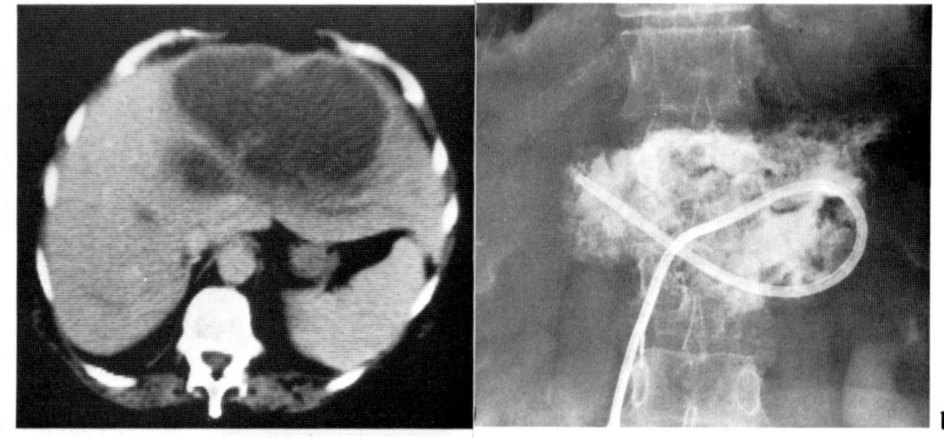

Fig. 36.2 a. Abscess in the left lobe of the liver. b. Percutaneous drainage with Ring–McLean sump coiled up within the abscess here injected with contrast

without damaging adjacent organs. A success rate of 70% to more than 90% is reported (Greenwood et al 1982, Scheinfeld et al 1982, van Sonnenberg et al 1982, Clark & Towbin 1983 (Fig. 36.2).

Technique

Guided by ultrasound or CT the abscess is punctured with a 0.9 mm needle. When the tip of the needle is in the correct position, aspiration of the contents is taken for aerobic and anaerobic culture. Contrast medium is injected into the cavity and the patient is moved to an examination room with fluoroscopic facilities. Guided by the previous direction of puncture and the contrast-stained cavity, the operator now uses a sheathed PTC-needle. When the tip of this needle is within the cavity, the stylet is removed and a guide wire is introduced through the sheath. The guide wire is coiled up within the cavity and the canal is dilated to the size of the drainage catheter which is to be used. At our institution we prefer to use sump drains (F14 or 16 Ring-McLean*). The sump drain is introduced over the guide wire with the stiffening cannula in place until the tip of the sump is within the cavity. The sump is then slid over the guide wire and cannula and coiled up within the abscess.

As much of the content as possible is aspirated from the abscess followed by irrigation with saline.

With the patient on i.v. antibiotic therapy the sump is irrigated twice a day with saline. If aspiration of injected saline suggests clogging of the catheter, 5 ml of Acetylcysteine** is injected through each of the canals of the sump. After 10 minutes the sump is again irrigated with saline and its function is usually restored. If, however, the sump remains clogged it is exchanged over a guide wire.

The healing of the abscess is followed with ultrasound, CT or injection of contrast medium under fluoroscopic control. When the cavity is reduced to a canal surrounding

* Cook, Bloomington, Indiana, USA
** Mead Johnson Pharmaceutical Div., Evansville, Indiana, USA

the drainage catheter this is slowly removed over a few days.

Complications

The complication rate is low when compared with open surgical drainage. In a review of the literature, Scheinfeld et al (1982) collected a total number of 59 liver abscesses drained percutaneously. Only one death was recorded and this was a patient who was finally surgically explored. Surgical exploration, on the other hand, has a mortality rate reported between 30 and 65%.

Ascites is a contraindication to percutaneous abscess drainage since peritonitis may ensue.

Complications may also be caused by unintentional perforation of a loop of the bowel. This is usually a minor complication and the bowel heals when the catheter is withdrawn.

Interventional procedures in liver trauma

Indications

Damage to the liver with haemorrhage caused either by blunt or penetrating trauma has usually been treated by surgery (Ch. 82, 84). During the last few years, however, a more conservative approach has been developed in selected cases. CT usually demonstrates the location and extent of the lesion and if immediate surgery is not necessary to stop life-threatening haemorrhage, angiography is often used to show the extent of the damage and whether bleeding has stopped.

The angiographic demonstration of extravasation from an hepatic artery or an hepatic artery-bile duct fistula (Ch. 85) does not necessarily mean that surgery is indicated. Angiography allows the possibility of transcatheter embolisation in the control of bleeding. (Rubin & Katzen 1977, Heimbach et al 1978, Schmidt et al 1980) (Fig. 36.3).

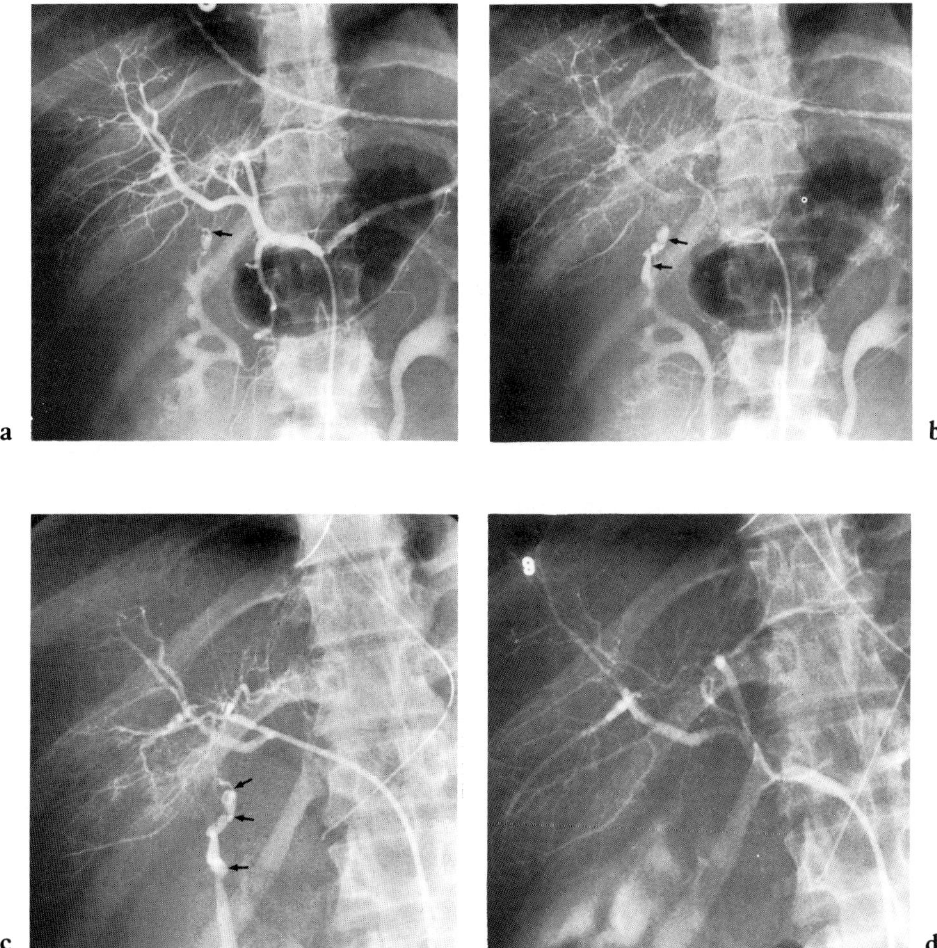

Fig. 36.3 Traffic accident with liver rupture. a. Angiography of common hepatic artery shows extravasation from an arterial branch in the liver (arrow). b. and c. The artery feeding the bleeding vessel is selectively catheterized giving better demonstration of extravasation (arrows). d. Common hepatic arteriogram after occlusion with pieces of gelfoam of the bleeding vessel. Other arterial branches of the liver still patent

Before any attempt to embolize the hepatic artery, one has to make sure that the portal blood flow is not seriously compromised, otherwise liver failure may ensue.

Technique

Liver angiography is usually performed via a transfemoral approach and, as soon as the bleeding artery has been demonstrated, a decision has to be made to catheterize this artery selectively for subsequent occlusion. In most cases the same transfemoral approach can be used but a change of catheter or guide wire may be necessary.

If the catheter cannot be advanced to the bleeding artery, a coaxial F3 Teflon catheter can be used in combination with a 0.53 mm guide wire. This thin catheter, however, limits the choice of embolization material to isobutyl 2-cyanoacrylate (Bucrylate) or absolute alcohol. Personally, I prefer Bucrylate as this material can be made radiopaque by mixing it with the same volume of Lipiodol (which also prolongs the hardening time and makes injection easier). The catheter has to be prefilled with 5.5% glucose solution to prevent occlusion of the catheter itself.

When, on the other hand, a F5 or larger catheter can be manipulated into the bleeding artery, particulate embolization material can be used. This material can be either resorbable or non-resorbable.

The most frequently used resorbable embolization material is gelfoam which is injected in pieces of a few mm in size through the catheter.

Non-resorbable embolization materials are polyvinyl alcohol foam (Ivalon®) and Gianturco steel coils. Pieces of Ivalon are selected when small arterial branches are to be occluded and the steel coils are used for larger arteries.

Whatever material is used for embolization of the bleeding artery the effect of the procedure is easily controlled by a repeat angiogram.

In a few cases the vascular anatomy makes transfemoral superselective catheterization impossible. In such cases it is advisable to use the transaxillary approach. When the hepatic artery is entered from above, the catheterization of small peripheral branches is often much easier and reduces the time of the procedure.

More expensive to use and requiring more technical expertise are the detachable balloons (White et al 1979). They are flow directed, can be advanced far out into peripheral arteries and do not need to be detached before a correct position and function is achieved.

Complications

These are few and limited to inadvertent deposition of the embolized material into the gastro-duodenal artery or its branches.

Embolization cannot be used to treat late complications such as traumatic hematoma or bile leak. These are best treated surgically when the patient has recovered from the haemorrhage.

Embolization of liver tumours (Ch. 94)

Indications

The only curative treatment of liver tumours is resection. When resection is not possible chemotherapy or other palliative measures may be employed. Patients with liver metastases from endocrine tumours have an approximate 20–30% five-year survival without treatment. Symptoms from released vasoactive amines, however, markedly reduce the quality of life especially in patients with carcinoid metastases. To reduce the tumour burden and thus the amount of released amines, enucleation of tumours has been tried (Stephen & Graham-Smith 1972). As most of the blood supply to hepatic neoplasms is provided by the hepatic artery and only to a minor degree by the portal vein, occlusion of the hepatic artery causes tumour necrosis to a varying degree. With this in mind surgical hepatic dearterialization (Idema et al 1977), and surgical temporary dearterialization (Bengmark et al 1982) have successfully been tried to reduce the symptoms in patients with carcinoid metastases (Ch. 95). It seems that transcatheter embolization of the hepatic artery provides the same positive effect as surgical dearterialization and avoids the surgical trauma (Lunderquist et al 1982) (Fig. 36.4).

Patients with multiple primary and secondary non-endocrine liver tumours may be treated with infusion chemotherapy (Ch. 96). Hepatic artery embolization has also been tried and there are indications that survival time may be increased (Chuang et al 1982, 1984). In primary tumours of the liver mixing of the embolization material with cytotoxic drugs has been tried. Marked reduction of tumour size and vascularity is reported (Yamada et al 1983, Konno et al 1983).

Cavernous haemangiomas of the liver may be large and cause life-threatening complications including rupture or heart failure (Ch. 87). Such lesions can be resected but transcatheter embolization may be the treatment of choice (Stanley et al 1983).

Patient preparation

To reduce the risk of abscess formation patients are given antibiotics from the day before and for one week following embolization. It has been suggested that patients should be well hydrated and be prepared with allopurinol and urine alkalinization to minimize the risk of the post-embolization syndrome (Clouse & Lee 1974).

Blumgart & Allison (1982) recommend pre-treatment of patients with metastasis to the liver from carcinoid tumours with cyprohepatidine and P-chlorophenylalanine for a day or two before and after the embolization to

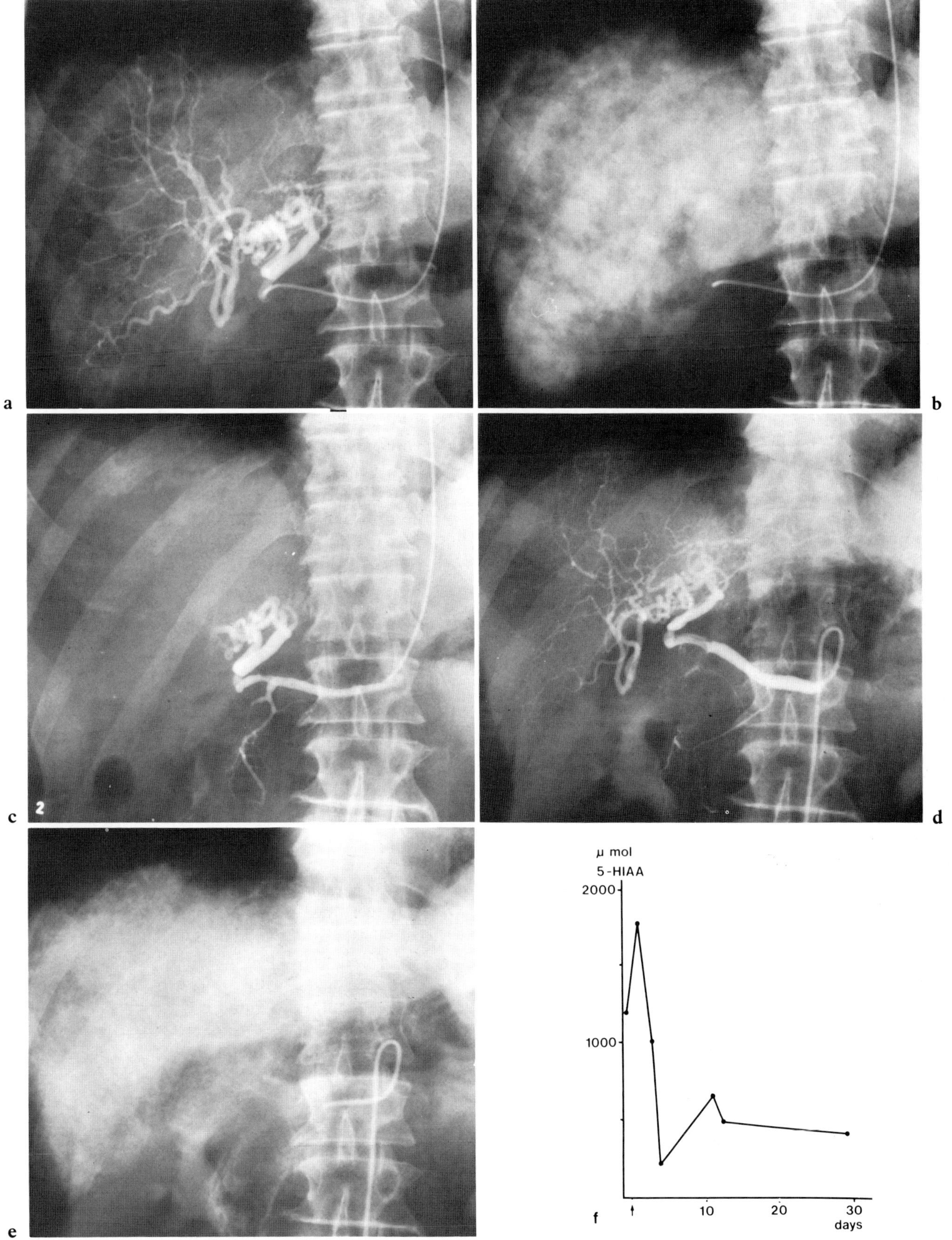

Fig. 36.4 Patient with carcinoid metastases to the liver and carcinoid syndrome. Right hepatic artery previously ligated. a. Left axillary catheterization of left hepatic artery. Arterial phase. b. Parenchymal phase shows multiple hypervascular metastases. c. Angiogram after gelfoam powder embolisation shows totally blocked blood flow. d. Angiogram one month later shows recanalization of the arteries. e. Parenchymal phase shows reduction of the hypervascularized metastases and liver size. f. Response of 5-HIAA in urine on embolisation. Arrow indicates embolisation

reduce the risk of side effects from released vasoactive amines (Ch. 94).

Embolization technique

After liver angiography has been performed to chart the vascular anatomy and patency of the portal vein, the left and right hepatic arteries are catheterized selectively one after the other. The catheter is placed as far out as possible to reduce the risk of spill-over of embolization material into the gastroduodenal artery. If necessary separate branches of the right and left hepatic artery are catheterized and occluded. At our institution we prefer gelatin foam powder* as embolization material since the arterial occlusion achieved in this way is often temporary and the procedure can be repeated when symptoms recur.

One ml of dry gelatin foam powder is aspirated in a 10 ml syringe and mixed with 9 ml of 60% water-soluble contrast medium and 1 g of Keflin.® After careful shaking the mixture is slowly injected under fluoroscopic control. It is seen clearly when the flow becomes stagnant and the injection is then stopped. When all branches to the liver have been treated in this way the catheter is withdrawn.

At some institutions other embolization materials such as Ivalon (pieces or powder) and Gianturco steel coils are used either alone or in combination (Chuang & Wallace 1981, Chuang et al 1982). The technique is the same but recanalization does not occur and the procedure cannot be repeated.

The advantage of using powdered material 0.1–0.2 mm in size is that it produces peripheral embolization of small hepatic arterial branches and in this way reduces the possibility of the development of collateral circulation (Lunderquist et al 1982). Collaterals, however, always develop to some degree even with peripheral embolization. Experimental studies have shown that collaterals over the bile duct plexus soon bypass occluded arterial branches (Stridbeck et al 1984).

It has also been suggested that absolute alcohol may be used as occlusion material in the liver in the same way as in the treatment of renal tumours. Experimental studies have shown, however, that injection of absolute alcohol into the hepatic artery produces fibrotic changes in the bile ducts mimicking those of sclerosing cholangitis (Doppman & Girton 1984).

Complications

If care is taken not to embolize the hepatic artery in patients with cirrhosis or with compromised portal blood flow (or when the portal vein is occluded from other causes) complications are few.

Right upper quadrant pain that needs medication appears half-an-hour to an hour after the embolization and lasts for up to 24 hours.

A febrile reaction (38.5–39°C) is generally observed lasting for 2–14 days. When post-embolization CT scans are performed one may see gas formation within large tumours. This, however, is not an indication of abscess but merely tumour necrosis (Bernardino et al 1981). Liver function tests, as estimated by levels of enzymes, show an elevation but return to normal within two weeks.

If the patients are not cholecystectomized prior to embolization there is a presumptive risk of necrosis of the gallbladder. Few cases have been reported (De Jode et al 1976) but patients have to be carefully watched for symptoms during the post-embolization period (Blumgart & Allison 1982).

Spill over of embolization material into the gastroduodenal artery may occur and can produce ischaemic changes of the duodenum with risk of perforation.

THE BILE DUCTS

Percutaneous transhepatic cholangiography (Ch. 19)

Indications

Percutaneous transhepatic cholangiography (PTC) has been used to visualize the bile ducts in non-jaundiced and jaundiced patients for more than 10 years. In patients without obstructive jaundice, fine needle PTC has been performed when endoscopic retrograde cholangiography (ERC) has been unsuccessful. Fine needle PTC has also been performed in jaundiced patients to visualize the bile ducts above an obstruction and followed either by surgery the same day or by a percutaneous drainage procedure (PTCD) (Ch. 68) to reduce the jaundice prior to a later operation.

Patients with non-resectable malignant tumours causing obstructive jaundice may be palliated by percutaneous drainage of the bile. There also may be an indication for PTCD in patients with post-surgical biliary fistulae (Ch. 60) which do not heal on conservative treatment (Fig. 36.5).

However it is debatable whether a drainage procedure prior to surgery really benefits the patient with obstructive jaundice. Denning et al (1981) showed that operative and postoperative complications were reduced if patients had a PTCD prior to surgery. Pitt et al (1980) made an analysis of 155 patients who underwent biliary tract surgery. They established five clinical and ten laboratory parameters as risk factors, the most significant of which were age above 60 years, malignancy, signs of infection, jaundice, elevation of creatinine, reduction of albumin and haematocrit. In patients with seven to eight risk factors the mortality associated with the surgery was 100%. However, obstruc-

* (Spongostan, Pharmacia, Denmark)

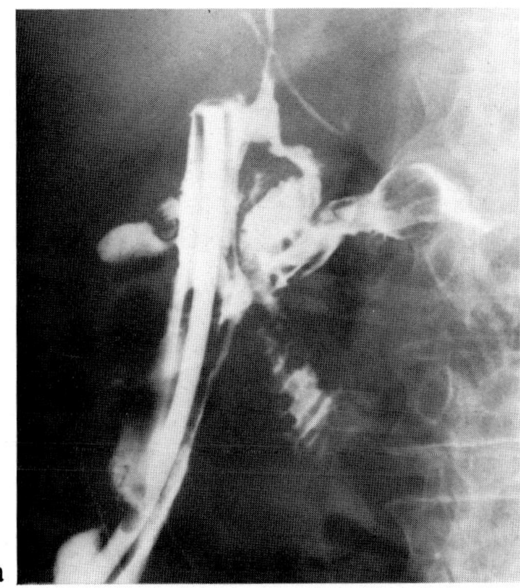

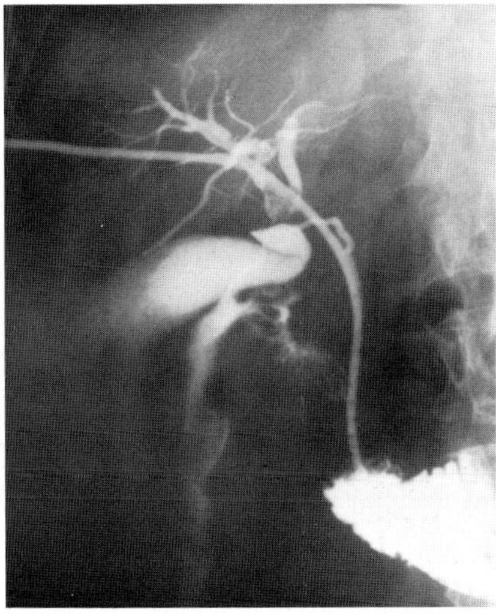

Fig. 36.5 Biliary fistula as complication to surgery for bleeding duodenal ulcer with continous bile leak for almost two months. a. Contrast injected through drain introduced subhepatically at the time of operation. Bile ducts as well as duodenum fill with contrast. b. The leak heals after PTC catheter has been introduced for combined internal–external drainage

tive jaundice was only one of several risk factors which could be corrected.

In 1978 Nakayama et al in an uncontrolled study reported a reduction in operative and postoperative mortality from 28.3% to 8.2% when PTCD was performed. Similarly Gundry et al (1984) found a reduction of mortality from 20% to 4% and of major morbidity (sepsis, abscess, renal failure, bleeding) from 52% to 8% when PTCD was used.

On the other hand, in a multicentre study Passariello (1984) (personal communication) has shown that PTCD does not confer any advantage with regard to operative and postoperative complications. The number of patients in all published series is, however, small and there is great variation in the severity of the illness at the time of referal. Complications after immediate surgery or after initial PTCD are therefore very difficult to compare.

As a result of the questionable advantages of PTCD, the relatively high complication rate from this procedure and recent advances with ERC and endoscopic catheterization (Ch. 117), the future will surely be marked by a reduction in the indications for PTC and PTCD. These indications and their relevance to endoscopic drainage procedures or surgical drainage are discussed in Chs 37, 68, 35.

Technique

Patient preparation. The patient's coagulation factors are checked and corrected if necessary. Diazepam (10 mg) and atropine (0.5 mg) are given 30 minutes before the procedure. The skin over the right lateral and upper ventral abdomen is prepared with an antiseptic solution.

Right lateral approach. Thin needle cholangiogram. Under local anaesthesia the liver is punctured with a thin needle (0.7–0.9 mm outer diameter) in the right midaxillary line below the visible costo-phrenic angle when the patient is normally breathing. Under fluoroscopic control the needle is directed slightly above the presumed position of the bifurcation. When the tip of the needle has reached that position a slow injection of 60% water-soluble contrast medium is started during continous retraction of the needle. It is clearly visible when a bile duct starts to fill with contrast and the retraction of the needle is stopped. At this moment a few ml of bile are aspirated for aerobic and anaerobic culture following by additional injection of contrast to allow for diagnostic cholangiography in a.p. and both oblique views.

The drainage procedure. There are two alternative methods for biliary drainage after the fine needle cholangiogram has demonstrated the bile ducts:

Alternative 1. With this technique we take advantage of the fine needle puncture of the bile duct if the angle of puncture is suitable for further catheterization of the duct. Care is taken not to inject too much contrast into the bile duct system so as not to render it too radio-opaque. An ultra-thin special guide wire (0.46 mm introduction wire*) is advanced through the needle into the bile duct and manipulated under fluoroscopic control as far down the common bile duct as possible. With the guide wire well positioned in the bile duct, the needle is removed and a 3F teflon catheter is advanced over the guide wire. After this a 5F radio-opaque polyethylene sheath is advanced over the teflon catheter. When the tips of the two catheters are in the same position, the guide wire and the teflon catheter are removed leaving the polyethylene catheter in the bile ducts.

* William Cook, Europe ApS, Denmark

A diagnostic cholangiogram is performed and the cause of the obstruction can be evaluated.

A torque control 0.9 mm guide wire is advanced through the polyethylene catheter and manipulated beyond the obstruction and on into the duodenum. The catheter is then slid over the guide wire until its tip also is positioned in the duodenum. Advance into the duodenum is not always necessary especially with tumours above the papilla and may be more readily open to ascending infection.

The torque control guide wire is exchanged to the stiff introduction guide wire* for the drainage catheter. When the tip of the introduction guide wire is in the duodenum the polyethylene catheter is removed, the canal is dilated up to 8F and the drainage catheter is introduced. This 8.3F Ring drainage catheter is placed with side-holes above and below the obstruction. The dilatation procedure and introduction of the drainage catheter are very painful and the patient is given appropriate intravenous analgesics.

The drainage catheter is sutured to half of a colostomy adhesive which is fixed to the skin above the entrance hole of the catheter. This way of fixing has been shown to markedly reduce skin infection.

It is important to make sure that the proximal side-holes of the drainage catheter are located within the bile ducts and not in the liver parenchyma. Side-holes at the level of the liver parenchyma can easily transmit infected bile to the blood stream (Fig. 36.6).

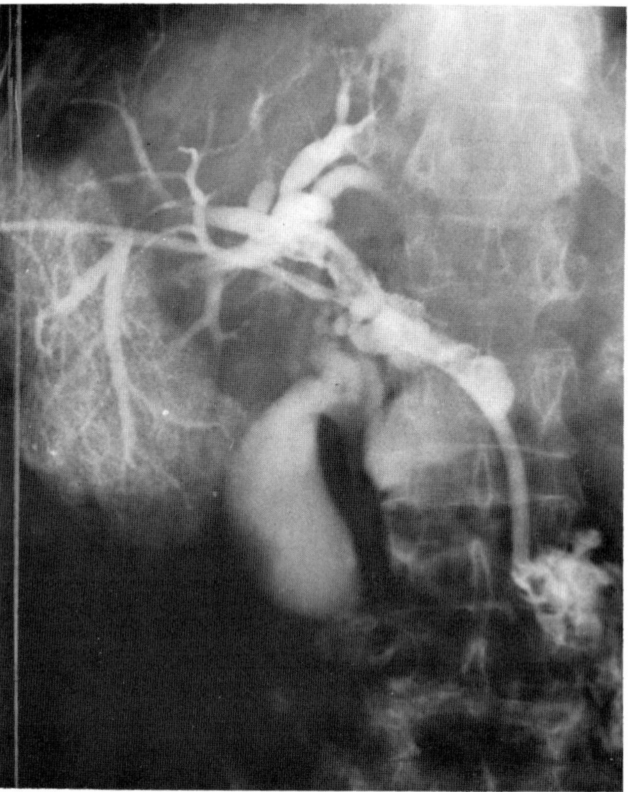

Fig. 36.6 PTC catheter with wrongly placed sideholes outside of the bile ducts. Injection of contrast gives simultaneous filling of bile ducts and a branch of the portal vein

Guided by the cholangiogram and the location of the catheter percutaneous fine needle aspiration cytology (Fig. 36.7) may be performed and allows a correct diagnosis in about 60% of cases.

Before the patient is returned to the ward 10 ml of Mucomyst®** is injected through the catheter to reduce the viscosity of the bile and increase the flow to the duodenum.

To reduce the backflow from the duodenum to the bile ducts we keep the drainage catheter capped from the first day of drainage.

Alternative 2. If the anatomy does not allow catheterization through the fine needle the bile ducts are well filled up with contrast medium before the needle is removed. With the contrast-filled bile ducts as a guide a second puncture is made with a polyethylene sheathed PTC needle. Availability of bi-plane fluoroscopy markedly increases the success rate of this puncture. If only one-plane fluoroscopy is available the puncture is directed slightly above the bifurcation into the right and left ducts, where they are closest together. After the needle is removed, the sheath is slowly pulled back during intermittent aspiration. As soon as bile can be aspirated, an injection of a small amount of contrast will indicate the exact position of the sheath in the duct. The torque control guide wire is then introduced through the sheath and the drainage procedure is continued as under alternative.

Anterior approach. An anterior approach has the advantage of less liver parenchyma to penetrate before a bile duct is reached. Theoretically this also reduces the number of complications. If the puncture is guided by ultrasound the ventral anterior approach is to be preferred.

The drawback with this approach is that it is difficult to prevent the hands of the operator being in the radiation field although this can be avoided with the new U- or C-arm angiographic units.

The puncture site is close to the xiphoid process and the needle is aimed slightly above the expected position of the liver hilum. If the puncture is guided by ultrasound the shortest route to the bile duct can be selected. Again the fine needle technique under alternative 1 or sheathed needle under alternative 2 can be used.

Complications

Major complications increase from about 3% of examined patients with the fine needle technique (Harbin et al 1980) to 7–23% when a drainage procedure is added (Stambuk et al 1983, Demas et al 1984). In addition, a number of minor complications occur.

* (Surgimed, Denmark; William Cook Europe, Denmark)
** (Mead Johnson, USA)

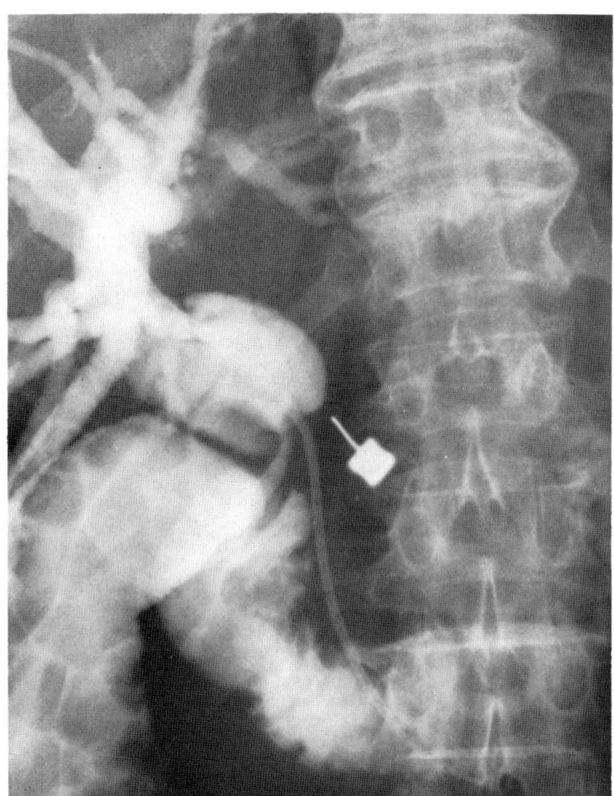

Fig. 36.7 Guided by the cholangiogram and PTC catheter, a percutaneous biopsy is performed

Intraperitoneal bleeding The most feared complication of PTCD is profuse intraperitoneal arterial bleeding. This may be caused by puncture of an intercostal artery or a branch of the hepatic artery. Damaging an intercostal artery can usually be prevented by making the puncture immediately above a rib and not below. It is almost impossible to exclude the possibility of damage to a branch of the hepatic artery. This damage probably happens much more often than we are aware of (Hoevels & Nilsson 1980) but significant bleeding is rare. When haemorrhage occurs it is usually combined with an unsuccessful puncture of a bile duct and the sheathed needle has been removed from the liver parenchyma for another puncture. This suggests that the catheter by itself is a good tamponade for the bleeding artery.

The system using an ultra-thin guide wire inserted through the fine needle reduces the number of punctures and also the complication rate.

Profuse arterial haemorrhage caused by the PTCD procedure can sometimes be life-threatening (Ferrucci et al 1980). If the bleeding does not stop on conservative treatment surgical ligation or transcatheter occlusion of the hepatic artery may be necessary. A liver already damaged by obstructive jaundice does not tolerate the same degree of arterial blood flow deprivation as does a normal liver. It is supposed that dilated bile ducts compress portal venous branches within the liver and reduce portal venous flow. Ligation or transcatheter occlusion of the proper hepatic artery may result in liver failure (Doppman et al 1982). If intrahepatic arterial bleeding does not stop on conservative treatment, transcatheter occlusion of only the bleeding branch of the hepatic artery is desirable.

Bleeding into the bile ducts is a common complication when PTCD is performed (Nakayama et al 1978, Ferrucci et al 1980, Berquist et al 1981) (Ch. 85). To the inexperienced radiologist the finding of blood clots in the contrast filled bile ducts (Fig. 36.8) might be frightening but there are usually no reasons to fear prolonged bleeding. As blood vessels and bile ducts are close together within the liver one can expect blood to enter the bile duct if both are punctured. However, as soon as the drainage catheter is introduced this will tamponade the vessel and prevent further bleeding. If, however, bleeding continues after introduction of a drainage catheter, this might not have been introduced far enough. Side-holes can be located both within the liver parenchyma, blood vessels, and the bile duct.

Subcapsular liver haematoma is a common complication of PTCD. In most cases it is of minor importance and causes no clinical symptoms. It is often an accidental finding when the patient is examined with CT within a few days of the procedure. If the CT examination is repeated one or two weeks later the haematoma is usually resorbed.

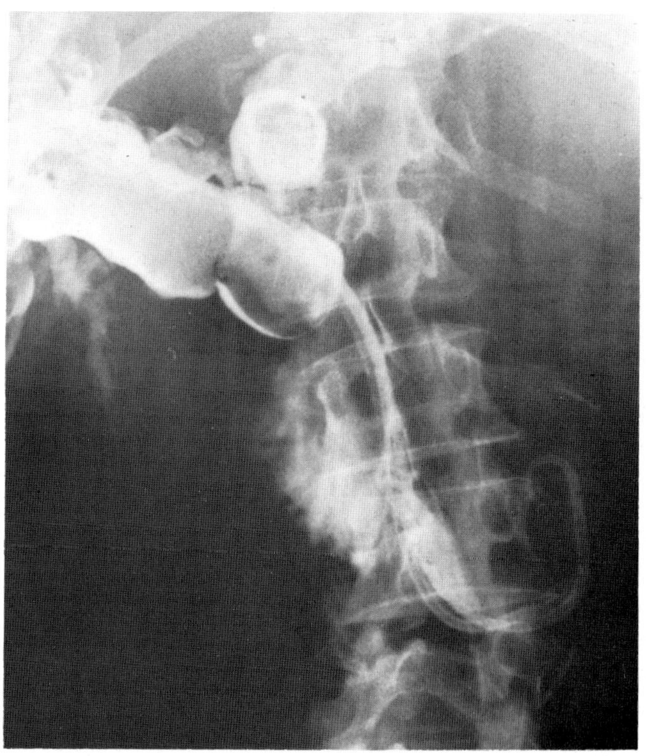

Fig. 36.8 PTC with tip of drainage catheter into the duodenum. Filling defects in the bile ducts are caused by blood clots

Infection Septicaemia may be an immediate result of the PTCD procedure. The bile is commonly infected in patients with obstructive jaundice (Berk et al 1978, Ferrucci et al 1980, Berquist et al 1981) (Ch. 11.) more often in patients with calculi than in those with a malignant lesion (Harbin et al 1980). In some cases multiple abscesses are scattered in the liver parenchyma with communications to the bile ducts (Fig. 36.9).

There are few ways to prevent septicaemia when pus is present within the bile ducts or when biliary abscesses are present in the parenchyma of the liver. One way to reduce the risk of septicaemia is not to overfill the bile ducts with contrast medium when the puncture has been performed. The elevated bile duct pressure may force infected bile through into the blood stream. As soon as a catheter is well anchored into the bile ducts, aspiration of bile should be performed in order to reduce the pressure. One has to check carefully that side-holes of the drainage catheter are not placed within the liver parenchyma and in that way produce direct communication between a bile duct and the vascular system (Fig. 36.6). It is also wise to have the patient on broad spectrum antibiotic treatment prior to the PTCD procedure. The number of complications may be reduced if a bile duct of the left lobe is punctured since there is less liver parenchyma to be traversed before the bile duct is reached.

Infection can also spread to a subcapsular or extrahepatic haematoma and an abscess may develop between the liver and the abdominal wall around the drainage catheter. This is not an unusual finding if the drainage catheter has been displaced or accidentally removed. Repuncture close to the previous puncture site then almost always results in septicaemia.

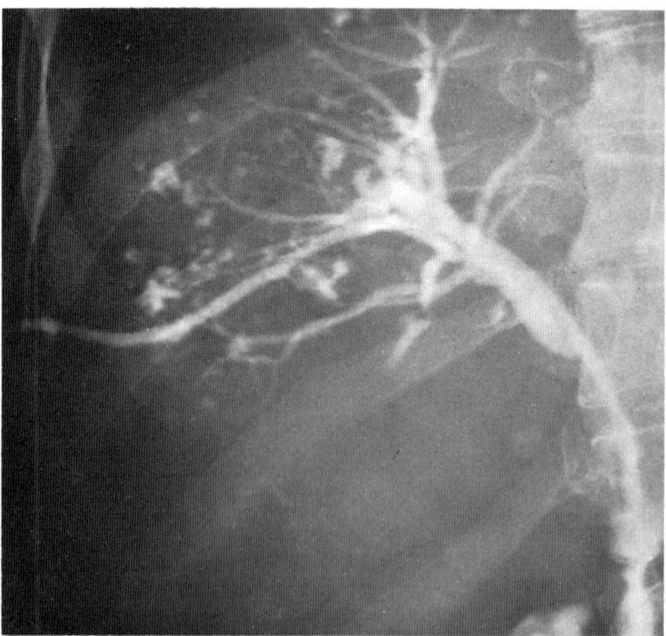

Fig. 36.9 Cholangiogram in patient with PTCD catheter demonstrates multiple abscesses within the liver

Cholangitis, if not present at the time of the PTCD procedure, may complicate the later course of the drainage (Hoevels et al 1978, Ferrucci et al 1980, Ring & McLean, McPherson et al 1982). The patient's temperature curve has to be closely observed and bile culture performed in order to supply him with adequate antibiotic.

In a consecutive series of 237 PTC and PTCD procedures, we found that during the drainage period the bile was more often infected when the catheter was placed with the tip in the duodenum than if it was above the papilla of Vater or above the obstruction (Nilsson et al 1983). We have also shown, by giving the patients an isotope juice to drink, that the isotope appears in the bag if the patient is on combined internal–external drainage. This latter finding has led us to exclude external drainage from the time of the introduction of the catheter if this has been passed down into the duodenum.

Bile leakage into the peritoneal cavity causes intense pain if the leak occurs during the PTCD procedure (Harbin et al 1980). If the leak occurs later as a consequence of a dislodged catheter severe pain is unusual but bile ascites may develop (Rosato et al 1970). In most cases intense pain because of bile leak is caused by inadvertent puncture of the gallbladder. This may be prevented by making the puncture horizontally and entering the liver at a point midway between the ventral and dorsal surface of the body. If, however, the sheathed needle goes too far ventrally and the gallbladder is punctured this becomes evident as soon as contrast medium is injected. If the needle is removed for another puncture, bile leak from the gallbladder will immediately result in intense abdominal pain. In most cases the pain reaction can be prevented by leaving the catheter in the gallbladder when the stylet is removed. After as much bile as possible has been removed from the gallbladder another sheathed needle is used for a repeat puncture. The first sheath in the gallbladder is removed when the drainage procedure is completed.

Insufficient drainage may cause bile to leak along the catheter to the peritoneal cavity. This can usually be handled by changing the drainage catheter to another with larger side-holes or by injection of Mucomyst to reduce the viscosity of the bile.

Pneumothorax, leak of bile, or bleeding into the right pleural cavity are rare complications (Hoevels et al 1978, Harbin et al 1980, Berquist et al 1981) but may occur as the PTCD catheter is often introduced through the obliterated pleural sinus (Nakayama et al 1978) (Fig. 36.10). In order to gain good access to the bile duct the puncture must be performed as directly as possible towards the hilum of the liver. If the puncture is performed too far caudally, the introduction of a drainage catheter is much more difficult. Bleeding at the time of the first PTCD procedure may find its way to the pleura rather than to the

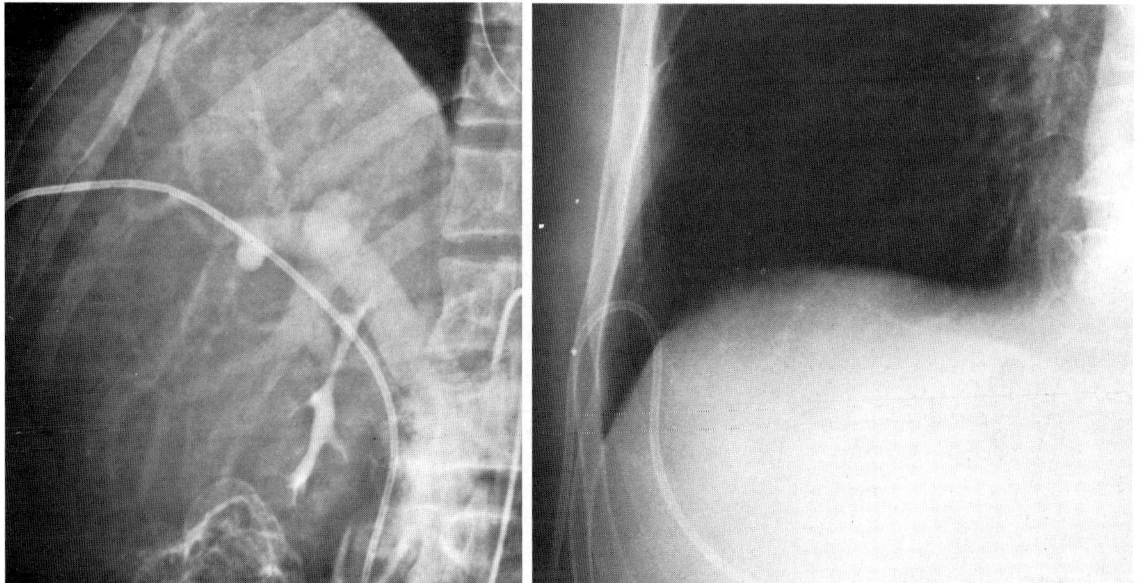

Fig. 36.10 Patient with PTCD for pancreatic carcinoma. a. With patient supine during angiography for resectability the catheter seems to be safe below the pleural sinus. b. With patient upright for chest film the catheter is seen to pass through the pleura

peritoneum, but in most cases pleural adhesions which form within days will prevent these complications. Pneumothorax can be caused by displacement of the drainage catheter leaving side-holes both outside the body of the patient and within the pleura. Bile leak as well as ascites can follow a similar route to the pleura (Fig. 36.11).

Displacement of the drainage catheter is common if the drainage catheter has not passed through the tumour obstruction and on to the duodenum. This displacement is the most common cause of complications such as septicaemia, abscess formation and bile leak. It is therefore important to try to pass the bile duct obstruction in every case in order to anchor the drainage catheter in the duodenum. In order to allow early recognition of catheter displacement a daily scout film of the right upper abdomen is taken during the first seven days following the PTCD procedure. As soon as even slight displacement is recognized the catheter is repositioned.

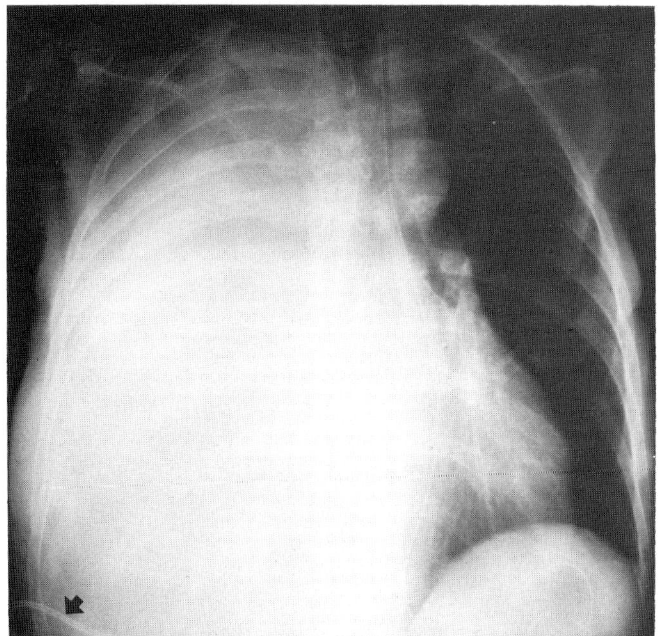

Fig. 36.11 Leak of ascites to the right pleural cavity after PTCD. PTCD catheter (Arrow)

It has been postulated that a drainage catheter in the region of the papilla of Vater might block the pancreatic duct and be the cause of pancreatitis. Pancreatitis is, however, rare in combination with PTCD and there is no indication that obstruction from the catheter is the causative factor (Berquist et al 1981). If for some reason the drainage catheter is accidentally dislodged the patient has to be treated immediately. Often it is possible to catheterize the tract through the abdominal wall and the liver with the aid of a guide wire after the tract has been visualized by injection of a small amount of contrast medium (Ring & McLean 1981) (Fig. 36.12).

Percutaneous removal of retained stones (Ch. 49.)

Indications

Retained stones in the bile ducts after cholecystectomy and/or choledocho-lithotomy are not very frequent when compared with the number of surgical procedures performed. However, it is always a severe setback to find residual stones in the bile ducts when postoperative cholangiography is performed.

For more than ten years a technique has been used to

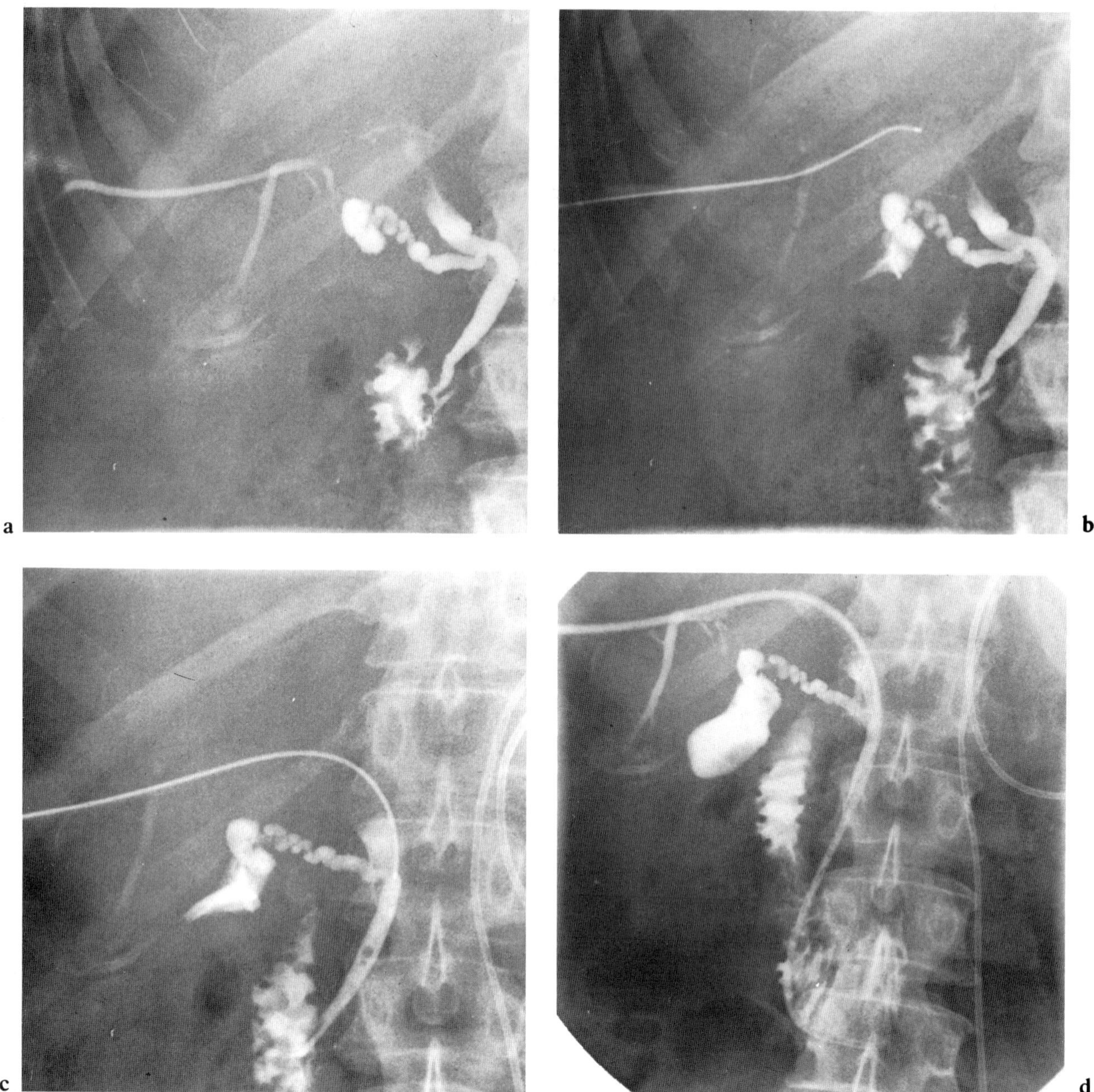

Fig. 36.12 PTCD catheter has been accidentally removed. a. Contrast injected through the cutaneous fistula fills the tract and bile ducts. b. A torque control guide wire is manipulated through the contrast filled tract and into the bile ducts (c). d. A new drainage catheter is inserted

remove retained stones percutaneously through the T-tube tract (Mazzariello 1970, Burhenne 1973, 1980) with a Dormia basket (Fig. 36.13). With the increased skill of the endoscopists this percutaneous technique of stone removal has been augmented by endoscopic sphincterotomy (Rösch et al 1981). The relationship of percutaneous and endoscopic approaches to surgical operation is discussed in Ch. 50.

Stones are sometimes found in the bile ducts when PTC is performed for obstructive jaundice. These stones can be removed either after endoscopic sphincterotomy or if for some reason this is contraindicated stones can be moved down into the duodenum after balloon dilatation of the papilla of Vater (Fig. 36.14). Cases are reported where the stones have been extracted through the parenchyma of the liver, but this is not advisable.

Technique

Stone removal through the T-tube tract (Ch. 48) The T-tube has to be left in place for four to six weeks to allow a granulation track to develop around the catheter. The

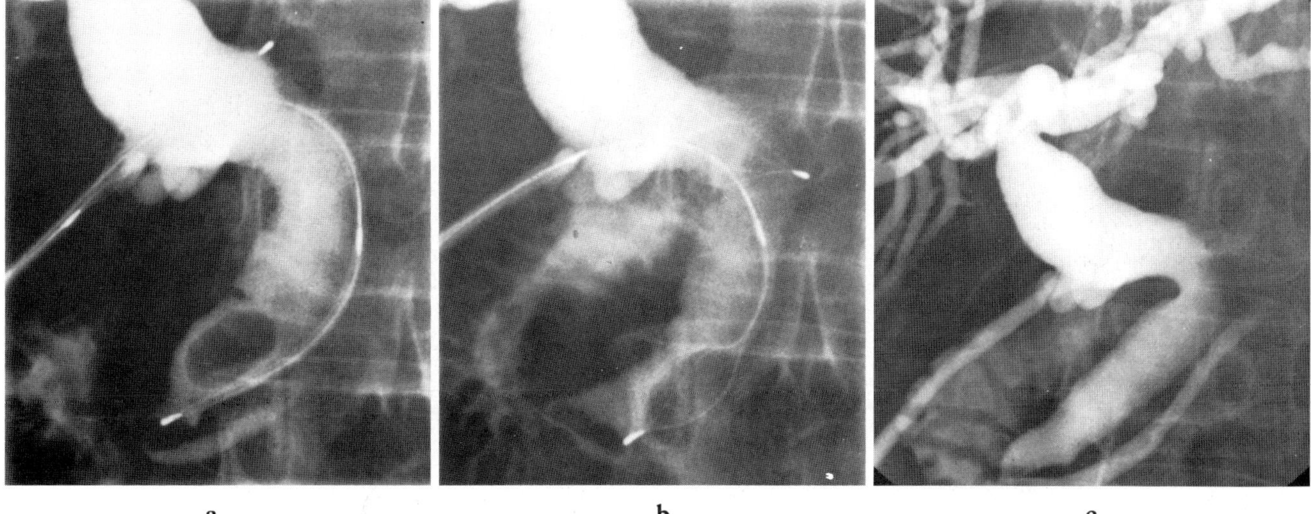

Fig. 36.13 Retained stone in common bile duct after cholecystectomy. a. Contrast injected through T-tube and two Dormia baskets are introduced; one with the tip at the papilla, the other higher up. b. The stone at the papilla is trapped in the basket and removed. c. Cholangiogram afterwards shows no filling defects

patient is kept on antibiotics from the day before and for three to four days after the procedure. Pain medication is usually not indicated and was needed in only four of 661 patients treated by Burhenne (1980).

After contrast has been injected into the bile ducts a teflon-coated torque control guide wire is manipulated through the T-tube into the bile duct. The T-tube is then removed leaving the guide wire in the bile duct. If the guide wire cannot be manipulated through the T-tube, this is removed. Contrast is injected into the fistula tract and guided by the contrast-filled tract, the operator manipulates the torque control guide wire into the bile duct under fluoroscopic control.

With the guide wire in place in the bile duct a teflon catheter is slid over the guide wire until also positioned in the bile duct. The guide wire is exchanged for a Dormia® basket which is placed at the level of the stone. By rotation of the basket the stone can be moved into its lumen and trapped by pulling the basket back. The catheter and basket with the trapped stone are then extracted through the old T-tube tract. If large stones are retained in the bile duct and a small sized T-tube has been used, it is wise to dilate the tract before the stone is extracted. Stones in intrahepatic bile ducts can be pulled down into the common bile duct with a small balloon catheter if they cannot be caught with a basket in the original position.

In cases with stones which cannot be trapped in the basket balloon, dilatation of the papilla of Vater can be successfully tried (Centola et al 1981).

Complications

When multiple stones are present in the bile duct the sinus tract can be damaged when the first stone is removed. This damage may prevent any further catheter guide wire introduction but is otherwise harmless, provided the residual stones are not blocking the bile flow to the duodenum. In that case a bile fistula may develop.

Bile is often infected in patients with biliary tract stones (Harbin et al 1980) and manipulations within the bile ducts can cause fever for a few days after the stone extraction. Sepsis is infrequent and was only reported in two of 612 patients reported by Burhenne (1976).

Stone removal after percutaneous transhepatic cholangiography

Technique When stones of a size to allow passage to the duodenum are found at PTC a guide wire is manipulated through the papilla of Vater into the duodenum. After dilatation of the canal through the liver parenchyma a vascular balloon catheter of appropriate size is advanced over the guide wire into the region of the papilla. The balloon is inflated for two to three minutes several times and the balloon catheter is then exchanged for a special type of Dormia basket* with a guide wire at the tip of the basket. With the guide wire tip of the basket in the duodenum the stone is caught in the basket and forcefully pushed through the previously dilated papilla. This manoeuvre may be extended over several minutes in order to distend the papilla enough to allow the basket with the stone to pass.

Complications have not been seen with this procedure. Dilatation of the papilla can cause pain and the patients need medication.

* (Schwarz biliary stone removal basket, William Cook Europe *Denmark*).

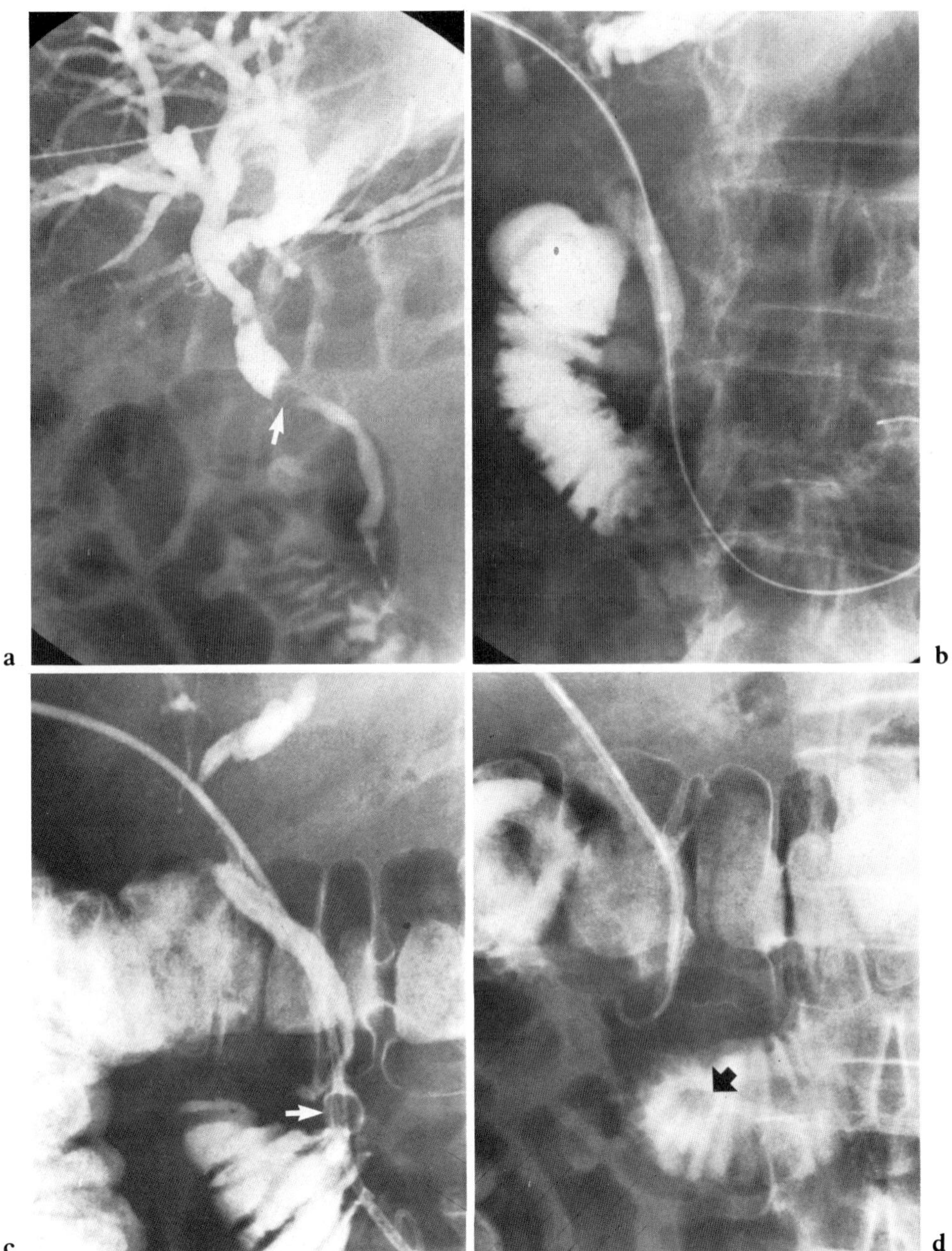

Fig. 36.14 a. PTC demonstrates a stone (arrow) in the common bile duct in patient with suppurative cholecystitis where cholecystectomy and choledochotomy was unsuccessful because of adhesions and haemorrhage. Stricture of common bile duct prevents the stone from moving down after sphincterotomy. b. Percutaneous balloon dilatation of the strictured bile duct makes it possible to move the stone down to the papilla (arrow in c) and push it into the duodenum (arrow in d)

Percutaneous insertion of bile duct endoprostheses (Ch. 68)

Indications

At our institution indications for biliary endoprostheses are patients with non-resectable malignant tumours and a presumptive survival of only a few months after the diagnosis (Fig. 36.15). We prefer, however, to leave these patients with a PTC catheter as this is easily exchanged if obliterated but if the patient feels very uncomfortable with the drainage catheter an endoprosthesis is introduced.

During the last year more and more endoscopically introduced transpapillary endoprostheses (Ch. 80) have been introduced and without doubt this technique will be important in the future (Huibregtse & Tytgat 1982).

Technique

Endoprostheses of many different sizes have been tried from small diameter 2 mm (Burcharth et al 1981) to

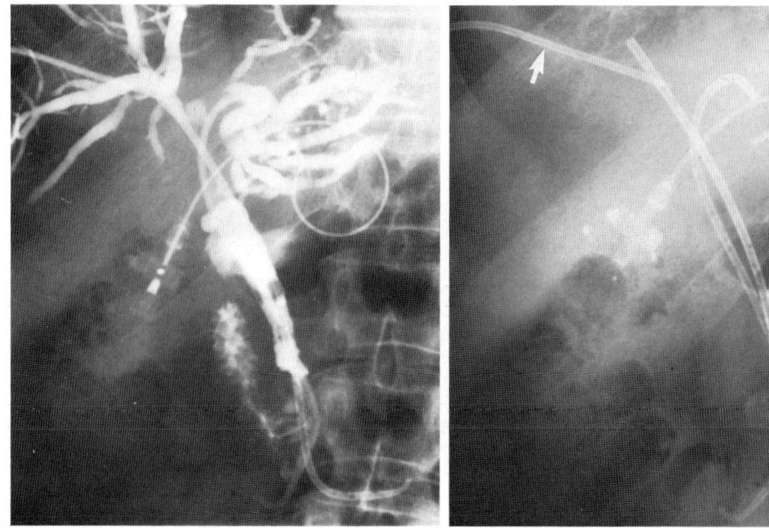

Fig. 36.15 Patient with tumour stricture at the bifurcation of the bile ducts into right and left lobe. Palliation with stents into the right and left bile ducts and their tip into duodenum. a. Contrast injected through catheter left for control of stent function shows the tumour stricture at bifurcation level. b. The stents in the bile ducts before the catheter (arrow) for control cholangiogram is removed

large 4 mm (Hoevels et al 1980, Dooley et al 1981). The smaller diameter has been used with the presumption that the increased flow rate of bile should reduce sludging within the endoprosthesis. Originally we used the 4-mm Teflon endoprosthesis but later changed to 3-mm in order to reduce parenchymal liver damage during the introduction.

We usually introduce the endoprosthesis after PTCD has been performed for one or two weeks and work-up of the patient has shown non-resectability of a malignant tumour.

The tract of the PTCD cathether is dilated up to the size of the endoprosthesis. The endoprosthesis supplied with multiple side-holes and a curved tip is positioned in the duodenum and its proximal end is well above the obstructing lesion. If the entrance of the PTC catheter is too low to allow enough length of the endoprosthesis above the tumour, a sling retraction technique can be used to accomplish an adequate position (Owman & Lunderquist 1983). An external catheter is usually left in the bile duct above the endoprosthesis for a few days to enable control of the function of the endoprosthesis (Fig. 36.15b).

Complications

Complications are mainly those connected with the PTCD procedure with a few additional ones specific to this kind of treatment (Hoevels et al 1980, Burcharth et al 1981, Dooley et al 1981, Gouma et al 1983).

Displacement of the endoprosthesis occurs in about 5% of cases. In most the stent is dislocated distally leaving the proximal end within the tumour. To prevent distal dislocation a technique has been tried to anchor the stent with a nylon line (Owman & Lunderquist 1983). This, however, will not prevent proximal displacement which has been reported in a few cases.

Clogging of the endoprosthesis is the main contraindication to the use of this technique in patients who are likely to survive a longer period of time. PTCD and insertion of a stent are both painful procedures and very few patients who have experienced this kind of treatment are willing to have it repeated.

Clogging of the stent may occur after one or two months in some patients but it can be expected in almost all patients surviving more than six months. Therefore it is advisable to retain a PTCD catheter in patients with expected long survival. To maintain a good function of this catheter it is exchanged for a new one every other month. This can be performed on an out-patient basis.

Duodenal perforation produced by pressure necrosis from a straight endoprosthesis extending too far into the duodenum is a rare complication. We have experienced one such case.

Transcatheter radiation of bile duct carcinoma (Ch. 65).

Indications

A new technique for palliative treatment of patients with bile duct carcinoma has recently been reported (Fletcher et al 1981, Herskovic et al 1981). The treatment was designed for non-resectable tumours at the bifurcation level of the bile ducts but can certainly be extended to tumours in any part of the bile duct system where a resection is not possible.

Technique

After PTCD has disclosed a tumour suitable for the treatment, a 0.3 mm iridium-192 wire of desired length is loaded into an angiographic guide wire after its core has been removed. Under fluoroscopic control the guide wire is inserted into the PTCD catheter until the iridium-192 wire is located at the level of the obstructing tumour. A radiation dose of 40–50 Gy is delivered over 48 hours. The wire is then removed leaving the PTCD catheter in place for drainage.

From the few patients treated so far with this technique it is impossible to tell how it might influence the survival of the patients. One advantage might be that the drainage catheter can be removed after the size of the obstructing tumour has been reduced.

Complications

Only one complication has been reported so far (E. Ring, personal communication). This was a patient where necrosis of the tumour and adjacent tissue caused a fistula between the bile duct and the portal vein.

Balloon dilatation of benign strictures of the bile ducts (Ch. 58)

Indications

Most benign strictures of the bile ducts are iatrogenic either as an effect of damage asociated with cholecystectomy or fibrotic scarring of a surgical bilio-digestive anastomosis.

When the diagnosis is made at PTC there is the possibility to extend the procedure to a therapeutic one and dilate the stricture with a balloon catheter (Martin et al 1980, Herskovic et al 1981). The place of these techniques is discussed in Ch. 58.

Balloon dilatation has also been successfully tried in

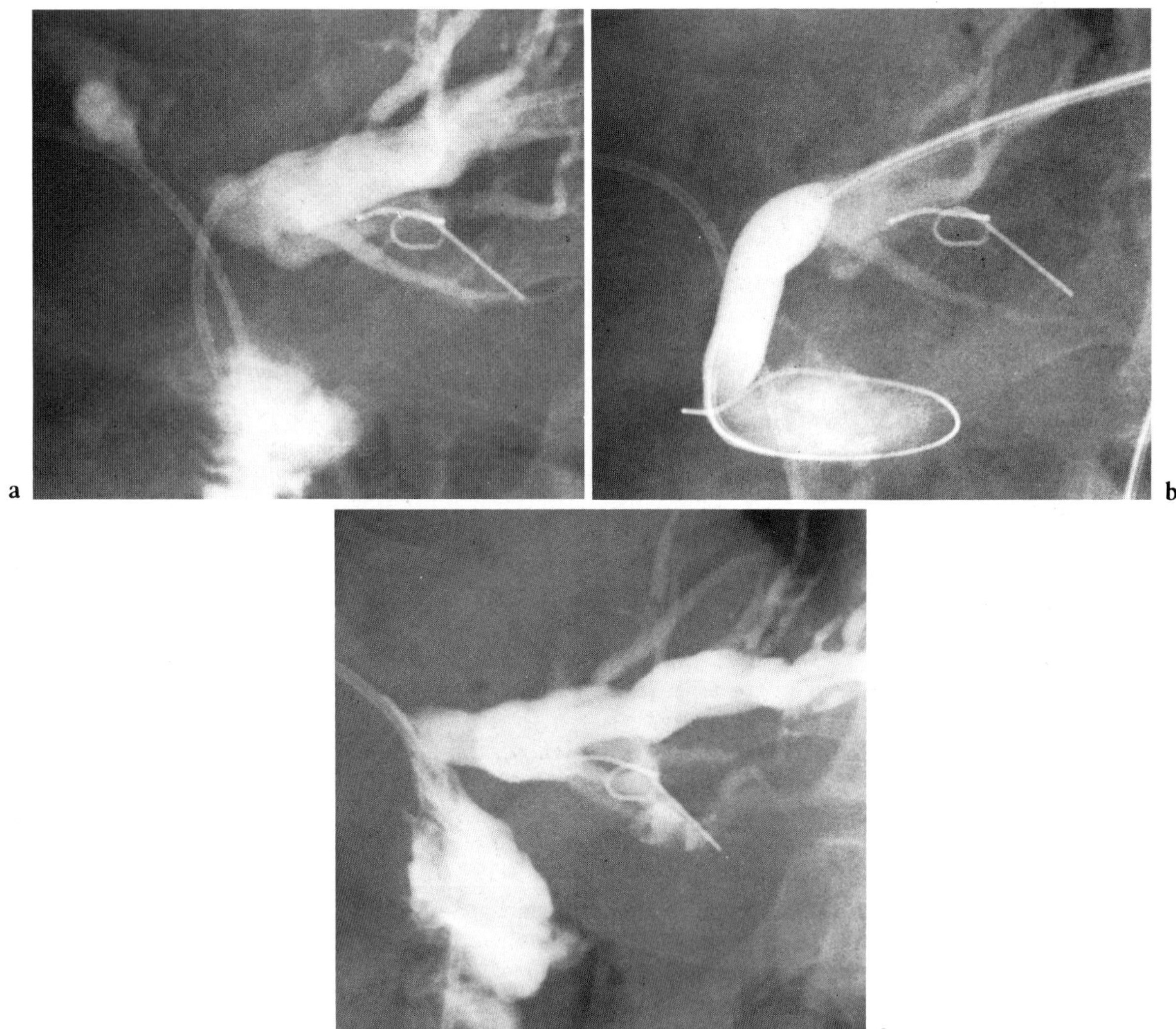

Fig. 36.16 a. Right and left PTCD through stricture of hepaticojejunostomy. b. Balloon dilatation of stricture. c. Wide anastomosis after dilatation

patients with strictures due to primary sclerosing cholangitis (Martin et al 1981).

Technique

As soon as a PTC catheter has been able to advance beyond the stricture, the canal through the liver is dilated to allow for the vascular balloon catheter of desired diameter to pass. Unlike the dilatation of vascular strictures the balloon has to be distended over a longer period of time. Alternating one hour inflation with deflation periods for 8–12 hours has been tried (Salomonowitz et al 1984).

It is advisable to leave a PTCD catheter in place after the dilatation for follow-up. In this way repeated dilatations can be performed at one to two monthly intervals until re-stenosis seems unlikely.

Complications

The dilatation procedure is painful to the patient and valium or narcotics are necessary. Serious complications are not reported. Experience is still too limited to allow assessment of the frequency of restenosis. There seems to be an indication that bilio-digestive anastomotic strictures respond better than other strictures within the bile duct system (Fig. 36.16) (Ch. 58).

Transhepatic obliteration of oesophageal varices

As this method of treating patients with portal hypertension and bleeding oesophageal varices is more extensively covered in Ch. 107, the reader is referred to that chapter.

REFERENCES

Bengmark S, Ericsson M, Lunderquist A, Mårtensson H, Nobin A, Sako M 1982 Temporary liver dearterialization in patients with metastatic carcinoid disease. World Journal of Surgery 6: 46–53

Berk R N, Ferrucci J T, Goldstein H M, Leopold G R, Loeb P M, Parkey R W, Stanley R J 1978 Diagnostic imaging of the liver and bile ducts. Investigative Radiology 13: 265–278

Berquist T H, May G R, Johnson C M, Adson M A, Thistle J L 1981 Percutaneous biliary decompression: Internal and external drainage in 50 patients. American Journal of Roentgenology 136: 901–906

Bernardino M E, Chuang V P, Wallace S, Thomas J L, Soo C S 1981 Therapeutically infarcted tumors: CT findings. American Journal of Roentgenology 136: 527–530

Blumgart L H, Allison D J 1982 Resection and embolization in the management of secondary hepatic tumours. World Journal of Surgery 6: 32–45

Burcharth F et al 1981 Nonsurgical internal biliary drainage by endoprosthesis. Surgery, Gynecology and Obstetrics 153: 857–860

Burhenne H J 1973 Nonoperative retained biliary tract stone extraction. A new roentgenologic technique. American Journal of Roentgenology 117: 388–399

Burhenne H J 1976 Complications of nonoperative extraction of retained common duct stones. American Journal of Surgery 131: 260–262

Burhenne H J 1980 Percutaneous extraction of retained biliary tract stones: 661 patients. American Journal of Roentgenology 134: 888–898

Centola C A P, Jander H P, Stauffer A, Russinovich N A E 1981 Balloon dilatation of the papilla of Vater to biliary stone passage. American Journal of Roentgenology 136: 613–614

Chuang V P, Wallace S 1981 Hepatic artery embolization in the treatment of hepatic neoplasms. Radiology 140: 51–58

Chuang V P, Wallace S, Soo C S, Charnsangavej C, Bowers T 1982 Therapeutic Ivalon embolization of hepatic tumours. American Journal of Roentgenology 138: 289–294

Chuang V P, Wallace S, Carrasco H, Charnsangavej C 1984 Embolization as a therapeutic modality. The Cancer Bulletin 36: 15–20

Clark R A, Towbin R 1983 Abscess drainage with CT and ultrasound guidance. Radiological Clinics of North America 21: 445–459

Clouse M E, Lee R G 1984 Management of the posthepatic artery embolization syndrome. Radiology 152:238

De Jode L R, Nicholls R D, Wright P L 1976 Ischaemic necrosis of the gallbladder following hepatic artery embolism. British Journal of Surgery 63: 621–623

Demas B E, Moss A A, Goldberg H I 1984 Computed tomographic diagnosis of complications of transhepatic cholangiography and percutaneous biliary drainage. Gastrointestinal Radiology 9: 219–222

Denning D A, Ellison C, Carey L C 1981 Preoperative percutaneous transhepatic biliary decompression lowers operative morbidity in patients with obstructive jaundice. American Journal of Surgery 141: 61–65

Dooley J S, Dick R, Irving D, Olney J, Sherlock S 1981 Relief of bile duct obstruction by the percutaneous transhepatic insertion of an endoprosthesis. Clinical Radiology 32: 163–172

Doppman J L, Girton M, Vermess M 1982 The risk of hepatic artery embolization in the presence of obstructive jaundice. Radiology 143: 37–43

Doppman J L, Girton M E 1984 Bile duct scarring following ethanol embolization of the hepatic artery: an experimental study in monkeys. Radiology 152: 621–626

Ferrucci Jr J T, Mueller P R, Harbin W P 1980 Percutaneous transhepatic biliary drainage. Radiology 135: 1–13

Fletcher M S, Dawson J L, Wheeler P G, Brinkley D, Nunnerley H, Williams R 1981 Treatment of high bile duct carcinoma by internal radiotherapy with iridium-192 wire. Lancet ii No. 8239: 172–174

Gouma D J, Wesdorp R I C, Oostenbroek R J, Soeters P B, Greep J M 1983 Percutaneous transhepatic drainage and insertion of an endoprosthesis for obstructive jaundice. American Journal of Surgery 145: 763–767

Greenwood L H, Collins T L, Yrizarry J M 1982 Percutaneous management of multiple liver abscesses. Case report. American Journal of Roentgenology 139: 390–392

Gundry S R, Strodel W E, Knol J A, Eckhauser F E, Thompson N W 1984 Efficacy or preoperatice biliary tract decompression in patients with obstructive jaundice. Archives of Surgery 119: 703–708

Harbin W P, Mueller P R, Ferrucci Jr J T 1980 Transhepatic cholangiography: complications and use patterns of the fine needle technique. Radiology 135: 15–22

Heimbach D M, Ferguson G S, Harley J D 1978 Treatment of traumatic hemobilia with angiographic embolization. Journal of Trauma 18: 221–224

Herskovic A, Heaston D, Engler M J, Fishburn R I, Jones R S, Noell K T 1981 Irradiation of biliary carcinoma. Radiology 139: 219–222

Hoevels J, Lunderquist A, Ihse I 1978 Perkutane transhepatische Intubation der Gallengänge zur kombinierten inneren und äusseren Drainage bei extrahepatischer Cholestase. Fortschritte auf dem Gebiete der Röntgenstrahlen 129: 533–550

Hoevels J, Nilsson U 1980 Intrahepatic vascular lesions following nonsurgical percutaneous transhepatic bile duct intubation. Gastrointestinal Radiology 5: 127–135

Hoevels J, Lunderquist A, Owman T, Ihse I 1980 A large-bore Teflon endoprosthesis with side holes for nonoperative decompression of the biliary tract in malignant obstructive jaundice. Gastrointestinal Radiology 5: 361–366

Huibregtse K, Tytgat G N, 1982 Palliative treatment of obstructive jaundice by transpapillary introduction of large bore bile duct endoprosthesis. Gut 23: 371–375

Idema A A J, Niermeyer P, Oldhoff J 1977 Hepatic dearterialization for carcinoid syndrome due to liver metastases. Archivum Chirurgicum Neerlandicum 27: 125–133

Konno T et al 1983 Effect of arterial administration of high-molecular-weight anticancer agent SMANCS with lipid lymphographic agent on hepatoma: a preliminary report. European Journal of Cancer and Clinical Oncology 19: 1053–1065

Lunderquist A, Ericsson M, Nobin A, Sandén G 1982 Gelfoam powder embolization of the hepatic artery in liver metastases of carcinoid tumour. Radiologe 22: 65–70

Martin E, Karlson K B, Fankuchen E I, Mattern R F, Casarella W J 1980 Percutaneous transhepatic dilatation of intrahepatic biliary strictures. American Journal of Roentgenology 135: 837–840

Martin E C, Fankuchen E I, Schultz R, Casarella W J 1981 Percutaneous dilatation in primary sclerosing cholangitis: two experiences. American Journal of Roentgenology 137: 603–605

McPherson G A D, Benjamin I S, Habib N A, Bowley N B, Blumgart L H 1982 Percutaneous transhepatic drainage in obstructive jaundice: advantages and problems. British Journal of Surgery 69: 261–264

Mazzariello R M 1970 Removal of residual biliary calculi without operation. Surgery 67: 566–573

Nakayama T, Ikeda A, Okuda K 1978 Percutaneous transhepatic drainage of the biliary tract. Technique and results in 104 cases. Gastroenterology 74: 554–559

Nilsson U, Evander A, Ihse I, Lunderquist A, Mocibob A 1983 Percutaneous transhepatic cholangiography and drainage. Risks and complications. Acta Radiologica: Diagnosis 24: 433–439

Owman T, Lunderquist A 1983 Sling retraction for proximal placement of percutaneous transhepatic biliary endoprosthesis. Radiology 146: 228–229

Pitt H A, Cameron J L, Postier R G, Gadacz T R 1981 Factors affecting mortality in biliary tract surgery. American Journal of Surgery 141: 66–72

Ring E J, McLean G K 1981 Interventional radiology. Principles and techniques. Little Brown, Boston

Rosato E F, Berkowitz H D, Roberts B 1970 Bile ascites. Surgery, Gynecology and Obstetrics 130: 494–496

Rösch W, Riemann J F, Lux G, Lindner H G 1981 Long-term follow-up after endoscopic sphincterotomy. Endoscopy 13: 152–153

Rubin B E, Katzen B T 1977 Selective hepatic artery embolization to control massive hepatic hemorrhage after trauma. American Journal of Roentgenology 129: 253–256

Salomonowitz E et al 1984 Balloon dilatation of benign biliary strictures. Radiology 151: 613–611

Scheinfeld A M, Steiner A E, Rivkin L B, Dermer R H, Shemesh O N, Dolberg M S 1982 Transcutaneous drainage of abscesses of the liver guided by computed tomography scan. Surgery, Gynecology and Obstetrics 155: 662–666

Schmidt B, Bhatt G M, Abo M N 1980 Management of post-traumatic vascular malformations of the liver by catheter embolization. American Journal of Surgery 140: 332–335

Stambuk E C, Pitt H A, Pais O, Mann L L, Lois J F, Gomes A S 1983 Percutaneous transhepatic drainage. Archives of Surgery 118: 1388–1394

Stanley P, Grinnell V S, Stanton R E, Williams K O, Shore N A 1983 Therapeutic embolization of infantile hepatic hemangioma with polyvinyl alcohol. American Journal of Roentgenology 141: 1047–1051

Stephen J L. Graham-Smith D G 1972 Treatment of the carcinoid syndrome by local removal of hepatic metastases. Proceedings of the Royal Society of Medicine 65: 444–445

Stridbeck H, Lörelius L E, Reuter S R 1984 Collateral circulation following repeated distal embolization of the hepatic artery in pigs. Investigative Radiology 19: 179–183

van Sonnenberg E, Ferrucci J T, Mueller P R, Wittenberg J, Simeone J F 1982 Percutaneous drainage of abscesses and fluid collections: Technique, results and application. Radiology 142: 1–10

White R I, Kaufman S L, Barth K H, De Capiro V, Strandberg J D 1979 Therapeutic embolization with detachable silicone balloons, Journal of the American Medical Association 241: 1257–1260

Yamada R, Sato M, Kawabata M, Nakatsuka H, Takashima S 1983 Hepatic artery embolization in 120 patients with unresectable hepatoma. Radiology 148:397–401

G. A. D. McPherson and L. H. Blumgart

Percutaneous transhepatic and endoscopic drainage and endoprosthesis — surgical relevance

The development of percutaneous and endoscopic intubation of the biliary tract provides new therapeutic options in the management of the patient with obstructive jaundice. Firstly, in patients who are either medically unfit for surgery or in whom surgical biliary bypass is not possible, non-operative intubation offers a therapeutic alternative to allow decompression of the biliary tract. Secondly, as a non-operative first stage in the management of biliary tract obstruction prior to definitive surgery, patients can be intubated either percutaneously or endoscopically. The results of these approaches should be considered in relation to the risks of surgery in the management of obstructive jaundice.

The mortality and morbidity for operations on the obstructed biliary tract are high. The pooled operative mortality for 1699 patients with malignant biliary tract obstruction drawn from eight reputable series published in the 1970s is 20% (Benjamin 1981). For benign biliary tract obstruction the mortality is much lower (McSherry 1982) although figures as high as 17% have been reported for gallstone obstruction in the presence of sepsis (Welch & Donaldson 1976). Recent retrospective studies of risk factors related to mortality in the jaundiced patient who undergoes surgery have produced broadly comparable results but failed to agree as to precisely which factors are the most important (Pitt et al 1981, Blamey et al 1983, Dixon et al 1982). Pitt et al (1981) analyzed the outcome of 155 consecutive patients undergoing biliary tract surgery. Of a total of 15 clinical and laboratory parameters that were examined no less than 10 were significantly correlated with surgical outcome. These factors are listed in Table 37.1. Blamey et al (1983) applied a linear discriminant analysis to a retrospective group of 186 patients and found four out of eight factors that might affect outcome which had a significant association with mortality. These were a raised serum creatinine, low serum albumin, age over 60 and a raised serum bilirubin. Indeed, the operative mortality for patients with a preoperative serum bilirubin concentration of less than 50 μmol/l was 2% in 97 patients compared with 24% for patients in whom the preoperative serum bilirubin was greater than 50 μmol/l. Dixon et al (1982) reported a series of 373 patients undergoing surgery for relief of bile duct obstruction and, using a multivariate analysis, identified only three independent factors associated with increased operative morbidity and mortality. These were an initial haematocrit of 30% or less, an initial plasma bilirubin of greater than 200 μmol/l and malignancy as the cause of the obstruction.

Table 37.1 Clinical and laboratory risk factors correlated with mortality in patients undergoing biliary tract surgery

Disease	Malignancy
Age	> 60 years
Fever	> 38°C
Haematocrit	< 30%
Wbc	> 10 000/mm^3
Blood urea nitrogen	> 20 g/100 ml
Creatinine	> 1.3 mg/100 ml
Albumin	< 3 g/100 ml
Bilirubin	> 10 mg/100 ml
Alkaline phosphatase	> 100 iu/1

(Pitt et al 1981)

Thus although there is broad agreement on the risk factors facing the jaundiced patient at operation, precise identification of the individual patient at high risk remains a problem. Indeed it is only by an ability to select such patients that the advantages and disadvantages of any technique for the relief of jaundice can be properly assessed. Furthermore, controlled or comparative studies examining the merits of one technical approach against another depend on the selection of patients at comparable risk.

These general factors in relation to the risks of treatment of obstructive jaundice must be taken into account in assessing the results of studies of percutaneous and endoscopic intubational techniques. The purpose of this chapter is to examine the relevance of non-operative intubation of the biliary tract as regards preliminary preoperative biliary decompression and in providing an alternative option to surgery.

INTUBATIONAL BILIARY DRAINAGE AND ENDOPROSTHESIS — AN ALTERNATIVE TO SURGERY IN MALIGNANT OBSTRUCTION

The essential features of treatment for suspected malignant disease obstructing the biliary tract are threefold. Firstly, it is desirable to obtain full diagnosis and in particular cholangiographic information. Histological confirmation of malignancy is desirable. Secondly, it is necessary to select cases for potential curative treatment by removal of the tumour. Thirdly, it is important to obtain adequate biliary enteric drainage. The ideal is of course to combine all three objectives, namely precise diagnosis, adequate biliary drainage and curative removal of the offending tumour.

It is not intended in this chapter to go into detail regarding cholangiography or the methods for obtaining confirmation of a diagnosis of malignancy by means of aspiration or exfoliative cytology (Okamura et al 1983, Dalton Clarke et al 1986) (Ch. 24) or operative biopsy (Blumgart et al 1984a) (Ch. 65). Suffice it to say that the accurate pathological diagnosis of the cause of obstruction is of considerable importance. Indeed benign bile duct stricture closely mimicking malignancy may occur in up to 8% of cases (Hadjis et al 1985) suspected to be malignant on clinical and radiological grounds (Ch. 65). Since such strictures are easily excised or bypassed with excellent results, patients should not be submitted to indiscriminate intubational techniques which have their own hazards. Tumours of the periampullary region and pancreas are notoriously difficult to diagnose with accuracy and there is probably a 10–15% rate of wrong diagnosis in this region. Adenocarcinoma of the pancreas or low bile duct may be mistakenly diagnosed in the presence of chronic pancreatitis, cystadenoma, lymphoma or some other pancreatic lesion (Jones et al 1985). Tumours of the papilla of Vater itself are more easily diagnosed and histological material obtained at endoscopy. Certainly the risks of endoscopic or percutaneous intubational drainage techniques must be taken into account along with the age and general condition of the patient before they are chosen as primary methods of treatment in undiagnosed cases which may be better served by traditional surgical approaches.

The preoperative assessment of resectability both in proximal and distal cancers obstructing the biliary tract has improved very considerably (Chs 65, 66), but laparotomy is still necessary in many cases. If the clinical team in charge of the patient's care considers that laparotomy might be necessary, then it is at present probably better to proceed without initial intubation with its attendant risks than to complicate the surgical procedure and surgical decision-making by the presence of a tube. Furthermore, should laparotomy be required and preoperative cholangiography indicate that adequate surgical bypass may be possible, then intubation should probably not be performed. In particular in high bile duct lesions intubation of the ducts of the right liver, which is not followed by subsequent insertion of endoprosthesis should be avoided, especially if surgical decompression of the Segment III duct of the left lobe (ligamentum teres approach) is possible (Ch. 70). In addition to the usual risks of intubation the passage of a tube in such a situation may leave the patient adequately decompressed by surgical means through the left ductal system, but with a persistent biliary fistula to the skin on the right (Ch. 60). The authors have encountered several such cases leading to considerable difficulties in management.

Should surgical excision for potential cure be seriously entertained in any given case, then intubation should probably be avoided unless deliberately used in a preoperative manner (see above). The current complication rate of intubation and the introduction of infection may not be serious when looked at simply in terms of the presence of an indwelling tube, but may become highly significant at subsequent operation. Thus, e.g. a positive bile culture obtained during a period of drainage and not accompanied by septic episodes may be considered insignificant by the radiologist or endoscopist, but will become of serious importance to the surgeon faced with major excisional surgery in the presence of established infection at the site of operation. There is indeed data to suggest that excisional or bypass surgery following initial intervention whether surgical, radiological or endoscopic is accompanied by fewer good results (Blumgart et al 1984a) (Table 37.2) (Ch. 65). However, it is apposite in this chapter to emphasize that local excision of hilar cholangiocarcinoma can be carried out with near to zero mortality (Ch. 65) and that pancreaticoduodenectomy should now have a mortality of 10% or less (Ch. 66). Even excision of hilar cholangiocarcinoma in the presence of jaundice and accompanied by hepatic resection probably has a mortality no greater than 15% (Ch. 65) and this indeed may be lower if there has been no previous intubation (Blumgart et al 1984a).

It is difficult to assess the value of percutaneous biliary drainage and endoprosthesis as compared to surgical bypass in the palliation of malignant bile duct obstruction. However to assess the success of a palliative procedure for obstructive jaundice a number of features must be considered. The objectives are to relieve the obstruction,

Table 37.2 Hilar cholangiocarcinoma. Effect of previous surgery or drainage on mortality

Procedure	No. of patients	Previous surgery or drainage	No previous intervention
Curative surgery	18	7 2 died (28.5%)	11 1 died (9%)
Palliative hepaticojejunostomy	46	24 8 died (33%)	22 4 died (18%)
Total		31 10 died (32%)	33 5 died (15%)

lower bilirubin, relieve itching and allow entry of bile salts to the duodenum, all with the minimum of distress, risk and cost to the patient. The method chosen should be assessed in terms of 'comfortable' time of survival. There are many publications regarding palliative surgery for biliary tract obstruction in malignant disease and particularly in the presence of irresectable pancreatic cancer. Representative of these reports is a review of over 8000 patients with irresectable pancreatic cancer reported in the English literature from 1965–1980, which shows that surgical bypass leads to clinical improvement in 56–85% of patients. There is relief of pruritus, improvement in liver function and return of appetite. Morbidity, particularly from cholangitis tends to be low, the incidence being 4% after cholecystojejunostomy. The mortality was 19% (Sarr & Cameron 1982). A similar figure for surgical mortality is reported by Benjamin (1981). Length of survival depends on the site and size of the tumour (Richards et al 1973).

Consideration of the results of percutaneous transhepatic biliary drainage, endoprosthetic drainage by the transhepatic route, or by endoprosthesis introduced endoscopically reveals a success rate for intubation of between 70 and 100% (Table 37.3) (Chs 35, 36, 68, 69). Successful intubation, however, does not necessarily equate with low risk or effective drainage. The 30-day mortality approaches 30% (whichever method is used) and reflects in part the nature of malignant biliary obstruction. This figure is higher than the generally accepted figure for surgical bypass. The complication rate for percutaneous methods is higher than for endoscopic approaches. None of the series reflected in Table 37.3 has a mean survival longer than 6.5 months. Fletcher et al (1983) at Kings College Hospital, London, have claimed a prolonged median survival of 11 months in 11 patients with hilar cholangiocarcinoma treated with PTBD combined with internal radiotherapy, using ^{192}Iridium wire. The Kings College Group have now treated 30 patients with hilar biliary obstruction in whom 23 are histologically confirmed cholangiocarcinoma with an overall mean survival of 16.8 months, 11 patients being alive at a mean time of 23.2 months (Nunnerley 1985). These preliminary results require confirmation in a prospective controlled trial. The best results are reported using a large bore endoscopically introduced endoprosthesis (Tytgat & Huibregtse 1983) (Ch. 69). For 279 patients they reported an overall 30-day mortality of 16% (Table 37.3) but the figure reached 24% for hilar obstruction. 140 patients were dead at a median time of three months for hilar obstruction and four months for distal common duct obstruction. These results for hilar obstruction, in a situation where surgical bypass is technically difficult, are not better than those reported by

Table 37.3 Palliative percutaneous and endoscopic drainage of malignant obstruction

Author	Year	Number of successful intubations/attempts	Mortality 30-day	Survival months
PTBD				
Molnar & Stockum	1974	5/5	80%	1 for 3 m
Hansson et al	1978	32/32	25%	median 2 m
Nakayama et al	1978	21/21	—	15 > 3 m (longest 24 m)
Ishikawa et al	1980	18	—	mean 2.5 m (longest 12 m)
Berquist et al	1981	34	—	mean 6.5 m (3 > 12 m)
Mueller et al	1982	51	—	mean < 7 m (16 > 7 m)
Percutaneous endoprosthesis				
Burcharth et al	1981	94/121	30%	median 2 m (13 > 3 m)
Lorelius et al	1982	18/25	—	mean 5 m (1 for 9 m)
Gouma et al	1983	24	20%	mean 4 m
Dooley et al	1984	40/47	25%	median 4 m (1 > 15 m)
Duodenoscopic endoprosthesis				
Riemann et al	1981	17	—	median 4 m (1 > 11/12)
Cotton	1982	15/20	33%	6 dead — median 4 m 6 alive — median 4 m
Hagenmüller & Soehendra	1983	58	31%	median 2 m (16 still alive)
Tytgat & Huibregtse	1983	279	16%	140 dead — median 3 m for hilar obstruction and 4 m for distal common duct obstruction

Blumgart et al (1984a) for surgically managed patients in whom no previous intervention had been carried out. In addition, the efficacy of endoscopic drainage for hilar tumours is almost certainly less than that of adequate surgery, although there is no controlled comparative study to prove or refute this point. A comparison of percutaneous transhepatic endoprosthetic drainage and surgical bypass to the segment III duct is presently being conducted by the authors at the Royal Postgraduate Medical School, Hammersmith Hospital.

At least as important to the patient as the mortality related to that procedure itself is the length of survival following a palliative procedure and the quality of life obtained. In a review of 15 papers examining non-operative drainage of the obstructed biliary tree (Table 37.4) the authors find a total of 17 (2%) deaths directly attributable to the intubation procedure, eight being due to uncontrollable bleeding and four due to sepsis. The incidence of tube dislodgement was reported in eight of these publications and varied between 4 and 22%. For the patient this of course represents a failure associated with a recurrence of jaundice and sometimes with intra-abdominal bile contamination. The major disabling complication of PTBD and endoprosthesis is cholangitis. Not all reports mention cholangitis and some quote a low incidence of 5–6% (Pollock et al 1979, Burcharth et al 1981). Two series specifically reporting on cholangitis as a complication found an incidence of 27 and 33% (McPherson et al 1982, Clouse et al 1983). The incidence of cholangitis in 12 reports examining percutaneous biliary drainage, percutaneous endoprosthesis, and duodenoscopic endoprosthesis was a median of 13.5%. Thus it is likely that at least one in every seven patients treated palliatively by non-surgical intubation for malignant biliary tract obstruction will suffer from cholangitis and the real figure may be somewhat higher. This is much higher than the figures reported for surgical bypass. Thus Richards et al (1973) in a series of 74 patients found a 0% incidence of cholangitis following choledochojejunostomy and 4% following cholecystojejunostomy for malignant biliary tract obstruction.

Table 37.4 Significant complications of PTBD and endoscopic drainage of the obstructed bile duct

Author	Year	Cholangitis frequency	Tube dislodgement frequency	Procedure related* deaths
PTBD				
Molnar & Stockum	1974	—	2/11 (18%)	—
Hansson et al	1978	9/68 (13%)	12/105 (11%)	1
Nakayama et al	1978	—	9/104 (9%)	1
Ring (Pollock) et al	1979	2/41 (5%)	—	—
Berquist et al	1981	7/50 (14%)	—	1
Mueller et al	1982	21/200 (10%)	11/200 (5%)	2
McPherson et al	1982	10/37 (27%)	4/37 (11%)	2
Clouse et al	1983	19/52 (36%)	—	2
Percutaneous endoprosthesis				
Burcharth et al	1981	7/123 (6%)	5/123 (4%)	1
Lorelius et al	1982	—	1/18 (6%)	—
Dooley et al	1984	5/53 (9%)	—	2
Duodenoscopic endoprosthesis				
Riemann et al	1981	3/17 (18%)	5/23 (22%)	—
Cotton	1982	5/15 (33%)	—	—
Hagenmüller & Soehendra	1983	22/176 (13%)	—	5
Tytgat & Huibregtse	1983	48/279 (16%)	—	—

* 17 (2%) Procedure related deaths

Although up to 30% of patients with malignant biliary tract obstruction will have infected bile ab initio the major source of cholangitis is exogenous infection after intubation. Blenkharn et al (1984) have successfully reduced the incidence of exogenous contamination by the introduction of a closed biliary drainage system (Ch. 11) and this reduction in cholangitis has been accompanied by a reduction in bacteraemia and postoperative wound sepsis.

It is somewhat surprising that the benefits of drainage have been poorly documented (Table 37.5). Ideally assessment should record at least relief of jaundice and pruritus, the incidence of cholangitis, the presence of bile leakage, the number of days spent in bed and a pain analogue chart. No single report has documented these details. Only four reports mention whether or not pruritus had improved. In most patients the serum bilirubin had fallen but this was not uniformly so and in only three series were normal values achieved. It would seem that the proponents of non-surgical intubation have concentrated on serum bilirubin values but this may not provide the best guide to effective palliation. Only two papers recorded in Table 37.5 mention whether there has been any improvement in renal function or any change in nutritional status during the period of drainage.

Clearly, while non-surgical intubational methods will have a place in selected cases they should not be used as a panacea and further evaluation and prospective controlled trials are required before the relevance of these techniques can be fully appreciated.

PREOPERATIVE PERCUTANEOUS BILIARY DRAINAGE

As long ago as 1935 Whipple proposed a staged approach to the jaundiced patient with a resectable pancreatic cancer. The first stage, cholecystjejunostomy, was carried out to relieve jaundice and improve hepatic function, the patient then being left for a period before proceeding to a second operation for definitive resection. With the introduction of vitamin K (Butt 1938) and of antibiotics, Whipple abandoned this approach (Whipple 1935) but the attraction of improving the status of the patient by means of an initial minor procedure before proceeding to a major resective operation have remained, and many have practised such an approach. Initial operation may be in the

Table 37.5 Benefits of PTBD and endoprosthesis drainage of biliary tract obstruction

Author	Year	Pruritus improved	Fall in serum bilirubin	Other changes
PTBD				
Molnar & Stockum	1974	8/8	9/11	Nutrition improved in 1/11
Hansson et al	1978	—	mean fall from 14.8–7.7 mg%	—
Nakayama et al	1978	—	mean fall from 12–10.8 mg%	—
Ishikawa et al	1980	—	69/69	—
Berquist et al	1981	44/48	44/48 (mean fall from 20–5 mg%)	—
Pollock et al	1979	—	30/36	—
McPherson et al	1982	Yes	30/37 (mean fall from 365–136 μmol/l)	Renal function improved 8/10 No improvement in nutrition
Clouse et al	1983	—	52/52	—
Percutaneous endoprosthesis				
Burcharth et al	1981	—	79/99 (64 to normal levels)	—
Lorelius et al	1982	—	13/18 (all to normal levels)	—
Dooley et al	1984	—	28/40	—
Duodenoscopic endoprosthesis				
Riemann et al	1981	—	17/23	—
Cotton	1982	Yes	10/15 (3 to normal levels)	—
Hagenmüller & Soehendra	1983	—	105/121	—
Tytgat & Huibregtse	1983	—	236/279	—

form of a biliary-enteric anastomosis, normally cholecystenterostomy or choledochoenterostomy, but some have practised temporary external drainage by means of a T-tube introduced high in the common hepatic duct (Blumgart 1978) or temporary cholecystostomy. Inherent in such approaches was the advantage of early operative definition of irresectability which indeed was the fate of the majority of patients, a small number being selected for subsequent definitive resection. In addition, a period of some six to ten weeks was usually allowed to elapse between the initial and subsequent operation, the patient coming to definitive surgery fully recovered from the effects of biliary tract obstruction.

Occasionally in benign biliary disease initial simple external biliary drainage was employed in desperately ill patients with cholangitis, a T-tube being placed and brought to the exterior until control of the situation was obtained, secondary operation then being carried out to treat the cause (usually common bile duct stones) at a later date (Benjamin & Blumgart 1979).

Preoperative percutaneous transhepatic or endoscopic biliary drainage can be performed for similar indications. In 1978 Nakayama suggested, as a result of a retrospective study, that preoperative percutaneous biliary drainage lowered the operative mortality for malignant obstructive jaundice. In a study group of 49 patients, all of whom had preoperative percutaneous drainage, the subsequent operative mortality was 8% compared with 28% for a series of 148 retrospective controls. There was no mention as to whether the drained patients were a high risk group nor indeed of any criteria employed in their selection and the study was not controlled.

Despite a number of enthusiastic anecdotal claims as to the efficacy of non-surgical preoperative drainage methods in lowering subsequent operative mortality, a review of the literature reveals surprisingly few studies of the impact of PTBD on surgical mortality. Both Dooley at the Royal Free Hospital, London, (Dooley et al 1979) and McPherson at the Royal Postgraduate Medical School, Hammersmith Hospital (McPherson et al 1982) found an operative mortality of 19% after preoperative PTBD in uncontrolled prospective studies. Denning et al (1981) reported an operative mortality of 16% in a similar group of patients. These studies and the possibility that the work of Nakayama (1978) might not be reproducible has resulted in a number of studies comparing the fate of patients who did or did not have preoperative percutaneous drainage. Norlander et al (1982) using retrospective non-randomized controls demonstrated a reduction of operative mortality from 33–18% following the introduction of preoperative percutaneous biliary drainage in malignant biliary tract obstruction. A trial conducted in Cape Town of preoperative percutaneous transhepatic biliary drainage found an operative mortality of 14% following drainage as compared with 15% following laparotomy alone (Hatfield et al 1982). This was a prospective controlled study but did include some patients with benign disease. The study was terminated after the entry of 55 patients and with a total of eight deaths, four in each group. There were insufficient numbers to conclude firmly that preoperative percutaneous drainage was ineffective (McPherson 1982b). The report did emphasize however some of the inherent risks of PTBD and is in broad agreement with the trial reported from the Hepatobiliary

Surgical Unit, Hammersmith Hospital (McPherson et al 1984).

Patients were entered to the Hammersmith Drainage Trial according to defined criteria: only patients with malignant biliary tract obstruction, with a serum bilirubin greater than 100 μmol/l on admission and who had not been previously drained, were accepted. Drainage was maintained for a median period of three weeks. It was found that the mortality for laparotomy was 19% (6/31) as compared with 32% (11/34) for patients submitted to drainage and subsequent laparotomy. Assessment of the 95% confidence limits suggests that the lowest estimate of mortality in the drainage group would be 15%, only slightly less than that of the control group. The trial was terminated when it became clear that there was no obvious benefit of PTBD in a high risk group of patients with malignant obstruction and indeed there was a chance that there was an actual increase in the surgical mortality due to the complications of the procedure (McPherson et al 1984).

A prospective randomized trial from Los Angeles reported similar results (Pitt et al 1985). Of 37 jaundiced patients undergoing preoperative PTBD the mortality was 8.1% compared with 5.3% for 38 patients who underwent operation without preoperative drainage. Only patients with a serum bilirubin greater than 10 mg/dl were included and approximately three-quarters of the total had a malignant obstruction. The overall morbidity was slightly higher (57% vs 53%) in the PTBD group. However, the total hospital stay was significantly longer (31.6 vs 23.1 days) in the drainage group. The cost of the prolonged hospital stay was over $8000/patient. The low overall mortality is explained by the exclusion of patients with widespread advanced malignancy.

It should be noted however, that the majority of the patients in the Hammersmith Trial were drained to the exterior, bile still being excluded from the gut, and that there is as yet no study of internal drainage via a large bore endoprosthesis introduced either percutaneously or endoprosthetically in the preparation of the patient with malignant biliary tract obstruction for subsequent surgery. A collaborative controlled study has, however, been commenced at the Middlesex Hospital and the Royal Postgraduate Medical School, London, in an attempt to answer this question.

The only trial to date which favours preoperative PTBD is the study from Ann Arbor (Grundy et al 1984). The groups of patients studied were not randomized and only 50 patients were included. 25 patients underwent drainage for a mean of nine days before operation and 25 underwent operation without preliminary drainage. There was one death (4%) in the drainage group and five deaths (20%) in the group without drainage. The mean hospital stay was shorter for the drainage group. The conclusion that preoperative PTBD reduces operative mortality is invalidated by inadequate trial design and insufficient numbers.

Thus, to date, no hard data can be found for the supposition that preliminary percutaneous or endoscopic drainage of the obstructed biliary tree in malignancy affords benefit. However, it should be clearly understood that a number of questions have yet to be answered. Firstly, it is not yet possible to select matched high risk patients for comparative studies by any one or set of agreed criteria. One approach to this problem has been the introduction of antipyrine clearance studies as a dynamic assessment of hepatic function in the jaundiced patient. Antipyrine clearance in a variety of jaundiced patients as compared with controls was found to be a useful predictor of outcome in a preliminary study of 46 patients (McPherson et al 1985). Studies of antipyrine clearance offer a more sensitive index of hepatic function than crude static tests and may prove to be a useful method of selection of high risk patients with impaired hepatic functional reserve. Secondly, not only is the selection of patients as yet imperfect, but the optimum timing of the duration of biliary drainage prior to subsequent surgery is unknown. Certainly, the period of time allowed to elapse between the institution of drainage and subsequent surgery in all studies reported to date is probably too short, but this has been occasioned by the need to keep patients in hospital for prolonged periods, the increasing risk of exogenous infection with time, and the increase in complication rate also noted to occur with the passage of time. As techniques improve, and this is already the case for endoscopic endoprosthesis, it will be possible to allow greater periods of time to elapse between initial intubation and subsequent operation. Such studies as are available have examined mitochondrial function and other aspects of dynamic liver activity and suggest that a minimum period of six weeks' drainage is probably necessary before proceeding to surgery (Koyama 1981). Antipyrine clearance studies may also be of value in the assessment of the duration of effective drainage (McPherson et al 1985).

Finally, it is important to acknowledge that in malignant disease which subsequently proves irresectable, a period of initial drainage especially if open to complications, possible mortality and prolonged hospitalization, which simply results in ultimate bypass surgery carried out with similar risks as if performed initially, is hardly in the best interest of the patient. It is for this reason that many have become dubious of the benefits of preliminary percutaneous or endoscopic drainage since these techniques, especially percutaneous drainage, appear to be associated with morbidity and a 30-day mortality very similar to, if not greater, than surgical bypass.

INTUBATIONAL METHODS IN BENIGN BILIARY OBSTRUCTION

Percutaneous and endoscopic methods for the relief of benign biliary tract obstruction have also been widely used. Methods employed are percutaneous biliary drainage or the placement of endoprosthesis, and endoscopic papillotomy with or without endoprosthesis or naso-biliary drainage.

The authors have reviewed the reported results from 15 centres published between the years 1974 and 1984 (Table 37.6). The commonest indication was postoperative benign biliary stricture although a large number of drainage procedures were done in the presence of common bile duct calculi and a smaller number for biliary obstruction associated with chronic pancreatitis. The findings of this review are broadly in line with the report of Hagenmüller & Classen (1983) who reviewed the collected data from 1602 patients although this latter report also included patients drained by endoscopic transpapillary external drainage (naso-biliary drainage) (Wurbs & Classen 1977).

The use of non-surgical means to drain the biliary tree in acute cholangitis has been the subject of sporadic reports. Suppurative cholangitis is almost always fatal unless biliary drainage is carried out (Ch. 72) and the peroperative mortality for surgery is also very considerable, being at least 17% if operation is carried out in the first 24 hours and rising to 50% with a 24-hour delay (Welch & Donaldson 1976). The reported results of percutaneous biliary drainage and endoprosthesis are but few. Benjamin & Blumgart published a successful case in 1979 and Dooley et al (1979) report one patient successfully treated. Ikeda et al (1981) report three patients with the same condition successfully treated by duodenoscopic cannulation with disimpaction of stones and Wurbs et al (1980) a group of 16 patients, average age more than 80 years, with suppurative cholangitis treated by endoscopic insertion of a naso-biliary drain, 25% of whom died.

The essential aim in acute suppurative cholangitis is complete and effective drainage of the biliary tree. Percutaneous and endoscopic methods have a place in this situation but each case should be judged on its merits. Certainly, for the management of gallstone obstruction in the presence of sepsis and associated medical risk factors, non-surgical methods and particularly endoscopic approaches will be appropriate for many, particularly in centres with the relevant expertise, but it is important to recognize that gangrenous cholecystitis and perforation of the gallbladder can be associated with suppurative cholangitis, are extremely difficult to diagnose, and cannot be treated by endoscopic intubational techniques (Ch. 50).

Table 37.6 PTBD and endoprosthesis for benign biliary tract obstruction

Cause of obstruction	All	PTBD	Percutaneous endoprosthesis	Duodenoscopic endoprosthesis
CBD stones	89	55	18	16
Postop/benign strictures	110	88	18	4
Chronic pancreatitis	17	1	5	11
Other	13	6	1	6
Total	229	150	42	37

Collected results from 15 centres: Hansson et al 1978, Nakayama et al 1978, Pollock et al 1979, Molnar & Stockum 1979, Ishikawa et al 1980, Berquist et al 1981, Reiman et al 1981, Burcharth et al 1981, McPherson et al 1982, Mueller et al 1982, Clouse et al 1983, Hagenmüller & Soehendra 1983, Zuidema et al 1983, Gouma et al 1983, Dooley et al 1984.

Naso-biliary drainage has also been used as a primary temporary drainage procedure where the drain is left in situ to prevent stone impaction after endoscopic papillotomy without stone removal (Wurbs & Classen 1977). The method may be used in association with chemical litholysis using stone solvents.

The treatment of biliary obstruction due to chronic pancreatitis by endoprosthesis was first described by Burcharth (1981) and has been reported by a number of other authors (Hagenmüller & Soehendra 1983). The indications are not clear cut and it would seem that there is no great place for the procedure in this situation.

Similarly, in the management of sclerosing cholangitis (Ch. 59) percutaneous biliary drainage and endoprosthesis may be used particularly in situations where there is a single stricture present and these methods may be combined with balloon dilatation of strictures (Toufanian 1978) (Ch. 58). However, the risk of introducing infection into an already compromised biliary tract is extremely high and surgical bypass is to be preferred in most cases.

There is much debate regarding the role of percutaneous biliary drainage and balloon dilatation and of percutaneously introduced endoprostheses in the treatment of postoperative biliary strictures. Although a large number of patients have been treated (Table 37.6) (Hagenmüller & Classen 1983) there are no long-term follow-up results for comparison with the results of surgical approaches. Following surgical repair the majority of recurrent strictures present within the first two to three years (Pitt 1982) and it has been established that good results are obtained in 80% of patients with benign bile duct stricture treated in reputable centres. Indeed even re-operation is not associated with greater risk in some reports (Blumgart et al 1984b, Pellagrini et al 1984) (Ch. 58). Zuidema et al (1983) suggest that percutaneous biliary drainage and endoprosthesis have a role in the management of postoperative stricture and claim that there were only transient episodes of sepsis related to catheter manipulation. However, 11 patients in this series required operative drainage of abscess. This is in conflict with a variety of other reports (Table 37.4) which emphasize that cholangitis may occur in up to 36% of cases (Clouse 1983) and that other periprocedural complications, e.g. arterioportodochal fistulae, bilious empyema and duodenal perforation (McPherson et al 1984, Armstrong 1982, Irving 1981) occur. It is important to appreciate that the risks for repair of bile duct stricture are related to sepsis, to the management of associated gastrointestinal bleeding and to portal hypertension and that deaths occur predominantly in patients with liver fibrosis. There are now several reports revealing a zero or near to zero mortality for biliary enteric mucosa-to-mucosa repair in the absence of these factors (Blumgart et al 1984, Bismuth 1982) (Ch. 58). It may well be that the risk in percutaneous biliary approaches is higher than that for surgical approaches. Some have attempted to obtain good long-term results after percutaneous approaches by combining passage of the catheter with transhepatic dilatation using a Grüntzig balloon (Toufanian et al 1978, Oleaga & Ring 1981). For such techniques to be successful the stricture must be circumferential (Oleaga & Ring 1981) and the method is more successful following biliary enteric anastomosis than with strictures in the line of the intact duct.

It is also important to realize that incomplete biliary obstruction may be associated with steadily progressive liver fibrosis resulting in portal hypertension and that this may occur in the patient who is asymptomatic or who is having only occasional attacks of mild fever. Such an incomplete decompression may be produced by the use of balloon dilatational methods.

It has been suggested that the application of these techniques in postoperative biliary stricture may be important in defined situations and probably will be of most value either as a preliminary or instead of surgery in postoperative strictures with coexistent portal hypertension where peroperative mortality may be high (Blumgart 1983) (Ch. 58). If a transanastomotic tube has been left in place after surgical repair, particularly in the instance of intrahepatic stones which could not be completely removed at initial surgery, the tubal tract may be used for postoperative choledochoscopy or postoperative intubation with a sterile catheter for stone removal and dilatation of stenoses (Gibson et al 1986).

REFERENCES

Armstrong C P, Taylor T V 1982 Complicating percutaneous transhepatic drainage of the obstructed biliary tree. Journal of the Royal College of Surgeons of Edinburgh 27: 308–309

Benjamin I S 1981 Tumour and host. Aims and decisions in pancreatic cancer. In: Cohn I, Hastings P R (eds) Pancreatic cancer. UICC, Geneva, p 103–113

Benjamin I S, Blumgart L H 1979 Biliary bypass and reconstructive surgery. In: Wright R, Alberti K G M M, Karran S, Millward-Sadler G H (eds) Liver and biliary disease: pathophysiology, diagnosis, management. 1st Edition W B Saunders, London, p 1219–1246

Berquist T H, May G R, Johnson C M, Adson M A, Thistle J L 1981 Percutaneous biliary decompression. Internal and external drainage in 50 patients. American Journal of Surgery 136: 901–906

Bismuth H 1982 Postoperative strictures of the bile duct. In: Blumgart L H (ed) The biliary tract. Clinical surgery international. Churchill Livingstone, Edinburgh, p 209–218

Blamey S L, Fearen K C H, Gilmour W H, Osborne D H, Carter D C 1983 Prediction of risk in biliary surgery. British Journal of Surgery 70: 535–538

Blenkharn J I, McPherson G A D, Blumgart L H 1984 Septic complications of percutaneous transhepatic biliary drainage. Evaluation of a new closed drainage system. American Journal of Surgery 147: 318–321

Blumgart L H 1978 Biliary tract obstruction — new approaches to old problems. American Journal of Surgery 135: 19–31

Blumgart L H 1983 Bile duct strictures. In: Fromm D (ed) Gastrointestinal surgery vol. I. Churchill Livingstone, New York p 755–811

Blumgart L H, Hadjis N S, Benjamin I S, Beazley R 1984a Surgical approaches to cholangiocarcinoma at the confluence of the hepatic ducts. Lancet i: 66–69

Blumgart L H, Kelley C J, Benjamin I S 1984b Benign bile duct stricture following cholecystectomy: critical factors in management. British Journal of Surgery 71: 836–843

Burcharth F, Efsen F, Christiansen L A, Pedersen J H, Pedersen G 1981 Non-surgical internal biliary drainage by endoprosthesis. Surgery, Gynecology and Obstetrics 153: 857–860

Butt H R, Snell A M, Osterberg A E 1938 The use of vitamin K and bile in the treatment of hemorrhagic diathesis in cases of jaundice. Proceedings Staff Meeting, Mayo Clinic 13:74

Clouse M E, Evans D, Costello P, Alday M, Edwards S A, McDermott S A 1983 Percutaneous transhepatic biliary drainage. Complications due to multiple duct obstructions. Annals of Surgery 198: 25–29

Cotton P B 1982 Duodenoscopic placement of biliary prosthesis to relieve malignant obstructive jaundice. British Journal of Surgery 69: 501–503

Dalton-Clarke H J, Pearse E, Krausz T, McPherson G A D, Benjamin I S, Blumgart L H 1986 Fine needle aspiration cytology and exfoliative biliary cytology in the diagnosis of hilar cholangiocarcinoma. European Journal of Surgical Oncology 12: 143–145

Denning D A, Ellison E C, Carey L C 1981 Preoperative percutaneous transhepatic biliary decompression lowers operative morbidity in patients with obstructive jaundice. American Journal of Surgery 141: 61–65

Dixon J M, Armstrong C P, Duffy S W, Davies G C 1982 Statistical analysis of the factors affecting mortality and morbidity in biliary tract surgery. Gut 23:A441

Dooley J S, Dick K, Olney J, Sherlock S 1979 Non-surgical treatment of biliary obstruction. Lancet ii: 1040–1044

Dooley J S, Dick K, George P, Kirk R M, Hobbs K E F, Sherlock S 1984 Percutaneous transhepatic endoprosthesis for bile duct obstruction. Gastroenterology 86: 905–909

Fletcher M S, Brinkley D, Dawson J L, Nunnerley H, Williams R 1983 Treatment of hilar carcinoma by bile drainage combined with internal radiotherapy using 192 Iridium wire. British Journal of Surgery 70: 733–735

Gibson R N, Adam A, Halevy A, Hadjis N S, Benjamin I S, Allison D J, Blumgart L H 1986 Benign biliary strictures: a proposed combined surgical and radiological management. (In press).

Gouma D J, Wesdap R I C, Oestenbroek R J, Soeters P B, Greep J M 1983 Percutaneous transhepatic drainage and insertion of endoprosthesis for obstructive jaundice. American Journal of Surgery 145: 763–768

Grundy S R, Strodel W E, Knoll J A, Eckhauser F E 1984 Efficacy of preoperative biliary tract decompression in patients with obstructive jaundice. Archives of Surgery 119: 703–708

Hadjis N C, Collier N A, Blumgart L H 1985 Malignant masquerade at the hilum of the liver. British Journal of Surgery 72: 659–661.

Hagenmüller F, Classen M 1983 Therapeutic endoscopic and percutaneous procedures. In: Popper H, Schaffer F (eds) Progress in liver diseases vol III. Grune and Strutton, New York, p 299–318

Hagenmüller F, Soehendra N 1983 Non surgical biliary drainage. Clinics in Gastroenterology 12: 297–315

Hansson J A, Hoevels J, Smert G, Tylen V, Vang J 1979 Clinical aspects of non-surgical percutaneous transhepatic bile drainage in obstructive lesions of the extrahepatic bile ducts. Annals of Surgery 189: 58–61

Hatfield A R W, Terblanche J, Fataar S, Kemoff L, Tobias R, Girdwood A H, Harris-Jones R, Marks I N 1982 Preoperative external biliary drainage in obstructive jaundice. Lancet ii 896–899.

Ikeda S, Tanaka M, Itoh H, Kishikawa H, Nakayama F 1981 Emergency decompression of bile duct in acute obstructive suppurative cholangitis by duodenoscopic cannulation: a life saving procedure. World Journal of Surgery 5: 587–593

Irving J D 1981 Interventional radiology. Relief of biliary obstruction. British Journal of Hospital Medicine 26: 329–338

Ishikawa Y 1980 Percutaneous transhepatic drainage. Experience in 100 cases. Journal of Clinical Gastroenterology 12: 305–314

Jones B A, Langer B, Taylor B R, Girotti M 1985 Periampullary tumours: which ones should be resected? American Journal of Surgery 149: 46–52

Koyama K, Takaqi Y, Hok Sato T 1981 Experimental and clinical studies on the effect of biliary drainage in obstructive jaundice. American Journal of Surgery 142: 293–299

Lorelius L E, Jacobson G, Swada S 1982 Endoprosthesis as an internal biliary drainage in inoperable patients with biliary obstruction. Acta Chirurgica Scandinavica 148: 613–616

McPherson G A D, Benjamin I S, Habib N A, Bowley N B, Blumgart L H 1982 Percutaneous transhepatic drainage in obstructive jaundice: advantages and problems. British Journal of Surgery 69: 261–264

McPherson G A D, Benjamin I S, Hodgson H J F, Bowley N B, Allison D J, Blumgart L H 1984 Pre-operative percutaneous transhepatic biliary drainage. The results of a controlled trial. British Journal of Surgery 71: 371–375

McPherson G A D, Benjamin I S, Boobis A R, Blumgart L H 1985 Antipyrine elimination in patients with obstructive jaundice: a predictor of outcome. American Journal of Surgery 149: 140–143

McSherry C K 1982 Cholecystectomy and common duct exploration. In: Blumgart L H (ed) The biliary tract. Clinical surgery international. Churchill Livingstone, Edinburgh, p 128–142

Molnar W, Stockum A E 1979 Relief of obstructive jaundice through a percutaneous transhepatic catheter — a new therapeutic method. American Journal of Roentgenology, Radiotherapy and Nuclear Medicine 122: 356–357

Mueller P R, Van Sonnenberg E, Ferrucci J T Jr 1982 Percutaneous biliary drainage: technical and catheter-related problems in 200 procedures. American Journal of Radiology 138: 17–23

Nakayama T, Ikeda A, Okuda K 1978 Percutaneous transhepatic drainage of the biliary tract. Gastroenterology 74: 554–559

Norlander A, Kalin B, Sundblad R 1982 Effect of percutaneous transhepatic drainage on liver function and post-operative mortality. Surgery, Gynecology and Obstetrics 155: 161–166

Nunnerley H 1985 Personal communication

Okamura J, Monden M, Haikawa S, Gotoh M, Kosaki G, Kuroda C, Sakinai M 1983 Exfoliative cytology and biliary biopsy using a percutaneous transhepatic biliary tube. Journal of Surgical Oncology 22: 121–124

Oleaga J A, Ring E J 1981 Interventional biliary radiology. Seminars in Roentgenology XVI:116

Pellagrini C A, Thomas M J, Way L W 1984 Recurrent biliary stricture. Patterns of recurrence and outcome of surgical therapy. American Journal of Surgical 147: 175–180

Pitt H A, Cameron J L, Postier R G, Gadacz T R 1981 Factors affecting mortality in biliary tract surgery. American Journal of Surgery 141: 66–72

Pitt H A, Miyamoto T, Parapatis S K, Tompkins R K, Longmire W P 1982 Factors influencing outcome in patients with postoperative biliary strictures. American Journal of Surgery 144: 14–21

Pitt H A, Gomes A S, Lois J F, Mann L L, Deutsch L S, Longmire W P 1985 Does preoperative percutaneous biliary drainage reduce operative risk or increase hospital cost? Annals of Surgery 201: 9–16

Pollock T W, Ring E R, Oleaga J A, Freiman D B, Muller J L, Rosato G F 1979 Percutaneous decompression of benign and malignant biliary tract obstruction. Archives of Surgery 114: 148–151

Richards A B, Sosin H 1973 Cancer of the pancreas, the value of radical and palliative surgery. Annals of Surgery 177: 325–331

Rieman J F, Lux G, Rosch W, Sterba B 1981 Nonsurgical biliary drainage technique. Indications and results. Lymphology 13: 157–161

Sarr M G, Cameron J L 1982 Surgical management of unresectable carcinoma of the pancreas. Surgery 91: 123–133

Toufanian A, Carey L C, Martin E T Jr 1978 Transhepatic biliary dilatation: an alternative to surgical reconstruction. Current Surgery 35: 70–73

Tytgat G N J, Huibregtse K 1983 Transpapillary introduction of a large bore biliary endoprosthesis in malignant bile duct obstruction. Experience in 300 patients. 3rd International Symposium of Digestive Surgery and Endoscopy, Rome, p 140–141

Welch J P, Donaldson G A 1976 The urgency of diagnosis and surgical treatment of acute suppurative cholangitis. American Journal of Surgery 131: 527–532

Whipple A O, Parsons W B, Mullins C R 1935 Treatment of carcinoma of the ampulla of Vater. Annals of Surgery 102: 763–799

Wurbs D, Classen M 1977 Transpapillary longstanding tube for hepatobiliary drainage. Endoscopy 9: 192–13

Wurbs D, Phillip J, Classen M 1980 Endoskopische Papillotomie mit Gallenwegsdrainage. Internist 21: 617–623

Zuidema G D, Cameron J L, Sitzmann J V 1983 Percutaneous transhepatic management of complex biliary problems. Annals of Surgery 197: 584–593

SECTION 5

Gallstones and gallbladder

Ian A. D. Bouchier

Gallstones: formation and epidemiology

Gallstone disease is an important cause of morbidity in the Western world. Operations on the biliary tree are more frequent than any other major surgical intervention in the abdomen. Significant advances have occurred in our understanding of the physico-chemical relationship of the biliary lipids providing insights into, if not complete elucidation of, the mechanism of gallstone formation. This in turn has heralded the era of the medical dissolution of gallstones.

In this chapter an account will be presented of the chemical nature of gallstones, the mechanism for their formation, and their epidemiology. Many of the known, and less well known, associations with gallstone formation can be explained from our understanding of biliary lipid interactions.

COMPOSITION OF GALLSTONES

In 1924 Aschoff proposed a classification of gallstones in which stones are grouped as *inflammatory*: multiple, faceted and yellow-brown; *metabolic*: solitary, yellow-white cholesterol stones, or multiple, nodular yellow-brown calcium bilirubinate stones, or multiple, irregular black pigment stones; *mixed*: stones with the features of both metabolic and inflammatory stones; and *stasis* stones which are oval, soft yellow-brown and formed predominantly in the common bile duct. This classification no longer has merit for it is unnecessarily complex and implies an aetiology which is uncertain and unproven.

A simpler and more useful classification of gallstones is into cholesterol and pigment types (Trotman et al 1974, Soloway et al 1977). This distinction can be made easily by inspection of a stone and chemically. It also has the merits of distinguishing those gallstones which should respond to medical dissolution therapy (cholesterol gallstones) and those that will not. *Cholesterol gallstones* are light brown, smooth or faceted, single or multiple, and on cross-section show a laminated and/or crystalline appearance. *Pigment stones* are smaller, black or brown in colour, more numerous, irregular in shape and amorphous or crystalline on cross-section. In Western communities about 75% of all gallstones are formed solely or predominantly of cholesterol (Sutor & Wooley 1971, Whiting et al 1983). We now appreciate that pigment gallstones are far more common in the West than the 10% originally believed and probably account for up to 30% of gallstones. The prediction of stone type at cholecystography or ultrasonography remains difficult. A cholesterol stone may be diagnosed when the stones are small and float on cholecystography (Dolgin et al 1981), or ultrasonography demonstrates floating stones with sonic shadowing without internal echoes (Good et al 1979).

The cholesterol in gallstones is mainly in the form of cholesterol monohydrate crystals and anhydrous cholesterol with lesser amounts of an alternative crystalline form of anhydrous cholesterol (Sutor & Wooley 1969). Most cholesterol stones contain small amounts of calcium salts either alone or in combination: calcium carbonate, calcium phosphate, calcium palmitate (Sutor & Wooley 1973). Calcium carbonate may be found as valerite, calcite and aragonite; calcium phosphate as apatite and whitlockite (Beer et al 1979). The calcium content is greater in stones with a low cholesterol content than those containing more than 80% by weight of cholesterol (Whiting et al 1983).

Much work has been expended on defining the core of gallstones and the majority of observations suggest that the centre contains pigmented material, calcium bilirubinate, often trapped in an organic matrix which is possibly glycoprotein. Analysis of the remainder of a stone shows the pigmented organic matrix to be present in a layered fashion alternating between planes of cholesterol crystals. This suggests that gallstones are built up step by step around a centre of bile pigment and/or glycoprotein (Sutor & Wooley 1974, Bills & Lewis 1975, Beer et al 1977, 1979). Electron probe analysis shows that stones contain varying amounts of Na, K, P, Fe Mg, Ma, Ca, Pb, S, Al, Ni Cr, Ag, and B (Markkanen & Aho 1972, Beer et al 1977, 1979).

The nature of the pigment material in gallstones has

Table 38.1 Black vs. brown pigment stones

Black	Brown
Shiny	Dull brown
Resist manual crushing	Easily crushable
Found in gallbladder	Alternating light and dark layers
Bile sterile	Bile infected
Associated with haemolysis, old age and cirrhosis	Found throughout biliary tract
40% calcium bilirubinate	60% calcium bilirubinate
Tr calcium palmitate	15% calcium palmitate
6% calcium carbonate	Tr calcium carbonate
2% cholesterol	15% cholesterol

Table 38.3 Biliary bile salt composition in human bile

Type	Bile salt	No. and position of hydroxyl groups	Percent in bile	
Primary	Glycocholate	3α, 7α, 12α	23	35
	Taurocholate		12	
Primary	Glycochenodeoxycholate	3α, 7α	23	35
	Taurochenodeoxycholate		12	
Secondary	Glycodeoxycholate	3α, 12α	16	24
	Taurodeoxycholate		8	
Secondary	Glycolithocholate	3α	4	6
	Taurolithocholate		2	
Tertiary	Glycoursodeoxycholate	3α, 7β	trace	
	Tauroursodeoxycholate		trace	

been intensively studied by many groups but particularly by R. D. Soloway and his colleagues in Philadelphia who have classified pigment gallstones as 'black' and 'brown' (Table 38.1). All pigment stones contain calcium bilirubinate. Black stones can be subdivided according to the presence of calcium carbonate as black carbonate and black non-carbonate pigment stones. As with cholesterol gallstones, pigment stones demonstrate layering of calcium bilirubinate salts and a glycoprotein matrix. Black and brown stones show differences in chemical composition and micro structure which might reflect different mechanisms of stone formation (Trotman et al 1977, Soloway et al 1982, Malet et al 1984).

CHOLESTEROL SOLUBILITY IN BILE

Cholesterol, which is the major component of most gallstones in Western communities, is sparingly soluble in water. It is held in solution in bile in the form of mixed micelles comprising cholesterol, phospholipids and bile salts. Table 38.2 indicates the average concentration of these lipids in normal hepatic and gallbladder bile. Phospholipids are present mainly in the form of lecithin and bile salts as the glycine or taurine conjugates of the primary bile salts, cholic and chenodeoxycholic acids, and the secondary bile acids deoxycholic and lithocholic acids (Table 38.3). Primary bile salts are formed in the liver and secondary in the gut by 7α-dehydroxylation of the primary bile salts. Ursodeoxycholic acid is a bacterial metabolite of chenodeoxycholic acid but also has other mechanisms of formation in the liver. Bile acids require to be conjugated either with glycine or taurine before excretion from the liver into bile. Cholesterol in bile is mainly in the free, unesterified form but cholesterol esters may comprise as much as 15% of biliary cholesterol.

Table 38.2 Lipids in human bile

	Hepatic mmol/litre	Gallbladder	% Solids
Cholesterol	3	15	4
Phospholipids	7	35	22
Bile salts	40	300	67

Bile salt secretion by the liver is the driving force for the hepatic secretion of cholesterol and phospholipids and these three molecules are excreted in a macromolecular complex known as a mixed micelle. The precise site for the formation of micelles has yet to be determined, being either in the liver cell or at the canalicular membrane to be released into the bile canaliculus by exocytosis, or in the canalicular lumen itself.

In normal gallstone-free bile, the ratio of cholesterol : phospholipids : bile salts is such that all the cholesterol is maintained in micellar solution. Should the amount of cholesterol increase either because of an excess of cholesterol or a lack of bile salts (phospholipids do not appear to play an independent role) cholesterol will be found in a liquid crystalline phase and when the capacity of the liquid crystalline phase, or liposome, to solubilize cholesterol is exceeded, cholesterol will form crystals. These relationships can be expressed in a phase diagram where cholesterol, phospholipids and bile salts are plotted on triangular coordinates (Admirand & Small 1968).

Not all bile which is supersaturated with cholesterol will contain crystals. Of much significance to the pathogenesis of cholesterol gallstones is the identification of a *metastable* zone in which bile is supersaturated with cholesterol, possibly in the liquid crystalline phase, which has not formed crystals. A metastable solution is relatively stable but will precipitate cholesterol crystals either spontaneously if the cholesterol content becomes markedly increased (homogeneous nucleation) or if nucleating factors are introduced into the supersaturated solution (heterogeneous nucleation) (Mufson et al 1974, Carey & Small 1978).

While in vitro studies suggest some differences in the

capacity of the major bile salts and phospholipid species to solubilize cholesterol, it is probable that such differences have no influence on solubility when cholesterol is dissolved in mixed micelles in bile. A variety of proteins is present in bile including apolipoproteins A-I, A-II, C-II, C-III and B in amounts up to 10% of plasma values (Sewell et al 1983). There is much discussion over the role of such biliary 'lipoproteins', whether they have a role in maintaining biliary cholesterol in solution, and whether there are some which are specific for bile. The interaction of calcium with bile salts and the mixed micelle is of considerable significance. The binding of calcium to bile salts limits the quantity of free Ca^{2+} which would be available to precipitate with anions such as bilirubinate, phosphate and carbonate, and act as the nucleating factor for the precipitation of cholesterol from supersaturated bile, as well as in the formation of pigment stones (Williamson & Percy-Robb 1980, Moore et al 1982).

The relative quantities of bile salts, phospholipids and cholesterol can be expressed as a percentage of the total of the three components in bile and plotted as a single point on triangular coordinates (Admirand & Small 1968). It is convenient to represent cholesterol saturation as a single number that takes into consideration the three biliary lipids, for which the term saturation index or lithogenic index is used. The saturation index of bile is most conveniently calculated by the method of Thomas & Hofmann (1973).

BILIARY LIPID CHANGES WITH CHOLESTEROL GALLSTONES

Supersaturated bile

Individuals with cholesterol gallstones secrete bile that is supersaturated with cholesterol, having a saturation index greater than one. The supersaturated bile originates from the liver (Vlahcevic et al 1970a). By measuring hourly hepatic secretory rates of cholesterol, bile salts and phospholipids in American Indian women, Grundy et al (1972) concluded that there was both a reduced rate of bile salt secretion and an increased biliary secretion of cholesterol in subjects with cholesterol gallstones. In another study in obese white females with gallstones, only an increased secretion of cholesterol was found (Grundy et al 1974).

The massive exercise on gallstone dissolution mounted in the USA by the National Cooperative Gallstone Study Group provided an outstanding opportunity to study biliary lipid composition in a large population with cholesterol gallstones and it provided confirmation of the increased saturation of bile with cholesterol. Using multiple regression analysis an attempt was made to ascertain whether it was possible to predict the cholesterol content in bile. Cholesterol saturation could not be predicted by age, previous pregnancies, smoking, clinical features, serum lipids and biliary bile acid composition. There was a correlation of percentage ideal body weight with some of the lipid classes: obese men tended to have bile with relatively less bile acids and obese females had proportionately more biliary cholesterol. But no characteristic correlated significantly with cholesterol saturation in either sex (Hofmann et al 1982). At present it is not possible to predict biliary cholesterol saturation, which can only be established by direct measurement on bile samples.

Bile acid pool size

Many patients with cholesterol gallstones have a diminished total bile acid pool size. Vlahcevic et al (1970b) reported the pool to be 2.38 g in non-stone formers and 1.29 in gallstone subjects; other authors have also observed the total body pool of bile salts to be about half that of normal individuals (Pomare & Heaton 1973, Northfield & Hofmann 1975), although there is an overlap between the two groups. It was also suggested that the reduced bile salt pool was important in the genesis of saturated bile (Vlahcevic et al 1972), but it now appears that this is unlikely for there is a poor correlation between the total bile salt pool and biliary cholesterol saturation (Mok et al 1980).

The reason for the reduced bile salt pool is not clear and might follow a variety of events (Table 38.4). Salen et al (1975) reported that there was increased hepatic activity of 3-hydroxy-3-methylglutaryl-CoA (HMGCoA) reductase (the rate-limiting enzyme for cholesterol synthesis) and a reduced activity of hepatic 7α-hydroxylase (rate-limiting for bile salt synthesis) in subjects with cholesterol gallstones. Carulli et al (1980) confirmed the decreased 7α-hydroxylase activity in gallstone patients but neither this group nor Ahlberg et al (1981) observed any difference between normals and gallstone subjects in the activity of HMGCoA reductase. The in vitro activity of HMGCoA reductase is not related to the hepatic cholesterol content, serum lipids or biliary cholesterol saturation and may not be a major determinant of the increased biliary cholesterol in cholesterol gallstone disease (Maton et al 1982).

The bile of subjects with cholesterol gallstones tends to have an increase in deoxycholic acid (Pomare & Heaton 1973, Ahlberg et al 1977) and this might be related to the increased biliary cholesterol saturation because an increased enterohepatic circulation of deoxycholate reduces the content of chenodeoxycholic acid in bile and increases

Table 38.4 Possible causes for the reduced total body pool of bile salts

Oversensitive feedback regulation
Decreased efficiency of intestinal absorption
Increased cycling frequency
Decreased steady-state synthesis

the amount of biliary cholesterol (Low-Beer & Pomare 1975, Pomare & Low-Beer 1975). While the influence of deoxycholate on cholesterol saturation is still controversial, the observations of the National Cooperative Gallstone Study Group favour the hypothesis of Pomare & Low-Beer (1975) although the tendency for deoxycholic acid to be associated with saturated bile was less potent than the desaturating effect of chenodeoxycholic acid (Hofmann et al 1982).

The bile salt pool normally makes from five to 10 cycles per day depending upon gallbladder contraction and intestinal transit. The enterohepatic circulation is interrupted during fasting when the gallbladder is not emptying and this is accompanied by increased cholesterol saturation in bile because biliary cholesterol output is not tightly coupled with biliary bile acid secretion (Metzger et al 1973). The biliary cholesterol : phospholipid ratio during fasting can vary greatly from subject to subject (Mok et al 1980, Hofmann et al 1982). Bile salt secretory rates are not significantly different in gallstone subjects and controls.

The essential feature however in cholesterol gallstone formation is an increased proportion of cholesterol in bile compared with bile salts and this may result from a variety of factors: defective bile salt synthesis, excessive intestinal loss of bile salts, oversensitive bile salt feedback, excessive cholesterol secretion and abnormal gallbladder function. But it should be emphasized that the basic mechanism is not known in the majority of patients in Western communities with cholesterol gallstones, who have both an excessive cholesterol secretion and reduced bile acid secretion.

Stratification of bile

If there is a variation in the saturation of bile during the 24 hours, and the gallbladder receives bile of differing cholesterol content, the degree of mixing within the gallbladder may be an important determinant of cholesterol crystal formation. Bile in the gallbladder may form layers of non-homogeneity (Campbell & Burton 1949, Tera 1960, Thureburn 1966), although Jazwari et al (1983) did not observe stratification in normal gallbladders. Gallbladder motility may be different in patients with gallstones, but the observations are conflicting, with some authors reporting increased emptying (Maudgal et al 1980) in association with a greater gallbladder sensitivity to cholecystokinin (Northfield et al 1980) and others finding diminished gallbladder emptying in patients with gallstones (Fisher et al 1982).

It is usually only in the gallbladder that supersaturated bile forms crystals because of the differences in metastability between dilute and concentrated bile. Thus gallbladder filling and emptying has relevance not only in interrupting the enterohepatic circulation and influencing bile salt pool size, but also in determining the mixing of bile. There is no correlation between a radiologically functioning gallbladder and bile saturation and it may be that the role of the gallbladder is more important in determining cholesterol crystal growth than in influencing bile salt kinetics.

Phospholipids in bile

Both quantitative and qualitative changes in the phospholipid content of bile have been reported in gallstone disease, but it is unlikely that they make an important contribution to the pathogenesis of gallstones (Bouchier 1983).

Metabolic function of the gallbladder

The role of the gallbladder in concentrating bile is well recognized but the extent to which mucosal metabolism and the release of mucosal enzymes into the lumen influences biliary lipids and their solubility remains to be clarified. Lysolecithin, derived from lecithin under the action of phospholipase A which is present in human gallbladder epithelial lysosomes, can adversely influence cholesterol solubility in bile (Neiderhiser & Roth 1970), and may also cause acute inflammation (Sjödahl & Wetterfors 1974). The human gallbladder mucosa contains a variety of esterases and hydrolases which could influence biliary lipid composition (Kouroumalis et al 1982, 1984).

Bile mucus glycoproteins

There has been much work on biliary glycoprotein. These proteins are increased in the gallbladder bile of patients with gallstones (Bouchier et al 1965), are present in gallstones (Womack 1971) and can be identified in the gallbladder wall (Lee et al 1979). Their precise composition and structure has yet to be determined. There is considerable animal experimental evidence to implicate glycoproteins in gallstone formation including the important observation that excessive production of glycoproteins by the gallbladder mucosa precedes stone formation (Freston et al 1969), but the recent studies on nucleation in human bile (Gollish et al 1983, Whiting & Watts 1984) cast doubt on the role of these proteins in the initiation of gallstones.

Nucleation of cholesterol crystals

Although the early studies on cholesterol solubility (Admirand & Small 1968) suggested that good separation of normal from cholesterol stone-containing bile could be achieved by relating solubility to the micellar zone on a phase diagram, it has become evident that no clear distinction between normal and abnormal bile can be made solely on the basis of the biliary lipid composition. Holzbach and his colleagues (1973) using data of their own and from an analysis of published work concluded that human bile is frequently supersaturated with cholesterol. Between 40–80% of normal persons have supersaturated bile. Bile from patients with cholesterol gallstones has a micellar zone similar to normals, but has a larger amount of cholesterol above saturation. Recent data derived from the National Cooperative Gallstone Study support this, the difference between the biliary lipid composition of normal and gallstone bile being 'astonishingly small' (Hofmann et al 1982) (Table 38.5). In general lithogenic bile has a higher degree of supersaturation than normal bile but the difference between normal and gallstone bile is not a question simply of supersaturation with cholesterol, rather it is that factor which causes the cholesterol to precipitate. All gallstone-forming bile must be supersaturated with cholesterol but not all supersaturated bile will necessarily have gallstones. A supersaturated bile may be non-lithogenic if it is sufficiently metastable because nucleation of crystals will be delayed.

Appreciation of the importance of the metastable phase and the initial stages of cholesterol crystal growth means that the emphasis has shifted from documenting bile chemistry to attempting to define and understand the phenomenon of nucleation in human bile. Holan et al (1979) studied the time it took stone-free bile and bile which had contained gallstones to form crystals: the nucleation time. The mean nucleation time for normal bile was 15 days but only three days for bile from cholesterol gallstone patients; this difference in nucleation time was much more striking than the difference in cholesterol saturation. The difference between supersaturated bile in forming crystals is in the nucleation capacity and not the ability of crystals to grow (Whiting & Watts 1984). The nature of the nucleating factor has yet to be defined. Indeed there is uncertainty whether the ease of nucleation, which is a feature of stone-forming biles, depends upon the addition of a nucleating agent, the lack of an agent in normal bile, or the absence of naturally occurring inhibitors of crystal formation. The nucleation phenomenon depends upon the gallbladder and not the liver, which explains why cholesterol stones rarely form in the bile ducts. Gallbladder bile shows a more rapid nucleation time than hepatic bile and this is not simply a reflection of concentration (Gollish et al 1983). A study of bile from patients with gallstones suggested that the nucleating factor is added by the gallbladder, and that it is probably either bilirubinate or mucus glycoproteins (Burnstein et al 1983), an observation supported by Whiting & Watts (1984) who also concluded that there are no inhibitors of crystal growth in bile.

In a different study Holzbach et al (1984) examined normal, stone-free bile for nucleating factors and demonstrated that a cholesterol crystal nucleation inhibitor is present which appears to be a bile protein. The nature of this protein is unclear; the effect is possibly specific, apparently residing in a protein associated with the bile proteins: possibly a bile lipoprotein complex. The present situation regarding nucleation is far from clear but it appears that the prolonged metastability of supersaturated normal bile depends upon an inhibitor which is one of the bile proteins. Bile in which nucleation occurs more readily may lack such an inhibitor, but might also possess a nucleation-promoting factor which has yet to be characterized; it is not obviously mucus or bilirubin or lecithin-cholesterol liquid crystals (Table 38.6). Both cholesterol saturation and nucleation factors (or a lack of inhibitors) must be present for cholesterol stones to form.

Table 38.5 Biliary lipid composition in normal and cholesterol stone bile

	Normal	Cholesterol gallstones
Number of subjects	196	545
Bile salts mol%	72.0 ± 5.4	70.5 ± 5.8
Phospholipids mol%	21.1 ± 4.6	20.6 ± 4.6
Cholesterol mol%	6.9 ± 2.3	8.8 ± 2.7
*Cholesterol saturation %	107 ± 34.3	137 ± 42.0
*Upper limit of micellar solubility 100%		

Hofmann et al 1982.

PIGMENT GALLSTONES

In contrast to the enormous amount of information about cholesterol solubility and cholesterol gallstones, comparatively little is known about the mechanism of formation of pigment gallstones. Black and brown pigment stones differ in composition and in their clinical associations (Table 38.1). The major component of these stones is calcium bilirubinate and it is probable that the ionized calcium is important in their formation (Moore et al 1982).

Bilirubin is present in bile as both the di- and monoglucuronide which are associated with micellar lipids. Free, unconjugated bilirubin precipitates as its insoluble calcium salt. One way in which calcium bilirubinate might form is following the action of β-glucuronidase of bacterial origin which hydrolyses conjugated bilirubin to its free form (Maki 1966). Glucuronidase is normally inhibited by glucuronic acid, a normal constituent of bile, but it is

Table 38.6 Nucleation in human bile

Stimulation	Inhibition
Present in stone-containing bile	Present in stone-free bile
?nature	? lipoprotein
No correlation with cholesterol saturation	

inadequate in the presence of gross bacterial infection. This hypothesis might apply to oriental pigment stones, but not those found in Western communities where infection with *E. coli* is an uncommon accompaniment of pigment stones. Excessive bilirubin secretion when haemolysis is present may play a role, but the majority of patients do not have haemolysis and those without haemolysis do not have an increased output of bilirubin in bile (Boonyapisit et al 1978). Stasis of bile and contact of conjugated bilirubin with hydrolytic enzymes from the gallbladder mucosa or pancreas might be important. Gallbladder mucus can bind to bilirubin and may be a factor in stone formation (Smith & LaMont 1983). The role of bilirubin mono-glucuronide is possibly critical because it is an unstable molecule and easily converted to unconjugated bilirubin.

BILIARY SLUDGE

The term 'biliary sludge' is used to describe bile which is in a gel form that contains numerous crystals of microspheroliths. Originally of limited interest and an occasional observation at cholecystectomy, biliary sludge has assumed greater importance since the advent of gallbladder ultrasonography and the finding that biliary sludge is a common phenomenon. It is recognized as a fluid substance that layers in the dependent portion of the gallbladder and produces low amplitude echoes, usually not associated with acoustic shadowing (Allen et al 1981).

The precise nature of biliary sludge has yet to be determined but it is probably a mixture of calcium bilirubinate granules, cholesterol crystals and glycoproteins (Allen et al 1981). Mucus cannot be degraded in bile and if there is any stasis in the gallbladder the accumulation of glycoprotein in the gallbladder bile will tend to induce gel formation which traps bile pigments. It is possible that this gel material interacts with calcium, bile salts, and cholesterol to reduce the solubility of bilirubin and cholesterol, forming calcium bilirubinate and cholesterol monohydrate crystals, and these become trapped in the gel. It is this physical state that is recognized on ultrasonography. Studies on patients who undergo prolonged fasting, e.g. when treated by total parenteral nutrition (Messing et al 1983), suggest that sludge is a reversible state and may disappear if normal feeding is resumed.

These observations suggest that the following conditions relate to and are pre-requisites for gallstone formation: biliary cholesterol supersaturation, an excess of glycoproteins, inadequate gallbladder emptying, an absolute or relative lack of protein inhibitors of nucleation, and the relative concentration of calcium ions. Almost certainly identical conditions do not apply to all situations in which gallstones are formed.

ANIMAL MODELS

Only human gallbladder bile is consistently supersaturated with cholesterol and therefore the observations on most animal models of gallstone disease are not immediately applicable to man. Of the many experimental forms of gallstones (Bouchier 1971, Van Der Linden & Bergman 1977) only two have provided relevant information: cholesterol gallstones in cholesterol-fed prairie dogs and pigment stones in mice with hereditary haemolytic anaemia.

The prairie dog model has provided a great deal of interesting information and enabled cholesterol gallstone formation to be observed from the precursor state through the nucleation of cholesterol and mucus hypersecretion to stone growth and subsequently stone dissolution with bile salts. Factors influencing stone growth, such as gallbladder motility and sphincterotomy, have also been studied (Lee et al 1981, Hutton et al 1981, Fridhandler et al 1983, Doty et al 1983). It seems that this model may have less relevance to the human situation than had been anticipated because of the failure to identify mucus as a nucleating factor in human bile, and the presence of inhibitors of nucleation in normal bile.

Mice of the genotype nb/nb have an hereditary haemolytic anaemia and regularly form calcium bilirubinate stones (Trotman et al 1980). Again this model has proved the importance of glycoprotein secretion by the gallbladder enabling pigment to be precipitated as stones (La Mont et al 1983). The increased mucus production may even precede stone formation. Thus an increased hepatic secretion of unconjugated bilirubin in bile (Trotman et al 1981) and an excessive secretion of mucus by glands in the gallbladder neck provide the circumstances under which mucus-calcium bilirubinate concretions form, aggregate and develop into stones.

EPIDEMIOLOGY OF GALLSTONES

Epidemiological studies on gallstone disease should provide not only an indication of the prevalence of the disease but also furnish important indicators to its aetiology. Until recently most information was obtained from autopsy studies but such studies are unrepresentative of free-living populations because of selection in hospital populations, cultural differences in autopsy rates and variations in recording information at post-mortem. Large population surveys using oral cholecystography are neither practicable nor desirable, but the widespread use of ultrasonography has dramatically introduced a new tool which should enable accurate data to be obtained about the prevalence of gallstones in large populations at all ages. Furthermore, this technique promises to shed light on the natural history of gallstones, their growth from biliary sludge, their existence as 'silent' stones and (in a small proportion) their progression to symptomatic stones with clinical disease and complications. The epidemiology and clinical associations of gallstones will be reviewed and where possible explained according to what is known of the pathogenesis of gallstone formation. Such information as is available relates almost entirely to biliary lipid analyses; there has been no large scale evaluation of nucleating factors. Furthermore many of the epidemiological studies relate only to the presence or absence of gallstones without identifying whether these are cholesterol or pigment in type.

General prevalence

It has been calculated that there are some five million persons in the UK and 25 million in the USA with gallstones. A single statistic for the prevalence of gallstones is misleading because of the large variation with age, but stones occur in 10–20% of persons at post-mortem (Table 38.7). Godfrey et al (1984) correlated both autopsy and cholecystectomy data and observed that the prevalence of gallstones in an adult English population is 17%. It is unclear whether the prevalence of gallstones is increasing. The data in Table 38.7 suggest a gradual increase in post-mortem prevalence over the years, while Brett & Barker (1976) reported the post-mortem prevalence in Europe to be 10.5% pre-1940 and 18.5% after 1940. Bateson (1984), on the basis of data derived from autopsy records in Dundee, Scotland, concluded that gallbladder disease was commoner in 1974–83 than 1953–73 and that this increase occurred in each year after 1974. The interpretation of cholecystectomy rates (Holland & Heaton 1972) should be made with caution and they may not indicate an increase in prevalence (Opit & Greenhill 1974).

There have been many studies on various associations with gallstone disease. These are summarized in Table 38.8, and discussed in detail below. Major American and British studies have shown that socio-economic factors are not critical determinants of gallstone disease (Friedman et al 1966, Barker et al 1979).

Racial and geographic prevalence

There have been many studies of the prevalence of gallstones in different racial groups and these are summarized in Table 38.9.

Certain American Indian communities have some of the highest prevalence rates in the world and this is due to the production of supersaturated bile (Grundy et al 1972, Williams et al 1981). Sampliner et al (1970) found the overall prevalence in Pima Indian females to be 48.6%. Apart from genetic factors which might determine gallstone formation, obesity, diet and diabetes mellitus may play a role in inducing saturated bile (Tucker et al 1982). Studies in Caucasian populations relate the increased prevalence to saturated bile.

There is a marked difference in prevalence between Indians living in the north of the Indian subcontinent who have prevalence rates seven times greater than persons living in South India (Malhotra 1968). An interesting change in the nature of gallstones has occurred in Japan. Pigment stones were very commonly found in the early part of this century but recent data indicate that cholesterol stones are now the predominant stone (Nakayama & Miyake 1970). This may be related to a reduction in biliary tract parasites and changing diet (Nagase et al 1980). The Masai of East Africa rarely develop gallstones and their bile has a low cholesterol content (Biss et al 1971).

Table 38.7 Frequency of gallstones at autopsy

Investigator	Date	%
Ehnmark	1939	11
Davidson	1962	14
Bouchier	1969	13
Bateson & Bouchier	1975	20
Lindstorm	1977	36

Table 38.8 Associations with gallstones

Definite	Probable	Possible
Race	Total parenteral nutrition	Hiatal hernia
Age	Diabetes mellitus	Coeliac disease
Sex	S.I. by-pass surgery	Pattern of eating
Obesity	Oestrogen therapy	Gastric surgery
Clofibrate	Type IV hyperlipoproteinaemia	Cystic fibrosis
Ileal disease		
Hepatic cirrhosis		
Haemolysis		
Refined carbohydrate diet		

Table 38.9 Racial/geographic prevalence of gallstones at autopsy

Very high	High	Moderate	Low
Pima Indians	USA (whites)	USA (blacks)	Greece
Micmac Indians	Britain	Singapore	Japan
Chippewa Indians	Norway	Germany	Singapore
Mexicans	Australia		India
Sweden			China
Czechoslovakia			
Chile (women)			

Familial frequency

There are few data on familial factors in gallstone disease. Studies claiming that cholelithiasis is an inherited disease tend to have inadequate control groups (Jackson & Gay 1959, Van Der Linden & Lindelof 1965, Wheeler et al 1970). A more satisfactory study undertaken in Israel using oral cholecystography demonstrated a two-fold increase of gallstones in first degree relatives compared with controls (Gilat et al 1983).

Age

All the studies on gallstone prevalence show a steady increase with age, the maximal frequency occurring in patients over 80 (Friedman et al 1966, Bateson & Bouchier 1975, Godfrey et al 1984). The age-related data for females in countries with a high to very high prevalence of gallstones is shown in Table 38.10. Studies on the change in biliary lipids with ageing suggest that the cholesterol content increases (Trash et al 1976, Valdivieso et al 1978, Fujiyama et al 1979). This effect is most marked in women and is unrelated to any influence of obesity. The increased lithogenicity of bile is due to an increased output of cholesterol rather than any change in bile acid metabolism. Normal infants and children have secretion ratios of cholesterol:bile salts that are lower than adults (Heubi et al 1982). Studies in Pima Indians show that cholesterol saturation increases significantly in both sexes at the time of puberty, being more marked in females than males (Bennion et al 1979). Many factors contribute to gallstones in children. About 25% of children with gallstones have haemolytic disease; other possible predisposing factors are cystic fibrosis, liver disease, bowel resection and heart disease (Henschke & Teele 1983).

Sex

There is consistent evidence that gallbladder disease is more common in females at all ages, although the female:male proportion decreases slightly with age (Friedman et al 1966, Bateson & Bouchier 1975). An increase in the number of pregnancies is associated with an increased risk of gallstones. Bile tends to be more saturated in women than men and this cannot be explained by differences in body weight or age (Hofmann et al 1982).

It is tempting to explain the increased frequency of gallstones in women as an effect of female sex hormones on hepatic function, bile secretion and gallbladder function. In contrast to earlier reports, recent studies of biliary lipids during the menstrual cycle show no effect on cholesterol saturation (Kern et al 1981, Whiting et al 1981). On the other hand, oral contraceptive therapy may be associated with an increase in cholesterol saturation (Bennion et al 1976, Down et al 1983). Down et al (1983) believe that it is the progestagen component rather than the oestrogens which are responsible for the changes in biliary lipids. Bile is more saturated during the second and third trimester of pregnancy (Kern et al 1981).

The use of oral contraceptives induces an increased risk of gallbladder disease (Boston Collaborative Drug Surveillance Program 1973), but the nature of the disorder is controversial. While Everson and colleagues (1982) observed an increased number of cholecystectomies in women taking oral contraceptives there was no increased tendency to gallstone disease. On the other hand, Scragg et al (1984a) recorded an increased risk of gallstones in young but not in older women.

Apart from an effect on bile chemistry, hormones also influence gallbladder function which, in turn, might affect biliary lipid secretion or predispose the organ to cholecystitis. In pregnancy the fasting and residual gallbladder volumes are larger and the emptying rate slower than in non-pregnant women (Braverman et al 1980). The decreased rate of bile salt return may stimulate the increased synthesis of primary bile salts and expand the bile salt pool; but in the latter stages of pregnancy there is a decrease in hepatic synthesis of chenodeoxycholic acid, possibly due to the hormonal effect on hepatic synthesis. This in turn might enable cholesterol output in bile to increase causing bile to become saturated in the third trimester. Nervi et al (1981) reported that the flux of lipoprotein cholesterol in Chilean females is increased. Oestrogens also decrease bile salt synthesis and secretion. Thus the effect of female sex hormones on the biliary system is complex and diverse but, by adversely influencing cholesterol and bile salt secretion into bile as well as gallbladder function, they do appear to predispose to cholesterol gallstone disease.

Table 38.10 Post-mortem prevalence of gallstones in women

Age (yrs)	Chile	Scotland	USA	Norway
10–19	7.2	2.8	0	0
20–29	25.1	3.8	4.2	1.9
30–39	40.8	6.2	8.6	2.5
40–49	46.5	12.0	12.1	8.4
50–59	55.6	15.8	23.3	16.9
60–69	65.3	25.4	27.5	24.0

Obesity

Obesity is an independent factor determining the development of gallstones which can be separated from any sex or ageing effect. Overweight is thought to be an important cause for the high prevalence of gallstones in Pima Indians. There is a three-fold increase in gallstone prevalence in obese Caucasian females with the majority of the obese women in the third decade having asymptomatic gallstones. In one study the prevalence ran from 23% in the third decade to 42% in the fifth (Tucker et al 1982). However, Scragg et al (1984b) found the risk to be increased only in obese women below 50. It is generally believed that the gallstones are cholesterol in type.

The obese individual produces bile which is supersaturated with cholesterol and this reflects an excessive secretion by the liver which is related to excessive production of

Table 38.11 Mechanism of gallstone formation in obese vs. non-obese individuals

Gross obesity	Moderate obesity	Non-obese
Increased cholesterol synthesis	Increased biliary cholesterol	Normal biliary cholesterol
Normal or raised bile salt output	Reduced bile salt output	Reduced bile salt output
Raised biliary cholesterol	Raised biliary cholesterol	Reduced biliary bile salts
Cholesterol saturation in bile	Cholesterol saturation in bile	Cholesterol saturation in bile

cholesterol by the liver and/or the intestine. Bile salt pool size and secretion is normal or increased in obesity. The mechanism of stone formation in obesity differs from that in the non-obese individual where either a reduction in bile acid pool size or a reduced hepatic secretion of bile salts and phospholipids, or a dual defect of both excessive cholesterol secretion and diminished bile salt secretion may be responsible (Table 38.11) (Bennion & Grundy 1975, Shaffer & Small 1977). Fasting is normally associated with an increased biliary cholesterol saturation and this phenomenon persists or even becomes more accentuated in obesity (Bennion & Grundy 1975, Mabee et al 1976).

The bile remains saturated during an acute period of calorie restriction and weight loss but once the weight has been stabilized at a lower level bile usually becomes less saturated.

Diabetes mellitus

There is still dispute as to whether diabetics are at risk of developing gallstones. Haber & Heaton (1979) list a number of publications claiming an increased prevalence of gallstones in diabetes mellitus but Diehl & Elford (1981) using multiple-cause mortality tables for diabetics in England and Wales were unable to confirm that these individuals are at increased risk of death from gallstone-related diseases. The prevalence of asymptomatic stones in diabetics is not known and ultrasonographic surveys of free-living populations will be of considerable interest.

There is also disagreement about whether the disturbed metabolism in diabetes mellitus is accompanied by an increased biliary cholesterol saturation. Bennion & Grundy (1977) reported an increased bile salt synthesis, expanded bile acid pool and reduced cholesterol saturation of bile in obese diabetics. The institution of insulin therapy effected a reduced synthesis of bile salts, a contraction of total body pool of bile salts and an increase in biliary cholesterol. In another study, Haber & Heaton (1979) found no difference in the cholesterol saturation of bile between diabetic and non-diabetic subjects. Both groups had supersaturated bile which was accounted for by obesity. It is probable that there is no specific biochemical defect in diabetes mellitus which will predispose to gallstone formation. The increased cholesterol saturation which occurs in the bile of diabetics is the consequence of associated obesity and possibly hypertriglyceridaemia. Gallbladder atony consequent upon an autonomic neuropathy may favour stone formation in supersaturated bile.

Clofibrate therapy

Clofibrate is a drug capable of reducing serum cholesterol levels but its use is accompanied by an increase in biliary cholesterol that persists throughout treatment (Pertsemlidis et al 1974, Bateson et al 1978). Persons taking clofibrate have an increased prevalence of gallstones (Bateson et al 1978) and an increased cholecystectomy rate (Coronary Drug Project Research Group 1977, Oliver et al 1978).

Diet

There has been much debate over the role of diet in cholesterol gallstone disease and an increased intake of cholesterol, fat, calories, refined carbohydrate or a lack of dietary fibre have all been blamed. The studies are confusing with conflicting results. Males taking a low cholesterol, low saturated fat but high polyunsaturated fat and high plant sterol diet have an increased frequency of gallstones (Sturdevant et al 1973). While there is experimental evidence that a high cholesterol intake in man can raise cholesterol saturation in the bile (Den Besten et al 1973) there are no dietary studies to support a major role for excess dietary cholesterol in lithogenesis. Dietary cholesterol normally makes only a small contribution to bile cholesterol.

Scragg et al (1984b) have conducted a large case-control study with carefully matched controls in Australia and demonstrated an association between simple refined sugar (mainly sucrose) taken in sweets and drinks, and gallstones. Metabolic studies have failed to show why sucrose should cause gallstones for a diet rich in sucrose does not cause cholesterol saturation (Werner et al 1984). Although a diet rich in fibre might reduce biliary cholesterol saturation (Thornton et al 1983a) Scragg and his colleagues could not demonstrate a decreased risk of gallstones in persons having a high fibre intake.

The Australian study also supported the view that a moderate intake of alcohol ($<$30 g/day, about $\frac{1}{2}$ a bottle of wine) is associated with a reduced risk of gallstones. This may be because alcohol reduces the cholesterol saturation in bile (Thornton et al 1983b). A brief report from France indicated that reduced meal frequency, with prolongation of fasting periods increases the risk of gallstone disease

(Capron et al 1981a). Fasting raises the cholesterol saturation in bile and is associated with retention of bile in the gallbladder and probably poor mixing of saturated and unsaturated bile in the gallbladder: all factors which will predispose to gallstone formation. The concept that the pattern of eating might be relevant to lithogenesis is imaginative and important and requires further study.

Hyperlipidaemia

There are a great many studies showing that there is no association between serum cholesterol concentrations and myocardial infarction and gallstones (Friedman et al 1966, Bateson & Bouchier 1975, Hofmann et al 1982). On the other hand there are data indicating that gallstone disease is more frequent in Type IV (hyper pre-beta) hyperlipoproteinaemia (Einarsson et al 1975, Kadziolka et al 1977) although this association could not be demonstrated by Bateson et al (1978). Individuals with Type IV hyperlipoproteinaemia have bile saturated with cholesterol. Their total body pool size of bile salts is often increased but it is significant that this is mainly due to an increase in cholic acid and there is a relative reduction in chenodeoxycholic acid (Ahlberg et al 1980) which could predispose to an increased secretion of biliary cholesterol.

Cirrhosis of the liver

Patients with cirrhosis of the liver have a prevalence of gallstones which is two to three times greater than a non-cirrhotic population and this tendency is present at all ages in contrast to the rising frequency with age that occurs in the general population. The increased risk of gallstones is not associated with any one type of cirrhosis and the gallstones are predominantly of the pigment variety (Bouchier 1969, Nicholas et al 1972).

Patients with moderately advanced, well compensated cirrhosis may have a reduced total body pool of bile salts but no major derangement of cholesterol metabolism, and their bile is no more supersaturated than normal (Von Bergmann et al 1979). There is a marked reduction of bile salt secretion in advanced cirrhosis but this is matched by diminished biliary lecithin and cholesterol so that bile is not lithogenic (Schwartz et al 1979). The stones in chronic liver disease are of the pigment type and probably result from the chronic haemolysis which occurs in cirrhosis. Interestingly, the stones are usually asymptomatic. Jaundice in cirrhosis is more likely to be due to hepatic decompensation than a stone in the common bile duct.

Inflammatory bowel disease

Gallstones are more than four times as frequent in patients with a disorder of the terminal ileum either from disease or because of resection (Heaton & Read 1969, Cohen et al 1971). The gallstones tend to be asymptomatic. The type of stone has not been adequately documented but the observation that at least 50% were calcified might indicate a higher proportion of pigment stones. However, patients with ileal dysfunction have bile which is more saturated with cholesterol than subjects with normal ileal function and this is due to a diminished total bile salt pool size (Dowling et al 1972). Jejuno–ileal bypass operations are associated with an increased saturation of bile and a risk of gallstone disease (Sørensen et al 1980).

Gastric surgery

Whether or not operations upon the stomach and the vagus predispose to gallstone formation remains uncertain (Fletcher & Clark 1968, Bouchier 1970), with the weight of evidence not supporting any association. Shaffer (1982) reported that truncal vagotomy did not adversely influence either gallbladder emptying or bile lipid composition. It has been suggested that gastric bypass surgery for gross obesity is complicated by an increased prevalence of gallstones (Wattchow et al 1983).

Total parenteral nutrition

Evidence is mounting to show that patients undergoing treatment by total parenteral nutrition might be at increased risk of developing gallstones. Roslyn et al (1983) reported that 23% of patients who had received total parenteral nutrition for a mean of 14 months developed gallbladder disease and that the risk was even greater in those patients who had ileal disorders. Total parenteral nutrition is accompanied by an increased tendency to develop biliary sludge as demonstrated at ultrasonography and on analysis of gallbladder bile, which is thick and contains cholesterol and calcium bilirubinate crystals. The tendency to sludge formation is reversed once oral feeding is instituted (Messing et al 1983). Precisely how sludge develops has still to be explained but doubtlessly reduced gallbladder motility is an important factor.

Haemolytic anaemia

Patients with haemolysis have an increased prevalence of pigment gallstones, the relative frequency probably depending upon the severity of haemolysis. In hereditary spherocytosis the prevalence is 43–66%, 10–37% in sickle-cell disease and about 10% in thalassaemia (Barrett-Connor 1968, Dewey et al 1970). Saudi Arabs with sickle-cell anaemia have milder manifestations of haemolysis because of a high level of alkali-resistant haemoglobin and they have a relative low (approximately 6%) prevalence of gallstones (Perrine 1973). The gallstones in haemolytic disease tend to be asymptomatic. Ultrasonic screening of a population with haemolysis indicates that around 12% of two to four-year-old children have stones, and-the prevalence rises to 42% in the 15–18-year-old group (Sarnaik et al 1980).

Miscellaneous associations

An association between gallstones and many other diseases has been implied. Firm evidence is wanting to implicate peptic ulcer and hyperparathyroidism. It is possible that an association does exist for both hiatal hernia and diverticular disease of the colon (Capron et al 1978, 1981b). There is controversy over an association between gallstones and colorectal cancer (Lowenfels 1980, Linos et al 1982) and gastric cancer (Lowenfels 1980, Kalima et al 1982). Children with cystic fibrosis may have an increased frequency of gallbladder disease (Rovsing & Sloth 1973) and the bile in untreated disease is saturated with cholesterol, probably reflecting the bile salt malabsorption which these children have. Treatment with pancreatic enzymes restores biliary lipids to more normal proportions (Roy et al 1977).

NATURAL HISTORY OF GALLSTONES

It is important to appreciate that the great majority of gallstones are asymptomatic and remain so (Table 38.12). When symptoms do occur they are usually moderate (Table 38.13). Early studies were based mainly on projections from post-mortem data but information is being accumulated by screening healthy populations and the data to be obtained by ultrasonographic surveys will be invaluable. It is essential, when determining the natural history of gallstones, to make a clear distinction between symptomatic and silent stones. At least 35% of patients with symptomatic gallstones will develop significant symptoms over 11 years (Wenckert & Robertson 1966). The National Cooperative Gallstone Study showed that 31% of patients who were free of biliary pain for one year prior to entering the study developed biliary pain whereas 69% of patients developed further pain if they had had biliary pain during the year prior to entering (Thistle et al 1982). In the only study of its kind Gracie & Ransohoff (1982) reported the follow-up of asymptomatic stones discovered by cholecystographic screening. The cumulative probability of developing biliary pain was 15% at 10 years and 18% at both 15 and 20 years. The yearly risk of biliary pain appeared to decrease with time.

It is apparent that people do not die because of the presence of gallstones and the risk of major complications is low. If symptoms do occur they generally appear soon after stones are diagnosed. The data from Gracie & Ransohoff indicate that around 87% of asymptomatic gallbladder stones remain silent, a figure similar to data obtained in a male Pima Indian population (Sampliner et al 1970). Thus both autopsy and prospective studies in free-living populations support the concept that the majority of gallstones are asymptomatic and remain so. The great majority of people with gallstones in the UK never undergo a cholecystectomy (Godfrey et al 1984).

Table 38.12 Prevalence of asymptomatic gallstones (data from autopsies)

Author	Date	%
Kehr	1901	95*
Baker	1920	90
Robertson	1945	61
Newman & Northop	1959	77
Sato & Matsushiro	1974	75

*data from laparotomies

Table 38.13 Natural history of gallstones

Remain asymptomatic	85–90%
Become symptomatic	
Moderate	10–7
Severe	5–3

REFERENCES

Admirand W H, Small D M 1968 The physicochemical basis of cholesterol gallstone formation in man. Journal of Clinical Investigation 47: 1043–1052

Ahlberg J, Angelin B, Einarsson K, Hellstrom K, Leijd B 1977 Influence of deoxycholic acid on biliary lipids in man. Clinical Science and Molecular Medicine 53: 249–256

Ahlberg J, Angelin B, Einarsson K, Hellstrom K, Lejid B 1980 Biliary lipid composition in normo- and hyperlipoproteinaemia. Gastroenterology 79: 90–94

Ahlberg J, Angelin B, Einarsson K 1981 Hepatic 3-hydroxy-3-methylglutaryl coenzyme A reductase activity and biliary composition in man: relation to cholesterol gallstone disease and effects of cholic and chenodeoxycholic acid treatment. Journal of Lipid Research 22: 410–422

Allen B, Bernhoft R, Blanckaert N, Svanvik J, Filly R, Gooding G et al 1981 Sludge is calcium bilirubinate associated with bile salts. American Journal of Surgery 141: 51–56

Aschoff L 1924 Lectures on pathology. New York

Barker D J P, Gardner M J, Power C, Hutt M S R 1979 Prevalence of gallstones at necropsy in nine British towns: a collaborative study. British Medical Journal 2: 1389–1392

Barrett-Connor E 1968 Cholelithiasis in sickle cell anaemia. American Journal of Medicine 45: 889–897

Bateson M C 1984 Gallbladder disease and the cholecystectomy rate are independently variable. Lancet ii: 621–624

Bateson M C, Bouchier I A D 1975 Prevalence of gallstones in Dundee: a necropsy study. British Medical Journal 4: 427–429

Bateson M C, Maclean D, Ross P E, Bouchier I A D 1978 Clofibrate therapy and gallstone induction. Digestive Diseases 23: 623–628

Beer J M, Bills P M, Lewis D 1977 Electron probe microanalysis in the study of gallstones. Gut 18: 836–842

Beer J M, Bills P M, Lewis D 1979 Microstructure of gallstones. Gastroenterology 76: 548–555

Bennion L J, Grundy S M 1975 Effects of obesity and caloric intake on biliary lipid metabolism in man. Journal of Clinical Investigation 56: 996–1011

Bennion L J, Grundy S M 1977 Effects of diabetes mellitus on cholesterol metabolism in man. New England Journal of Medicine 296: 1365–1371

Bennion L J, Ginsberg R L, Garnick M B, Bennett P H 1976 Effects of oral contraceptives on the gallbladder bile of normal women. New England Journal of Medicine 294: 189–192

Bennion L J, Knowles W C, Mott D M, Spangola A M, Bennett P H 1979 Development of lithogenic bile during puberty in Pima Indians. New England Journal of Medicine 300: 873–876

Bills P M, Lewis D 1975 A structural study of gallstones. Gut 16: 630–637

Biss K, Ho K-J, Mikkelson B, Lewis L, Taylor B C 1971 Some unique biologic characteristics of the Masai of East Africa. New England Journal of Medicine 284: 694–699

Boonyapisit S T, Trotman B W, Ostrow J D 1978 Unconjugated bilirubin, and the hydrolysis of conjugated bilirubin, in gallbladder bile of patients with cholelithiasis. Gastroenterology 74: 70–74

Boston Collaborative Drug Surveillance Program 1973 Oral contraceptives and thromboembolic disease, surgically confirmed gallbladder disease, and breast tumours. Lancet i: 1399–1404

Bouchier I A D 1969 Postmortem study of the frequency of gallstones in patients with cirrhosis of the liver. Gut 10: 705–710

Bouchier I A D 1970 The vagus, the bile, and gallstones. Gut 11: 799–803

Bouchier I A D 1971 Experimental cholelithiasis. In: the Scientific Basis of Medicine. Annual Reviews, p 232–243

Bouchier I A D 1983 Biochemistry of gallstone formation. Clinics in Gastroenterology 12: 25–48

Bouchier I A D, Cooperband S R, El Kodsi B M 1965 Mucus substances and viscosity of normal and pathological human bile. Gastroenterology 49: 343–353

Braverman D Z, Johnson M L, Kern F Jr 1980 Effects of pregnancy and contraceptive steroids on gallbladder function. New England Journal of Medicine 302: 362–364

Brett M, Barker D J P 1976 The world distribution of gallstones. International Journal of Epidemiology 5: 335–341

Burnstein M J, Ilson R G, Petrunka C N, Taylor R D, Strasberg S M 1983 Evidence of a potent nucleating factor in the gallbladder bile of patients with cholesterol gallstones. Gastroenterology 85: 801–807

Campbell B A, Burton A C 1949 Stratification of bile in the gallbladder and cholelithiasis. Surgery, Gynecology and Obstetrics 88: 731–738

Capron J-P, Payenneville H, Dumont M, Dupas J-L, Lorriaux A 1978 Evidence of an association between cholelithiasis and hiatus hernia. Lancet ii: 329–331

Capron J-P, Delamarre J, Herve M A, Dupas J L, Poulain P, Descombes P 1981a Meal frequency and duration of overnight fast: a role in gall-stone formation? British Medical Journal 283:1435

Capron J-P, Piperaud R, Dupas J-L, Delamarre J, Lorriaux A 1981b Evidence for an association between cholelithiasis and diverticular disease of the colon. A case-controlled study. Digestive Diseases and Sciences 26: 523–527

Carey M C, Small D M 1978 The physical chemistry of cholesterol solubility in bile. Relationship to gallstone formation and dissolution in bile. Journal of Clinical Investigation 61: 998–1026

Carulli N, Ponz De Leon M, Zironi F, Pinetti A, Smerieri A, Iori R, Loria P 1980 Hepatic cholesterol and bile acid metabolism in subjects with gallstones: comparative effects of short term feeding of chenodeoxycholic and ursodeoxycholic acid. Journal of Lipid Research 21: 35–43

Coronary Drug Project Research Group 1977 Gallbladder disease as a side effect of drugs influencing lipid metabolism. New England Journal of Medicine 296: 1185–1190

Cohen S, Kaplan M, Gottlieb L, Patterson J 1971 Liver disease and gallstones in regional enteritis. Gastroenterology 60: 237–245

Davidson J F 1962 Alcohol and cholelithiasis: a necropsy survey of cirrhotics. American Journal of Medical Sciences 244: 703–705

Den Besten L, Connor W E, Bell S 1973 The effect of dietary cholesterol on the composition of human bile. Surgery 73: 266–273

Dewey K W, Grossman H, Canale V C 1970 Cholelithiasis in thalassemia major. Radiology 96: 385–388

Diehl A K, Elford J 1981 Gallstone disease in diabetes: analysis using multiple-cause mortality tables. Public Health, London 95: 261–263

Dolgin S M, Schwartz J S, Kressel H Y, Soloway R D, Miller W T, Trotman B W et al 1981 Identification of patients with cholesterol or pigment gallstones by discriminant analysis of radiologic features. New England Journal of Medicine 304: 808–811

Doty J E, Pitt H A, Kachenbecker S L, Den Besten L 1983 Impaired gallbladder emptying before gallstone formation in the prairie dog. Gastroenterology 85: 168–174

Dowling R H, Bell G D, White J 1972 Lithogenic bile in patients with ileal dysfunction. Gut 13: 415–420

Down R H L, Whiting M J, Watts J McK, Jones W 1983 Effect of synthetic oestrogens and progesterones in oral contraceptives on bile lipid composition. Gut 24: 253–259

Ehnmark E 1939 The gallstone disease: a clinical–statistical study. Acta Chirurgica Scandinavica Suppl 37

Einarsson K, Hellström K, Kallner M 1975 Gallbladder disease in hyperlipoproteinaemia. Lancet i: 484–487

Everson R B, Byar D P, Bischoff A J 1982 Estrogen predisposes to cholecystectomy but not stones. Gastroenterology 82: 4–8

Fisher R S, Stelzer F, Rock E, Malmud L S 1982 Abnormal gallbladder emptying in patients with gallstones. Digestive Diseases and Sciences 27: 1019–1024

Fletcher D M, Clark C G 1968 Gall-stones and gastric surgery. A review. British Journal of Surgery 55: 895–899

Freston J W, Bouchier I A D, Newman J 1969 Biliary mucus substances in dihydrocholesterol-induced cholelithiasis. Gastroenterology 57: 670–678

Fridhandler T M, Davison J S, Shaffer E A 1983 Defective gallbladder contractility in the ground squirrel and prairie dog during the early stage of cholesterol gallstone formation. Gastroenterology 85: 830–836

Friedman G D, Kannel W B, Dawber T R 1966 The epidemiology of gallbladder disease: observations in the Framingham Study. Journal of Chronic Disease 19: 273–292

Fujiyama M, Kajiyama G, Maruhashi A, Mizumo T, Yamada K, Kawamoto T et al 1979 Changes in lipid composition of bile with age in normal subjects and patients with gallstones. Hiroshima Journal of Medical Sciences 28: 23–29

Gilat T, Feldman C, Halpern Z, Dan M, Bar-Meir S 1983 An increased familial frequency of gallstones. Gastroenterology 84: 242–246

Godfrey P J, Bates T, Harrison M, King M B, Padley N R 1984 Gallstones and morbidity. A study of all gallstone-related deaths in a single health district. Gut 25: 1029–1033

Gollish S H, Burnstein M J, Ilson R G, Petrunka C N, Strasberg S M 1983 Nucleation of cholesterol monohydrate crystals from hepatic and gall-bladder bile of patients with cholesterol gallstones. Gut 24: 836–844

Good L I, Edell S L, Soloway R D, Trotman B W, Mulhera C, Arger P A 1979 Ultrasonic properties of gallstones. Effect of stone size and composition. Gastroenterology 77: 258–263

Gracie W A, Ransohoff D F 1982 The natural history of silent gallstones. The innocent gallstone is not a myth. New England Journal of Medicine 307: 798–800

Grundy S M, Metzger A L, Adler R D 1972 Mechanisms of lithogenic bile formation in American Indian women with cholesterol gallstones. Journal of Clinical Investigation 51: 3026–3043

Grundy S M, Duane W C, Adler R D, Aron J M, Matzger A L 1974 Biliary lipid outputs in young women with cholesterol stones. Metabolism 23: 67–73

Haber G B, Heaton K W 1979 Lipid composition of bile in diabetics and obesity-matched controls. Gut 20: 518–522

Heaton K W, Read A E 1969 Gall stones in patients with disorders of the terminal ileum and disturbed bile salt metabolism. British Medical Journal 3: 494–496

Henschke C I, Teele R L 1983 Cholelithiasis in children. Journal of Ultrasound Medicine 2: 481–484

Heubi J E, Soloway R D, Balistreri W F 1982 Biliary lipid composition in healthy and diseased infants, children, and young adults. Gastroenterology 82: 1295–1299

Hofmann A F, Grundy S M, Lachin J M, Lan S-P, Baum R A,

Hanson R F et al 1982 Pretreatment biliary lipid composition in white patients with radiolucent gallstones in the National Cooperative Gallstone Study. Gastroenterology 83: 738–752

Holan K R, Holzbach R T, Hermann R E, Cooperman A M, Claffey W J 1979 Nucleation time: a key factor in the pathogenesis of cholesterol gallstone disease. Gastroenterology 77: 611–617

Holland C, Heaton K W 1972 Increasing frequency of gall bladder operations in the Bristol clinical area. British Medical Journal 3: 672–675

Holzbach R T, Marsh M, Olszewski M, Holan K 1973 Cholesterol solubility in bile. Evidence that supersaturated bile is frequent in healthy man. Journal of Clinical Investigation 52: 1467–1479

Holzbach R T, Kibe A, Thiel E, Howell J H, Marsh M, Hermann R E 1984 Biliary proteins. Unique inhibitors of cholesterol crystal nucleation in human gallbladder bile. Journal of Clinical Investigation 73: 35–45

Hutton S W, Sievert C E Jr, Vennes J A, Duane W C 1981 The effect of sphincterotomy on gallstone formation in the prairie dog. Gastroenterology 81: 663–667

Jackson C E, Gay B-C 1959 Inheritance of gall-bladder disease. Surgery 46: 853–857

Jazwari R P, Kupfer R M, Bridges C, Joseph A, Northfield T C 1983 Assessment of gall-bladder storage function in man. Clinical Science 65: 185–191

Kadziolka R, Nilsson S, Scherstén T 1977 Prevalence of hyperlipoproteinaemia in men with gallstone disease. Scandinavian Journal of Gastroenterology 12: 353–355

Kalima T, Sipponen J, Kivilaakso E, Sipponen P 1982 Decreased prevalence of gallstones in gastric cancer. American Journal of Surgery 144: 531–533

Kehr H 1901 Introduction to the differential diagnosis of the separate forms of gallstone disease. Blakiston, Philadelphia

Kern F Jr, Everson G T, De Mark B, Mckinley C, Showalter R, Erfling W et al 1981 Biliary lipids, bile acids, and gallbladder function in the human female. Effects of pregnancy and the ovulatory cycle. Journal of Clinical Investigation 68: 1229–1242

Kouroumalis E, Hopwood D, Ross P E, Milne G, Bouchier I A D 1982 Gallbladder epithelial and hydrolases in human cholecystitis. Journal of Pathology 139: 179–191

Kouroumalis E, Hopwood D, Ross P E, Bouchier I A D 1984 Human gallbladder epithelium: non-specific esterases in cholecystitis. Journal of Pathology 142: 151–159

LaMont J T, Turner B S, Bernstein S E, Trotman B W 1983 Gallbladder glycoprotein secretion in mice with hemolytic anaemia and pigment gallstones. Hepatology 3: 198–200

Lee S P, Lim T H, Scott A J 1979 Carbohydrate moieties of glycoproteins in human hepatic and gall-bladder bile, gall-bladder mucosa and gall stones. Clinical Science 56: 533–538

Lee S P, La Mont T, Carey M C 1981 Role of gallbladder mucus hypersecretion in the evolution of cholesterol gallstones. Journal of Clinical Investigation 67: 1712–1723

Lindström C G 1977 Frequency of gallstone disease in a well-defined Swedish population. Scandinavian Journal of Gastroenterology 12: 341–346

Linos D A, O'Fallon W M, Thistle J L, Kurland L T 1982 Cholelithiasis and carcinoma of the colon. Cancer 50: 1015–1019

Low-Beer T S, Pomare E W 1975 Can colonic bacterial metabolites predispose to cholesterol gall stones? British Medical Journal 1: 438–440

Lowenfels A B 1980 Gallstones and the risk of cancer. Gut 21: 1090–1092

Mabee T M, Meyer P, Den Besten L, Mason E E 1976 The mechanism of increased gallstone formation in obese human subjects. Surgery 79: 460–468

Maki T 1966 Pathogenesis of calcium bilirubinate gallstones. Annals of Surgery 164: 90–100

Malet P F, Takabayashi A, Trotman B W, Soloway R D, Weston N E 1984 Black and brown pigment gallstones differ in microstructure and microcomposition. Hepatology 4: 227–234

Malhotra S L 1968 Epidemiological study of cholelithiasis among railroad workers in India with special reference to causation. Gut 9: 290–295

Markkanen T, Aho A J 1972 Metabolic aspects of trace metal content of gallstones and gallbladders. Acta Chirugica Scandinavia 138: 301–305

Maton P N, Reuben A, Dowling R H 1982 Relationship between hepatic cholesterol synthesis and biliary cholesterol secretion in man: hepatic cholesterol synthesis is not a major regulator of biliary lipid secretion. Clinical Science 62: 515–519

Maudgal D P, Kupfer R M, Zentler-Munro P L, Northfield T C 1980 Postprandial gall-bladder emptying in patients with gall-stones. British Medical Journal 280: 141–143

Messing B, Boris C, Kunstlingen F, Bernier J J 1983 Does total parenteral nutrition induce gallbladder sludge formation and lithiasis? Gastroenterology 84: 1012–1019

Metzger A L, Adler R, Heymsfield S, Grundy S M 1973 Diurnal variation in biliary lipid composition. Possible role in cholesterol gallstone formation. New England Journal of Medicine 288: 333–336

Mok H Y I, von Bergmann K, Grundy S M 1980 Kinetics of the enterohepatic circulation during fasting: biliary lipid secretion and gallbladder storage. Gastroenterology 78: 1023–1033

Moore E W, Celic L, Ostrow J D 1982 Interactions between ionized calcium and sodium taurocholate: bile salts are important buffers for the prevention of calcium-containing gallstones. Gastroenterology 83: 1079–1089

Mufson D, Triyanond K, Zarembo J E, Ravin L J 1974 Cholesterol solubility in model bile systems: implications in cholelithiasis. Journal of Pharmaceutical Sciences 63: 327–332

Nagase M, Hikasa Y, Soloway R D, Tanimura H, Setoyama M, Kato H 1980 Gallstones in Western Japan. Factors affecting the prevalence of intrahepatic gallstones. Gastroenterology 78: 684–690

Nakayama F, Miyake H 1970 Changing state of gallstone disease in Japan. Composition of stones and treatment of condition. American Journal of Surgery 120: 794–799

Neiderhiser D H, Roth H P 1970 Effect of phospholipase A on cholesterol solubilization by lecithin in a bile salt solution. Gastroenterology 58: 26–31

Nervi F O, Covarrubias C F, Valdivieso V D, Ronco B O, Solari A, Tocornal J 1981 Hepatic cholesterogenesis in Chileans with cholesterol gallstone disease. Gastroenterology 80: 539–545

Nicholas P, Rinaudo P A, Conn H O 1972 Increased incidence of cholelithiasis in Laënnec's cirrhosis. Gastroenterology 63: 112–121

Northfield T C, Hofmann A F 1975 Biliary lipid output during three meals and an overnight fast. I: Relationship to bile acid pool size and cholesterol saturation of bile in gallstone and control patients. Gut 16: 1–17

Northfield T C, Kupfer R M, Maudgal D P, Zentler-Munro P L, Meller S T, Garvie N W et al 1980 Gall-bladder sensitivity to cholecystokinin in patients with gallstones. British Medical Journal 280: 143–144

Oliver M F, Heady J A, Morris J N, Cooper J 1978 A co-operative trial on the primary prevention of ischaemic heart disease using clofibrate. British Heart Journal 40: 1069–1118

Opit L J, Greenhill S 1974 Prevalence of gallstones in relation to differing treatment rates for biliary disease. British Journal of Preventive and Social Medicine 28: 268–272

Perrine R P 1973 Cholelithiasis in sickle cell anemia in a Caucasian population. American Journal of Medicine 54: 327–332

Pertsemlidis D, Panveliwalla D, Ahrens E H Jr 1974 Effects of clofibrate and of an estrogen-progestin combination on fasting biliary lipids and cholic acid kinetics in man. Gastroenterology 66: 565–573

Pomare E W, Heaton K W 1973 Bile salt metabolism in patients with gallstones in functioning gallbladders. Gut 14: 885–890

Pomare E W, Low-Beer T S 1975 Selective suppression of chenodeoxylate synthesis by cholate metabolites in man. Clinical Science and Molecular Medicine 48: 315–321

Robertson H E 1945 Silent gallstones. Gastroenterology 5: 345–372

Roslyn J J, Pitt H A, Mann L L, Ament M E, Den Besten L 1983 Gallbladder disease in patients on long-term parenteral nutrition. Gastroenterology 84: 148–154

Rovsing H, Sloth K 1973 Micro-gallbladder and biliary calculi in mucoviscidosis. Acta Radiologica 14: 588–592

Roy C C, Weber A M, Morin C L, Combes J-C, Nusslé D, Mégevand

A et al 1977 Abnormal biliary lipid composition in cystic fibrosis. New England Journal of Medicine 297: 1301–1305

Salen G, Nicolau G, Shafer S, Mosbach E H 1975 Hepatic cholesterol metabolism in patients with gallstone. Gastroenterology 69: 676–684

Sampliner R E, Bennett P H, Commess L J, Rose F A, Burch T A 1970 Gallbladder disease in Pima Indians. Demonstration of high prevalence and early onset by cholecystography. New England Journal of Medicine 283: 1358–1364

Sarnaik S, Slovis T L, Corbett D P, Enami A, Whitten C F 1980 Incidence of cholelithiasis in sickle cell anemia using the ultrasonic gray-scale technique. Journal of Pediatrics 96: 1005–1008

Sato T, Matsushiro T 1974 Surgical indications in patients with silent gallstones. American Journal of Surgery 128: 368

Schwartz C C, Almond H R, Vlahcevic Z R, Swell L 1979 Bile acid metabolism in cirrhosis: V. Determination of biliary lipid secretion rates in patients with advanced cirrhosis. Gastroenterology 77: 1177–1182

Scragg R K R, McMichael A J, Seamark R F 1984a Oral contraceptives, pregnancy, and endogenous oestrogen in gall stone disease — a case control study. British Medical Journal 288: 1795–1799

Scragg R K R, McMichael A J, Baghurst P A 1984b Diet, alcohol, and relative weight in gall stone disease: a case-control study. British Medical Journal 288: 1113–1119

Sewell R B, Mao S J T, Kawamoto T, La Russo N F 1983 Apolipoproteins of high, low, and very low density lipoproteins in human bile. Journal of Lipid Research 24: 391–401

Shaffer E A 1982 The effect of vagotomy on gallbladder function and bile composition in man. Annals of Surgery 195: 413–418

Shaffer E A, Small D M 1977 Biliary lipid secretion in cholesterol gallstone disease. The effect of cholecystectomy and obesity. Journal of Clinical Investigation 59: 828–840

Sjodahl R, Wetterfors J 1974 Lysolecithin and lecithin in gallbladder wall and bile, their possible roles in the pathogenesis of acute cholecystitis. Scandinavian Journal of Gastroenterology 9: 519–525

Smith B F, La Mont J T 1983 Bovine gallbladder mucin binds bilirubin in vitro. Gastroenterology 85: 707–712

Soloway R D, Trotman D W, Ostrow J D 1977 Pigment stones. Gastroenterology 72: 167–182

Soloway R D, Fayasal E B, Trotman B W, Weston N E, Ficca J F Jr 1982 Water content of gallstones: location and contribution to a hypothesis concerning stone structure. Hepatology 2: 223–229

Sørensen T I A, Jensen I, Klein H C, Andersen B, Petersen O, Laursen K et al 1980 Risk of gallstone formation after jejunoileal bypass increases more with a 1 : 3 than with a 3 : 1 jejunoileal ratio. Scandinavian Journal of Gastroenterology 15: 979–984

Sturdevant R A L, Pearce M L, Dayton S 1973 Increased prevalence of cholelithiasis in men ingesting a serum-cholesterol-lowering diet. New England Journal of Medicine 288: 24–27

Sutor D J, Wooley S E 1969 X-ray diffraction studies of the composition of gallstones from English and Australian patients. Gut 10: 681–683

Sutor D J, Wooley S E 1971 A statistical survey of the composition of gallstones in eight countries. Gut 12: 55–64

Sutor D J, Wooley S E 1973 The nature and incidence of gallstone containing calcium. Gut 14: 215–220

Sutor D J, Wooley S E 1974 The organic matrix of gallstones. Gut 15: 487–491

Tera H 1960 Stratification of human gallbladder bile in vivo. Acta Chirugica Scandinavica Supplementum 256

Thistle J C, Cleary P A, Lachin J M, Tyor M P, Hersh T 1982 The natural history of untreated cholelithiasis during the National Cooperative Gallstone Study (NCGS). Gastroenterology 82:1197 (abstract)

Thomas P J, Hofmann A F 1973 A simple calculation of the lithogenic index of bile: expressing biliary lipid composition on rectangular coordinates. Gastroenterology 65: 698–700

Thornton J R, Emmett P M, Heaton K W 1983a Diet and gall stones: effects of refined and unrefined carbohydrate diets on bile cholesterol saturation and bile acid metabolism. Gut 24: 2–6

Thornton J, Symes C, Heaton K 1983b Moderate alcohol intake reduces bile cholesterol saturation and raises HDL cholesterol. Lancet ii: 819–822

Thureborn E 1966 On the stratification of human bile and its importance for the solubility of cholesterol. Gastroenterology 50: 775–780

Trash D B, Ross P E, Murison J, Bouchier I A D 1976 The influence of age on cholesterol saturation of bile. Gut 17:394

Trotman B W, Ostrow J D, Soloway R D 1974 Pigment vs cholesterol cholelithiasis: comparison of stone and bile composition. American Journal of Digestive Diseases 19: 585–590

Trotman B W, Morris T A III, Sanchez H M, Soloway R D, Ostrow J D 1977 Pigment versus cholesterol cholelithiasis: identification and quantification by infrared spectroscopy. Gastroenterology 72: 495–498

Trotman B W, Bernstein S E, Bove K E, Wirt G D 1980 Studies on the pathogenesis of pigment gallstones in hemolytic anemia. Description and characteristics of a mouse model. Journal of Clinical Investigation 65: 1301–1308

Trotman B W, Bernstein S E, Balistreri W F, Wirt G D, Martin R A 1981 Hemolysis-induced gallstones in mice: increased unconjugated bilirubin in hepatic bile predisposes to gallstone formation. Gastroenterology 81: 232–236

Tucker L E, Tangedahl T N, Newmark S R 1982 Prevalence of gallstones in obese Caucasian American women. International Journal of Obesity 6: 247–251

Valdivieso V, Palma R, Wünkhmus R, Antezana C, Severin C, Contreras A 1978 Effect of ageing on biliary lipid composition and bile acid metabolism in normal Chilean women. Gastroenterology 74: 871–874

Van Der Linden W, Lindelöf G 1965 The familial occurrence of gallstone disease. Acta Genetica Basel 15: 159–164

Van Der Linden W, Bergman F 1977 Formation and dissolution of gallstones in experimental animals. International Review of Experimental Pathology 17: 173–233

Vlahcevic Z R, Bell C C Jr, Swell L 1970a Significance of the liver in the production of lithogenic bile in man. Gastroenterology 59: 62–69

Vlahcevic Z R, Bell C C Jr, Buhac I, Farrar J T, Swell L 1970b Diminished bile acid pool size in patients with gallstones. Gastroenterology 59: 165–173

Vlahcevic Z R, Bell C C Jr, Gregory D H, Baker G, Jattijudata P, Swell L 1972 Relationship of bile acid pool size to the formation of lithogenic bile in female Indians of the southwest. Gastroenterology 62: 73–83

Von Bergmann K, Mok H Y, Handison W G M, Grundy S M 1979 Cholesterol and bile acid metabolism in moderately advanced, stable cirrhosis of the liver. Gastroenterology 77: 1183–1192

Wattchow D A, Hall J C, Whiting M J, Bradley B, Iannos J, Watts J McK 1983 Prevalence and treatment of gallstones after gastric bypass surgery for morbid obesity. British Medical Journal 286:763

Wenckert A, Robertson B 1966 The natural course of gallstone disease. Eleven-year review of 781 nonoperated cases. Gastroenterology 50: 376–381

Werner D, Emmett P M, Heaton K W 1984 Effects of dietary sucrose on factors influencing cholesterol gallstone formation. Gut 25: 269–274

Wheeler M, Hills L L, Laby B 1970 Cholelithiasis: a clinical and dietary survey. Gut 11: 430–437

Whiting M J, Down R A L, Watts J McK 1981 Precision and accuracy in the measurement of the cholesterol saturation index of duodenal bile. Lack of variation due to the menstrual cycle. Gastroenterology 80: 533–538

Whiting M J, Bradley B M, Watts J McK 1983 Chemical and physical properties of gallstones in South Australia: implications for dissolution treatment. Gut 24: 11–15

Whiting M J, Watts J M 1984 Supersaturated bile from obese patients without gallstones supports cholesterol crystal growth but not nucleation. Gastroenterology 86: 243–248

Williams C N, Johnston J L, McCarthy S, Field C A 1981 Dietary lipid, bile acid composition, and dietary correlations in Micmac Indian women. A population study. Digestive Diseases and Sciences 26: 42–49

Williamson B W A, Percy-Robb I W 1980 Contribution of biliary lipids to calcium binding in bile. Gastroenterology 78: 696–702

Womack N A 1971 The development of gallstones. Surgery, Gynecology and Obstetrics 133: 937–945

J. McK. Watts, M. J. Whiting

Dissolution of gallbladder stones

INTRODUCTION

Until recent years, cholecystectomy was the only available treatment for stones in the gallbladder. However, in 1972 hope of a non-surgical treatment for gallbladder stone disease was raised when orally administered chenodeoxycholic acid (CDCA) was shown to be capable of dissolving cholesterol stones (Danzinger et al 1972). Three years later, ursodeoxycholic acid (UDCA) was also shown to be effective as a dissolution agent (Makino et al 1975).

The idea of dissolving gallstones by medical treatment originated long ago and claims of successful dissolution of gallstones by oral medication are found throughout recorded history (Rains 1964). In 1863, Thudichum noted that a mixture of ether and turpentine was able to disintegrate and dissolve cholesterol calculi which had been removed from the gallbladder. Rewbridge first reported the successful dissolution of gallstones in patients after prolonged oral treatment with mixed bile salts and olive oil (Rewbridge 1937). This report was not confirmed, although it was later reasoned that a non-toxic substance which could be excreted in bile in concentrations sufficient to dissolve cholesterol readily would be an ideal drug for gallstone dissolution (Johnston & Nakayama 1957).

Over a decade has now passed since the first reports of gallstone dissolution by CDCA and UDCA. The experience gained with these two bile acids as dissolution agents for gallbladder stones is discussed in this chapter.

TREATMENT WITH CHENODEOXYCHOLIC ACID AND URSODEOXYCHOLIC ACID

Patient selection

For dissolution therapy with bile acids to be contemplated for a patient with gallbladder stones, several conditions should apply. Firstly, patients of any age or sex can be treated, but women capable of becoming pregnant should have adequate contraception. Secondly, potential patients for dissolution therapy must not have persistent, severe symptoms. If symptoms are mild and tolerable, they may improve after taking CDCA or UDCA. Thirdly, the patient must agree to comply with a prolonged course of treatment. As a minimum requirement, it is usually necessary to take around eight capsules a day for at least six months, when the response to treatment is first assessed. Finally, the gallbladder must opacify on oral cholecystography and the stones must be radiolucent with the largest stone not exceeding 15 mm in diameter.

All patients selected according to these criteria have a reasonable chance of successful dissolution treatment. However, as is discussed later in considering the efficacy of bile acid therapy, other patient factors which affect the probability of a favourable outcome have been identified. These include sex, weight, and the level of serum cholesterol (Schoenfield et al 1981).

Bile acid dose

Chenodeoxycholic acid

A dose of CDCA of 750 mg/day was originally thought to be sufficient to effect gallstone dissolution. However, later studies indicated that better overall results were obtained using 1000 mg/day (Bateson et al 1978) or 13–15 mg per kg/day (Maton et al 1982). The currently recommended dose is 12–15 mg per kg/day.

As well as the actual amount of CDCA ingested per day, the timing of administration of CDCA may be important. Although CDCA is usually prescribed to be taken in divided doses three times a day with meals, evidence has recently been presented that CDCA given at a single dose at bedtime, plus a low cholesterol diet, can approximately double the dissolution rate (Kupfer et al 1982).

Ursodeoxycholic acid

Compared to CDCA, UDCA has not been as extensively studied in clinical trials and is still not available in countries such as Australia and the USA. Nevertheless, available evidence suggests that UDCA is as equally effective as CDCA in dissolving gallstones at slightly lower doses, such as 10–12 mg per kg/day or 600 mg/day taken at bedtime (Conte et al 1981).

Mechanism of action

The rationale for administering bile acids to dissolve gallstones was to reduce the cholesterol saturation of gallbladder bile by increasing bile acid secretion from the liver. However, the fact that there was a specificity in the action of bile acids, in that CDCA and UDCA were effective in dissolving gallstones while cholic acid was not (Thistle & Hofmann 1973), indicated a different mechanism of action. It is now known that CDCA and UDCA decrease biliary cholesterol saturation by decreasing the hepatic secretion of cholesterol into bile. Exactly how this is achieved is uncertain (Andersen 1979), although both these bile acids suppress the activity of 3-hydroxy-3-methyl glutaryl CoA (HMGCoA) reductase, the rate limiting enzyme of hepatic cholesterol synthesis (Maton et al 1980). However, it is doubtful whether secretion of cholesterol into bile is closely linked to the rate of hepatic synthesis (Andersen 1979).

The dissolution rate of cholesterol in vitro is significantly faster in CDCA solutions than in UDCA solutions (Igimi & Carey 1981) and yet the results of clinical trials indicate that these two bile acids are comparable with respect to the rate of gallstone dissolution in vivo. This discrepancy can be explained by in vitro studies of cholesterol gallstone dissolution in bile acid–lecithin solutions (Corrigan et al 1980). Cholesterol release from gallstones into a UDCA-lecithin solution continued far beyond the apparent equilibrium solubility by the formation of a turbid, liquid-crystalline phase. In comparison cholesterol release from stones in a CDCA-lecithin medium stopped once the apparent equilibrium solubility was reached. Thus, CDCA- and UDCA-rich bile may act by different mechanisms in dissolving cholesterol gallstones.

Patient monitoring

Patients undergoing dissolution therapy are treated as outpatients and supervision of their treatment may be restricted to an initial monthly and subsequent two-monthly clinic visit. Before treatment is commenced, liver function tests are performed. Then the patient is instructed to start ingesting the bile acid tablets or capsules and to increase the dose of bile acid to the prescribed level over several days. If diarrhoea occurs, as is sometimes the case with CDCA, one or more doses of the drug are omitted. After one month, liver function tests are repeated. If transaminase levels are raised to greater than twice the pre-treatment values, these tests are repeated after a further two weeks and treatment is discontinued if elevated levels persist.

Oral cholecystography or ultrasound is used to check for gallbladder stone dissolution at six-monthly intervals during treatment. Both investigations are required to confirm complete gallstone dissolution (Shapero et al 1982, Somerville et al 1982). Partial gallstone dissolution is best assessed using oral cholecystography, but only if cholegrams are taken in a standardized manner to avoid changes in the magnification of stone images between X-rays. When a patient's gallstones have been judged as completely dissolved, bile acid therapy is continued for a further three months in case very small residual stones may have escaped detection.

Specialized treatment centres consider it valuable to obtain pre- and post-treatment samples of fasting gallbladder bile to ensure that bile has become unsaturated with cholesterol during treatment. The bile is collected by duodenal intubation after stimulation of gallbladder contraction by intravenous administration of cholecystokinin. The pre-treatment sample of fasting gallbladder bile may also be analysed microscopically to exclude some patients who are likely to have pigment stones. If pigment granules are found by microscopy and the biliary cholesterol saturation index is less than 1.0, the chance of the stones being composed of cholesterol is less than 50% (Whiting et al 1982, Bruusgaard et al 1977). Conversely, the finding of cholesterol crystals in the bile indicates a 99% probability that the stones are cholesterol in type (Whiting et al 1982). An estimate of greater than 1.0 for the cholesterol saturation index of fasting duodenal bile after several weeks of CDCA treatment may indicate an inadequate dose of bile acid, especially in an obese patient (Iser et al 1978). However, the cholesterol saturation index is subject to considerable biological variation and this must be borne in mind in interpreting changes in saturation index values (Whiting et al 1981). Furthermore, most patients do not readily tolerate repeated duodenal intubations to obtain bile.

A novel way of monitoring patient compliance during CDCA treatment has been developed by analysing serum for its CDCA content relative to the other bile acids and predicting the percentage of CDCA present in gallbladder bile (Whiting & Watts 1980, Whiting et al 1983a). When bile contains greater than 70% CDCA, it is usually unsaturated with cholesterol. This method has the advantage of avoiding duodenal intubation, but it does require specialized laboratory facilities to perform serum bile acid analyses.

Efficacy of treatment

Results of clinical trials

Chenodeoxycholic acid Around the world, thousands of gallstone patients have now been treated with CDCA.

However, only a few clinical trials involving a large number of patients (around 100 or more) have been carried out to determine the efficacy of CDCA (Table 39.1).

To date, by far the most extensive and well controlled study is the American National Cooperative Gallstone Study (NCGS). This study was carried out over eight years at a cost of over $11 million. When completed, 916 patients with radiolucent gallbladder stones had been treated for two years at 10 centres. Patients were allocated randomly to one of three treatment groups. These received 750 mg/day CDCA, 375 mg/day CDCA or placebo, and the incidence of complete gallstone dissolution in each group was 14%, 5% and 1% respectively. These results include 15% of the total group who failed to complete the course of treatment for various reasons.

In a second large study by Maton et al in the UK, 125 patients with radiolucent gallbladder stones were treated with CDCA at a dose of 13 to 15 mg per kg/day, which is approximately 1000 mg/day for a patient of normal weight. Stones were less than 15 mm in diameter in most patients. The incidence of complete gallstone dissolution was 38% (Table 39.1). Again, this result includes some patients (17%) who withdrew from the study before completing a satisfactory course of treatment.

Other clinical trials, each involving nearly 100 patients, have been carried out in Australia (Watts & Iser 1983) and the USA (Tangedahl et al 1983). These studies both used a dose of CDCA of 15 mg per kg/day and found complete gallstone dissolution in around 30% of all patients recruited for the study (Table 39.1).

Ursodeoxycholic acid Clinical experience with the use of UDCA has been less extensive than with CDCA, although UDCA is now widely prescribed in Europe and Japan. Results from the largest studies reported to date are summarized in Table 39.2. A variety of doses of UDCA have been used in the different studies, and in general smaller doses of UDCA have been used than for CDCA. The incidence of complete gallstone dissolution in the studies presented in Table 39.2 ranges from 8% to 30%. In a review of world experience with UDCA to 1980, Bachrach & Hofmann (1982) reported that gallstone dissolution occurred in 148 of 852 patients (17%) treated with different doses of UDCA, usually for periods of one year or less.

Table 39.1 The efficacy of treatment with CDCA to achieve complete gallstone dissolution

Reference	No. of patients	CDCA dose	Incidence of complete dissolution
Schoenfield et al 1981	305	750 mg/day	41 (14%)
	306	375 mg/day	15 (5%)
	305	placebo	2 (1%)
Maton et al 1982	125	13–15 mg/kg/day	47 (38%)
Watts & Iser 1983	94	15 mg/kg/day	30 (32%)
Tangedahl et al 1983	97	15 mg/kg/day	27 (28%)

Table 39.2 The efficacy of treatment with UDCA to achieve complete gallstone dissolution

Reference	No. of patients	UDCA dose	Incidence of complete dissolution
Okumura et al 1977	89	450 mg/day	16 (18%)
Kameda et al 1980	106	150–600 mg/day	9 (8%)
Sugata et al 1980	83	6–12 mg/kg/day	25 (30%)
Polli et al 1980	78	5–12 mg/kg/day	14 (18%)
Neligan et al 1983	84	500 or 1000 mg/day	16 (19%)

The above results of clinical trials consider all patients entering the trials. It is now apparent that with more careful patient selection for factors favourable to the outcome of dissolution treatment, efficacy can be markedly improved to 70–80%.

Factors affecting response to treatment

Bile acid dose and timing of dose Although there are individual variations in response to bile acid therapy, the overall response is dose-related. For CDCA, the recommended dose is 13–15 mg per kg/day. Dissolution has been successful with doses of CDCA as low as 3 mg per kg/day (Danzinger et al 1980) or 375 mg/day (Schoenfield et al 1981), but it has not been possible to predict the lowest CDCA dose for each individual patient. With this aim in mind, we have used serum bile profiling to monitor the proportion of CDCA in the bile acid pool. A level of 70% CDCA appears sufficient to bring about gallstone dissolution in those patients likely to respond to treatment (Whiting et al 1984).

The timing of the dose of bile acid appears important. Because gallbladder bile reaches its most saturated state overnight during fasting, it was reasoned that bedtime

Table 39.3 Factors influencing the outcome of gallbladder stone dissolution treatment

Factor	Favourable	Unfavourable
Bile acid dose — CDCA	12–15 mg/kg/day	5 mg/kg/day
— UDCA	10–12 mg/kg/day	5 mg/kg/day
Treatment duration	⩾ 12 months	< 6 months
Stone size (diameter)	< 5 mm	> 15 mm
Volume of stones	< 2 ml	> 8 ml
Radiographic appearance	Radiolucent, floating	Radio-opaque, irregular shape
Patient weight	⩽ 100% I.B.W.*	> 120% I.B.W.*
Serum cholesterol	> 227 mg/dl	< 227 mg/dl

*I.B.W. = Ideal Body Weight

dosage of bile acids would be more effective. Indeed, there is evidence that bedtime administration of CDCA will desaturate gallbladder bile to a greater degree than bile acid taken in divided doses with meals (Maudgal et al 1979) and lead to a faster rate of gallstone dissolution when combined with a low cholesterol diet (Kupfer et al 1982).

UDCA is thought to be as effective as CDCA at slightly lower doses, and the optimum dose appears to be 10–12 mg per kg/day or 750 mg/day. If taken as a single dose at bedtime, 600 mg of UDCA may give similar results.

Treatment duration If the stones are of suitable chemical composition for dissolution, a response to therapy is almost always observed after six to nine months of treatment (Maton et al 1982, Schoenfield et al 1981). Treatment should not be prolonged unless there is a definite reduction in stone volume after nine months (Schoenfield et al 1981). The dissolution rate is dependent on the degree of unsaturation of gallbladder bile achieved during bile acid treatment (Maudgal et al 1983).

In clinical trials, approximately 15% of patients have withdrawn from treatment before completing six months therapy. These cases lower the overall treatment efficacy and need to be excluded when evaluating the drug efficacy of bile acid therapy.

Stone size and volume There is no doubt that stone size and volume affect the rate of dissolution. The duration to dissolution may vary from two to three months for very tiny, 'pinhead' stones to 12 to 24 months for large 'cherry' stones (Bachrach & Hofmann 1982). The larger the stone, the smaller the surface area available for dissolution in relation to stone volume. In the NCGS, a single stone with a total volume less than 1.75 ml was nine times more likely to dissolve completely than a single large stone with a volume greater than 1.75 ml (Schoenfield et al 1981). In general, stones with a total volume of less than 2 ml should dissolve, whereas this is unlikely to occur in a reasonable time if the total stone volume exceeds 8 ml (Table 39.3). The efficacy of bile acid treatment for stones greater than 15 mm in diameter is so poor and the time necessary for dissolution therapy so long that, except in very unusual circumstances, dissolution therapy should not be contemplated. Furthermore, there is the possibility that large stones are older than small stones and may contain inhibitory deposits of calcium salts on their surface (Whiting et al 1980).

Stone composition A gallbladder stone rich in cholesterol and containing low amounts of calcium salts will be radiolucent on an oral cholecystogram. However, not all radiolucent stones are rich in cholesterol. Between 14 and 20% of radiolucent stones are low in cholesterol content (Whiting et al 1983b, Bell et al 1975) and will not respond to dissolution therapy with bile acids. In a study of the gallbladder stones of 14 patients who had been treated unsuccessfully with CDCA, two patients (14%) were found to have pigment-type stones (Whiting et al 1980).

There is no completely reliable method for distinguishing patients with cholesterol stones from those with pigment stones. However, careful analysis of radiographic features (Dolgin et al 1981) and microscopic examination of duodenal bile for cholesterol crystals or pigment granules (Whiting et al 1982) can help. Small radiolucent stones which float in the gallbladder when visualized by oral cholecystography are invariably composed of cholesterol and are very amenable to dissolution therapy (Schoenfield et al 1981).

Aside from pigment stones, some radiolucent stones of high cholesterol content may not respond to treatment because they contain calcium salts. These salts can form a thin dissolution-resistant layer, either on the surface of the stone (Whiting et al 1980) or in the interior, resulting in partial stone dissolution until the layer is reached. Thus partial stone dissolution may not necessarily lead to complete dissolution and cannot be regarded as a successful outcome of treatment. Gallstone calcification with cessation of the dissolution process has been reported in several cases during treatment with UDCA (Bateson et al 1981, Gleeson et al 1983) and in two cases during treatment with CDCA (Whiting et al 1980). In the NCGS, calcification of gallstones occurred equally among patients receiving CDCA or placebo (Schoenfield et al 1981), indicating that the process may not be dependent on bile acid administration.

Other factors A number of other factors have been shown to influence the outcome of dissolution treatment with bile acids. Probably the most important of these is obesity. Most reported studies with CDCA have found that obese patients are less likely to have their stones dissolved than patients of normal weight (Schoenfield et al 1981, Maton et al 1982). This resistance to treatment is probably due to gallbladder bile remaining supersaturated with cholesterol during therapy (Iser et al 1978). Higher bile acid doses appear to be necessary in obese patients.

Because of their potential influence on the frequency of dissolution of gallbladder stones, many factors were examined in the NCGS (Schoenfield et al 1981). Apart from those already discussed, patient sex and serum cholesterol levels were found to have a significant effect. Dissolution occurred more often in women than men and inexplicably more often in patients with serum cholesterol levels greater than 227 mg/dl (Schoenfield et al 1981). Table 39.3 summarizes the effect of various factors influencing the outcome of gallbladder stone dissolution treatment.

Gallbladder stone recurrence

It is not surprising that gallstones should recur after bile acid treatment because nothing has been done to alter irreversibly the abnormal biochemical mechanism leading to their formation. The frequency of recurrence will depend on the duration of follow-up since dissolution, but

Table 39.4 Gallstone recurrence after dissolution treatment with bile acids

Reference	Bile acid	Number of patients	Duration of follow-up (months)	Number of patients with recurrence	Time for recurrence (months)
Ponz de Leon et al 1980	CDCA	29	6–48	5 (17%)	8–24
Sugata et al 1980	UDCA	25	–60	3 (12%)	
Thistle 1981	CDCA	24	6–90	11 (46%)	12–90
Ruppin and Dowling 1982	CDCA UDCA	37 9	3–90	22 (59%) 3 (33%)	3–90
Marks et al 1984	CDCA	48*	24–42	13 (27%)	6–42

* Patients were randomly allocated to receive CDCA (375 mg/day) or placebo after successful dissolution therapy

it is clear that up to 50% of patients will redevelop gallbladder stones, usually within two years of ceasing treatment (Table 39.4). It is likely that recurrence can be prevented by continuation of treatment after dissolution has occurred, although the bile acid dose required is not known. Extended studies from the NCGS have suggested that 375 mg/day of CDCA is not sufficient to prevent the recurrence of gallstones (Marks et al 1984). Lifelong treatment with a high dose of bile acids would be too expensive for most patients. It is hoped that simpler measures such as dietary manipulation may prevent recurrence. A multicentre trial is now being conducted in the UK to compare the effects of low-dose bedtime UDCA treatment with those of placebo and a bran-supplemented, low refined-carbohydrate diet on gallstone recurrence.

Side effects

The main side effects of bile acid therapy to consider are diarrhoea and hepatotoxicity. However, experience has shown that these side effects are specific to CDCA and do not occur with UDCA. On these grounds at least, UDCA is preferable to CDCA for treating gallstones.

Diarrhoea is a common side effect of oral CDCA treatment and occurs in more than 50% of patients treated with 15 mg per kg/day (Maton et al 1982). It is dose-related and responds to temporary cessation of treatment or a reduction in drug dose. In the NCGS, diarrhoea was observed in 41% of patients receiving 750 mg/day of CDCA compared to 20% of patients receiving placebo, but treatment was never required to be suspended (Schoenfield et al 1981). In patients receiving higher doses of CDCA, severe persistent diarrhoea only occasionally results in cessation of treatment.

Because CDCA is converted by intestinal bacteria to lithocholic acid, a known hepatotoxin, it was originally feared that CDCA might cause liver damage in man. Lithocholic acid is toxic to the liver in many animal species, but humans have enzyme systems which are able to sulphate lithocholic acid, thus inhibiting its absorption and preventing toxicity (Allan et al 1976). Nevertheless, reports indicate that around 30% of patients taking CDCA for gallstone dissolution therapy develop elevated serum transaminase levels, although this is only slight and often transient (Shoenfield et al 1981). It is usual for increases in serum hepatic enzyme levels to return to normal, even during treatment with the drug. Occasionally, the elevated levels persist and then the drug should be discontinued. In the NCGS, clinically significant hepatotoxity occurred in only 3% of patients treated with 750 mg/day (Schoenfield et al 1981). As part of this study, detailed analysis by light and electron microscopy of liver biopsies obtained from 126 patients before and during CDCA therapy revealed no major changes in liver cell morphology (Fisher et al 1982). The effect of bile acids on the liver of the human foetus is not known, so that these drugs should not be given to women who can become pregnant during the course of therapy.

Although it was predicted that prolonged bile acid administration might lead to hypercholesterolaemia by suppressing cholesterol catabolism and biliary excretion, this has not proved to be the case. Fasting levels of serum cholesterol are either unchanged (Hoffman et al 1974, Bachrach & Hofmann 1982) or only slightly elevated (Schoenfield et al 1981). On the other hand, fasting levels of serum triglyceride are lowered during CDCA therapy and this bile acid has been used to treat patients with hypertriglyceridaemia (Camarri et al 1978).

Many patients undergoing dissolution treatment with bile acids report improvement in their symptoms. This improvement may take the form of a reduction in the frequency of biliary pain or a reduction in minor gastrointestinal symptoms, which are common in patients with gallstones. In the case of CDCA, prospective appraisal of this effect in the NCGS showed no differences in the frequency of biliary pain, dyspepsia or nausea between patients treated with CDCA or placebo (Schoenfield et al 1981). This would indicate that the symptomatic improvement during CDCA treatment is simply a placebo effect. However, another report of a double-blind controlled trial, involving 762 patients, claimed that UDCA showed significant therapeutic effects with respect to dyspepsia and biliary pain when compared to placebo (Frigerio 1979).

OTHER POTENTIAL DISSOLUTION AGENTS

Several other chemicals have been tried as cholesterol gallstone dissolving agents, but with little or no success. Agents examined include Rowachol, glycerophosphate, lecithin, cholic acid, cholic acid plus lecithin, phenobarbitone, choline, β-sitosterol, clofibrate and thyroid hormones. None of these agents compares with CDCA and UDCA, although Rowachol does seem capable of dissolving gallstones in a few patients. This inexpensive preparation contains six cyclic monoterpenes, which inhibit HMGCoA reductase and alter biliary cholesterol saturation (Doran et al 1979). Complete gallstone dissolution was reported in three out of 24 patients after six months' treatment with this agent, which was well tolerated and free from side effects (Bell & Doran 1979). When used in combination with a low (375 mg) dose of CDCA, Rowachol appeared to enhance the frequency of gallstone dissolution (Ellis et al 1981).

IMPACT OF DISSOLUTION THERAPY FOR GALLBLADDER STONES

Given that there are limitations to the use of bile acids for gallbladder stone dissolution, it may be questioned whether this form of therapy constitutes a major advance in the treatment of gallstone disease. Since the large NCGS was completed with poor overall results in terms of dissolution efficacy, there has been much scepticism. Isselbacher wrote in 1972: 'Can we dissolve gallstones? Yes, but right now the best way probably is to perform a cholecystectomy and put the stones in a beaker of ethyl ether.' Some critics argue that this statement is still true, while other investigators have a more optimistic viewpoint (Palmer & Carey 1982).

In our own hospital, we have estimated that around one third of all gallstone patients presenting for treatment fulfil the primary criteria for dissolution therapy; that is, they have radiolucent stones in a functioning gallbladder. Since gallbladder stone disease is very common, this represents a large number of patients who could potentially be treated by bile acid dissolution therapy. However, the criterion of the stone size must also be considered, since large stones usually require a long (over two years), expensive course of therapy, which is not acceptable to most patients. In a study of 406 consecutive gallstone patients, we found 77 (19%) had functioning gallbladders which contained radiolucent stones 15 mm or less in diameter (Whiting et al 1983b). The gallstones of most of these patients were available for chemical analysis and 85% were found to be rich in cholesterol (over 80% by weight). When the criterion for acceptable stone size was made more stringent at 10 mm or 5 mm maximum stone diameter, the number of patients suitable for dissolution therapy fell sharply (Table 39.5). In addition, the proportion of these patients who had stones rich in cholesterol also decreased, because pigment stones tend to be smaller than cholesterol stones (Table 39.5). Thus, although small cholesterol gallbladder stones less than 5 mm in diameter are very suitable for dissolution treatment, patients with such stones are not common and make up less than 3% of the gallstone population presenting to our hospital.

Table 39.5 Estimated proportion of gallstone patients suitable for dissolution therapy in South Australia, according to the diameter of the largest stone

	Stone diameter (mm)		
	≤5	≤10	≤15
Patients suitable for dissolution (%)	4	11	19
Proportion with cholesterol stones (%)	62	76	85

In summary dissolution therapy in its present form is a viable alternative to surgery in a small proportion of gallstone patients, who are carefully selected to have a high probability of successful treatment. It is particularly valuable for those patients who represent a poor surgical risk because of other diseases.

FUTURE PROSPECTS

In principle at least, an oral gallstone dissolution agent could be excreted in bile and act as solvent to increase the solubility of cholesterol or, as is the case for the bile acids CDCA and UDCA, it could act by reducing hepatic cholesterol secretion. CDCA and UDCA can be regarded as the first generation dissolution agents, which show that gallstone dissolution is possible. The way is now open for second and third generation drugs with improved efficacy. Dissolution therapy would be much more attractive if the rate of dissolution could be increased. More research is required on substances which can accelerate the dissolution of cholesterol stones. One approach that has been described recently is to infuse a good cholesterol solvent, such as methyl butyl ether, directly into the gallbladder via a percutaneous transhepatic catheter. By continuous infusion and aspiration of the ether, rapid progressive stone dissolution was achieved in a few hours (Allen et al 1985). Further work is in progress to establish the efficacy and safety of this procedure.

Unfortunately, it seems unlikely that the cost of bile acid therapy will allow it to be used prophylactically for preventing gallstone formation, although this could be justified in high-risk groups. If gallstones could be detected soon after their formation, while they were still small and the gallbladder was still fully functional, dissolution therapy would be more successful. Further progress in the control of gallstone disease is likely only when more is known of the early events which lead to the production of macroscopic stones in the gallbladder.

REFERENCES

Allan R N, Thistle J L, Hofmann A F 1976 Lithocholate metabolism during chemotherapy for gallstone dissolution. 2. Absorption and sulfation. Gut 17: 413–419

Allen M J, Borody T J, Bugliosi T F, May G R, LaRusso N F, Thistle J L 1985 Rapid dissolution of gallstones by methyl tert-butyl ether. New England Journal of Medicine 312: 217–220

Andersen J M 1979 Chenodeoxycholic acid desaturates bile — but how? Gastroenterology 77: 1146–1151

Bachrach W H, Hofmann A F 1982 Ursodeoxycholic acid in the treatment of cholesterol cholelithiasis. Digestive Diseases and Sciences 27: 833–858

Bateson M C, Ross P E, Murison J, Bouchier I A D 1978 Comparison of fixed doses of chenodeoxycholic acid for gallstone dissolution. Lancet i: 1111–1114

Bateson M C, Bouchier I A D, Maudgal D P, Trash D B, Northfield T C 1981 Calcification of radiolucent gallstones during treatment with ursodeoxycholic acid. British Medical Journal 283: 645–646

Bell G D, Dowling R H, Whitney B, Sutor D J 1975 The value of radiology in predicting gallstone type when selecting patients for medical treatment. Gut 16: 359–364

Bell G D, Doran J 1979 Gallstone dissolution in man using an essential oil preparation, Rowachol. British Medical Journal 1:24

Bruusgaard A, Malver E, Pedersen L R, Schlichting P, Sylvest J 1977 Criteria for selection of patients for medical treatment (chenodeoxycholic acid therapy) of gallstones. Scandinavian Journal of Gastroenterology 12: 97–102

Camarri E, Fici F, Marcolongo F 1978 Influence of chenodeoxycholic acid on serum triglycerides in patients with primary hypertriglyceridaemia. International Journal of Clinical Pharmacology and Biopharmacy 16: 523–526

Conte D, Bozzani A, Sironi L, Rocca F, Camassa L, Bianchi P A 1981 Radiolucent gallstone dissolution with bedtime UDCA administration. Digestion 22: 302–304

Corrigan O L, Su C C, Higuchi W I, Hofman A F 1980 Mesophase formation during cholesterol dissolution in ursodeoxycholate-lecithin solutions: a new mechanism for gallstone dissolution in humans. Journal of Pharmaceutical Science 69: 869–874

Danzinger R G, Hofmann A F, Schoenfield L J, Thistle J L 1972 Dissolution of cholesterol gallstones by chenodeoxycholic acid. New England Journal of Medicine 286: 1–5

Danzinger R G, Kurtas T K, Torchia M E 1980 Low-dose chenodeoxycholic acid for gallstone dissolution: a randomised trial in poor operative risk patients. Digestive Diseases and Sciences 25: 785–789

Dolgin S M, Schwartz J S, Kressel H Y, Soloway R D, Wallace T M, Trotman B W, Soloway A S, Good L I 1981 Identification of patients with cholesterol or pigment stones by discriminant analysis of radiographic features. New England Journal of Medicine 304: 808–811

Doran J, Keighley M R B, Bell G D 1979 Rowachol — a possible treatment for cholesterol gallstones. Gut 20: 312–317

Ellis W R, Bell G D, Middleton B, White D A 1981 Adjunct to bile-acid treatment for gallstone dissolution: Low-dose chenodeoxycholic acid combined with a terpene preparation. British Medical Journal 282: 611–612

Fisher R L, Anderson D W, Boyer J L, Ishak K, Klatskin G, Lachin J M, Phillips M J et al 1982 A prospective morphologic evaluation of hepatic toxicity of chenodeoxycholic acid in patients with cholelithiasis: The National Cooperative Gallstone Study. Hepatology 2: 187–201

Frigerio G 1979 Ursodeoxycholic acid in the treatment of dyspepsia: Report of a multicentre controlled trial. Current Therapeutic Research 26: 214–223

Gleeson D, Ruppin D C, Murphy G M, Dowling R H 1983 Second look at ursodeoxycholic acid: high efficacy for partial but low efficacy for complete gallstone dissolution, and a high rate of acquired stone opacification. Gut 24: 999 (Abstract)

Hoffman N E, Hofmann A F, Thistle J L 1974 Effect of bile acid feeding on cholesterol metabolism in gallstone patients. Mayo Clinic Proceedings 49: 236–239

Igimi H, Carey M C 1981 Cholesterol gallstone dissolution in bile: dissolution kinetics of crystalline (anhydrate and monohydrate) cholesterol with chenodeoxycholate, ursodeoxycholate and their glycine and taurine conjugates. Journal of Lipid Research 22: 254–263

Iser J H, Maton P N, Murphy G M, Dowling R H 1978 Resistance to chenodeoxycholic acid (CDCA) treatment in obese patients with gallstones. British Medical Journal 1: 1509–1512

Johnston C G, Nakayama F 1957 Solubility of cholesterol and gallstones in metabolic material. Archives of Surgery 75: 436–442

Kameda H and the Tokyo Co-operative Gallstone Study Group 1980 Efficacy and indications of ursodeoxycholic acid treatment for dissolving gallstones. A multi-centre double-blind trial. Gastroenterology 78: 542–548

Kupfer R M, Maudgal D P, Northfield T C 1982 Gallstone dissolution rate during chenic acid therapy. Digestive Diseases and Sciences 27: 1025–1029

Makino I, Shinozaki K, Yoshino K, Nakagawa S 1975 Dissolution of cholesterol gallstones by ursodeoxycholic acid. Japanese Journal of Gastroenterology 72: 690–702

Marks J W, Shu-Ping L. The Steering Committee. The National Co-operative Gallstone Study Group 1984 Low-dose chenodiol to prevent gallstone recurrence after dissolution therapy. Annals of Internal Medicine 100: 376–381

Maton P N, Ellis J H, Higgins M J, Dowling R H 1980 Hepatic HMGCoA reductase in human cholelithiasis: effects of chenodeoxycholic and ursodeoxycholic acids. European Journal of Clinical Investigation 10: 325–332

Maton P N, Iser J H, Reuben A, Saxton H M, Murphy G M, Dowling R H 1982 Outcome of chenodeoxycholic acid treatment in 125 patients with radiolucent gallstones. Medicine 61: 86–97

Maudgal D P, Bird R, Northfield T C 1979 Optimal timing of doses of chenic acid in patients with gallstones. British Medical Journal 1: 922–923

Maudgal D P, Kupfer R M, Northfield T C 1983 Factors affecting gallstone dissolution rate during chenic acid therapy. Gut 24: 7–10

Neligan P, Bateson M C, Trash D B, Ross P E, Bouchier I A D 1983 Ursodeoxycholic acid for the dissolution of radiolucent gallbladder stones. Digestion 28: 225–233

Okumura M, Tanikawa K, Chuman Y, Koji T, Nakagawa S, Nakamura Y, Iino H, Yamasuki S, Hisatsugu T 1977 Clinical studies on dissolution of gallstones using ursodeoxycholic acid. Gastroenterology Japan 12: 469–475

Palmer R H, Carey M C 1982 An optimistic view of the National Cooperative Gallstone Study. New England Journal of Medicine 306: 1171–1174

Polli E E, Bianchi P A, Conte D, Sironi L 1981 Treatment of radiolucent gallstones with CDCA or UDCA. A multicentre trial. Digestion 22: 185–191

Ponz de Leon M, Carulli N, Iori R, Loria P, Smerieri A, Zironi F 1980 Medical treatment of gallstones with chenodeoxycholic acid: Follow up report at four years. Italian Journal of Gastroenterology 12: 17–22

Rains A J H 1964 Gallstones: Causes and treatment. Heinemann Medical Books, London

Rewbridge A G 1937 Disappearance of gallstone shadows following prolonged administration of bile salts. Surgery 1: 395–400

Ruppin D C, Dowling R H 1982 Is recurrence inevitable after gallstone dissolution by bile acid treatment? Lancet i: 181–185

Schoenfield L J, Lachin J M, National Co-operative Gallstone Study Group 1981 Chenodiol (chenodeoxycholic acid) for dissolution of gallstones: the National Co-operative Gallstone Study. Annals of Internal Medicine 95: 257–282

Shapero T F, Rosen I E, Wilson S R, Fisher M M 1982 Discrepancy between ultrasound and oral cholecystography in the assessment of gallstone dissolution. Hepatology 2: 587–590

Somerville K W, Rose D H, Bell G D, Ellis W R, Knapp D R 1982 Gallstone dissolution and recurrence: are we being misled? British Medical Journal 284: 1295–1297

Sugata F, Kobayashi A, Yamamura M, Shimizu M 1980 Five year follow-up study on UDCA therapy for cholelithiasis with special

reference to recurrence. XI International Congress of Gastroenterology, Hamburg, E 34.11 (abstract)
Tangedahl T, Carey W D, Ferguson D R, Forsythe S, Williams M, Paradis K, Hightower N C 1983 Drug and treatment efficacy of chenodeoxycholic acid in 97 patients with cholelithiasis and increased surgical risk. Digestive Diseases and Sciences 28: 545–551
Thistle J L 1981 Medical treatment of gallstones. Practical Gastroenterology 5: 31–38
Thistle J L, Hofmann A F 1973 Efficacy and specificity of chenodeoxycholic acid therapy for dissolving gallstones. New England Journal of Medicine 289: 655–659
Watts J McK, Iser J H 1983 Chenodeoxycholic acid for gallstone dissolution. (unpublished observations).
Whiting M J, Watts J McK 1980 Prediction of the bile acid composition of bile from serum bile acid analysis during gallstone dissolution therapy. Gastroenterology 78: 220–225
Whiting M J, Jarvinen V, Watts J McK 1980 Chemical composition of gallstones resistant to dissolution therapy with chenodeoxycholic acid. Gut 21: 1077–1081
Whiting M J, Down R H L, Watts J McK 1981 Precision and accuracy in the measurement of the cholesterol saturation index of duodenal bile. Gastroenterology 80: 553–558
Whiting M J, Down R H L, Watts J McK 1982 Biliary crystals and granules, the cholesterol saturation index and the prediction of gallstone type. Surgical Gastroenterology 1: 17–21
Whiting M J, Down R H L, Watts J McK 1983a Chenodeoxycholic acid administration monitored by serum bile acid profiles: a dose-response study. Annals of Clinical Biochemistry 20: 336–340
Whiting M J, Bradley B M, Watts J McK 1983b Chemical and physical properties of gallstones in South Australia: implications for dissolution treatment. Gut 24: 11–15
Whiting M J, Bradley B M, Hall J C, Watts J McK 1984 Comparison of a monitored dose with a standard dose of chenodeoxycholic acid for gallstone dissolution. Digestion 30: 211–217

L. Den Besten

Asymptomatic gallstones

OVERVIEW

The definition and therapy of asymptomatic gallstones continue to evoke controversy. Seminars and courses dealing with hepatobiliary disease almost invariably include a discussion of 'silent gallstones'. A number of recent, careful, prospective studies have generated important data on the incidence, natural history, and risk factors of asymptomatic gallstones. However, the validity and clinical application of these data continue to be debated. As a result, clearly stated algorithms for patient management are not currently available. This chapter will summarize the current state of our knowledge on the definition, incidence, natural history, risk factors, and recommended therapy for asymptomatic gallstones.

Historical vignettes

Gallstones were described long before the modern era of cholecystectomy was ushered in by Langenbuch in the late 19th century (1882). Numerous calculi were found in the gallbladder of the mummy of a priestess of Amenen in the 21st Egyptian Dynasty (1500 b.c.) (Schwartz 1981). The Greek physician, Alexander Trallianus, described calculi within the hepatic radicles of a human liver (Glenn & Grafe 1966). By the 16th century, both Vesalius and Fallopius described gallstones found in the gallbladders of dissected human bodies (Schwartz 1981). The codification of the Talmud, about the same time, provides additional insight into the frequency with which gallstones were observed in animals. The dietary laws included the admonition that 'if hard things are found in the gallbladder, which are like the pits of dates, without sharp edges, the animal is Kosher; but if the edges are sharp as in the pits of olives, the animal is terefah (unfit for eating)' (Schwartz 1981). These observations suggest a clear recognition of the phenomenon of cholelithiasis. The pathogenesis and clinical significance of gallstones are seldom referred to, probably because of the absence of interventions to deal with the problem.

Definitions

Two quite different definitions have been used to describe the patient with asymptomatic or silent gallstones. The traditional definition included gallstones discovered in patients contacting a physician with nonspecific abdominal complaints. The current definition includes only those gallstones discovered during screening examinations. The broader, traditional definition included patients whose symptoms were vague or who were unable to articulate their complaints clearly. Gallstones discovered in patients with non-specific abdominal complaints were classified as 'silent gallstones'. The diagnosis of stones was based on an oral cholecystogram which showed stones, or failed to concentrate dye in the gallbladder. The incidence of gallstones was almost certainly underestimated, and patients diagnosed by these methods often had a more advanced disease. The data emanating from studies using the restrictive, current definition provided a more accurate statistical sampling of the incidence of gallstones and their natural history. These data derive from ultrasound screening of all members of defined populations.

STATEMENT OF THE PROBLEM

As perceived by the medical epidemiologist

A realistic assessment of the problem of gallstones in general and asymptomatic gallstones more particularly is illustrated by data describing the population of the USA. An estimated 20 million people in the United States have gallstones. Each year 300 000 patients undergo cholecystectomy. Slightly less than one-third of all patients who develop gallstones in any given year have an operation. Of the two-thirds of patients who do not have an operation, 50% are asymptomatic. Algorithms to deal with this vast reservoir of patients with stones and the large number of new stone-bearing patients are a justifiable concern of the medical epidemiologist.

As perceived by the medical economist

Any recommendation to eradicate all gallstones would have staggering implications for medical economics. For instance, if the backlog of asymptomatic stones in the United States was decreased by ten million at a cost of six thousand dollars per operation, the initial cost would equal sixty billion dollars. Additionally, new cases arising each year would cost billions of dollars for diagnosis and therapy. Even gallstone dissolution at two to three dollars per day is costly because of the low dissolution and high recurrence rates. Given the finite financial resources for health care, a Spartan attitude towards the elective treatment of asymptomatic gallstones seems reasonable.

As perceived by the clinician-scientist

Although the incidence and natural history of gallstones differ throughout the world, extrapolation from US data underscores a potentially staggering public health problem. Prior to the era of ultrasonography, most patients with asymptomatic stones failed to be diagnosed. With the advent of ultrasonography safe, rapid screening for gallstones is possible. Furthermore, many patients given ultrasound examinations for complaints remote from the gallbladder are having asymptomatic stones diagnosed. The cost, morbidity, mortality, and days lost from the work force all support the thesis that treatment will have to be individualized. Data are therefore necessary to identify those patients with asymptomatic gallstones who are most likely to suffer morbidity or mortality from withholding therapy. Way & Sleisenger (1983) have categorized the types of data necessary to determine ideal treatment for asymptomatic stones:

1. The rate at which symptoms develop (e.g. colic, dyspepsia);
2. The rate at which complications develop (acute cholecystitis, cholangitis, pancreatitis, carcinoma, etc.);
3. The likelihood that a complication rather than uncomplicated symptoms will be the initial clinical manifestation;
4. The mortality for elective cholecystectomy in asymptomatic patients;
5. The mortality from complications following elective cholecystectomy;
6. The cost of treatment.

These data are available in part from several recent studies.

NATURAL HISTORY OF ASYMPTOMATIC GALLSTONES

Old data

Until recently data quoted to describe the natural history of gallstones were largely from studies more than 20 years old. Typical of these are articles published in 1960 and 1966, respectively, by Lund (1960) and Wenckert & Robertson (1966) which describe the natural history of 1307 unoperated patients followed for five years. In these studies only 50% remained asymptomatic and 20% developed complications. These essayists recommended elective cholecystectomy for asymptomatic stones. However, many of their patients were not 'asymptomatic' since all were diagnosed to have cholelithiasis during hospitalization, and 70% had non-functioning gallbladders, an indication of more severe disease.

New data

Recent publications suggest that patients with stones found during 'screening' examinations have a 2% chance per year of experiencing colic. Complications such as acute cholecystitis occur as the first symptom in less than 10% of those who become symptomatic. Many of these studies strongly recommend expectant therapy.

The more substantive publications during the past three years are summarized as follows: Ransohoff et al (1983) carried out a decision analysis to compare the consequence of prophylactic cholecystectomy with expectant management for silent gallstone disease. Probability values were derived from a study of the natural history of the silent gallstone disease, published cholecystectomy mortality rates, and life tables. The two strategies were compared by calculating cumulative numbers of person-years lost for hypothetical cohorts of men and women. Prophylactic cholecystectomy slightly decreases survival. A 30-year-old man choosing prophylactic cholecystectomy instead of expectant management would lose, on average, four days of life; a 50-year-old man would lose 18 days. Sensitivity analysis showed that differences between the two strategies remain small over a broad range of probability values both for men and women. This analysis is an extension from data on a group of university faculty members with silent gallstones previously published (Gracie & Ransohoff 1982). A study from Italy (GREPCO 1984) reports the results of real time ultrasonography screening for gallstones in a population of female civil servants in Rome. The prevalence of gallstone disease increased with age from 2.5% in the 20- to 29-year-old age group to 25% in the 60- to 64-year-old age group, based on both presence of gallstones and the history of cholecystectomy. Only one-third of the women with gallstones had complained of at least one episode of biliary pain in the last five years. The frequency of 'minor' dyspeptic symptoms was not different between women with and without gallstones. A study by Massarrat et al from West Germany (1982) reports the incidence of gallstones in autopsy patients and outpatients in West Germany. The incidence of cholelithiasis and rate of cholecystectomy were studied in three differently selected groups. The first group consisted of 3842 autopsies between the years 1969 and 1977, the second group were 6564 patients undergoing X-ray examination for various reasons between 1970 and 1974, and the third group were 163 patients over 50 referred for reasons other than abdominal discomfort. The incidence of dyspeptic symptoms was registered in the patients of the last group. The rate of cholelithiasis and cholecystectomy in the first (autopsy) group corresponded well to that of the second group (X-ray examinations for non-specific complaints). In men and women over 60 who had been referred to the Outpatient Clinic for reasons not related to abdominal pain, the rate of cholelithiasis was 33 and 42%, respectively. These findings correspond to those of the first and second groups. The authors observe that the incidence of silent stones increases with age, but the rate of cholecystectomy does not.

RISK FACTORS IN PATIENTS WITH SILENT GALLSTONES

Genetic

The incidence of gallstones varies markedly among world populations and is exceptionally high or low in certain well described groups. The Pima Indians of the United States, especially females (Sampliner et al 1970), have an unusually high incidence of gallstones. Stones develop at a young age and complications requiring cholecystectomy occur in the majority of those who survive for longer than 50 years. In contrast, the Masai of East Africa (BISS et al 1971) have a very low incidence of cholelithiasis and a very low frequency of complications. Studies contrasting the prevalence of gallstones in Sweden and Japan (Van der Linden & Nakayama 1973) clearly document a statistically greater frequency of gallstones in the former population. In populations of relative genetic homogeneity the incidence of cholelithiasis has a rather clearly established familial relationship. Gilat and colleagues (1983) studied, in a prospective manner, the frequency of gallstones in 171 first-degree relatives of patients with proven gallstones compared with 200 matched controls. All subjects were studied by oral cholecystography, and their height, weight, blood glucose, cholesterol, and other parameters were measured. Gallstones were found in 22.8% of the female and 16.7% of the male family members (20.5% overall), as opposed to 10.3% of the female and 8.0% of the male controls (9.0% overall). All these differences were statistically significant. Gallstones in populations at high risk develop at an earlier age, and data from numerous studies show that the risk of acute symptoms and/or acute complications is cumulative. Perhaps the indications for cholecystectomy should be liberalized in these high risk populations.

Related to the biliary tract

Although asymptomatic gallstones have a relatively benign prognosis and usually present with indigestion or colic rather than life-threatening complications, specific subgroups are at increased risk. Non-visualization of the gallbladder during oral cholecystography is indicative of more advanced disease and suggests a high likelihood for development of symptoms (Wenckert & Robertson 1966, Wilbur & Bolt 1959). Similarly, gallstones greater than 2.5 cm in diameter are more likely to precipitate an attack of acute cholecystitis than are smaller stones (Carveth et al 1959). Calcification of the wall of the gallbladder, although uncommon, is frequently associated with gallbladder carcinoma and should be treated as a premalignant condition (Ashur et al 1978).

Unrelated to the biliary tract

Numerous risk factors both for increased incidence and complications of gallstones have been identified. These risk factors can be classified as major on the basis of a marked increase in incidence and risk of complications, or minor because of minimal increase in these categories.

Major risk factors

The most important major factors are 1. prolonged parenteral nutrition; 2. diabetes mellitus; 3. immunosuppression; 4. certain drugs. Both paediatric and adult patients receiving prolonged parenteral nutrition have been shown in retrospective and prospective studies to have both an increased incidence of cholelithiasis and risk of having complications at first presentation (Pitt et al 1983a, 1983b, Roslyn et al 1983a, 1983b, 1984). Patients receiving total parenteral nutrition without oral alimentation to stimulate gallbladder emptying develop sludge within weeks (Messing et al 1983) which is composed primarily of calcium bilirubinate (Allen et al 1981). The mortality from operation for acute cholecystitis in patients on parenteral nutrition exceeds 30%, and the benefits of prophylactic cholecystectomy seem strongly supported. Patients with diabetes mellitus have a well establised increase in both mortality and morbidity from cholecystectomy for acute cholecystitis (Turrill 1961). The increased risk from diabetes mellitus can be brought to a level approaching normal patients with normal risk factors if elective operation is carried out. The immunosuppressed patient often presents without significant temperature elevation or physical findings until the disease is far advanced. The patient with gallstones who is immunosuppressed from steroids in the treatment of inflammatory bowel disease or organ transplantation, or immuno-incompetent from disseminated neoplasm has a similar presentation and an unacceptably high mortality from cholecystectomy. A number of drugs, including exogenous oestrogens, (Boston Collaborative Drug Surveillance Program 1973, 1974, Coronary Drug Project Research Group 1977) and certain agents to decrease serum lipids (Friedman et al 1966) have the capacity both to increase the incidence of gallstones and to decrease gallbladder emptying, thereby inducing stasis and increased risk of acute symptoms.

Minor factors

An almost unlimited number of minor factors increase the incidence of gallstones, and several of these also increase the incidence of complications at the time of presentation. Morbid obesity is associated with a three-fold increased incidence of cholesterol cholelithiasis, probably related to the marked increase in hepatic cholesterol secretion (Freeman et al 1975, Mabee et al 1976, Tucher et al 1982). Ileal resection or bypass is associated with a similar three-fold increase in cholelithiasis (Coyle et al 1980). Gallstones associated with ileal disease are usually calcium bilirubinate stones, and the patients, by virtue of their underlying illness, have a frequent delay in diagnosis suggesting that elective prophylactic cholecystectomy is indicated. Several other minor risk factors, including haemolytic anaemia (Bates & Brown 1952), sickle-cell anaemia (Jordan 1957), and vagotomy (Clave & Gaspar 1969, Ihasz & Griffith 1981, Sapala et al 1979), are associated with a higher incidence of gallstones. However, gallstones developing in this group of patients have a risk of complications which is no greater than observed in other patients with gallstones.

GALLSTONE DISSOLUTION FOR ASYMPTOMATIC STONES

The use of gallstone dissolving agents such as chenodeoxycholic and ursodeoxycholic acid should be reserved for a carefully selected group of patients. Given the large reservoir of patients with asymptomatic gallstones, the cost, even at two to three dollars per day, would be prohibitive, especially in view of the high rate of failure of dissolution and recurrence after therapy. A study reported by Sonnenberg and colleagues (1982) tested three therapeutic strategies in patients with asymptomatic or mildly symptomatic cholesterol gallstones. These therapies included cholecystectomy, medical gallstone dissolution, and expectant non-treatment. The course of cholelithiasis under these three strategies was evaluated by three decision trees using the incidence of complications from the literature. For every complication the cost of drugs, absenteeism, and treatment as outpatient and inpatient was listed. The costs were multiplied by the likelihood of the complication. The total costs due to the initial treatment and the expected costs of all anticipated complications were taken to represent the expected costs of the various therapeutic strategies. Although costs were similar, this study is unique in that the projected cost for expectant therapy was slightly higher than that of cholecystectomy or dissolution therapy. These conclusions are at variance with those observed for expectant therapy by other investigators (Gracie & Ransohoff 1982, Ransohoff et al 1983, Way & Sleisenger 1983).

RECOMMENDATIONS

Prophylactic cholecystectomy for asymptomatic gallstones is recommended for patients with increased major risk factors, or those undergoing laparotomy for another indication. Patients, especially those in the paediatric age group, who will require lifetime parenteral nutrition should have cholecystectomy even in the absence of cholelithiasis if laparotomy is being performed for another indication. Because the presentation is so frequently atypical, the accompanying physiological derangement so complex, and the mortality and morbidity from emergency cholecystectomy so prohibitively high in the paediatric patient on lifelong parenteral nutrition, we have come to recommend cholecystectomy in the absence of cholelithiasis when life expectancy is greater than five years.

Prophylactic cholecystectomy cannot be recommended for silent stones in healthy adults because of the risks of morbidity and mortality from cholecystectomy and the cost of operative or dissolution therapy. The majority of available data suggests that mortality from operation, the cost of operative intervention, and cost from lost employment are equal to, or exceed that which results from expectant therapy.

A 'grey zone' remains in some patients with silent gallstones. In these patients individual decisions must be made based on the data we have summarized. Included among these are patients who desire cholecystectomy or dissolution because of concern with developing acute cholecystitis during travelling or who will be isolated from optimal medical and surgical care for prolonged periods of time.

SUMMARY

Asymptomatic gallstones are best defined as those discovered during screening examinations. The risk of symptoms from those stones is estimated at 2% per year with 10% of these first presenting with complications requiring urgent medical therapy. Prophylactic cholecystectomy cannot be recommended for asymptomatic gallstones in healthy patients because the risk of cholecystectomy exceeds the risk of expectant therapy, and the cost of operative intervention for all patients in this category would deplete the resources for medical care in most countries. Prophylactic cholecystectomy is recommended in patients with increased risk factors. Although the choice of cholecystectomy or dissolution therapy will continue to be influenced by physician choice, the low dissolution and frequent recurrence rates would suggest that cholecystectomy is the preferred therapy.

REFERENCES

Allen B, Bernhoft R, Blanckaert N, Svavik J, Filly R, Gooding G, et al 1981 Sludge is calcium bilirubinate associated with bile stasis. American Journal of Surgery 141: 51–56

Ashur H, Siegal B, Oland Y, Adam Y G 1978 Calcified gallbladder (porcelain gallbladder). Archives of Surgery 113: 594–596

Bates G L, Brown C H 1952 Incidence of gallbladder disease in chronic hemolytic anemia (spherocytosis). Gastroenterology 21: 104–109

Biss K, Ho K J, Mikkelson B, Lewis L, Taylor C B 1971 Some unique biologic characteristics of the Masai of East Africa. New England Journal of Medicine 284: 694–699

Boston Collaborative Drug Surveillance Program 1973 Oral contraceptives and venous thromboembolic disease, surgically confirmed gallbladder disease and breast tumours. Lancet i:1399

Boston Collaborative Drug Surveillance Program 1974 Surgically confirmed gallbladder disease, venous thromboembolism and breast tumors in relation to postmenopausal estrogen therapy. New England Journal of Medicine 290: 15–19

Carveth S W, Priestley J T, Gage R P 1959 Size and number of gallstones in acute and chronic cholecystitis. Mayo Clinic Proceedings 34: 371–374

Clave R A, Gaspar M R 1969 Incidence of gallbladder disease after vagotomy. American Journal of Surgery 118: 169–176

Coronary Drug Project Research Group 1977 Gallbladder disease as a side effect of drugs influencing lipid metabolism: Experience in the coronary drug project. New England Journal of Medicine 296: 1185–1190

Coyle J J, Hoyt D B, Sedaghat A 1980 Relationship of intestinal bypass operations and cholelithiasis. Surgical Forum 31: 139–141

Freeman J B, Meyer P D, Printed K J, Mason E E, DenBesten L 1975 Analysis of gallbladder bile in morbid obesity. American Journal of Surgery 129: 163–166

Friedman G D, Kannel W B, Dawber T R 1966 The epidemiology of gallbladder disease: Observations in the Framingham study. Journal of Chronic Diseases 19: 273–292

Gilat T, Feldam C, Halpern Z, Dan M, Bar-Meir S 1983 An increased familial frequency of gallstones. Gastroenterology 84: 242–246

Glenn F, Grafe W R Jr 1966 Historical events in biliary tract surgery. Archives of Surgery 93: 848–852

Gracie W A, Ransohoff D F 1982 The natural history of silent gallstones: The innocent gallstone is not a myth. New England Journal of Medicine 307: 798–800

Ihasz M, Griffith C A 1981 Gallstones after vagotomy. American Journal of Surgery 141: 48–50

Jordan R A 1957 Cholelithiasis in sickle cell disease. Gastroenterology 33: 952–958

Langenbuch C 1882 Ein fall von exstirpation der gallenblase wegen chronischer cholelithiasis. Berliner Klinische Wochenschrift 48: 725–727

Lund J 1960 Surgical indications in cholelithiasis: Prophylactic cholecystectomy elucidated on the basis of long-term followup on 526 nonoperated cases. Annals of Surgery 151: 153–162

Mabee T M, Mayer P, DenBesten L, Mason E E 1976 The mechanism of increased gallstone formation in obese human subjects. Surgery 79: 460–468

Massarrat S, Klinsemann H G, Kappert J, Jaspersen D, Schmitz-Moormann P 1982 Incidence of gallstone disease in autopsy material and outpatients from West Germany. Gastroenterology 20: 341–345

Messing B, Bories C, Kunstlinger F, Bernier J J 1983 Does total parenteral nutrition induce gallbladder sludge formation and lithiasis? Gastroenterology 84: 1012–1019

Pitt H A, Berquist W E, Mann L L, Porter-Fink V, Fonkalsrud E W, Ament M E et al 1983a Parenteral nutrition induces calcium bilirubinate gallstones. Gastroenterology 84:1274 (abstract)

Pitt H A, King W III, Mann L L, Roslyn J J, Berquist W E, Ament W E 1983b Increased risk of cholelithiasis with prolonged total parenteral nutrition. American Journal of Surgery 145: 106–112

Ransohoff D F, Gracie W A, Wolfenson L B, Neuhauser D 1983 Prophylactic cholecystectomy or expectant management for silent gallstones. A decision analysis to assess survival. Annals of Internal Medicine 99: 199–204

Rome Group for the Epidemiology and Prevention of Cholelithiasis (GREPCO) 1984 Prevalence of gallstone disease in an Italian adult female population. American Journal of Epidemiology 119: 796–805

Roslyn J J, Berquist W E, Pitt H A, Mann L L, Kangarloo H, DenBesten L et al 1983a Inceased risk of gallstones in children receiving total parenteral nutrition. Pediatrics 71: 784–789

Roslyn J J, Pitt H A, Mann L L, Ament M E, DenBesten L 1983b Gallbladder disease in patients on long-term parenteral nutrition. Gastroenterology 84: 148–154

Roslyn J J, Pitt H A, Mann L L, Fonkalsrud E W, DenBesten L 1984 Parenteral nutrition induced gallbladder disease: A reason for early cholecystectomy. American Journal of Surgery 148: 58–63

Sampliner R E, Bennett P H, Comess L J, Rose F A, Burch T A 1970 Gallbladder disease in Pima Indians. Demonstration of high prevalence and early onset by cholecystography. New England Journal of Medicine 283: 1358–1364

Sapala M A, Sapala J A, Soto A D, Bouwman D L 1979 Cholelithiasis following subtotal gastric resection with truncal vagotomy. Surgery, Gynecology and Obstetrics 148: 36–38

Schwartz S I 1981 Sequence of stones. Contemporary Surgery 18:9

Sonnenberg A, Leuschner U, Leuschner M 1982 Expected costs in the conservative and surgical treatment of uncomplicated cholecystolithiasis. Zeitschrift fur Gastroenterologie 20: 66–77

Tucker L E, Tansedahl T N, Newmark S R 1982 Prevalence of gallstones in obese Caucasian American women. International Journal of Obesity 6: 247–251

Turrill F L, McCarron N M, Mikkelsen W P 1961 Gallstones and diabetics: An ominous association. American Journal of Surgery 102: 184–190

Van der Linden W, Nakayama F 1973 Gallstone disease in Sweden versus Japan. Clinical and etiologic aspects. American Journal of Surgery 125: 267–272

Way L W, Sleisenger M H 1983 Cholelithiasis and chronic cholecystitis. In: Sleisenger M H, Fortrand J S (eds) Gastrointestinal Disease, 3rd edn. W B Saunders p 1383

Wenckert A, Robertson B 1966 The natural course of gallstone disease. Gastroenterology 50: 376–381

Wilbur R S, Bolt R J 1959 Incidence of gallbladder disease in 'normal' men. Gastroenterology 36: 251–255

Acute cholecystitis

Britain, North America, Australia and Europe have a high prevalence of gallstones (Lieber 1952, Cleland 1953, Torvik & Hoivik 1960, Barker et al 1979). With few exceptions the alleged differences between most Western countries disappear when figures are standardized (Opit & Greenhill 1974). Nonetheless some countries such as Sweden, Czechoslovakia and Chile, and certain ethnic groups e.g. the Pima and Chippewa tribes of American Indians have an undoubted greater incidence of gallstone disease (Ch. 38).

In Britain gallstones are expected to develop in one in three females and one in five males and there is evidence for a moderate increase since 1974. In a recent prospective study of gallstone related deaths, the prevalence of gallstones in the adult population was found to be 17.1%. However, in this study nine out of 10 subjects with gallstones had not had a cholecystectomy and females were three times more likely to have had their gallstones removed than males (Godfrey et al 1984).

The incidence of gallstones rises with age in both sexes but the cholecystectomy rate per head of population declines sharply after the age of 70 years. There are major differences in the cholecystectomy rates between different countries (70–79/100 000 in the UK). In the USA and Canada the figure is three to four times higher (Bunker 1970, Vayda 1970). As these rates cannot be explained on the basis of different disease prevalence, it seems likely that the indications for cholecystectomy differ between Britain and North America and Canada. Figures for Scotland demonstrate a rising cholecystectomy rate since 1961 (Fig. 41.1). This cannot be accounted for fully by increased incidence of the disease and has not been accompanied by a reduced overall mortality. The rise in the cholecystectomy rate in the UK has been attributed to the gradual improvement in diagnostic and surgical resources (Bateson 1984) although there is no evidence for this assertion. The available evidence suggests that in the UK, cholecystectomy rate and gallstone prevalence are linked (McPherson et al 1984). In the author's view this apparent anomaly may be explained by a higher percentage of patients who are symptomatic or develop acute disease because of their gallstones and there is evidence that diuretic therapy may be a factor (see below).

Gallstone disease either causes chronic symptoms or presents acutely with biliary colic/acute cholecystitis.

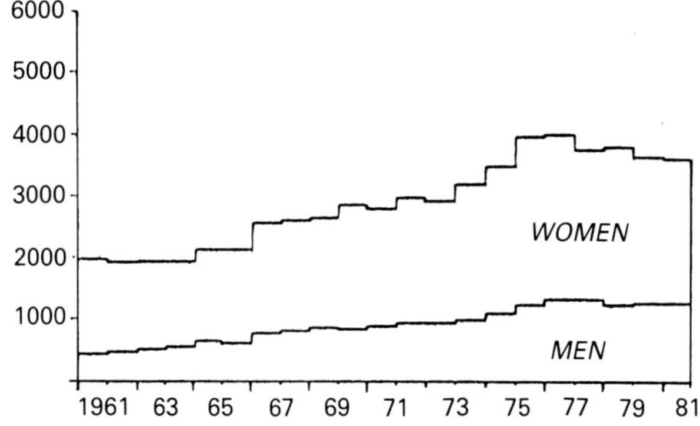

Fig. 41.1 Rising cholecystectomy rate in Scotland between 1961 and 1981. This was attributed by Bateson to the gradual improvement in the diagnosis and surgical resources. The evidence available within the UK is against this assertion and analysis from several districts within the UK indicate that gallstone prevalence and cholecystectomy rate are linked. In the author's view, although the overall increase in gallstone prevalence does not match the increase in the cholecystectomy rate, the percentage of patients who are symptomatic or develop acute disease is probably higher than it was in the early sixties. Reproduced by permission of the Lancet ii, 1984 p 623

Table 41.1 Cholecystectomies in Scotland

	No of cholecystectomies (by age-group)						
	0–14	15–24	25–44	45–64	65–74	75+	All ages
Women							
1961	—	32	435	1119	332	85	1993
1971	—	106	828	1212	526	163	2835
1981	3	161	1168	1443	638	256	3669
Increase	—	503%	269%	129%	198%	301%	184%
Men							
1961	—	5	80	261	86	24	456
1971	1	4	156	448	210	67	886
1981	1	11	197	596	348	114	1267
Increase	—	—	246%	228%	404%	475%	278%

Symptomless gallstones are often encountered during investigation of patients for unrelated disorders. The arguments for cholecystectomy in this group have included the risk of gallbladder cancer and the eventual development of acute life threatening disease. There are no prospective studies on symptomless gallstones which clearly document the long term risk for acute disease but obviously this must be age related. The incidence of primary carcinoma of the gallbladder in two recent necropsy surveys of gallstone disease was 17/4499 (0.38%) and 1/291 (0.34%) (Bateson 1984, Godfrey et al 1984). There is clearly no benefit from cholecystectomy for symptomless gallstone disease in the prevention of gallbladder cancer since the overall mortality of elective surgery would certainly exceed this figure (Ch. 64).

An inverse relationship between death from gallstone disease and coronary artery occlusion has been reported (Barker et al 1979) but this has not been confirmed by other studies (Bateson & Bouchier 1975, Bateson 1984). A high incidence of gallstones has been documented in epileptics on chronic anticonvulsant therapy (Fleming 1930, Bateson & Bouchier 1975). This is unexpected since phenobarbitone might have been expected to protect against stones by improving bile composition or enhancing stone dissolution. Although the chronic administration of thiazide diuretics is not associated with development of gallstones (O'Fallon et al 1975), two studies have implicated this therapy with the subsequent development of acute cholecystitis (Rosenberg et al 1980, van der Linden et al 1984). Thus thiazide diuretic therapy may induce acute cholecystitis in patients at risk and caution should be exercised in the prescription of these drugs to patients known to harbour gallstones. The widespread use of diuretic therapy in the treatment of hypertension may well be a factor in the rising cholecystectomy rate for gallstone disease in the UK.

SPECTRUM OF CHOLECYSTITIS

Inflammation of the gallbladder can be acute, acute on chronic or chronic. Furthermore, the inflammatory process is either associated with stones (calculous cholecystitis) or occurs in their absence (acalculous). The term chronic acalculous cholecystitis is often extended to include conditions such as cholesterolosis and adenomyomatosis (cholecystitis glandularis proliferans). This chapter deals with acute cholecystitis and is based on a consecutive series of 510 patients undergoing early surgery for acute cholecystitis at Ninewells Hospitals, Dundee, Scotland (Table, 41.2).

Table 41.2 Operative findings in 534 patients undergoing early surgery for acute cholecystitis

Operative pathology	n	%
Acute/acute on chronic calculous cholecystitis	495	97.0
Acute acalculous cholecystitis	12	2.4
Acute emphysematous cholecystitis	3	0.6
Empyema	14	2.7
Patchy gangrene	37	7.3
Perforation — localized	25	4.9
Perforation — free	8	1.6
Ductal calculi	57	11.2
Cholecysto-duodenal fistula	3	0.6
Cholecysto-choledochal fistula	1	0.2
Carcinoma of gallbladder + stones + acute cholecystitis	2	0.4
Misdiagnosis	24	4.5

ACUTE OBSTRUCTIVE (CALCULOUS) CHOLECYSTITIS

This is by far the commonest form of the disease and accounts for 90–95% of cases. It results from cystic duct obstruction by a stone impacted in Hartman's pouch. The obstruction of the cystic duct is thus more often due to compression than intra-luminal occlusion.

Pathology

The gallbladder becomes acutely inflamed with transmural oedema. The current consensus is that the initial inflammation is chemically induced and not of bacterial origin although sepsis is an important feature of the complications of the disease. The currently held hypothesis is that mucosal trauma releases phospholipase which converts the lecithin in the gallbladder bile to lysolecithin, a known mucosal toxin. At the time of surgery approximately 50% of cultures of gallbladder contents are sterile. Aerobic enteric organisms account for 94% of positive cultures and anaerobes for the remainder (Lou et al 1977). Bacterial lysosomal enzymes have been implicated in the initiation of the disease. Usually however infected gallbladder bile is encountered later on, during the second week of the disease. The role of prostaglandins as mediators of the inflammation has been suggested but not established.

Patchy gangrene (Fig 41.2), usually of the gallbladder fundus, was observed in 7% in the Ninewells series. Often this becomes obvious only after the omental wrap around the inflamed gallbladder is detached from the organ. Localised perforation with peri-cholecystic collection/abscess was encountered in 25 patients (4.9%) and free perforation with established generalized peritonitis in 1.6%. However three out of the eight patients with free perforations had emphysematous cholecystitis with gangrene of the gallbladder. Positive cultures of gallbladder contents were obtained in 39% of patients. Anaerobic (clostridial) infections were encountered in four patients. Histological

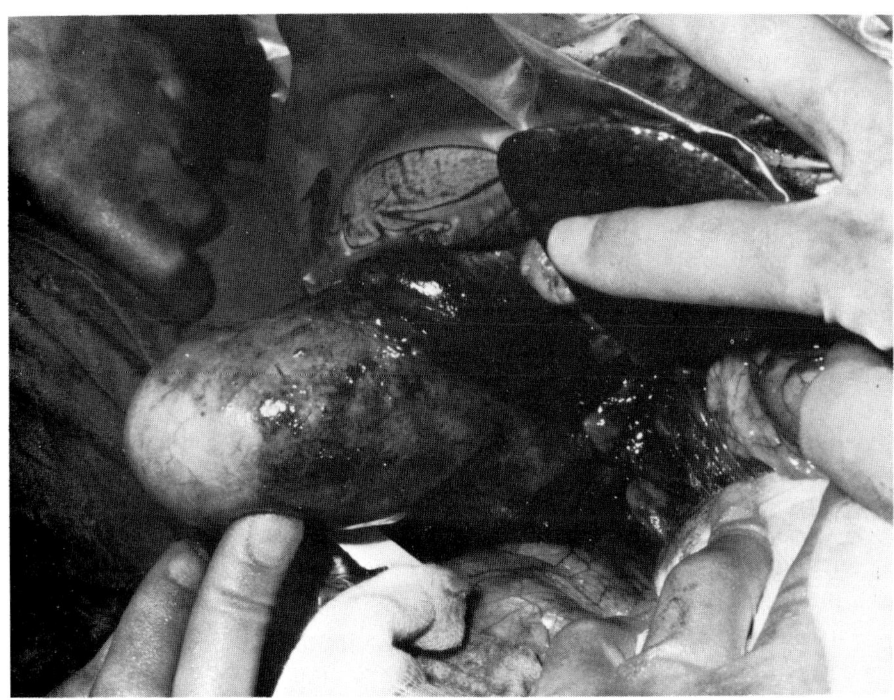

Fig. 41.2 Patchy gangrene of the gallbladder fundus encountered during early cholecystectomy. This has been observed in 7.0% of the Ninewells series

evidence of chronic cholecystitis (acute on chronic) indicating previous episodes of inflammation was found in 31% of excised gallbladders.

Clinical features

The clinical picture varies with the severity of the inflammatory process. Known pre-existing gallbladder disease may be present or chronic symptoms over several months to years may precede the acute presentation. Pain is usually in the right hypochrondrium although it can be mid-epigastric and less commonly in the right chest or back. The condition of 'biliary colic' has been ascribed to those patients who are restless from the pain, especially when this is of short duration (30 minutes to three hours) and is unaccompanied by evidence of inflammation such as fever and leucocytosis. In the author's experience differentiation between biliary colic and acute cholecystitis is often impossible and absence of fever, leucocytosis and minimal signs do not exclude gallbladder inflammation, particularly in the elderly. Nausea is a common feature of the disease but vomiting is infrequent.

Physical signs include pyrexia, tenderness with rebound in the right hypochondrium, positive Murphy's sign (inspiratory arrest), ileus and mild abdominal distension. A tender palpable mass in the right hypochondrium is found in 25% of patients and may signify any of the following: empyema of the gallbladder, abscess due to localized perforation, carcinoma of the gallbladder or hepatic flexure.

Jaundice occurs in 20–25% of patients with acute cholecystitis but the incidence of common duct stones averages 12% (Pitluk et al 1979, Stryker et al 1983). These recent studies have shown no correlation between the level of serum bilirubin and ductal calculi. This is contrary to the findings in a previous report which documented a high incidence of ductal calculi (69%) in patients with a serum bilirubin exceeding 80 μmol/l (Dumont 1976). The level of serum alkaline phosphatase activity is a poor predictor of ductal calculi in patients with acute cholecystitis. Clinical jaundice (bilirubin > 50 μmol/l) was observed in 103 patients in the present series and ductal calculi were found at operation in 57 of these with an overall incidence of 11.2% in patients with acute cholecystitis. In the absence of ductal calculi, jaundice has been ascribed to reactive hepatitis or oedema of the common bile duct.

Other laboratory findings include raised transaminases, leucocytosis and an elevated serum amylase. In a preliminary analysis of the operative findings in patients with 'acute gallstone pancreatitis' randomized to early surgery, acute or acute on chronic cholecystitis without any obvious pancreatic inflammation at the time of operation was found in 10 out of 16 patients (Mackie et al 1985). It is thus clear that hyperamylasaemia exceeding 1200 I.U. (Phadebas) is found in some patients with acute obstructive cholecystitis.

Imaging tests

Plain X-rays of the abdomen may show gallstones (15%), gas in the gallbladder lumen and biliary tree (in emphysematous cholecystitis, biliary-enteric fistula) or an enlarged gallbladder shadow. However, the main practical value of this investigation is to exclude free air under the diaphragm particularly when peritonism is marked.

Ultrasound examination has been advocated as the initial diagnosis procedure for acute cholecystitis (Ulreich et al 1980). It permits the determination of tenderness over the sonographically identified gallbladder and is able to detect stones, sludge and gallbladder thickening in 80–90%. However, the sensitivity and specificity for the diagnosis of acute cholecystitis (as opposed to gallbladder disease) is low (Zeman et al 1981, Krishnamurthy et al 1982). Moreover this investigative modality is highly observer dependent and the diagnostic yield will therefore vary from centre to centre depending on local expertise.

Gallbladder scintiscanning (Ch. 15) (99m Tc HIDA, IDA, iprofenin) (Fig 41.3) is nowadays regarded as the most accurate test of acute cholecystitis (Hall et al 1981, Freitas et al 1980, Zeman 1981, O'Callaghan et al 1980, Ralls et al 1982) and has a sensitivity of 91–97% and a specificity of 87%. False positives are due to chronic cholecystitis and are also encountered in patients with gallstone pancreatitis (Glazer et al 1981). A normal gallbladder scintiscan is virtually 100% accurate in excluding acute cholecystitis.

Intravenous cholangiography is a time honoured method for the detection of acute cystic duct obstruction particularly when the infusion technique is used. However, it is less accurate than biliary scintigraphy for the diagnosis of acute cholecystitis (Hall et al 1981) and cannot be used when the serum bilirubin exceeds 50 μmol/1. There is no good reason to use oral cholecystography for the diagnosis of acute cholecystitis as the test is unpredictable in the ill patient who is nauseous and may vomit. The method is however useful after the acute episode has subsided and in patients with mild attacks.

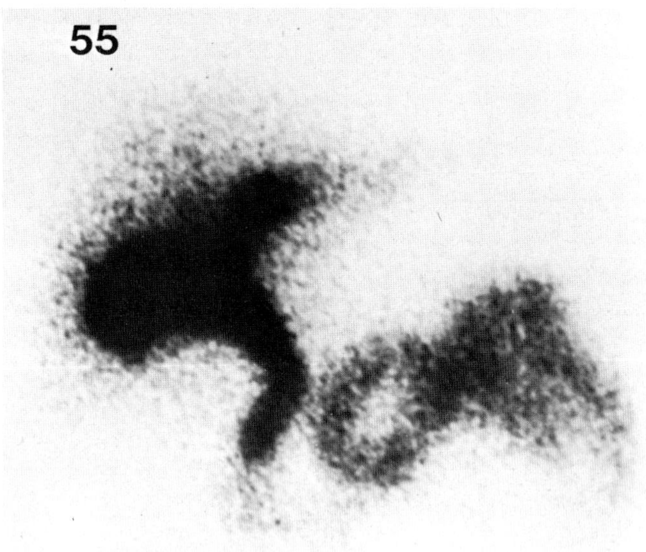

a

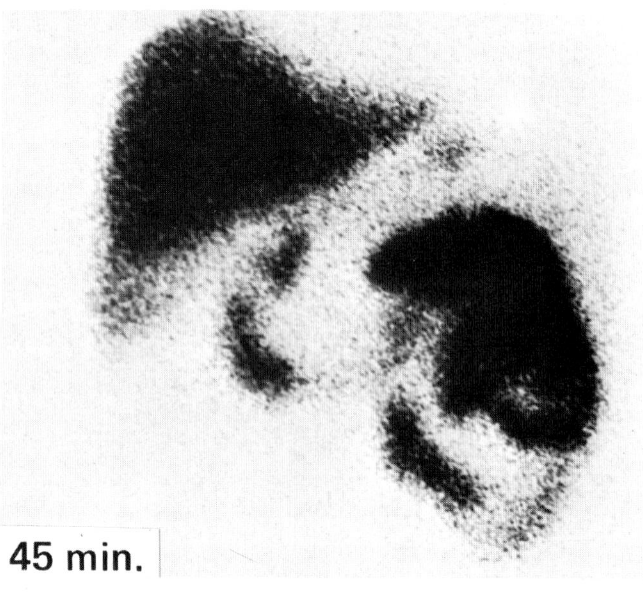

b

Fig. 41.3 a. E-Hida scintiscan in a patient with acute pain and tenderness in the right hypochondrium. A normal gallbladder and bile duct system is imaged thereby excluding the possibility of acute cholecystitis. The patient was found to have a small sealed perforated DU at operation. b. E-HIDA scintiscan in patient with acute cholecystitis. The typical features are absence of gallbladder image with visualization of a normal free draining common bile duct

Complications

1. Empyema (suppurative cholecystitis) This is an uncommon complication with a 2.4% incidence of all patients with gallbladder disease. Typically it affects elderly patients and in a recent reported series, the mean age at presentation was 71 years (Thornton et al 1983). The gallbladder is invariably obstructed by stones and aerobic cultures of the gallbladder contents are positive in 80%. The condition is usually characterized by intermittent fever, abdominal pain, tender mass in the right hypochrondium and marked leucocytosis. However, empyema of the gallbladder may be painless, unaccompanied by fever and pronounced tenderness, and present solely with a minimally tender mass in the right hypochrondrium. This is especially the case in the elderly and debilitated.

2. Gangrene and perforation Patchy gangrene of the gallbladder wall is not uncommon and typically affects the fundus. It may lead to localized or free perforation. Gangrene is more frequently found in the elderly, in diabetics, in patients who develop an empyema, in acalculous cholecystitis and especially in emphysematous cholecystitis.

Perforation into the duodenum results in a cholecystoduodenal fistula with resolution of the cholecystitis but the condition may then progress to gallstone ileus (Ch. 61). Free perforation into the general peritoneal cavity with the development of generalized peritonitis carries a high mortality variously reported between 30 and 50%.

ACUTE ACALCULOUS CHOLECYSTITIS

This must be distinguished from acalculous chronic gallbladder disease and accounts for up to 8% of acute cholecystitis (Keddie et al 1976, Glenn et al 1981). Acute acalculous cholecystitis usually occurs in critically ill patients with an equal sex distribution and at an average age of 60 to 70 years (Roslyn et al 1984), but the condition has been reported in children (Ternberg et al 1975). The disease usually develops on a background of prolonged illness, e.g., multiple trauma, extensive burns, severe sepsis, major surgery and drug overdosage. The risk factors suspected in precipitating the onset of the gallbladder inflammation include volume depletion, prolonged ileus, morphine administration exceeding six days, hyperalimentation, multiple transfusions, infected wounds and starvation (Long et al 1978, Petersen et al 1979). Whilst long term parenteral nutrition (TPN) appears to predispose to the development of biliary tract disease, only 17% of 35 patients receiving TPN were found to have acalculous cholecystitis whereas the majority had gallstone associated disease (Roslyn et al 1984).

Pathogenesis

The aetiology of acute acalculous cholecystitis remains unknown. The presumed pathophysiology involves gallbladder distension, bile stasis and inspissation together with a mucosal injury and vascular occlusion leading to acute inflammation of the gallbladder. Pathological examination of excised specimens demonstrates marked oedema of the serosa and muscular coat with focal necrotic areas and thrombosis of arterioles and venules. However the mucosa is usually spared except in gangrenous areas. Glenn has postulated the activation of factor XII by trauma leading to injury and thrombosis of the blood vessels of the sero-muscular layer (1982).

Clinical features

The presentation is often insidious and diagnosis is often made at laparotomy. The most common features are pyrexia, right upper quadrant pain and tenderness, leucocytosis and jaundice. A palpable tender mass in the right upper quadrant is present in 25%. In addition to hyperbilirubinaemia, elevations of the serum amylase, alkaline phosphatase and transaminases are frequently observed. Thus the clinical picture is virtually indistinguishable from acute obstructive cholecystitis and differentiation between the two is only possible at laparotomy.

The two most useful preoperative tests which carry a high diagnostic yield are ultrasound examination (thickened, distended, tender gallbladder) and 99mTc HIDA scintiscanning (Fox et al 1984). Treatment necessitates emergency cholecystectomy. Although patchy gangrene is common (40–50%), frank perforation is rare. The reported mortality varies from 4–35% depending on the nature and severity of the antecedent illness.

ACUTE EMPHYSEMATOUS CHOLECYSTITIS

This is a severe and fulminant form of acute cholecystitis which is caused by a mixed infection including gas-forming organisms. It is usually but not always acalculous. Acute emphysematous cholecystitis has a predilection for males (70% of reported cases) and diabetic individuals (Mentzer et al 1975).

The disease is acute and rapidly progressive with marked deterioration in the general condition of the patient and onset of peripheral circulatory failure. It is best diagnosed by a plain X-ray of the abdomen which outlines gas in the gallbladder lumen, its wall or the biliary ducts. Not infrequently, these radiological findings are interpreted as evidence of a cholecysto-enteric fistula. The gallbladder is usually gangrenous at operation with free perforation and generalized peritonitis in 15%. Adjacent gas in the hepato-duodenal ligament was encountered in two patients in the Ninewells series. Bile cultures are positive in 90% of cases and clostridial organisms are present in 50%. The reported mortality exceeds 20%.

CHOLECYSTITIS IN THE ELDERLY

Acute cholecystitis in the elderly (>60 years) is a serious condition. The disease tends to be severe in this age group and is often diagnosed late because of minimal signs. Furthermore, it is associated with a high complication rate (empyema perforation) and carries an appreciable mortality (10–14% as opposed to 1–2% in patients below 60 years) contributed in part by co-existing cardio-respiratory disease (Glenn et al 1976, Morrow et al 1978, Huber et al 1983). The common intercurrent medical illnesses are coronary disease, pulmonary disorders, hypertension and diabetes.

The clinical features are often nondescript and bear little relation to the severity of the underlying gallbladder inflammation. Thus the temperature may not be elevated, peritoneal irritation may be absent and the white cell count may be normal (Wilson et al 1978). At operation, gangrene or perforation is found in 10–15% of cases. Bile cultures are positive in 80% of cases. Thus elderly patients in whom the diagnosis of acute cholecystitis is entertained should be operated early if clinical improvement is not witnessed after conservative management for 16 to 24 hours (Sullivan et al 1982).

CHOLECYSTITIS IN CHILDREN

Although uncommon, acute cholecystitis is well documented in children and is associated with gallstones in 50–75% of cases (Pieretti et al 1975, Ternberg et al 1975). Acute acalculous cholecystitis is encountered as a complication of a severe childhood infection associated with vomiting and dehydration. In a review of 100 patients aged 14 months to 18 years, non-haemolytic cholelithiasis accounted for 74 patients, cholelithiasis due to haemolytic disease (spherocytosis, sickle-cell anaemia) 11, acalculous cholecystitis for seven and stenosis of the common duct in six patients (Holcomb et al 1980).

TREATMENT OF ACUTE CHOLECYSTITIS

Opinions still differ regarding the treatment of acute cholecystitis. Three options are available: emergency surgery, early cholecystectomy and delayed (interval) cholecystectomy. The controversy centres on the surgical management of mild or resolving disease.

Initial management

This consists of nasogastric suction, intravenous fluid and electrolyte therapy, systemic antibiotics and analgesic medication. Most centres now favour a third generation cephalosporin as the antibiotic of choice. Metronidazole is added in severe infections particularly in elderly patients and those with an empyema.

Opiates are the most commonly used analgesics despite theoretical objections concerning spasm of the sphincter of Oddi induced by these drugs. Contrary to popular belief pethidine constricts the sphincter as much as morphine or omnopon. Indomethacin is used in some centres to control pain but the use of this non-steroidal analgesic may be complicated by the development of erosive gastritis particularly in the elderly. Glucagon has been shown to be an effective agent in relieving biliary colic in a placebo controlled trial (Stower et al 1982). Pentazocine which is frequently prescribed for the condition induces hallucinatory episodes in the elderly.

Surgical treatment

Progressive/life threatening disease

The need for emergency or urgent surgical intervention is unquestioned for the following categories:

1. Deterioration in the patient's general condition and physical signs.
2. Evidence of generalized peritonitis.
3. Development of an inflammatory mass in the right hypochondrium.
4. Gas in the gallbladder lumen, wall or biliary ducts.
5. Onset of intestinal obstruction.

The approach in these patients should be via a right paramedian incision which can be easily extended if necessary. The objective is to remove the inflammed, perforated or gangrenous gallbladder, close any biliary-enteric fistula, exclude the presence of calculi from the extra-hepatic biliary tract by operative cholangiography and perform thorough peritoneal lavage with saline-antibiotic solution (tetracycline or cefuroxime). In patients with a tense non-perforated empyema, preliminary decompression of the gallbladder contents is performed by means of a suction trocar cannula inserted through a purse string suture at the fundus of the gallbladder. In the presence of oedema and inflammatory adhesions, the cholecystectomy is best carried out in a retrograde fashion (fundus first) as this leads to a better identification of the cystic duct junction with the common bile duct and thereby minimizes the risk of iatrogenic bile duct trauma. In poor risk patients who are haemodynamically unstable, excision of gangrenous patches of gallbladder wall, removal of gallstones and cholecystostomy are performed together with saline-antibiotic lavage.

Mild resolving disease

Two options are available: delayed (interval) or early cholecystectomy. The interval approach is the traditional one and entails discharge from hospital after resolution of the attack by conservative treatment with subsequent re-admission some two to three months later for elective cholecystectomy.

The early cholecystectomy approach has become increasingly popular and must be distinguished from emergency cholecystectomy. Supportive therapy with nasogastric suction, antibiotics and analgesics is initiated on admission. The diagnosis is then confirmed by appropriate imaging tests and the patient is then operated on the next available elective list. The duration of the disease from its onset does not influence this policy. There have now been several clinical prospective clinical trials comparing the results of early versus delayed cholecystectomy for acute cholecystitis (van der Linden & Sunzel 1970, McArthur et al 1975, Lathinen et al 1978, Jarvinen & Hästbacka 1980, Van der Linden & Edlund 1981, Norrby et al 1983). The results of these trials have shown a clear benefit from early cholecystectomy. No statistical difference in the overall mortality has been observed although deaths have only occurred in the delayed group (Table 41.3). Patients allocated to the delayed cholecystectomy group spend on average an extra 10 days in hospital (Table 41.4). The incidence of missed stone has been the same for both types of management (Table 41.5). In addition delayed cholecystectomy incurs a number of disadvantages. These

Table 41.3 Early versus delayed cholecystectomy — mortality rate

Trial	Mortality (%)	
	Early cholecystectomy	Delayed cholecystectomy
Van der Linden & Sunzel 1979	0	0
McArthur, Cuschieri, Sells et al 1975	0	0
Lathinen, Alhava & Aukes 1978	0	8
Jarvinen & Hästbacka 1980	0	1.3
Norrby, Herlin, Holminet et al 1983	0	1.1

Table 41.4 Early versus delayed cholecystectomy — hospital stay

Trial	Mean hospital days saved by early cholecystectomy
Van der Linden & Sunzel 1970	8.8
McArthur, Cuschieri, Sells et al 1975	11.1
Lathinen, Alhava & Aukes 1978	12.0
Järvinen & Hästbacka 1980	7.5
Norrby, Herlin, Holmin et al 1983	6.4

Table 41.5 Early versus delayed cholecystectomy — residual stone rate

Trial	Residual stone rate (%)	
	Early cholecystectomy	Delayed cholecystectomy
Van der Linden & Sunzel 1970	0	0
McArthur, Cuschieri, Sells et al 1975	0	0
Lathinen, Alhava & Aukes 1978	2	7
Järvinen & Hästbacka 1980	1.3	1.3
Norrby, Herlin, Holmin et al 1983	2.0	0

include failure of medical treatment which has averaged 13%, premature readmission with further attack whilst waiting for elective cholecystectomy (13%) and patient defaulting after discharge (10%). Despite these unequivocal results in favour of early cholecystectomy, many surgeons continue to practise the delayed approach largely because they remain sceptical of the safety in terms of bile duct injury when cholecystectomy is performed early in the course of acute cholecystitis. In this context it is important to stress certain criteria which are necessary for safe early cholecystectomy. In the first place, the procedure should be carried out by a surgeon experienced in biliary tract surgery. The operation should not be delegated to a junior surgical trainee. It has been our practice to adopt the method of retrograde (fundus first) cholecystectomy (Ch. 44) as this procedure is safe and permits ready identification of the cystic artery and duct and in particular the cystic duct–common bile duct junction even in the presence of oedema and adhesion of the gallbladder neck to the extra-hepatic biliary tract. A gallbladder neck/Hartman's pouch adherent to the common bile duct is gently teased away from it by pledget dissection. In the event of a cholecysto-choledochal fistula, the gallbladder may be divided a few millimetres away from the fistulous opening which can then be used for CBD exploration if indicated. Thereafter the fistula is closed with interrupted sutures after the insertion of a T-tube. With this surgical approach, there has been one instance of partial (non-circumferential) damage to the common bile duct in 510 cases. The injury was recognized at operation and primary repair effected.

Peroperative cholangiography is necessary as a routine in all patients undergoing early cholecystectomy. Hold up of contrast medium at the lower end does not necessarily indicate calculous obstruction since it may result from peri-ampullary oedema. Nevertheless CBD exploration is usually warranted in these cases.

There is a small cohort of patients (1–2%) in whom cholecystectomy is found to be technically impossible. In these patients a cholecystostomy is performed. However any stones in the gallbladder should be removed especially those impacted in the neck of the organ. The subsequent management after cholecystostomy depends on the age and general condition of the patient. It is advisable wherever possible to remove the gallbladder a few months later as more than 50% of these patients will develop recurrent biliary symptoms within five years. However, in the elderly patient with intercurrent disease, cholecystectomy should not be performed unless pain and other symptoms recur.

In the Ninewells series cholecystectomy alone was performed in 81%, cholecystectomy and exploration of the common bile duct in 17%, cholecystectomy and closure of fistula in 0.5% and cholecystostomy in 1.5%. The overall mortality for early cholecystectomy was 3.4% for patients < 60 yrs and 6.1% in patients > 60 years.

Another argument voiced against early cholecystectomy is the high misdiagnosis rate (Essenhigh 1966, Halazs 1975). However, with the institution of appropriate imaging tests, the misdiagnosis rate was reduced to 3% in one study (Norrby et al 1983) and averaged 4.5% in the Ninewells Series (Table 41.2).

Drainage after cholecystectomy

The author considers it necessary to insert a subhepatic pouch drain (silicone tube leading to a closed drainage system) in all patients after cholecystectomy (Cuschieri & Berci 1984). Although the argument against drainage appears to have been strengthened by the results of two prospective clinical trials (Gordon et al 1976, Towbridge 1982) these studies have one severe limitation which precludes safe conclusion, i.e. the number of patients entered into the study, 50 in each group. As the incidence of unexpected bile leakage after cholecystectomy without bile duct exploration averages 0.5%, it is obvious that with the numbers concerned, it is not possible to detect a difference; indeed in both studies not a single case of bile leak was observed in the drainage and non-drainage groups. In the author's opinion, the avoidance of drainage of the subhepatic pouch can expose the occasional patient to an otherwise avoidable complication particularly when cholecystectomy is undertaken early during the initial hospital admission.

REFERENCES

Barker D J P, Gardner H J, Power C and Hutt M S R 1979 Prevalence of gallstones at necropsy in nine British towns. A collaborative study. British Medical Journal ii: 1389–1392

Bateson M C 1984 Gallbladder disease and cholecystectomy rate are independently variable. Lancet ii: 621–624

Bateson M C, Bouchier I A D 1975 Prevalence of gallstones in Dundee: a necropsy study. British Medical Journal ii: 427–430

Bunker J P 1970 Surgical manpower: a comparison of operations and surgeons in the United States and in England and Wales. New England Journal of Medicine 222: 135–139

Cleland J B 1953 Gallstones in seven thousand post-mortem examinations. Medical Journal of Australia 2: 488–490

Cuschieri A, Berci G 1984 Common bile duct exploration. Martinus Nijhoff, Dondrecht, p 7–17

Dumont A E 1976 Significance of hyperbilirubinaemia in acute cholecystitis. Surgery, Gynecology and Obstetrics 142: 855–857

Essenhigh D M 1966 Management of acute cholecystitis. British Journal of Surgery 53: 1032–1038

Fleming G W T H 1930 Cholelithiasis in the insane. Journal of Pathology and Bacteriology Vol i 33: 197–201

Fox M, Wilk P J, Weissman H S, Freeman L M and Gliedman M L 1984 Acute acalculous cholecystitis. Surgery, Gynecology and Obstetrics 159: 13–16

Freitas J E, Gulati R M 1980 Rapid evaluation of acute abdominal pain by hepatobiliary scanning. Journal of American Medical Association 224: 1585–1587

Glazer G, Murphy F, Clayden G S, Lawrence R G, Craig 1981 Radionuclide biliary scanning in acute pancreatitis. British Journal of Surgery 68: 766–770

Glenn F 1976 Acute cholecystitis. Surgery, Gynecology and Obstetrics 143: 56–60

Glenn F 1981 Surgical management of acute cholecystitis in patients 65 years of age and older. Annals of Surgery 193: 56–59

Glenn F, Becker C G 1982 Acute acalculous cholecystitis. An increasing entity. Annals of Surgery 195: 131–136

Godfrey P J, Bates T, Harrison H, King M B, Padley N R 1984 Gall stones and mortality: a study of all gallstone related deaths in a single health district. Gut 25: 1029–1033

Gordon A B, Bates T, Fiddian V 1976 A controlled trial of drainage after cholecystectomy. British Journal of Surgery 63: 278–282

Halaz S N A 1975 Counterfeit cholecystitis. American Journal of Surgery 130: 189–192

Hall A W, Wisbey M L, Hutchinson F, Wood R A B, Cuschieri A 1981 The place of hepatobiliary scanning in the diagnosis of gallbladder disease. British Journal of Surgery 68: 85–90

Holcomb G W Jr, O'Neill J A Jr, Holcomb G W 3rd 1980 Cholecystitis, cholelithiasis and common duct stenosis in children and adolescents. Annals of Surgery 191: 626–635

Huber D F, Martin E W Jr, Cooperman M 1983 Cholecystectomy in elderly patients. American Journal of Surgery 146: 719–722

Jarvinen J H, Hästbacka J 1980 Early cholecystectomy for acute cholecystitis. A prospective randomized study. Annals of Surgery 191: 502–505

Keddie N C, Gough A L, Galland R B 1976 Acalculous gallbladder disease: A prospective study. British Journal of Surgery 63: 797–798

Krishnamurthy G T 1982 Acute cholecystitis: the diagnostic role for current imaging tests. Western Journal of Medicine 137: 87–94

Lathinen J, Alhava E M, Aukes 1978 Acute cholecystitis treated by early and delayed surgery. Scandinavian Journal of Gastroenterology 13: 673–678

Lieber M M 1952 The incidence of gallstones and their correlation with other diseases. Annals of Surgery 135: 37–42

Long T N, Heimbach D M, Carrico C J 1978 Acalculous cholecystitis in critically ill patients. American Journal of Surgery 136: 30–36

Lou M A, Mandal A K, Alexander H L 1978 Bacteriology of the human biliary tract and the duodenum. Archives of Surgery 112: 965–967

Mackie C R, Wood R A B, Preece P E, Cuschieri A 1985 Surgical pathology at early elective operation for suspected acute gallstone pancreatitis: preliminary report of a prospective clinical trial. British Journal of Surgery (in press)

McArthur P, Cuschieri A, Sells R A, Shields R 1975 Controlled clinical trial comparing early with interval cholecystectomy for acute cholecystitis. British Journal of Surgery 62: 850–852

McPherson K, Strong P M, Jones L, Britton B J 1984 Do cholecystectomy rates correlate with geographic variations in prevalence of gallstones? Lancet ii: 1092–1093

Mentzer R M Jr, Golden G T, Chandler J G 1975 A comparative appraisal of emphysematous cholecystitis. American Journal of Surgery 129: 10–15

Morrow D J, Thompson J, Wilson S F 1978 Acute cholecystitis in the elderly: a surgical emergency. Archives of Surgery 118: 1492–1152

Norrby S, Herlin P, Holmin T, Sjödahl R, Tagesson C 1983 Early or delayed cholecystectomy in acute cholecystitis? A clinical trial. British Journal of Surgery 70: 163–165

O'Callaghan J D, Verow P W, Hopton D, Craven J L 1980 The diagnosis of acute gallbladder disease by technetum-99 m-labelled HIDA hepatobiliary scanning. British Journal of Surgery 67: 805–808

O'Fallon W M, Labarthe D W, Kurland L T 1975 Rauwolfia derivatives and breast cancer. A case control study in Olmsted County, Minnesota. Lancet ii: 292–296

Opit L T, Greenhill S 1974 Prevalence of gallstones in relation to differing treatment rates for biliary disease. British Journal of Preventive and Social Medicine 28: 269–272

Petersen S R, Sheldon G F 1979 Acute acalculous cholecystitis. A complication of hyperalimentation. American Journal of Surgery 138: 814–817

Pieretti R, Auldist A W, Stephens C A 1975 Acute cholecystitis in children. Surgery, Gynecology and Obstetrics 140: 16–18

Pitluk H C, Beal J M 1979 Choledocholithiasis associated with acute cholecystitis. Archives of Surgery 114: 887–888

Ralls P W, Colletti P M, Halls J M, Siemsen J K 1982 Prospective evaluation of 99mTC-IDA cholescintigraphy and gray-scale ultrasound in the diagnosis of acute cholecystitis. Radiology 144: 369–371

Rosenberg L, Shapiro S, Sloane D, Kaufman D W, Miethinen O S, Stolley P D 1980 Thiazides and acute cholecystitis. New England Journal of Medicine 303: 546–548

Roslyn J J, Pitt H A, Mann L, Fonkalsrud E W, DenBesten L 1984 Parenteral nutrition in induced gallbladder disease: a reason for early cholecystectomy. American Journal of Surgery 148: 58–63

Stower M J, Foster G E, Hardcastle J D 1982 A trial of glucagon in the treatment of painful biliary tract disease. British Journal of Surgery 69: 591–592

Stryker S J, Beal J M 1983 Acute cholecystitis and common duct calculi. Archives of Surgery 118: 1063–1064
Sullivan D M, Ruffin Hood T, Griffen W O 1982 Biliary tract surgery in the elderly. American Journal of Surgery 143: 218–220
Ternberg J L, Keating J P 1978 Acute acalculous cholecystitis: Complication of other illnesses in childhood. Archives of Surgery 110: 543–547
Thornton J, Heaton K W, Espiner H J, Eltringham W K 1983 Empyema of the gallbladder: reappraisal of a neglected disease. Gut 24: 1183–1185
Torvik A, Hoivik B 1960 Gallstones in an autopsy series. Incidence, complications and correlations with carcinoma of the gallbladder. Acta Chirurgica Scandinavica 120: 168–174
Trowbridge P E 1982 A randomized study of cholecystectomy with and without drainage. Surgery, Gynecology and Obstetrics 155: 171–176
Ulreich S, Foster K W, Stier S A, Rosenfield A T 1980 Acute cholecystitis: comparison of ultrasound and intravenous cholangiography. Archives of Surgery 115: 158–160
Vayda E 1970 A comparison of surgical rates in Canada and in England and Wales. New England Journal of Medicine 289: 1224–1234
Van der Linden W, Sunzel H 1970 Early versus delayed operations for acute cholecystitis. American Journal of Surgery 120: 7–13
Van der Linden W, Edlund G 1981 Early versus delayed cholecystectomy. The effect of a change in management. British Journal of Surgery 68: 753–757
Van der Linden W, Ritter B, Edlund G 1984 Acute cholecystitis and thiazides. British Medical Journal ii: 654–655
Zemen R K, Burrell M I, Cahow C E, Caride V 1981 Diagnostic utility of cholescintography and ultrasonography in acute cholecystitis. American Journal of Surgery 141: 446–451

R. E. Hermann, S. Grundfest-Broniatowski

Chronic cholecystitis

INTRODUCTION — INCIDENCE

Biliary inflammatory disease presents in a variety of ways. Experience at the Cleveland Clinic is that approximately 20% of patients with symptomatic gallstones present with signs and symptoms of acute cholecystitis, 10% to 15% of patients have complicated cholecystitis (jaundice, cholangitis or pancreatitis, and from 65% to 70% of patients are diagnosed as having chronic cholecystitis. Of the group of patients with chronic cholecystitis, approximately 20% have mild, vague symptoms which are difficult to diagnose but, since the symptoms persist and are distressing, and since the patient has gallstones, cholecystectomy is eventually performed.

The authors have reviewed their experience with cholecystectomy for acute and chronic cholecystitis at the Cleveland Clinic during two time periods: the years from 1962 to 1978 and, most recently, from January 1981 to December 1982. In these reviews the incidence and patterns of disease, their relationship to the age of the patient, methods of diagnosis and treatment, and results of therapy were examined.

In an initial review in 1978, overall experience with cholecystitis in approximately 1600 patients with biliary disease was studied and correlated with the age of patients. It was found that the incidence of acute versus chronic cholecystitis appeared to remain reasonably stable throughout all age groups (Hermann 1983). Approximately 20% of patients in all age groups presented with acute cholecystitis, although there was evidence that in patients of 75 or older, the incidence of acute disease rose slightly. The interesting fact is that acute and chronic cholecystitis appear to have a relationship which remains constant. In contrast to this finding, in the same study, bile duct stones and complicated cholecystitis increased dramatically after 60 years of age, from an average of 15% up to age 60, to higher than 90% above age 80 (see Table 27.I).

During a recent two-year study, approximately 450 cholecystectomies were performed. Cholecystectomy was performed for symptoms of chronic cholecystitis in 51% of the patients, for acute cholecystitis in 24%, for complicated cholecystitis (jaundice, cholangitis, pancreatitis) in 11%, and as an incidental procedure at the time of another operation in 14% of patients.

DIAGNOSIS

The diagnosis of chronic cholecystitis can be difficult. We define chronic cholecystitis to include patients who have had a series of mild, acute episodes of pain, usually of short duration (less than 12 hours), as well as those who have had recurrent, low-grade symptoms which persist over a longer time. These symptoms include, typically, right upper quadrant abdominal pain which occurs in association with or shortly after a heavy or fatty meal, radiates around to the right subscapular area, and is associated with some degree of nausea or vomiting. Other, less typical symptoms include pain in the epigastrium, mid-abdomen, or left upper quadrant; a feeling of gaseous bloating or indigestion, often described as a sense of heaviness or 'like a balloon blown up in my upper abdomen'; fever as an isolated symptom; back pain alone; pancreatitis without evidence of cholecystitis; or weight loss without obvious cause. In patients with mild or vague symptoms, atypical pain, or lack of correlation of symptoms with heavy meals or fatty foods, the presence of gallstones on radiographic studies may be the only indication of chronic cholecystitis or biliary disease.

Occasionally, patients with no symptoms of biliary disease are found at operation for some other problem to have gallstones. If the patient's general health and the conduct of the operative procedure permits it, an incidental cholecystectomy may be performed. When the gallbladder specimen is examined by the pathologist, the pathologic diagnosis of chronic cholecystitis is often returned. Thus a pathological diagnosis of chronic cholecystitis does not always correlate with symptoms.

Physical examination of the patient with chronic cholecystitis is usually normal. Occasionally, there may be some tenderness in the right upper abdomen or tenderness when palpating the liver edge. Rarely, in less than 1% to 2% of patients, a chronic hydrops of the gallbladder may be palpated as a right upper quadrant abdominal mass. Occasionally, there may be evidence of mild jaundice.

Confirmatory diagnostic studies for patients suspected to have chronic cholecystitis should include an ultrasound image of the gallbladder and biliary system to identify the presence of gallstones (Fig. 42.1). A plain abdominal roentgenogram may show opaque or calcified stones in about 10% of patients (Fig. 42.2). Since the advent of ultrasonography, the use of oral cholecystography (Ch. 18) has diminished. The oral cholecystogram is rarely used in the diagnosis of acute cholecystitis at the present time, except occasionally for the diagnosis of patients with chronic cholecystitis seen in an asymptomatic interval or when ultrasound is equivocal. Although ultrasonography has been shown to be sensitive and accurate (95%) in the diagnosis of gallstones, it does not give information about gallbladder function (Bartrum, Crow & Foote 1977, Sterioff et al 1977). Oral cystography provides this information and, if there is poor visualization or nonvisualization of the gallbladder, the diagnosis of gallbladder disease or chronic cholecystitis can be established with increased certainty (Mujabed, Evans & Whalen 1974). The sensitivity and specificity of oral cholecystography is in the range of 90% to 95%.

Radio-isotope technetium (HIDA, DISIDA, PIPIDA) (Ch. 15) scans were not used in the diagnosis of chronic cholecystitis, but exclusively for the diagnosis of acute cholecystitis. Radio-isotope technetium scans are not reliable in the diagnosis of chronic cholecystitis (Saurex et al 1980, Zeman et al 1981).

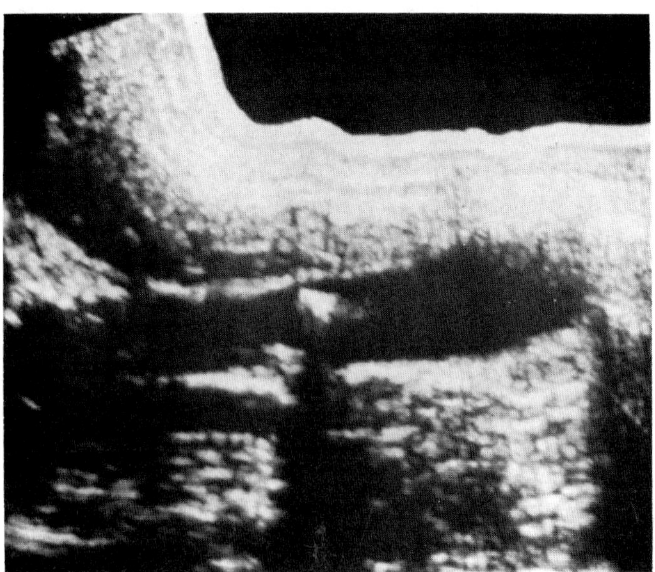

Fig. 42.1 Ultrasound study of the gallbladder shows a single stone in the lumen of the gallbladder with an echogenic acoustical shadow below the stone

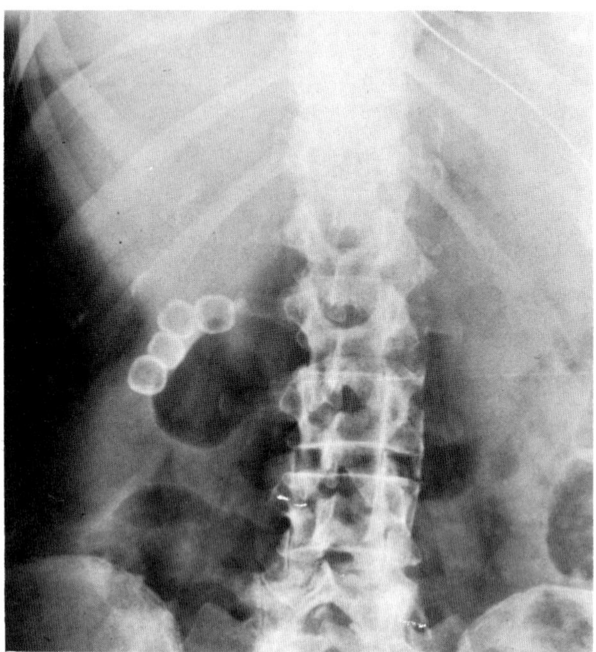

Fig. 42.2 A plain abdominal roentgenogram shows multiple opaque gallstones in the right upper abdomen

The differential diagnosis in patients considered to have chronic cholecystitis should include peptic ulcer disease, symptomatic hiatal hernia, hepatitis, recurrent episodes of pancreatitis, a right renal calculus, irritable bowel syndrome or other functional symptoms. In patients with atypical symptoms, other studies such as an upper gastrointestinal X-ray series using barium, upper gastrointestinal endoscopy, intravenous urography, or a barium enema may be helpful.

Occasionally, patients have typical symptoms of chronic cholecystitis but the ultrasound scan and oral cholecystogram appear to be normal. In spite of multiple other diagnostic studies, no other cause for the symptoms can be found. In such patients, a duodenal drainage study with cholecystokinin stimulation of gallbladder function may be rewarding. If cholesterol crystals or white blood cells are seen in the duodenal drainage, the diagnosis of chronic cholesterolosis or chronic cholecystitis can be made with reasonable certainty and cholecystectomy recommended (Porterfield, Cheung & Berenson 1977).

TREATMENT

Medical therapy is often tried for patients with mild symptoms of chronic cholecystitis or for patients who are a poor operative risk. This should include a low-fat diet, avoidance of heavy meals, and the use of an antispasmodic medication. If the episodes of cholecystitis are severe, however, or recurrent or progressive in their intensity, most patients will wish to consider operative treatment without delay. Cholecystectomy is the operative treatment of choice, and should be carried out as soon as the diagnosis of chronic cholecystitis is made. However, some patients procrastinate, especially in the presence of mild symptoms, and it is not unusual for the occasional patient to wait one or more years before going ahead with cholecystectomy.

One of the major risks in delaying cholecystectomy is the development of an acute episode of cholecystitis or a complication of the disease, such as jaundice, cholangitis or pancreatitis. It has been well shown in almost all studies of patients with biliary disease, that the operative risk associated with cholecystectomy is least in the patient having an elective operation for chronic cholecystitis and highest for patients having an emergency operation for acute cholecystitis or for some complication of the disease (see below).

Another risk of permitting gallstones to remain in the patient with mild symptoms of cholecystitis is the potential for developing cancer of the gallbladder. Cancer of the gallbladder (Ch. 64), while uncommon, is the fifth most common malignancy of the gastrointestinal tract and accounts for 4% of all cancer deaths. Approximately 80%–90% of all patients with carcinoma of the gallbladder have gallstones (McLaughlin 1964). No definite causal relationship between carcinoma of the gallbladder and gallstones has been established, but their association makes this relationship likely. It is not known, however, whether the presence of stones and the chronic irritation or inflammation they cause predisposes to cancer or whether the development of cancer causes the precipitation of gallstones in the affected gallbladder.

Cancer of the gallbladder is found predominantly in elderly patients, age 65 or older, often with a long history of diagnosed gallstones or symptoms of mild cholecystitis. Since the prognosis of carcinoma of the gallbladder is almost uniformly grave, there is an argument for removing the chronically inflamed organ as soon as mild symptoms begin. However, the incidence of carcinoma of the gallbladder is sufficiently low to make prophylactic cholecystectomy in asymptomatic patients with gallstones seem unwarranted (Wenckert & Robertson 1966). The only long-term survivals recorded in patients with carcinoma of the gallbladder are among patients who have had cholecystectomy for acute or chronic cholecystitis, in whom the carcinoma was early or confined to the mucosal or submucosal layers of the gallbladder and had not infiltrated or extended beyond the wall of the gallbladder (Ch. 64) (Bergdahl 1980).

OPERATIVE RISK

A number of risk factors have been identified in patients with both acute and chronic cholecystitis. Almost all studies reported have shown an increased morbidity and mortality for biliary surgery in association with the age of the patient, the presence of acute inflammation and the presence of other coexisting illness, especially vascular disease (Glenn 1975, Ibach et al 1968, Seltzer et al 1970). A review of morbidity and mortality from cholecystitis at the Cleveland Clinic shows that the major causes of severe morbidity or death in patients are those of cardiac and respiratory disease, renal failure and hepatic failure. The major risk factors identified by the authors in patients undergoing cholecystectomy include: age over 65 years; vascular disease, especially symptomatic coronary artery disease; presence of acute cholecystitis or complicated cholecystitis (pancreatitis, jaundice, cholangitis); chronic obstructive pulmonary disease; cirrhosis of the liver; and patients on long-term, high dose steroids or other immunosuppressive agents.

The overall operative risk of patients having cholecystectomy for chronic cholecystitis is much less than that for patients operated upon for acute or complicated cholecystitis. The morbidity of cholecystectomy for chronic cholecystitis, in most series, is in the range of 5% or less and consists predominantly of local wound problems or respiratory complications; the overall mortality of patients undergoing elective cholecystectomy for chronic cholecystitis is less than 0.5% (Ch. 44) (McSherry & Glenn 1980). Many reports, however, assess morbidity and mortality statistics for patients undergoing cholecystectomy and add together acute, complicated, and chronic cholecystitis. Therefore, the greater the number of patients in a series with acute or complicated cholecystitis, the higher the morbidity and mortality. With increased severity of disease, operating time is longer and the magnitude of the surgery required to correct the problem is greater.

Of 1600 patients undergoing biliary surgery at the Cleveland Clinic during the period of 1962 to 1978, 38 patients died, an overall mortality rate of 2.4% (Hermann 1983). In patients under 60, the hospital mortality rate was 1.2%, among patients over 60 it was 5.7%, and among patients over 70 years it was 12.5%. For all patients with acute cholecystitis the mortality rate was 5.2% and for all patients with chronic cholecystitis it was 1.1%. For patients with benign inflammatory disease hospital mortality was 1.8%, while for those with carcinoma it was 14%.

Glenn & Hays (1955) reviewed the hospital mortality after cholecystectomy at the New York Hospital and found a mortality of 0.65% in patients under 50, 2.5% in patients aged 50–64, and 6.7% in patients over 65. They related this increased hospital mortality predominantly to the problems of acute cholecystitis, finding no significant difference in morbidity or mortality related to age among patients undergoing elective cholecystectomy for chronic cholecystitis.

Ibach, Hume & Erb (1968) studied 151 patients

undergoing cholecystectomy who were over 60 years of age and found an overall operative mortality of 4%, with a 2.3% mortality rate after elective cholecystectomy and a 16.7% mortality rate after emergency cholecystectomy. These studies emphasize the importance of performing cholecystectomy, if at all possible, under elective circumstances rather than waiting for an acute attack which might require an emergency operation under less than optimal circumstances. This is especially important in elderly patients.

The risk of diabetes mellitus for patients with cholecystitis was investigated by Mundth (1962) who reviewed 145 patients with diabetes and cholelithiasis undergoing cholecystectomy. There was no increase in mortality for patients having elective cholecystectomy, but for patients undergoing emergency cholecystectomy a high incidence of complications (67%) and operative mortality (47%) was found. A recent review of data at the Cleveland Clinic showed an insignificant difference in morbidity and mortality (Ransohoff, Miller & Hermann 1985).

Several recent reports have shown that cirrhotic patients have an increased operative risk, with operative mortality rates as high as 80% in one series of patients with severe cirrhosis of the liver (Doberneck, Sterling & Allison 1983). The complications of excessive intra-abdominal bleeding, difficult to control, and progressive liver and renal failure makes even elective cholecystectomy in these severely cirrhotic patients a hazardous operative procedure (Castaing et al 1983). Some surgeons have suggested cholecystostomy with removal of the stones from the gallbladder only, avoiding cholecystectomy in patients with severe cirrhosis of the liver.

The question of whether peroperative antibiotics should be given prophylactically for patients undergoing elective cholecystectomy for chronic cholecystitis has been controversial. It has been shown, in several studies, that patients with chronic cholecystitis have positive gallbladder bile cultures in from 5% to 15% of cases, whereas among patients with acute cholecystitis positive bile cultures occur in from 55% to 65% (Keighley 1977, Traedson, Elmros & Holm 1983). Several authors have reviewed the risk of developing infection in patients undergoing biliary surgery and have found that those patients at high risk of infection include patients: aged over 70 years, with acute cholecystitis, with obstructive jaundice due to gallstones and/or common bile duct stones. Chetlin & Elliott (1971), Keighley (1977), and Stone et al (1976) have all recommended prophylactic antibiotics only for patients at high risk of developing infection. Other authors, including Stubbs (1983) Conte, Jacob & Polk (1984) and Ausobsky & Polk (1983) have pointed out that a short course of prophylactic antibiotic therapy is unlikely to cause any problems. It cannot be predicted exactly which patients may harbour stones in the common bile duct, requiring common bile duct exploration during elective cholecystectomy for chronic cholecystitis and placing these patients in a higher risk group; therefore it is probably wise to cover all patients with a prophylactic broad spectrum antibiotic, started preoperatively and continued during the 24 hours surrounding the operative procedure. It is the author's policy to cover all patients undergoing biliary surgery with prophylactic antibiotics for 24 hours, using a broad spectrum first or second generation cephalosporin, since any patient having cholecystectomy could have a potentially contaminated biliary system.

OPERATIVE TECHNIQUE

An operating table which permits intraoperative cholangiography (Ch. 27) should always be used for the patient having cholecystectomy. The patient is placed in the supine position with the left side of the abdomen slightly elevated so that the common bile duct will not be superimposed upon the spine during the operative cholangiogram.

A right upper quadrant, subcostal incision is preferred for most patients having cholecystectomy or other biliary surgery (Fig. 42.3). Most patients with biliary disease have a wide costal margin and this incision gives optimal access to the right upper abdomen and subhepatic space. In thin patients or in patients with a narrow costal angle, a midline upper abdominal incision or right paramedian incision provides adequate exposure.

The abdominal cavity is entered through a muscle transecting incision. Immediately after entering the abdominal cavity, a thorough intra-abdominal examination is performed. This includes careful inspection and palpation of the gallbladder itself, the porta hepatis and common bile duct, liver, stomach, spleen, duodenum, pancreas, both kidneys and small and large intestines. A hand is passed into the lower abdomen and pelvis to assess any pelvic disease.

Adhesions to the undersurface of the liver or gallbladder are dissected free to expose the gallbladder, cystic duct and porta hepatis. A self-retaining retractor is used, with the bar of the retractor placed inferiorly so as not to pass over the bile duct and potentially obscure the bile duct on the operative cholangiogram (Fig. 42.4). A flat Doyen or Harrington retractor is placed against the liver, medial to the gallbladder for exposure. A large laparotomy pad is placed in the right gutter to depress the hepatic flexure of the colon and to prevent any bile spillage from draining into the lower abdomen. Another laparotomy pad is placed over the duodenum and the first assistant's left hand is used to provide exposure downwards, further exposing the subhepatic space.

There are two methods of removing the gallbladder (Ch. 44). The safest technique, the one the authors employ in all cases, is dissection of the gallbladder from the liver bed starting at the fundus of the gallbladder and carrying

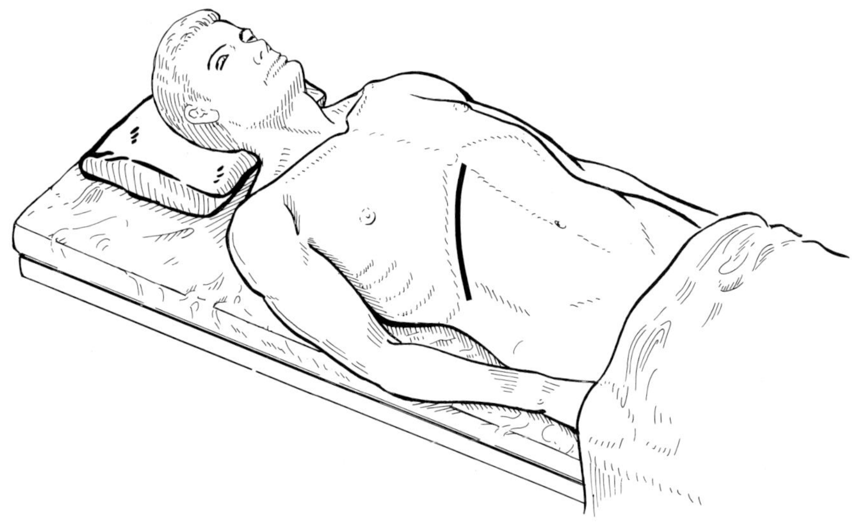

Fig. 42.3 Artist's drawing shows a right subcostal incision which parallels the right costal margin and extends up to the xiphoid process

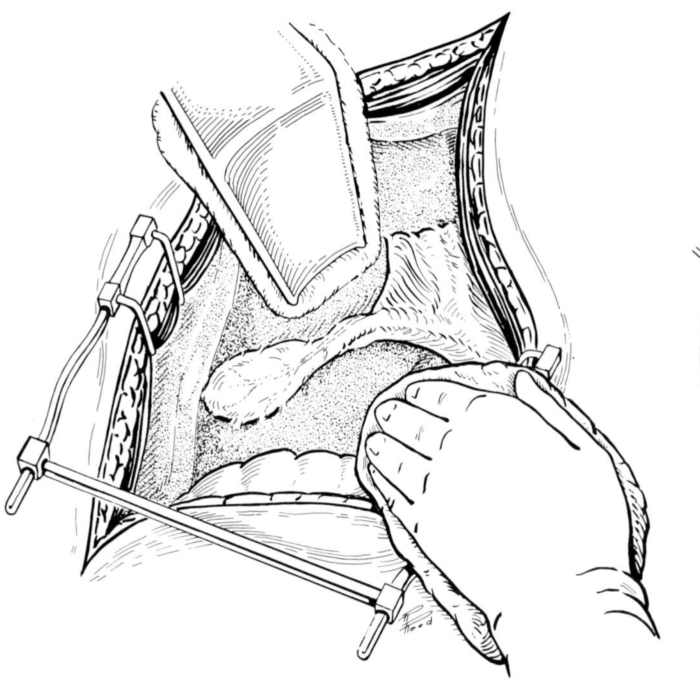

Fig. 42.4 Exposure of the subhepatic space. The retractor is placed upside down so the cross bar is below the liver and does not obscure the anatomy during operative cholangiography

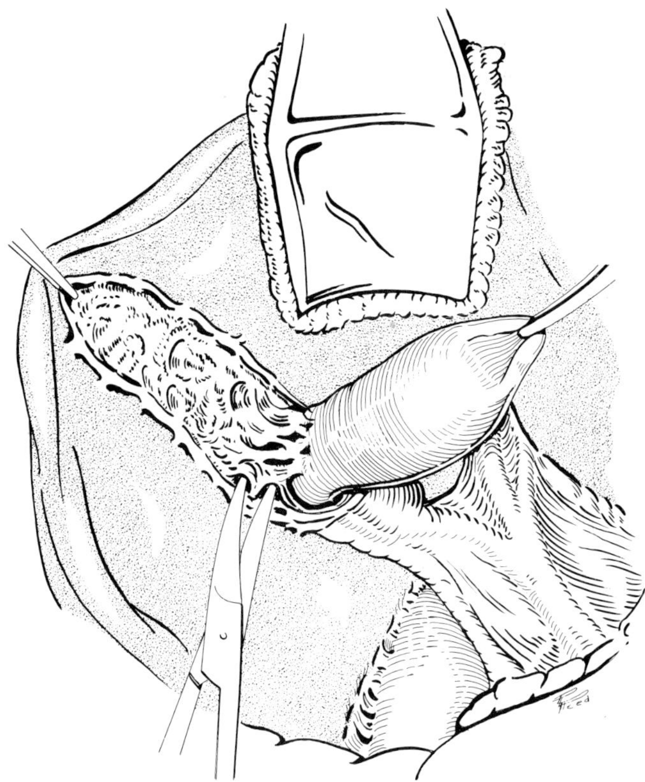

Fig. 42.5 Dissection of the gallbladder from the liver bed is carried from the fundus towards the cystic duct–common bile duct junction

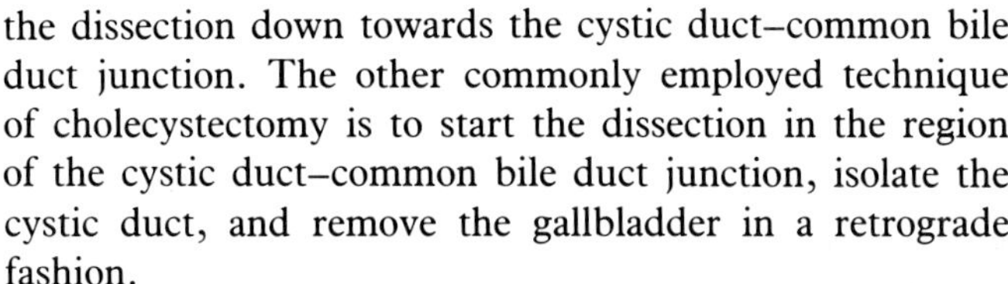

the dissection down towards the cystic duct–common bile duct junction. The other commonly employed technique of cholecystectomy is to start the dissection in the region of the cystic duct–common bile duct junction, isolate the cystic duct, and remove the gallbladder in a retrograde fashion.

The safest technique of cholecystectomy is to start the dissection at the fundus of the gallbladder and carry the removal down to the cystic duct–common bile duct junction (Fig. 42.5). The gallbladder resection can be terminated at any time and converted to a cholecystostomy if the anatomy becomes unclear or the dissection becomes difficult or hazardous. A Kelly clamp is placed on the fundus of the gallbladder for traction, and with a scissors, the gallbladder is sharply dissected from the liver bed. Small bleeding vessels in the liver bed or on the gallbladder may be cauterized as the dissection progresses. The cystic artery is identified as traction is placed on the gallbladder (Fig. 42.6), isolated, clamped, divided and ligated with 2-0 silk. A segment of cystic duct is isolated and its junction with the common bile duct is identified. Any stones in the cystic duct are milked back into the gallbladder. A ligature is placed around the junction of the gallbladder with the cystic duct, and another ligature is placed loosely around the distal cystic duct. The cystic duct is then partially divided and an operative cholangiogram performed (Fig. 42.7) (see Ch. 27). Once a satisfactory cholangiogram has been obtained, the cystic duct is clamped, divided and ligated with 2-0 silk approximately 1.5 cm from its junction with the common bile duct. The gallbladder is removed.

At this point, the operating room nurse is asked to open the gallbladder specimen and obtain aerobic and anaerobic bile cultures. The stones in the gallbladder are inspected and several stones extracted to give to the patient. The right upper quadrant is then irrigated with saline and the liver bed reassessed for any further bleeding or oozing and these vessels cauterized. The gallbladder bed may be closed with interrupted 3-0 silk sutures or left open (Fig. 42.8).

Within five minutes, the intraoperative cholangiograms are returned to the operating room for viewing by the surgeon and his team (Fig. 42.9 & 42.10). These films are

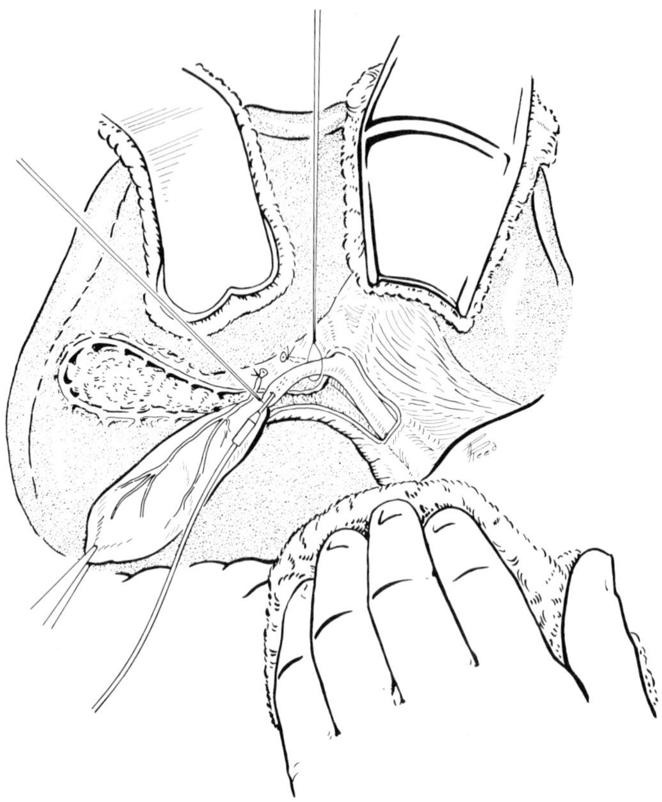

Fig. 42.7 The cystic duct has been isolated and a blunt needle-catheter is inserted for an intraoperative cholangiogram

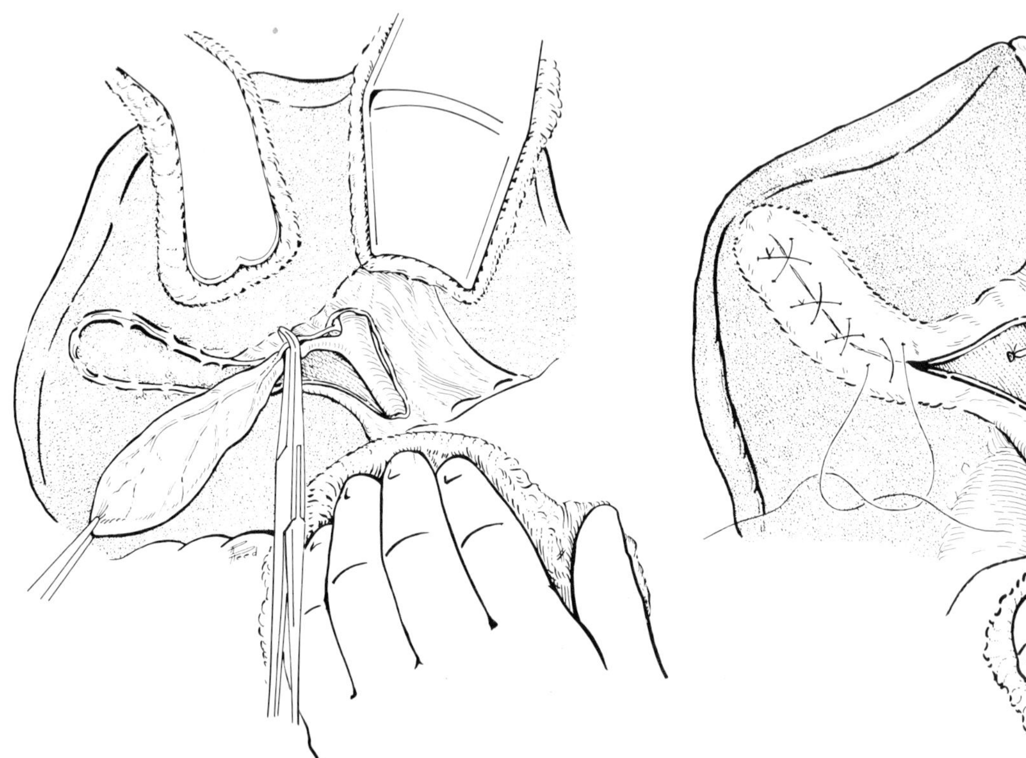

Fig. 42.6 With traction on the fundus of the gallbladder, the cystic artery can be palpated and isolated for division and ligation

Fig. 42.8 The completed cholecystectomy. The peritoneum can be closed over the gallbladder bed or this area can be left open

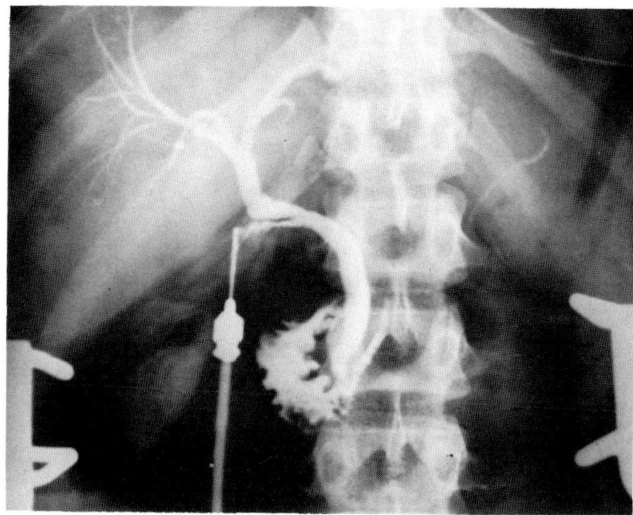

Fig. 42.9 Operative cholangiogram shows a normal bile duct with flow of contrast medium into the duodenum. No stone or other ductal pathology is seen. The pancreatic duct is partially visualized on this study (seen in 45% of the intraoperative cholangiograms) and appears normal

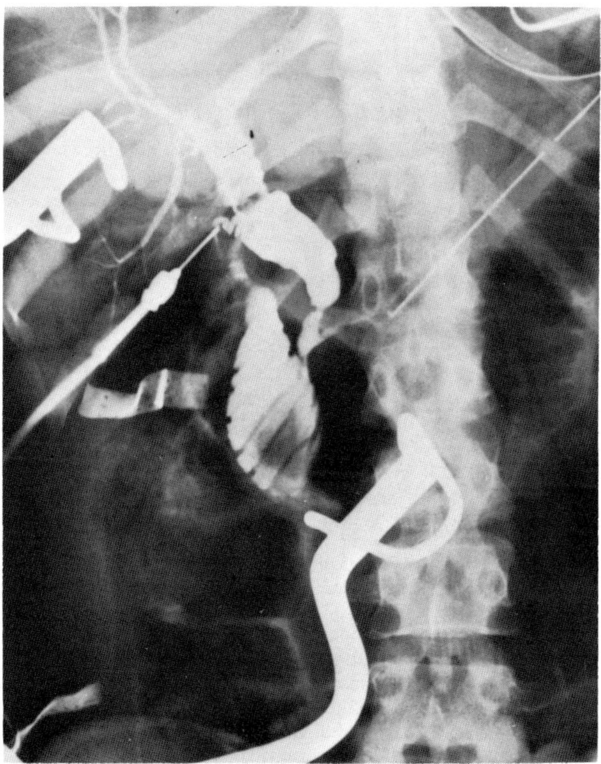

Fig. 42.10 Operative cholangiogram shows an abnormal study. The common bile duct is dilated, contains at least one or two stones, and there is a stricture of the distal bile duct. This stricture is most likely congenital, but if one is found in an older patient, carcinoma of the bile duct must be considered

reviewed to look for bile duct anomalies, to assess patency of the biliary system with flow of contrast media into the duodenum, to look for unsuspected pathology in the ducts (stones, tumours, sclerosing cholangitis, strictures), and are used as the principal indication to explore the common bile duct. Intraoperative choledochoscopy is used occasionally during routine cholecystectomy, if a suspicious filling defect is seen in the common bile duct or upper bile ducts, not easily accessible by common bile duct exploration, so that biopsy of this area could be performed.

During the past ten years, the authors have abandoned drainage of the abdomen after an uncomplicated, elective cholecystectomy in patients with chronic cholecystitis. During this time, there has been no single complication which could be attributed to lack of subhepatic drainage. In fact, there are studies which show that postoperative drainage in uncomplicated cases is associated with a higher incidence of postoperative infection (Mittelman & Doberneck 1982). Drainage is continued for patients after cholecystectomy for acute cholecystitis and patients who have had a complicated operation, including common bile duct exploration. The authors prefer to use, in all such patients, a closed system suction drain brought out through a separate stab incision, rather than the open, Penrose type of drain which was used in years past. Infiltration of the incision with 50 ml of 0.25% bupivacaine hydrochloride is used frequently to decrease incisional pain and improve pulmonary function in the postoperative period (Patel et al 1983).

In recent years, the length of hospitalization after elective cholecystectomy for chronic cholecystitis has gradually been reduced and now averages between four and five days for patients with no other complicating illness.

RESULTS

As previously mentioned, the authors have reviewed their experience with elective cholecystectomy for chronic cholecystitis in two time periods at the Cleveland Clinic. During the years 1962 to 1978, the operative or hospital mortality rate was 1.1%. All deaths occurred in patients over 60 and were associated with other complicating problems, such as vascular or coronary artery disease, chronic lung disease or cirrhosis of the liver. In a recent survey during 1981–1982, no operative deaths were noted in patients having elective cholecystectomy for chronic cholecystitis. Complications were found in 6% and included a postoperative bile leak which lasted one week and closed spontaneously, a non-fatal pulmonary embolus, a wound haematoma, a wound seroma, one patient with postoperative pneumonia and one patient with postoperative atelectasis. No retained common bile duct stones were noted; 12% of the group had a common bile duct exploration.

DeMarco, Nance & Cohn (1967) in a review of 695 patients operated upon for chronic cholecystitis, found a 1.3% mortality and noted that the mortality rate in the decade 1900–1910 was in the range of 10% to 15% and that by 1934 it had fallen to 6.6%. Haff, Butcher & Ballinger

(1969) in a review of 1000 patients reported a mortality rate of 2% for patients with chronic cholecystitis undergoing elective cholecystectomy. By contrast, the mortality rate for patients having cholecystectomy for acute cholecystitis was 20%. In 1975, Glenn reported the New York Hospital experience from 1932 to 1974 and reviewed 6367 patients with chronic cholecystitis. The mortality rate for elective cholecystectomy in this group was 0.5%.

Late complications of cholecystectomy for chronic cholecystitis include retained or recurrent bile duct stones, stricture of the bile duct and the postcholecystectomy syndrome. The authors' incidence of retained or recurrent bile duct stones is less than 2% at five years of follow-up. Stricture of the bile duct usually relates to an intraoperative injury or direct trauma to the duct, causing jaundice or prolonged bile leakage in the early postoperative period and the authors' incidence of this serious complication has, fortunately, been zero.

The postcholecystectomy syndrome (Ch. 55), recurrent symptoms of upper abdominal or right upper abdominal pain which mimic the preoperative symptoms of chronic cholecystitis, are generally reported to occur in from 10% to 15% of patients (Cooperman 1979). At the Cleveland Clinic this complication has been uncommon (5% to 7%) and has seemed to relate more to chronic incisional or wound pain, which persisted up to six months or longer in the few patients who had this problem. With careful preoperative selection of patients for operation and complete evaluation of the entire biliary system at cholecystectomy by intraoperative cholangiography, the incidence of the postcholecystectomy syndrome can be markedly diminished.

Review of the results of cholecystectomy for chronic cholecystitis, both at the Cleveland Clinic and from the experience of others, indicates that the operation is safe and effective. Careful evaluation of patients preoperatively to be certain that symptoms are those of chronic cholecystitis, an assessment of operative risk with the correction of any potentially controllable risk factors preoperatively, the prophylactic use of broad spectrum antibiotics given perioperatively, and the safe conduct of the operative procedure including operative cholangiography to assess the entire biliary system, all contribute to the success of the operative procedure.

REFERENCES

Ausobsky J R, Polk H C Jr 1983 Aspects of biliary sepsis. (Ch. 17 p 133–146) In: Moody F G (ed) Advances in diagnosis and surgical treatment of biliary tract disease. Masson Publishing, New York

Bartrum R J Jr, Crow H C, Foote S R 1977 Ultrasonic and radiographic cholecystography. New England Journal of Medicine 296: 538–541

Berghall L 1980 Gallbladder carcinoma first diagnosed at microscopic examination of gallbladder removed for presumed benign disease. Annals of Surgery 171: 19–22

Castaing D, Houssin D, Lemoine J, Bismuth H 1983 Surgical management of gallstones in cirrhotic patients. American Journal of Surgery 146: 310–313

Chetlin S H, Elliot D W 1971 Biliary bacteremia. Archives of Surgery 102: 303–307

Conte J E, Jacob L S, Polk H C Jr 1984 Surgery of the alimentary tract. Chapter 2, pp. 27–57, In: Antibiotic prophylaxis in surgery. Lippincott, Philadelphia

Cooperman A M 1979 Post cholecystectomy syndrome and biliary dyskinesia (Ch. 3 p 60). In: Hermann R E (ed) Manual of surgery of the gallbladder, bile ducts, and exocrine pancreas. Springer-Verlag, New York

DeMarco A, Nance F C, Cohn I 1968 Chronic cholecystitis: Experience in a large charity institution. Surgery 63: 750–756

Doberneck R C, Sterling W A Jr., Allison D C 1983 Morbidity and mortality after operation in nonbleeding cirrhotic patients. American Journal of Surgery 146: 306–309

Glenn F 1975 Trends in surgical treatment of calculous disease of the biliary tract. Surgery, Gynecology and Obstetrics 140: 877–884

Glenn F, Hays D M 1955 The age factor in the morbidity rate of patients undergoing surgery of the biliary tract. Surgery, Gynecology and Obstetrics 100: 11–18

Haff R C, Butcher H R Jr, Ballinger W F 1969 Biliary tract operations — Overview of 1000 patients. Archives of Surgery 98: 428–434

Hermann R E 1983 Biliary disease in the aging patient (Chapter 5 p 27). In: Texter E C (ed), The aging gut. Masson Publishing, New York

Ibach J R Jr, Hume H A, Erb W H 1968 Cholecystectomy in the aged. Surgery, Gynecology and Obstetrics 126: 523–528

Keighley M R B 1977 Micro-organisms in the bile: A preventable cause of sepsis after biliary surgery. Annals of the Royal College of Surgeons 59: 328–324

Martin L F, Zinner S H, Kogan J P, Zametkin A J, Garrity F L, Fry D E 1983 Bacteriology of the human gallbladder in cholelithiasis and cholecystitis. American Surgeon 49: 151–154

McLaughlin C W Jr 1964 Carcinoma of the gallbladder, an added hazard in untreated calculous cholecystitis in older patients. Surgery 56: 755–759

McSherry C K, Glenn F 1980 The incidence and causes of death following surgery for non-malignant biliary tract disease. Annals of Surgery 191: 271–275

Mittelman J J, Doberneck R C 1982 Drains and antibiotics peroperatively for elective cholecystectomy. Surgery, Gynecology and Obstetrics 155: 653–654

Mujabed Z, Evans J A, Whalen J P 1974 The non-opacified gallbladder on oral cholecystography. Diagnostic Radiology 112: 1–3

Mundth E D 1962 Cholecystitis and diabetes mellitus. New England Journal of Medicine 267: 642–646

Patel J M, Lanzafame R J, Williams J S, Mullen B V, Hinshaw J R 1983 The effect of incisional bupivacaine hydrochloride upon pulmonary functions, atelectasis, and narcotic need following elective cholecystectomy. Surgery, Gynecology and Obstetrics 157: 338–340

Porterfield G, Cheung L Y, Berenson M 1977 Detection of occult gallbladder disease by duodenal drainage. American Journal of Surgery 134: 702–704

Ransohoff D F, Miller G, Hermann R E 1985 Unpublished data.

Saurex C A, Bloch F, Bernstein D, Serafini A, Rodman G Jr, Zeppa R 1980 The role of HIDA/PIPIDA scanning in diagnosing cystic duct obstruction. Annals of Surgery 191: 391–396

Seltzer M H, Steiger E, Rosato F E 1970 Mortality following cholecystectomy. Surgery, Gynecology and Obstetrics 130: 64–66

Sterioff S, Smith G W, Oppel W C, Nugyn V C 1977 Comparison of oral and ultrasound cholecystography. Surgery, Gynecology and Obstetrics 145: 898–900

Stone H H, Hooper C A, Kolb L D, Geheber C E, Dawkins E J 1976 Antibiotic prophylaxis in gastric, biliary, and colonic surgery. Annals of Surgery 184: 443–450

Stubbs R S 1983 Wound infections after cholecystectomy. A case for routine prophylaxis. Annals of the Royal College of Surgeons of England 65: 30–31

Truedson H, Elmros T, Holm S 1983 The incidence of bacteria in gallbladder bile at acute and elective cholecystectomy. Acta Chirurgica Scandinavica 149: 307–313

Wenckert A, Robertson B 1966 The natural course of gallstone disease. Gastroenterology 50: 376–381

Zeman R, Burrell M I, Cahow C E, Caride V 1981 Diagnostic utility of cholescintigraphy and ultrasonography in acute cholecystitis. American Journal of Surgery 141: 446–451

43

C. W. Imrie

Gallstone acute pancreatitis

INTRODUCTION

The two most common aetiological factors associated with acute pancreatitis are gallstones and alcohol abuse. These two factors together account for over 80% af all patients with acute pancreatitis described in prospective studies of the disease. The major importance in identifying the presence of gallstones is the almost 100% success rate in eliminating further attacks of pancreatitis when all stones are removed. This efficient treatment contrasts markedly with the results in the treatment of alcohol abuse pancreatitis in which recurrent attacks are so common.

In Great Britain most studies have found that approximately half the patients with acute pancreatitis have gallstones. However, it has been recently claimed that, by sieving of the faeces to identify gallstones that have passed, this figure is actually around 60% (Mayer et al 1984). On this basis a significant proportion of so-called idiopathic cases are of biliary origin.

MECHANISM OF DISEASE

Although the classic paper by Opie in 1901 illustrated the association between a small stone impacted at the ampulla of Vater and the presence of acute pancreatitis, it was not until 1974 that Acosta and Ledesma highlighted the frequent phenomenon of the transient migration of stones from the biliary tree, through the lower bile duct, and into the duodenum in patients with gallstone associated pancreatitis. Other groups in the US (Kelly 1976, Kelly & Swaney 1982) and Great Britain (Mayer et al 1984) have supported the evidence that transient migration of small gallstones is the hallmark of gallstone associated acute pancreatitis. The task of faecal sieving to identify gallstones is not likely to prove popular unless a simple and reliable machine is designed to carry out this work, which is unpleasant but very valuable in defining the aetiology of pancreatitis.

A recent study from Manchester (Armstrong et al 1985) emphasized the importance of several features in the biliary and pancreatic duct systems which were specifically associated with gallstone pancreatitis (Fig. 43.1). The frequent finding of stones in the biliary tree not exceeding 3 mm in diameter in 90% of 59 patients with gallstone associated pancreatitis, compared to less than 40% of 710 patients with gallstones and no pancreatitis, is important. In addition to patients with pancreatitis having smaller stones they also harbour stones which are more numerous and associated with a larger diameter cystic duct (McMahon & Shefta 1980, Armstrong et al 1985). Furthermore, the diameter of thc common bile duct (CBD) tends to be larger and pancreatic duct reflux is seen much more frequently at operative cholangiography than in patients with biliary disease and no pancreatitis. Two other anatomical features were noted, the first of these being that the interductal angle between the lower CBD and pancreatic duct was larger in patients prone to pancreatitis. Secondly the common channel of the two ducts was at least 5 mm in 73% of these patients when compared to less than 20% of those patients with gallstones and no pancreatitis

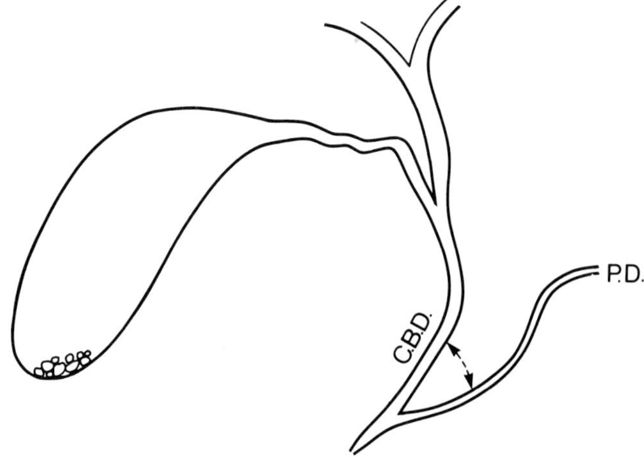

Fig. 43.1 Diagram illustrating features favouring gallstone pancreatitis (Arrows indicate interductal angle): Larger angle; small stones; large cystic duct and long common channel (Armstrong et al 1985) CBD = common bile duct; PD = pancreatic duct

(Armstrong et al 1985). There are therefore anatomical features which predispose to the presence of pancreatitis, but none of these fully explain the mechanism. The possible events at the lower end of the CBD and pancreatic duct are represented in Figure 43.2a where hold-up of a stone in the common channel may permit reflux of bile; a stone impacted in the exit of the pancreatic duct may facilitate reflux of pancreatic juice (Fig. 43.3); and a small irregular shaped stone stuck at the ampulla may cause pain and subsequent vomiting with duodenal juice potentially refluxing past the stone and into the pancreas.

In the situation of the reflux of bile initiating acute pancreatitis it is known that bile lecithin and in some circumstances bile salts damage the mucosal barrier of the pancreatic duct and that potentiation by bacterial infection and drugs such as aspirin is also important. Pancreatic juice refluxing under pressure back up the duct system may well cause pain but is relatively unlikely, on the basis of experimental studies, to initiate an attack of acute pancreatitis. The final situation depicted in Figure 43.2c would permit enterokinase in duodenal juice to be forced at high pressure along the pancreatic duct activating trypsinogen and potentially initiating an attack of pancreatitis. It is even possible, when a stone is impacted at the ampulla, that a combination of bile reflux and duodenal reflux under pressure could occur simultaneously and so initiate an attack of pancreatitis. Partial or complete obstruction of the pancreatic duct outflow, either within the common channel or at the duodenal orifice would possibly explain episodes of acute pancreatitis following operative or endoscopic instrumentation in this area; a similar mechanism may explain the acute pancreatitis which may occur if a long limb surgical T-tube is allowed to pass through the lower CBD and on into the duodenum.

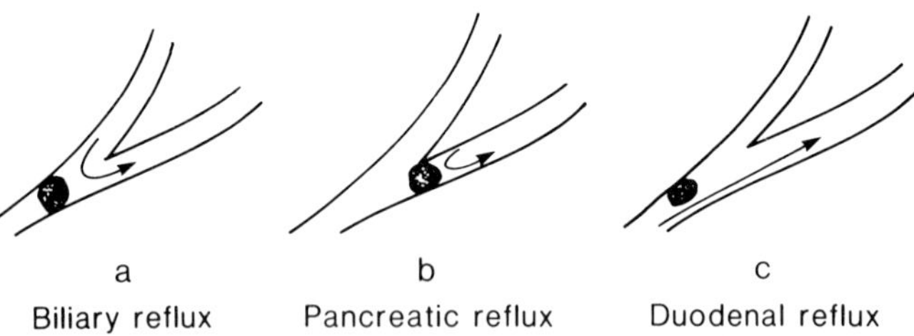

Fig. 43.2 The various ways in which stone 'hold up' may facilitate reflux

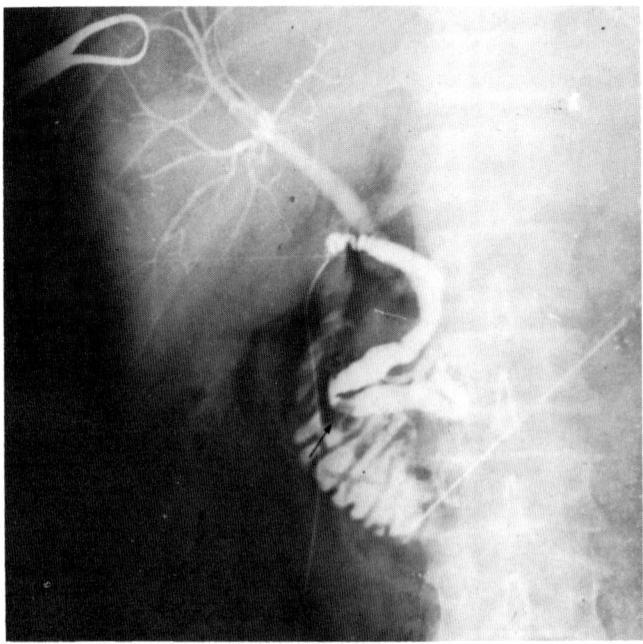

Fig. 43.3 Operative cholangiogram. Example of a gallstone impacted in the pancreatic duct (arrow) in a patient operated upon within 12 hours of admission

Of the many patients who suffer biliary associated pancreatitis it is a relative rarity to find a stone truly impacted at the ampulla of Vater. Those surgeons who advocate immediate operation (within 48 hours of diagnosis) find many more stones in the lower CBD than those who advocate a longer delay before initiating active measures to eradicate stones. This supports the contention of Acosta that stones usually pass spontaneously into the duodenum (Acosta & Ledesma 1974).

It has been well shown that very small stones, or even biliary sand, may precipitate episodes of acute pancreatitis, but some authors have suggested that even tiny biliary crystals might initiate disease, although this view is less widely accepted.

It is worthy of note that the association between pregnancy and acute pancreatitis is probably gallstone related. 90% of the pregnancy associated cases of acute pancreatitis in one study had gallstones present as the only identifiable explanation of their problem. Subsequent eradication of stones not only gave freedom from further attacks of pancreatitis beyond pregnancy but during each subsequent pregnancy as well (McKay et al 1980).

It is important to remember that both biliary disease and alcohol abuse are increasing in frequency in most Western societies. For this reason it is not unusual to find that 2–10% of patients will have both of these aetiological factors present (Trapnell & Duncan 1975, Imrie et al 1978a).

Finally in the consideration of possible factors initiating an attack of gallstone pancreatitis, it is noteworthy that recent manometric studies at the sphincter of Oddi suggest that motility disorders of this area (found in patients with and without gallstones) may be implicated in the mechanism of acute pancreatitis (Toouli et al 1985).

INVESTIGATION FOR THE PRESENCE OF STONES

Straight abdominal X-ray will reveal the presence of radio-opaque stones in between 10% and 16% of patients; for the remaining 84% to 90% other methods will be necessary. It has already been stated that faecal sieving has made the biggest single impact on defining the size of the idiopathic group of patients with acute pancreatitis (Acosta & Ledesma 1974, Kelly 1976, Mayer et al 1984). Ultrasound scanning has a very important role to play in the identification of gall-stones which are often not well visualized by the more expensive CT-scanner. Isotope scanning has been less helpful than in the patient with cholecystitis and intravenous cholangiography tends to be unreliable. Although bowel gas can be troublesome there can be little doubt that ultrasound has become a very important diagnostic modality in this disease (McKay et al 1982). In the situation where ultrasound is equivocal ERCP will provide a valuable indication of the presence or absence of stones and is preferred to percutaneous transhepatic cholangiography (Fig. 43.4).

Finally it has been suggested that measurement of liver function tests would prove valuable in differentiation between acute pancreatitis of biliary and alcohol origin (McMahon & Pickford 1979). Good data is accumulating to confirm that the levels of transferase enzymes, alkaline phosphatase and bilirubin are accurate indicators of the presence of gallstones (Blamey et al 1983) but surgeons have a natural reluctance to accept such data, preferring the more direct evidence of imaging modalities. However, initially liver function tests may well have value in indicating the patients who justify an ERCP with a likely high yield of positive information (Goodman et al 1985). This area is likely to be the focus of further clinical studies as the Glasgow group (Blamey et al 1983) found the addition of the simple data of age and sex of patients to the knowledge of alkaline phosphatase, transferase enzymes and bilirubin resulted in a very high rate of identification of gallstone aetiology. Older patients of both sexes and younger females bias the likelihood of acute pancreatitis being due to gallstones (Blamey et al 1983).

MANAGEMENT

It frequently takes some time to identify the aetiology in a particular episode of pancreatitis and in the initial phases it is more important to identify the severity of the attack. The group of patients who do not have severe acute pancreatitis may be graded mild or moderate, but it is important to identify the group at maximum risk of death and major complications. In order to achieve this a number of grading systems have been devised. An initial system (Ranson et al 1974) was more geared to patients with alcohol associated disease. Indeed Ranson subsequently introduced a modified grading system for the patient with biliary disease. This has complicated the system since a dilemma exists as to which to utilize when the patient is initially admitted. This has not proved a problem with the Glasgow grading system which has been increasingly utilized in the UK and elsewhere (Imrie et al 1978a, Osborne et al 1981). The system comprises eight factors; the presence of any three or more within 48 hours of admission defines the patient as having severe disease (Table 43.1).

A recent prospective study comparison of three methods of assessment of prognosis in acute pancreatitis reveals that this multiple laboratory grading system (Fig. 43.4) is equally good for patients with either alcohol or gallstone related pancreatitis (Corfield et al 1985). The system is superior to clinical assessment alone and to peritoneal aspiration in grading patients with gallstone pancreatitis but less good in grading the alcohol related group when compared to peritoneal aspiration. Indeed, clinical assessment and peritoneal aspiration/lavage approaches were found especially poor in assessing the severity of gallstone related pancreatitis (Corfield et al 1985). Both identified less than 35% of such patients with severe disease while the Glasgow grading system was twice as accurate. In the clinical situation it is impossible to exclude the clinician's assessment, and combining this with the Glasgow assessment system is the method of choice in grading severity of disease in those with biliary associated pancreatitis.

In patients with *mild pancreatitis* it is usually sufficient to simply provide analgesia in the form of pethidine (Demerol®), intravenous fluids, nasogastric suction and hourly urine volume monitoring, the last two often being discontinued after 24 hours. This contrasts with the problem of *severe acute pancreatitis* where multi-system organ failure is the major initial problem. At particular risk are the heart, lungs and kidneys. The haemodynamic upset closely mimics the problems encountered in septic shock with an elevation in cardiac index and a decrease in peripheral resistance (Bradley et al 1983). The respiratory problem is complex and may well necessitate assisted ventilator therapy. Simple measures to combat the risk of renal insufficiency in terms of ensuring adequate intravenous fluid replacement, with or without an osmotic diuretic such as mannitol, usually suffice. Occasionally low

Table 43.1 Glasgow system of prognostic factors

TWBC	> 15 000
PaO_2	< 60 mmHg (8 KPa)
Glucose	> 10 mmol/l (excludes diabetics)
Urea	> 16 mmol/l (despite i.v. fluids)
Calcium	< 2.0 mmol/l
Albumin	< 32 g/l
LDH	> 600 international units/l
AST	> 200 international units/l

The presence of any three or more of these within 48 hours of admission indicates severe acute pancreatitis. (Osborne et al 1981)

dose dopamine and frusemide have an important place. These patients are best initially managed in an intensive care area, and if renal failure is incipient or established then peritoneal dialysis is the treatment of choice.

Other phenomena which tend to occur include haematological and biochemical abnormalities. Blood loss into and around the pancreas is rarely sufficient itself to require transfusion, but the effect of haemodilution from the correction of hypovolaemia requires careful observation. A degree of intravascular coagulation is common but disseminated intravascular coagulation is a rare occurrence. In terms of biochemical upsets, the most frequent and important is the rapid and sustained loss of albumin from the intravascular space with high albumin levels being found in the pleural effusion fluid as well as the fluid in the peritoneal cavity. This is the major factor leading to the occurrence of hypocalcaemia, and when correction is made for the low levels of serum albumin true falls in blood calcium are much less common than previously thought. Occasionally there is a justification for the infusion of calcium gluconate solution but the parathyroid response is usually brisk, resulting in the restoration of any depression in calcium levels within a short time (Imrie et al 1978b).

The policy which has been followed in the management of acute pancreatitis with regard to antibiotic therapy in Glasgow Royal Infirmary has been to withhold these drugs entirely unless there are any specific indications. One indication would be accompanying cholangitis which should be covered with intravenous third generation cephalosporins, a newer penicillin such as mezlocillin, or an aminoglycoside combined with ampicillin. The need for metronidazole is infrequent based on the knowledge of the organisms which are usually found in the bile. Cholangitis complicating acute pancreatitis is a very serious entity and is an indication for early intervention. This may be performed by endoscopic sphincterotomy although the alternative of surgical exploration with clearance of the common bile duct (and possible surgical sphincterotomy or sphincteroplasty) is also valuable. In a recent UK multicentre study of management of severe acute pancreatitis, peritoneal lavage was found of no clear benefit (Mayer et al 1985), but a small number of patients who developed cholangitis ran a hazardous course, despite the initial attack being only moderately severe. Two of these patients died (Corfield et al 1985) and consideration of early endoscopic sphincterotomy or surgery is clearly important.

The success of management of gallstone pancreatitis (Fig. 43.4) in mild or moderate acute pancreatitis should result in a 97% patient survival although present studies have shown the mortality in severe acute pancreatitis to be in the region of 27% to 35%. Nearly all fatal cases are in patients over 50 years of age (Corfield et al 1985). Areas for future improvement include a greater understanding of the mechanisms of respiratory and cardiac insufficiency. Of particular value would be the identification of factors which facilitate albumin loss from the intravascular space. Correction of this problem would have implications for many other similar situations such as occur in severe burns and septic shock. Another recent development may affect the speed with which patients with acute pancreatitis commence resuscitation by favourably improving accuracy of diagnosis. This is the introduction of test 'paper strips' for amylase in urine and lipase in blood, abnormally high levels causing a characteristic colour change. The application of these as a biochemical screen may result in earlier hospital admission and hence earlier therapy for a proportion of patients with acute pancreatitis.

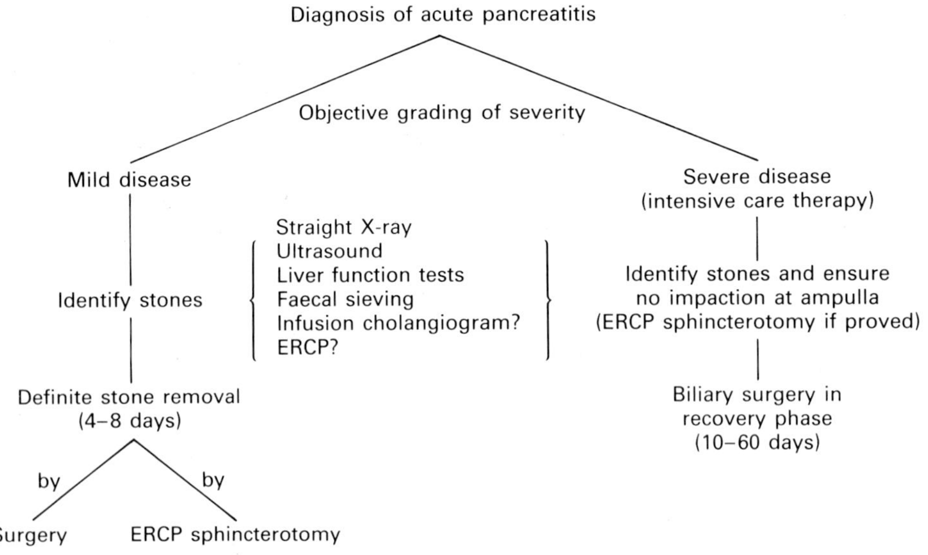

Fig. 43.4 Suggested optimum therapy in gallstone pancreatitis

THE TIMING OF SURGICAL OR ENDOSCOPIC INTERVENTION

During the last five years a number of approaches in timing of interventional procedures have been advocated. These can be subdivided into three categories:

1. Immediate intervention (within 48 hours of hospital admission) This timing has been championed by Acosta and Stone who advocate a surgical approach (Acosta et al 1978, Stone, Fabian & Dunlop 1981), while a number of groups have suggested that immediate endoscopic sphincterotomy is also effective (Safrany & Cotton 1981, Rosseland & Solhaug 1984).

2. Early intervention (between two and seven days) This allows more time for verification of the presence of gallstones and is favoured by Ranson, Kelly, Tondelli and our own group in Glasgow (Ranson 1979, Kelly 1980, Osborne et al 1981, Tondelli et al 1982).

3. Delayed intervention This traditional approach allows the patient a complete recovery from the episode of pancreatitis with subsequent planned admission for elective biliary surgery.

In the discussion and controversy which surrounds this subject some authors have not made it clear whether their policy applies 'across the board' to patients with mild and moderate pancreatitis as well as to the most severe forms of the disease in which intensive care (including assisted ventilator therapy) is often required within hours of hospital admission. Furthermore, it is not always clear whether those who advocate the earlier surgical approaches apply them to the older group of patients. With these points in mind it is reasonable to cover the problems associated with each of these lines of management.

If *immediate intervention* is chosen one of the major problems is being sure that the aetiology is attributable to gallstones. The Atlanta group (Stone et al 1981) relied heavily on an absence of a history of alcohol intake. While Acosta's group took this into account they put great weight on the findings of liver function tests (Acosta et al 1978). The surgical approach of Stone and his colleagues was a little unusual in that the only opening into the proximal area of the biliary tree was created via the cystic duct through which the cholangiogram catheter and subsequently a Fogarty balloon catheter was passed. They created a surgical sphincteroplasty extending 2.0 cm to 2.5 cm and also divided the septum with the pancreatic duct. Reliance was then placed on retrieval of stones within the biliary tree from below using balloon catheters. Although mortality and morbidity were not significantly improved by immediate surgery compared to the group of patients who had delayed therapy, the total stay in hospital was significantly reduced with obvious advantages both to the patient and the community in terms of hospital economy (Stone et al 1981). Acosta and his colleagues did not have a control group in their study but relied on historical controls and claimed an advantage for immediate surgical intervention (Acosta et al 1978).

Controlled studies of endoscopic sphincterotomy in acute pancreatitis are in progress in various parts of the world and a preliminary report from Leicester in Great Britain (Leese et al 1985) suggests that this may prove to be a valuable option which will obviously be associated with less upset than a major surgical operation. Nevertheless, it must be remembered that this is an interventional procedure which carries its own complications (Ch. 47). One major advantage over operative surgery is that the endoscopist can check whether or not gallstones are present by a diagnostic cannulation prior to any attempt at diathermy sphincterotomy. In addition, the respiratory upset of severe hypoxaemia, which is a hallmark of acute pancreatitis, is considerably less after the intravenous sedation required to carry out ERCP as compared to that which follows a general anaesthetic and a full surgical procedure. On balance therefore, it seems that clinicians who favour an early interventional approach may be more likely to utilize the choice of endoscopic sphincterotomy, depending on the availability of local expertise and in the knowledge that cholecystectomy will be necessary in most patients at a subsequent time (Fig. 43.4).

Those who favour *early operation* (two to seven days) have an advantage regarding the investigation and delineation of the presence of gallstones. In addition, a selective policy is possible with regard to the timing of intervention in patients with the most severe forms of acute pancreatitis. In the author's retrospective study it was clear that these patients represented particular problems and in some instances surgery was delayed until much later on account of severe illness due to various system failures (Osborne et al 1981). At present it is difficult to be dogmatic about the optimum timing of intervention for these severely ill patients. While those who advocate immediate intervention and point to some patients who do exceptionally well, there is a tendency to forget that it is *transient* migration of gallstones which precipitate an attack of pancreatitis. True impaction of stones at the ampulla is a relatively uncommon entity, although a case for checking whether or not impaction is present by diagnostic ERCP has already been implied. A report from Switzerland (Tondelli et al 1982) makes it clear that immediate surgery is associated with a much higher mortality. For this reason both the author and others (Ranson 1979, Kelly 1980) favour delay of a few days before operation. All are in agreement that the advantages to the patient with mild or moderate pancreatitis in having eradication of stones from the biliary tree during the same admission are considerable but doubts remain regarding an 'across the board' policy for those with the most severe forms of the disease.

All who have reported on biliary surgery or endoscopic sphincterotomy within 48 hours of hospitalization have found a much higher incidence of stones within the common bile duct than in patients in whom operation is delayed for a few days or for many weeks. The incidence of CBD stones is in the region of 70% to 95% with the immediate approach as compared with 15% to 20% for delayed intervention.

The older school of thought, which favours an *appreciable time interval* between the episode of pancreatitis and elective biliary surgery, cannot be discounted since all studies indicate that the risk, in terms of mortality and morbidity, is no higher, provided that a recurrent attack of acute pancreatitis does not supervene in the interval period. Prediction of the onset of such further attacks is impossible and this, combined with the increased efficiency of the earlier surgical approaches, has resulted in a greater interest in stone eradication at the first admission to hospital.

GALLSTONES AND LATER COMPLICATIONS OF ACUTE PANCREATITIS

In the author's personal experience the incidence of *pancreatic pseudocyst* associated with gallstone induced pancreatitis is approximately one-fifth of that associated with alcohol associated disease. However it is important to note that patients with pseudocysts as a complication of gallstone pancreatitis have a much greater tendency to both haemorrhage and sepsis than those with alcohol associated disease, especially if a delay in drainage is permitted. Antibiotic cover is a prerequisite to either surgical or percutaneous drainage. It is important to realize that a pancreatic slough, often present in the depth of a pseudocyst, is usually sterile but may become infected by needle or percutaneous catheter drainage of the pseudocyst. In addition the biliary tree should be cleared of stones at the same operation as surgical pseudocyst drainage and a cholecystectomy performed. Data from Glasgow Royal Infirmary indicates the greatly increased risk of death from a pancreatic pseudocyst in gallstone related acute pancreatitis (Table 43.2). While it must be conceded that the patients with biliary associated disease tend to be older than those with alcohol abuse (mean age of 60 years versus mean age of 40 years for alcohol related disease) there appears to be a marked difference in the predisposition to both haemorrhage and sepsis where gallstones are present.

Table 43.2 Mortality of pseudocyst and aetiology (Data from consecutive series of 88 patients)

Aetiology	Number	Died (%)
Alcohol	51	2 (3.9)
Gallstones	26	6 (23.1)
Trauma	6	1
Unknown	5	1
Total	88	10 (11.4)

Abscess formation and peripancreatic sepsis are two of the most feared phenomena associated with the late complications of acute pancreatitis and are much more common in biliary associated disease. Both have an exceptionally high mortality ranging from 60% to 100%. Failure of adequate drainage invariably results in the death of the patient. The challenge of the well circumscribed abscess is not nearly so great as the diffuse infection associated with necrosis of the gland or of the surrounding tissue which subsequently becomes infected. It is relatively easy to detect a well circumscribed abscess by ultrasonic scanning while the other forms may warrant percutaneous guided needle aspiration using a modern CT-scanner to enable the diagnosis to be made. In addition to the diagnostic difficulties, treatment of a localized collection is considerably easier and more effective. Adequate surgical drainage of the peripancreatic tissue and removal of slough in and around the pancreas is very difficult. Extension of the necrotic process in the retroperitoneal planes towards the diaphragm and behind the colon represents one of the greatest problems encountered in abdominal surgery. It is usual for multiple procedures to be required in these patients. Indeed some have advocated non-closure of the abdominal wall at the first operation in order to facilitate subsequent daily antiseptic lavage and change of packs. Since the majority of patients are in intensive care units with assisted ventilator therapy, management problems using this approach are not as great as might be envisaged.

In most cases necrosis of the pancreatic parenchyma does not occur, peripancreatic necrosis being much more frequent. While most surgeons believe this necrotic tissue warrants removal, there is no conclusive evidence that uninfected tissue must be excised. However, the danger of infection, especially adjacent to the mid and distal transverse colon, is ever present and a great concern. Future advances in imaging the pancreas with computerized tomography and magnetic resonance techniques, allied with percutaneous aspiration, may clarify diagnosis and management of this serious complication.

REFERENCES

Acosta J M, Ledesma C L 1974 Gallstone migration as a cause of acute pancreatitis. New England Journal of Medicine 290: 484–7

Acosta J M, Rossi R, Galli O M R, Pellegrini C A, Skinner D B 1978 Early surgery for acute gallstone pancreatitis: Evaluation of a systematic approach. Surgery 83: 367–80

Armstrong C P, Taylor T V, Jeacock J, Lucas S 1985 The biliary tract in patients with acute gallstone pancreatitis. British Journal of Surgery 72: 551–5

Blamey S L, Osborne D H, Gilmour W H, O'Neill J, Carter D C, Imrie C W 1983 The early identification of patients with gallstone associated pancreatitis using clinical and biochemical factors only. Annals of Surgery 198: 574–8

Bradley E L, Hall J R, Lutz J, Hamner L, Lattouf O 1983 Haemodynamic consequence of severe acute pancreatitis. Annals of Surgery 198: 130–133

Corfield A P, Cooper M J, Williamson R C N, Mayer A D, McMahon M J, Dickson A P, Shearer M G, Imrie C W 1985 Predication of severity in acute pancreatitis: Prospective comparison of three prognostic indices. Lancet ii: 403–7

Goodman A J, Neoptolemos J P, Carr-locke D L, Finlay D B L, Fossard D P 1985 Detection of gallstones after acute pancreatitis. Gut 26: 125–32

Imrie C W, Benjamin I S, Ferguson J C et al 1978a A single centre double-blind trial of Trasylol® therapy in primary acute pancreatitis. British Journal of Surgery 65: 337–41

Imrie C W, Beastall G H, Allam B F, O'Neill J, Benjamin I S, McKay A J 1978b Parathyroid hormone and calcium homeostasis in acute pancreatitis. British Journal of Surgery 65: 717–20

Kelly T R 1976 Gallstone pancreatitis: pathophysiology. Surgery 80: 488–92

Kelly T R 1980 Gallstone pancreatitis: the timing of surgery. Surgery 88: 345–9

Kelly T R, Swaney P E 1982 Gallstone pancreatitis: the second time around. Surgery 92: 571–4

Leese T, Neoptolemos J P, Carr-Locke D L 1985 Successes, failures, early complications and their management following endoscopic sphincterotomy: Results in 394 consecutive patients from a single centre. British Journal of Surgery 72: 215–9

Mayer A D, McMahon M J, Benson E A, Axon A T R 1984 Operations upon the biliary tract in patients with acute pancreatitis: Aims, indications and timing. Annals of the Royal College of Surgeons of England 66: 179–83

Mayer A D, McMahon M J, Corfield A P, Cooper M J, Williamson R C N, Dickson A P et al 1985 Controlled clinical trial of peritoneal lavage for the treatment of severe acute pancreatitis. New England Journal of Medicine 312: 399–404

McKay A J, O'Neill J, Imrie C W 1980 Pancreatitis, pregnancy and gallstones. British Journal of Obstetrics and Gynaecology 87: 47–50

McKay A J, Imrie C W, O'Neill J, Duncan J G 1982 Is an early ultrasound scan of value in acute pancreatitis? British Journal of Surgery 69: 369–72

McMahon M J, Pickford I R 1979 Biochemical prediction of gallstones early in an attack of acute pancreatitis. Lancet ii: 541–543

McMahon M J, Shefta J R 1980 Physical characteristics of gallstones and the calibre of the cystic duct in patients with acute pancreatitis. British Journal of Surgery 67: 6–9

Opie E L 1901 The etiology of acute hemorrhagic pancreatitis. Bulletin of the Johns Hopkins Hospital 12: 182–188

Osborne D H, Imrie C W, Carter D C 1981 Biliary surgery in the same admission for gallstone-associated acute pancreatitis. British Journal of Surgery 68: 758–61

Ranson J H C, Rifkind K M, Roses D F, Fink S D, Eng K, Spencer F C 1974 Prognostic signs and the role of operative management in acute pancreatitis. Surgery, Gynecology and Obstetrics 139: 69–81

Ranson J H C 1979 The timing of biliary surgery in acute pancreatitis. Annals of Surgery 189: 654–63

Rosseland A R, Solhaug J H 1984 Early or delayed endoscopic papillotomy (EPT) in gallstone pancreatitis. Annals of Surgery 199: 165–7

Safrany L, Cotton P B 1981 A preliminary report: urgent duodenoscopic sphincterotomy for acute gallstone pancreatitis. Surgery 89: 424–8

Stone H H, Fabian T C, Dunlop W E 1981 Gallstone pancreatitis. Biliary tract pathology in relation to time of operation. Annals of Surgery 194: 305–12

Tondelli P, Stutz K, Harder F, Schupisser J-P, Allgower M 1982 Acute gallstone pancreatitis: best timing for biliary surgery. British Journal of Surgery 69: 709–710

Toouli J, Roberts-Thomson I C, Dent J, Lee J 1985 Sphincter of Oddi motility disorders in patients with idiopathic recurrent pancreatitis. British Journal of Surgery 72: 859–863

Trrapnell J E, Duncan E H L, 1975 Patterns of incidence in acute pancreatitis. British Medical Journal 2: 179–83

J. M. Ham

Cholecystectomy

Cholecystectomy is one of the commonest operations in general surgery. There is no doubt that its risks have been reduced considerably in recent years, with mortality rates close to zero in many units. Nevertheless, the operation may be associated with damage to important structures in the porta hepatis and consequent short- and long-term morbidity and mortality. Such damage should be preventable in most patients (Ch. 38), and this chapter will therefore emphasize the principle of 'defensive cholecystectomy'. It will also be emphasized that anatomical variations are so common that they should be regarded as normal, and not termed congenital abnormalities. The implication from the last two statements is that no structure should be ligated or divided during the operation until it has been positively identified.

INDICATIONS

The indications have been covered in Chapters 41, 42. The great majority of cholecystectomies are performed for acute or chronic calculous disease and their complications. A small number are required for acute acalculous cholecystitis and adenomyomatosis (Le Quesne & Ranger 1975, Ham 1980a) and for carcinoma or are carried out as part of a more extensive operation such as pancreaticoduodenectomy. The indications for operation in patients who appear to have disorders of gallbladder function are controversial as are those for patients who should have gallstones on clinical evidence, but in whom none can be demonstrated by cholecystography or ultrasonography (Ham 1980a, Lennard et al 1984).

It must also be emphasized that the presence of gallstones in a patient with upper abdominal pain does not necessarily mean that the former are the cause of the latter. Gallstones are so common that they are frequently associated by chance with gastroduodenal and pancreatic disease, and other hepatobiliary disorders (Ch. 55).

PREOPERATIVE ASSESSMENT

There are certain preoperative clinical features which are a guide to the difficulty of the operation. Patients who have had one or more attacks of biliary pain lasting only a few hours usually have a relatively uninflamed gallbladder and the operation is usually technically straightforward. By contrast, those patients who have had one or more major attacks of pain and a slow response to treatment usually have gross acute and/or chronic inflammation at the time of operation. Unfortunately, these clinical patterns are not always reliable in predicting the biliary pathology.

Patients with cirrhosis often present major problems as a result of excessive bleeding and postoperative liver decompensation and there is a significant morbidity and even mortality (Schwartz 1981). Similarly, cholecystectomy in patients with thalassaemia may be technically difficult due to bleeding.

Preoperative investigations should include liver function tests and a prothrombin time. Elevation of the serum alkaline phosphatase and γ-glutamyl transpeptidase may suggest the presence of a stone in the common bile duct; if none is found a liver biopsy should be performed since the patient may have primary liver disease. A prolonged prothrombin time which does not return to normal after parenteral vitamin K is strong evidence that the patient has serious liver disease and that the operation carries significant risks.

THE OPERATION

Position on the operating table

The positioning of the patient on the operating table must permit rotation, approximately 15 degrees to the right, when cholangiography is performed. The image of the common bile duct does not then overlap that of the vertebral column. A preliminary film should be taken before the operation is commenced to ensure correct exposure and positioning.

The incision

This is a matter of personal choice and of patient configuration; the options are the midline, right paramedian, Kocher and transverse incisions. The author's own preference is for a midline or transverse incision.

Initial assessment

A full laparotomy should be performed in all patients, but with particular reference to the liver, biliary tract and pancreas, since multiple pathology in these areas is common. Bimanual examination of the pancreatic head, distal common bile duct and ampulla must be delayed until after operative cholangiography has been performed, since the latter may be affected by Kocher's manoeuvre.

If there was doubt preoperatively about the presence of stones and none can be felt in the gallbladder, then the latter should be aspirated to permit accurate palpation. Gallstones are often difficult to feel in a tense gallbladder and inability to feel stones does not exclude them.

Finally, a decision is taken as to whether the standard operation is possible, or whether some modification may be necessary (see below).

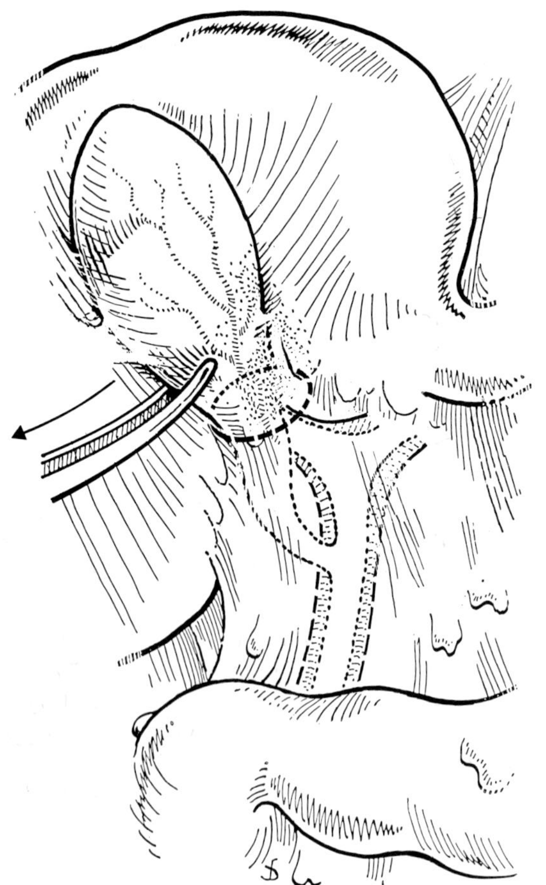

Fig. 44.1 Placement of clamp on gallbladder near Hartmann's pouch to open up Calot's triangle. The dotted circle signifies the area of the gallbladder neck to be subsequently dissected

Exposure of the operative field

The following points are important:

1. Ensure that the incision is of sufficient length.
2. Insert a self-retaining retractor.
3. Retraction of the right costal margin may be facilitated by using a single Goligher retractor (such as used in the operation of highly selective vagotomy). This is especially helpful if there is only one assistant.
4. Divide any attachments between the colon and the liver and insert a pack deep to the right side of the wound to keep the colon and small intestine out of the field.
5. Place a pack over the stomach and transverse colon. A nasogastric tube may have to be inserted temporarily if the stomach is distended with gas.

The first assistant's hand is then placed over this pack to produce tension along the line of the common bile duct, with fingers on either side of the duct and on top of the duodenum.

6. The liver is retracted anterior to the porta and Calot's triangle (see below) using a Deaver retractor.
7. Divide any attachments between the gallbladder and the duodenum or colon.
8. The surgeon may stand on either the right or left side of the patient, or perhaps on alternate sides at different stages of the operation. The exposure of Calot's triangle is often easier from the left side. The view from the right side may be improved if the patient is rotated to the right.

Steps in the standard operation

1. If a liver biopsy is indicated, it should be carried out as the first step in the operation, since biopsies performed late in the operation will contain leucocyte infiltrates as a result of the anaesthesia and operative manipulation (Edlund & Zettergren 1957). The indications and technique have been discussed previously (Ham 1980b). A wedge biopsy is preferable provided it is not superficial and avoids areas of capsular fibrosis. It should be taken from the left lobe so that the site is well away from the operative area.
2. The anatomy of the porta and Calot's triangle is assessed.
3. The gallbladder should be aspirated after insertion of a purse-string suture if it is so enlarged as to obscure the anatomy, or if it is so tense that a clamp cannot be safely applied.
4. A Duval Harrison-Cripp or similar forceps is placed on the gallbladder in the region of Hartmann's pouch (Fig. 44.1). The direction of pull is towards the right iliac fossa, so as to open up Calot's triangle. The latter is the triangle bounded by the cystic duct and gallbladder, the liver and the common hepatic duct (Wood 1970, Northover & Terblanche 1983) (Ch. 2). A second clamp may be placed near the fundus if necessary.

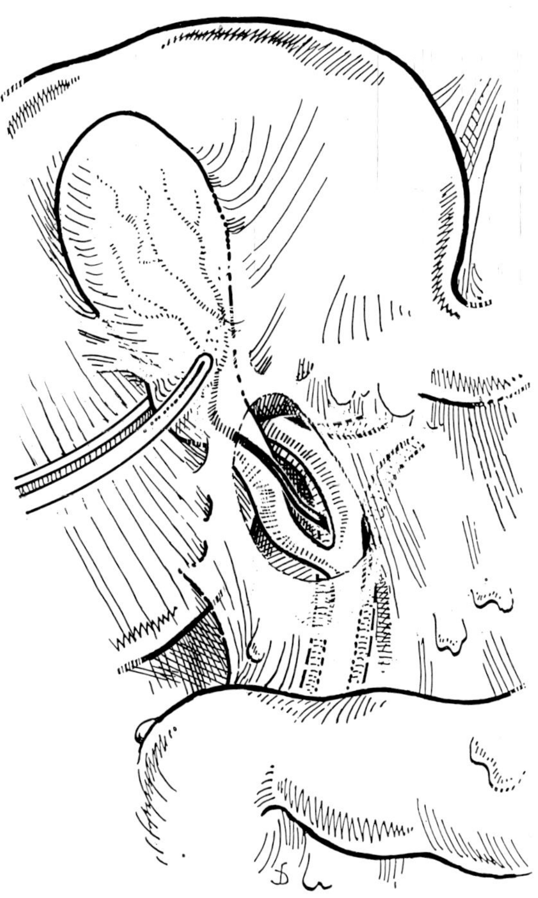

Fig. 44.2 The initial peritoneal incisions are made anteriorly *and posteriorly* near the apex of Calot's triangle

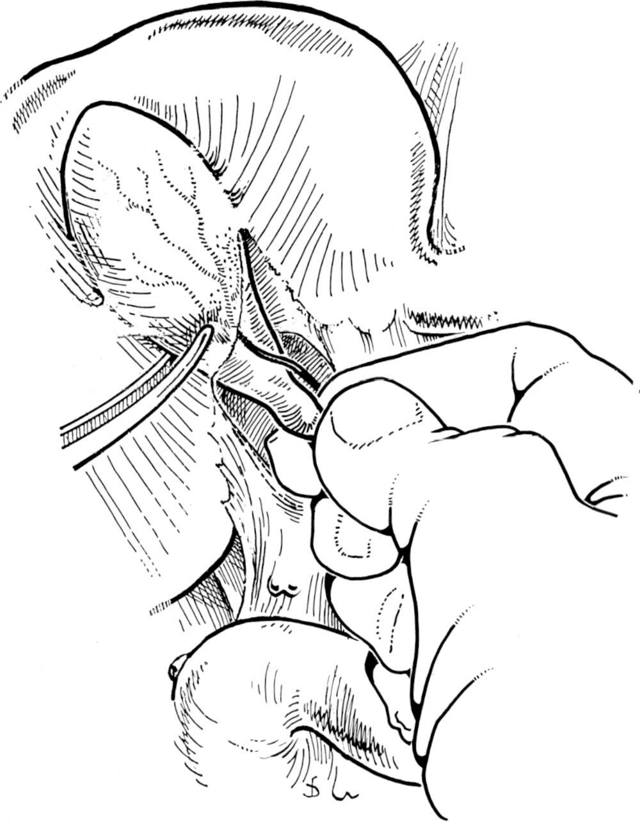

Fig. 44.3 Palpation reveals a stone in the cystic duct, which may be 'milked' back into the gallbladder

5. The initial peritoneal incisions are best placed away from the main structures in the porta. It is recommended that the first be transversely across the region of Hartmann's pouch towards the liver anteriorly, linked with a second similar incision posteriorly (Fig. 44.2). The reason for the posterior incision (and dissection) is that it greatly facilitates the dissection of Calot's triangle, there being no rigid posterior peritoneum.

The next objective is to define the triangle bounded by the presumed cystic duct and common hepatic or right hepatic duct, and the liver. This is achieved by a combination of blunt and sharp dissection, the direction of the latter being towards the gallbladder fundus and towards the porta hepatis.

Within the triangle are usually found the cystic artery (passing diagonally across it to the gallbladder), the cystic node and one or more small veins. There may also be part of the right hepatic artery and a bile duct from the right lobe of the liver (Ch. 2). Palpation during this dissection may identify the former; palpation may also detect a stone in the cystic duct, and this may be 'milked' back into the gallbladder (Fig. 44.3), taking care not to dislodge a stone into the common bile duct.

Loose ties may then be placed around the presumed cystic artery and cystic duct, but their identification cannot be confirmed until dissection is complete. The gallbladder should be dissected from the liver to a point about 5 cm or more from the porta hepatis and traction then converts Calot's triangle to an irregular quadrilateral (Fig. 44.4). The presumed cystic artery and cystic duct are dissected towards the porta so that there is now a large space between the gallbladder and the liver, with a small artery crossing it to the gallbladder (i.e. the cystic artery). This may then be ligated *on or close to the gallbladder wall* (Fig. 44.4) and divided, and the space will then open up even more. Small veins crossing it to be gallbladder are then divided.

The presumed cystic duct is then dissected to its apparent junction with a duct running in the free edge of the lesser omentum or close to it, and this should be either the common hepatic duct, the right hepatic duct or a major sectoral right hepatic duct (Ch. 2). The apparent junction is displayed further by dissection of the peritoneum on the anterior aspect of the duct as it runs up towards the liver and down to the duodenum. The junction is termed 'apparent', since the true junction cannot be determined by external examination.

At the end of this dissection, there should be clearly

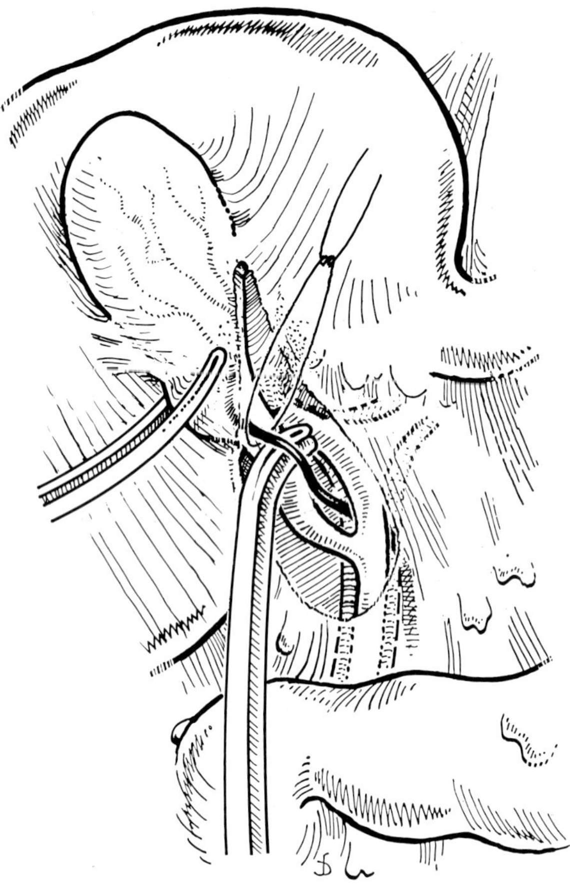

Fig. 44.4 Calot's triangle is converted into an irregular quadrilateral. The cystic artery is ligated on, or close to, the gallbladder wall

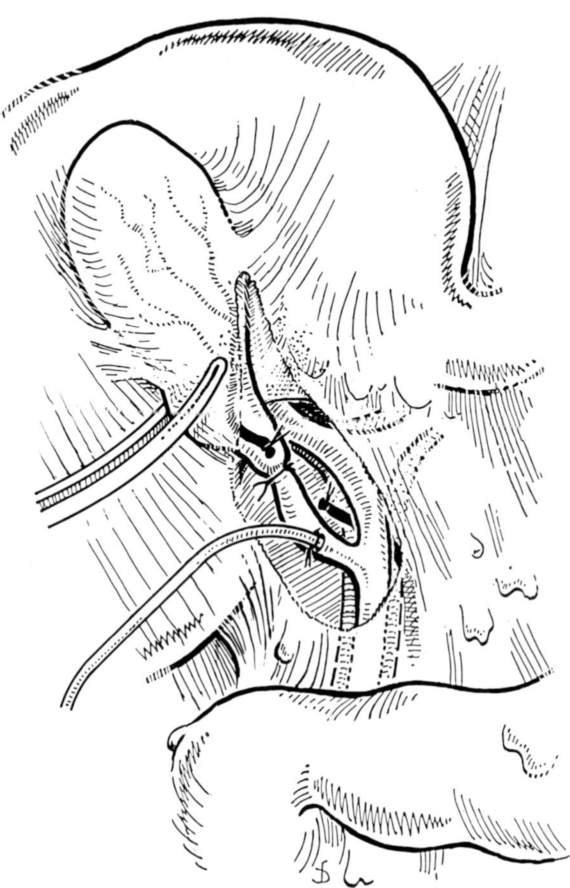

Fig. 44.5 The cystic duct is ligated at its junction with the gallbladder. A Stoke-on-Trent catheter has been inserted

visible a duct joining the gallbladder to a T or Y junction with a duct running from the liver towards the duodenum. The former can only be the cystic duct. Operative cholangiography should then be performed.

6. The junction of the cystic duct and gallbladder is ligated, and a loose tie placed round the former; it is then incised about 2 cm from the apparent junction with the 'common hepatic duct' and the bile flowing out is checked for the presence of 'mud' or small calculi.

A Stoke-on-Trent or similar catheter is then inserted so that it just reaches the junction and is fixed in position with a tie (Fig. 44.5). Cholangiography is performed using the technique described by Le Quesne & Bolton (1980). It is important to check that all packs and instruments have been removed, that the patient is rotated to the right, and that neither the catheter nor a gastric tube overlie the region of the common bile duct.

7. Whilst awaiting the films, remove the gallbladder; the cystic duct is divided leaving the catheter in place, and the gallbladder is then dissected from its fossa using a combination of traction, gentle finger dissection, sharp dissection and diathermy. There may be further branches of the cystic artery and very occasionally small bile ducts. The dissection should keep close to the gallbladder wall to avoid damage to the cystic plate or the liver.

8. The gallbladder should then be opened and checked for the following: the type and size of stones; the presence of a tumour or fundal adenoma; the presence of a stricture associated with adenomyomatosis. Culture of the bile is advisable.

9. The duodenum and pancreatic head are then mobilized by Kocher's manoeuvre, and the common bile duct, pancreatic head and ampulla carefully palpated.

10. The radiographs are then assessed according to the criteria of Le Quesne & Bolton (1980). If there is any doubt about the technical quality or about the normality of the bile ducts, a further set of three films should be obtained. If the entry of the cystic duct is low, the film should be checked even more carefully since a stone in a long cystic duct may easily be missed. The anatomy of the duct system is assessed; lack of filling of the common hepatic duct or intrahepatic ducts suggests the possibility that the cannula is placed within the common bile duct or of damage to the duct system. On occasion, leakage of dye from a right hepatic duct, either in the porta or in the gallbladder bed, will be observed (Hopkinson et al 1983).

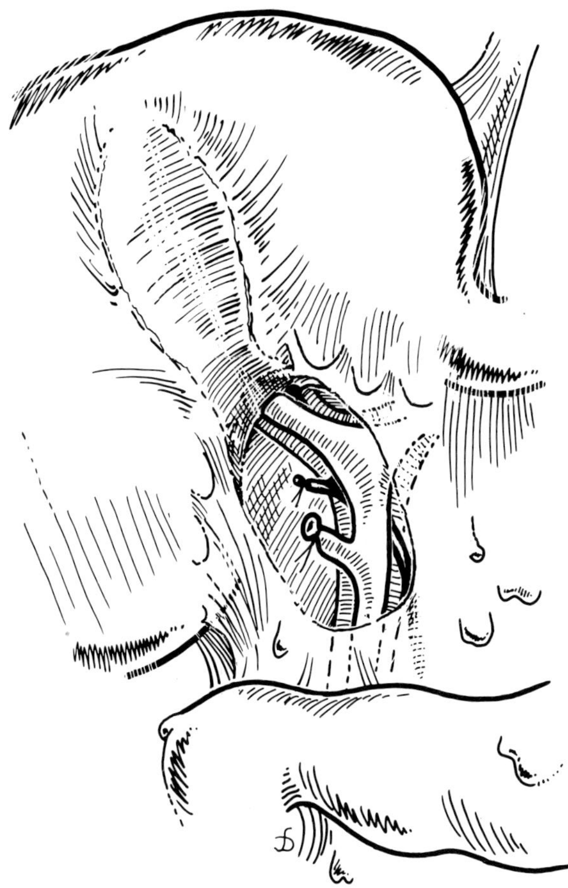

Fig. 44.6 The cystic duct is ligated about 1 cm from its apparent junction with the common hepatic duct.

Such a leak must be identified and carefully repaired.

11. The catheter is then removed from the cystic duct, and the latter ligated about 1 cm from the apparent junction (Fig. 44.6). Some recommend transfixion of the cystic duct and ligation using this suture. This site of ligation avoids the possibility of damage to the blood supply to the common bile duct running on its right side (Northover & Terblanche 1979). It is usually recommended that this tie (or ties) be of absorbable material, since non-absorbable ties may act as a nidus for stones (Gunn 1977). However, the author has also seen stones formed on chromic catgut ties.

12. The gallbladder bed and porta hepatis are then checked for haemostasis and bile leaks. The peritoneum of the gallbladder bed may be sutured, but this is not essential. The question of drainage of the region is controversial (Kune & Sali 1980), some authors favouring routine drainage, some no drainage and some selective drainage.

The author favours the last option, with a soft Portex tube drain being inserted in most patients. The drain is positioned in the region of the opening into the lesser sac, and passes to the exterior along the line of the gallbladder fossa. Externally, the drain should be connected to a closed collection system. Usually, only about 50 ml of haemoserous fluid drains in the first 24 hours, and the drain may then be removed. It should be retained if there is excessive oozing, or leakage of bile.

Variations in technique

There are a number of variations in the standard technique. These will be discussed, followed by a consideration of the situations in which they may be applicable.

'Fundus-down' cholecystectomy

This method is used by many surgeons as a routine. The gallbladder is first separated from the liver beginning at the fundus (Fig. 44.7), and this provides good exposure of the region of Calot's triangle. This approach has much in common with that described above, but it must be stressed that the dissection of Calot's triangle must be carried out in the same fashion and particular care must be taken to avoid damage to structures reached unexpectedly. The method allows identification of variations of normal

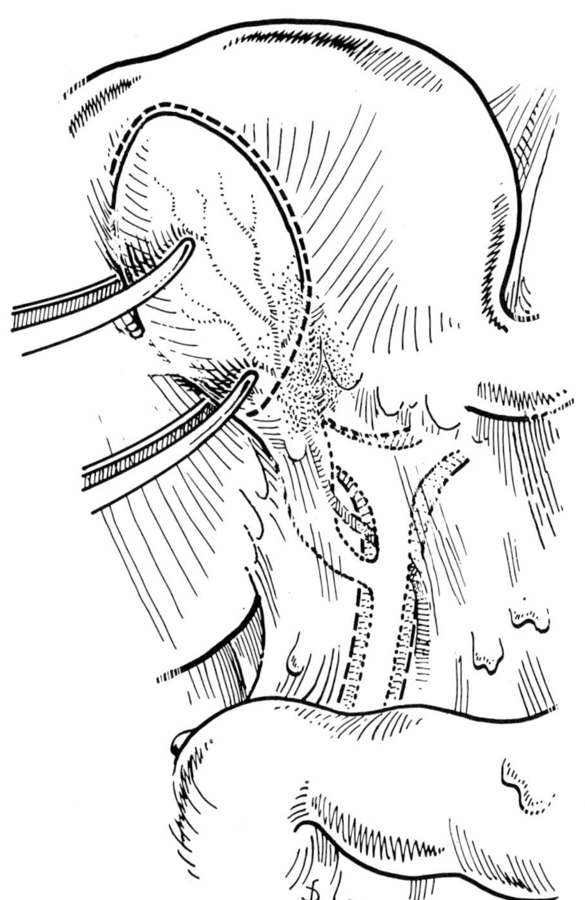

Fig. 44.7 The dissection may commence with separation of the gallbladder from the liver at the fundus

anatomy. On occasion bleeding from the gallbladder fossa may obscure the deeper field.

Opening the common bile duct

In some patients, the anatomy of the bile ducts is difficult to determine; it may then be wise to open the presumed common bile duct and, by the passage of probes, establish the location of the various ducts.

Cholecystostomy

This option may be taken if it is felt that cholecystectomy would be technically very difficult or when the condition of the patient is such that the simplest and quickest procedure should be performed.

In brief, the procedure begins with the insertion of a purse-string suture in the fundus; the gallbladder contents are then aspirated using a trochar and cannula attached to a suction apparatus. The gallbladder is then opened, and all stones are removed paying particular attention to those which may be in Hartmann's pouch or in the cystic duct. Preferably, a free flow of bile should be obtained from the latter but this is not always possible. A De Pezza or Foley catheter is then placed in the gallbladder and fixed in position with the purse-string. Usually a second purse-string is inserted. The catheter is then brought to the exterior by the shortest possible route through a small window in the omentum.

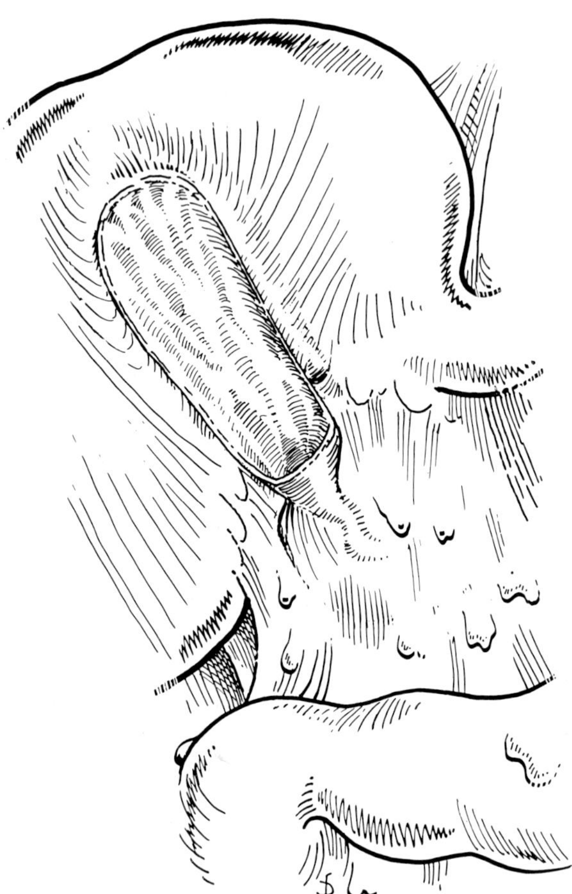

Fig. 44.8 Partial cholecystectomy. Portion of the gallbladder wall has been left overlying the liver and right side of the porta hepatis

Partial cholecystectomy

This technique is a useful alternative to the standard one for situations in which dissection of the gallbladder from the region of the common hepatic duct would be hazardous (Ch. 58). It may also be used when dissection of the gallbladder from the liver is likely to be followed by bleeding which would be difficult to control.

The cystic duct and common bile duct are exposed, and then the gallbladder is opened near the fundus and its contents evacuated. The gallbladder wall is then excised from the fundus towards the cystic duct, leaving in situ part or all of the gallbladder wall which lies directly in relation to the liver and porta. If the cystic duct is patent, then a standard cholangiogram may be performed but this is seldom possible if the procedure is indicated; if not, cholangiography may be done by needle puncture of the common bile duct. The cystic duct is then ligated.

Figure 44.8 shows the operation field after completion of the partial gallbladder excision. The exposed gallbladder mucosa may then be diathermied but this is probably not essential.

UNUSUAL CLINICAL OR PATHOLOGICAL PROBLEMS

Gross inflammation or empyema

Cholecystectomy is usually possible — and safe — after gallbladder aspiration. The other alternatives are cholecystostomy or partial cholecystectomy.

Perforation

This usually follows gallbladder ischaemia and cholecystectomy is necessary.

Abscess

An abscess extending from the fundus or body of the gallbladder into the liver may mimic gallbladder carcinoma and frozen section may be necessary to resolve the dilemma.

An abscess, or gross chronic inflammation, in Calot's triangle (Fig. 44.9) will create considerable difficulties in displaying the anatomy. The options are common bile duct exploration to identify the hepatic ducts, cholecystostomy or partial cholecystectomy (Ch. 58). The choice will

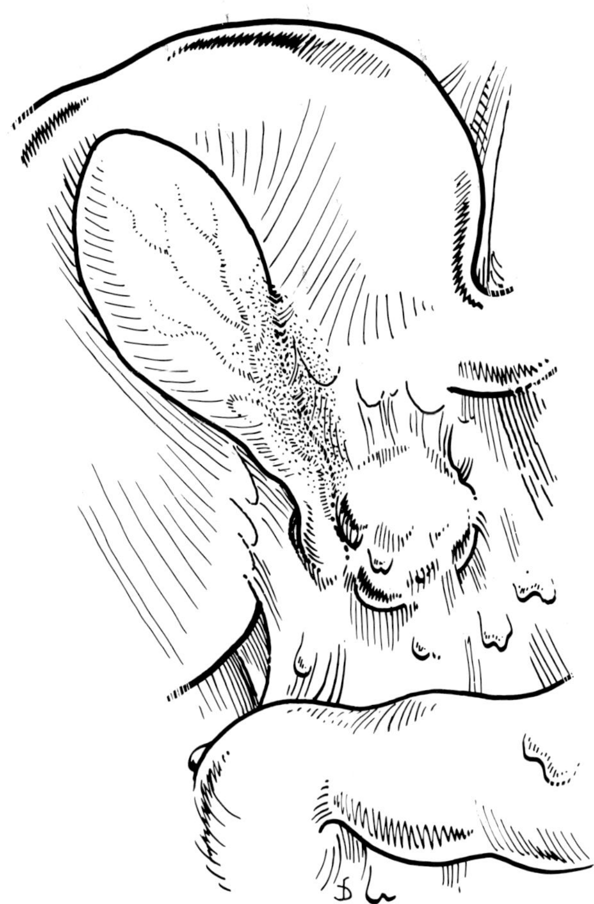

Fig. 44.9 An inflammatory mass obscures the right side of the porta and Calot's triangle. The standard technique may be dangerous

depend on the pathology and on the experience of the surgeon. Of the three options, cholecystostomy is the safest.

Fistulae

Fistulae from the gallbladder or cystic duct to the common bile duct, hepatic ducts, duodenum or colon may be found. They are usually associated with considerable fibrosis and the operation is correspondingly difficult. In the case of fistulae involving the common bile duct or hepatic ducts, exploration of the common bile duct may be necessary to identify the site of entry of the fistula and to repair it safely or alternatively partial cholecystectomy with subsequent cholecystduodenostomy may be indicated (Ch. 61). Fistulae into the bowel should be divided and the site of entry into the bowel oversewn.

A large fistula into the duodenum should prompt careful examination of the small bowel for a gallstone which may obstruct the ileum.

Cholecystectomy after previous cholecystostomy

The exposure of the gallbladder is more difficult than usual because of adherent omentum and because the gallbladder is usually shrunken and fibrotic. After adequate exposure is achieved, the remaining steps in the operation are usually straightforward.

Cholecystectomy in the patient with cirrhosis

The operation may be done for symptomatic gallbladder disease or it may be performed as part of another procedure, e.g. a shunt procedure for portal hypertension. The presence of cirrhosis does not create any particular difficulties apart from restricted access to the porta hepatis in some patients due to regenerative nodules or liver enlargement. However, associated portal hypertension may make control of bleeding in the gallbladder fossa extremely difficult. Partial cholecystectomy is an excellent alternative to the standard procedure. If the cholecystectomy is performed in conjunction with a shunt operation, it should be done after the shunt is completed, since control of bleeding will probably be much easier. Liver functional reserve is an important determinant of prognosis.

It should be noted that external biliary drainage (by cholecystostomy or T-tube) in the cirrhotic patient may result in problems with fluid and electrolyte therapy. The reason is that these patients often have high bile flow and 2–3 litres of bile per day may be lost through the drain.

Drainage of the operative area is best avoided in the cirrhotic patient, especially if there is associated portal hypertension. If the patient develops ascites postoperatively, then an ascitic fistula may result; this is a potentially lethal complication. For the same reason, wound closure should be meticulous.

Unsuspected carcinoma

Carcinoma of the gallbladder may be encountered unexpectedly at the time of cholecystectomy in two main ways. Firstly, the patient has gallstones but the cause of the symptoms is cystic duct obstruction by the tumour. Secondly, the patient has gallstones and these are the cause of symptoms; the carcinoma is found on external examination of the gallbladder or, more commonly, after it has been opened. Indeed suspect areas of gallbladder wall should be submitted to frozen section (Ch. 64).

In the first situation, there is usually tumour involvement of the structures in the porta hepatis, and radical removal is almost always impossible. Some form of common bile duct or common hepatic duct decompression is required (Ch. 64). It may also be necessary to relieve symptoms due to the cystic duct obstruction. Cholecystectomy is often difficult or impossible, and decompression may be achieved by cholecystoduodenostomy or cholecystjejunostomy.

In the second situation, the carcinoma is usually in the body or fundus of the gallbladder. Simple cholecystectomy may achieve adequate clearance for early tumours (Ch. 64). However, the depth of invasion of the tumour through the gallbladder wall should be checked by frozen section. If invasion of liver tissue is possible, or likely, then the options are either to excise liver tissue in the region of the tumour or to perform an hepatic resection (Ch. 64).

THE HANDLING OF PROBLEMS WHICH MAY ARISE DURING THE OPERATION

Bleeding

Excessive bleeding is of two main types. Firstly, there may be bleeding from multiple areas, including the wound margins. This is usually due to an unrecognized acquired coagulation disorder (e.g. prolonged prothrombin time, subcutaneous heparin overdose), to a congenital disorder such as Von Willebrand's syndrome or to chronic liver disease especially with portal hypertension. The management includes local haemostasis and administration of appropriate coagulant factor(s) if the cause is identified, or fresh frozen plasma and platelets if it is not. The operation may usually be completed with these measures. A drain is mandatory, except in the patient with portal hypertension, for reasons given earlier.

Secondly, there may be bleeding due to damage to the cystic artery or right hepatic artery. Control of bleeding from the cystic artery is usually straightforward, using direct pressure with packs or compression of the hepatic artery and suction. Bleeding from the right hepatic artery is a more difficult problem. It usually follows avulsion of the cystic artery due to excessive traction, or may be caused by direct injury. A combination of compression of the artery, or the common hepatic artery in the free edge of the lesser omentum (Pringle manoeuvre), and adequate suction should demonstrate the injury; the artery may then be precisely clamped with a vascular clamp and the laceration repaired. Ligation of the right hepatic artery should be considered only if reasonable attempts at control fail. It cannot be sufficiently emphasized that good visualisation and precise control is necessary if ductal damage is to be avoided (Ch. 58).

Damage to major bile ducts

Damage to the major bile ducts is not often recognized at the time it occurs. Appropriate management of these injuries is discussed in Ch. 58.

Stone in a low entry cystic duct

Such a stone may be difficult to diagnose, and difficult to retrieve. The diagnosis may be made by palpation or by cholangiography. However, the view of the termination of the cystic duct on the cholangiogram may be obscured by the dye in the common bile duct making identification difficult. The possibility of such a stone should be considered if the cholangiogram shows a stone apparently in the common bile duct, and yet none is found at exploration.

The stone may sometimes be retrieved by 'milking' it back, but usually it must be manipulated into the common duct and then removed from the latter.

Bile leakage identified at the end of the operation

Leakage of bile at the end of the procedure should prompt

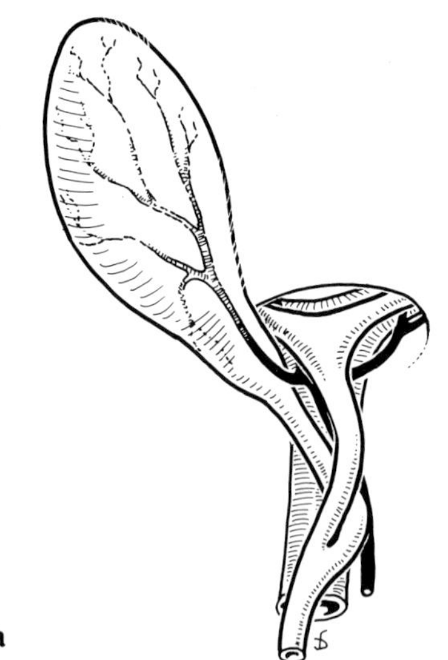

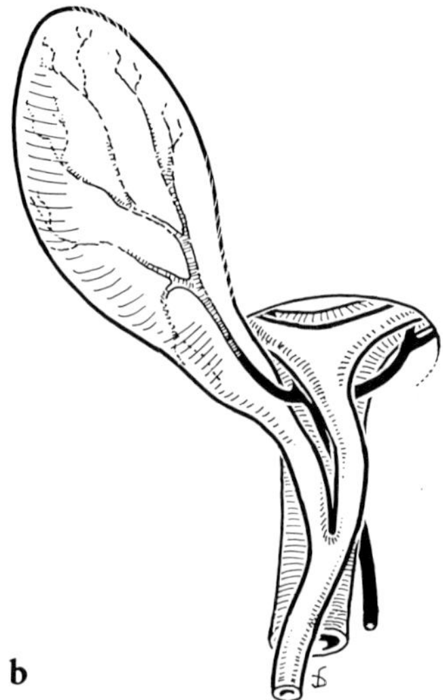

Fig. 44.10 a & b. Two anatomical variations in which the common hepatic duct may be mistaken for the cystic duct, particulary if the dissection begins near the free edge of the lesser omentum. The common hepatic duct runs less vertically than usual, and is similar in size to the cystic duct. The cystic duct may spiral about the common duct

a detailed examination of the operative area and review of the cholangiograms. There may be a major duct injury, but the usual site of leakage will be from the gallbladder fossa, or from the region of the right hepatic duct high in the porta. The former may be safely sutured, but repair of the latter will require careful identification of the site of leakage. If necessary, cholangiography should be repeated.

CONCLUDING REMARKS

There are a number of excellent descriptions of the variations in the ductal and arterial anatomy which are important in cholecystectomy and other hepatobiliary operations (Ch. 2) (Flint 1923, Michels 1951, Maingot 1980, Puente & Bannura 1983, Northover & Terblanche 1983). However, anatomical variations may not always be easily recognized and damage to important structures may result. It has therefore been the purpose of this chapter to describe a method which takes account of the variety of operative findings.

One of the common types of damage to the major bile ducts is excision of a length of common hepatic duct in mistake for the cystic duct. Figure 44.10 illustrates two situations in which this might occur. False identification of the common hepatic duct for the cystic duct is more likely if the dissection is commenced at the base of Calot's triangle (the common hepatic duct) rather than near its apex (junction of gallbladder and liver) and if ligation or division of duct is performed before complete dissection of the triangle.

Thus the two major points in the technique are: complete dissection of Calot's triangle commencing near its apex, with divison of the peritoneal coverings of the structures in the triangle both anteriorly and posteriorly; secondly, avoidance of ligation or division of any structure until it is positively identified. Every patient should be assumed to have a variation from the 'standard' anatomy.

Finally, if the identification of the major ducts or vessels is difficult or impossible, one of the variations in the technique should be considered.

REFERENCES

Edlund Y A, Zettergren L S W 1957 Microstructure of the liver in biliary tract disease and notes on the effect on the liver of anaesthesia, intubation and operation trauma. Acta Chirurgica Scandinavica 113: 201–210

Flint E R 1923 Abnormalities of the right hepatic, cystic, and gastroduodenal arteries, and of the bile-ducts. British Journal of Surgery 10: 509–519

Gunn A A 1977 Cholecystectomy and cholecystostomy. In: Dudley H, Rob C, Smith R (eds) Operative surgery, abdomen 3rd edn. Butterworths, London, p 329

Ham J M 1980a Acalculous benign biliary disease. In: Kune G A, Sali A The practice of biliary surgery 2nd edn. Blackwell, Oxford, ch 12, p 344

Ham J M 1980b The liver in biliary disease. In: Kune G A, Sali A The practice of biliary surgery 2nd edn. Blackwell, Oxford, ch 17, p 442

Hopkinson G B, Woodward D A K, Prasad N, Bullen B R 1983 Identification of accessory bile ducts at cholecystectomy. Annals of the Royal College of Surgeons of England 64: 323–324

Kune G A, Sali A 1980 The practice of biliary surgery 2nd edn. Blackwell, Oxford, p 143

Lennard T W J, Farndon J R, Taylor R M R 1984 Acalculous biliary pain: diagnosis and selection for cholecystectomy using the cholecystokinin test for pain reproduction. British Journal of Surgery 71: 368–370

Le Quesne L P, Ranger I 1975 Cholecystitis glandularis proliferans. British Journal of Surgery 44: 447–458

Le Quesne L P, Bolton J P 1980 Choledocholithiasis: incidence, diagnosis and operative procedures. In: Maingot R Abdominal operations 7th edn. Appleton-Century-Crofts, New York, ch 66, p 1055

Maingot R 1980 Anatomical abnormalities of the biliary tract and the hepatic and cystic arteries. In: Maingot R Abdominal operations 7th edn. Appleton-Century-Crofts, New York, ch 61, p 979

Michels N A 1951 The hepatic, cystic and retroduodenal arteries and their relations to the biliary ducts. Annals of Surgery 133: 503–524

Northover J M A, Terblanche J 1979 A new look at the arterial supply of the bile duct in man and its surgical implications. British Journal of Surgery 66: 379–384

Northover J M A, Terblanche J 1983 Applied surgical anatomy of the biliary tract. In: Blumgart L H (ed) Clinical surgery international, Vol 5. The biliary tract, Churchill Livingstone, Edinburgh, ch I, p 1

Puente S G, Bannura G C 1983 Radiologic anatomy of the biliary tract: variations and congenital anomalies. World Journal of Surgery 7: 271–276

Schwartz S I 1981 Biliary tract surgery and cirrhosis: a critical combination. Surgery 90: 577–582

Wood M 1979 Eponyms in biliary tract surgery. American Journal of Surgery 138: 746–754

45

P. B. Cotton

Endoscopic management of gallbladder stones

INTRODUCTION

Endoscopic methods are being used to treat patients with gallbladder stones in two different circumstances. The first concerns per-oral endoscopic sphincterotomy in patients (with gallbladders) who present with symptoms due to stones in the bile duct (Ch. 50). Endoscopic clearance of the duct stones deals with the immediate problem, and simple cholecystectomy can be performed electively in relative safety. However, it is becoming clear that cholecystectomy is necessary in less than 20% of elderly and frail patients. The second context concerns direct endoscopic attack on the stones in the gallbladder. At duodenoscopy, baskets and catheters can be passed through the cystic duct into the gallbladder. Fibrescopes have been used to extract gallbladder stones percutaneously, via the drain track after emergency cholecystostomy. A laparoscopic approach to gallbladdder stones is theoretically possible.

ENDOSCOPIC SPHINCTEROTOMY IN THE PRESENCE OF A GALLBLADDER

The rationale and techniques for duodenoscopic management of duct stones are described in detail in Chapter 47. The popularity of the method indicates that physicians and surgeons alike have welcomed the development of a treatment which has major advantages over conventional surgery. Endoscopic sphincterotomy was introduced for patients with retained or recurrent stones following cholecystectomy, but the indications have been extended now to include patients who have not undergone biliary surgery (Cotton 1984) (Fig. 45.1). Most European centres report that such patients constitute about 50% of their referrals (Cotton & Vallon 1982). This has developed because it is clear that the endoscopic approach is substantially safer (as well as being simpler) than surgical exploration, in two groups of patients. The first group are those who (at any age) are acutely ill because of the duct stones, suffering with acute cholangitis, jaundice, septicaemia or gallstone pancreatitis. Simple cholecystectomy can be performed safely once the acute illness has subsided, with substantially less risk than an emergency cholecystectomy and duct exploration. The second group of patients are those whose general condition renders surgery undesirable or hazardous. This contraindication may be temporary (such as pregnancy or recent cardiac incident), or permanent (such as severe cardio-respiratory insufficiency). Recurrent attacks of biliary pain due to duct stones can be dealt with endoscopically, in the hope that the gallbladder stones will remain quiescent. Indeed, some gallbladder stones may pass spontaneously through the cystic duct and out the duodenum through the sphincterotomy.

Certain questions must be answered in order to justify these approaches.

1. Is it possible to exclude acute cholecystitis in patients with acute cholangitis?

2. Is endoscopic treatment indeed safer than surgical intervention in patients with acute cholangitis and gallstone pancreatitis?

3. Are the complications of endoscopic sphincterotomy different in the presence of a gallbladder? Is there a substantial risk of provoking cholecystitis?

4. What is the incidence of gallbladder symptoms and cholecystitis in those patients who are not submitted to cholecystectomy soon after endoscopic sphincterotomy. Is it possible to define a group of patients at high risk?

Several of these questions can only be answered with accuracy by suitable randomized controlled trials. None have been published.

Those centres offering urgent endoscopic management for cholangitis do not appear to have difficulties in differential diagnosis. However, this may partly reflect the fact that most of the acutely ill patients are admitted under the care of surgeons, who refer to their endoscopic colleagues only those patients in whom there is little or no suspicion of acute gallbladder disease.

The risks of surgical intervention in patients with acute cholangitis are well documented (Thompson, Tompkins

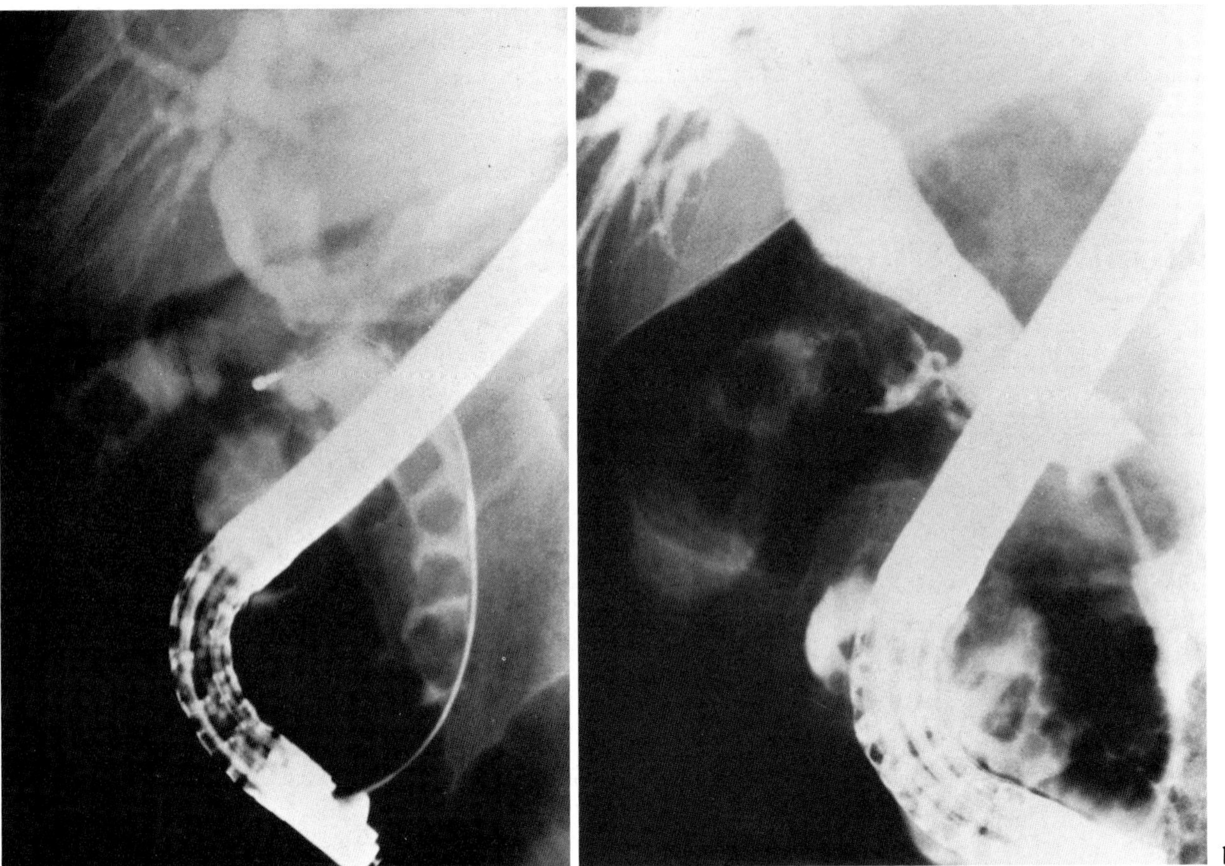

Fig. 45.1 Endoscopic treatment of stones in a patient who has not undergone cholecystectomy: a. basket in place after sphincterotomy; b. check cholangiogram using a balloon occlusion catheter after endoscopic duct clearance

& Longmire 1982). Many surgeons have assumed that acute cholangitis is a contraindication for endoscopic treatment, since it is a recognized complication of ERCP and sphincterotomy. However, those active in the field are convinced that the reverse is true. Endoscopic sphincterotomy with stone extraction (or naso-biliary drainage) is the simplest and safest method of dealing with a patient with acute suppurative cholangitis (Vallon, Shorvon & Cotton 1982). The endoscopic method will fail in about 10% of patients, who should be treated immediately by an alternative method of drainage (percutaneous or surgical). Endoscopic treatment has been shown to be safe and effective also in patients with jaundice (Neoptolemos et al 1984) and in those with acute gallstone related pancreatitis (Safrany & Cotton 1981, Rosseland & Solhang 1984).

The complications of endoscopic sphincterotomy are detailed in Chapter 47. The only possible additional complication in patients with gallbladders in place is that of provoking acute cholecystitis by injection of contrast (with infected bile) into the gallbladder, and inadvertent instrumentation of the cystic duct. This complication is rare. Acute cholecystitis occurred within one week of sphincterotomy in two of our initial series of 71 patients (Cotton & Vallon 1982). At that time antibiotics were not being given routinely. Subsequently we have used prophylactic antibiotics routinely, and have seen no early cholecystitis in at least 200 further cases. Escourrou et al (1984) reported no episodes of cholecystitis amongst 234 patients undergoing sphincterotomy with a gallbladder in place. Two out of 59 patients reported by Neoptelemos et al (1984) required early cholecystectomy for empyema of the gallbladder.

The main interest in this context is the risk of leaving the gallbladder in place after endoscopic duct clearance. It is possible that some patients will pass their gallbladder stones through the cystic duct and into the duodenum. An expectant approach can be justified if follow-up studies show that the risk of gallbladder symptoms is small. However, prophylactic cholecystectomy would be the best treatment (with the patient in optimum condition) if most patients develop gallbladder symptoms, especially if there is a risk that they will require emergency treatment for cholecystitis or empyema.

Some guidance can be gained from the recent reviews and controversy concerning the treatment of gallbladder stones in general (Bouchier 1983). The often quoted study by Wenckert & Robertson (1966) concerned 781 patients with symptomatic gallbladder stones; follow-up without surgery showed that only 30% developed substantial complaints. Subsequent studies of patients with *asymptomatic* gallbladder stones indicate a much lower incidence (Gracie & Ransohoff 1982). These risks have to be placed in the context of the patient's age and general condition, and specifically the expectation of life. Most of the patients so far treated endoscopically (with the gallbladder in place) have been poor risks, either because of advanced age or general medical illness; usually they are patients deemed unlikely to survive more than five or 10 years. Thus, relatively short term follow-up data are relevant.

We have recently reviewed 145 patients who underwent endoscopic duct clearance with a gallbladder in place, at The Middlesex Hospital between 1975 and 1981. 19 (11.5%) proceeded to interval cholecystectomy within a matter of weeks, once health status had improved. The mean age of these patients was 62 years, and there were no deaths. Half of these patients had no stones in the gallbladder at the time of cholecystectomy. 125 patients were discharged with the gallbladder in place, and follow-up has been obtained (at 2–8 years) in 118 of these. The mean age was 75 years. At the time of follow-up, 32 patients had already died after a mean interval of 20 months. Only one of these deaths may have been related to biliary disease. Of the 86 survivors at a mean interval of three years, only 19 (22%) have reported any symptoms referable to the biliary tree. None presented on an emergency basis. Eight have required interventional treatment (six had cholecystectomy, two further endoscopic stone extraction), without mortality.

Several other authors have reported that less than 10% of their patients have required cholecystectomy at intervals after endoscopic sphincterotomy (Escourrou et al 1984, Neoptolemos et al 1984, Seifert, Gail & Weismuller 1982). Further long-term data are required. The number of patients who do require cholecystectomy is sufficiently small to make it difficult at present to define any predictive factors. It was suggested initially that patients with cystic duct obstruction were at greater risk. However, in our own series, the incidence of further biliary symptoms was similar in those whose gallbladder filled at the initial ERCP to those in whom it did not.

It is also difficult to determine the likelihood of stones passing spontaneously from the gallbladder after sphincterotomy. Further investigations are often difficult to justify and to arrange in the elderly and frail patients with whom we are concerned. However, follow-up ultrasound scans of the gallbladder in 30 of our patients has shown that 12 appear to have no residual stones.

These data together clearly justify the use of endoscopic treatment for selected patients in whom the presenting symptoms are due to stones in the bile duct, despite the presence of a gallbladder. There can be no argument about the patients at highest risk, e.g., those beyond the age of 75 with serious medical disabilities, and it is a logical approach when there is a temporary contraindication to surgery, such as recent myocardial infarction or pregnancy. Orthodox surgical management remains the treatment of choice for young and fit patients. The interest and discussion concerns the correct approach for those patients in the middle of the spectrum, e.g. those in relatively good health, perhaps close to the age of retirement. Any comments will remain a matter of opinion until facts are provided from long-term follow-up studies and randomized trials. Central to this discussion is the precise documentation of risk factors (Cotton 1984).

It has been suggested that even young and fit patients should be treated by endoscopic duct clearance, combined with a cholecystectomy. This is based on the belief that the combined morbidity and mortality of the two procedures is less than that of cholecystectomy with duct exploration. This controversial hypothesis is now being tested in a randomized controlled trial. Patients in the study will have to be followed up for many years, since the potential long-term disadvantages of destroying the sphincter must be included in the evaluation.

DIRECT DUODENOSCOPIC EXTRACTION OF GALLBLADDER STONES

At ERCP it is sometimes possible to pass baskets and catheters through the cystic duct and into the gallbladder. Balloon dilatation of the cystic duct has been performed by radiologists, working down a cholecystostomy drain track. We have dilated the cystic duct with similar balloon catheters passed endoscopically (Fig. 45.2), to facilitate extraction of stones from the cystic duct, and from the gallbladder (Figs. 45.3 and 45.4). By similar techniques, a naso-biliary tube can be placed in the gallbladder, and left in situ for drainage or infusion of chemicals (Fig. 45.5).

These manipulations might be more easily performed under direct vision, with the latest generation of per-oral baby choledochoscopes (Fig. 45.6). Presumably someone will attempt to perform an endoscopic cholecystectomy, by grasping the gallbladder wall and inverting it through the cystic duct.

Endoscopic invasion of the gallbladder is experimental. No one has yet reported a systematic study; success rates and the obvious potential hazards have not been assessed.

PERCUTANEOUS CHOLECYSTOSCOPY AND STONE EXTRACTION

Cholecystostomy is used for emergency treatment of acutely ill and frail patients. Cholangiograms taken post-operatively via the drainage tube may show stones remaining in the gallbladder (and bile duct). Further

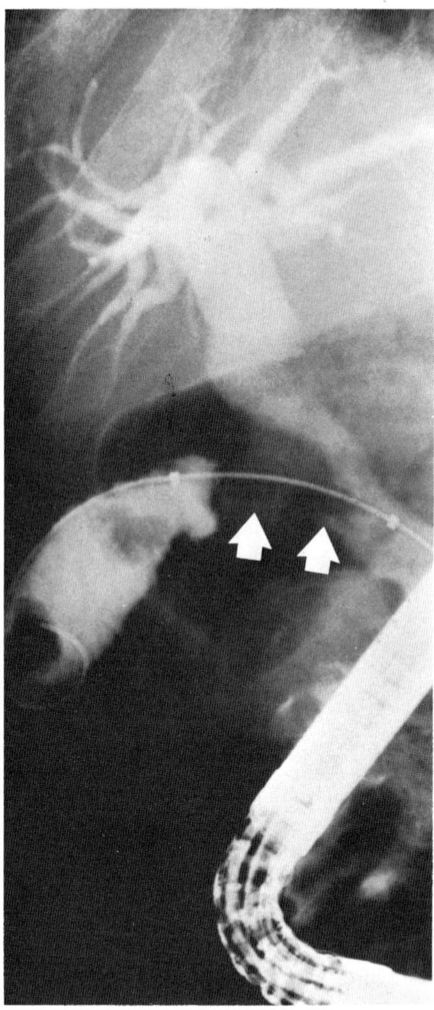

Fig. 45.2 Endoscopic dilatation of the cystic duct with a balloon catheter (arrow)

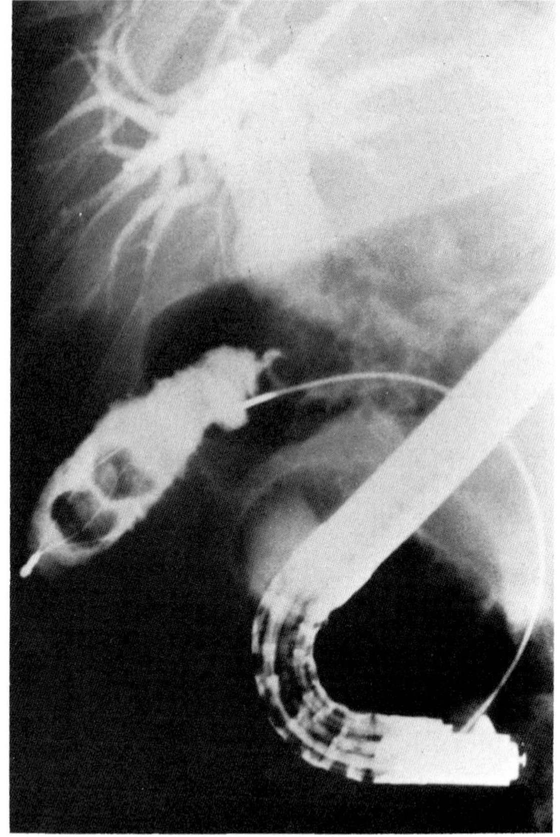

Fig. 45.3 Attempted basket extraction of gallbladder stones

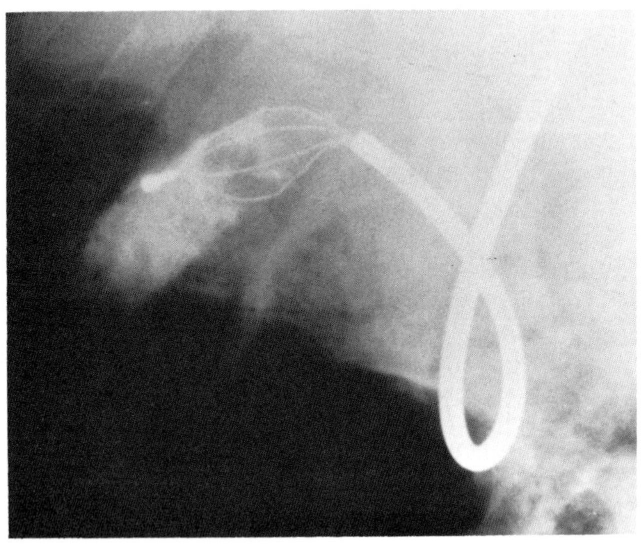

Fig. 45.4 Use of a crushing basket placed endoscopically in the gallbladder

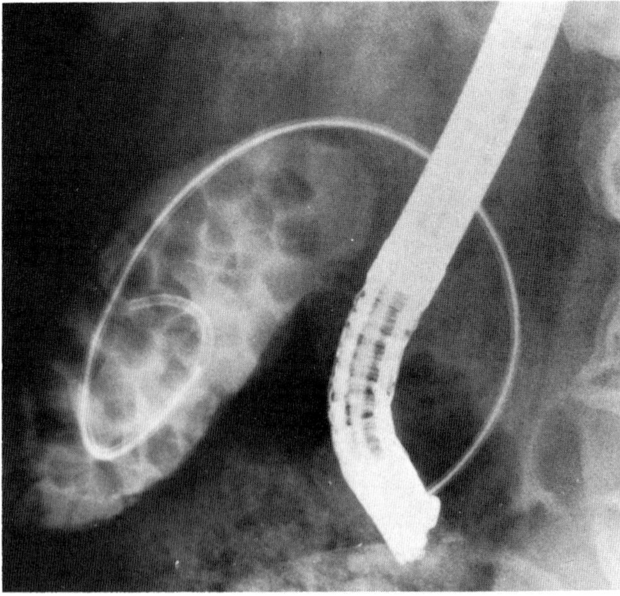

Fig. 45.5 Placement of a naso-biliary drain in the gallbladder

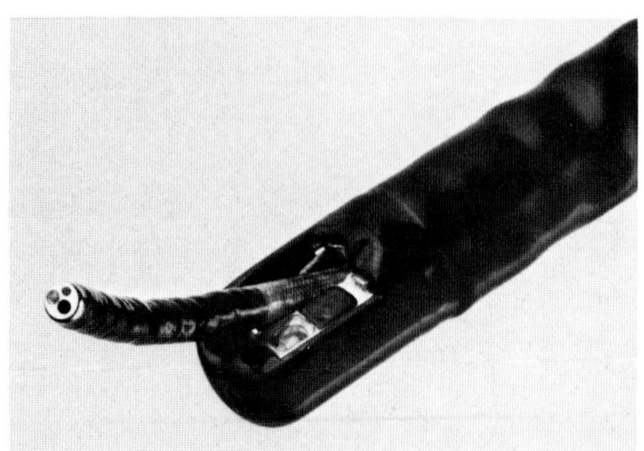

Fig. 45.6 Tip of a 'mother and baby' per-oral choledochoscope

operation can be avoided by percutaneous manipulation once the drain track has matured, using baskets under radiological control or under direct vision with a small choledochoscope.

Patients with these indications are rare, and should be referred to special centres once their general condition has improved.

LAPAROSCOPIC CHOLECYSTOTOMY

Simple removal of gallbladder stones by surgical cholecystotomy was soon replaced by cholecystectomy, in the belief that a diseased stone-containing gallbladder would always give further problems. Extrapolation from data given earlier in this chapter indicates that this is not necessarily the case, at least in patients with a relatively short life expectancy. Laparoscopes are used extensively to perform surgical procedures in the pelvis. Experiments are currently being undertaken to test the feasibility and safety of laparoscopic cholecystotomy.

REFERENCES

Bouchier I A D 1983 Brides of quietness; silent gall stones. British Medical Journal 286: 415–416

Cotton P B 1984 Endoscopic management of bile duct stones; (Apples and Oranges) Gut 25: 587–597

Cotton P B, Vallon A G 1982 Duodenoscopic sphincterotomy for removal of bile duct stones in patients with gall bladders. Surgery 91: 628–630

Escourrou J, Cordova J A, Lazorthes F et al 1984 Early and late complications after endoscopic sphincterotomy for biliary lithiasis, with and without the gallbladder 'in situ'. Gut 25: 598–602

Gracie W A, Ransohoff D F 1982 The natural history of silent gall stones. The innocent gall stone is not a myth. New England Journal of Medicine 307: 798–800

Neoptolemos J P, Carr-Locke D L, Fraser I, Fossard D P 1984 The management of common bile duct calculi by endoscopic sphincterotomy in patients with gallbladders in situ. British Journal of Surgery 71: 69–71

Rosseland A R, Solhaug J H 1984 Early or delayed endoscopic papillotomy (EPT) in gallstone pancreatitis. Annals of Surgery 199: 165–167

Safrany L, Cotton P B 1981 A preliminary report. Urgent duodenoscopic sphincterotomy for acute gall stone pancreatitis. Surgery 89: 424–428

Seifert E, Gail K, Weismuller J 1982 Langzeitresultate nach endoskopischer sphinktertomie, follow-up studie aus 25 centren in der Bundesrepublik. Deutsch Med wochenschr 107: 610–614

Thompson J E, Tompkins R K, Longmire W P 1982 Factors in the management of acute cholangitis. Annals of Surgery 195: 137–145

Vallon A G, Shorvon P J, Cotton P B 1982 Duodenoscopic treatment of acute cholangitis (Abstract) Gut 23:A915

Wenckert A, Robertson B 1966 The natural course of gall stone disease. 11 year review of 781 non operated cases. Gastroenterology 50: 376–381

SECTION 6

Stones in the bile ducts

R. M. Girard, G. Legros

Stones in the common bile duct — surgical approaches

Detection and removal of common bile duct stones as well as prevention of retained and recurrent stones remain a major challenge to contemporary biliary surgeons. The common bile duct is explored in approximately 15% of all cholecystectomies and stones are removed in approximately 65% of these explorations. The incidence of concomitant choledocholithiasis varies between 8 to 15% (Table 46.1). While retained stones after common bile duct exploration were usually reported in the range of 4 to 7% (Way et al 1972, Bartlett 1972, Glenn 1974, Bergdahl & Holmlund 1976), the adjunct of routine post-exploratory cholangiography and/or choledochoscopy has contributed to a decreased incidence of less than 5% (Nora et al 1977, Berci et al 1978, Kappes et al 1982, Dayton et al 1984, LeQuesne 1980).

ORIGIN OF CHOLEDOCHOLITHIASIS

It is generally accepted that the majority of common bile duct stones form originally in the gallbladder and later pass down through the cystic duct into the common bile duct. Usually patients with choledocholithiasis also have cholelithiasis but when they do not the gallbladder almost always shows chronic inflammatory change suggesting that it previously contained stones. Stones may also form primarily in the common bile duct and, when found in patients with congenital absence of the gallbladder, provide an absolute proof of their origin. However proving that a stone had its origin in the common duct in the presence of a gallbladder is difficult.

The incidence of primary common duct stones is controversial and varies from 4% (Saharia et al 1977) to 56% (Madden 1973). Madden defined them as solitary ovoid, light brown in colour, soft and easily crushable. More than 50% of primary stones in this study were noted at cholecystectomy and 21% of gallbladders contained no stones. However, Saharia et al (1977) classified patients as having primary stones if they met all the following criteria: previous cholecystectomy with or without common duct exploration; at least a two-year asymptomatic period after initial biliary tract surgery; presence of soft, friable, light brown stones or sludge in the common duct and absence of a long cystic duct or biliary stricture due to previous surgery.

CLINICAL FEATURES

The natural history of choledocholithiasis is unpredictable. Small stones may pass spontaneously into the duodenum without causing symptoms or they may temporarily obstruct the pancreatic duct, induce an episode of pancreatitis and then pass into the duodenum with relief of symptoms. Stones that do not pass spontaneously may reside in the bile duct for long symptom free periods and then suddenly precipitate an episode of jaundice or cholangitis. Clinical manifestations are manifold, ranging from an absence of symptoms and signs to acute obstructive suppurative cholangitis. Most frequently common bile duct stones are an unanticipated finding during elective cholecystectomy for gallstones. Symptoms can be non-specific and result in general ill health, nausea and fever and are usually the result of complications, the most common being obstruction of the bile duct.

If stones obstruct the common duct and the bile becomes infected, acute cholangitis ensues. The classic triad of fever, chills and jaundice leads to the suspicion of choledocholithiasis and, when associated with known cholelithiasis, the diagnosis is almost certain. When this triad is associated with hypotension and mental confusion, it confirms the presence of an acute obstructive suppurative cholangitis with impending bacteraemic shock.

If a stone obstructs the common bile duct in the absence of infected bile, asymptomatic jaundice, often fluctuating, will ensue and in many patients there will be spontaneous complete resolution. This will happen if, as ductal dilatation develops, the stone floats back up the common bile duct and away from the narrow distal end as oedema subsides; thus it should not be assumed that the common duct is free of stones when jaundice clears. However, occasionally jaundice is relieved because the stone indeed passes into the duodenum. Should incomplete obstruction persist for years before a definitive diagnosis is made and therapy instituted secondary biliary cirrhosis with hepatic failure and portal hypertension may develop.

Pancreatitis (Ch. 43) is the second most frequent complication of choledocholithiasis whereas choledocho-enteric fistula and common duct stricture are uncommon.

PREOPERATIVE DIAGNOSIS

As the diagnosis of choledocholithiasis is usually made at operation by careful inspection, palpation, and importantly operative cholangiography, routine preoperative radiological investigation of the biliary tree is unnecessary (DenBesten & Doty 1981). In most patients, preoperative indicators of choledocholithiasis such as age, duration of the disease and a careful history suggestive of obstruction or pancreatitis, rather than expensive preoperative studies, should alert the surgeon to the need for accurate intra-operative assessment.

The jaundiced patient presents a different problem. Even when there is known cholelithiasis, the presence or absence of obstruction and the nature of the obstructing lesion must be determined prior to laparotomy. Although ultrasonography infrequently detects common duct stones, it has evolved as the primary screening examination because of its reliability to demonstrate gallbladder stones and to detect dilated bile ducts (Thomas et al 1982). Evidence of duct dilatation at ultrasonography is almost always indicative of obstruction but failure to detect dilated ducts does not rule out choledocholithiasis.

If bile duct dilatation is clearly identified in a patient with gallstones, preoperative evaluation may be judged adequate. However, the ideal is to display more accurately the degree, site and cause of obstruction. Either percutaneous or endoscopic cholangiography are usually successful in this respect.

Our approach to the investigation of the jaundiced patient with suspected choledocholithiasis is to attempt to confirm the presence of gallstones and eliminate other causes of obstruction. If dilated ducts are demonstrated by ultrasonography in patients with known choledocholithiasis, whether associated with previous pancreatitis, transient jaundice or cholangitis, we proceed with surgery; however in jaundiced patients with cholelithiasis where other causes of obstruction cannot be excluded, percutaneous cholangiography is performed.

This will usually confirm the diagnosis but if doubt remains endoscopic cholangiography may be undertaken in addition. Endoscopic retrograde cholangiopancreatography is preferred to percutaneous cholangiography in the post-cholecystectomy situation (Ch. 55), since in this circumstance, pathology unrelated to the biliary tract may be present and information available from oesophagogastroduodenoscopy and biopsy or retrograde pancreatography may be important.

INDICATIONS FOR COMMON BILE DUCT EXPLORATION AT CHOLECYSTECTOMY

The purpose of common bile duct exploration for choledocholithiasis is to detect and remove all stones within the bile duct system as safely as possible. It is however not without risk. While cholecystectomy alone may be performed with little morbidity, and a mortality of less than 0.5%, the addition of an exploration of the bile duct increases the morbidity and mortality may rise by three to seven times (Table 46.2). Indeed common bile duct exploration is currently the most important factor in influencing the morbidity and mortality of cholecystectomy since the procedure is more often necessary in patients of advanced age and consequently with associated diseases. In addition the longer duration of operation and the increase in sepsis in patients with common duct stones influence morbidity.

Thus it is desirable that *all those and only those* with choledocholithiasis should have bile duct exploration at cholecystectomy. Accurate diagnosis is therefore essential. In the past, many patients were selected for bile duct exploration on the basis of clinical and operative findings such as a previous history of jaundice or pancreatitis, a dilated common bile duct, a single faceted stone in the gallbladder or multiple small gallstones. There are important observations which should alert the surgeon to the possibility of choledocholithiasis but the use of these criteria alone to predict the presence of common duct stones has led to negative choledochotomy in a high percentage of patients (Way et al 1972, Kakos et al 1972). Clearly, the decision to explore the common bile duct must be based on the most accurate methods to confirm choledocholithiasis.

Indications for common bile duct exploration

The absolute indications for common bile duct exploration are: 1. palpable stones in the common bile duct; 2. jaundice with cholangitis; 3. a stone visualized at intra-operative cholangiography and 4. preoperative radiographic demonstration of choledocholithiasis.

Palpation of the common bile duct is often underestimated as it is the most reliable indication for choledochotomy, having an accuracy of 98% if a stone is judged palpable (Way et al 1972, Kakos et al 1972). Palpation should be performed from the liver hilum to the papilla after a Kocher maneouvre. Obstructive jaundice with fever and chills is indicative of either cholangitis or acute cholecystitis. If patients with acute cholecystitis are excluded, this triad will be associated with choledocholithiasis in approximately 97% of the patients (Way et al 1972).

For the non-jaundiced patient, intraoperative cholangiography (Ch. 27) is, with palpation of stones, the most reliable determinant of the presence of choledocholithiasis and should be performed routinely at cholecystectomy (Tompkins & Pitt 1982, Doyle et al 1982, Stubbs et al 1983). Its accuracy is between 85 and 98%. When technically satisfactory, the incidence of false positive and false negative examinations are 4 and 0.2% respectively (Stark & Loughry 1980). The main reasons to perform routine intraoperative cholangiography are: exclusion from common bile duct exploration of patients who have clinical indications for choledochotomy, yet may not harbour stones at the time of surgery; detection of unsuspected common duct stones in 3 to 7% of patients undergoing cholecystectomy (Tompkins & Pitt 1982); pre-exploratory identification of the number and location of bile duct stones and their size; visualization of the ampullary region and biliary anatomy. For these reasons, when technically possible, we perform cystic duct cholangiography on every patient prior to choledochotomy.

Specific diagnostic tests used preoperatively to demonstrate ductal stones should not be employed routinely in patients with proven gallstones. However, demonstration of choledocholithiasis by preoperative percutaneous or endoscopic cholangiography should be an absolute indication for common bile duct exploration since the accuracy rate for both investigations is greater than 90% (Thomas et al 1982).

Other intraoperative indications based on positive ultrasonography or intraoperative manometry are discussed in Ch. 28, 30).

Technical considerations

Routine exploration of the common bile duct should be through a supraduodenal choledochotomy (Ch. 52) and the transduodenal route should be reserved for patients in whom stones cannot be readily removed from above. Although impacted stones at the ampulla may be broken down and removed by a supraduodenal approach, they should probably be removed by means of a transduodenal sphincteroplasty (Ch. 53) since this is less traumatic in such circumstances.

The only reliable method to confirm complete clearance of stone from the biliary tree is post-exploratory choledochoscopy (Ch. 29) or cholangiography. The value of choledochoscopy has been confirmed by many (Nora et al 1977, Berci et al 1978, Kappes et al 1982, Dayton et al 1984). Post-exploratory cholangiography can also be used and should be obtained before closure of the abdomen not only because it can locate occasional missed stones but also since it may reveal unsuspected disruption of the biliary ductal system. While often regarded as unreliable because of the failure of contrast material to enter the duodenum and the difficulty of eliminating air bubbles, post-exploratory cholangiography can be carried out reliably with attention to detail. Myat et al (1973) described a reliable technique which does not involve suture of the choledochotomy before post-exploratory films are obtained (Ch. 52). A small balloon catheter is introduced proximally and distally into the choledochus as the film is being taken after the introduction of the contrast material. Post-exploratory choledochoscopy or cholangiography are mandatory in all patients following exploration of the common bile duct.

Following exploration a T-tube (at least 14 French gauge) is left within the common bile duct so as to permit postoperative cholangiography and percutaneous extraction of retained stones if necessary (Ch. 48).

In addition to routine post-exploratory choledochoscopy or cholangiography, the selective use of biliary enteric drainage procedures is another method of decreasing the incidence of subsequently symptomatic retained stones (Ch. 53, 54). While we do not recommend routine biliary enteric decompression at initial operation it should be carefully considered in patients with one or more of the following:

1. multiple or primary duct stones, particularly in dilated ducts in elderly patients;
2. one or several large stones within a dilated duct.

If these conditions pertain in an elderly or poor risk patient then choledochoduodenostomy or transduodenal sphincteroplasty may avoid re-exploration. Other indications are:

3. irretrievable intrahepatic stones;
4. proven ampullary stenosis;
5. an impacted ampullary stone.

Choledochoduodenostomy (Ch. 54) and transduodenal sphincteroplasty (Ch. 53) both have their advocates. When the common duct is less than 1.5 cm diameter in a young, low-risk patient with a solitary impacted ampullary stone, sphincteroplasty is preferable. However, in elderly and high-risk patients with dilated ducts, choledochoduodenostomy is the procedure of choice (Thomas et al 1971) (see below).

Results of clinical experience

We have reviewed the course of 819 consecutive patients who underwent cholecystectomy and bile duct exploration for presumed choledocholithiasis at Maisonneuve-Rosemont Hospital between April 1971 and April 1982. They constituted 11% of 7436 patients who had cholecystectomy during this period and common duct stones were recovered in 588 patients (71.8%) (Table 46.1). The age and sex distribution of the patients are shown in Table 46.2. The most reliable clinical indicator of choledocholithiasis was jaundice associated with chills and fever (92%). The accuracy of preoperative intravenous cholangiography was 70%

Table 46.1 Incidence of choledocholithiasis in patients with gallstones

Authors	Total cases of gallstones	Explorations of common duct %	Explorations yielding stones %	Overall incidence of common duct stones %
Way et al 1972	952	21	65	14
Kakos et al 1972	753	25	62	15
McSherry & Glenn 1980	8791	15.6	59.7	9.3
Hampson et al 1981	2889	15	51	7.8
Doyle et al 1982	4000	22	52.5	11.5
Lygidakis 1983	3710	11.6	80	9.4
Coelho et al 1984	908	21	72	14.9
Own series	7436	11	71.8	7.9
Total	29439	15.3	62.5	9.6

Table 46.2 Age and sex distribution of patients who had common duct exploration

Age (years)	Number of Patients Men	Women	Total
0–19	2	21	23
20–29	12	97	109
30–39	31	58	89
40–49	61	74	135
50–59	57	105	162
60–69	86	85	171
70–79	42	63	105
>80	5	20	25
Total	296	523	819

while preoperative percutaneous or endoscopic cholangiography was 100% accurate. Intraoperative findings that proved most reliable were palpation of common duct stones (96%) and positive cholangiography which was 88% accurate in the demonstration of stones.

The surgical procedures performed are shown in Table 46.3. Post-exploratory T-tube cholangiography was done intraoperatively in 637 patients. The examination was in all respects normal in 519 of these and in 56, despite an absence of flow of contrast into the duodenum, there was no filling defect and the appearances were accepted as indicating a stone free duct. In 43 patients the examination revealed a stone which was removed in 31, whereas in 12 stones were abandoned within the ducts. Subsequent postoperative examination shows a missed stone in 19 cases. Since 1978 operative choledochoscopy has been used and

Table 46.3 Surgical procedures performed in addition to cholecystectomy

	Number	%
Choledochotomy with T-tube drainage	685	83.6
Choledochotomy with T-tube drainage and other intra-abdominal procedures	80	9.8
Choledochotomy with transduodenal sphincteroplasty	29	3.5
Choledochotomy with choledochoduodenostomy	25	3.1

in a consecutive series of 102 patients only one was subsequently found to have a retained stone.

Of the 819 patients, 11 died (1.3%). This mortality rate is significantly higher than the 0.36% mortality rate recorded for 6617 cholecystectomies without common bile duct exploration performed during the same period. This confirms the increased risk associated with choledochotomy as reported by others (Table 46.4). The mortality rate was higher in patients with a positive duct exploration (1.5%) than in those with negative exploration of the duct (0.9%) and increased with age (Table 46.5). All patients who died had either jaundice and/or acute pancreatitis at the time of operation. The major cause of death was cardiac (seven patients). A massive haemorrhage from a duodenal ulcer occurred in the eighth patient. The remaining three died of a perforated duodenal ulcer associated with acute pancreatitis, bacteraemic shock and a prolonged biliary fistula respectively.

The morbidity rate (4% in 6617 cholecystectomies) increased to 14% in patients with common bile duct exploration. The incidence of complications was higher in positive than in negative duct exploration (15.3% vs 10.8%) and increased with age (Table 46.6). The most frequent complications were retained stones and pulmonary in nature (Table 46.7). 37 patients (4.5%) had retained stones shown on the postoperative T-tube cholangiography. Five (2.2%) of the 231 patients with negative choledochotomy had retained stones whereas they were found in 32 (5.4%) of 558 patients with initial choledocholithotomy (positive exploration). Moreover six patients had residual or recurrent stones diagnosed nine months to eight years after the initial operation giving an overall incidence of retained and recurrent stones of 5.25%.

Of the 37 patients with retained stones, spontaneous evacuation confirmed at T-tube cholangiography occurred in seven at intervals from one to seven months after operation. 14 were successfully extracted via the T-tube tract and nine underwent surgical choledocholithotomy three weeks to six months after the initial operation. In five patients, a stone was abandoned in the bile duct and two further patients were lost to follow-up.

Table 46.4 Mortality of biliary surgery for calculous diseases

Authors	Number of patients	Overall mortality %	Mortality: Cholecystectomy alone %	Mortality: Cholecystectomy with common bile duct exploration %
Bartlett & Waddel 1958	2243	1.1	0.6	1.8
Chetlin & Elliot 1971	1421	1.5	1.0	4.8
Vellacott & Powell 1979	630	2.2	1.0	7.4
McSherry & Glenn 1980	10775	1.2	0.6	4.1
Doyle et al 1982	4000	2.8	1.8	6.6
Own series	7436	0.47	0.36	1.3

Table 46.5 Age related mortality in common bile duct exploration

Age (years)	Number of patients	Number of deaths	%
<50	356	1	0.3
50–70	333	7	2.1
>70	130	3	2.3
Total	819	11	1.3

Table 46.6 Age related morbidity in common bile exploration

Age (years)	Number of patients	Number of patients with complications	%
< 50	356	36	10
50–70	333	43	12.9
> 70	130	36	27.7
Total	819	115	14

Table 46.7 Complications in 819 patients with exploration of the common bile duct

	Number
Retained stone	37
Pulmonary complications	25
Wound infection	23
Wound dehiscence	4
Biliary fistula	20
Intra-abdominal abscess	4
Haemobilia	1
Haematemesis (DU)	1

POSTCHOLECYSTECTOMY CHOLEDOCHOLITHIASIS

Incidence

Although most initial operations for gallstone disease with or without demonstrated choledocholithiasis are curative, a small percentage of patients is found at some later date to have additional stones in the bile duct. The overall incidence of residual and recurrent calculi is estimated at 1 to 2% in patients operated upon for calculous biliary tract disease (Glenn 1974, White & Bordley 1978). While retained or overlooked calculi following cholecystectomy without common bile duct exploration are rare (Bergdahl & Holmlund 1976), their incidence following cholecystectomy with concomitant common bile duct exploration is estimated to range from 1.3 to 7% (Bartlett 1972, Way et al 1972, Glenn 1974, Nora et al 1977, Feliciano et al 1980, Rattner & Warshaw 1981) with higher frequency in positive than in negative exploration. After a second operation on the biliary tract, a recurrence rate of approximately 20% has been reported (Way 1973, Saharia et al 1977) with even higher rates following subsequent reoperation (Allen et al 1981).

Prevention

Prevention of retained and recurrent bile duct stones is a very important goal and there is every reason to believe that most such stones can be prevented. Retained calculi are either knowingly left in the ductal system (abandoned stones) or inadvertently discovered on postoperative T-tube cholangiography thus representing a failure in detection at the time of operation. Bergdahl & Holmlund (1976) reported that stones were retained in their patients for the following reasons:

1. lodged inextricably in the intrahepatic duct (50%);
2. overlooked because of technically inadequate post-exploratory cholangiography (23%);
3. not visualized despite good quality post-exploratory cholangiography (19%);
4. misinterpreted as air bubbles on post-exploratory cholangiography (8%).

The incidence of retained stones is almost certainly less if better techniques of post-exploratory cholangiography (Myat et al 1973) (Ch. 52) and post-exploratory choledochoscopy are used. The best treatment for retained and recurrent stones is undoubtedly: prevention through routine cystic duct cholangiography to discover the 3 to 7% common duct stones unsuspected at cholecystectomy; knowledge of when and how to explore the common bile duct; routine post-exploratory choledochoscopy or cholangiography; and finally the selective use of adjunctive biliary enteric drainage procedures when indicated.

Treatment

Contrary to practice in previous years, when reoperation was usually necessary to remove retained or recurrent stones, therapeutic alternatives have evolved over the last two decades. These include:

1. mechanical non-operative extraction through the T-tube tract (Ch. 48);
2. dissolution of stones by infusion of various solvents into the T-tube (Ch. 49);
3. stone extraction after endoscopic sphincterotomy (Ch. 47).

Choice of management is determined by clinical presentation, the condition of the patient, available expertise and the presence or absence of a T-tube (Ch. 50).

Retained stones in the presence of a T-tube

In the absence of biliary obstruction or infection, no treatment should be attempted for four to six weeks. During this period 10 to 20% of retained stones found on post-operative cholangiography can be expected to pass spontaneously into the duodenum and no further treatment will be required (Way 1973). Occasionally a radiological artifact (pseudocalculus) strongly suggests the presence of a stone which is then not seen on repeated examination.

If after four to six weeks the stone persists, active treatment should be instituted. Because of its high success rate, low morbidity and mortality, non-operative mechanical extraction is currently the treatment of choice in this situation. A success rate of 95% has been reported with a morbidity of only 4 to 5% (Mazzariello 1978, Burhenne 1980). When complications do occur they can be treated medically in most instances and only 0.2% require surgery (Mazzariello 1978) (Ch. 48).

If mechanical extraction fails, chemical dissolution should be considered (Ch. 49). Probably the most effective agent is mono-octanoin and a success rate of 66% has been reported (Hofman et al 1981). Although from a theoretical point of view chemical dissolution is the most attractive method of solving the problem, the authors reserve it only for elderly or poor-risk patients with retained radiolucent stones which cannot be extracted percutaneously. Although side effects are few, the long hospitalization required for successful dissolution and its low efficacy limit a more liberal use of the approach.

When retained stones have not been removed mechanically it is the authors' practice in young and low risk patients to proceed to reoperation eight to 10 weeks after initial surgery. Occasionally it may be necessary to reoperate sooner if biliary obstruction or infection is not adequately controlled. In patients with high surgical risk dissolution through the T-tube should be attempted first and, if unsuccessful, endoscopic sphincterotomy employed (Ch. 47).

Retained or recurrent stones in the absence of a T-tube

For the patient without a T-tube in place, the choice of therapy lies between reoperation and stone extraction by means of endoscopic sphincterotomy (Ch. 50).

In expert hands endoscopic sphincterotomy achieves a success rate of approximately 90% (Safrany 1978, Cotton & Vallon 1981). Complication rates vary from 7 to 10% with a mortality of 0.5 to 2% (Safrany & Cotton 1982). Haemorrhage, cholangitis, pancreatitis, retroperitoneal perforation and stone impaction are the most frequent complications and it is in this group of patients that the mortality is highest. Emergency surgical intervention is required in nearly one-third of the patients developing complications and up to 50% of these patients die (Cotton & Vallon 1981). The long-term results, efficacy and possible late complications of endoscopic sphincterotomy are difficult to evaluate since there is a paucity of reports regarding long-term follow-up. Nevertheless in many centres the technique is increasingly replacing surgery for the treatment of retained and recurrent stones (Allen et al 1981, Ghazi & McSherry 1984). While endoscopic sphincterotomy may be preferable to surgery in elderly and high risk patients, there is no doubt that it is a procedure which carries risk. Its use in young and fit patients remains controversial (Cotton & Vallon 1981). Moreover there seems little justification for endoscopic sphincterotomy in those patients with recurrent or retained primary common duct stones, retained impacted stones, large stones (>2 cm) or retained stones with a long-segment ampullary stenosis in whom concurrent ductal drainage procedure is indicated.

On the other hand, it is important to recognize that reoperation on the common bile duct for retained stones is possible with a mortality rate of less than 2% (Girard & Legros 1981). Thus the immediate risks of surgery and endoscopy are not dissimilar, and it is necessary to balance the convenience and simplicity of endoscopic sphincterotomy against the unknown risk of longer-term complications. This argument is further developed in Chapter 50. As far as our present practice is concerned the authors consider that reoperation is still the treatment of choice in the majority of patients with retained stones. The success, morbidity and mortality rates of surgery are comparable to those of endoscopic sphincterotomy which appears preferable for patients who are poor surgical risks.

The most common surgical procedure for treatment of retained stones is choledocholithotomy, choledochoscopy, placement of a T-tube and completion cholangiography. This procedure is probably adequate for the majority of patients at second operation and indeed the authors' overall failure rate following choledochotomy for residual recurrent stones was only 3.2%. However, others have reported failure rates as high as 18 and 33% (Saharia et al

1977, Allen et al 1981). Because of this some (Allen et al 1981, Lygidakis 1982a) recommend a biliary enteric drainage procedure in all patients with previous choledocholithotomy. The authors' view is that the addition of such a procedure probably results in an additional risk and that the surgeon should identify those patients in whom the benefit to risk ratio for drainage procedures is high enough to warrant it. Several authors (Saharia et al 1977, DenBesten & Doty 1981, Tompkins & Pitt 1982) emphasize that concomitant biliary drainage should not be carried out as mandatory in all patients with retained stones. The authors agree with this but do carry out biliary enteric drainage at reoperation if any of the following occur:

1. stricture of the distal bile duct or sphincter of Oddi
2. marked dilatation of the duct (2 cm or more)
3. multiple or primary bile duct stones
4. inability to remove all stones from the duct
5. a third operation.

Either transduodenal sphincteroplasty, choledochoduodenostomy or choledochojejunostomy are effective (Jones 1978, Johnson & Harding Rains 1978, Braasch et al 1980). Sphincteroplasty allows direct inspection of the papilla and extraction of an impacted stone but is not adequate to treat a long stricture of the distal duct. It is the treatment of choice in patients with a duct smaller than 1.5 cm in diameter to avoid possible stricture formation at the anastomosis but carries a greater risk of postoperative pancreatitis. Side-to-side or end-to-side choledochoduodenostomy, or end-to-side Roux-en-Y choledochojejunostomy are suitable for common ducts larger than 1.5 cm and offer better decompression of a very large duct. The mortality rate of choledochoduodenostomy is lower than that attending transduodenal sphincteroplasty and it has been shown to be a safe and simple operation with low morbidity and mortality especially in elderly patients (Schein & Gliedman 1981, Lygidakis 1982b) (Ch. 54). Occasionally recurrent or primary stones are seen in patients with dilated ducts and a widely patent sphincter. In such cases, which have also been reported after endoscopic papillotomy, side-to-side choledochoduodenostomy or end-to-side Roux-en-Y choledochojejunostomy is necessary.

Results of clinical experience with reoperation

The course of all patients who had a reoperation for retained or recurrent choledocholithiasis at Maisonneuve-Rosemont Hospital between January 1969 and April 1984 was reviewed. 83 patients underwent a total of 86 operations: 83 were secondary operations and three patients needed a third operation. Common bile duct stones were confirmed in all patients before reoperation by either intravenous cholangiography, percutaneous cholangiography, endoscopic cholangiography or postoperative T-tube cholangiography. 74 associated conditions which can be identified with increased operative risk were present in 44 patients (Table 46.8).

There were 59 female and 24 male patients (age range 20 to 86 years; mean 57 years). 42 of the 86 reoperations were performed in patients over the age of 60. The initial biliary operations performed are shown in Table 46.9. The mean interval between the first and second operation was 81 months (range: one month to 20 years) (Table 46.10) and the interval between the second and third operation in the three patients was 2, 48 and 72 months.

There were three types of bile duct reoperation: choledocholithotomy with T-tube drainage (62 patients); choledocholithotomy with side-to-side choledochoduodenostomy (15 patients); choledocholithotomy with transduodenal sphincteroplasty (six patients). Choledocholithotomy with T-tube drainage in one patient and choledocholithotomy

Table 46.8 Risk factors in 83 patients submitted to reoperation for retained or recurrent choledocholithiasis

	Number
Cardiac atherosclerosis	18
Septic cholangitis	15
Obesity	10
High blood pressure	8
Chronic pulmonary obstructive disease	7
Diabetes	5
Acute pancreatitis	5
Atrial fibrillation	3
Posthepatic cirrhosis	1
Chronic renal failure	1

Table 46.9 Initial biliary operation performed

Type of operation	Number
Cholecystectomy with operative cholangiography	6
Cholecystectomy without operative cholangiography	47
Cholecystectomy with choledocholithotomy	27
Cholecystectomy with choledocholithotomy and sphincterotomy	3

Table 46.10 Interval between first and second operation for retained or recurrent stones

Type of operation	Total	<1 year	1–5 years	>5 years	Mean interval (months)
Cholecystectomy with operative cholangiography	6	1	3	2	53
Cholecystectomy without operative cholangiography	47	10	12	25	98
Cholecystectomy with choledocholithotomy	27	13	7	7	46
Cholecystectomy with choledocholithotomy and sphincterotomy	3	0	0	3	152

Table 46.11 Complications of 86 common bile duct reoperations

Type	Number of complications
Lung atelectasis	2
Partial wound disruption	1
Stitch abscess	1
Wound infection	1
Pancreatic fistula	1
Total	6 (6.9%)

with side-to-side choledochoduodenostomy in two patients were performed at a third operation. Choledochoscopy was used during the last 15 operations performed since 1979.

The average hospital stay was 9.3 days (range: five to 24 days) and was approximately the same (9.7 days) for patients over 60 years of age. No patient died. There were only six minor complications and none of them necessitated urgent surgery (Table 46.11). In 42 reoperations performed in patients over 60 years of age, there were two (4.7%) complications (wound infection and pancreatic fistula). It is noteworthy that there was not a single complication in the last 15 operations. Two patients (3.2%) of the 62 who had choledocholithotomy with T-tube drainage developed recurrent bile duct stones four and five years after a second operation and side-to-side choledochoduodenostomy was performed. To date, no patient has needed a fourth operation.

Taking our experience with that of other recently reported series there were 13 deaths among 766 patients submitted for reoperation for recurrent bile duct stones (Table 46.12). In one of these series (McSherry & Glenn 1980), 331 patients were reported in whom choledocholithotomy was carried out for retained or recurrent stones. Of these patients, 2.1% died but, if those with cholangitis and acute pancreatitis were excluded (as is done by many endoscopists performing sphincterotomy), only four patients (1.2%) died after secondary choledocholithotomy.

These results show that the overall mortality rate for retained or recurrent stones is probably less than 2%, with most deaths occurring in elderly patients. This mortality rate is comparable with that of endoscopic sphincterotomy.

Table 46.12 Mortality rate of biliary reoperation for retained or recurrent bile duct stones

Authors	Number of operations	Mortality rate
Stuart & Hoerr (1972)	24	0
Freund et al (1977)	16	0
Saharia et al (1977)	30	0
Jones (1978)	22	0
Kaminski et al (1979)	26	1 (3.8%)
McSherry & Glenn (1980)	341	7 (2.1%)
Allen et al (1981)	47	1 (2.1%)
Choi et al (1982)	34	1 (2.9%)
Lygidakis (1982b)	116	2 (1.7%)
De Almeida et al (1984)	24	1 (4.1%)
Own series	86	0
Total	776	13 (1.7%)

CONCLUSION

The goal of surgeons performing common bile duct exploration for calculous disease is to explore all and only all patients with choledocholithiasis, to detect and remove all stones within the bile ducts safely and to prevent retained and recurrent stones.

Before exploring a common duct, surgeons must make accurate diagnosis of choledocholithiasis which should be confirmed by pre-exploratory intraoperative cholangiography. The only reliable methods to confirm complete clearance of stones from the biliary tree at operation are post-exploratory choledochoscopy and/or cholangiography and these are mandatory procedures in all patients. Biliary enteric drainage procedures should be used selectively when indicated.

Patients with residual or recurrent bile duct stones should be managed on an individual basis depending on the general condition of the patient, available expertise and the presence or absence of a T-tube. The discovery of a retained or recurrent bile duct stone after biliary tract surgery is a signal for a thorough evaluation and subsequent decision. For a further discussion of the factors concerned, the reader is referred to Ch. 50.

REFERENCES

Allen B, Shapiro W, Way L W 1981 Management of recurrent and residual common duct stones. American Journal of Surgery 142: 41–47

Bartlett M K 1972 Retained and recurrent common duct stones. American Surgeon 38: 63–68

Bartlett M K, Waddel W R 1958 Indications for common-duct exploration. Evaluation in 1000 cases. The New England Journal of Medicine 258: 164–167

Berci G, Shore J M, Morgenstern L, Hamlin J A 1978 Choledochoscopy and operative fluorocholangiography in the prevention of retained bile duct stones. World Journal of Surgery 2: 411–427

Bergdahl L, Holmlund D E W 1976 Retained bile duct stones. Acta Chirurgica Scandinavica 142: 145–149

Braasch J W, Fender H R, Boneval M M 1980 Refractory primary common bile duct stone disease. American Journal of Surgery 139: 526–530

Burhenne H J 1980 Percutaneous extraction of retained biliary tract stones: 661 patients. American Journal of Roentgenology 134: 889–898

Chetlin S H, Elliot D W 1971 Biliary bacteremia. Archives of Surgery 102: 303–307

Choi T K, Lee N W, Wong J, Ong G B 1982 Extraperitoneal sphincteroplasty for residual stones. An update. Annals of Surgery 196: 26–29

Coelho J C U, Buffara M, Pozzobon C E, Altenburg F L, Artigas G V 1984 Incidence of common bile duct stones in patients with acute and chronic cholecystitis. Surgery, Gynecology and Obstetrics 158: 76–80

Cotton P B, Vallon A G 1981 British experience with duodenoscopic

sphincterotomy for removal of bile duct stones. British Journal of Surgery 68: 373–375
Dayton M T, Conter R, Tompkins R K 1984 Incidence of complications with operative choledochoscopy. American Journal of Surgery 147: 139–145
De Almeida A M, Cruz A G, Aldeia F J 1984 Side-to-side choledochoduodenostomy in the management of choledocholithiasis and associated disease. Facts and fiction. American Journal of Surgery 147: 253–259
DenBesten L, Doty J E 1981 Pathogenesis and management of choledocholithiasis. Surgical Clinics of North America 61: 893–907
Doyle P J, Ward-McQuaid J N, McEwen-Smith A 1982 The value of routine peroperative cholangiography: a report of 4000 cholecystectomies. British Journal of Surgery 69: 617–619
Feliciano D V, Mattox K L, Jordan G L 1980 The value of choledochoscopy in exploration of the common bile duct. Annals of Surgery 191: 649–654
Freund H, Charuzi P, Granit G, Berlatzky Y, Eyal Z 1977 Choledochoduodenostomy in the treatment of benign biliary tract disease. Archives of Surgery 112: 1032–1034
Ghazi A, McSherry C K 1984 Endoscopic retrograde cholangiopancreatography and sphincterotomy. Annals of Surgery 193: 150–154
Girard R M, Legros G 1981 Retained and recurrent bile duct stones. Surgical or nonsurgical removal? Annals of Surgery 199: 21–27
Glenn F 1974 Retained calculi within the biliary ductal system. Annals of Surgery 179: 528–539
Hampson L G, Fried G M, Stets J, Ayeni O R, Bourdon-Conochie F 1981 Common bile duct exploration: indications and results. Canadian Journal of Surgery 24: 455–457
Hofmann A F, Schmack B, Thistle J L, Babayan V K 1981 Clinical experience with monooctanoin for dissolution of bile duct stones. An uncontrolled multicenter trial. Digestive Diseases and Sciences 26: 954–955
Johnson A G, Harding Rains A J 1978 Prevention and treatment of recurrent bile duct stones by choledochoduodenostomy. World Journal of Surgery 2: 487–496
Jones S A 1978 The prevention and treatment of recurrent bile duct stones by transduodenal sphincteroplasty. World Journal of Surgery 2: 473–485
Kakos G S, Tompkins R K, Turnipseed W, Zollinger R M 1972 Operative cholangiography during routine cholecystectomy. A review of 3012 cases. Archives of Surgery 104: 484–488
Kaminski D L, Barner H B, Codd J E, Wolfe B M 1979 Evaluation of the results of external choledochoduodenostomy for retained, recurrent or primary common duct stones. American Journal of Surgery 137: 162–166
Kappes S K, Adams M B, Wilson S D 1982 Intraoperative endoscopy. Mandatory for all common duct operations? Archives of Surgery 117: 603–607
Le Quesne L P, Bolton J P 1980 Choledocholithiasis: incidence, diagnosis, and operative procedures. In: Maingot R (ed) Abdominal operations 7th edn, Vol I. Appleton-Century-Crofts, New York, p 1055–1102
Lygidakis N J 1982a A prospective randomised study of recurrent choledocholithiasis. Surgery, Gynecology and Obstetrics 155: 679–684
Lygidakis N J 1982b Surgical approaches to postcholecystectomy choledocholithiasis. Archives of Surgery 117: 481–484
Lygidakis N J 1983 Incidence and significance of primary stones of the common bile duct in choledocholithiasis. Surgery, Gynecology and Obstetrics 157: 434–436
McSherry C K, Glenn F 1980 The incidence and causes of death following surgery for nonmalignant biliary tract disease. Annals of Surgery 191: 271–275
Madden J L 1973 Common duct stones: their origin and surgical management. Surgical Clinics of North America 53: 1095–1113
Mazzariello R M 1978 A fourteen-year experience with nonoperative instrument extraction of retained bile duct stones. World Journal of Surgery 2: 447–455
Myat Thu Ya, Robinson D, Gunn A A 1973 Peroperative cholangiography. British Journal of Surgery 60: 711–712
Nora P F, Berci G, Dorazio R A, Kirshenbaum G, Shore J M, Tompkins R K et al 1977 Operative choledochoscopy. Results of a prospective study in several institutions. American Journal of Surgery 133: 105–110
Rattner D W, Warshaw A L 1981 Impact of choledochoscopy on the management of choledocholithiasis. Experience with 499 common duct explorations at the Massachusetts General Hospital. Annals of Surgery 194: 76–79
Safrany L 1978 Endoscopic treatment of biliary tract disease. An international study. Lancet ii: 983–985
Safrany L, Cotton P B 1982 Endoscopic management of choledocholithiasis. Surgical Clinics of North America 62: 825–836
Saharia P C, Zuidema G D, Cameron J L 1977 Primary common duct stones. Annals of Surgery 185: 598–602
Schein C J, Gliedman M L 1981 Choledochoduodenostomy as an adjunct to choledocholithotomy. Surgery, Gynecology and Obstetrics 152: 797–804
Stark M E, Loughry W 1980 Routine operative cholangiography with cholecystectomy. Surgery, Gynecology and Obstetrics 151: 657–658
Stuart M, Hoerr S O 1972 Late results of side-to-side choledochoduodenostomy and of transduodenal sphincterotomy for benign disorders. A twenty-year comparative study. American Journal of Surgery 123: 67–72
Stubbs R S, McCloy R F, Blumgart L H 1983 Cholelithiasis and cholecystitis: surgical treatment. Clinics in Gastroenterology 122: 179–201
Thomas C G, Nicholson C P, Owen J 1971 Effectiveness of choledochoduodenostomy and transduodenal sphincterotomy in the treatment of benign obstruction of the common duct. Annals of Surgery 173: 845–856
Thomas M J, Pellegrini C A, Way L W 1982 Usefulness of diagnostic tests for biliary obstruction. American Journal of Surgery 144: 102–108
Tompkins R K, Pitt H A 1982 Surgical management of benign lesions of the bile ducts. Current Problems in Surgery 19: 327–398
Vellacott R K, Powell P H 1979 Exploration of the common bile duct. A comparative study. British Journal of Surgery 66: 389–391
Way L W 1973 Retained common duct stones. Surgical Clinics of North America 53: 1139–1147
Way L W, Admirand W H, Dunphy J E 1972 Management of choledocholithiasis. Annals of Surgery 176: 347–359
White T T, Bordley J 1978 One per cent incidence of recurrent gallstones six to eight years after manometric cholangiography. Annals of Surgery 188: 562–569

47

D. L. Carr–Locke

Endoscopic approaches

INTRODUCTION

In the same way that ERCP has transformed the diagnostic approach to suspected biliary problems and jaundice, so endoscopic sphincterotomy (ES), in the ten years since it was first performed in man (Kawai et al 1974, Classen & Demling 1974), has, more than any other therapeutic development, had a dramatic impact on the management of biliary disease in general and the treatment of bile duct stones in particular (Ch. 35). It has undoubtedly influenced surgical decision-making about patients with biliary problems where the technique is readily available and it is, therefore, more than appropriate to discuss this topic in a textbook devoted to 'surgery' of the biliary tract. Although early understandable resistance by surgeons to the concept of endoscopic therapy of bile duct stones ostensibly performed by physicians has, to a great extent, disappeared there is still a great need (Cotton 1984) to define accurately the place of ES and its associated techniques in the management of biliary problems in comparison with previously available and long-established principles of surgical treatment (Ch. 46, 50). A number of variable risk factors are present in all patients with biliary disease which, when combined together as a clinical judgement, allows a decision to be made in favour of one or other mode of therapy. It is the precise documentation of such factors and how they determine outcome from different treatments which needs to be examined carefully in relation to ES and its surgical alternatives and which until now has only been possible by retrospective analysis. A number of randomized clinical trials are currently in progress which are attempting to answer these questions and some preliminary results will be cited.

Interest in ERCP and ES both as a preoperative and definitive therapy for bile duct stones has grown enormously. The author's practice over the last nine years and at present provides a referral rate of over 600 ERCP requests per annum of which more than a quarter are for therapeutic considerations. This has allowed a personal experience of over 700 endoscopic sphincterotomies to date and the views expressed in this chapter are based on this work as well as comments derived from collected reports of recognized experts. Only peroral endoscopic techniques developed from diagnostic ERCP will be considered here and no discussion of peroperative choledochoscopy, percutaneous choledochoscopy, per-laparoscopic biliary procedures nor peroral choledochoscopy will be included although these represent additional endoscopic approaches.

BILE DUCT STONES — GENERAL CONSIDERATIONS

Endoscopic techniques

The endoscopist now offering an ES service for the treatment of bile duct stones must be suitably equipped and have access to a radiology suite providing high quality image intensification and permanent radiographs. The team must be fully cognisant of all the basic procedures and lesser used techniques as well as potential complications and their management and must include medical, nursing and technical endoscopy staff together with radiography and portering personnel, all of whom allow the smooth running of an ERCP/ES session and facilitate any decisions which must be made during an examination.

Details of patient preparation, sedation, use of drugs during endoscopy, endoscope equipment, its handling and disinfection and endoscopic techniques now employed for ERCP and ES have been described in Chapters 20 and 35, but brief mention here of the author's practice will permit clearer interpretation of the clinical data presented. It is essential for the endoscopy staff to explain the nature of the procedure to the patient, outlining the purpose, advantages and possible hazards of the examination and therapy. It will happen occasionally that a severe complication, such as haemorrhage, will occur too rapidly after ES for prolonged explanations to take place with the patient and forewarning, however small the risk, should be mandatory.

The majority of patients undergoing ES, immediately following diagnostic ERCP which delineates the problem

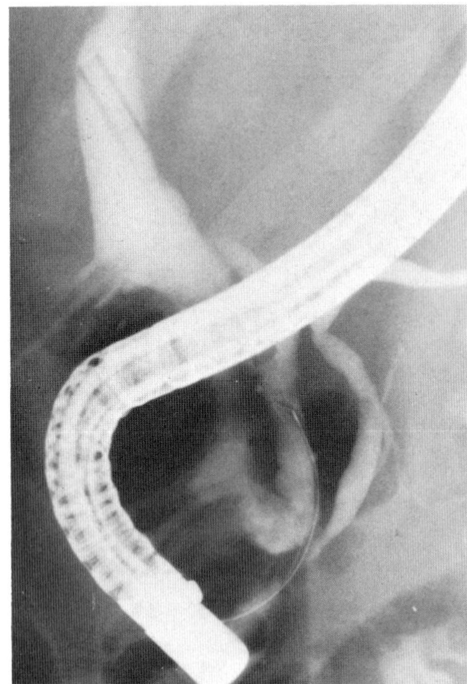

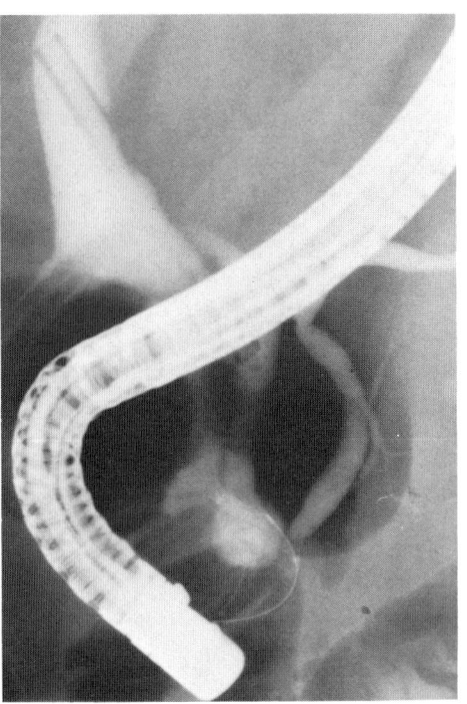

Fig. 47.1 Radiography showing a. sphincterotome in position with tip deeply inserted in bile duct (below T-tube); b. sphincterotome wire fully bowed during performance of sphincterotomy

to be treated and allows accurate placement of instruments within the common bile duct (CBD), will have a standard vertical incision made from the papillary orifice of the CBD in a cephalad direction along the intramural course of the CBD for a variable length (on average 10 to 15 mm) depending on local anatomy, the degree of CBD dilatation and the size of stone to be removed (Fig. 47.1). The incision is produced by the controlled application of a blended cutting/coagulating diathermy current delivered by a power source specifically made for endoscopic use which will not exceed 100 watts and connected to a sphincterotome which has changed little from the original design of Classen & Demling (1974). It is fundamental to good ES technique that complete control of wire tension and diathermy current be maintained at all times whether or not the ES incision is made as a single continuous movement or in incremental steps. More recently developed diathermy power units incorporate a timed/pulsed generator which may be safer. Radiographic confirmation of correct sphincterotome placement is mandatory to avoid pancreatic trauma (Fig. 47.1). Occasionally a 'precut' sphincterotome is needed to initiate ES when the standard instrument cannot be deeply inserted but more often cannulation is prevented by an impacted stone and the author finds the 'needle-knife' more useful in this situation as the intramural common bile duct (CBD) is usually grossly distended and easily incised to form a choledochoduodenal fistulotomy. Patients with Billroth II partial gastrectomy (Fig. 47.2) present special problems to the endoscopist and a number of methods have been described to overcome them when ES is required (Carr-Locke & Cotton 1985).

It is our practice and that of most other centres to attempt stone extraction from the CBD immediately after ES as this decreases the likelihood of subsequent complications due to retained stones and removes the need to repeat the ERCP to check on ductal clearance at a later date. The two accessory instruments used most commonly for this are the Dormia-type basket (Fig. 47.2, 47.3) and the Fogarty-type balloon (Fig 47.4) which although successful in clearing the CBD in over 90% of attempts, are not without difficulty of handling and may produce complications (see below).

It is also possible now to extract stones from the CBD without a preliminary ES either using a balloon dilators (Staritz 1983a) or after the lingual application of glyceryl trinitrate to relax the sphincter of Oddi (Staritz et al 1985) (Fig. 47.5) and both techniques are highly successful for small stones.

In the 10% or less where extraction of stones is incomplete or impossible because of stone number, size or unfavourable bile duct anatomy, and spontaneous passage is thought unlikely, most endoscopists would now insert a nasobiliary catheter (Cotton et al 1979) (Fig. 47.6). This allows temporary bile drainage and permits repeat cholangiography and solvent infusion for dissolution if stone passage has not occurred (Hoffman et al 1981, Allen et al 1985) (see Ch. 49). In some patients surgery will be the most appropriate course of action with either an improved

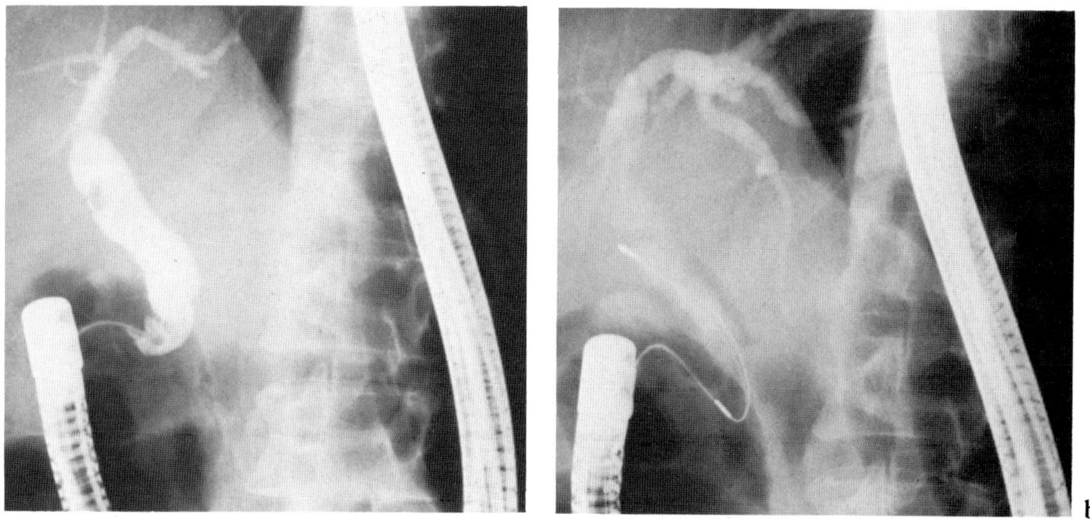

Fig. 47.2 Radiographs showing a. duodenoscope within afferent loop of Billroth II gastrectomy and single bile duct stone; b. basket extraction after ES

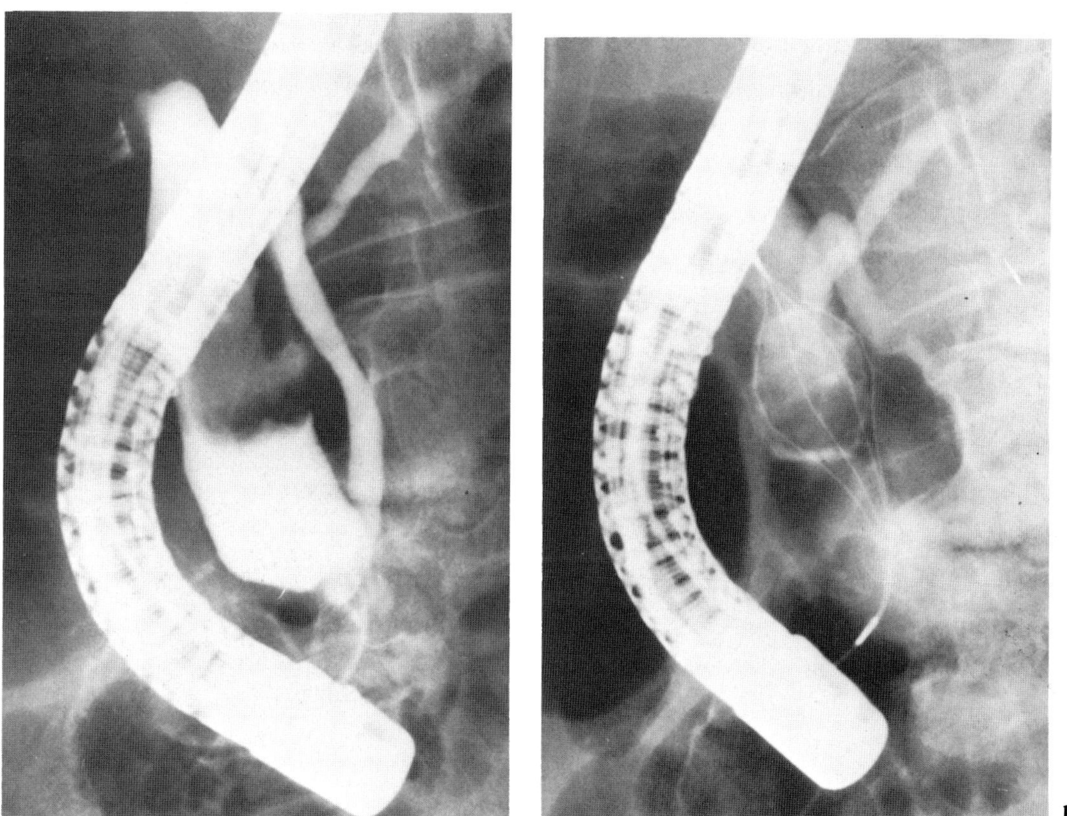

Fig. 47.3 Radiographs showing a. large stone in lower bile duct and b. basket extraction after ES.

general state, in those with adequate bile drainage or, conversely, continuing biliary sepsis and stasis when drainage has not been sufficiently achieved. Mechanical lithotripsy has recently been added to the endoscopic armoury (Staritz 1983b) and provides a welcome improvement to the success in treating large or difficult stones where fragmentation can be achieved (Fig. 47.7). In exceptional circumstances when all endoscopic manoeuvres have failed and surgical intervention is contraindicated the insertion of an endoprosthesis may seem justified to maintain bile flow although no long-term results of this technique are yet available.

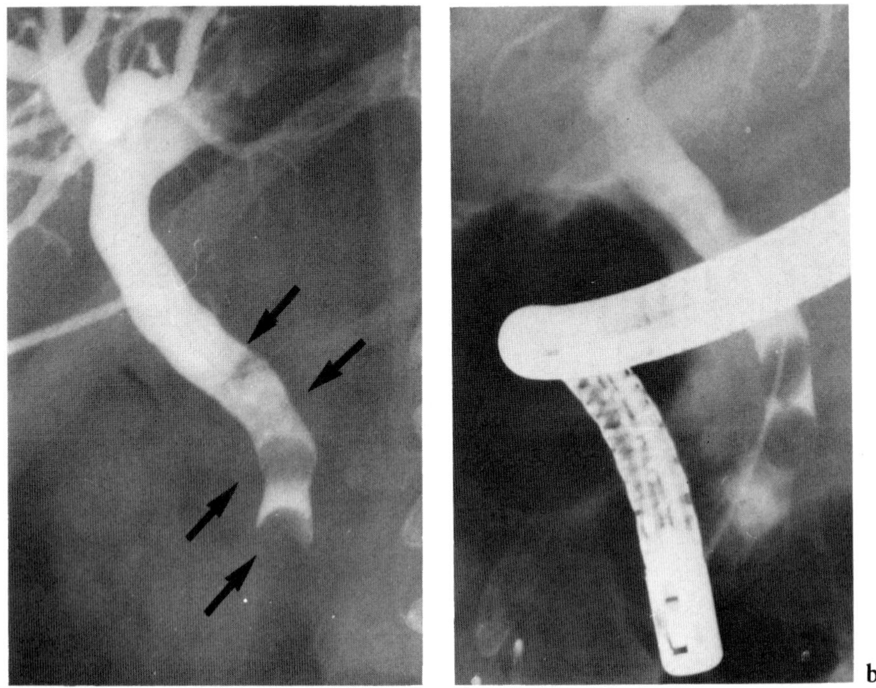

Fig. 47.4 Radiographs showing a. several retained stones (Arrows) on T-tube cholangiogram and b. balloon extraction of remaining stone after ES

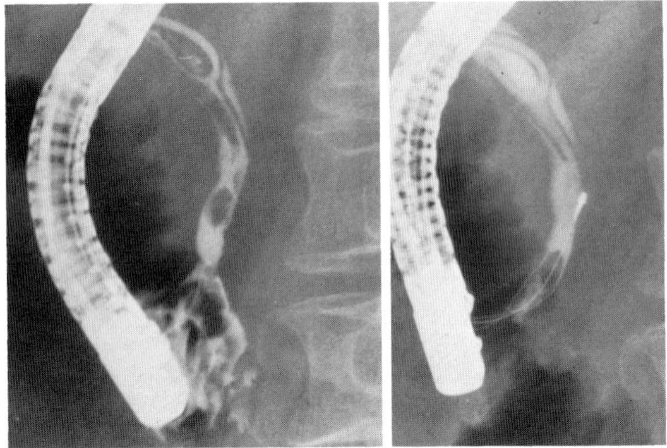

Fig. 47.5 Radiographs showing (left) small stone below T-tube and (right) extraction after lingual application of glyceryl trinitrate

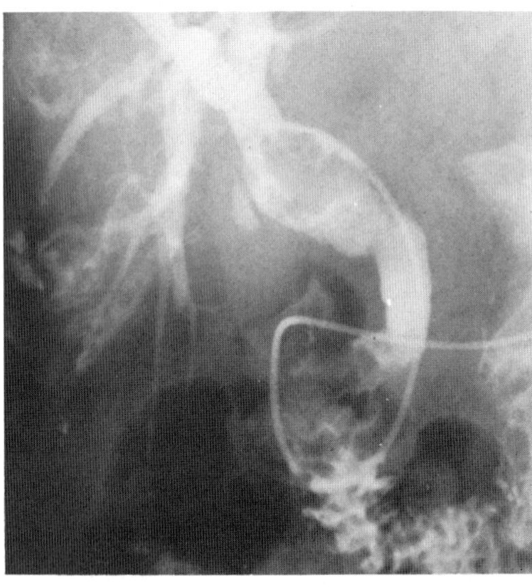

Fig. 47.6 Radiograph showing nasobiliary catheter in place with large stone in CBD above narrow lower bile duct segment

Indications for endoscopic therapy

Patients with bile duct stones present with a variety of clinical problems either alone or in combination, namely, cholestasis, pain, cholangitis, pancreatitis, or as asymptomatic demonstration on T-tube cholangiography. It has become increasingly possible, feasible and, seemingly, acceptable to treat patients in all of these categories endoscopically.

How and why has this come about? Endoscopic sphincterotomy was initially considered justifiable only in elderly post-cholecystectomy patients with recurrent or retained CBD stones who were at high risk of serious complications from orthodox surgical CBD exploration or re-exploration, at a time when few endoscopy centres could offer the technique and criticisms by surgical experts were common (Blumgart & Wood 1978). The impressive successes of ES in this group, however, and an expansion of units practising ES, together with a reasonably low level of complications and a strong patient preference, led many centres to widen their indications for the procedure to include

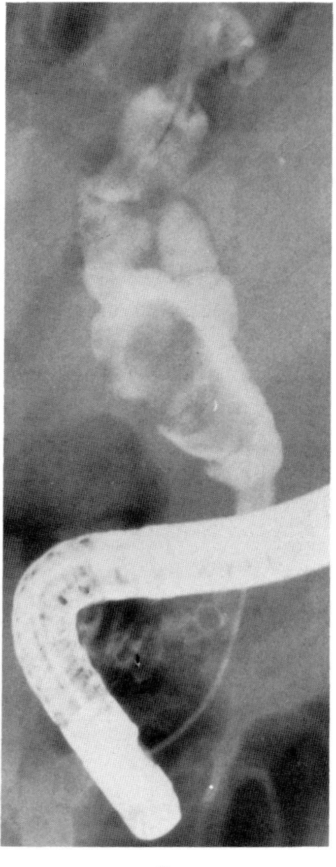

a

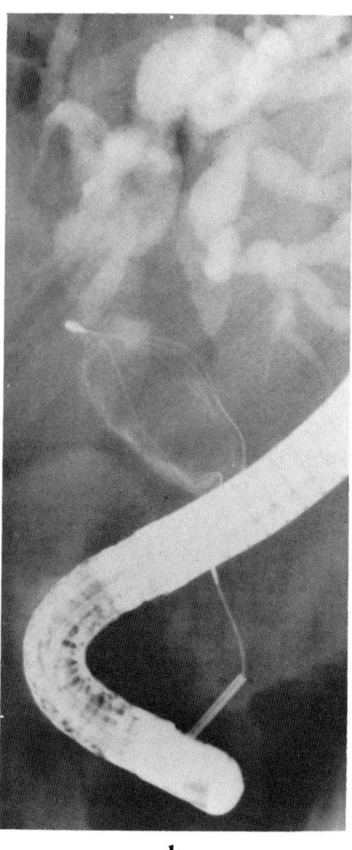

b

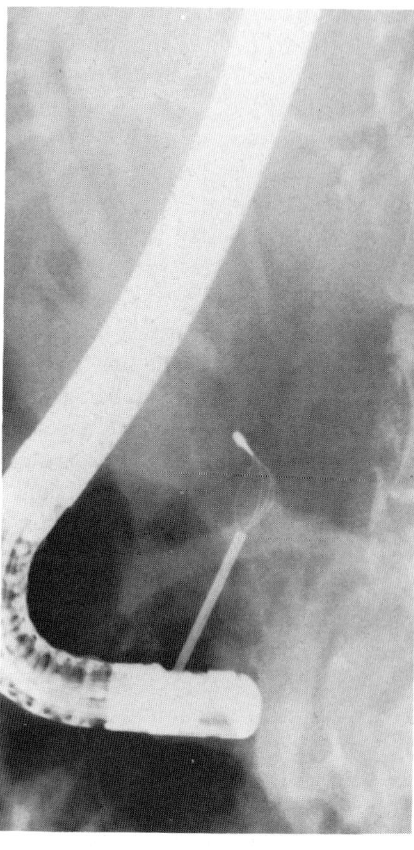

c

Fig. 47.7 Radiographs in post-cholecystectomy patient showing a. large stone with narrow lower bile duct segment, b. lithotriptor basket in place around stone and c. appearance after closing handle with fragementation of stone

younger and fitter post-cholecystectomy patients, and more recently, a range of patients in whom the gallbladder is still in situ but in whom CBD stones give rise to the principal clinical problem. Much of this has occurred in the complete absence of any clinical comparative trial data to aid decision-making and, indeed, there has been such enthusiasm for ES that the establishment of randomized trials has been difficult to organize. Nevertheless, they are essential to settle arguments about relative morbidity and mortality risks as different groups of patients are likely to be treated by either endoscopic or surgical means and these will not necessarily be comparable (Cotton 1984).

The endoscopist is now faced with the prospect of referral of a number of clearly defined groups of patients with confirmed or suspected bile duct stones for whom ES may be indicated:

- post-cholecystectomy, retained stone(s), T-tube in situ
- post-cholecystectomy, later presentation, variable risk factors for surgical CBD (re)exploration
- post-cholecystostomy, stone(s) shown on tubogram
- gallbladder in situ, variable risk factors for surgical CBD exploration, ?need for subsequent cholecystectomy
- acute gallstone-associated pancreatitis irrespective of gallbladder status

These groups are dealt with in detail later in this chapter.

Until such time as trials are available to guide our decisions for ES or surgery it is the responsibility of endoscopists to review their own successes, failures and complications and, more importantly, for surgeons to do the same, in order to make representative comparisons possible and worthwhile and in order to offer patients the best alternatives.

Results of endoscopic therapy

Successful endoscopic treatment of bile duct stones requires an adequate ES and this is now achieved in over 90% of attempts in most reported series, with noticeable improvement as experience increases (Cotton 1984, Blumgart & Wood 1978, Safrany 1978, Reiter et al 1978, Nakajima et al 1979, Siegel 1981, Geenen et al 1981, Cotton & Vallon 1981, Seifert et al 1982, Leese et al 1985a). Failure to achieve an ES or one of sufficient size for the clinical situation is usually due to inaccessibility of the papilla (e.g. pyloric or duodenal stenosis, papilla within a duodenal diverticulum or in the afferent loop of a Billroth II partial gastrectomy) and occasionally difficulties due to a previous surgical duodenotomy or surgery to the papilla itself; technical failure resulting from cannulation difficulties; or poor patient co-operation.

Although success rates for achieving ES are fairly uniform, rates for complete clearance of the CBD vary as not all endoscopists use extraction methods routinely and follow-up ERCP may be incomplete. Most experts would now expect to extract or confirm spontaneous passage of stones in at least 90% of successful sphincterotomies, making an overall successful therapeutic rate of over 80% and often over 90%. Failure to extract or pass stones may be due to size and/or number of stones within the duct or unfavourable duct diameter, usually in its retropancreatic segment (Fig. 47.6, 47.7). Stones up to 10 mm in diameter will not give rise to many problems but, in general, with increasing size above 15 to 20 mm chance of retention rises.

Interpretation of success rates needs care as centres with greater expertise are more likely to be referred difficult cases who may be failures from attempts elsewhere and this will bias some results. Patient groups will also vary considerably from unit to unit and country to country reflecting different referral patterns, selection of patients and attitudes to endoscopic therapy.

In the author's unit, of the 694 ES procedures performed over an eight-year period, 577 (83%) were for bile duct stones with a successful ES performance rate of 98%, extraction rate of 85% of the total group, with spontaneous passage in 5%, and in a further 2% success was achieved after a period of nasobiliary drainage followed by infusion of glyceryl-l-mono-octanoate. This gives an overall successful therapeutic rate of 92% for all patients in whom a decision was taken to attempt ES but excludes those who were amenable to ES treatment but who were randomized to surgery as part of a comparative trial (see below). In the earlier years of our experience some patients with unfavourable biliary anatomy or other potentially complicating problems were also excluded from analysis as there was no 'intention to treat' these endoscopically, but more recently with improvements in accessory instruments and expertise more of these difficult cases have been included. Results from other centres around the world (Cotton 1984, Safrany 1978, Reiter et al 1978, Nakajima et al 1979, Siegel 1981, Geenen et al 1981, Cotton & Vallon 1981, Seifert et al 1982, Leese et al 1985a) with individual and collected series of from 430 to 7585 patients ranged from 78% to 94% for duct clearance with a median value of 87%, figures very similar to our own. There does not appear to be any difference in technical success after ES in patients with and without gallbladders.

An equivalent assessment of surgical success in the same terms is more difficult. In the first few years after the introduction of endoscopic therapy the vast majority of patients treated by this means were those with bile duct stones following a previous cholecystectomy (with or without bile duct exploration). There was a predominance of elderly unfit cases but, with time, younger patients with less risk factors were treated. Endoscopic success rates of over 90%, and thus, conversely, a retained stone rate of less than 10%, must, therefore, be put into the same context as secondary biliary operations and not primary duct procedures as these patients represent 'failures' of previous surgery. Reported results for retained stones after second bile duct explorations are as impressively low as 2.9% (Girard & Legros 1981) but other series have not reported such good results, despite the use of post-exploration cholangiography and choledochoscopy (Kune 1972, Allen et al 1981). With these results in mind many surgeons would now add a biliary drainage procedure to exploration in appropriate circumstances when the bile duct has not been completely cleared or when transpapillary bile flow is thought to be inadequate and this will increase the success rate of bile duct clearance. In addition, secondary operations are potentially more difficult to perform and there must be a failure rate for exploration of the bile duct due, e.g. to limitations of access in some patients but quantification of this is not possible. Non-comparability between endoscopically-treated and surgically-treated patients in this category is compounded by the selection of referrals to specialist centres when complicated biliary surgery is contemplated. A full discussion of this problem is to be found in Chapter 50.

Most endoscopy centres are now referred increasing numbers of patients in whom the gallbladder is still in situ and at Leicester the proportion has risen from under 50% in 1977 to 74% in 1985 of all ES cases. It is in this group that primary bile duct surgery needs to be compared by randomized trial (see below) to define comparability. Excellent surgical series are reported (Ch. 50) but some suggest retained stone rates of from 4.3% (Glenn 1974) to 10% or higher (Way et al 1972) and, even with the use of choledochoscopy, figures of 6% to 8% are reported (Rattner & Warshaw 1981, Feliciano et al 1980). Some primary duct explorations may prove to be difficult or impossible and many surgeons in centres where alternative methods are available may now desist from further attempts and merely provide temporary biliary drainage by T-tube. This attitude is now common where surgeons and endoscopists work closely together and will add further selection difficulties to any retrospective analysis of surgical results.

Management of failures of surgical bile duct exploration will depend on the availability of local expertise but many surgeons would now rather refer patients some distance for endoscopic treatment than carry out a second or subsequent biliary operation. Failures of ES, however, tend to be treated at the endoscopic centre as some patients will require emergency surgery for complications or the rapid relief of a pre-existing problem for which ES was undertaken but has been unsuccessful. A close liaison between the endoscopist and resident surgical teams is important in order that severe and potentially life-threatening complications are recognized and managed effectively. Of a series of 577 patients whose bile duct stones we attempted to treat endoscopically, there were 11 in whom ES was unsuccessful or incomplete (1.9%) and 35 in whom the bile duct could not be cleared (6.1%). Of these, five required urgent surgery; three for continuing cholangitis and retained stones of whom two elderly patients, aged 72 and 84, died, and two for impacted baskets although one was found to be lying free in the duodenal lumen and was removed by the anaesthetist! Six patients had no further treatment; four were moribund on admission and died before any intervention could be undertaken and two elderly frail patients who were left with biliary endoprostheses acting to prevent stone impaction at the papilla and both continue to be well. The remaining 35 were all operated upon successfully without complication and it is probable that many of these were rendered fitter by a period of preoperative bile drainage either through the ES or a nasobiliary catheter.

Complications of endoscopic therapy

Early complications of endoscopic sphincterotomy have been well documented and, despite the disparate indications and selection of patients between centres, the incidence seems to be remarkably consistent at 8 to 10% (Cotton 1984, Safrany 1978, Reiter et al 1978, Nakajima et al 1979, Siegel 1981, Geenen et al, 1981, Cotton & Vallon 1981, Seifert et al 1982, Leese et al 1985a) The expected higher complication rate during early experience of the technique is reflected in a personal series comparing the results of the first 394 procedures in the author's Unit (Leese et al 1985a), which carried an overall morbidity of 10.4%, with a subsequent consecutive group of 300 sphincterotomies in which this rate has fallen to under 6%. The respective proportions of individual complications, however, remain similar in most reports with acute haemorrhage from the sphincterotomy site representing 2.3 to 2.9%, acute pancreatitis 1.5 to 3.3%, cholangitis 1.2 to 2.7% and retroperitoneal perforation about 1%, with small numbers of other problems such as impacted basket, gallstone ileus and acute cholecystitis. Emergency surgery is required in 1 to 2.5% of cases for bleeding, cholangitis, perforation and pancreatitis in descending order of frequency. There must be reservations about some figures, however, as definitions of haemorrhage, acute pancreatitis, cholangitis and perforation are often not given. We have always included any episode of overt bleeding (haematemesis and/or melaena) and/or fall in haemoglobin of 2 g/dl or more following ES as significant haemorrhage although some have included only those requiring transfusion. Pancreatitis and cholangitis must depend on the presence of clinically recognizable syndromes rather than asymptomatic hyperamylasaemia or transient elevation of temperature alone but these events may be under-reported. There does not appear to be an influence on significant complication rate or type by the initial presentation of the bile duct stone event (pain alone, jaundice alone, pancreatitits, a combination of these) except that cholangitis is more likely post-ES if it pre-exists. Present evidence does not suggest that complications are more likely in older patients nor after previous biliary surgery and duodenal diverticula, although sometimes rendering ERCP and ES technically more difficult, do not seem to add any further risk. In addition, many series do not include non-endoscopic complications occurring after ES, such as cardiovascular, cerebrovascular or respiratory ones, and although surgery for the treatment of complications is usually documented, that for failed endoscopic therapy is often not and these factors are important if comparative data from surgical reports are to be interpreted correctly (Ch. 50).

The management of complications by the centres performing ES will be clear and well standardized but many patients are referred from other hospitals and are returned there shortly after the procedure. It is therefore vital that appropriate advice be given and experience recorded (Leese et al 1985a). Of all the complications, haemorrhage requires surgical intervention most commonly (in up to one-third of cases) to control bleeding when the ES is usually converted to a formal surgical sphincteroplasty, as the bleeding artery is nearly always at the apex of the endosopic incision. Attempts to circumvent this feared event are being made by the development of Doppler probes which can be applied endoscopically to the intended sphincterotomy site in order to map the vascular anatomy. This may be particularly helpful when ES is contemplated after a previous ES or surgical sphincter procedure when aberrant vessels are more likely. Alternative methods for haemorrhage control have been tried with variable success and include direct diathermy coagulation, washing the area with adrenaline solution, application of laser coagulation, superselective arterial catheterisation and embolisation, and infiltration with sclerosant (Grimm & Soehendra 1983). It should be stated, however, that the endoscopic view of the papillary area is often completely obscured by blood in these circumstances and further endoscopic therapy may not be possible.

Acute pancreatitis is managed along standard lines and, although many attacks will be mild and self-limiting, clinicians should not be complacent as some will be more severe and should therefore be graded and treated intensively as appropriate. There is no evidence that pre-ES or post-ES administration of Trasylol® or glucagon influences the incidence or severity of pancreatitis. Unlike haemorrhage, the onset of pancreatitis may be delayed for several hours and, rarely, one or two days.

Cholangitis is almost completely confined to those

patients in whom bile duct clearance has not been achieved and measures should be directed at providing adequate bile drainage, e.g. by nasobiliary catheter, as well as provision of parenteral antibiotics. Emergency surgery carries high risks when performed for cholangitis but will be indicated in those patients who do not improve within 24 hours (see below).

Perforation may be asymptomatic and noticed only as retroperitoneal gas or extravasation of radiographic contrast but even in the symptomatic patient conservative treatment may be effective with spontaneous resolution and avoidance of potentially difficult surgery. Occasionally this complication presents late after ES with a retroperitoneal collection of bile or pus pointing in the flank or inguinal region (Leese et al 1985a, Neoptolemos et al 1984a) and will require surgical drainage.

Gallstone ileus should be treated along standard surgical lines but its recognition needs to be emphasized as symptoms may be obscure in elderly patients and present many days after ES and stone release (Ch. 61). Although a complication of ES, the operation required to treat it may be considerably more straightforward than the biliary procedure which has been avoided.

The impaction of an extraction basket now occurs rarely in experienced hands as many endoscopic manoeuvres have been learned by operators to prevent or save this embarrassing situation. Techniques are available to help the endoscopist, such as: non-closing of the basket during initial attempts to extract a large stones to avoid impaling the basket wires in the stone surface; removal of the duodenoscope over an impacted basket catheter and reintroduction of it alongside the catheter to increase the ES incision; introduction of a second duodenoscope to enlarge the ES; passage of a sphincterotome down the same instrument channel as the impacted basket catheter when using large channel (3.7 or 4.2 mm) endoscopes in order to enlarge the ES; and conversion of the standard basket into a crushing type by replacement of the handle with a ratchet device. Complications affecting the gallbladder and the outcome of endoscopic failures are mentioned below in other sections.

Mortality after ES has, unfortunately, not been reported in a standardized way by different centres. Those deaths directly attributable to the procedure are fairly constant at 0.8 to 1.5% (Cotton 1984, Safrany 1978, Reiter et al 1978, Nakajima et al 1979, Seigel 1981, Geenen et al 1981, Cotton & Vallon 1981, Seifert et al 1982, Leese et al 1985a) with almost equal causation distributed between haemorrhage, pancreatitis, cholangitis and perforation with many being postoperative. These deaths as a proportion of complications, however, range from 7% to 17% which presumably reflects the comprehensive reporting of all complications by some but only more severe ones by others. The accepted method of reporting surgical mortality within one month of the operation should be applied to ES results also. Treatment of our own data in this way (Leese et al 1985) produces a mortality of 0.8% resulting from ES itself in 394 patients but an overall 3.3% within one month of ES. The additional deaths were due to a variety of vascular, respiratory, renal, infective and malignant conditions in a group whose mean age was 79 years. A further series of 59 elderly patients considered unfit for surgery (by surgeons) underwent ES (Neoptolemos et al 1984b) with only one death (1.7%) (see below).

Long-term morbidity after ES cannot be fully assessed until follow-up data probably extend well beyond ten years. This will not be possible for another five years at least since it is important to include sufficient numbers of younger patients as it is in this group that long-term results may eventually determine choice of therapy. Results in post-cholecystectomy patients already available, with follow-up information from one to seven years after ES (Cotton 1984, Seifert et al 1982, Escourrou et al 1984, Rosch et al 1981, Vallon et al 1986) shows in excess of 90% of patients to be well on symptomatic review alone and about 8% with significant symptoms found to be due to recurrent stones (5%) and/or stenosis of the ES (3%) site on investigation. Radiological review of all patients after ES by plain abdominal radiograph for detecting air cholangiograms, repeat ERCP, barium studies for duodenobiliary reflux, or radionuclide scanning does not seem justified outside clinical trials but a higher rate of asymptomatic stones and stenosis might be the result. The majority of these long-term complications are amenable to further endoscopic treatment. An air cholangiogram on plain radiography is present in half to two-thirds of patients after ES but does not exclude recurrent bile duct stone formation. Bacteria in the bile aspirated endoscopically long after ES (Vallon et al 1986, Gregg et al 1985) shows almost universal contamination with bowel organisms but the significance of this is unknown at present as there does not seem to be any long-term effect of this on liver function, bile flow or symptoms.

Complications, mortality rates and long-term results of bile duct surgery have been well documented (Girard & Legros 1981, Kune 1972, Allen et al 1981, Glenn 1974, Way et al 1972, McSherry & Glenn 1980, Pitt et al 1981, Blamey et at 1983, Dixon et al 1983, Glenn 1975, Vellacott & Powell 1979, Doyle et al 1982) with more recent interest in specific risk factors (Pitt et al 1981, Blamey et al 1983, Dixon et al 1983) allowing some prediction of likelihood of complications and perhaps the need for preoperative biliary drainage. Direct comparison with the endoscopic data already discussed is not scientifically accurate as it is clear that very different groups of patients are being treated by these modes of therapy. This highlights the concept of 'apples and oranges' succinctly stated by Cotton (1984) but mention must be given here of published surgical figures to enable some clinical judgements to be made in the absence of randomized trials. It is immediately apparent that, unlike endoscopic therapy, surgical morbidity and mortality is very much determined by patient age, presence of other medical conditions (McSherry & Glenn 1980, Glenn 1985, Vellacott & Powell 1979, Doyle et al 1982), both acute and chronic, certain haematological and biochemical factors (Pitt et al 1981, Blamey et al 1983, Dixon et al 1983), and whether or not the operation is elective (Sullivan & Ruffin-Hood 1982, Houghton & Donaldson 1983) or an emergency (Thompson et al 1982, Boey & Way 1980). Mortality rates range from 1% in relatively fit younger patients to 5%, 12% and 28% in the unfit and elderly, and 12 to 14% in younger patients undergoing emergency surgery for cholangitis. These practically all refer to primary bile duct operations which, as already discussed, should only be compared with results of ES when the gallbladder is in situ (see below). Equivalent results for secondary bile duct explorations are less well recorded but mortality rates of 0 to 2% are possible for elective surgery (Girard & Legros 1981, McSherry & Glenn 1980) presumably in relatively fit patients.

Consideration must also be given to biliary drainage operations which will avoid problems of stone retention but this may be at the expense of an increased postoperative morbidity and mortality. Average mortality rates of 1 to 5% for choledochoduodenostomy (CDD) and transduodenal sphincteroplasty (TDS) are reported (Madden et al 1970, Capper 1961, Jones 1978, Lygidakis 1981, Stuart & Hoerr 1972, Speranza et al 1982). We have recently completed a review of 246 such operations (Baker A R, Neoptolemos J P, Leese T, Fossard D P, unpublished observations) carried out between 1972 and 1981 in which one of these drainage procedures was employed and a mortality of 5.4% was found for each of the two types of operation with major morbidity of 12% for CDD and 21% for TDS.

Long-term follow-up of surgically explored and re-explored bile ducts is surprisingly lacking (Ch. 50). The wide variation in reported recurrent stone rates has been mentioned (see above) but morbidity and the need for further surgery has been found in 5% after 5 years (Larson et al 1966), 10% after 12 years (Peel et al 1985), and 21% after six to 11 years (Lygidakis 1983) when exploration without biliary drainage has been performed. Following CDD there may be no morbidity in a six to 11 year follow-up (Lygidakis 1983) with similar results for TDS (Stuart & Hoerr 1972, Degenshein 1974). Follow-up of 90% of the survivors of our series of 246 patients (see above) from one to 12 years postoperatively (mean 4.4 years) revealed that complications had been treated in 3% of the CDD group (mainly sump syndrome) and 6% of the TDS group (mainly cholangitis) with additional symptoms on interview in 8% of the CDD and 5% of the TDS groups.

BILE DUCT STONES — SPECIFIC CLINICAL PROBLEMS

Post-cholecystectomy with T-tube in situ

Bile duct stones detected in the early postoperative period on T-tube cholangiography occur in 4 to 15% of patients and, although those less than 10 mm in diameter may pass spontaneously or after flushing the T-tube, most will be retained and require mechanical removal (Fig. 47.4 & 47.5). The increased morbidity, mortality and retained stone rate after secondary bile duct explorations (see above) has stimulated the development of alternative techniques such as hydraulic T-tube irrigation with or without pharmacological relaxation of the sphincter of Oddi with glucagon or caeruletide, T-tube infusion of cholesterol solvents which are successful in less than 50% (see Ch. 49) to date, and percutaneous extraction via a mature T-tube track which requires a delay of four to six weeks to form (Ch. 48). Advocates of this technique, pioneered by Burhenne (1980), obtain extraction rates of 90% or more but this has not been emulated in Britain where reports

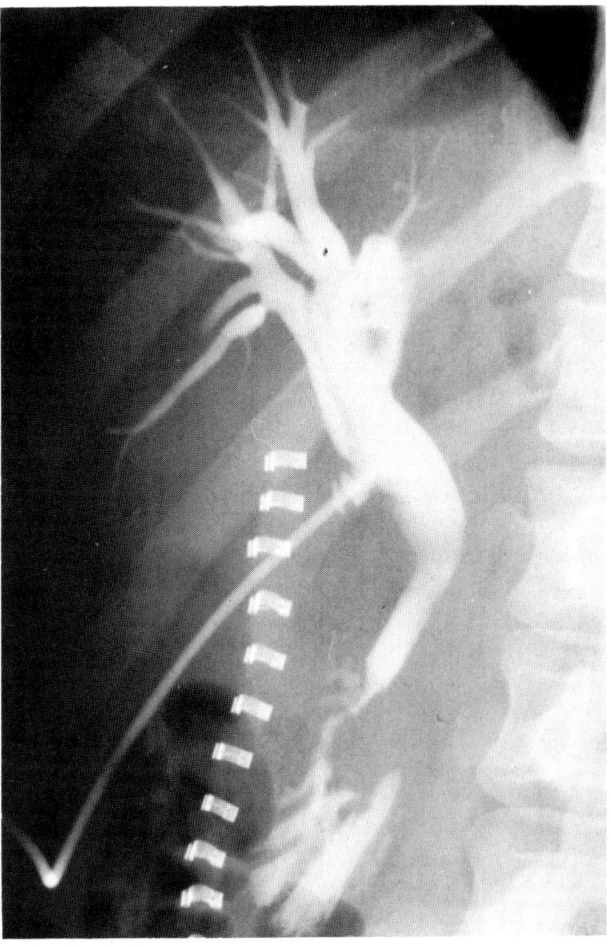

Fig. 47.8 Cholangiogram showing single stone retained above T-tube

of 70 to 78% success are more usual; multiple sessions may be required in a third of cases and be complicated by sepsis, biliary trauma and leakage in up to 12% (Mason 1985, Leese et al 1985b). We have recently reported (O'Doherty et al 1986) our results of ES in 39 patients with T-tubes in place in whom 76 stones were present, 53 distal (Fig. 47.4 and 47.5) and 23 proximal (Fig. 47.8) to the T-tube. Stones ranged in diameter from 5 to 15 mm and were single in 25, two to four in 11 and more than four in three patients (one with eight stones). Endoscopic sphincterotomy was successful in all and the bile duct was cleared in 38 (97.4%), requiring two attempts in two. Complications occurred in three (7.7%): an impacted basket in one, removed surgically, mild pancreatitis in one and transient cholangitis in another. Most patients were treated within four weeks of their operation but this reflected delays in referral as ES can be carried out immediately stones are demonstrated, usually on the tenth postoperative day allowing discharge from hospital the following day. There have been no long-term complications to date and we have continued to apply this technique when requested in all patients with the new addition of stone extraction after lingual application of gluceryl trinitrate (Staritz et al 1985) in younger patients if stones are small (Fig. 47.5).

Post-cholecystectomy without T-tube in situ

Patients presenting from a few weeks to many years after cholecystectomy with symptoms and signs suggesting biliary disease are best investigated by ERCP when bile duct stones will be the commonest finding (Ch. 55). Few would now question the use of ES in the treatment of elderly patients in this context who are at high risk for abdominal surgery but there may remain doubts when surgeons are faced with younger and fitter patients. The successes, failures and complications of secondary bile duct operations have been discussed (see above and Ch. 50) from which it may be deduced that, if endoscopic therapy can achieve the high success rates published by most established centres, this should be the treatment of first choice. It is most unlikely that any comparative trials of surgery against ES will be performed in post-cholecystectomy patients in the light of current medical and surgical opinion but critical assessment of long-term morbidity following ES should be continued as this will determine whether or not the endoscopic approach should remain the correct one in this group.

Gallbladder in situ

There has been an increasing trend over the last few years for patients who have not previously undergone biliary surgery to be referred for endoscopic therapy for bile duct stones. The reasoning behind this is twofold. Firstly, the elderly patient with pain, jaundice, cholangitis, pancreatitis or a combination of these may best be served by endoscopic clearance of the bile duct to relieve the acute biliary problem and not proceed to cholecystectomy unless symptoms dictate in view of the expected short life expectancy and the low possibility of gallbladder complications (Fig. 47.9). Secondly, younger patients presenting with these same acute biliary conditions may fare better with initial biliary decompression by ES followed by elective cholecystectomy when the acute problem has subsided (Fig. 47.10). What is the present evidence that either of these propositions is justified?

The short- and long-term results and complications of ES in patients with gallbladders seem no different from those without. The same arguments in favour of endoscopic bile duct clearance therefore apply equally in these patients as to those who are post-cholecystectomy. The difference in the elderly group, in whom a deliberate decision is made to leave the gallbladder in situ, is the incidence of subsequent complications referrable to the residual gallbladder itself. Careful follow-up of 59 such patients for up to four years (Neoptolemos et al 1984), 130 for up to five years (Escourou et al 1984) and 260 for up to six years (Cotton 1984) has shown that 4.6%, 6% and 10% respectively have developed gallbladder symptoms or complications sufficient to warrant cholecystectomy and nearly all were required within the first year. There do not appear to be any predictors of subsequent gallbladder complications definable at the time of ES, and in particular, non-filling of the gallbladder with radiographic contrast at ERCP does not confer a higher likelihood of problems. A small subgroup probably have empyema of the gallbladder at the time of presentation or develop it shortly after endoscopic treatment and all must be aware

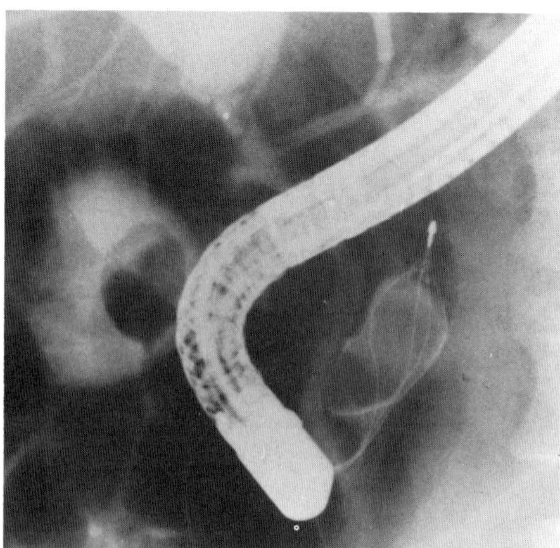

Fig. 47.9 Radiograph showing endoscopic extraction of large bile duct stone after ES in an elderly patient whose gallbladder contains a single stone

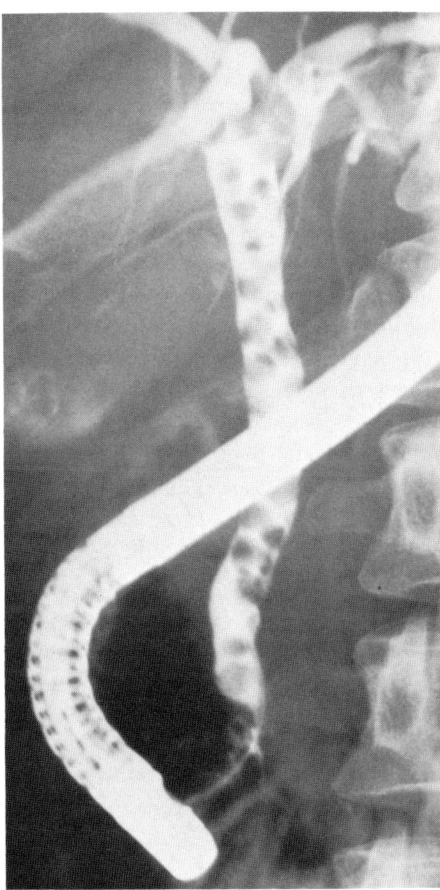

Fig. 47.10 ERCP showing multiple bile duct stones, all removed after ES, in 45-year-old male with cholangitis whose gallbladder contains multiple stones (early filling only shown here)

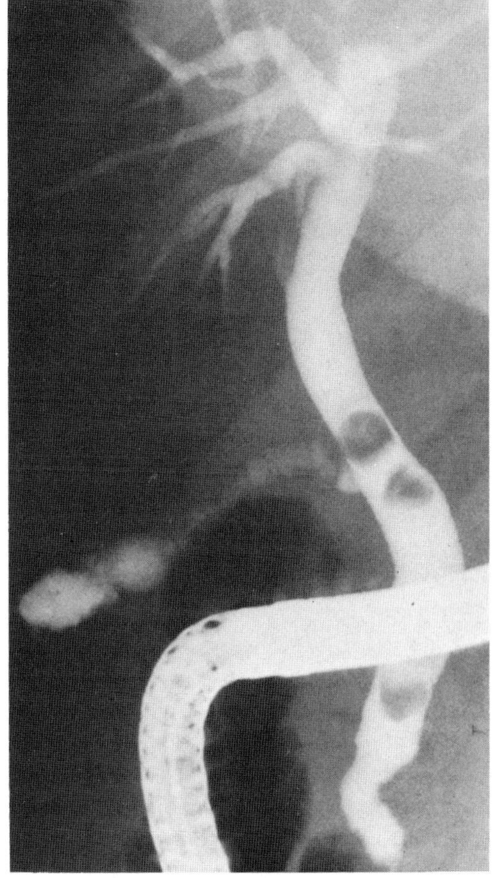

Fig. 47.11 ERCP showing bile duct stones and contracted empty gallbladder

of this in view of the difficulty in diagnosis and high mortality connected with this condition if left untreated. One patient aged 76 years in our series (Neoptolemos 1984b) died from this condition five weeks after ES but all other late deaths were due to non-biliary causes as would be expected in this age group. Some patients are found to have empty gallbladders at the time of initial ES (Fig. 47.11) and others with gallbladder stones have certainly passed them following ES. These results suggest that the low risk of subsequent gallbladder complications after ES and bile duct clearance outweighs the known higher mortality for cholecystectomy in the elderly (Sullivan & Roffin-Hood 1982). The low but definite risk of neoplastic change in the residual gallbladder becomes irrelevant in view of the short life expectancy in this group of elderly patients.

Emergency surgery in younger patients with acute biliary tract disease may carry a high risk although elective bile duct exploration is relatively safe (see above). The place of preliminary ES in these patients can only be decided by controlled trial. A pilot study was undertaken in 38 patients (Neoptolemos et al 1984b), with a mean age of 63 years, considered fit for surgery but presenting with combinations of jaundice in 95%, recent cholangitis in 45%, active cholangitis in 26%, and acute pancreatitis in 10%. Thirty-three (87%) were successfully treated by ES and extraction of stones, with failure of performing ES in two and extraction in three. All were subsequently operated upon apart from one patient who felt well and refused further treatment and remains well with the gallbladder in situ. Of the remainder, all 37 had a cholecystectomy, three with negative bile duct explorations owing to misinterpretation of the perioperative cholangiogram from the presence of air in the duct, and five with positive explorations representing the five failures of endoscopic therapy. There were no postoperative deaths within one month and all are alive and well with no late complications. With these encouraging results a prospective trial was established entering patients with bile duct stones shown on endoscopic or percutaneous cholangiography who were considered treatable by either endoscopy or surgery and whose gallbladders were still intact. Clinicians were asked to offer patients for the study but could elect to exclude them and request one or other mode of therapy, usually ES, when the reasons for this were recorded. Trial patients were randomized either to preliminary ES followed by elective cholecystectomy (Group I) or surgery (cholecystectomy, bile duct exploration and any additional procedure considered appropriate, Group II) with failures of either mode of therapy treated by the other or by an alternative method as indicated by the clinical situation. Preliminary analysis of the first 98 patients entered is currently available. The two groups are comparable in their demographic characteristics with 48 in Group I and 50 in Group II. There were four failures of endoscopic treatment in Group I, two failed sphincteromies and two failed duct clearances, all of whom underwent subsequent successful surgical duct exploration together with cholecystectomy. The remaining 44 (92%) in Group I underwent elective cholecystectomy after successful endoscopic clearance of bile duct, usually within one month of ES and many during the same admission when jaundice had subsided. No unsuspected bile duct stones were detected at operation and there were no postoperative deaths. No serious complications of ES were encountered but two patients experienced exacerbations of their cholangitis after ES despite prophylactic antibiotics and 16 (33%) developed adverse postoperative events of which the most important were septic e.g. wound infections in four (8.3%), two of whom sufferred burst abdomens, chest infections in seven (14.6%) and septicaemia in one (2.1%). Significant blood loss occurred in two (4.2%) and a bile leak following surgical bile duct damage in one. In Group II, all patients had a positive bile duct exploration combined with cholecystectomy and there was one postoperative death in a patient with Nelson's syndrome following previous adrenalectomy for Cushing's disease. Complications occurred in 25 patients (50%) with sepsis in a similar number to Group I, namely, wound infections in six (12%), one of whom suffered of a burst abdomen, chest infections in six (12%), and septicaemia in one (2%). Other postoperative events were acute pancreatitis in the one patient who died, significant blood loss in four (8%), bile leakage in two (4%), early sump syndrome complicating a choledochoduodenostomy in one and retained bile duct stones in five (10%). Thus the principal differences in early outcome between the two groups to date are the failures of endoscopic treatment (8%) in Group I and the failures of surgical bile duct clearance in Group II (12%, retained stones and sump syndrome) all of the latter being subsequently treated by ES. There does not appear to be a significant difference between the two groups in terms of other postoperative complications. Analysis of risk factors (Pitt et al 1981, Blamey et al 1983, Dixon et al 1983), however, reveals patients in the trial to be younger and fitter than a similar number referred specifically for ES at the clinicians' request during the trial period. This 'para-trial' group is being analyzed separately as are patients who have undergone cholecystectomy with bile duct exploration for stones found unexpectedly on perioperative cholangiography during the trial period. It is hoped that comparison of these four groups will allow conclusions to be drawn concerning the risks and benefits of preoperative ES in younger patients. No firm recommendations can yet be given.

Acute cholangitis

Acute cholangitis due to bile duct stones is traditionally treated by initial supportive measures with parenteral antibiotics followed by early surgery (Ch. 72) if improvement is slow or absent. The mortality from emergency surgery can be as high as 12 to 16% with higher rates for elderly patients (Cotton 1984, Thompson et al 1982, Boey 1980). We have analysed the results of treatment of 82 patients with severe acute cholangitis with bile duct stones admitted to our hospital over a seven year period during which ES was available (Leese et al 1985b). There were 28 males and 54 females with a mean age of 71 years (range 19 to 88). 87% were aged over 60 and 23% over 80 years. Overall 30-day mortality was 14.6% but varied considerably with different modes of therapy. Eleven received conservative treatment only. Of these, seven responded to antibiotics alone but four were moribund and died (36.4%) before any treatment could be instituted. Seventy-one underwent early biliary decompression surgically (28) or endoscopically (43). Of the eleven who were post-cholecystectomy, four had early surgery with bilio-digestive bypass and two died within 30 days (50%) and seven had early ES with no mortality. Of the 60 with gallbladders, 24 were treated surgically (mean age 62 years) with a mortality of 16.7%, 13 had an ES followed by elective cholecystectomy (mean age 64 years) with no mortality and 23 had an ES with gallbladders left in situ (mean age 79 years) with a mortality of 8.7%. During follow-up of the 21 survivors with gallbladders, six have died from unrelated causes, two have required surgery for empyema of the gallbladder at 19 days post-ES in one and recurrence of cholangitis at five months in the other. Complications after ES occurred in 10: haemorrhage in five, exacerbation of cholangitis in three, mild acute pancreatitis in one and gallstone ileus in one with only the latter requiring surgical intervention. Bile duct clearance was achieved in 40 out of 43 patients (93%). Of the three failures, one died without further therapy, one underwent surgery four weeks later and one remains asymptomatic having declined further treatment. Thus the 30-days mortality for patients treated by early surgery was 21.4% (six out of 28) and that for early ES irrespective of subsequent treatment was 4.7% (two out of 43). We have concluded that patients not responding to standard initial therapy within 24 hours or those who have already developed extra-biliary complications should be offered for endoscopic biliary decompression and bile duct clearance if this is locally available.

Gallstone-associated acute pancreatitis

There have been advocates for early biliary surgery in

acute gallstone-associated pancreatitis both to prevent progression of the current attack to one of more severity and also to reduce the incidence of further attacks (Neoptolemos et al 1986) (Ch. 43). This aggressive management has been criticized as carrying too high a risk of mortality (Neoptolemos et al 1986). The application of ES in this situation seems logical although ERCP has long been regarded as contraindicated in the presence of active pancreatitis. After an encouraging pilot study in 16 patients we set up a prospective controlled trial of ERCP and ES in patients admitted with acute pancreatitis whose initial ultrasound examination, biochemical criteria (Goodman et al 1985, Neoptolemos et al 1984c) or absence of other identifiable causes allowed selection in favour of a biliary association. To date from a consecutive series of 112 patients with acute pancreatitis, 70 have been included in the study with 35 randomized to urgent ERCP (performed within 72 hours) and ES if bile duct stones were present (Group I) and 35 to conventional treatment (Group II). Fifty were found to have a biliary aetiology of whom 24 were in Group I and 26 in Group II. All but one in Group I had a successful ERCP and 11 were found to have bile duct stones, all of which were removed endoscopically. The proportion of patients with bile duct stones was greater in those with severe attacks on prognostic grading (40%) compared to those with mild attack (23%) and the overall complication rates were 35% and 10% respectively. The two deaths in the trial occurred in Group II patients (7.7%) one of whom had an impacted stone at the duodenal papilla at autopsy and may therefore have been saved by early biliary intervention. There were no adverse events attributable to ERCP or ES and three patients in each of Group I and II developed local pancreatic complications: pseudocyst in three and abscess in three. Two subjects with coexistent cholangitis in Group I made a dramatic improvement following ES and stone extraction. In the 20 patients suspected of gallstone-associated pancreatitis but in whom no biliary pathology was found, ERCP was performed in 11 without complication. Forty-two patients from the original 112 did not fulfil the trial entry criteria and were not randomized. Eight of these, however, had an urgent ERCP and one, with bile duct stones, pancreatic and hepatic abscesses, an ES with rapid improvement. There were seven deaths (16.7%) in this para-trial group of whom two had biliary disease making an overall mortality of 8% (9 out of 112) but 6.8% (4 out of 59) for gallstone-associated pancreatitis. No deaths occurred in patients undergoing ERCP and/or ES. Although no statistical differences can yet be demonstrated between Group I and II patients, our trial is continuing in the hope that clear guidelines for selection of cases likely to benefit from early endoscopic therapy may be formulated.

CONCLUSIONS

Endoscopic sphincterotomy (ES) has been conceived and matured in a very short space of time with wide acceptance as a respectable and highly effective therapy for bile duct stones. Endoscopic technique is now well established but accessory equipment and other adjuncts will undoubtedly develop to enhance the endoscopists' success and safety record in treating patients with gallstone disease. This review has summarized the author's views of current successes, failures and complications of ES in his own practice and that of others around the world and has attempted to put this into the context of alternative surgical methods of treatment. A further detailed argument is presented in Ch. 50. There would seem to be little argument against the use of ES in preference to surgery in the management of elderly high risk patients with bile duct stones in the majority of clinical situations, irrespective of the presence or absence of the gallbladder and in all patients presenting with bile duct stones late after previous biliary surgery where the only alternative is further surgical intervention. The removal of retained stones in the early postoperative period with a T-tube in place with depend on 'local' expertise but ES has been shown to be effective in this situation, carries a small risk of complications and allows early discharge from hospital without the continuing need for T-tube access. In addition, patients of all ages with acute cholangitis not responding to conventional therapy should be considered for ES before emergency surgery if this is logistically feasible. The case for ES in the treatment of all patients with acute gallstone-associated pancreatitis and younger patients with bile duct and gallbladder stones has not yet been made but early trial results suggest that it will have a place in management when selection criteria are accurately defined. Integrated endoscopic therapy for biliary disease is now well advanced in those centres where surgical and endoscopic clinicians work closely together and where each provides the other with a suitable forum for critical evaluation of alternative therapeutic techniques.

REFERENCES

Allen B, Shapiro H, Way L W 1981 Management of recurrent and residual common duct stones. American Journal of Surgery 142: 41–47

Allen M J, Borody T J, Bugliosi T F, May G R, Larusso N F, Thistle J L 1985 Rapid dissolution of gallstones by methyl tert-butyl ether. New England Journal of Medicine 312: 217–220

Blamey S L, Fearon K C H, Gilmore W H, Osborn D H, Carter D C 1983 Prediction of risk in biliary surgery. British Journal of Surgery 70: 535–538

Blumgart L H, Wood C B 1978 Letter on: Endoscopic treatment of biliary tract diseases. Lancet ii: 1249

Boey J H, Way L W 1980 Acute cholangitis. Annals of Surgery 190: 264–270
Burhenne J H 1980 Percutaneous extraction of retained biliary tract stones. American Journal of Roentgenology 134: 888–898
Capper W M 1961 External choledochoduodenostomy, an evaluation of 125 cases. British Journal of Surgery 49: 292–300
Carr-Locke D L, Cotton P B. 1985 Endoscopic Surgery: Biliary Tract and Pancreas. British Medical Bulletin 42: 257–264
Classen M, Demling L 1974 Endoscopische Sphinkterotomie der papilla Vater. Deutsche Medizinische Wochenschrift 99: 496–497
Cotton P B, 1984 Endoscopic management of bile duct stones; (apples and oranges). Gut 25: 587–597
Cotton P B, Burney P G J, Mason R R 1979 Transnasal bile duct catheterisation after endoscopic sphincterotomy. Gut 20: 285–287
Cotton P B, Vallon A G 1981 British experience with duodenoscopic sphincterotomy for removal of bile duct stones. British Journal of Surgery 68: 373–375
Degenshein G A 1974 Choledocho-duodenostomy; an 18 year study of 175 consecutive cases. Surgery 76: 316–324
Dixon J M, Armstrong C B, Duffy S W, Davies G C 1983 Factors affecting morbidity and mortality after surgery for obstructive jaundice; a review of 373 patients. Gut 24: 845–852
Doyle P J, Ward-McQuaid J N, McEwen-Smith A 1982 The value of routine per-operative cholangiography — a report of 4000 cholecystectomies. British Journal of Surgery 69: 617–619
Escourrou J, Cordova J A, Lazorthes F, et al 1984 Early and late complications after endoscopic sphincterotomy for biliary lithiasis, with and without the gallbladder 'in situ'. Gut 25: 598–602
Feliciano D W, Mattox K L, Jordan G L 1980 The value of choledochoscopy in exploration of the common bile duct. Annals of Surgery 191: 649–653
Geenen J E, Vennes J A, Silvis S E 1981 Resume of a seminar on endoscopic retrograde sphincterotomy (ERS). Gastrointestinal Endoscopy 27: 31–38
Girard R M, Legros G 1981 Retained and recurrent bile duct stones: surgical or non-surgical removal? Annals of Surgery 193: 150–154
Glenn F 1974 Retained calculi within the biliary ductal system. Annals of Surgery 179: 528–539
Glenn F 1975 Trends in surgical treatment of calculus disease of the biliary tract. Surgery, Gynecology and Obstetrics 140: 877–884
Goodman A J, Neoptolemos J P, Carr-Locke D L, Finlay D B L, Fossard D P 1985 Detection of gallstones after acute pancreatitis. Gut 26: 125–132
Gregg J A, de Girolami P, Carr-Locke D L 1985 Effects of sphincteroplasty and endoscopic sphincterotomy on the bacteriologic characteristics of the common bile duct. American Journal of Surgery 149: 668–671
Grimm H, Soehendra N 1983 Unterspritzung zur Behandlung der Papillotomie-Blutung. Deutsche Medizinische Wochenschrift 108: 1512–1514
Hoffman A F, Schmack B, Thistle J L, Babayan V K 1981 Clinical experience with mono-octanoin for dissolution of bile duct stones. Digestive Diseases and Sciences 26: 954–957
Houghton P J W, Donaldson L A 1983 Elective biliary surgery — a safe procedure Geriatric Medicine 13: 814–816
Jones S A 1978 The prevention and treatment of recurrent bile duct stones by transduodenal sphincteroplasty. World Journal of Surgery 2: 473–485
Kawai K, Akasaka Y, Murakami K, Tada M, Kohli Y, Nakajima M 1974 Endoscopic sphincterotomy of the ampulla of Vater. Gastrointestinal Endoscopy 20: 148–151
Kune G A 1972 Current practice of biliary surgery. Little Brown, Boston, p 221–223
Larson R E, Hodgson J R, Priestley J T 1966 The early and long term results of 500 consecutive explorations of the common duct. Surgery Gynecology and Obstetrics 122: 744–750
Leese T, Neoptolemos J P, Carr-Locke D L 1985a Successes, failures, early complications and their management following endoscopic sphincterotomy: results in 394 consecutive patients from a single centre. British Journal of Surgery 72: 215–219
Leese T, Neoptolemos J P, Baker A R, Carr-Locke D L 1985b Management of acute cholangitis and the impact of endoscopic sphincterotomy. Gut 26:A553
Lygidakis N J 1981 Choledochoduodenostomy in calculous biliary tract disease. British Journal of Surgery 68: 762–765
Lygidakis N J 1983 Surgical approaches to recurrent choledocholithiasis. American Journal of Surgery 145: 633–639
McSherry C K, Glenn F 1980 The incidence and causes of death following surgery for non-malignant biliary tract disease. Annals of Surgery 191: 271–275
Madden J L, Chun J Y, Kandalaft S, Parekh M 1970 Choledochoduodenostomy, an unjustly maligned surgical procedure? American Journal of Surgery 119: 45–54
Mason R 1980 Percutaneous extraction of retained gallstones via the T-tube tract — British experience of 131 cases. Clinical Radiology 1: 497–499
Mason R 1985 Percutaneous extraction of retained gallstones. Clinical Gatroenterology 14: 403–419
Nakajima M, Kizu M, Akasaka Y, Kawai K 1979 Five years experience of endoscopic sphincterotomy in Japan: a collective study from 25 centres. Endoscopy 2: 138–141
Neoptolemos J P, Harvey M H, Slater N D, Carr-Locke D L 1984a Abdominal wall staining and 'biliscrotum' after retroperitoneal perforation following endoscopic sphincterotomy. British Journal of Surgery 71: 684
Neoptolemos J P, Carr-Locke D L, Fraser I, Fossard D P 1984b The management of common bile duct calculi by endoscopic sphincterotomy in patients with gallbladders in situ. British Journal of Surgery 71: 69–71
Neoptolemos J P, Hall A W, Finlay D B, Berry J M, Carr-Locke D L, Fossard D P 1984c The urgent diagnosis of gallstones in acute pancreatitis: a prospective study of three methods. British Journal of Surgery 71: 230–233
Neoptolemos J P, London N, Slater N D, Carr-Locke D L, Fossard D P, Moossa A R 1986 A prospective study of ERCP and endoscopic sphincterotomy in the diagnosis and treatment of gallstone acute pancreatitis. Archives of Surgery (in press)
O'Doherty D P, Neoptolemos J P, Carr-Locke D L 1986 Endoscopic sphincterotomy for retained common bile duct stones in patients with T-tube in situ in the early post-operative period. British Journal of Surgery (in press)
Peel A L G, Bourke J B, Hermon Taylor J, et al 1975 How should the common bile duct be explored? Annals of the Royal College of Surgeons of England 56: 124–134
Pitt H A, Cameron J L, Postier R G, Gadacz T R 1981 Factors affecting mortality in biliary tract surgery. American Journal of Surgery 141: 66–72
Rattner D W, Warshaw A L 1981 Impact of choledochoscopy in the management of choledocholithiasis. Annals of Surgery 194: 76–79
Reiter J J, Bayer H P, Mennicken C, Manegold B C 1978 Results of endoscopic papillotomy: A collective experience from nine endoscopic centers in West Germany. World Journal of Surgery 2: 505–511
Rosch W, Riemann J F, Lux G, Lindner H G 1981 Long term follow-up after endoscopic sphincterotomy. Endoscopy 13: 152–153
Safrany L 1978 Endoscopic treatment of biliary tract diseases. Lancet ii: 983–985
Seifert E, Gail K, Weismuller J 1982 Langzeitresultate nach endoskopischer Sphinkterotomie: follow-up-Studie aus 25 Zentren in der Bundesrepublik. Deutsche Medizinische Wochenschrift 107: 610–614
Siegel J H 1981 Endoscopic papillotomy in the treatment of biliary tract disease: 258 procedures and results. Digestive Diseases and Sciences 26: 1057–1064
Speranza V, Lezoche E, Minervina S, Carlei F, Basso N, Simi M 1982 Transduodenal papillostomy as a routine procedure in managing choledocholithiasis. Archives of Surgery 117: 875–878
Staritz M 1983a Endoscopic papillary dilatation. Endoscopy 15: 197–198
Staritz M 1983b Mechanical gallstone lithotripsy. Endoscopy 15: 316–318
Staritz M, Poaralla T, Dormeyer H H, Meyer zum Buschenfelde K H 1985 Endoscopic removal of common bile duct stones through the intact papilla after medical sphincter dilation. Gastroenterology 88: 1807–1811
Stuart M, Hoerr S O 1972 Late results of side to side choledochoduodenostomy and of transduodenal sphincterotomy for benign disorders. American Journal of Surgery 123: 67–72

Sullivan D M, Ruffin-Hood T, Griffin W O 1982 Biliary tract surgery in the elderly. American Journal of Surgery 143: 218–220
Thompson J E, Thompkins R K, Longmire W P 1982 Factors in management of acute cholangitis. Annals of Surgery 195: 137–145
Vallon A G, Holton J M, Cotton P B 1986 Follow-up after duodenoscopic sphincterotomy for recurrent duct stones. (unpublished observations)
Vellacott K D, Powell P H 1979 Exploration of the common bile duct; a comparative study. British Journal of Surgery 66: 389–391
Way L W, Admirand W H, Dunphy J E 1972 Management of choledocholithiasis. Annals of Surgery 176: 347–359

Interventional radiology

GENERAL CONSIDERATIONS

Radiology of the biliary tract owes its beginnings to contributions from surgery with the original description of transhepatic gallbladder puncture in 1921 (Burckhardt & Mueller 1921), cholecystography in 1923 (Cole 1960), and post-surgical cholangiography in 1924 (Cotte 1925). The two specialties of radiology and surgery have had a close and important relationship ever since in the diagnosis of biliary disease and, in the last decade, in therapy. This specialty of interventional radiology is expanding rapidly with non-operative retained biliary stone extraction popularized in 1973 (Mazzariello 1973) and radiologic interventional dilatation of biliary tract strictures initiated in 1975 (Burhenne 1975a). The growing body of manipulative radiological biliary tract procedures entails clinical judgement, manual skill and responsibility to the patient before, during, and after the procedure. It requires close co-operation between the surgeon and the radiologist to set indications, evaluate results and treat complications.

EQUIPMENT AND RADIATION PROTECTION

Image intensification fluoroscopy and its superb image resolution make interventional radiology of the biliary tract possible. Modern equipment is required with at least single plane imaging and good spot film facilities. Small retained stones of 2 mm or less are better seen with radiographic than with fluoroscopic imaging. The roentgen ray tube should be under the couch in order to decrease scatter to the radioiogist. Under table collimation is ideal for the same purpose. A lead shield or apron with a window can be draped over the patient, leaving the area of interest free. The radiologist's fingers should never be in the primary beam and collimation should be to the smallest possible field, preferably to a 3 × 5 cm opening. This is facilitated if the fluoroscopic equipment carries a magnification device. Periodic exposure measurements should be obtained for table top radiation.

The equipment for instrumentation of the biliary tract via postoperative tracts or percutaneous transhepatic access includes standard angiographic guide wires and catheters. A 30 cm steerable catheter (Medi-Tech, Watertown, Massachusetts) has made rapid catheterization of sinus tracts feasible (Burhenne 1973). Steerable catheters are available in sizes 8, 10, and 13 French gauge. The 13 French steerable catheter lumen is large enough to permit passage of all types of baskets and of the biopsy wire forceps. If the surgeon has placed a T-tube smaller than 14 French, dilatation of the tract with angiographic balloon catheters is required. These are passed over a guide wire after an 8 French steerable catheter has been placed into the duct system (Burhenne & Morris 1980).

It is important to have a variety of stone extraction baskets available. The Dormia ureteral stone basket without filament leader is adequate for most stone extraction procedures, but larger baskets are required for larger stones. Even a small retained stone in an enlarged common duct is more easily engaged if a large basket is used as stone entrapment is facilitated if the retracting open basket touches the walls of the dilated common duct. Baskets are available up to 3.5 cm size (Cook, Indianapolis). Medi-Tech® baskets employ a softer stainless steel wire which provides little opening force in the bile duct but these baskets are available in three sizes.

INTERVENTIONAL ACCESS ROUTES

Access to the biliary tract for interventional procedures is gained via postoperative sinus tracts from a T-tube or cholecystostomy tube or percutaneously through the liver.

T-tube tract

Instrumentation of a T-tube tract is the easier technical procedure and has implications for surgical T-tube placement. The long arm of the rubber T-tube should be at least of a 14 French calibre (Fig. 48.1). If the common

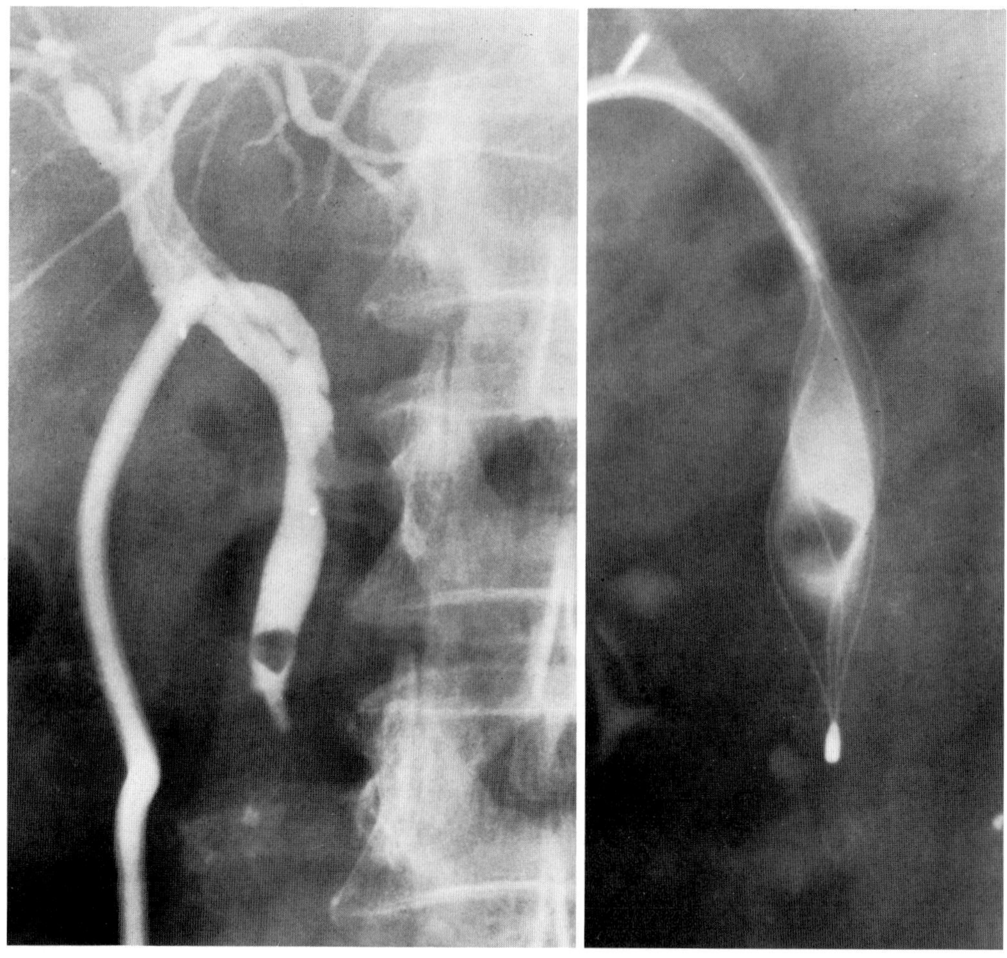

Fig. 48.1 a. Faceted retained distal common duct stone on T-tube cholangiography one week after operation. Note that the T-tube is inserted in the common hepatic duct above the confluence of the cystic duct. b. The retained common duct stone is ensnared in the wire basket before extraction. This stone measured 5 mm in diameter and was extracted intact through the sinus tract of a 14 French T-tube

duct is small in calibre, the short arms of the T-tube should be trimmed appropriately. 14 French T-tubes are also commercially available now with 10 or 12 French small arms (Darvol). The T-tube should exit through a stab wound in the right flank antero-laterally. Anterior T-tube placement through surgical incisions makes radiological instrumentation considerably more difficult and the operator's hands are often in the field of radiation.

If the postoperative T-tube cholangiogram demonstrates retained stones, the T-tube is left in place for another four weeks to permit formation of a fibrous tract. This permits access with a steerable catheter to the extrahepatic ducts for stone extraction. A T-tube tract with a less than 14 French tube may require more than a four week interval for tract formation, particularly if the patient is obese. Fibrous reaction in adipose tissue occurs more slowly.

If the postoperative T-tube cholangiogram demonstrates retained biliary stones, the patient is usually discharged. Multiple high resolution spot radiographs may be required to ascertain the diagnosis and differentiate choledocholithiasis from a blood clot or tumour (Fig. 48.2). Radiological stone extraction is accomplished in the ambulatory patient as a routine. Re-admission is only required in complicated cases.

Transhepatic route

A percutaneous transhepatic approach to the biliary tract for stone removal may occasionally be used if a postoperative drainage tract is not available and when surgical or endoscopic stone removal is contraindicated. This interventional radiological procedure is a further development of percutaneous transhepatic cholangiography (Dotter et al 1979). The technique is analogous to biliary drainage procedures but carries a higher complication rate than instrumentation through a T-tube tract. The stone must be fragmented with a basket in the bile duct and the fragments are then expelled from the duct into the duodenum. More serious complications must be expected if the stone cannot be fragmented as hepatic injury can occur during transhepatic stone extraction (Ellman & Berman 1981).

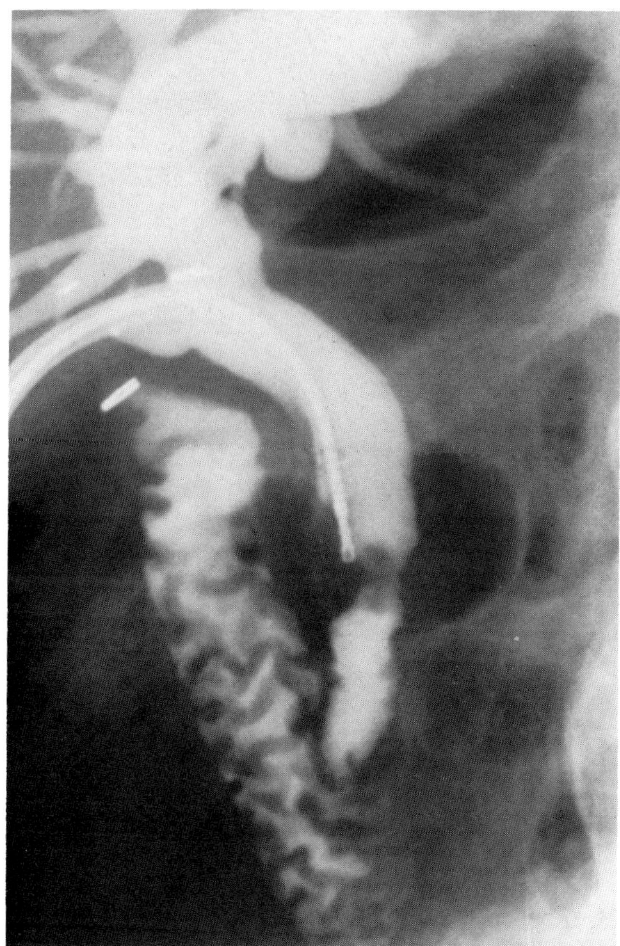

Fig. 48.2 Patient referred for retained common duct stone removal. The filling defect was immobile on instrumentation. A flexible biopsy wire was positioned on the lesion with the steerable catheter and tissue was obtained. Histopathological diagnosis revealed cholangiocarcinoma of the common duct

Cholecystostomy tract

Similar to the use of the postoperative T-tube tract, radiological instrumentation through a cholecystostomy is feasible in order to gain access to the gallbladder or common duct for stone extraction.

A five-week waiting period after surgical cholecystostomy is required before instrumentation. If deliberate cholecystostomy is performed in high-risk patients with cholelithiasis, it is advisable to stitch the gallbladder fundus to the peritoneum behind the rectus sheath. This permits radiological instrumentation for gallstone removal one week after operation.

Jejunostomy

Presence of a jejunostomy facilitates radiological intervention for stone removal in patients with intrahepatic stones proximal to a hepatojejunostomy. We have used the same approach for repeated intrahepatic stone removal and stricture dilatation in patients with Caroli's disease (Ch. 80) and recurrent pyogenic cholangitis, particularly when stones recur after surgical left hepatojejunostomy for decompression of the obstructed biliary tract.

EXTRACTION OF STONES FROM THE BILE DUCTS

Bile duct stones retained after operation continue to be an exasperating problem (Ch. 46). Operative cholangiography has reduced the number of retained stones (Jolly, Baker & Schmidt 1968), but the incidence of false negative completion cholangiograms remains about 5% after common duct exploration (Longmire et al 1979). The additional use of intraoperative choledochoscopy may reduce this figure (Ch. 29).

The problem is not new. More than 70 years ago, William Halstead, who performed one of the earliest operations on the gallbladder, stated that a simple reliable method was needed to determine accurately the presence of stones in the common bile duct. 20 years later, Dr. Halstead was himself to die of complications after the removal of a retained common duct stone (Longmire et al 1979).

Non-operative radiological intervention for retained bile duct stone removal has greatly helped in the treatment of this surgical complication. The technique is not technically demanding and is now widely employed.

Technique

Radiological intervention for retained stone removal is usually done in the ambulatory patient five weeks after cholecystectomy and common duct exploration. The T-tube is removed and a steerable catheter is introduced through the fibrous tract into the common duct. A stone extraction basket is then manoeuvred through the steerable catheter in a closed position alongside the stone and opened behind it. The retained material is ensnared with the basket under fluoroscopic vision during cholangiography. The stones are then extracted through the sinus tract. The tract of a 14 French T-tube will permit extraction of the intact stone if it measures 6 or 7 mm in diameter. Larger stones require fragmentation before the fragments are extracted. The radiologist must allow for a 30% magnification factor when measuring stones on cholangiograms. This magnification factor is larger in the distal common duct and less for intrahepatic stones.

We no longer close the stone basket after the stone has been engaged since closure often results in fragmentation or disengagement of the stone. Even small stones will remain in the basket tip during continuous extraction through the duct system and sinus tract. Hesitant with-

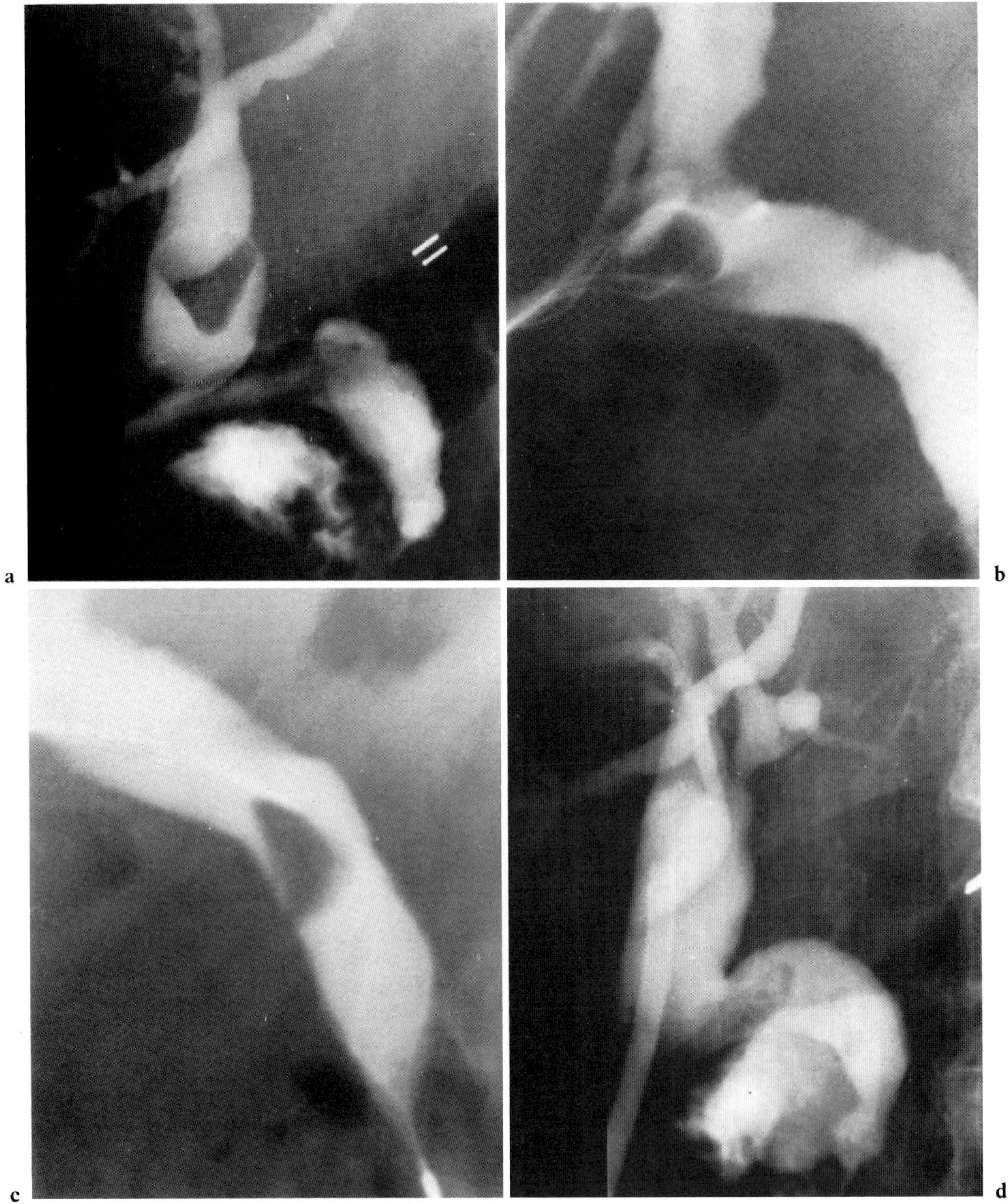

Fig. 48.3 a. Large retained common hepatic duct stone. b. The retained stone was fragmented at the junction of bile duct and sinus tract. Note deformity of the wire basket due to traction c. Major fragments remaining are extracted. Note the straight cut margin of this fragment due to fragmentation with a basket wire. d. The major fragments have been extracted. A few very small fragments remain but passed spontaneously into the duodenum as confirmed on cholangiogram three days later

drawal, however, may permit small stones to fall outside the basket.

Small stones and fragments of about 3 mm size and smaller frequently pass spontaneously through the ampulla. If the short arm of the T-tube prevents retained small stones in the common hepatic duct from moving distally, the T-tube should be exchanged for a straight tube early in the postoperative period to permit spontaneous passage of small stones. Small stones and fragments of 1 or 2 mm in size are difficult to identify on the fluoroscopic screen. Intermittent spot films are then indicated to assess stone location. If the steerable catheter does not advance beyond the retained stone, the closed basket is moved alongside it. The tip of the basket is never directed against the wall of the common duct but is manoeuvred in an axial direction by steering the catheter tip.

Large stones (over 6 to 8 mm in diameter) cannot be extracted intact through the sinus tract of a 14 French T-tube (Fig. 48.3). Fragmentation is then required. This was indicated in 98 out of 661 patients reported by the author (Burhenne 1980). Fragmentation, however, was possible in all these patients because large retained stones are almost always relatively soft. The stone is brought with the basket to the junction of the bile duct and the sinus tract, where strong resistance is felt. Increased and steady traction on the end of the basket wire is then applied over one to two minutes. No more than a pulling force of about 10 kg is necessary. The steady and increasing pull results in the stone being cut by the wire basket. No common duct injury has been experienced. Stones may also be fragmented by closing the basket within the duct. The open basket with the stone within it is pulled against the catheter tip. As the steerable catheter is quite soft, catheter exchange over the wire end of the basket may be required. Stiff dilatation catheters are useful for this purpose. After a fragmentation procedure, only the major fragments are extracted during the same session. Small fragments will usually pass spontaneously.

Partially impacted stones in the distal end of the common duct are often difficult to engage in the wire basket since the basket must be opened beyond the papilla of Vater, there being insufficient space between the stone and the papilla. Impacted stones must therefore be moved to a more proximal position in the duct to permit satisfactory opening of the basket. Suction through the catheter or a forcible contrast injection with a small 8 French steerable catheter distal to the stone are sometimes of help. If the stone cannot be moved the author proceeds to the use of a vascular Fogarty balloon catheter. This is distended

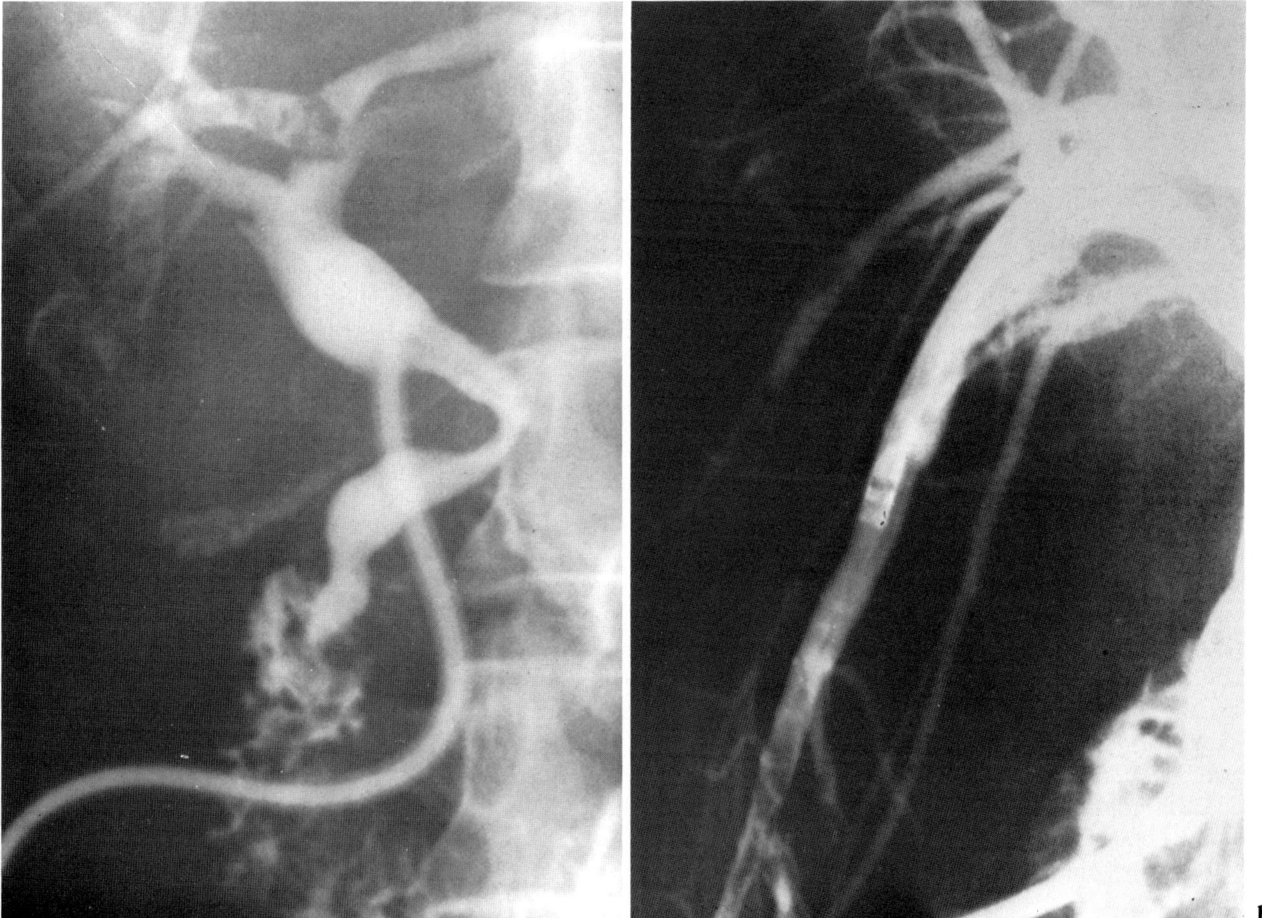

Fig. 48.4 a. Postoperative T-tube cholangiogram shows the dorso-caudal branch entering the left hepatic radicle completely filled with impacted retained stones. b. The steerable catheter has been manoeuvred into the dorso-caudal branch which is now almost completely free of retained material

with contrast material for exact visualization of size and position under the fluoroscope. The inflated balloon catheter is manipulated behind the stone and then eased centrally with a gentle pull. If the balloon is seen to wedge the stone sideways, no undue traction should be applied.

Intrahepatic stones

Biliary stones in intrahepatic radicles are often multiple and may be impacted (Figs. 48.4, 48.9). As the steerable catheter cannot be passed alongside, the closed stone basket is moved beyond the stone for extraction. This is technically more demanding and represents a greater challenge than extraction of extrahepatic stones. Intrahepatic stones, however, may move spontaneously into an extrahepatic location if the T-tube is exchanged. It is often the case that the short arm of a T-tube lying within the common hepatic duct or in one hepatic radicle prevents distal migration of stones. The T-tube is extracted and exchanged for a straight catheter and the patient is then recalled after one or two weeks of ambulation.

Use of the Fogarty balloon is often required if intrahepatic stones are lodged in position. The balloon is inflated with contrast for fluoroscopic identification and gentle traction is applied. Over-distension of the balloon may lead to extravasation. Manipulation and extraction of intrahepatic stones, however, is more readily accomplished under postoperative fluoroscopy than during surgery. Not infrequently, review of the operative cholangiogram will demonstrate evidence of iatrogenic liver injury resulting from ductal instrumentation with a Fogarty biliary balloon catheter (Eaton et al 1971).

Radiological intervention for intrahepatic biliary stones usually requires multiple sessions. A straight catheter is introduced through the sinus tract into the common duct in order to maintain access between sessions.

RESULTS

The author's experience now involves 1955 patients with an overall success rate of 96%. About one-half of the patients with failure to remove all stones had intrahepatic stones. Failure has also occurred with some impacted distal common duct stones. Other causes were inability to catheterize the sinus tract of a small T-tube or inability to recatheterize the tract on a return visit. Cystic duct remnant stones are sometimes impossible to remove, particularly when the stone does not migrate from the cystic duct into the distal common duct with the patient in the erect position. The steerable catheter is then used in an attempt to mobilize the cystic duct stone by transmural pressure exerted on the common hepatic and cystic ducts.

Twelve patients with known impacted distal common duct stones had residual stones after surgical exploration. Four of these twelve patients underwent a second surgical exploration and the surgeon was again unable to disimpact the distal common duct stone even after opening the duodenum. The author was able to dislodge all stones in these twelve patients successfully and extract them. Indeed radiological intervention for impacted stones is technically easier and more successful than operation in selected patients. In a review of the first 661 patients with retained intrahepatic stones after surgery, 80% were in extrahepatic location, 15% were in intrahepatic location, and 5% were combined (Burhenne 1980).

It probably takes at least 20 extraction procedures for a radiologist to become sufficiently experienced in this technique. Nevertheless the author's results have been duplicated by other investigators with large experience.

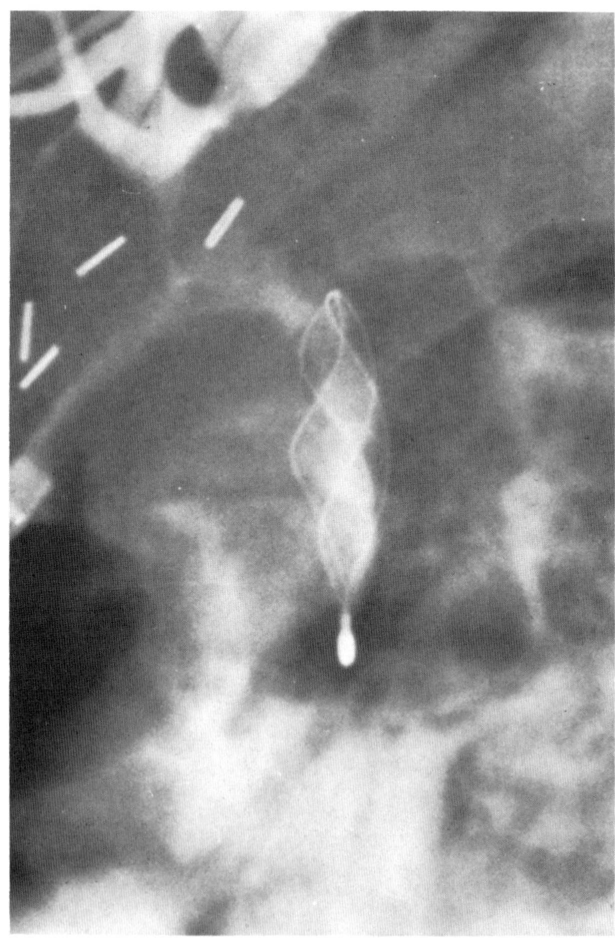

Fig. 48.5 The stone basket became detached from the wire stem during extraction procedure for retained distal common duct stone. A guide wire sling manoeuvred through the steerable catheter in the T-tube tract was then employed to ensnare the end of the wire basket and remove it successfully. Cholangiograms demonstrated no subsequent extravasation from the bile ducts. The retained common duct stone was also removed

Complications

No perforation of the biliary tract and no mortality occurred in any of the 1955 patients referred for retained stone extraction. The morbidity rate has been 4.1%. A survey of 39 institutions reporting a total of 612 stone extraction procedures showed a morbidity of 5% and no mortality (Burhenne 1976). A review of the same procedure performed in 26 British hospitals showed a complication rate of 9.2%, including pancreatitis, fever and perforation of the sinus tract. No perforation of the biliary tract has been reported (Mason 1980) (Fig. 48.5).

Perforation of the sinus tract may render recatheterization impossible and does result in stone extraction failure. Patients with perforation of the sinus tract are placed on antibiotics. In the author's series signs and symptoms subsided within 48 hours. Patients with a history of post-operative pancreatitis are placed on prophylactic antibiotics. One patient reported by the author required surgical drainage of an extrahepatic bile collection after extraction intervention (Burhenne 1976).

One death has been reported with percutaneous stone extraction (Polack, Fainsinger & Bonnano 1977). The patient died of acute pancreatitis after radiological manipu-

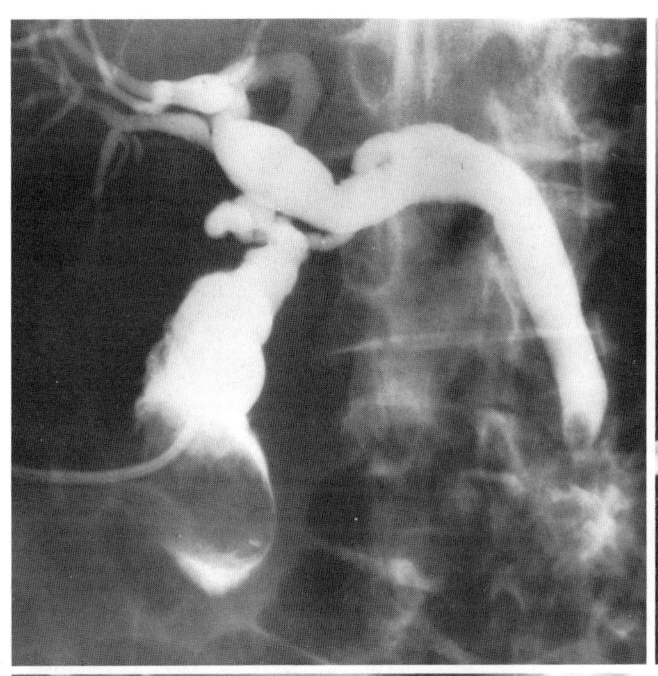

a

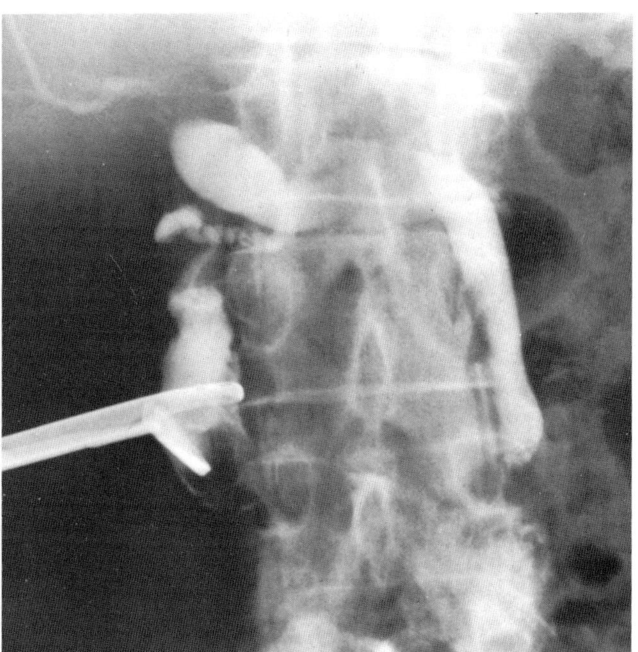

b

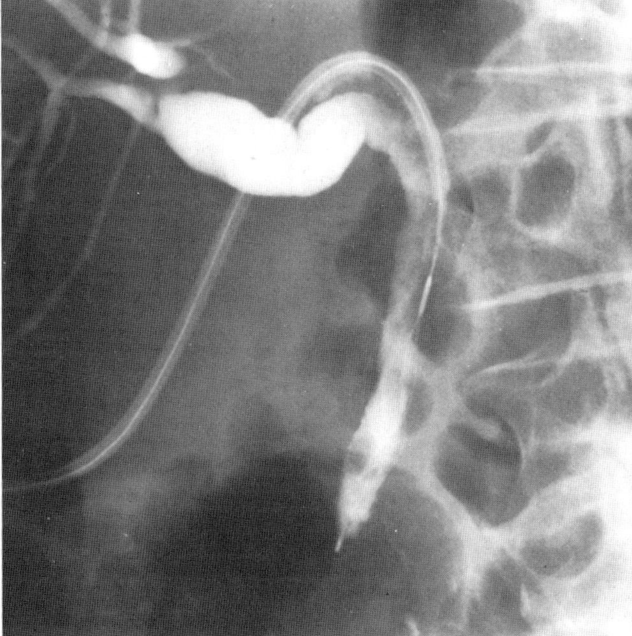

c

Fig. 48.6 a. Solitary 4 × 6 cm gallbladder stone and single distal common duct stone after cholecystotomy drainage for acute cholecystitis. b. Stortz bladder stone crushing forceps was introduced through the cholecystostomy tract for fragmentation and complete removal of the gallbladder stone. c. Steerable catheter was manipulated through the cystic duct and the distal common duct stone was engaged and removed through the cystic duct and gallbladder after balloon dilatation of the cystic duct. Following removal of all stones in multiple interventional sessions in this 93-year-old male, the cholecystostomy tube was removed and the gallbladder was left in place

lation of a retained stone. The case involved a small distal common duct stone and difficult instrumentation. The radiologist had had previous experience with four stone extractions. It is of interest that this patient had a previous history of acute pancreatitis. In addition, this patient was transferred with the instruments in place from one fluoroscopic room to another with spot film facilities. Fluoroscopic visualization alone is insufficient, particularly with small stones, since identification of small stones on the fluoroscopic screen alone can be impossible. A spot film device is mandatory.

EXTRACTION OF GALLBLADDER STONES

Radiological instrumentation through cholecystostomy tracts permits removal of stones from the gallbladder, the cystic duct and the common duct (Burhenne 1983). Large stones in the gallbladder require fragmentation with a bladder stone crushing forceps. Fragments are then extracted with the stone basket or with a Mazzariello forceps (Fig. 48.6). The same subhepatic interventional approach through the cholecystostomy tract may be used for removal of common bile duct stones. This usually requires dilatation of the cystic duct with an angioplasty balloon catheter.

Surgical cholecystostomy and subsequent radiological stone removal is an alternative to cholecystectomy in high-risk elderly patients where cholecystectomy for acute cholecystitis carries a 9.8% operative death rate in patients over 65 (Glenn 1981). 21 high risk patients in our institution underwent mini-cholecystostomy under local anaesthetic followed by radiological stone extraction without mortality (Burhenne and Stoller 1985) (Fig. 48.7). The gallbladder was left in place except in one young pregnant patient who underwent subsequent cholecystectomy.

EXTRACTION OF STONES PROXIMAL TO STRICTURES

Intrahepatic stones are often situated above hepatic duct strictures. This is usually the case in recurrent pyogenic cholangitis and a complicating factor in Caroli's disease. Hepatic duct stones may also be present proximal to a stenosed hepato-jejunostomy (Ch. 58). Stone extraction in these patients cannot be accomplished without preceding stricture dilatation, another interventional

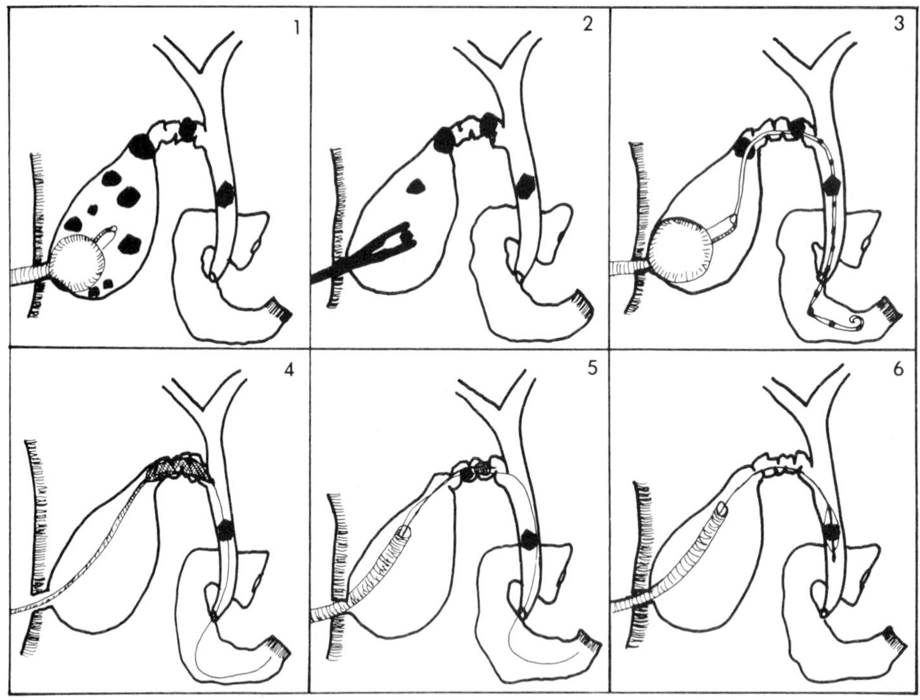

Fig. 48.7 Cholecystostomy intervention for cholelithiasis. 1. Balloon catheter is in place after mini-cholecystostomy with the gallbladder fundus sutured to the abdominal wall. Cholelithiasis affects gallbladder, cystic duct and common duct. 2. Ten days after mini-cholecystostomy, stones are removed from the gallbladder with Mazzariello forceps under fluoroscopic control. 3. A drainage catheter with side holes has been placed through the cystic and common ducts into the duodenum after manipulation with an 8 French steerable catheter and guide wire. The drainage catheter is placed through the 24 French cholecystostomy balloon catheter between procedures. 4. A guide wire is introduced through the drainage catheter into the duodenum and an angiographic balloon catheter is use for cystic duct dilatation. 5. Stones in the cystic duct are now retrieved into the gallbladder after inflation of a Fogarty balloon distally to the stone. A guide wire remains in place alongside the Fogarty balloon for access. 6. A final session involves catheter placement into the common duct followed by stone extraction basket positioning and extraction of the common duct stone through the cystic duct and gallbladder. The cholelithiasis treatment is completed

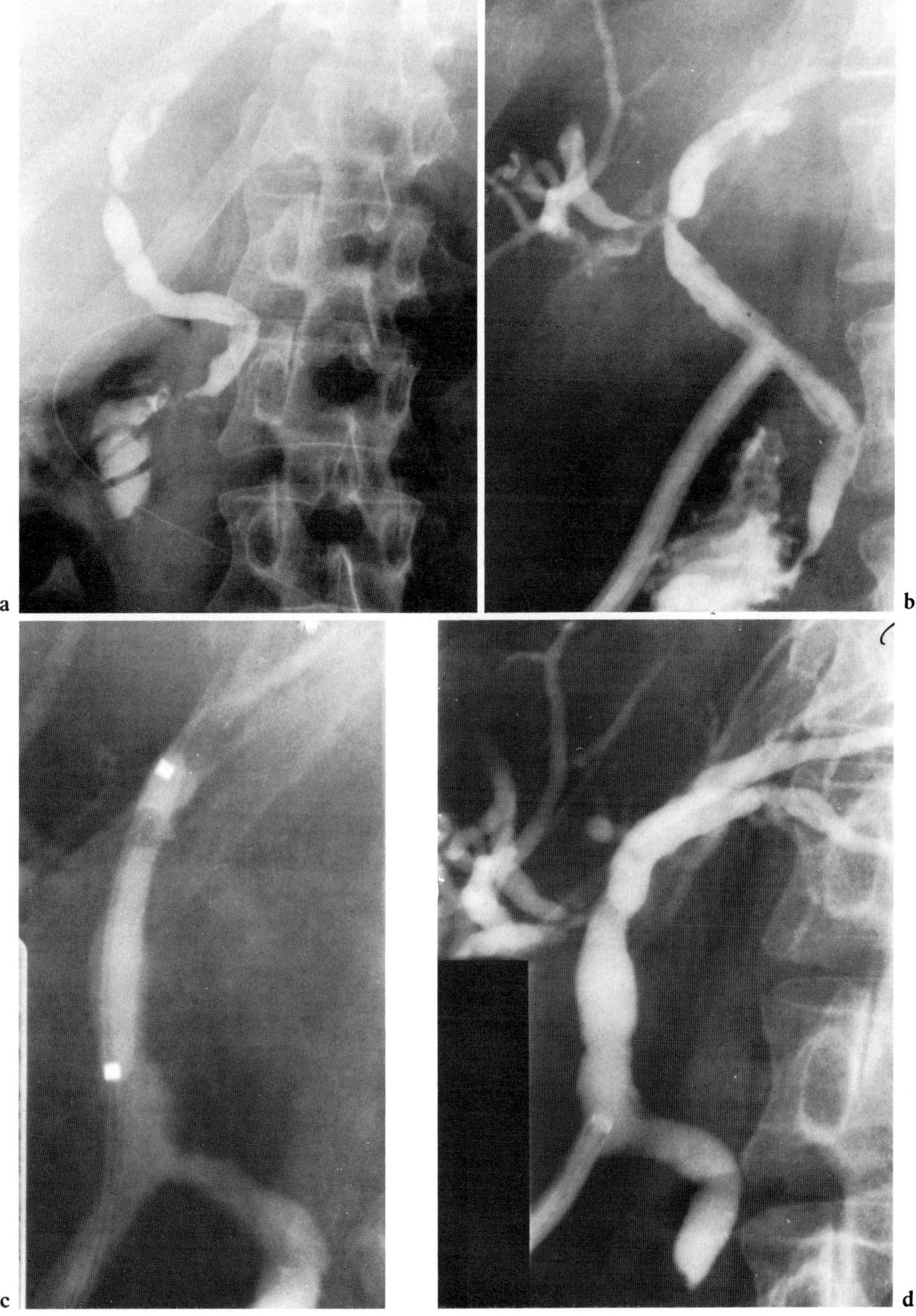

Fig. 48.8 a. The operative cholangiogram before common duct exploration shows a single common duct stone. This stone was removed surgically. There is also a stricture at the porta hepatis with stones proximal to it in the distended left hepatic duct. b. Five weeks after operation, the T-tube is removed in the ambulatory patient. The cholangiogram shows multiple duct strictures at the porta hepatis. A needle was placed percutaneously and histopathology revealed inflammatory changes with no evidence of carcinoma. c. Dilatation balloon is placed in the left hepatic duct for stricture dilatation. d. Completion cholangiogram shows all stones removed. The left hepatic stricture has been dilated to a normal calibre. Right hepatic duct strictures remain

radiological technique of recent origin (Burhenne 1975) (Fig. 48.8).

Similar to percutaneous stone extraction, the subhepatic approach through postoperative drain tracts or via a jejunostomy is used to position angioplasty balloon catheters across the stricture for dilatation. Manual injection pressure usually suffices to obtain satisfactory stricture dilatation (Burhenne 1983). If postoperative drain tracts are not available for instrumentation, percutaneous puncture of the dilated and stone-containing ducts is accomplished under ultrasonography. Guide wires are placed through the stricture, followed by a dilatation balloon (Fig. 48.9). It is our experience, however, that most strictures will recur without a stent placed through the duct or anastomosis after dilatation. End or side holes are placed in the stenting catheter above and below the

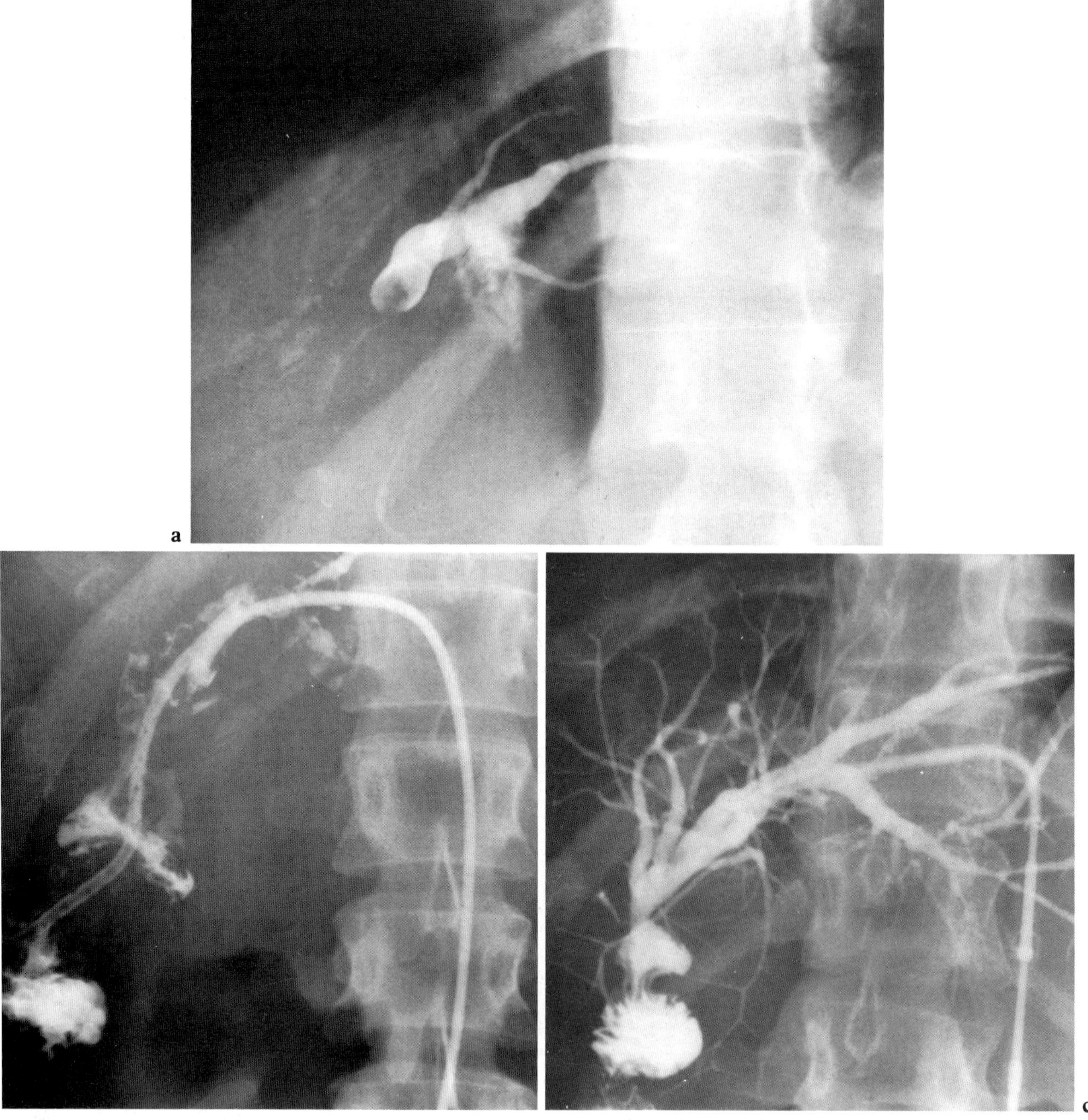

Fig. 48.9 a. Deeply jaundiced patient 16 months after hepatojejunostomy shows impacted intrahepatic stone in left radicle on subxiphoid transhepatic cholangiography. b. An internal drainage catheter was placed over a guide wire after balloon dilatation of a stricture at the hepato-jejunostomy anastomosis. Innumerable intrahepatic stones are now identified. c. Cholangiogram demonstrates that all stones were extracted or expelled and the anastomotic dilatation was maintained after three months of catheter stenting

stricture site for internal drainage. The stenting catheter is then closed externally.

REPLACEMENT OF T-TUBES

Indwelling postoperative drainage tubes often require replacement because of obstruction or inadvertent extraction. Restoration of tube patency may be accomplished by passing guide wires through the obstructed tube but obstruction of draining tubes by sediment is a recurrent problem and tube exchange over a guide wire is preferable. This can be accomplished even in the case of T-tubes. Two separate guide wires are placed through the drainage tract into the proximal and distal bile duct with the use of steerable catheters (Burhenne 1983). The two short arms of the T-tube are then inserted over the guide wires separately, whereas both guide wires are fed through the long arm of the T-tube. The critical catheter width is at the junction of the short and long arms of the tube at the point where the two short arms are folded alongside each other. Dilatation of the sinus tract with balloon catheters may be required before T-tube insertion (Burhenne & Morris 1980).

RADIOLOGIC CONVERSION OF T-TUBE INTO U-TUBE

T-tubes may be converted into transhepatic U-tubes if multiple intrahepatic stones require multiple sessions for removal or in patients with bile duct strictures requiring long-term stenting (Burhenne & Peters 1978).

With the use of a percutaneous puncture technique analogous to transhepatic cholangiography, a guide wire is inserted through the intrahepatic ducts to the porta hepatis and into the common hepatic duct. A stone removal wire basket is then positioned by means of a steerable catheter passed through the subhepatic drainage tract. The tip of the proximal transhepatic guide wire is engaged in the wire basket and the guide wire is pulled through the drainage tract in a U fashion (Fig. 48.10). A drainage tube is then placed over the guide wire and the two ends are connected externally. This prevents inadvertent removal and provides for internal drainage with properly positioned side holes in the catheter.

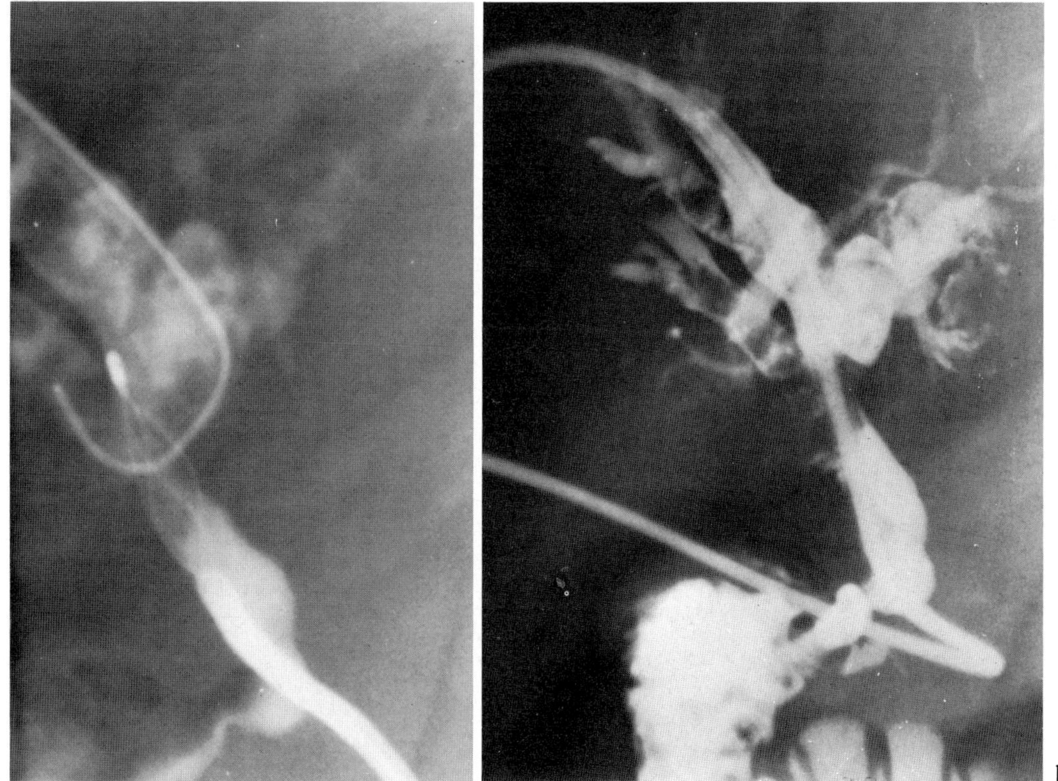

Fig. 48.10 a. T-tube has been extracted and a transhepatically placed guide wire is engaged in a wire basket from below in order to place a U-tube. b. The U-tube is in place for long-term stenting of an iatrogenic stricture in the common hepatic duct and for removal of intrahepatic stones ultilizing multiple interventional sessions

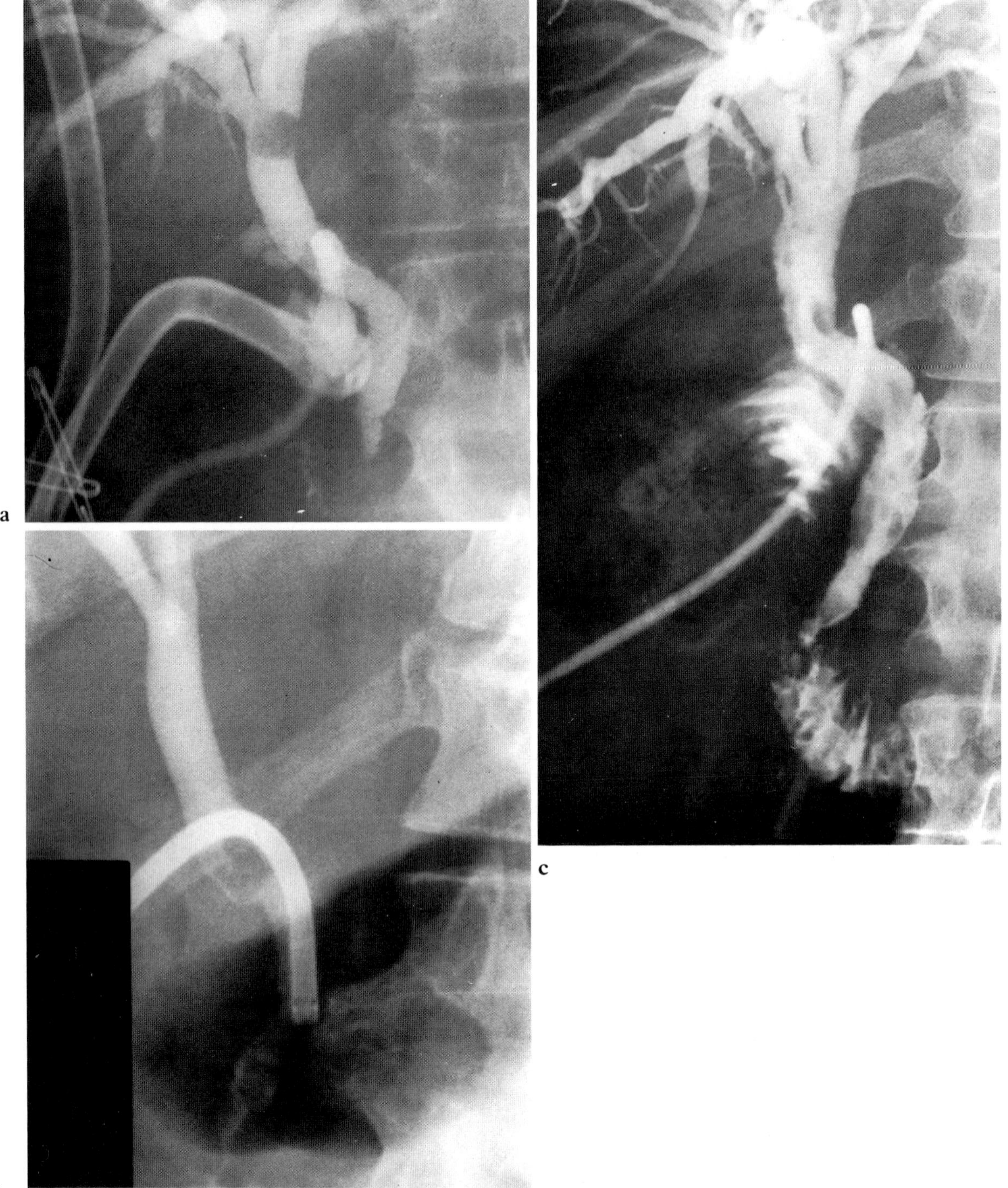

Fig. 48.11 a. Postoperative T-tube cholangiogram demonstrates retained common hepatic duct stone. b. The patient experienced septicaemia after 10 days of Capmul (monooctanoin, Ascot Pharmaceuticals, Inc., Skokie, Illinois) infusion in hospital. Note changes of cholangitis on T-tube cholangiogram. Attempts at chemical dissolution were discontinued and the patient recovered after 10 days of antibiotic therapy. He was discharged and referred for ambulatory radiological stone extraction eight weeks after surgery. c. The T-tube has been extracted and cholangiography with the steerable catheter in place in the common duct shows that the retained stone has increased in size. There is now a second stone in the distal common duct. Both stones were successfully extracted in the ambulatory patient

CONSIDERATIONS COMPARING RADIOLOGIC INTERVENTION TO OTHER TECHNIQUES FOR BILIARY STONE REMOVAL

Non-operative stone extraction techniques have almost replaced re-operation for retained stones. The latter procedure carries a higher mortality and morbidity than the initial operative procedure. The author has had no mortality in 1955 patients undergoing radiological intervention for retained stones.

Endoscopic retrograde sphincterotomy (Ch. 47) and stone extraction is useful in patients without radiological access through postoperative drain tracts. If a postoperative T-tube is in place, however, radiological intervention is the procedure of choice (Classen and Ossenberg 1977), as endoscopic stone removal has a lower success rate and a higher complication rate. Endoscopic removal of intrahepatic stones, fragmentation of large stones in the bile ducts and stricture dilatation is not very successful. Percutaneous transhepatic removal of biliary stones should be reserved for the unusual case where endoscopic sphincterotomy and surgery are contraindicated.

Stone lithotripsy for retained common duct stones (Burhenne 1975b) should only be attempted if calcified biliary stones are present which cannot be fragmented with the wire basket. Infusion of various chemicals for dissolution of bile duct stones has been reported but with a limited success. The treatment requires hospitalization and therapeutic results do not compare favourably with instrumentation techniques at the present time (Fig. 48.11) (Ch. 49). Stone dissolution is not recommended as the initial procedure of choice.

REFERENCES

Burckhardt H, Mueller W 1921 Versuche über die Punktion der Gallenblase und ihre Röntgendarstellung; Deutsche Zeitschrift für Chirurgie 162: 168–197

Burhenne H J 1973 Nonoperative retained biliary tract stone extraction: a new roentgenologic technique. American Journal of Roentgenology 117: 388–399

Burhenne H J 1975a Dilatation of biliary tract strictures. Radiologia Clinica 44: 153–159

Burhenne H J 1975b Electrohydrolytic fragmentation of retained common duct stones. Radiology 117: 721–722

Burhenne H J 1976 Complications of nonoperative extraction of retained common duct stones. American Journal of Surgery 131: 260–262

Burhenne H J 1980 Percutaneous extraction of retained biliary tract stones: 661 patients. American Journal of Roentgenology 134: 888–898

Burhenne H J 1983 Biliary tract. In: Margulis A R, Burhenne H J (eds) Alimentary tract radiology; 3rd edn. C V Mosby, St. Louis, ch. 90, p 2318–2352

Burhenne H J, Peters H E 1978 Retained intrahepatic stones: use of the U tube during repeated nonoperative stone extraction. Archives of Surgery 113: 837–841

Burhenne H J, Morris D C 1980 Biliary stricture dilatation: use of the Grüntzig balloon catheter. Journal of the Canadian Association of Radiologists 31: 196–197

Burhenne H J, Stoller J L 1985 Mini-cholecystostomy and radiological stone extraction in high risk cholelithiasis patients: preliminary experience. American Journal of Surgery 149: 632–635

Classen M, Ossenberg F W 1977 Nonsurgical removal of common bile duct stones. Gut 18: 760–769

Cole W H 1960 The story of cholecystography. American Journal of Surgery 99: 206–222

Cotte G 1925 Sur l'exploration des voies biliares au lipiodal en case de fistule. Bulletin et Memories de la Société nationalie de Chirurgie 23: 759–764

Dotter C T, Bilbao M K, Katon R M 1979 Percutaneous transhepatic gallstone removal by needle tract. Radiology 133: 242–243

Eaton S B Jr, Wirtz R D, Eyck J R et al 1971 Iatrogenic liver injury resulting from ductal instrumentation with a Fogarty biliary balloon catheter. Radiology 100: 581–584

Ellman B A, Berman H L 1981 Treatment of a common duct stone via transhepatic approach. Gastrointestinal Radiology 6: 357–359

Glenn F 1981 Surgical management of acute cholecystitis in patients 65 years of age and older. Annals of Surgery 193: 56–59

Jolly P C, Baker J W, Schmidt H M 1968 Operative cholangiography: a case for its routine use. Annals of Surgery 168: 551–556

Longmire W P Jr, Goldstein L I, Sample W F, Kadell B, Tompkins R K 1979 The treatment of retained gallstones. Western Journal of Medicine 130: 422–434

Mason R 1980 Percutaneous extraction of retained gallstones via the T-tube track: British experience of 131 cases. Clinical Radiology 31: 497–499

Mazzariello R 1973 Review of 220 cases of residual biliary tract calculi treated without reoperation: an eight-year study. Surgery 73: 299–306

Polack E P, Fainsinger M H, Bonnano S V 1977 A death following complications of roentgenologic nonoperative manipulation of common bile duct calculi. Radiology 123: 585–586

E. Mack

Dissolution of common duct stones

Approximately 700 000 cholecystectomies are performed every year in the United States. If one assumes that 15–20% of these operations include exploration of the common duct for removal of biliary calculi, and that 2–9% of choledochotomies are complicated by retained common duct stones, one can appreciate the number of patients who need additional treatment for this problem. This chapter is strictly confined to dissolution of common duct stones. The reader is referred to chapters 46 to 48 in this book for the radiological, endoscopic and surgical management of common duct calculi.

Dissolution of common duct stones has been attempted with varying degrees of success for almost 100 years. However, during the past 20 years, due to a clearer understanding of the pathogenesis and composition of gallstones in general and common duct stones in particular, significant progress has been achieved in the treatment of common duct stones by dissolution. Most common duct stones are secondary; that is, these stones are formed within the gallbladder and then pass through the cystic into the common duct. In sharp contrast are primary common duct stones, which form within the common duct itself often many years following previous biliary tract surgery, and which are composed primarily of calcium bilirubinate with a cholesterol content of less than 25% (Heiss et al 1984).

The purpose of this chapter is to review the various agents used for dissolution of common duct stones, to report the techniques employed and the results achieved, and to place the dissolution of common duct stones in proper clinical perspective.

DISSOLUTION AGENTS

The major chemical solvents used for common duct stone dissolution include ether, chloroform, additive drugs such as lidocaine, sphincter relaxants, bile acids, heparin, clofibrate, flushing with normal saline, monooctanoin, and bile acid-EDTA mixtures (Table 49.1).

Table 49.1 Examples of major solvents used for dissolution of common duct stones

Year	Agent	Principal investigator
1891	ether	Walker
1930–39	ether	Pribram
1953	chloroform	Best
1971	heparin	Gardner
1972	sodium cholate 100 mM	Admirand & Way
1974	sodium cholate 200 mM	Toouli
1977	monooctanoin in vitro	Thistle & Hofmann
1978	monooctanoin in man	Mack & Thistle

Ether

In 1891, only two years after the first successful choledochotomies had been performed, Walker first attempted the dissolution of a retained stone. To dissolve an impacted gallstone, he used a mixture of ether and glycerine which he instilled drop by drop through a glass tube into the fistulous tract to the gallbladder of a patient who had already had 27 stones removed by cholecystostomy. Two days after this treatment, Walker could no longer palpate the stone and believed that ether had accomplished the dissolution.

Walker's idea did not attract much attention until the 1930s when Pribram (1939) rekindled interest in dissolution of gallstones with ether. For historical interest, it seems appropriate to quote from Pribram's 1938 lecture delivered at the British Postgraduate Medical School, London describing his first attempt to dissolve stones remaining in the common bile duct after operation, and published in the Lancet the following year.

A man, age 68, had had gall-stones for many years, and a fresh attack had been followed by jaundice lasting several weeks. His general state was deteriorating, and he was having chills and rigors. Signs of acute pancreatitis appeared.

The diagnosis was confirmed at operation. The badly inflamed inner coats of the gall-bladder were quickly electrocoagulated (mucoclasis). A supraduodenal opening was made into the common duct, and many stones were extracted, but it was impossible to empty the ampulla completely through this incision. Further manipulation by the retroduodenal or the transduodenal route would have been risky, especially in the presence of acute pancreatitis, and I did nothing more than introduce a small drain into the common duct. The drain reached the stones, and the common duct was tightly sewn around it, my idea being that, if the patient survived, I would try to dissolve or soften the stones by injecting suitable solvents through the drain. The operation was thus performed very quickly, and the recovery of the patient was so satisfactory that on the fifth day we could begin our experiment.

In the hope of dissolving the cholesterol that forms the nucleus of the stones, we injected a few drops of ether through the drain several times daily. This procedure was followed by injection of a small quantity of liquid paraffin to facilitate the passage of the softened stones through the papilla. The course of the treatment was followed radiographically by injecting Lipiodol. The first radiogram showed the stone lying over the papilla, while the small amount of Lipiodol was already passing into the duodenum. After a fortnight's ether treatment a cholangiogram showed that the stones were already partly dissolved and that the remaining pulp had passed into the duodenum. It was relatively easy, as the next radiogram showed, to introduce the drain through the papilla into the duodenum.

Since then I have applied the ether method in further 37 cases of gall-stones impacted in the papilla and, as confirmed by cholangiography, I have in all cases surviving the operation (38 out of 40) succeeded in emptying the papilla. This conservative treatment has proved a real advance in lowering the operation risk and improving the results. The fatality-rate in these serious cases has dropped from 20 to 5 percent. By routine radiography after injection of Lipiodol into the bile-duct we can make certain that no stones are left and the whole bile-duct system is clear. This certainty we never had before, and its importance is shown by the observation at Kirschner's Clinic that in half the cases with recurrent trouble after operation the cause is stones left behind.

In a follow-up publication in 1947, Pribram reported that in 51 cases treated with his ether method, there were no failures and he was not forced to resort to reoperation. In his earlier publication in 1939, Pribram described the procedure. Since ether boils at body temperature (one cc ether vaporizes to about 222 cc of ether gas), sudden distension of the common duct with resulting pain usually follows its instillation. Therefore, Pribram stressed the importance of a drop by drop introduction of ether for small ducts, and 0.5–1.00 cc of ether for large ones. He emphasized the need to aspirate the bile prior to ether instillation, and to aspirate again should pain occur, repeating the process several times daily, thereby doing an actual lavage. At the end of each session, 1–2 cc of liquid paraffin were injected into the common duct and the tube clamped until the next treatment. Occasionally he added adrenaline, atropine or procaine as relaxants for the sphincter of Oddi. The time required for dissolution ranged from one to eight weeks.

Strickler et al (1951) summarized the modifications made by numerous other investigators of Pribram's ether flush method. Such modifications include a mixture of two-thirds ethyl ether to one-third ethyl alcohol followed by warm oil, the addition of nitroglycerin and atropine on alternate days with bile salts, magnesium sulphate and cream or olive oil as stimulants. Strickler and co-authors performed detailed in vitro experiments and found that only ether or ether-alcohol mixtures proved to be highly effective in dissolving or fragmenting gallstones. They did not find any solvent activity in ox bile, dog bile, sodium taurocholate, 0.5% acetic acid or papain.

Chloroform

The most detailed description of the usefulness of chloroform is given by Best et al (1953). These authors systematically tested 113 different solutions such as fat solvents, surface tension-lowering agents, calcium binding agents, naturally occurring fatty acids, hydrotropic agents (bile salts, dog and ox bile), hydrolytic and dispersing agents, and some miscellaneous substances such as acetic, hydrochloric and nitric acid. On the basis of their experiments, they found ether and chloroform to be the only satisfactory solvents. These investigators studied a group of 10 patients in whom retained common duct stones were seen by cholangiogram performed one week after surgery. These patients were placed on a three-day biliary flush regimen which included three tablets of dehydrocholic acid with belladonna after each meal and at bedtime; one-half bottle of magnesium citrate (6 oz) each morning before breakfast; three tablespoonsful of pure cream or olive oil before noon and evening meals each day; and one tablet of nitroglycerin dissolved under the tongue before the evening meal each day. On days one and two, 4 or 5 ml of heated chloroform were injected into the side arm of a double lumen T-tube. Prior to the chloroform treatment, the common duct was irrigated with warm saline and then its contents aspirated. On the third day of the flush, 5 ml of ethyl ether were injected, with pressure released as needed. Nitroglycerin was given sublingually five minutes prior to the instillation of the ether. This regimen succeeded in 80% of cases. In three patients the first injection series was successful; the remaining patients required several repeat injections before the duct system was free of stones. There were two failures. These authors point out that a heated solution of chloroform should be injected just under the vaporization point of chloroform, which is 61°C.

Lidocaine and isoproterenol

McCarthy (1969) injected lidocaine under pressure into the biliary tree as a manoeuvre to relax the sphincter of Oddi and to facilitate the passage of a retained calculus. In two patients, toxic side effects in the liver occurred and one patient died. Therefore, McCarthy recommended that lidocaine should not be used for this purpose.

Dardik et al reported in 1971 the effect of beta receptor stimulation by isoproterenol on ampullary flow and passage of intracholedochal foreign bodies in dogs. The mean irrigation pressures required for the passage of a foreign body into the duodenum decreased by 46% from control values when isoproterenol was infused at a rate of 10 μg/ml/min. Commenting on their results in 10 dogs, these authors conclude that the stimulation of beta receptors may serve as a valuable adjunct in the management of patients with retained choledochal calculi by decreasing ampullary resistance.

Bile acids

In 1972 Admirand & Way reported the successful dissolution of retained common duct stones in patients with a continuous infusion of sodium cholate. One hundred millimoles of commercial grade sodium cholate were dissolved in one litre of 0.5% normal saline. The solution was buffered to pH 8 with sodium bicarbonate and sterilized by millipore filtration. This sterile bile salt solution was infused continuously into a T-tube at a rate of 30 ml/hour with a calibrated intravenous set as pressure manometer. In 11 out of 17 patients studied, the gallstones completely disappeared, a success rate of 65%. The average time for stone disappearance was six days with a range of three to 14 days. Oral cholestyramine was given as necessary for control of bile salt-induced diarrhoea.

In a more extensive paper, Way et al (1972) reported success in treating retained common duct stones in 12 out of 22 patients using a sodium cholate solution (100 mM in saline buffered to pH 7.5) infused by gravity drip at 30 ml/hour for a maximum of 14 days. A manometer was placed in the line between the drip bottle and the patient and the zero level was adjusted to correspond with the approximate position of the bile duct. If the duct was unobstructed, the pressure usually varied between 15 and 20 cm of solution during treatment.

Proximal stones or those on the hepatic side of the T-tube could not be handled satisfactorily by this method. In these cases the authors threaded a small polyethylene catheter (PE-50) through the lumen of the T-tube and, with fluoroscopic control, placed the tip in the vicinity of the stone. The bile salt solution was administered through the polyethylene tube and allowed to escape from the duct in the residual lumen of the long arm of the T-tube. The same pressure-monitoring arrangement and follow-up cholangiograms were employed. Cholestyramine, 4 gm every two hours during the day, was given to control bile salt-induced diarrhoea.

Two years later Toouli et al (1974) successfully dissolved common duct stones in 13 out of 16 patients. These authors doubled the concentration of sodium cholate to a 200 mM solution. They essentially employed the same technique as Way & Admirand.

In 1974 Lansford and co-authors reported good results in dissolving retained common duct stones with sodium cholate according to the method of Way et al (1972). Five out of six patients were treated successfully because the stones were between the distal end of the T-tube and the ampulla. The failure occurred in a patient whose stone was between the T-tube and the liver. In contrast to Way's report, these authors observed side effects of the therapy in three out of five successfully treated patients. One stone became transiently impacted in the distal bile duct associated with a rise in intraductal pressure and pain in the epigastrium and back. Mild pancreatitis developed in two patients as evidenced by elevated amylase levels in serum and urine.

In a controlled trial, reported by LaRusso et al (1975), a solution of 75 mM sodium cholate or a 150 mM sodium chloride solution was infused into six patients at 30 ml/hour in a randomly assigned, sequential four-day schedule. Sodium cholate infusion dissolved stones in two out of six patients, but during infusion with saline no change in size or number of stones occurred in any of their six patients. Acute cholangitis occurred in one patient during cholate infusion, moderate transient abnormalities in liver function in three patients and moderate to severe diarrhoea in all patients.

To find a more effective contact dissolution solvent, Toouli et al (1975) tested the in vitro efficacy of bile salts with added lecithin and heparin solutions. They found that heparin solutions were ineffective in dissolving or fragmenting gallstones, and that a combination of deoxycholate and cholate was more effective than a cholate solution alone. The most effective combination in their study was a solution of 200 mM taurocholate plus 100 mM lecithin.

Christiansen et al (1978) succeeded with a combined instrument and chemical treatment of retained common duct stones in 18 patients with an indwelling T-tube. The chemical dissolution regimen consisted of a continuous infusion of a heparin-saline solution alternating with sodium cholate. Only three out of seven patients were successfully treated with the chemical method. In a combination of chemical dissolution and instrumentation, the authors successfully removed common duct stones in 16 of their 18 patients.

Sohrabi et al (1979) successfully used a sodium cholate infusion following the regimen of Admirand & Way (1972) to dissolve stones in six out of eight patients. The authors noted a mucosal deformity of the common duct in one patient during the cholate infusion which was no longer apparent on a subsequent cholangiogram.

In experiments in the Rhesus monkey (Mack et al 1977), sodium cholate infusion caused significant toxicity to the common duct. A 316 mM sodium cholate solution was infused in one group of monkeys and a 158 mM sodium cholate solution in a second group. All monkeys in the first group died within 24 hours. Common histological findings in both groups were severe acute inflammation and necrosis involving the mucosa and submucosa of the treated hepatic duct. In one monkey infused with the lower sodium cholate concentration of 158 mM, the ampulla of Vater revealed an impressive oedema with focal haemorrhage. On the basis of these findings, the authors cautioned against the possible long-term effects of this treatment with regard to common duct scarring or stricture formation.

Heparin

In 1971, Gardner et al reported the successful use of a heparinized saline solution in a patient with four retained common duct stones. Initially, the heparinized saline contained 10 000 units per 250 ml and was infused as a drip through the T-tube every six hours. Since the patient's clotting studies remained normal, the dose of heparin was increased to 20 000 units per 250 ml of saline. There were no side effects from this infusion and follow-up cholangiograms revealed that within one week, the patient's stones had disappeared. The use of this heparinized saline solution was based on previous in vitro work by Ostrowitz & Gardner (1970) who found that heparin uniformly increased the zeta potential of particles suspended in bile and therefore suggested that this compound might be useful in the treatment of retained common duct stones.

In 1974, Cheung et al reported their results from in vitro studies with bile salts, lecithin and heparin. They concluded that a solution consisting of 100 mM unconjugated deoxycholate and 100 mM lecithin was the most effective solution for dissolving human cholesterol gallstones. They point out that the addition of heparin at a concentration of 1000 units/10 ml did not increase the solubilizing capacity of deoxycholate. On the other hand, Chary (1977) reported the dissolution of retained bile duct stones in five patients with a heparinized saline solution. This author increased the concentration of heparin to 50 000 units in 500 ml of normal saline.

In a series of 26 patients treated with a sodium cholate infusion and a mixture of 20 000 units of heparin in 1000 ml of saline per 24 hours, Christiansen et al (1977) reported that stones disappeared in 19 patients (a success rate of 73%). No complications were encountered. It is interesting to note that in the same year, Hardie et al (1977) published their opinion that heparinized saline appeared unsuitable for gallstone dissolution based on in vitro studies with bile salt solutions and heparinized saline.

Clofibrate

Garcia-Romero and co-authors (1978) completely dissolved 22 human gallstones in vitro within 25 days with a clofibrate solution. They studied human gallstones in concentrations of 250, 500, 1000 and 1500 mg of clofibrate in 5 ml ethyl alcohol. From their results, these authors proposed clofibrate as a solvent for common duct stone dissolution.

Monooctanoin — Capmul 8210

In 1977, Thistle, Carlson, Hofmann & Babayan reported the usefulness of medium chain glycerides in dissolving gallstones in vitro. These authors had screened over 100 compounds (oral communication, Hofmann) to find a more potent and less toxic cholesterol solvent. Matched pairs of cholesterol stones from 15 patients were incubated at 37°C for 72 hours in 150 mM sodium cholate solution and in medium chain monoglycerides. At 24-hour intervals, the solutions were gently mixed, then 2 ml aliquots were removed for analysis. The sodium cholate solution was exchanged daily to decrease the possibility of a saturation effect. The results indicated that medium chain monoglycerides were invariably more effective than sodium cholate. During each 24 hour period, the amount of cholesterol dissolved by medium chain monoglycerides was about 2.5 times that dissolved by sodium cholate. Fortunately, Capmul 8210, a commercial emulsifier, contains predominantly monooctanoin (glyceryl-1-mono-octanoate) and other medium chain glycerides, obviating the need for costly synthesis of monooctanoin.

The following year Thistle et al (1978), as well as Mack et al (1978), reported the first successful use of monooctanoin in man. In Thistle's abstract, seven patients with radiolucent extra- and/or intrahepatic duct stones were studied at least two weeks after biliary tract surgery. Monooctanoin was infused through a T-tube or an intraductal catheter either continuously or intermittently at a rate of 5–10 ml per hour. A spectrum of laboratory studies including serum hepatic and pancreatic enzyme determinations and cholangiograms were performed initially and at four-day intervals. Thistle et al (1978) found that infusion of monooctanoin for 7–21 days decreased the stones in size and/or number in six out of the seven patients. In four patients the stones progressively decreased in size and completely dissolved in three. In the fourth patient the decrease in size was sufficient to permit extraction with a Dormia basket. The stones decreased in number during monooctanoin infusion in two other patients such that they could be removed by basket extraction or surgery. The treatment with monooctanoin was well-tolerated and serum hepatic and pancreatic enzyme levels remained stable.

In collaboration with researchers at the Mayo Clinic, the author performed toxicity studies in a primate model with monooctanoin and was able to compare those studies with the results obtained from sodium cholate infusion (Mack et al 1978). Histological studies showed only mild to moderate inflammatory changes in the common duct for up to one and a half months after monooctanoin infusion. Encouraged by these favourable results, we embarked on our own clinical series (1978) in 11 patients with a total of 20 retained common duct stones; the stones in eight patients dissolved in five to seven days. Some patients complained of nausea and vomiting which were controlled medically. The infusion rate was continuous at about 4.5 ml/hour. Figures 49.1, 49.2, and 49.3 illustrate a typical dissolution sequence as displayed at T-tube cholangiography.

It was our belief that an infusion catheter, passed alongside the T-tube directly to the stone surface would shorten the dissolution time because of greater contact of the solvent with the stone. Therefore, we elected from the onset of our study to place such a catheter as described by Crummy & Mack (1981) and to use the T-tube as a vent, adjusting the drainage bag to 15 cm above the common duct location to avoid pressure increases in the common duct (Fig. 49.4).

The following year, Leuschner et al (1979) reported success with monooctanoin in a 74-year-old high-risk patient who had undergone a cholecystectomy in 1965 and two common duct explorations. After the second common duct exploration 36 stones were still present in the right hepatic duct and two in the common duct. These authors threaded a catheter through the T-tube into the right hepatic duct and infused monooctanoin at a constant rate of 5 ml per hour for 72 hours. Side effects were nausea and

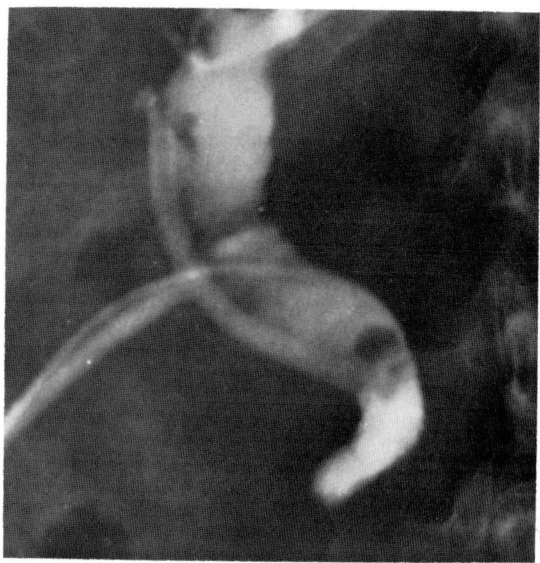

Fig. 49.2 Intermediate stage of dissolution (stone irregular and smaller). Reproduced with permission from the Archives of Surgery 1981

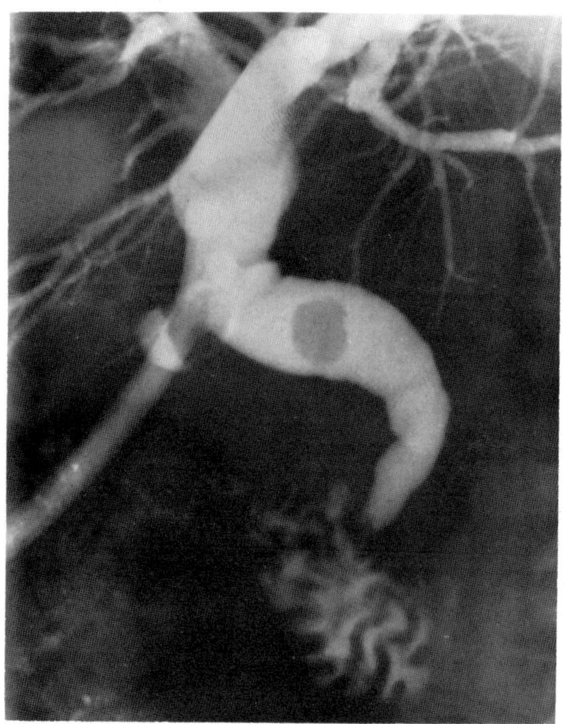

Fig. 49.1 Typical sequence of dissolution. Preinfusion cholangiogram (large stone). Reproduced with permission from the Archives of Surgery 1981

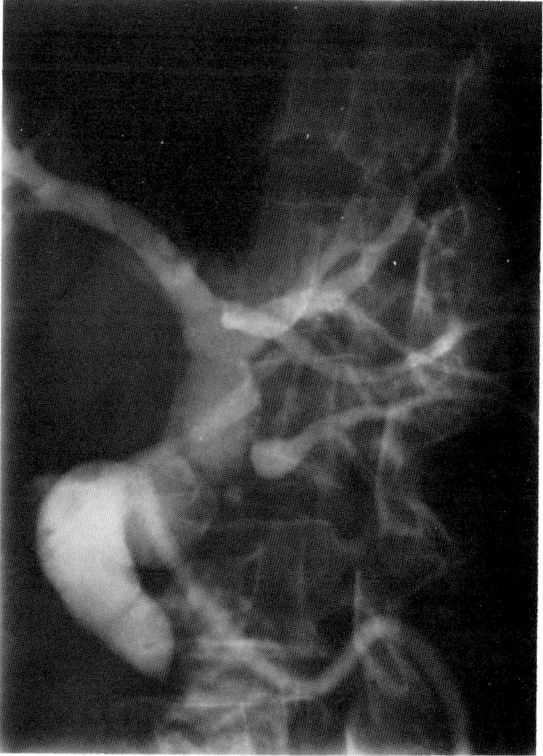

Fig. 49.3 Post-dissolution normal cholangiogram. Reproduced with permission from the Archives of Surgery 1981

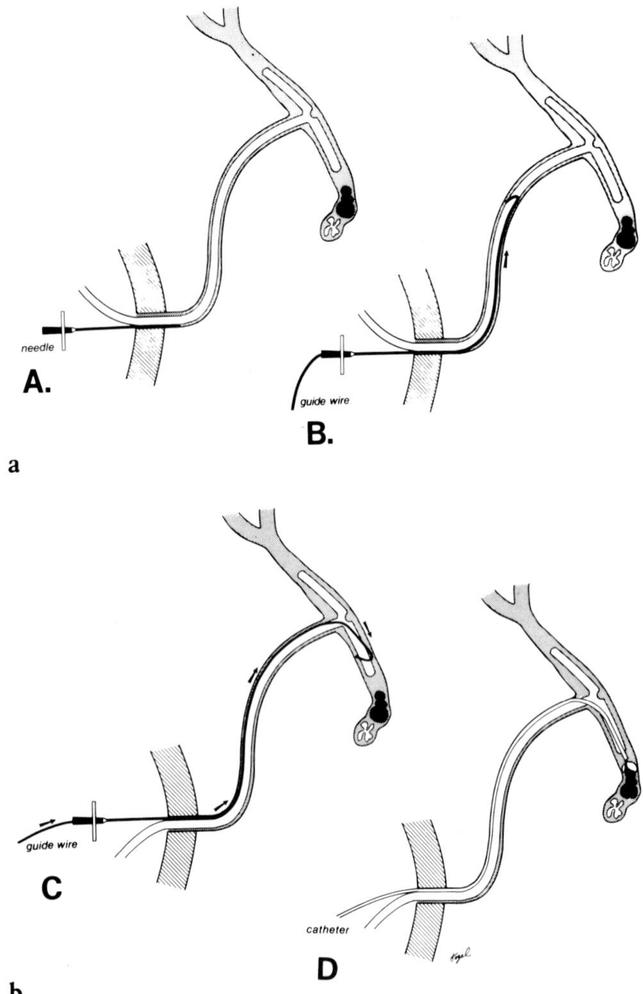

Fig. 49.4(a) A. Needle without obturator passes through body wall adjacent to T-tube; B. 3 mm Teflon-coated J guide wire advances through tract. (b) C. Guide wire enters biliary tree and catheter is advanced over it; D. Guide wire is removed with catheter in place. Reproduced with permission from the American Journal of Radiology 1981

diarrhoea but no changes occurred in liver enzymes, serum amylase, electrolytes or the blood count. After 72 hours there was a 60% reduction in stone number. The same treatment was repeated for 100 hours three weeks later. After that therapy, only four small stones were found incarcerated in a recess.

Gadacz (1979) reported the efficacy of Capmul in dissolving biliary tract stones. Cholesterol gallstones from six patients were matched and incubated in three different solutions: Capmul 8210 (or monooctanoin), sodium cholate and heparin. He observed that Capmul 8210 reduced the weight of the stones more rapidly than either sodium cholate or heparin.

In 1980, Thistle et al published a detailed discussion on the physicochemical properties of monooctanoin, and their clinical results in 12 patients. Side effects during treatment included mild anorexia, some nausea and occasional emesis. Upper abdominal, lower thoracic or back discomfort were similar to that associated with previous biliary tract pain. All of these symptoms could be relieved by decreasing the dosage of monooctanoin or by aspiration of the biliary tract. In several patients, a mild increase in stool frequency was observed. There were no changes in serum GOT, alkaline phosphatase, bilirubin, serum or urinary amylase. Infusion time was four to 21 days, and success was obtained in 10 out of their 12 patients.

Schenk et al (1980a) successfully dissolved common duct stones in three out of six patients. There was one failure. In two additional patients monooctanoin infusion had to be discontinued due to nausea, vomiting, colicky pain and diarrhoea.

Jarrett et al (1981) reported that 15 out of 24 patients no longer had stones after monooctanoin instillation into their bile ducts. In five patients the stones were smaller or reduced in number and in four of those patients the stones were extracted through the T-tube tract. These authors report that monooctanoin was well tolerated and only one patient complained of diarrhoea.

Gadacz (1981) reported a 62% success rate in using monooctanoin for retained common duct stones in eight patients. The only side effects were abdominal cramps and diarrhoea which resolved after temporary cessation of infusion or a decrease in the rate of infusion.

In the same year Mack et al (1981a) reported a 79% success rate using monooctanoin to treat 20 patients who had a total of 43 retained common duct stones. The dissolution time for a single stone averaged four days. Elevations in hepatic or pancreatic enzymes returned to normal after cessation of dissolution therapy and side effects such as nausea and vomiting, epigastric pain or diarrhoea were controlled medically.

In a multi-centre trial, Hofmann et al (1981) reported only a 45.8% success rate in 118 patients. Stone size was reduced in 20.3% of those patients, and no changes occurred in 33.9%.

Teplick et al (1982) tested the in vitro dissolution of gallstones from 43 patients and compared the efficacy of monooctanoin, sodium dehydrocholate, heparin and saline. The biliary calculi completely dissolved in monooctanoin, although bilirubinate stones did not.

Steinhagen & Pertsemlidis (1983) reported successfully using monooctanoin to dissolve common duct stones in high-risk patients. Their infusion rate was between 5 and 10 ml/hour and their patients' mean age was 76 years. The average infusion time was six days. The stones in two patients were completely dissolved. In two patients in their series in whom dissolution was unsuccessful, the recovered stones at reoperation were composed of less than 5% cholesterol. These authors emphasize that mechanical extraction when feasible is still the treatment of choice for retained biliary stones, although chemical dissolution should be attempted before undertaking reoperation.

In a prospective controlled study (Velasco 1983), comparing monooctanoin and heparin to treat retained common duct stones, monooctanoin was clearly more effective. Three patient groups were entered into the study. The first group of 54 patients was treated with a saline washout technique without any chemical additives resulting in a 20.4% (or 11 patients) success rate. Of 15 other patients infused with heparinized saline, only five were treated successfully. By contrast, 13 of 20 patients infused with monooctanoin were successfully treated, a statistically significant result. Recently Tritapepe et al (1984) reported a 69% success rate in 16 patients treated with monooctanoin.

Clinical toxicity of monooctanoin

Several publications have indicated that Capmul 8210 (or monooctanoin) may be toxic to the biliary tree or to gastric mucosa. Schenk et al (1979) studied the tissue compatibility of Capmul 8210 in 17 adult cats. A Teflon tube was inserted into the gallbladder and Capmul was infused at a continuous rate of 3 ml/hour for four, six or eight hours once (Group A), or intermittently for four hours daily over a period of four days at a rate of 0.6 ml/hour (Group B). Depending on the contact time, acute oedematous disruption of the biliary and papillary mucosa occurred in group A and cellular infiltration of the submucous layer as well as acute pancreatitis occurred in two animals in group B.

Uribe et al (1981) encountered one out of 12 patients in whom diarrhoea persisted despite discontinuation of monooctanoin infusion. Gastric bleeding and hyponatraemia resulted in death of the patient.

In 1982, Crabtree et al described a 72-year-old patient with choledocholithiasis and necrotizing choledochomalacia after treatment with monooctanoin to dissolve bile duct stones. The infusion rate of monooctanoin was 7.5 ml/hour and pressure monitoring was performed. The perfusion was carried out for 60 hours, but could not be continued because of abdominal pain, nausea and vomiting. This treatment was followed by progressive jaundice, anorexia and fever. The patient died five weeks after the perfusion. It is indeed debatable whether or not the perfusion with monooctanoin caused the death of this patient. The infusion rate was high and it is possible that a pre-existing cholangitis flared up.

In 1982, Minuk et al described a 25-year-old patient who had cirrhosis secondary to chronic active lupoid hepatitis and developed what the authors believed were systemic side effects of monooctanoin. The patient developed right upper quadrant pain as well as a sensation of tightness in her chest and difficulty in breathing during monooctanoin infusion. At that point the intrabiliary pressure had risen to 24 cm of water. In addition, at a rechallenge, facial flushing and a metallic taste in the mouth developed. The authors speculate that the systemic effects may have been caused by prior damage to the biliary tract epithelium from the attacks of cholangitis which led to a denuding of the biliary epithelium.

Lillemoe et al (1982) studied the effect of monooctanoin on gastric mucosa in dogs with Heidenhain pouches. Their results demonstrated an increased net hydrogen ion flux and a loss of electronegativity of transmucosal electrical potential difference, indicating mucosal injury.

In 1983, Train et al described duodenal ulcerations associated with monooctanoin infusion. A 57-year-old patient with obstructive jaundice secondary to common duct stones had signs of portal hypertension and had undergone a sphincteroplasty at the time of his cholecystectomy 16 years prior to monooctanoin treatment. The patient also had extensive duodenal varices secondary to portal hypertension. Monooctanoin infusion was begun via a percutaneous catheter at a rate of initially 5 ml/hour, increased to 10 ml/hour. On the eleventh day of monooctanoin infusion, haematemesis was demonstrated to be due to multiple deep ulcerations in the duodenum adjacent to the tip of this previously placed Ring catheter. We do not know if these ulcerations in the duodenum were caused by monooctanoin or by mechanical trauma from the catheter.

Endoscopic naso-biliary use of monooctanoin

In 1979, Schmack et al reported that three patients were treated with Capmul 8210 (monooctanoin) at a rate of 6 ml/hour through an endoscopically placed Teflon catheter through the intact papilla of Vater and delivered to the exterior via the nose. This naso-biliary perfusion was unsuccessful and an endoscopic papillotomy was performed to remove the stones.

Schenk et al (1980b) attempted naso-biliary dissolution therapy with monooctanoin in five patients. Although the stones did not dissolve completely, following treatment with 90, 550, and 700 ml of Capmul 8210 solution, the consistency of the stones had changed sufficiently during a three to six day treatment to allow the stones in two patients to be extracted with a Dormia basket. Another patient's stone fragmented and passed spontaneously into the duodenum. In one patient the infusion of monooctanoin had to be discontinued because of side effects.

Wurbs et al (1980) used a specially designed catheter to facilitate the naso-biliary approach. These authors successfully dissolved common duct stones in six out of ten patients with their retrograde naso-biliary technique.

Witzel et al (1980) administered Capmul 8210 through a nasal Teflon catheter introduced endoscopically into the bile ducts of ten patients. They infused Capmul 8210 into an additional six patients through a T-tube. Stone dissolution and the side effects of Capmul in both groups were considered together. In 12 patients 16 stones were dissolved within six to 25 days with a mean of 15.6 days. In two patients, the stones did not dissolve and in two other patients fever and leukocytosis developed during perfusion.

Cotton et al (1981) reported that as early as 1977 they had treated three patients with monooctanoin through a transnaso-biliary catheter placed at the time of duodenoscopy into the common duct. A detailed description of technique was reported in 1979. The infusion rate in those three patients was 10 ml/hour. The infusion had to be discontinued in all three patients within 72 hours because of severe pain, nausea and vomiting. The author later applied the same technique successfully and reduced the infusion rate to 3 ml/hour.

Venu et al (1982) partially or completely dissolved stones in seven out of nine patients by infusing monooctanoin through a naso-biliary catheter. In the remaining two patients, the stones could be crushed and extracted.

Modified monooctanoin

Leuschner et al (1981a) observed by in vitro experiments that a modified Capmul preparation (GMOC) was much more effective as a dissolution agent than Capmul alone as was a bile acid-EDTA solution. (For composition of solutions see Table 49.2.)

Infusion therapy for common duct stones in 20 patients was begun one week after placement of a naso-biliary tube. A total of 250 ml of GMOC was continuously infused at a rate of 5 ml/hour, alternating with a bile acid-EDTA solution (250 ml) at 20 ml/hour. Total stone dissolution occurred in eight and partial dissolution in four patients in an average time of 12 days. Diarrhoea was the main side effect. A better patient tolerance of GMOC as opposed to monooctanoin (or Capmul) alone was attributed to a more alkaline pH, the use of carnosine, Palmidrol®, and Pluronic F68®.

Percutaneous transhepatic use of monooctanoin

In four patients, we successfully dissolved common duct stones using a percutaneous catheter technique (Mack et al 1981b). Three of these patients presented with clinical signs of biliary tract obstruction. One patient was not jaundiced. Two transhepatic catheters were placed in two of these patients: one for infusion of Capmul 8210 and the other catheter for venting of the obstructed biliary system. Stone dissolution occurred in four to eight days. In one of these patients, two stones dissolved completely and the third stone was reduced in size. This stone was percutaneously crushed with a basket and the fragments irrigated (Fig. 49.5a-d). Since then, we have successfully treated four additional patients by this approach (unpublished data).

Table 49.2 Composition of modified Capmul and bile acid-EDTA solutions as utilized by Leuschner et al (1981)

GMOC	
Glyceryl-mono- and dioctanoin	92.8%
Pluronic F68 (nonionic surfactant polymer)	2.5–3.0%
Palmidrol	0.3–0.6%
Cholic acid	0.4%
Carnosine	0.3–0.45%
EDTA	0.18–0.24%
Water	2.8–5.8%
Bile acid-EDTA	
Ursodeoxycholic acid	0.5%
Cholic acid	0.5%
EDTA-sodium salt	1.0%
Carnosine	0.27%

Pigment stones (primary common duct stones)

Primary common duct stones are associated with biliary tract infections, advanced age, a long history of symptoms of the disease, and with previous biliary operations (Lygidakis 1983). Dissolution of such stones is difficult due to the low cholesterol content of the stones and a mixture of calcium, bilirubinate and other components. Leuschner et al (1981b) updated their experience with alternating GMOC and bile acid-EDTA solutions in 24 patients. A naso-biliary tube, tolerated up to 84 days, was used to achieve a 65% success rate with total dissolution of stones in 10 patients, and partial dissolution in six others. These authors observed that pigment matrix stones dissolved in an in vitro solution of bile acid-EDTA.

PRACTICAL RECOMMENDATIONS

Based on experience with 45 patients treated with monooctanoin for stone dissolution either through the T-tube tract, via the percutaneous transhepatic approach, or through a cholecystostomy catheter, the author recommends that Capmul 8210 should be infused slowly at approximately 3–5 ml/hour, depending on the size of the common duct and the presence or absence of obstruction in the distal common duct. It is helpful to use a catheter along the T-tube tract beside the tube for infusion of Capmul 8210 and to utilize the T-tube as a pressure controllable vent. Teplick et al (1984) concur that with this arrangement a close drug-stone contact is achieved, improving overall results and minimizing the side effects of Capmul 8210. Dissolution therapy in a postoperative patient with a T-tube in place should not be started until a good tract has formed (usually two to three weeks postoperatively) to avoid intra-abdominal leakage. Liver functions as well as serum amylase should be monitored continually and follow-up cholangiograms performed every three or four days, or sooner if severe pain develops during Capmul 8210 infusion, possibly indicating catheter dislodgement or stone impaction.

Special caution is advised when infusing patients who

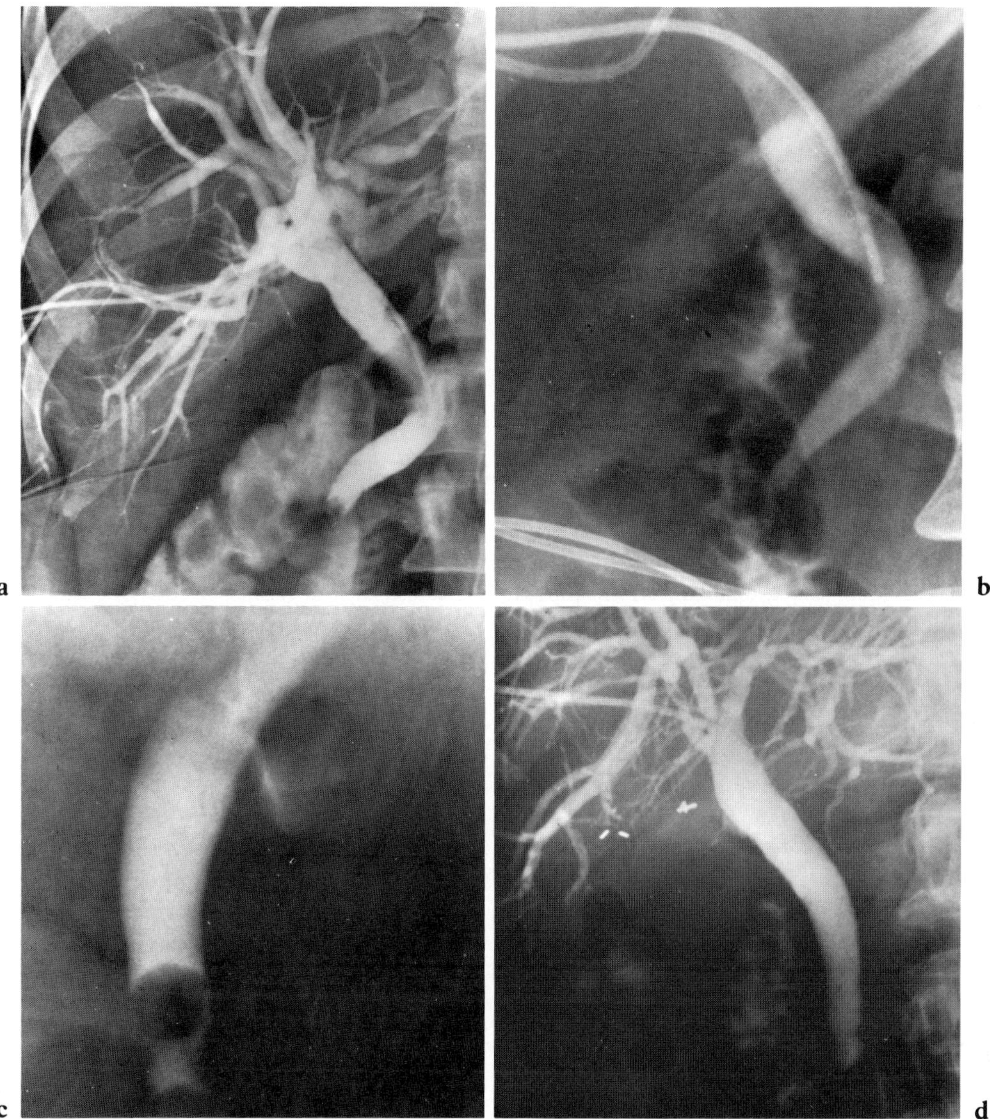

Fig. 49.5a. Percutaneous transhepatic cholangiogram demonstrates a single obstructing calculus in the distal common duct. b. Cholangiogram after dissolution of stone. c. Cholangiogram demonstrates two calculi in the distal common bile duct. A third, more proximal stone, is not shown in this film. d. Cholangiogram after dissolution of stones. Reproduced with permission from Surgery 1981

have obstructive jaundice or signs of sepsis. Antibiotic therapy and proper fluid replacement should be accomplished first, followed by a very slow Capmul 8210 infusion rate, perhaps 3 ml/hour. In four patients we hand-instilled 8–10 ml of Capmul 8210 every two hours after previous aspiration of bile from the bile duct. This manual method has succeeded and is helpful when no infusion pump is available. At present, the viscosity of Capmul 8210 is too high for administration through available hospital infusion pumps and the need for millipore filtration for antisepsis still exists. However, as soon as monooctanoin is approved for clinical use by the Food and Drug Administration in the United States, these problems will have been overcome, and a self-contained unit as planned by Ethitek Pharmaceuticals, Skokie, Illinois (Moctanin™)* may facilitate stone dissolution therapy to the point of home use (Fig. 49.6).

In 2700 operations for biliary tract stones, Simi et al (1979) have found intrahepatic lithiasis (stones located proximal to the confluence of the main hepatic ducts) in 36 patients (1.3%). It might indeed be this group of patients who may benefit from dissolution therapy with monooctanoin to avoid traumatic instrumentation or surgical intervention to retrieve such stones. We have expanded the indications for monooctanoin infusion for

* Moctanin ™ was released in November 1985 and is marketed by Ethitek Pharmaceuticals.

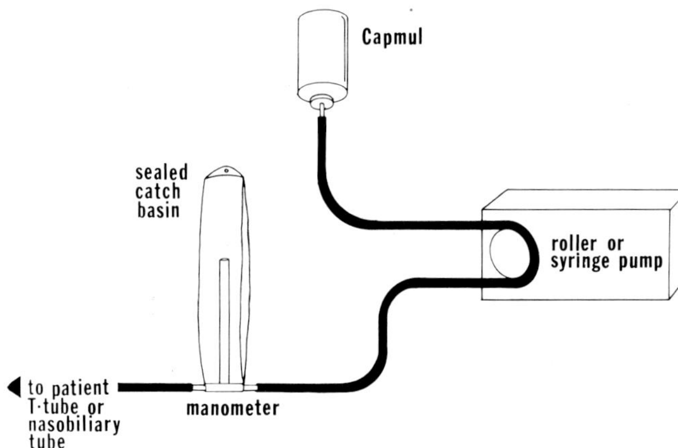

Fig. 49.6 Diagram of self-contained unit for Capmul 8210 infusion

partial or complete dissolution therapy in high-risk patients such as those with previous myocardial infarction, general debility or severe chronic obstructive pulmonary disease; and to minimize the extent of or to eliminate the need for a future surgical intervention. Gallstones and common duct stones removed at the initial surgical intervention should be saved so that if retained common duct stones develop, the stones originally removed can be either analyzed for their cholesterol content or simply incubated in a 37°C monooctanoin solution to assess dissolution time. We have saved gallstones in our patients with common duct explorations since Capmul 8210 became available and are thereby able to predict the time required for dissolution therapy adding one or two days to the in vitro dissolution time. Pain, diarrhoea, and nausea are treated if necessary.

CONCLUSIONS

1. Ether and chloroform were displaced as common duct stone solvents in the early 1970s by bile acids. As Motson (1981) points out, ether most likely caused a forceful expulsion of the common duct stone into the duodenum as it expanded during vapourization rather than truly dissolving the stone. Chloroform indeed has been a true solvent, but has caused duodenal ulceration, haematemesis and anaesthesia.
2. Additive drugs such as lidocaine, isoproterenol or lecithin are no longer used as stone solvents.
3. Heparin solutions and clofibrate seem to be ineffective and are no longer used.
4. Flushing of the common duct with normal saline may be helpful although distension of the biliary tree by the injection may cause significant side effects and pain for the patient (Catt et al 1974).
5. Bile acids (mainly sodium cholate) as single agents have been abandoned because of side effects and a longer dissolution time than with monooctanoin.
6. Currently, monooctanoin is the best cholesterol solvent for clinical use either instilled through a T-tube tract, through an endoscopically placed naso-biliary catheter, or by a percutaneous transhepatic route.

REFERENCES

Admirand W H, Way L 1972 Medical treatment of retained gallstones. Transactions of the Association of American Physicians 85: 382–387

Allen B L, Deveney C W, Way L W 1978 Chemical dissolution of bile duct stones. World Journal of Surgery 2: 429–437

Best R R, Rasmussen J A, Wilson C E 1953 An evaluation of solutions for fragmentation and dissolution of gallstones and their effect on liver and ductal tissue. Annals of Surgery 138: 570–581

Catt P B, Hogg D F, Clunie G J A, Hardie I R 1974 Retained biliary calculi: Removal by a simple non-operative technique. Annals of Surgery 180: 247–251

Chary S 1977 Dissolution of retained bile duct stones using heparin. British Journal of Surgery 64: 347–351

Cheung L Y, Englert E, Moody F G, Wales E E 1974 Dissolution of gallstones with bile salts, lecithin, and heparin. Surgery 76: 500–503

Christiansen L A, Schersten T, Burcharth F, Bruusgaard A, Lindblad L, Cahlin E 1977 Treatment of retained bile duct calculi with T-tube infusion of sodium cholate and heparin. Scandinavian Journal of Gastroenterology 12: 337–339

Christiansen L A, Nielsen O V, Efsen F 1978 Non-operative treatment of retained bile duct calculi in patients with an indwelling T-tube. British Journal of Surgery 65: 581–584

Cotton P B, Burney P G J, Mason R R 1979 Transnasal bile duct catheterization after endoscopic sphincterotomy. Gut 20: 285–287

Cotton P B, Vallon A G, Mason R 1981 Intra-ductal infusion of monooctanoin for common duct stones. Lancet i: 436–437

Crabtree T S, Dykstra R, Kelly J, Preshaw R M 1982 Necrotizing choledochomalacia after use of monooctanoin to dissolve bile-duct stones. Canadian Journal of Surgery 25: 644–646

Crummy A B, Mack E 1981 Infusion therapy of choledocholithiasis: technique for catheter placement. American Journal of Radiology 136: 622–623

Dardik H, Beneventano T, Rosen R, Gliedman M L, Schein C J 1971 Experimental management by nonoperative adrenergic stimulation of simulated common duct stones. Digestive Diseases 16: 321–326

Gadacz T R 1979 Efficacy of Capmul and the dissolution of biliary stones. Journal of Surgical Research 26: 378–380

Gadacz T R 1981 The effect of monooctanoin on retained common duct stones. Surgery 89: 527–531

Garcia-Romero E, Lopez-Cantarero M, Arcelus I M 1978 Dissolution of human gallstone with clofibrate. Journal of Surgical Research 24: 62–64

Gardner B, Ostrowitz A, Masur R 1971 Reappraisal of the possible role of heparin in solution of gallstones: A clinical extension of laboratory studies in removal of retained common duct stones. Surgery 69: 854–857

Hardie I R, Green M K, Burnett W, Walland D R, Hall-Brown A 1977 In vitro studies of gallstone dissolution using bile salt solutions and heparinized saline. British Journal of Surgery 64: 572–576

Heiss F W, Rossi R L, Scholz F J, Shea J A, Braasch J W 1984 Common bile duct calculi. Postgraduate Medicine 75: 88–117

Hofmann A F, Schmack B, Thistle J L, Babayan V K 1981 Clinical experience with monooctanoin for dissolution of bile duct stones. An uncontrolled multicenter trial. Digestive Diseases and Sciences 26: 954–955

Jarrett L N, Balfour T W, Bell G D, Knapp D R, Rose D H 1981 Intraductal infusion of mono-octanoin: experience in 24 patients with retained common-duct stones. Lancet i: 68–70

Lansford C, Mehta S, Kern F 1974 The treatment of retained stones in the common bile duct with sodium cholate infusion. Gut 15: 48–51

LaRusso N F, Thistle J L, Hofmann A F, Fulton R E 1975 Treatment of retained common bile duct stones by intraductal infusion of a cholate solution: A controlled trial. Gastroenterology 68:932

Leuschner U, Wurbs D, Landgraf H 1979 Dissolution of biliary duct stones with mono-octanoin. Lancet ii: 103–104

Leuschner U, Wurbs D, Baumgärtel H, Helm E B, Classen M 1981a Alternating treatment of common bile duct stones with a modified glyceryl-1-monooctanoate preparation and bile acid-EDTA solution by nasobiliary tube. Scandinavian Journal of Gastroenterology 16: 497–503

Leuschner U, Baumgärtel H, Phillip J, Hagenmüller F 1981b Dissolution of cholesterol and pigment matrix stones in the common bile duct. Gastroenterology 80:1208

Lillimoe K D, Gadacz T R, Weichbrod R H, Harmon J W 1982 Effect of mono-octanoin on canine gastric mucosa. Surgery, Gynecology and Obstetrics 155: 13–16

Lygidakis N J 1983 Incidence and significance of primary stones of the common bile duct in choledocholithiasis. Surgery, Gynecology and Obstetrics 157: 435–436

Mack E, Saito C, Goldfarb S, Carlson G L, Hofmann A F 1977 Local toxicity of T-tube-infused cholate in the Rhesus monkey. Surgical Forum 28: 408–409

Mack E A, Saito C, Goldfarb S, Crummy A B, Thistle J L, Carlson G L, Babayan V K, Hofmann A F 1978 A new agent for gallstone dissolution: experimental and clinical evaluation. Surgical Forum 29: 438–439

Mack E, Patzer E M, Crummy A B, Hofmann A F, Babayan V K 1981a Retained biliary tract stones: Nonsurgical treatment with Capmul 8210, a new cholesterol gallstone dissolution agent. Archives of Surgery 116: 341–344

Mack E, Crummy A B, Babayan V K 1981b Percutaneous transhepatic dissolution of common bile duct stones. Surgery 90: 584–587

McCarthy J D, Picazo J G 1969 Lidocaine in the common bile duct. Effects and possible toxicity. JAMA 209: 1904–1905

McGowan J M, Keeley J K, Henderson F 1974 Pathological physiology of biliary drainage: The use of a new type of T-tube and the criteria for its removal. Surgery, Gynecology and Obstetrics 84: 174–180

Minuk G Y, Hoofnagle J H, Jones E A 1982 Systemic side effects from the intrabiliary infusion of monooctanoin for the dissolution of gallstones. Journal of Clinical Gastroenterology 4: 133–135

Motson R W 1981 Dissolution of common bile duct stones. British Journal of Surgery 68: 203–208

Ostrowitz A, Gardner B 1970 Studies of bile as a suspending medium and its relationship to gallstone formation. Surgery 68: 329–333

Pribram B O C 1939 Ether treatment of gall-stones impacted in the common duct. Lancet 236: 1311–1313

Pribram B O C 1947 The method for dissolution of common duct stones remaining after operation. Surgery 22: 806–818

Schenk J, Koch H, Stolte M, Schmack B 1979 Tissue compatibility of the gallstone solubilizer Capmul 8210 — A study in cats. Gastroenterology 76:1237

Schenk J, Schmack B, Riemann J F, Rösch W 1980a Treatment of choledocholithiasis using the transpapillary perfusion technique. Endoscopy 12: 224–227

Schenk J, Schmack B, Rösch W, Riemann J F, Koch H, Demling L 1980b Spülbehandlung von Choledochussteinen mit Octanoat (Capmul 8210). Deutsche Medizinische Wochenschrift 105: 917–921

Schmack B, Schenk J, Riemann J, Koch H, Rösch W 1979 Dissolution of biliary-duct stones with mono-octanoin. Lancet ii: 423–424

Sharp K W, Gadacz T R 1982 Selection of patients for dissolution of retained common duct stones with mono-octanoin. Annals of Surgery 196: 137–139

Simi M, Loriga P, Basoli A, Leardi S, Speranza V 1979 Intrahepatic lithiasis: Study of thirty-six cases and review of the literature. The American Journal of Surgery 137: 317–322

Sohrabi A, Max M H, Hershey C D 1979 Cholate sodium infusion for retained common bile duct stones. Archives of Surgery 114: 1169–1172

Steinhagen R M, Pertsemlidis D 1983 Monooctanoin dissolution of retained biliary stones in high risk patients. American Journal of Gastroenterology 78: 756–760

Strickler J H, Muller J J, Rice C O, Baronofsky I D 1951 Nonoperative treatment of retained postoperative common duct stones. Annals of Surgery 133: 174–183

Teplick S K, Pavlides C A, Goodman L R, Babayan V K 1982 In vitro dissolution of gallstones: comparison of monooctanoin, sodium dehydrocholate, heparin, and saline. American Journal of Radiology 138: 271–273

Teplick S K, Haskin P H, Matsumoto T, Wolferth C C, Pavlides C A, Gain T 1984 Interventional radiology of the biliary system and pancreas. Surgical Clinics of North America 64: 87–119

Thistle J L, Carlson G L, Hofmann A F, Babayan V K 1977 Medium chain glycerides rapidly dissolve cholesterol gallstones in vitro. Gastroenterology 72:1141

Thistle J L, Carlson G L, LaRusso N F, Hofmann A F 1978 Effective dissolutions of biliary duct stones by intraductal infusion of mono-octanoin. Gastroenterology 74:1103

Thistle J L, Carlson G L, Hofmann A F, LaRusso N F, MacCarthy R L, Flynn G L, Higuchi W I, Babayan V K 1980 Monooctanoin, a dissolution agent for retained cholesterol bile duct stones: physical properties and clinical application. Gastroenterology 78: 1016–1022

Toouli J, Jablonski P, Watts J McK 1974 Dissolution of stones in the common bile duct with bile-salt solutions. Australian and New Zealand Journal of Surgery 44: 336–340

Toouli J, Jablonski P, Watts J McK 1975 Dissolution of human gallstones: The efficacy of bile salt, bile salt plus lecithin and heparin solutions. Journal of Surgical Research 19: 47–53

Train J S, Dan S J, Cohen L B, Mitty H A 1983 Duodenal ulceration associated with monooctanoin infusion. American Journal of Radiology 141: 557–558

Tritapepe R, DiPadova C, Pozzoli M, Rovagnati P, Montorsi W 1984 The treatment of retained biliary stones with monooctanoin: report of 16 patients. Gastroenterology 79: 710–714

Uribe M, Uscanga L, Sanjurjo J L, Lagarriga J 1980 Medium chain glycerides for the dissolution of retained gallstones: success and side effects. Gastroenterology 78:1281

Uribe M, Uscanga L, Farca S, Sanjurjo J L, Lagarriga J, Ortiz J H 1981 Dissolution of cholesterol ductal stones in the biliary tree with medium-chain glycerides. Digestive Diseases and Sciences 26: 636–640

Velasco N, Braghetto I, Csendes A 1983 Treatment of retained common bile duct stones: a prospective controlled study comparing monooctanoin and heparin. World Journal of Surgery 7: 266–270

Venu R P, Geenen J E, Toouli J, Hogan W J, Kozlov N, Steward E T 1982 Gallstone dissolution using mono-octanoin infusion through an endoscopically placed nasobiliary catheter. American Journal of Gastroenterology 77: 227–230

Walker J W 1891 The removal of gallstones. Lancet i: 874

Way L W, Admirand W H, Dunphy J E 1972 Management of choledocholithiasis. Annals of Surgery 176: 347–359

Witzel L, Wiederholt J, Wolbergs E 1980 Dissolution of gallstones by perfusion with Capmul via a catheter introduced endoscopically into the bile duct. New England Journal of Medicine 303:465

Wurbs D, Phillip J, Classen M 1980 Experiences with the long standing nasobiliary tube in biliary disease. Endoscopy 12: 219–223

D. E. F. Tweedle, L. H. Blumgart

Stones in the common duct — which approach when?

Stones occur in the common bile duct in a variety of circumstances, most frequently in patients with co-existing stones in the gallbladder, or as residual stones following cholecystectomy. However, choledocholithiasis may also occur in the stagnant bile proximal to benign bile duct stricture in papillary stenosis and in the lower common bile duct distal to choledochoduodenostomy. Choledocholithiasis and intrahepatic stones without coexistent cholecystolithiasis is common in Asian countries (Ch. 44, 51), but is unusual in Western countries. When it occurs the stones have usually migrated from the gallbladder.

This chapter is concerned with stones in the common bile duct which have formed in association with stones in the gallbladder and addresses the question as to whether surgery, endoscopy, interventional radiology or stone dissolution may be the most appropriate therapy in any given situation.

The incidence of choledocholithiasis increases with age. In many patients there is a single stone in the common bile duct and impaction, if it occurs, is usually at the lower end of the duct. If the patient has undergone previous cholecystectomy, stones discovered within the common bile duct were almost certainly present at the time of operation although primary (stasis) stones may develop following operations upon the bile duct, in situations where there is inadequate biliary flow. Stones in the common bile duct may remain asymptomatic for long periods of time, but acute pancreatitis, cholangitis, obstructive jaundice, biliary fibrosis and choledochoduodenal fistulae may develop.

WHICH APPROACH WHEN? GENERAL CONSIDERATIONS

The choice of optimum therapy for the management of choledocholithiasis in any particular patient is dependent upon a number of factors. However, the 'best buy' for the patient is often difficult to define since there is a lack of adequate data based on prospective or controlled observations in comparable groups of patients.

The age of the patient is relevant since increasing age is associated with an increase in the incidence of cardiac, respiratory and renal disease, diabetes and other diseases which increase the risks of treatment. Many studies have shown that jaundice at the time of presentation has an adverse effect upon mortality and morbidity, as does cholangitis or acute pancreatitis. Cirrhosis of the liver also militates against facile surgery and compromised liver function is associated with a high operative morbidity and mortality. Local factors are also important and in particular the presence or absence of the gallbladder, whether or not a drainage tube is present within the common bile duct, the size of the stones and the presence of any stenotic lesions within the ductal system influence the choice of therapy. The size of the stones and the presence of a grossly dilated duct with the possibility of further stone development is a feature which is of considerable importance in choosing the method of treatment. Finally, previous surgical operations not only render further surgery difficult, but may, e.g. after gastrectomy, make endoscopic papillotomy more difficult and often impossible.

The factors listed above pertain to the patient, but other general features are important in choosing particular methods of therapy. Not every institution has the facilities for all methods of treatment and in particular the expertise required to fulfil these treatments on a regular and successful basis.

Because of the many factors which influence results, conclusions drawn regarding comparisons of differing therapies are open to question. In many initial studies alternative techniques were used either when the patient was considered unfit for surgery, and in whom the results might naturally be poor, or in patients with retained stone in situations in which the referring surgeon wished to avoid further operations. Much of the information needed for comparative study is not available. Ideally the morbidity and mortality for up to one month following each procedure in patients matched for age, sex and other risk factors should be compared. However, it may prove impossible to conduct randomized trials and indeed many surgeons and endoscopists are unwilling to participate in such studies. Reasons for cross referral and acceptance of patients within a treatment programme are not always based on clinical facts but may be related to questions of status, practice procedure or financial considerations. The long-term consequences of recent innovations are not yet available, and in many surgical studies were never obtained.

Consequently it is not possible to be dogmatic in the assessment of available data and the contents of this chapter will undoubtedly require modification with the passage of time. Nevertheless, an attempt will be made to assess the current situation. In practice patients present in three main therapeutic groups: those who have been submitted to cholecystectomy and exploration of the duct with a T-tube in place; those with previous cholecystectomy without a T-tube in situ; and patients with common bile duct stones in association with cholecystolithiasis. The choice of therapy is influenced by the success rates for any particular treatment, its complications and by the risk factors outlined above.

CHOLEDOCHOLITHIASIS — PREVIOUS CHOLECYSTECTOMY AND NO T-TUBE

This is the most common combination of features observed in patients admitted to centres with expertise in endoscopic sphincterotomy and in patients entered into a prospective multicentre British study (Frost 1984). There are four main options in the management of such stones:

Leave stone(s) in situ
Stone dissolution
Surgical choledocholithotomy
Extraction of stones following endoscopic sphincterotomy.

Stones left in situ

In a small minority of patients it may be reasonable to leave the stone in situ, particularly in the very elderly patient or those with severe generalized disease in whom the stone is causing minimal symptoms. In patients with such a stone remaining above an associated stricture, impaction of the stone at the stricture can be prevented by the endoscopic insertion of a 'pig-tail' endoprosthesis.

Stone dissolution

In the absence of the gallbladder, chenodeoxycholic acid and ursodeoxycholic acid are not concentrated in the bile and their concentration in the common bile duct does not reach that in functioning gallbladders. Furthermore in many such patients the stones have been present for a number of years and contain quantities of calcium which make dissolution impossible. Gallstones in the common bile duct can be dissolved by oral therapy with chenodeoxycholic acid (Sue et al 1981), but the success rate is low and many patients require surgical or endoscopic intervention for obstruction or infective complications. In practical terms therefore the majority of patients require a therapeutic choice between surgical or endoscopic choledocholithotomy.

Surgical treatment

The literature is replete with information concerning the results of surgical exploration of the common bile duct. Unfortunately careful scrutiny reveals a dearth of precise data pertinent to the group of patients considered here. Frequently, figures of less than 2% are reported for retained stones but careful reading reveals that this refers to all biliary operations and retained stones are almost always found in patients who have undergone positive duct exploration (Kune 1972). Glenn (1974) recorded an average figure of 4.3% retained stones in such patients. Recent experience however is better, particularly with the use of post-exploratory cholangiography and choledochoscopy. Thus Girard & Legros (Ch. 46) reported a consecutive series of 102 patients in whom choledoscopy was used after exploration of the common bile duct for stone, with only one retained stone. The figures shown in Table 50.1 include some old and recent data and are taken from series in which choledocholithotomy was performed with or without cholecystectomy. In some of the series it is not always clear that the stones subsequently observed in the duct following choledocholithotomy were retained (residual) rather than recurrent stones, but we believe that the vast majority of stones subsequently identified are retained. It can be seen that a success rate for surgical choledocholithotomy of 90 to 96% is achievable and that with the use of post-exploratory radiology and/or choledochoscopy the retained stone rate is probably 4% or less in patients with positive duct exploration (see also Ch. 27, 28, 29, 46). Of course such data are influenced by the methods of assessment and length of follow-up. The identification of retained stones following choledocholithotomy is usually by means of postoperative T-tube cholangiography, a

Table 50.1 Choledocholithotomy — success rate

	Patients	Successful No	Successful %
Way et al 1972	141	127	90.1
Moller & Santavirta 1972	250	230	92.0
Bartlett 1972	744	658	88.5
Glenn 1974	47	43	91.5
Vellacott & Powell 1979	78	71	91.0
Kappes et al 1982	117	113	96.6
Stubbs & Blumgart 1984	41	39	95.1

method which excludes those patients who do not have a duct exploration at cholecystectomy and those in whom the duct is closed without T-tube drainage. In addition in our experience T-tube cholangiography is inaccurate in a proportion of cases. For this and for statistical reasons, successful surgical clearance of stones in the common bile duct may be lower than is often reported. The figures given in Table 50.1 differ considerably from those originally reported by the authors quoted. While most reported the incidence of retained stones (unsuccessful clearance) in those patients who underwent exploration of the common bile duct it is known that the incidence of negative exploration may be as great as 30 to 35% in specialist centres (Way, Admirand & Dunphy 1972, Madden 1973, Glenn 1974). The figures shown in Table 50.1 are calculated using only those patients who had a positive exploration and assuming that all the residual stones found occurred in these patients. Obviously some of the residual stones will have been found in some of the patients who underwent negative exploration. Consequently, the success rate shown in Table 50.1 may well be lower than the actual success recorded by the authors but is more likely to reflect the true success rate.

Another feature which must be taken into account is that endoscopic sphincterotomy is used increasingly in patients for retained or recurrent stones after cholecystectomy. As suggested by Cotton (1984) these patients are already failures of surgery and the results of endoscopic treatment should really be compared with those of a second or third operative procedure. In this context, Girard & Legros reported a rate of 2.9% for recurrent stones but the fact that such good results are not always obtainable has encouraged some surgeons to perform a biliary drainage procedure, such as choledochoduodenostomy, at least in patients with large ducts and multiple stones (Ch. 46, 54) (Allen, Shapiro & Way 1981, Lygidakis 1981, Degenshein 1974, Madden et al 1970). The results of such biliary drainage have not been compared with endoscopic treatment in the context of the patient with a large duct and large stones.

The *hazards* of biliary surgery have also been extensively documented and there are excellent studies of specific risk factors (McSherry & Glenn 1980, Pitt et al 1981, Blamey et al 1983, Dixon et al 1983). The morbidity and mortality for exploration of the common bile duct has often been assessed by the collection of data from groups of patients undergoing cholecystectomy alone and others undergoing cholecystectomy and exploration of the common bile duct and then considering the difference in the results as representing the morbidity and mortality of exploring the common bile duct. This is not only mathematically but also biologically incorrect. It is well known in other fields of surgery that the mortality and morbidity following two procedures performed on the same occasion may be lower or higher than the combined mortality and morbidity recorded when the two procedures are performed on different occasions. In the majority of reports concerning cholecystectomy and exploration of the common bile duct there is a high incidence of negative exploration and the mortality for such procedures may well be different from the mortality for those in which stones were present in the ducts. In patients undergoing choledochotomy following cholecystectomy one would expect perhaps an occasional negative exploration.

The mortality of choledocholithotomy alone is reflected by the data in Table 50.2. It can be seen that the average mortality of 521 patients in this collected series is 1.6%. As might be expected, the large series of McSherry & Glenn (1980) also demonstrates that mortality is higher in those patients with cholangitis and pancreatitis. In many of the patients included in Table 50.2, additional procedures such as choledochoduodenostomy and transduodenal sphincteroplasty were performed in order to ensure adequate future drainage of the duct. From the studies reported it is not possible to identify risk factors such as age, but by analogy with the result of patients undergoing combined cholecystectomy and choledocholithotomy (see below) the mortality for patients older than 50 and particularly older than 65 (Vellacot & Powell 1979, Glen 1975, Doyle et al 1982, Spohn et al 1973) is likely to be high.

In short, surgical exploration of the common bile duct following previous choledocholithotomy can be performed with an overall mortality of 1 to 2% and with a success rate of 90% or more. Increasing age, associated disease, cholangitis, jaundice and pancreatitis will make the risk considerably higher.

There are surprisingly few adequate studies of long-term assessment after surgical exploration of the common bile duct. Bordley & White (1979) suggest that at least 3 to 10% of patients can expect to undergo at least one further procedure on the biliary tract, but such figures refer to the whole range of operations. A five-year follow-up of 208 patients who underwent cholecystectomy and duct exploration at the Mayo clinic revealed 5.3% with recurrent biliary problems (Larson, Hodgson & Priestley 1966) and

Table 50.2 Mortality of choledocholithotomy alone

	No. of patients	Deaths	
		No.	%
Stuart & Hoerr 1972	24	0	0
Freund et al 1977	16	0	0
Jones 1978	22	0	0
Kaminski et al 1979	26	0	0
McSherry & Glenn 1980	341	7	2.1
cholangitis & panc.	72	3	4.3
no chol. & no panc.	269	4	1.5
Girard & Legros 1981	69	0	0
Tweedle 1984	22	1	4.5
TOTAL	520	8	1.6

Peel et al (1975) reported a 10% incidence of complications in a period of up to 12 years. A six- to eight-year follow-up of 198 patients reported by White & Bordley (1978) showed only three with residual problems and other studies of transduodenal duct exploration have documented residual problems in up to 3% of patients (Thomas, Nicholson & Owen 1971, Stefanini et al 1974, Jones 1978).

Those surgeons who have carried out choledochoduodenostomy report a low incidence of late problems (Degenshein 1974, Lygidakis 1983, Moesgaard et al 1982, Stewart & Herr 1972). Some patients have late symptoms of cholangitis without the presence of stones although this is unusual (Goldman, Steer & Silen 1983).

Endoscopic management

The success rate for the endoscopic treatment of retained common bile duct stones is also difficult to analyse. Data require careful scrutiny since some reports refer only to the success rate of performing sphincterotomy and others to that for performing sphincterotomy and extraction of stones. Thus data from 15 institutions around the world show that of 3070 patients with choledocholithiasis, spontaneous passage of calculi after sphincterotomy occurred in 1795 cases (58.5%) and extraction of stones was possible in 984 patients (32%), a success rate of 90.5%. However these data were confined to patients in whom a successful sphincterotomy had been performed (Safrany 1978). In a subsequent analysis of results from 25 centres in West Germany, successful clearance was achieved in 6376 (88.4%) of 7209 patients (Seifert 1982). These figures relate to retrospective studies.

Not all patients initially referred with stones in the common duct are suitable for endoscopic sphincterotomy (e.g. those with oesophageal or pyloric stenosis, and those with a Roux-en-Y gastrectomy). A prospective study in 30 centres in Britain has recently been completed and successful clearance of the duct was obtained in 80% of patients entered into the study with known choledocholithiasis (Frost 1984). Recently, successful clearance of the common bile duct in patients known to have choledocholithiasis has been achieved in 91–93% (Martin & Tweedle 1984, Leese, Carr-Locke & Neoptolemos 1984, Winstanley et al 1985).

It may be difficult to be certain that all stones have been cleared, particularly in patients with dilated ducts. Those who do not attempt to extract all stones at the time of sphincterotomy, believing that most will pass spontaneously, cannot quote technical success rates, as not all patients are checked later. Lack of success may be anticipated due to difficulty in performing sphincterotomy in patients who have previously undergone a Polya-gastrectomy, in those in whom the papilla is within or adjacent to a duodenal diverticulum and in those in whom there is a large stone (particularly a stone greater than 1.5 cm diameter). The finding of a narrow segment of duct below the stone is also a significant difficulty. In many patients initial failure may be overcome by crushing stones in baskets or by irrigation with or without dissolution through a trans-nasal biliary cannula. Indeed, in two patients the authors have been successful in clearing the duct after seven and eight endoscopic procedures (Tweedle & Martin 1985).

In essence the success rate for performing a sphincterotomy and subsequent extraction of stones with duct clearance is some 80–93% (Siegel 1981, Safrany 1979, Koch et al 1977, Geenen, Vennes & Silvis 1981, Reiter et al 1978, Escourrou et al 1984, Cotton 1984, Frost 1984, Leese, Carr-Locke & Neoptolemos 1984, Martin & Tweedle 1984, Winstanley et al 1985).

The *risk* of endoscopic papillotomy for removal of retained stones from the common bile duct is remarkably consistent with a mortality rate of 1 to 1.5% reported world-wide (Siegel 1981, Safrany 1978, Koch et al 1977, Geenen, Vennes & Silvis 1981, Reiter et al 1978, Escourrou et al 1984, Cotton & Vallon 1981, Frost 1984). Immediate post-sphincterotomy problems of bleeding, pancreatitis, cholangitis and retroperitoneal perforation occur in 8 to 10% of patients and surgery is needed urgently in 1 to 2%.

Some of these figures are not directly comparable with surgical data since most early reports exclude non-endoscopic complications and deaths from incidental problems such as myocardial infarction and pneumonia and do not include the risks of surgery done for endoscopic complications. A prospective multicentre British study (Frost 1984) has taken these points into account and has so far recorded 80 complications (11%) and 9 deaths (1.2%) following sphincterotomy in 721 patients. Two of these were caused by cardiopulmonary problems.

While few endoscopic, or indeed, surgical series provide a detailed analysis, it is probably true that recently patients referred for endoscopic treatment are generally older and more sick than those referred for surgery. Striking data provided by Neoptolemos et al (1984) reports one death in an elderly patient after endoscopic treatment out of 59 patients judged to be unsuitable for surgery, 90% of whom were jaundiced, 32% of whom had cholangitis and the mean age of whom was 78 years. Thus unlike surgical choledochotomy, patients undergoing endoscopic sphincterotomy may not be at greater risk because of old age, nor is there evidence of increased risk in patients who are jaundiced or suffering from cholangitis and pancreatitis (Cotton 1984).

Large sphincterotomies done for large stones are probably more dangerous and less effective and the risk of bleeding appears to be greater when a sphincterotomy is enlarged within a week or so. It may be expected that sphincterotomy is more hazardous in patients with portal hypertension and abnormalities of coagulation but few cases have been reported.

There are few *long-term studies* of follow-up after endoscopic sphincterotomy. In addition, some of the evidence that is available is based only on partial follow-up; relatively few patients have been followed for more than five years. Most of the studies reported cover ranges of one to seven years (Escourrou et al 1984, Seifert, Gail & Weismuller 1982, Rosch et al 1981, Von Brandstatter et al 1983, Safrany, Schott & Vallon 1982, Vallon & Cotton 1982) (Ch. 47). The results available suggest that about 10% of patients will have major symptoms and of these 4–10% will develop sphincteric stenosis, new stones or both. Some two-thirds of patients studied (Cotton 1984) had gas in the biliary tree and free reflux of barium up the bile duct and all submitted to repeat endoscopy had bacterial overgrowth in the bile, whether or not symptoms were present (Ch. 45) (Cotton 1984). Cotton makes the point that most patients followed-up for longest are elderly and that this is important for two reasons. Firstly, detailed follow-up studies are difficult to do in such patients and most reports are based mainly on questionnaires. The second is that observations made in the elderly may not reflect those in the young patient in whom longer follow-up may ultimately lead to the revelation of further late complications.

Choice of treatment

The ensuing comments assume that both procedures can be performed with competence and without unnecessary delay and that the physician has a choice. It should be emphasized that the indications for one or other form of treatment are more often relative than absolute and that sometimes not all details may be available before one or other procedure is undertaken (e.g. the presence of intrahepatic stones or of a biliary stricture).

In general the aged patient with retained stones present in the common bile duct after cholecystectomy should be treated by endoscopic sphincterotomy and stone extraction. While age in itself is not the important factor, it is true that the older the patient the more likely it is that he or she will have some other important coincident disease rendering the patient unfit for general anaesthesia and thus a greater surgical risk.

The presence of jaundice increases surgical risk, particularly if accompanied by cholangitis or pancreatitis but, as outlined above and provided that prophylactic antibiotics are given, there is as yet no evidence of increased morbidity and mortality following endoscopic sphincterotomy. In these patients endoscopic approaches may be preferable. Some authors (Vagar et al 1983) have not observed significantly better results following endoscopic treatment when compared with surgery in the acute situation. Other factors such as previous treatment, access to the ducts and the size of the ducts may influence the choice of therapy in acute cases. The authors would emphasize that in these patients urgent relief of obstruction is essential and if endoscopic therapy is not initially successful, surgery should not be delayed.

The role of endoscopic treatment for retained bile duct stones in the young and fit has yet to be established. The results of surgery are good with a 90 to 95% success rate in competent hands, a figure directly comparable with endoscopy (see above). Mortality and morbidity figures are also very similar but many surgeons are concerned about the possible long-term effects of division of the choledochal sphincter in young patients. In future endoscopic removal of stones without the need for endoscopic sphincterotomy may be possible in patients in whom the sphincter may be relaxed with sub-lingual nitroglycerine or dilated with a balloon catheter.

Local factors affecting access may dictate therapy. Thus patients with oesophageal stricture, pylotic stenosis or those with a previous Polya-gastrectomy are best treated surgically. Similarly, patients with cervical spondylosis are difficult to intubate and indeed it may be dangerous to attempt to do so. In patients who have previously undergone surgical mobilization of the duodenum and duodenotomy there may be distortion of the second part of the duodenum rendering cannulation difficult. Previous surgery of the sphincter of Oddi may result in sphincteric stenosis which precludes cannulation.

The finding of a large stone or stones within a dilated duct is in the authors' opinion a relatively strong index for a surgical approach rather than endoscopic sphincterotomy, since the latter has a much higher failure rate in the presence of large stones and does not offer the opportunity for definitive surgical bypass.

Finally, it is, in the authors' opinion, unwise to attempt to remove stones above a definite biliary stricture by means of a transduodenal endoscopic approach. Almost all such strictures require surgical treatment which can be carried out with an operative mortality of less than 2% (Ch. 58), and with good results. The likelihood of removing stones successfully above a significant stricture and without reformation of stones is small and the danger of introducing infection above such a stricture considerable.

Decisions as to surgical or endoscopic treatment should be carefully considered in the full knowledge of the likely success rate and risks so that the best possible advice in the circumstances is given to the patient. Treatment should not be selected on the basis of the avoidance of the embarrassment of a second operation for the surgeon who has left a stone in the common bile duct, nor on the basis of surgical or endoscopic pride in results. The discovery of a retained common bile duct stone is not an indication for immediate referral to an endoscopist nor is it an index for immediate re-operation without consideration of what endoscopic sphincterotomy can achieve.

CHOLECYSTOLITHIASIS AND CHOLEDOCHOLITHIASIS

If the gallbladder is functioning as shown by oral cholecystography and contains small non-opaque stones, then, in the western hemisphere, in 90% of patients these stones will be composed predominantly of cholesterol and might be considered suitable for dissolution therapy (Ch. 39). However, the method gives very poor results for the treatment of common bile duct stones and there are three possibilities for the management of patients with choledocholithiasis and cholecystolithiasis:

1. Cholecystectomy and surgical choledocholithotomy
2. Endoscopic sphincterotomy with clearance of the duct and elective cholecystectomy at a later date
3. Endoscopic sphincterotomy with clearance of the duct alone.

Cholecystectomy and surgical choledocholithotomy

Until recently, this was the only method used in the treatment of such patients and, in the great majority of institutions throughout the world, is still the only method chosen. The major concern regarding surgical therapy has been in relation to morbidity and mortality. As discussed above, addition of choledocholithotomy to the operation of cholecystectomy appears to increase the morbidity and mortality more than might be expected from the mortality of choledocholithotomy alone (Table 50.3). The findings of Vellacott & Powell (1979) suggested that there was no difference in mortality rate in those patients in whom stones were found at exploration when compared to those in whom no stones were discovered. However, in the series reported by McSherry & Glenn (1980) the mortality rate in those undergoing negative exploration was only half that of those in whom stones were recovered from the common bile duct. As might be expected there was a much higher mortality in patients with acute cholecystitis undergoing choledocholithotomy when compared with those with chronic cholecystitis undergoing choledocholithotomy (Table 50.3). In this large series, the mortality in patients under the age of 50 undergoing non-urgent cholecystectomy and choledocholithotomy was only 0.8% compared

Table 50.3 Cholecystectomy and choledocholithotomy: mortality

	Patients	Deaths No.	%
Way et al 1972	160	5	3.0
Vellacott & Powell 1979	78	6	7.6
McSherry & Glenn 1980			
chronic cholecystitis	1368	44	3.2
acute cholecystitis	351	27	7.7
Lygidakis 1982*	182	2	1.1
Stubbs & Blumgart 1984	62	1	1.6

* majority also underwent choledochoduodenostomy

with 4.4% in patients over the age of 50. The effect of age upon mortality following combined cholecystectomy and duct exploration has been well documented in other series, although results are difficult to assess since the majority of patients are elderly (a maximum incidence in the eighth decade). Girard & Legros (Ch. 46) examined 819 patients submitted to common bile duct exploration constituting 11% of 7436 patients submitted to cholecystectomy. 588 patients (71.8%) had a positive exploration. In this important series, there were a large number of relatively young patients with a peak incidence within the sixth decade. The mortality for cholecystectomy alone was 0.36% and for cholecystectomy with common bile duct exploration 1.3%. The mortality rate was higher in patients with a positive duct exploration (1.5%) than in those with negative exploration of the duct (0.9%) and increased with age, being 0.3% in patients less than 50 years of age, 2.1% in patients 50 to 70 years of age, and 2.3% in patients 70 years of age or older. All patients who died had either jaundice and/or acute pancreatitis at the time of operation and the major cause of death was cardiac disease accounting for seven out of 11 deaths.

Houghton, Jenkinson & Donaldson (1985), in a prospective study of cholecystectomy in the elderly, reported an overall mortality of 3.3% in 151 patients 64 years of age or older. The mortality for elective cholecystectomy was 0.7% but 19% for surgery undertaken as an emergency. In spite of the fact that 77% of the emergency group had a gangrenous gallbladder, a complication difficult to predict preoperatively, the majority of deaths were from cardiovascular disease. The overall incidence of common bile duct exploration was 36% in the study and was similar in the elective and emergency groups. A comparison was made between old patients (65 to 74 years) and aged patients (over 74 years of age) and revealed twice the number of emergency cases in the aged group. The mortality for elective surgery in old patients (65–74 years) was 1.3% and there were no deaths in 50 patients treated electively in those over 74 years of age. This study suggested that elective biliary surgery was safe, even in the aged. The very high incidence of gangrenous cholecystitis in the patients with acute cholecystitis in this study is of considerable importance in relation to arguments for the use of endoscopic sphincterotomy alone for elderly patients with stones in the common bile duct who present acutely with symptoms suggestive of cholangitis but with few features to suggest the presence of a gangrenous gallbladder (see below).

The mortality for cholecystectomy or cholecystectomy and choledocholithotomy in the elderly appears to be associated with two major causes, namely cardiovascular disease and sepsis. The morbidity is also predominantly related to sepsis. Organisms are particularly likely to be found in the bile in patients with acute cholecystitis or those with choledocholithiasis (Ch. 11). Infective complications which are often remote from the operative sites still appear to be due to the organisms found in the bile at operation and are presumably disseminated in the blood stream (Ch. 11). Although the use of a variety of prophylactic antibiotics has greatly reduced such complications, the incidence is still higher than the infective complications observed after endoscopic removal of stones from the common bile duct (Tweedle 1984a). The majority of trials of prophylactic antibiotics in association with biliary surgery have been confined to a single dose of antibiotic and it may well be necessary to prescribe antibiotics for a more prolonged period (five days) postoperatively in patients with stones in the common bile duct or in those with established complications.

Endoscopic sphincterotomy, endoscopic choledocholithotomy and delayed cholecystectomy

It was probably inevitable that soon after the removal of gallstones from the common duct by endoscopic means, patients with cholecystitis and choledocnolithiasis who were considered poor surgical risks should be submitted to initial endoscopic choledocholithotomy. However, even enthusiasts of the technique were surprised to note that by 1978, no less than 29% of patients with choledocholithiasis presenting for endoscopic choledocholithotomy in 15 gastroenterology centres throughout the world, fell into this category (Safrany 1978). By 1981 the data collected from 25 centres in West Germany showed that 2238 (34%) or 7585 patients undergoing endoscopic removal of stones from the common bile duct, had not undergone a previous cholecystectomy (Seifert 1978). By 1984 data from 13 British centres showed that no less than 358 (41%) of 866 patients undergoing endoscopic removal of gallstones, had not undergone prior cholecystectomy (Frost 1984). Of course while these numbers loom large in the figures gathered from specialist endoscopy centres, they still form a small proportion of the total number of patients with stones in the bile duct. Nevertheless, it seems likely that in the future this group may be the commonest of those patients undergoing endoscopic choledocholithotomy.

There are two main reasons for this change in attitude. Firstly patients with acute biliary disease other than acute cholecystitis (jaundice, cholangitis, gallstone pancreatitis) can be treated initially with endoscopic decompression and come to cholecystectomy electively in reasonable condition. Indeed as a consequence of experience in Manchester, it was suggested that the mortality of treatment of combined cholecystolithiasis and choledocholithiasis in patients without acute cholecystitis might be reduced by preliminary endoscopic choledocholithotomy and subsequent cholecystectomy (Tweedle & Martin 1981). No controlled clinical trial was undertaken and the authors are unaware of any controlled trial. Nevertheless in 32 patients in whom this sequence of endoscopic choledocholithotomy followed by elective cholecystectomy was completed, there were no operative or late deaths (Neoptolemos et al 1984). The second reason, discussed in detail below, is that in the elderly and frail whose chronic symptoms settle after complete endoscopic clearance of the duct, cholecystectomy may be avoided altogether.

The contention of the authors is that very much more information is necessary before endoscopic choledocholithotomy followed by cholecystectomy at a later date is accepted as a reasonable approach. The studies of Donaldson (Houghton, Jenkinson & Donaldson 1985) and others (Ch. 46) reveal that elective cholecystectomy and choledocholithotomy is a safe operation in district hospitals even in the elderly. The majority of deaths are related to cardiovascular disease and occur in patients treated as emergencies and with severe local septic complications. While endoscopic sphincterotomy may have a role in elective cases, its potential in the emergency situation is much less clear. It might prove beneficial in those patients who are jaundiced with cholangitis, but the main problem in this situation is the differentiation and selection of those patients with gangrenous cholecystitis, a complication which can only be treated, or indeed prevented, by early surgical intervention. A recent study of endoscopic sphincterotomy (Neoptolemos et al 1984) in patients with the gallbladder in situ, noted a significant incidence of both cholangitis and pancreatitis following the procedure and that some patients still required cholecystectomy because of empyema. Indeed Houghton, Jenkinson & Donaldson (1985) suggest that, since the major cause of mortality and morbidity in the elderly is related to the occurrence of sepsis and to cardiovascular causes in association with the treatment of the acute case, a more aggressive approach to gallstones in an elective fashion might reduce the incidence of subsequent gangrenous cholecystitis and its associated high risk.

At present caution should be exercised in advocating endoscopic sphincterotomy for the treatment of a group of patients in whom the highest risk may be due to complications which endoscopic sphincterotomy is unlikely to affect.

Endoscopic sphincterotomy with clearance of the duct alone

There is a group of patients who are elderly and frail presenting with *chronic symptoms* which settle completely after endoscopic clearance of the common bile duct. It is suggested that in these patients, cholecystectomy may never be necessary since life expectancy is short and that the incidence of problems arising from cholecystolithiasis is small. Indeed some patients in whom elective cholecystectomy was planned following urgent endoscopic sphincterotomy and choledocholithotomy subsequently refused to undergo operation since their symptoms had disappeared.

In 1982, of 2238 patients undergoing endoscopic sphincterotomy with the gallbladder in situ, only 9.8% came to subsequent cholecystectomy (Seifert 1982), the majority as part of a planned two-stage approach. However, the length of follow-up in this series is uncertain and obviously comparatively short. One of the authors (Martin & Tweedle 1985) has performed this procedure in 56 elderly patients and, four years later, there were three patients who required subsequent cholecystectomy, two for recurrent colic and one for acute cholecystitis. Thirteen of these patients have subsequently died from cardiovascular accidents and other diseases unrelated to biliary pathology. In two elderly patients in whom endoscopic sphincterotomy for choledocholithiasis was carried out and in whom it proved impossible to remove large stones, the referring surgeon elected to observe these patients following sphincterotomy alone. Safrany & Cotton (1982) found that only 10% of 260 such patients (mean age 76 years) required cholecystectomy for pain or cholecystitis during a follow up period of one to six years. Escourrou et al (1984) reports similar figures, with only eight (6%) developing late cholecystitis and other biliary problems in a similar number. In all the series quoted above, virtually all patients coming to cholecystectomy required it within one year. Interestingly, as pointed out by Cotton (1984) these figures lie somewhere between those reported for the follow-up of asymptomatic (Gracie & Ransohoff 1982) and symptomatic (Wenckert & Robertson 1966) gallstones. However patients with a blocked cystic duct should probably be approached particularly cautiously in this regard and one patient has been reported with gallbladder cancer four years after endoscopic sphincterotomy (Escourrou et al 1984).

There is thus a case for the *early* management of choledocholithiasis in the elderly (see above), and particularly those with cardiac or respiratory disease, since there is an increased mortality for surgical choledocholithotomy if acute symptoms develop. In the great majority of cases so treated symptoms disappear or are so abated that cholecystectomy will be unnecessary in many whose life expectancy is indeed short.

CHOLEDOCHOLITHIASIS, PREVIOUS CHOLECYSTECTOMY AND T-TUBE IN SITU

It is for these patients that the greatest number of methods of treatment is available, since they may be treated by reoperation, endoscopic sphincterotomy, by dissolution using the T-tube track (Ch. 49) or finally by interventional radiological techniques using the T-tube track (Ch. 48). Again, there are no controlled clinical trials on which to base definitive statements.

Detailed discussions of the indications for, methods and results of dissolution therapy or T-tube extraction are given in Chapters 48 and 49. The majority of patients with retained common bile duct stones and a T-tube in situ do not suffer from concurrent cholangitis or pancreatitis and, if bile is draining from the T-tube (as occurs in nearly all patients), then obstructive jaundice, if present, will be resolving. Consequently, there is no urgency and the least invasive procedures should be adopted first. It is the authors' opinion that in elderly patients, the duct should be irrigated and an X-ray repeated in order to ascertain whether the stone is still apparent. If so then the patient might be discharged with the T-tube in situ. It is the authors' practice not to institute therapy immediately in the majority of cases, but to allow a two-week period to elapse. Further cholangiography is then carried out to establish the continued presence of the stone. At this point an approach can be chosen and will frequently be determined by the expertise available.

Dissolution therapy is effective in a proportion of patients (Ch. 49), is safe, and does not require any further intervention. Percutaneous extraction along the track of the T-tube is very effective in expert hands, the success rate being in excess of 95%. However, sometimes the track is not suitable for this purpose and it is necessary for a period of some six weeks to elapse to allow maturation of the track before extraction is performed. In some circumstances this may not be practical. Nevertheless, employment of one of the above techniques is very much safer than either surgery or endoscopic sphincterotomy and leaves the paient with an intact choledochal sphincter and freedom from late complications. Of course, the presence of concurrent cholangitis or pancreatitis demand urgent treatment and as emphasized above in the authors' experience, if there is obstruction to the passage of the stone and it cannot be removed percutaneously, it is probably best removed either endoscopically or surgically.

CONCLUSION

The presence of stones in the common bile duct usually demands treatment, although in some elderly and infirm patients with minimal symptoms, there may be little hazard in leaving them in situ (Gracie & Ransahoff 1982).

While there may be reason to undertake endoscopic sphincterotomy as a preliminary measure in patients with chronic disease especially in the elderly and frail, this approach requires much further definition. Surgical options may be safe, even in the elderly, the majority of complications and deaths being associated with cardiovascular disease and with sepsis. There are dangers in adopting endoscopic sphincterotomy in acute disease because of the risk of a gangrenous or perforated gallbladder. For patients under the age of 60 who are otherwise fit, modern surgical approaches have a good record and offer not only clearance of the bile ducts but removal of the diseased gallbladder. There may be a good case for a more aggressive approach in terms of elective surgery for elderly patients with choledocholithiasis, since this may prevent many of the late complications of sepsis which are associated with high morbidity and mortality.

For patients with a retained or residual bile duct stone after cholecystectomy, there is a strong case to be made for the use of endoscopic methods in many patients. Successful endoscopic treatment is preferred by patients and often by the surgeon who missed the stone at initial surgery. It is substantially cheaper than surgery. Because there is at present no clear evidence that the risks of endoscopic treatment increase with age, it is the treatment of choice in the elderly patient and in the patient at high risk; but the arguments for its use in the young and fit patient require further substantiation, particularly since it appears to be associated with no better results than surgery and the long-term effects of endoscopic sphincterotomy are unknown. Surgery is preferable in patients with biliary strictures or stenosis, and in patients with previous gastrectomy. Endoscopic removal of large stones within large ducts is much more difficult and these patients may be best managed by surgical choledochotomy and possible choledochoduodenostomy. Ideally, therapy should be selected in a team setting, the surgeon and endoscopist discussing each individual case and selecting the most appropriate treatment based on the known facts.

For the patient with a stone discovered in the post-cholecystectomy period and with a T-tube still in situ, dissolution methods or percutaneous extraction of the stone along the T-tube track have obvious advantages and will succeed in the majority of instances. However, dissolution may be slow and it may be that surgical or endoscopic options are selected in some patients.

REFERENCES

Allen B, Shapiro H, Way L W 1981 Management of recurrent and residual common duct stones. American Journal of Surgery 142: 41–47

Bartlett M K 1972 Retained and recurrent common duct stones. American Journal of Surgery 38:63

Blamey S L, Fearon K C H, Gilmore W H, Osborne D H, Carter D C 1983 Prediction of risk in biliary surgery. British Journal of Surgery 70: 535–538

Bordley J, White T T 1979 Causes for 340 re-operations on the extra-hepatic bile ducts. Annals of Surgery 189: 442–446

Brandstatter G von, Kratochvil P, Stupnicki Th, Justich E, Kopp W 1983 Langzeitergebnisse nach endoskopischer papillotomie. Forstchr Med 101: 1237–40

Cotton P B 1984 Endoscopic management of bile duct stones (apples & oranges) Gut 25: 587–597

Cotton P B, Vallon A 1981 British experience with duodenoscopic sphincterotomy for removal of bile duct stones. British Journal of Surgery 68: 373–375

Degenshein G A 1974 Choledocho-duodenostomy; an 18 years study of 175 consecutive cases. Surgery 76: 316–24

Dixon J M, Armstrong C B, Duffy S W, Davies G C 1983 Factors affecting morbidity and mortality after surgery for obstructive jaundice; a review of 373 patients. Gut 24: 845–852

Doyle P J, Ward-McQuaid J N, McEwen-Smith A 1982 The value of routine per-operative cholangiography — a report of 4000 cholecystectomies. British Journal of Surgery 69: 617–619

Escourrou J, Cordova J A, Lazorthes F, Frexinos J, Ribet A 1984 Early and later complications after endoscopic sphincterotomy for biliary lithiasis with and without gall bladder 'in situ'. Gut 25: 598–602

Freund H, Charuzi I, Granit I, Berlatzky Y, Eyal Z 1977 Choledochoduodenostomy in the treatment of benign biliary tract disease. Archives of Surgery 112: 1032–34

Frost R A 1984 (for British Collaborative study of ERCP) Prospective multi-centre study of British sphincterotomy: initial results and complications. Gut 25:A549

Geenen J E, Vennes J A, Silvis S E 1981 Resumé of a seminar on endoscopic retrograde sphincterotomy (ERS). Gastrointestinal Endoscopy 27: 31–38

Girard R M, Legros G 1981 Retained and recurrent bile duct stones. Surgical or non-surgical removal. Annals of Surgery 193: 150–154

Glenn F 1974 Retained calculi within the biliary ductal system. Annals of Surgery 179: 258–539

Glenn F 1975 Trends in surgical treatment of calculus disease of the biliary tract. Surgery, Gynecology and Obstetrics 140: 877–884

Goldman L D, Steer M L, Silen W 1983 Recurrent cholangitis after biliary surgery. American Journal of Surgery 123: 67–72

Gracie W A, Ransohoff D F 1982 The natural history of silent gall stones, the innocent stone is not a myth. New England Journal of Medicine 307: 798–800

Houghton P W J, Jenkinson L R, Donaldson L A, 1985 Cholecystectomy in the elderly — a prospective study. British Journal of Surgery 72: 220–222

Jones S A 1978 The prevention and treatment of recurrent bile duct stones by transduodenal sphincteroplasty. World Journal of Surgery 2: 473–485

Kaminski D L, Barner H B, Codd J E, Wolfe B M 1979 Evaluation of the results of external choledochoduodenostomy for retained, recurrent or primary common duct stones. American Journal of Surgery 137: 162–166

Kappes S K, Adams M B, Wilson S K 1982 Intraoperative biliary endoscopy. Archives of Surgery 117: 603–607

Koch H, Rosch W, Schaffner O, Demling L 1977 Endoscopic sphincterotomy. Gastroenterology 73: 1393–1396

Kune G A 1972 Current practice of biliary surgery. Little Brown, Boston, p 221–223

Larson R E, Hodgson J R, Priestley J T 1966 The early and long term results of 500 consecutive explorations of the common duct. Surgery, Gynecology and Obstetrics 122: 744–750

Lygidakis N J 1981 Choledocho-duodenostomy in calculous biliary tract disease. British Journal of Surgery 68: 762–765

Lygidakis N J 1982 Infective complications after choledochotomy. Journal of the Royal College of Surgeons of Edinburgh 27: 233–237

Lygidakis N J 1983 Surgical approaches to recurrent choledocholithiasis. American Journal of Surgery 145: 633–639

McSherry C K, Glenn F 1980 The incidence and causes of death following surgery for non-malignant biliary tract disease. Annals of Surgery 191: 271–275

Madden J L, Chun J Y, Kandalaft S, Parekh M 1970 Choledocho-duodenostomy. An unjustly maligned surgical procedure? American Journal of Surgery 119: 425–454

Madden J L 1973 Common duct stones, their origin and surgical management. Surgical Clinics of North America 5: 1095–1113

Martin D F, Tweedle D E F 1984 Value of precut papillotomy at ERCP and endoscopic sphincterotomy. Gut 25:A549

Moesgaard F, Nielsen M L, Pedersen T, Hansen J B 1982 Protective choledochoduodenostomy in multiple common duct stones in the aged. Surgery, Gynecology and Obstetrics 154: 232–234

Moller C, Santavirta S 1972 Residual common duct stones. Acta Chirurgica Scandinavica 138:183

Neoptolemos J P, Carr-Locke D L, Fraser I, Fossard D P 1984 The management of common bile duct calculi by endoscopic sphincterotomy in patients with gallbladders in situ. British Journal of Surgery 71: 69–71

Peel A L G, Bourke J B, Hermon Taylor J, MacLean A D W, Mann C V, Ritchie H D 1975 How should the common bile duct be explored? Annals of the Royal College of Surgeons 56: 124–134

Pitt H A, Cameron J L, Postier R G, Gadacz T R 1981 Factors affecting mortality in biliary tract surgery. American Journal of Surgery 141: 66–72

Reiter J J, Bayer H B, Mennicken C, Manegold P C 1978 Results of endoscopic papillotomy: a collective experience from 9 endoscopic centres in West Germany. World Journal of Surgery 2: 505–507

Rosch W, Riemann J F, Lux G, Lindner H G 1981 Long term follow-up after endoscopic sphincterotomy. Endoscopy 13: 152–153

Safrany L 1978 Endoscopic treatment of biliary tract disease. Lancet ii: 983–985

Safrany L, Cotton P B 1982 Endoscopic management of choledocholithiasis. Surgical Clinics of North America 62: 825–836

Safrany L, Schott B, Vallon A G 1982 Endoscopic sphincterotomy: The long term results in choledocholithiasis (Abstract) Gastrointestinal Endoscopy 28:152

Seifert E 1978 Endoscopy and biliary disease. In: Blumgart L H (ed) The biliary tract. Churchill Livingstone, Edinburgh, p 72

Seifert E, Gail K, Weismuller J 1982 Langzeitresultate nach endoskopischer sphinkterotomie, follow-up studie aus 25 centren in der Bundersrepublik. Deutcher Medizinitcher Wochenschrift 107: 610–614

Siegel J H 1981 Endoscopic papillotomy in the treatment of biliary tract disease; 258 procedures and results. Digestive Diseases and Sciences 26: 1057–1064

Spohn K, Fux H D, Mehnert U, Muller-Kluge M, Tewes G 1973 Cholecystektomie und choledochotomie — Taktik und Techniken. Langenbecks Archives fur Chirurgie 334: 249–254

Stefanini P, Carboni M, Patrassi N et al 1974 Transduodenal sphincteroplasty: its use in the treatment of lithiasis and benign obstruction of the common duct. American Journal of Surgery 128: 672–677

Stuart M, Hoerr S O 1972 Late results of side to side choledocho-duodenostomy and of trans-duodenal sphincterotomy for benign disorders. American Journal of Surgery 123: 67–72

Stubbs R S, Blumgart L H 1984 Exploration of the common bile duct. Journal of the Royal College of Surgeons of Edinburgh 29: 76–79

Sue S O, Taub M, Pearlman B J, Marks J W, Bonorris G G, Schoenfield L J 1981 Treatment of choledocholithiasis with oral chenodeoxycholic acid. Surgery 90: 32–34

Thomas C G, Nicholson C P, Owen J 1971 Effectiveness of choledochoduodenostomy and transduodenal sphincterotomy in the treatment of benign obstruction of the bile duct. Annals of Surgery 173: 845–856

Tweedle D E F 1984 (unreported data: Table 50.2)

Tweedle D E F, Martin D F 1985 (unreported data)

Tweedle D E F, Martin D F, 1981 Choledocholithiasis — surgical or endoscopic lithotomy. Gut 22:A888

Vallon A G, Cotton P B, Holton J 1982 Clinical endoscopic follow-up after duodenoscopic sphincterotomy. Gut 22:A889

Vallon A G, Holton J M, Cotton P B 1985 personal communication British Journal of Surgery.

Vellacott K D, Powell P H 1979 Exploration of the common bile duct: A comparative study. British Journal of Surgery 66: 389–391

Way L W, Admirand W H, Dunphy J E 1972 Management of choledocholithiasis. Annals of Surgery 176: 347–359

Wenckert A, Robertson B 1966 The natural course of gallstone disease. 11-year review of 71 non-operated cases. Gastroenterology 50: 376–381

White T T, Bordley J 1978 One per cent incidence of recurrent gallstones six to eight years after manometric cholangiography. Annals of Surgery 188: 562–569

51

F. Nakayama

Intrahepatic stones

INTRODUCTION

The majority of gallstones are present in the gallbladder and less frequently are found in the extrahepatic bile ducts. Gallstones also occur in the intrahepatic ducts (Fig. 51.1) but much less frequently. In spite of their relatively rare occurrence, intrahepatic calculi have attracted much attention. The reasons for this are the difficulty of management and the intractable course of intrahepatic stones. In ordinary cholelithiasis, the treatment is reasonably straightforward. Cholecystectomy and common bile duct exploration usually lead to complete cure and operative mortality is less than 1–2%. Indeed even medical treatment may occasionally offer a complete cure in the form of gallstone dissolution (Nakayama 1980; Rupin & Dowling 1982).

In contrast the treatment of intrahepatic stone disease or hepatolithiasis must be surgical and it is not unusual to require multiple operations. Even then recurrence is not exceptional. Operative intervention frequently fails because of the complicated pathology inherent in hepatolithiasis. In addition, the recent rapid advance of hepatobiliary imaging techniques has facilitated the establishment of the diagnosis of hepatolithiasis since imaging displays not only the presence of gallstones in the gallbladder and extraheptic bile ducts but also in the intrahepatic bile ducts. The case shown in Fig. 51.2 was diagnosed by ultrasound-guided percutaneous transhepatic cholangiography with the demonstration of intrahepatic calculi in the inferior branch of the right anterior sectoral hepatic duct which would otherwise have been missed.

The aetiology of intrahepatic stones or heptolithiasis is far from clear and therefore no satisfactory treatment can be devised nor adequate preventative measures defined. In the present chapter the state of our knowledge of the cause, diagnosis and treatment of the disease is presented.

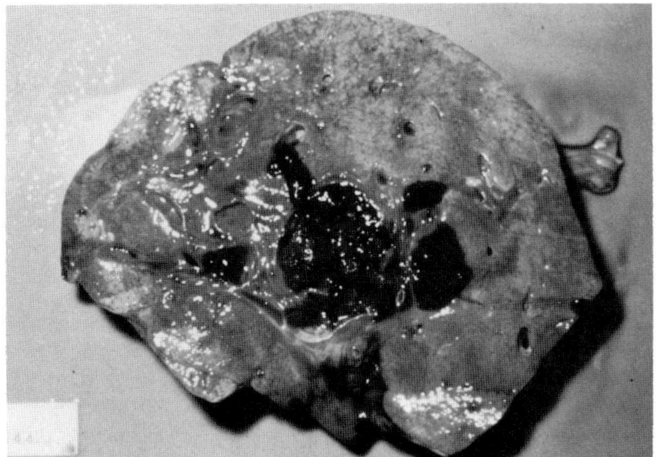

Fig. 51.1 Resected liver specimen showing dilated intrahepatic duct filled with stones

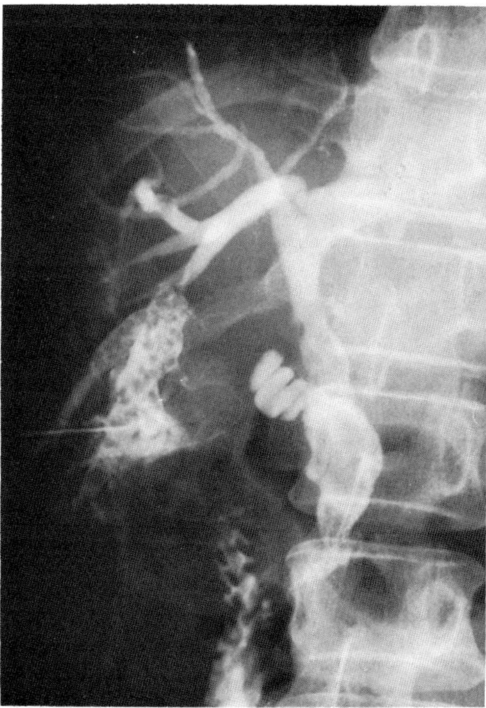

Fig. 51.2 PTC cholangiogram showing stones in inferior branch of the right anterior segmental duct

DEFINITION AND CLASSIFICATION

Intrahepatic stones are those concretions found in the intrahepatic bile ducts defined as any bile duct peripheral to the junction of right and left hepatic ducts even though the confluence is outside the liver substance (Mishima et al 1982). Stones may also be present coincidentally in the extrahepatic bile ducts, having passed down either from the intrahepatic bile ducts or, as a result of accumulation, from extrahepatic ducts to the intrahepatic biliary ductal system.

Numerous classifications of intrahepatic stones have confused understanding of the disease. Recently a standardized classification of hepatolithiasis was proposed (Nakayama 1982) (Table 51.1), based solely on the pathological findings. This classification is as follows: Hepatolithiasis is defined as gallstones present in intrahepatic bile ducts. The intrahepatic ducts are defined as including the right and left hepatic ducts distal to the confluence. The segmental ducts are divided into central and peripheral ducts. The former denotes that part between the first and second branches counting from the bifurcation of the hepatic ducts and the latter peripheral to the second branches. Stricture is defined as a decrease in the diameter of the bile ducts relative to the adjacent parts and is designated as S. S_0 denotes absence of stricture; S_1 slight stricture (diameter >2 mm); and S_2 marked stricture (<2 mm diameter).

Dilatation, D, is defined as an increase of the diameter of the bile duct beyond physiological range. D_0 denotes the absence of dilatation; D_1 slight dilatation; and D_2 marked dilatation. In the extrahepatic bile duct, D_2 denotes dilatation > 20 mm and D_1 <20 mm. In the intrahepatic bile duct, 10 mm is chosen to divide D_1 and D_2.

The sites of stricture and dilatation should be described as in Table 51.1. When stricture or dilatation involves A to B in continuity, they should be connected with the sign ~B, but if they are present in more than two sites separately, they should be expressed as A, B. The code describing the pathology is given in large parentheses. Presence or absence of stones in all parts of the biliary tract should be noted and described in code, preceding those describing the pathology. In addition, the kind of gallstones present is noted. G denotes gallbladder; B extrahepatic bile duct; and H intrahepatic duct. When no stone is present in the gallbladder, it is expressed as Go. If a cholesterol stone is present, it is designated as Gc; if a calcium bilirubinate stone is present, Gb. If stones other than cholesterol and calcium bilirubinate stones are present, types are given. If the presence or absence of stones is uncertain, x is added. When the presence of stone is known but its kind is uncertain, x is the designation. Presence or absence of stenosis of the duodenal papilla is treated separately. If absent, it is expressed as Spo; if present, Sp; and if uncertain, Spx. Passage of a bougie with 3 mm diameter, findings in the endoscopic retrograde cholangiopancreatography (ERCP) and pressure studies are criteria for the presence or absence of stenosis of the duodenal papilla. If cholecystectomy has already been performed, it is expressed as $\not{G}$.

Table 51.1 Classification of hepatolithiasis

Location of stones[a]		Stenosis of bile duct		Dilatation of bile duct	
Type	Lobe	Grade	Site[b]	Grade	Site[b]
Intrahepatic-I	Left-L	No stenosis-S_0	Peripheral: Sa-p[c] Sp-p Sl-p Sm-p	No dilatation-D_0	Peripheral: Da-p Dp-p Dl-p Dm-p
Intra- and extrahepatic-IE	Right-R	Slight stenosis-S_1	Central: Sa-c Sp-c Sl-c Sm-c	Slight dilatation-D_1	Central: Da-c Dp-c Dl-c Dm-c[d]
IE	Left and right: LR	High-grade stenosis-S_2	Hepatic duct-Slh or Srh	High-grade dilatation-D_2	Hepatic duct-Dlh or Drh
IE	LR		Common hepatic duct-Sch		Common hepatic duct-Dch
IE	LR LR		Common bile duct-Scb		Common bile Duct-Dcb

a Predominant location is underlined.
b p: peripheral; c: central; l: lateral segmental duct; m: medial segmental duct; a: anterior segmental duct; p: posterior segmental duct; rh: right hepatic duct; lh: left hepatic duct; ch: common hepatic duct; cb: common bile duct
c Stenosis of peripheral portion of anterior segmental duct
d Dilatation of central portion of medial segmental duct
Example: $\not{G}_o$ Bb Hb- [IE.LR.S_0.D_1cb~], Sp, two cdeg
No stone was present in gallbladder. Calcium bilirubinate stones were present in extrahepatic and intrahepatic bile duct. Intra-and extrahepatic ducts were involved, the latter predominating. Left and right lobes were involved: no stricture present. Slight dilatation of whole bile duct. Stenosis of duodenal papilla present. One previous operation, i.e., cholecystectomy. Present operation: choledochotomy, choledochostomy and sphincteroplasty done

In hepatolithiasis, it is not unusual to have multiple operations. It is quite possible for the pathology to change as further operative interventions are added. Therefore, it is useful to have previous and present operations listed at the end of the code. The operations are listed from the simplest to the more complicated procedures. These are assigned a letter alphabetically and consecutively. The code denoting the present operation is underlined.

This classification offers several advantages. It is based on the exact description of the prevailing pathological findings and is, therefore, devoid of subjective bias for the designation of stones as primary or secondary, or of conditions as congenital or acquired. The coding used offers easier compilation of the data which can be stored in a computer for later retrieval.

PATHOLOGY

Intrahepatic stones are mostly calcium bilirubinate stones composed mainly of bilirubin, cholesterol, fatty acid and calcium. They are dark brown, soft and friable. On the broken surface layer formation can be seen. Because of the low content of calcium they are usually radiolucent. In addition, it is usual to find sludge of similar composition but of higher water content among the stones. Intrahepatic stones are found in dilated intrahepatic bile ducts with stricture of the bile duct present proximally as shown cholangiographically (Fig. 51.3). The wall of the dilated bile duct is composed of dense fibrous tissue with tubular intramural and tubulo-glandular extramural glands which secrete mucinous fluid (Ohta et al 1983). The strictures are of similar histological appearance. No specific features can be found to suggest congenital origin. The disease appears from the third to the sixth decades but the highest prevalence is in the fifth decade. In the younger age group, stones are mostly confined to intrahepatic bile ducts but there is gradual involvement of extrahepatic bile ducts in older subjects. In one third of cases, the stones are confined to the intrahepatic ducts and associated with bile duct stricture. Left hepatic involvement predominates and in half the cases bile duct stricture can be demonstrated. Dilatation of bile ducts is almost always present.

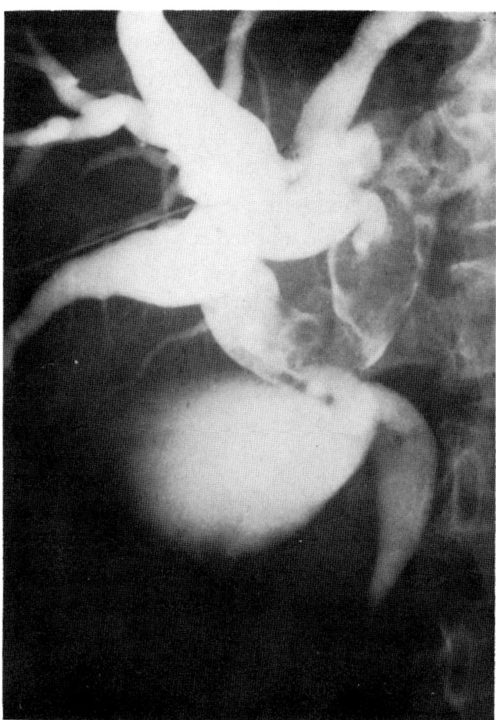

Fig. 51.3 Cholangiogram showing the presence of intrahepatic stones and proximal stricture of bile duct

EPIDEMIOLOGY

Hepatolithiasis occurs more frequently in East Asia including Japan, China, Korea, Taiwan, Philippines, Thailand, Malaysia and Indonesia. The prevalence varies considerably according to the area. For instance in Taiwan the proportion of hepatolithiasis is 50% greater than all cases of cholelithiasis (Ket et al 1981). Comparable figures for China are 38% (Huang 1976), South Korea 9% (Kwon et al 1982), Malaya 11% (King 1971, Balasegaram 1972) (Table 51.2). A recent nationwide survey in Japan of hepatolithiasis gives a prevalence rate of 3.9% (that is 1590 cases of hepatolithiasis in 38 606 cases of cholelithiasis) (Nakayama et al 1980). The prevalence was found to vary according to the area of Japan. The lowest prevalence was recorded in urban Tokyo and Osaka while the highest rate was found in more or less rural areas such as Tohoku, Shikoku and Hokkaido.

Although a description of hepatolithiasis is said to have been found in about the 16th century (Rufanov 1936), the prevalence of the disease in the West is low, being reported recently as between 0.6% and 3% (Lindström 1977, Simi et al 1979). However occasional cases have been described (Vachell & Stevens 1906) of an advanced nature with numerous stones filling both the intrahepatic and extrahepatic ducts. The largest calculus weighed 270 g. It is therefore possible that the nature and prevalence of the disease may have changed in the West over the years. Indeed the prevalence of hepatolithiasis in Japan seems to

Table 51.2 Prevalence of hepatolithiasis world-wide

	prevalence (%)
Taiwan	50
People's Republic of China	40
Korea	20
Hong Kong	10
Malaya	10
Japan	4–5
West	1–3

be declining. Thus in 1913, Miyake found 20 cases of hepatolithiasis and 257 cases of cholelithiasis among 8406 autopsy records at the three leading universities in Japan (Tokyo, Kyoto and Kyushu) — a prevalence of 7.7%. At present the prevalence of hepatolithiasis in Japan ranges from 3–4% (Nakayama et al 1980). The increase of ordinary cholelithiasis may have partly contributed to the apparent decrease in the prevalence of hepatolithiasis. Furthermore the pathology of hepatolithiasis is also changing. We no longer see extremely dilated intrahepatic ducts filled with large numbers of numerous intrahepatic calculi as in the immediate post–war period, 40 years ago.

In Latin America the prevalence of hepatolithiasis seems to be high, having been reported at between 2 and 7% (Bove et al 1963, Cobo et al 1964, Faintuch 1983). Admittedly the reported prevalence is unreliable because of the difficulty in making a correct diagnosis. This, despite modern hepatobiliary imaging techniques, depends somewhat upon the familiarity of the surgeons with the disease and this in turn depends on the local occurrence rate.

AETIOLOGY

Possible factors responsible for the geographical difference in the prevalence of intrahepatic stones may be divided conceptually into ethnic and environmental factors. In a recent survey conducted in South East Asia, the prevalence of hepatolithiasis in Taiwan, Hong Kong and Singapore has been compared with that in Japan (Nakayama et al 1986). In spite of a similar ethnic background (the majority of the population is Chinese or of Chinese descent) the prevalence of hepatolithiasis is markedly different, being over 50% in Taiwan and 2 to 4% in Hong Kong and Singapore. The explanation must therefore be environmental. Of the environmental factors, infestation with parasites has often been cited (Fung 1961) (Ch. 77). However, in Taiwan, which has a high prevalence of hepatolithiasis, infestation with *Clonorchis sinesis* is found mainly in Southern Taiwan (Chow 1961) and *Clonorchis* and its ova are found only infrequently in cases with intrahepatic stones. Even the demonstration of *Clonorchis* ova in intrahepatic calculi does not incriminate infection as responsible for the formation of intrahepatic stones since they may merely be associated with stones in endemic areas of infection such as Hong Kong and Southern China. For instance, in spite of the absence of *Clonorchis sinensis* infestation, Malaya has a high prevalence of hepatolithiasis.

The factors responsible for the formation of intrahepatic stones are not well defined but are thought to be due to bacterial infection and stasis. The incidence of bacteria in bile in cases of hepatolithiasis is almost 100% (Tabata & Nakayama 1984) suggesting a close association between bacterial colonization of bile and the presence of intrahepatic calculi. Among the bacteria present, *Escherichia coli* (Maki 1966), *Clostridium*, and *Bacteroides* show β-glucuronidase activity (Table 51.3) which are thought to be responsible for the hydrolysis of bilirubin glucuronide, the water soluble form of bilirubin in bile, to free unconjugated bilirubin. The latter is water insoluble and combines with ionized calcium in bile to form calcium bilirubinate leading to the formation of calcium bilirubinate stones of which the majority of intrahepatic stones are formed. However, recent analysis of intrahepatic stones showed, in addition to the usual calcium bilirubinate stones, the presence of calculi rich in cholesterol and fatty acid (Nakayama 1984). Therefore, when considering the aetiology of intrahepatic calculi, the solubilization of cholesterol and fatty acid in bile should be considered.

Table 51.3 Incidence of bacteria in hepatolithiasis and β-glucuronidase activity

Bacterial species	β-glucuronidase activity
Escherichia coli	+
Klebsiella	+
Pseudomonas	−
Streptococcus Group D	+
Morganella	−
Enterobacter	−
Aeromonas	−
Citrobacter	−
Bacteroides fragilis	+
Clostridium perfringens	+

Bile stasis is caused by the presence of stenosis and stricture formation usually associated with areas of ductal dilatation. Such stenosis may occur either in the left or right hepatic duct branches but left hepatic duct involvement predominates (Nakayama & Koga 1984). The stenosis is sometimes found at the liver hilum, involving both hepatic ducts. However, in some cases, in spite of the presence of stones not only in the intrahepatic but also the extrahepatic bile ducts, no stenosis can be demonstrated in the bile duct. The duodenal papilla may be patulous and no mechanical stenosis demonstrated in such cases.

CLINICAL FEATURES

Symptoms and signs

Abdominal pain either in the right upper quadrant or in the upper abdomen is the most frequent initial symptom. Jaundice and fever follow and indeed are present in 60 to 70% of cases. In a quarter of cases, jaundice and fever appear as the initial symptoms. Other abdominal complaints include abdominal discomfort, vomiting and lethargy. All of these symptoms are not pathognomonic to intrahepatic stone disease and are similar to those of choledocholithiasis.

Diagnosis

The presence of intrahepatic calculi should be suspected in endemic areas when there is a long history of abdominal pain especially from a young age. Continuing abdominal symptoms after cholecystectomy, especially in those in whom no gallstones could be demonstrated in the gallbladder despite the presence of highly suggestive symptoms are frequently found.

In 80% of cases, abnormality can be demonstrated in one of the liver function tests, which may therefore be used as initial screening procedures. However, ultrasound survey is non-invasive and a reliable, inexpensive and easily performed screening procedure. It is preferable to ERCP, PTC, CT or to scintigraphy. When diagnostic efficacy is compared among these diagnostic modalities, percutaneous transhepatic cholangiography (PTC) is found to be the most accurate (88.6%). In cases of suspected intrahepatic stones a diagnosis was obtained in 97% by PTC, 87% ERC, 81% by CT and in 75% by ultrasound (Kameda & Koga 1983). When the presence of intrahepatic calculi is suspected by non-invasive diagnostic procedures (ultrasound, computed tomography) the next procedure to be employed is direct cholangiography, such as percutaneous transhepatic cholangiography or endoscopic retrograde cholangiography (Fig. 51.4). When jaundice and fever are absent, endoscopic retrograde cholangiography should first be tried followed by PTC, if necessary, for more thorough visualization of the bile ducts. If jaundice and fever is present, suggestive of severe bacterial infection, PTC is the first choice procedure which can then be converted to percutaneous transhepatic cholangiodrainage (Ch. 36) for biliary decompression.

In 20% of cases the diagnosis is first established at laparotomy. In such cases intraoperative diagnostic procedures including operative cholangiography and intraoperative ultrasound should be carried out (Ikeda et al 1981a) in order to locate the dilated intrahepatic segments of the hepatic bile duct and stones. A search for scar tissue on the surface of the liver, especially the left lobe, and careful palpation of the liver substance to reveal the presence of intrahepatic stones are also important.

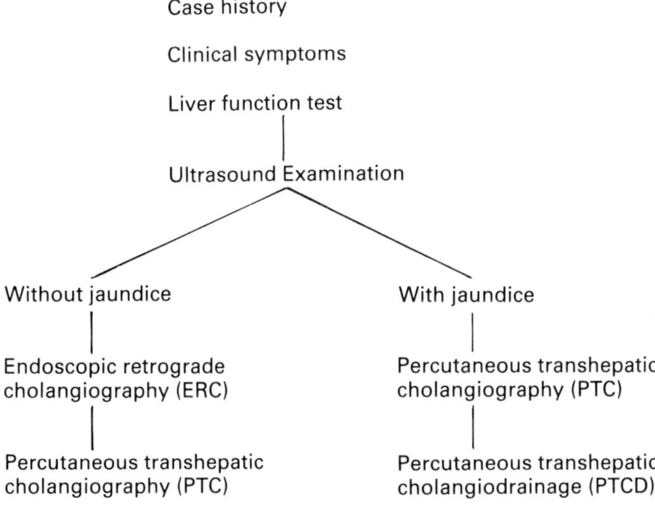

Fig. 51.4 Diagnostic steps in hepatolithiasis

TREATMENT

In two-thirds of cases of hepatolithiasis, asymptomatic stones are also present in the extrahepatic bile ducts. However, should a stone impact in the distal common duct, the rise of intraductal pressure accompanied by bacterial infection aggravates the situation leading to acute obstructive cholangitis. The condition of the patient rapidly deteriorates and in such circumstances immediate decompression of the biliary tree with the least risk to the patient is mandatory. Endoscopic decompression (Ch. 35) offers the best chance of relief by cannulating the distal common duct, dislodging impacted stones and providing continuous bile drainage (Ikeda et al 1981b).

If a stricture is present at the liver hilum, percutaneous transhepatic cholangiodrainage is more effective than endoscopic drainage but runs the risk of haemorrhage, cholangiovenous reflux and haemobilia. Although the recent introduction of the ultrasound guided percutaneous transhepatic cholangiography technique has greatly aided the accurate placement of drainage tubes in dilated intrahepatic bile ducts, the risks are still present.

Whether or not preoperative decompression of the biliary tract lessens the risk of operative mortality and morbidity in the presence of obstructive jaundice is at present controversial (Ch. 37) and a prospective controlled trial is necessary. However, in cases of hepatolithiasis, biliary tract infection is always present and the author considers it safer to perform preoperative biliary tract decompression as soon as possible to alleviate the occurrence of acute obstructive cholangitis and septicaemia. In addition, cholangiography can be done using the drainage route so as to provide accurate information on the pathology of the intrahepatic bile ducts.

The principles of the definitive treatment of intrahepatic stones are firstly to remove intrahepatic stones and secondly to treat bile duct strictures which result in dilatation and bile stasis. Hepatic resection offers the best chance of cure if the stones are confined to the left lobe (Ch. 77). However, owing to the presence of cirrhosis and of collaterals, the extent of liver resection may have to be limited and a strictured part of the intrahepatic bile duct may have to be left in situ. In such cases, to avoid formation of infected persistent fistula, the resected surface of the liver can be covered by a Roux-en-Y defunctionalized jejunal loop. Stones in the extrahepatic ducts can be removed at supraduodenal choledochotomy. If the stones are confined to the right hepatic duct, right hepatectomy is not usually undertaken since the risk is much greater than left hepatic resection.

As the pathology of intrahepatic stones is often quite complicated, the operative procedures should be tailored to suit the prevailing conditions. Additional procedures are often required in order to remove intrahepatic stones as completely as possible and prevent intrahepatic stones descending into the extrahepatic bile ducts. Sphinctero-plasty may be effective for the latter. However, the so-called narrow segment of distal common duct should be divided as extensively as possible so as to provide a wide enough opening for the stones to pass to the duodenum. When a stricture is present at the liver hilum, resection of the stricture of the bile duct followed by extended longitudinal division of the left hepatic duct and cholangio-jejunostomy side-to-side to a Roux-en-Y loop of jejunum (Ch. 70) is done (Fig. 51.5). End-to-end anastomosis without extended longitudinal division of the left hepatic duct may lead to narrowing of the anastomosis. If mucosa to mucosa anastomosis is not possible at the liver hilum because of the presence of extensive scarring, the end of the jejunal loop can be sutured around the exposed intra-hepatic bile ducts at the liver hilum in the form of a portojejunostomy. Side-to-side choledochoduodenostomy and choledochojejunostomy are not recommended because of the danger of ascending infection of the biliary tree due to the presence of a blind pouch at the distal end of the common duct.

Removal of intrahepatic calculi can be accomplished endoscopically via several routes. The use of a duodeno-scope via the duodenal papilla is not practical because of the long route to be traversed. An endoscope can be inserted via the choledochotomy drainage tract and used efficiently to remove intrahepatic stones remaining post-operatively (Yamakawa et al 1980). As the recurrence of intrahepatic stones is frequent, the end of the Roux-en-Y jejunal limb is placed subcutaneously after cholangiojejun-ostomy to provide for the subsequent insertion of the endoscope (Fig. 51.6) (Ch. 70). Alternatively a percutaneous transhepatic tract can be dilated using serially larger drainage tubes to allow accommodation of the endoscope for the removal of intrahepatic stones (Nimura et al 1984). This method offers the additional advantage of permitting observation of the duct peripheral to the stricture. This is important since as many as 5% of patients with hepato-lithiasis develop cholangiocarcinoma (Koga et al 1984). Biopsy can be taken if desired. Numerous attempts to dissolve intrahepatic stones have been made. However, the majority being calcium bilirubinate stones are not readily dissolved. In order for the solvent to be useful in clinical practice, it should dissolve stones readily yet not have injurious effects on the bile ducts. Such solvents are yet to be found. Even after an apparently complete removal of intrahepatic stones recurrence is usual rather than excep-tional, since the factors responsible for their formation may still be present. Therefore, removal of bile stasis and bacterial infection is mandatory in achieving complete cure.

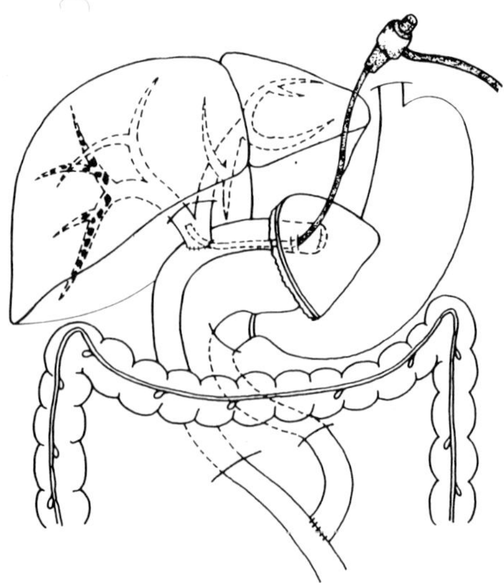

Fig. 51.6 Hepaticojejunostomy (Roux-en-Y), end to side, with subcutaneous anchoring of jejunal limb for later insertion of fibrescope to remove remaining intrahepatic stones

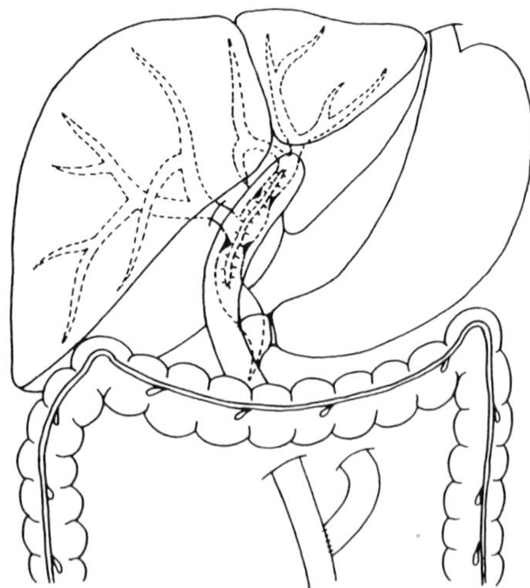

Fig. 51.5 Hepaticojejunostomy (Roux-en-Y) side-to-side following extended longitudinal division of left hepatic duct

Prognosis

Complete cure can only be achieved by hepatic resection with the removal of stones as well as the bile duct pathology which leads to the formation of further intra-hepatic stones. However, not all cases are amenable to such a radical approach. Usually half the cases still have intrahepatic calculi remaining in situ at the time of discharge; 30–40% of patients continue to have abdominal discomfort (Koga & Nakayama 1984). When the relief of bile duct stricture and dilated bile duct together with biliary infection is not achieved, recurrence of intrahepatic stones is usual rather than exceptional. The worst cases are those with stricture at the liver hilum involving both hepatic ducts. Even after the removal of stricture and cholangiojejunostomy, recurrence of stricture and intrahepatic stones is frequent.

REFERENCES

Balasegaram M 1972 Hepatic calculi. Annals of Surgery 175: 149–154

Bove P, de Oliveira M R, Sparanzini M 1963 Intrahepatic lithiasis. Gastroenterology 44: 391–410

Chow L 1960 Epidemiological studies of clonorchiasis at Meinung township in southern Taiwan. Formosan Science 14: 134–166

Cobo A, Hall R C, Torres E, Cuello C J 1964 Intrahepatic calculi. Archives of Surgery 89: 936–941

Faintuch J 1983 Personal communication

Fung J 1961 Liver fluke infestation and cholangiohepatitis. British Journal of Surgery 48:404–415

Huang Z 1976 Biliary tract surgery. People's Health Publishing Company, Beijing, p 161

Hur K B, Rice R G, Hong S S 1973 Cholelithiasis in Koreans. Yonsei Medical Journal 4: 103–118

Ikeda S, Tanaka M, Itoh H, Kishikawa H, Nakayama F 1981a Emergency decompression of bile duct in acute obstructive suppurative cholangitis by duodenoscopic cannulation: A life saving procedure. World Journal of Surgery 5: 587–593

Ikeda S, Tanaka M, Yoshimoto H, Itoh H, Nakayama F 1981b Improved visualisation of intrahepatic bile ducts by endoscopic retrograde balloon catheter cholangiography. Annals of Surgery 194: 171–175

Kameda H, Koga A 1983 Report on diagnosis of Hepatolithiasis. In: Annual report 1982 of research group for the study of hepatolithiasis. Ministry of Health (Head Prof. Fumio Nakayama), Japanese Government, Counter Measure Project for Intractable Diseases, Tokyo, p 17 (in Japanese)

Ker C G, Huang T J, Sheen P C 1981 Intrahepatic stones: I. Etiological study (in Chinese with English summary). Journal of Formosan Medical Association 80: 698–711

King M S 1971 Biliary tract disease in Malaya. British Journal of Surgery 58: 829–832

Koga A, Nakayama F 1984 Choice of treatment for hepatolithiasis based on pathological findings. World Journal of Surgery 8: 36–40

Koga A, Ichimiya H, Yamaguchi K, Miyazaki K, Nakayama F 1985 Hepatolithiasis associated with cholangiocarcinoma: Possible etiological significance. Cancer 55: 2826–2829

Kwon O J, Park Y H, Kim J P 1982 A clinical study of cholelithiasis in Korean. Journal of the Korean Surgical Society 24: 1052–1058 (In Korean with English abstract)

Lindström C G 1977 Frequency of gallstone disease in a well-defined Swedish population. A prospective necropsy study in Malmo. Scandinavian Journal of Gastroenterology 12: 311–346

Maki T 1966 Pathogenesis of calcium bilirubinate gallstones: Role of *E. coli*, β- glucuronidase and coagulation by inorganic ions, polyelectrolytes and agitation. Annals of Surgery 169: 90–100

Min P C, Cho M H, Im H N, Kim J H, Chin B O, Hahn S S 1966 Biliary tract diseases among Koreans: Analysis of 100 consecutive cases (in Korean with English summary). Journal of Korean Surgery Society 8:1

Mishima Y, Atomi Y, Danno M, Kuroda S 1982 Clinic and pathology of hepatolithiasis. In: Research group for the study of hepatolithiasis. Annual report 1981, Ministry of Health, Japanese Government, Counter Measure Project for Intractable Disease, Tokyo, p 15 (in Japanese)

Miyake H 1913 Statistische, klinische and chemische studien zur Aetiologie der Gallensteine mit besonderer Berücksichtigung der japanischen und deutschen Verhältnisse. Archiv für Klinischen Chirurgie 101: 54–117

Nakayama F 1980 Oral cholelitholysis — cheno versus urso: Japanese experience. Digestive Diseases and Science 25: 129–134

Nakayama F 1982 Intrahepatic calculi: A special problem in East Asia. World Journal of Surgery 6: 802–804

Nakayama F 1984 Report of Subcommittee for chemical study. Committee for etiological study. In: Annual report 1983 of research group for the study of hepatolithiasis. Ministry of Health, Japanese Government, Counter Measure Project for Intractable Diseases, Tokyo, p 2 (in Japanese)

Nakayama F, Furusawa T 1980 Hepatolithiasis: Present status. American Journal of Surgery 140: 216–220

Nakayama F, Soloway R, Nakama T, Miyazaki K, Ichimiya H, Sheen P C, Ker G B, Ong G B, Choi T K, Boey J, Foong W C, Tan E C, Tung K H, Lee C N 1986 Hepatolithiasis in East Asia. Retrospective study. Digestive Diseases and Science 31: 21–26

Nimura Y, Hayakawa N, Hasegawa Y, Kamiya J 1984 Treatment of hepatolithiasis: Place of endoscopic lithotomy. I to Cho (Stomach and Intestine) 19: 437–444 (In Japanese with English summary)

Ohta G 1983 Morphological study on hepatolithiasis and its etiological significance — Nation wide survey. In: Report of Subcomittee for pathological study, Committee for Etiological Study, Research Group for the Study of Hepatolithiasis (Head Prof. Fumio Nakayama) Ministry of Health, Japanese Government, Counter Measure Project for Intractable Diseases, Tokyo (in Japanese)

Rufanov I G 1936 Liver stones. Annals of Surgery 103: 321

Ruppin D C, Dowling R H 1982 Is recurrence inevitable after gallstone dissolution by bile acid treatment? Lancet i: 181–185

Simi M, Loriga P, Basoli A, Leardi S, Speranza V 1979 Intrahepatic lithiasis. Study of thirty-six cases and review of the literature. American Journal of Surgery 137: 317–322

Tabata M, Nakayama F 1984 Bacteriology of hepatolithiasis. In: Okuda K, Nakayama F, Wong J (eds) Intrahepatic calculi. Alan R Liss New York, pp 163–174

Vachell H R, Stevens W M 1906 Case of intrahepatic calculi. British Medical Journal 1: 434–436

Yamakawa T, Komaki F, Shikata J 1980 The importancce of postoperative choledochoscopy for management of retained biliary tract stones. Japanese Journal of Surgery 10:302

52

A. A. Gunn

Supraduodenal choledochotomy

The classic indications for choledochotomy have been shown to be unreliable (Table 52.1). This has resulted in many unnecessary common bile duct explorations with a resulting increase in the morbidity and mortality of operation for cholecystectomy (Ch. 46). The accepted absolute indications for duct exploration are the presence of a stone or stricture on the operative cholangiogram and a stone which can be palpated. However, even an experienced surgeon fails to palpate a significant percentage of stones. Some surgeons consider that drainage of the common bile duct is necessary during exploration for gallstone pancreatitis and operative exploration of the duct has, until recently, been the standard procedure for residual benign pathology in the biliary ducts after cholecystectomy.

Table 52.1 Classical indications for choledochotomy

Indications	% patients	% with stones in duct
Previous jaundice	17.9	34.4
Raised bilirubin	21.4	43.0
Small stones in gallbladder	58.3	16.9
Dilated cystic duct		
5–10 mm	18.5	31.2
10+ mm	4.4	86.9
Dilated common bile duct		
10–15 mm	14.3	21.6
15 + mm	15.6	72.8
Indurated pancreas	13.1	27.9
Palpable stone in duct	12.9	18.9*
Positive cholangiogram	18.3	18.9

* note surgeon error
This information was collected prospectively on punch cards.

These indications imply that the patients coming for exploration of the common bile duct have more serious pathology and, as a result, a higher morbidity than patients having cholecystectomy alone (Tables 52.2, 52.3).

Choledochotomy normally implies the subsequent use of T-tube drainage and this will be discussed later. However, the bile in these patients is more likely to contain bacteria than in those who do not require choledochotomy. It is recognized that some bile is likely to leak around the T-tube in a significant number of patients. This situation could be likened to a fistula with the connection between two potentially contaminated surfaces across the peritoneal cavity and the implied possibility of postoperative complications.

The operation of choledochotomy is not advised unless absolutely necessary and with the advent of endoscopic techniques, may be required much less often in the future, particularly in the management of retained stones after cholecystectomy (Ch. 47).

PREOPERATIVE PREPARATION

Preoperative preparation should be aimed at reduction of

Table 52.2 Clinical features

Parameters	Cholecystectomy* $n = 955$	Choledochotomy* $n = 216$
Age-mean (years)	48.3	57.1
Sex ratio M/F	1/3.2	1/2.2
	%	%
History of		
–jaundice	19.1	52.3
–acute pancreatitis	1.4	13.0
Presentation:		
acute	5.4	7.9
acute & chronic	14.1	13.4
acute & jaundice	1.2	6.0
acute, chronic, jaundice	4.4	14.8
chronic	61.6	26.4
chronic & jaundice	12.9	22.7
jaundice	0.4	8.8
Pathology:		
acute	3.3	7.7
acute & chronic	12.2	29.9
chronic	84.5	62.5
Positive bile culture	12.1	46.2

* no additional procedure
This information was collected prospectively on punch cards.

Table 52.3 Postoperative complications

Parameters	Cholecystectomy* n = 955 %	Choledochotomy* n = 216 %
Atelectasis	21.8	37.5
Pulmonary embolus	0.9	1.4
Deep vein thrombosis	0.4	1.9
Wound haematoma	1.6	0.9
infection	1.4	6.0
failure	0.8	1.4
Biliary fistula	0.4	3.2
peritonitis	0.3	0.5
Waltman Walters syndrome	0.1	0.5
Pancreatitis	0.4	0.0
Hypovolaemic shock	0.7	0.1
Bacteriogenic shock	0.3	1.4
Subphrenic collection	1.5	0.9
Renal failure	0.0	0.5
Other minor complications	6.3	11.6
Death	0.2	1.8
No complications	57.2	47.2

* no additional procedure
This information has been collected prospectively but is dependent on the definition of each category.

morbidity which is the base of the pyramid whose apex is death. This includes the following procedures:

Reduction of obesity, while difficult, can be more successful if a target is set with a limited period leading to prompt operation thereafter. The compliance of most patients can only be held for a short period. Preoperative measures include maximal improvement of any cardio-respiratory dysfunction, including the cessation of smoking, physiotherapy and appropriate treatment for any pre-existing lesions. This would include some delay in the operation if the patient has had a recent myocardial infarct.

It is necessary to discontinue the use of the contraceptive pill to reduce the risk of deep vein thrombosis. This is a more common problem now in Western countries where over 70% of the women under 40 years may be taking the pill. Opinion seems to have settled on a preoperative gap of six weeks. Full prophylactic measures including low dose heparin are essential.

Peroperative cover with antibiotics has been shown to reduce the risk of complications (Ch. 11) from infection of patients at risk (Gunn 1982, Haw & Gunn 1973, Keighley 1982). The risk factors include: age over 50, a history of jaundice, a non-functioning gallbladder on oral cholecystography, abnormal liver function tests, a clinical diagnosis of an acute empyema of the gallbladder, a dilated common duct and a stone or stricture in the duct. If three factors are present, 50% of the patients will have a positive bile culture and four or more make a positive result almost certain. These patients require peroperative antibiotic cover. Many patients requiring choledochotomy fall into this group and the antibiotic selected should be known to be effective against the organisms found in previous patients.

Some of the patients will be clinically or biochemically jaundiced and are at risk from renal failure. These patients should have a fluid load followed by mannitol infusion so that they come to operation during a diuresis (Dawson 1965).

The prothrombin activity may be altered in jaundiced patients and it is wise to prescribe Vitamin K preoperatively.

INCISION

The choice lies between a Kocher's, a paramedian, a Mayo-Robson, a midline or a transverse incision. The build of the patient, the shape of the costal margin and the possibility of an additional procedure for other pathology may modify the selection of incision but the main factor is the personal choice of the surgeon.

This contributor prefers the Kocher's incision which can be extended laterally, medially in a vertical direction for gastric procedures or converted into a 'roof-top' incision for more extensive procedures such as resection of the pancreas.

PROCEDURE

Exposure (Fig. 52.1–52.3)

The liver is retracted superiorly and to the right with a broad bladed slightly curved retractor. This retractor should be deep enough to displace the liver but not so curved as to traumatize it. A pack should be put over the hepatic flexure of the colon down to the hepato-renal pouch and the medial part over the first part of the duodenum. This pack is retracted by a similar broad bladed retractor to prevent the colon or duodenum obscuring vision. Care should be taken not to compress the vena cava as this results in reduction of venous return and a consequent change in the vital signs being monitored by the anaesthetist.

The lesser omentum and stomach are retracted to the left and slightly superiorly in a plane parallel to the free border of the lesser omentum. This retractor can be of the appropriate length but not as broad as those already used. The assistant should be warned not to pull unduly as there is a risk that the retractor might slip to the left and damage the spleen. (Fig. 52.1).

The need for choledochotomy becomes apparent during

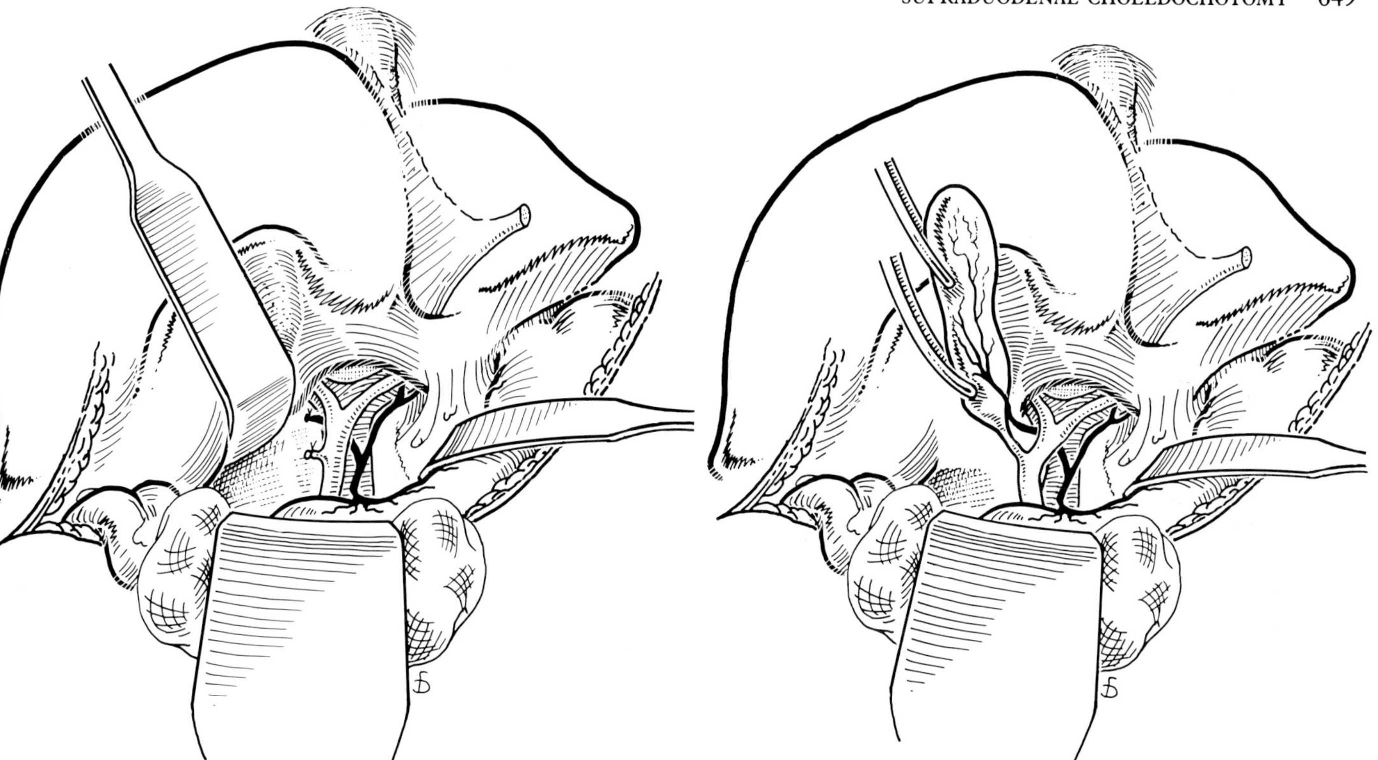

Fig. 52.1 Exposure of the common duct by packs and retractors

Fig. 52.2 Traction on the gallbladder with counter traction on duodenum to put the common bile duct on the stretch, facilitating dissection

cholecystectomy and intraoperative cholangiography prior to palpation of the common duct. This order is important as palpation can produce spasm at the ampulla and failure of the contrast to pass into the duodenum. This can lead to unnecessary exploration (Ch. 27, 46). A decision is necessary as to the wisdom of removing the gallbladder before or after exploration of the common bile duct. This will depend on the anatomy and pathology present. At times the gallbladder can be a useful aid to retraction (Fig. 52.2), but it can also obstruct vision in other patients. An alternative is to leave a long cystic duct for traction (Fig. 52.3) and after exploration of the common bile duct to remove the excess length of cystic duct.

The site of the choledochotomy (Fig. 52.4, 52.5)

This decision depends on three main factors:

Choledochoduodenostomy may become necessary and therefore the opening must be in the lowest part of the supraduodenal common bile duct that would be consistent with an easy subsequent anastomosis (Fig. 52.4).

A distal choledochotomy is advocated so that as much as possible of the common duct is left proximally in case the duct is needed for some further procedure, e.g. repair of a stricture in this part of the duct.

The anatomy of the cystic duct is so variable that care must be exercised to open the correct duct. A cystic duct lying anterior (Fig 52.5a) or closely applied to (Fig. 52.5b) the common bile duct can easily be opened in error.

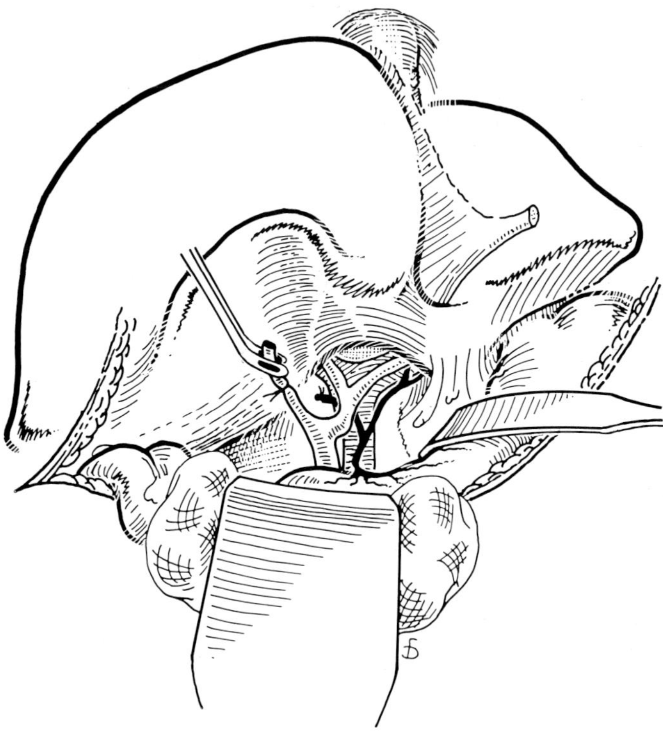

Fig. 52.3 Traction on the duct using the cystic duct if the gallbladder has been removed

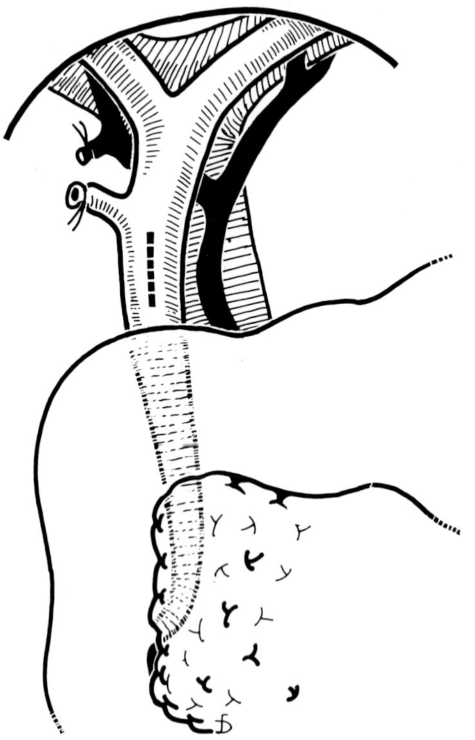

Fig. 52.4 The common bile duct is opened just above the duodenum leaving room for a choledochoduodenostomy if this is found to be necessary

Opening the common bile duct (Fig. 52.6)

It is helpful to use two fine stay sutures (Fig. 52.6) to lift and render the common bile duct tense for incision and exploration. A small knife is used to open the anterior wall in the mid point of the duct and to make an incision about 1–2 cm long depending on the size of the duct and the size of the stones. If the duct is not made tense then damage can be done to the posterior wall or an irregular incision made.

A specimen of the common duct bile should be sent for culture and the duct system emptied by gentle suction to prevent spilling of bile into the peritoneal cavity.

Exploration of the duct (Fig. 52.7–52.10)

The surgeon should aim at being as atraumatic as possible so as to prevent damage to the duct. The use of rigid instruments, such as Desjardin's forceps, is to be avoided (Orloff 1978, Gunn 1982). Grasping forceps of any type may catch the wall of the duct with possible damage and later stricture formation. Bougies have been used traditionally but metal instruments can create a false passage into the duodenum (Ch. 55) or even into the peritoneal cavity with serious consequences. Endoscopic techniques have revealed a significant proportion of false passages at examination subsequent to choledochotomy. Some surgeons

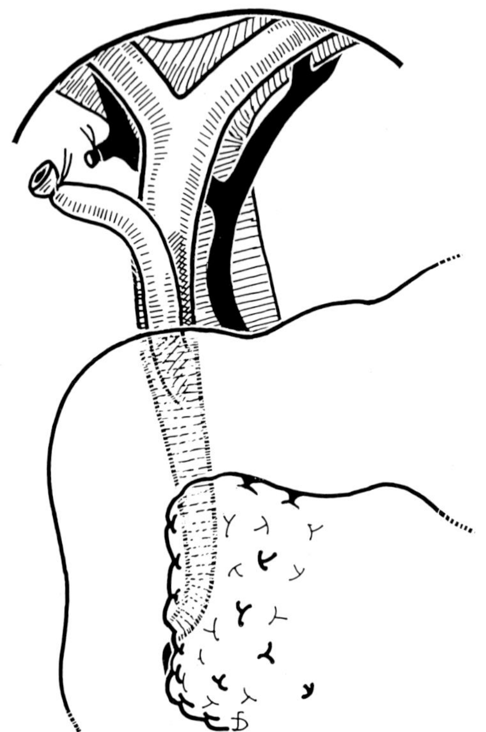

a

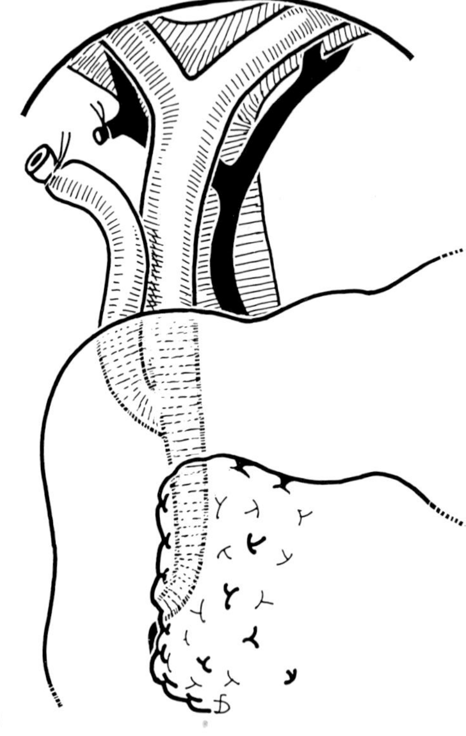

b

Fig. 52.5 a. The cystic duct may lie anterior to the common duct and may be opened in error. b. The cystic duct may run parallel to the common duct with a low entrance mimicking a dilated duct

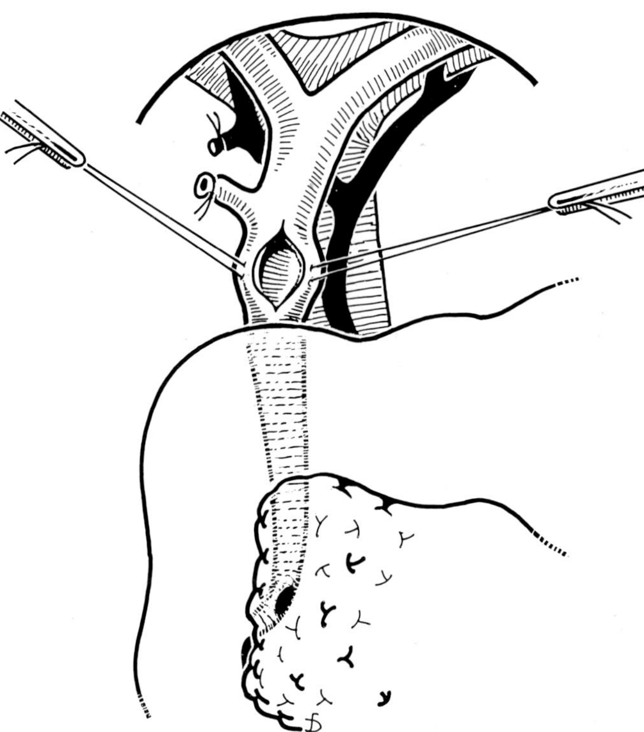

Fig. 52.6 Stay sutures aid the opening of the duct and allow clear vision of the contents

experienced in choledochoscopy advocate routine exploration of the common duct and removal of stone under direct vision using the choledochoscope (Ch. 29).

The Fogarty biliary probe has been found to be suitable and, in this contributor's experience, no stone which has been immoveable with a Fogarty balloon catheter has been removed using a metallic instrument (Fogarty et al 1968, Fox & Gunn 1984).

The Fogarty probe, with stylette in position, is held in cholecystectomy forceps and introduced into the common duct. The forceps are then transferred to the surgeon's left hand and the Fogarty probe grasped with long forceps nearer to the duct and held in the surgeon's right hand (Fig. 52.7). The cholecystectomy forceps are removed and the catheter is passed into the duodenum (Fig. 52.8a)

The balloon is inflated and the catheter withdrawn until it impinges against the papilla (Fig. 52.8b). The duct is normally about 7 cm from the point of choledochotomy to the duodenum but this may vary according to the point of entry into the duodenum. The second part of the duodenum is palpated and the balloon identified to determine the site of the papilla in case duodenotomy is necessary. Any stone can be felt against the shaft of the catheter.

The balloon is deflated and gently withdrawn through

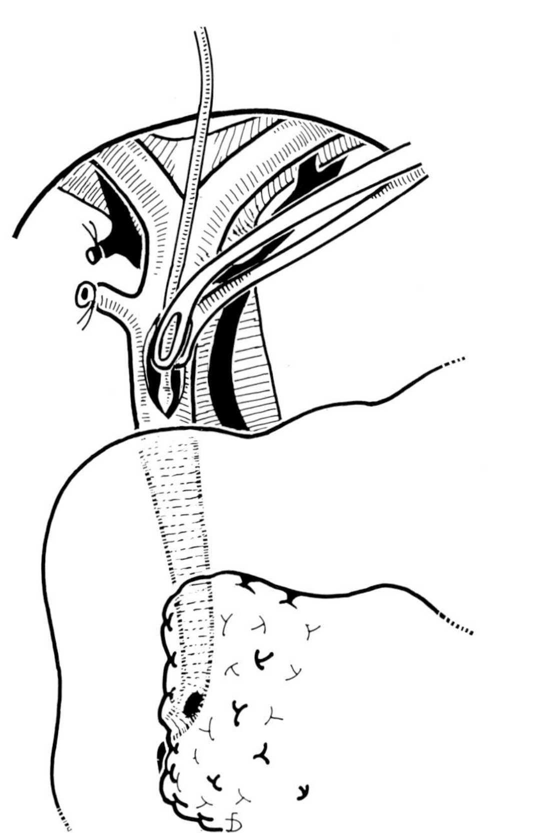

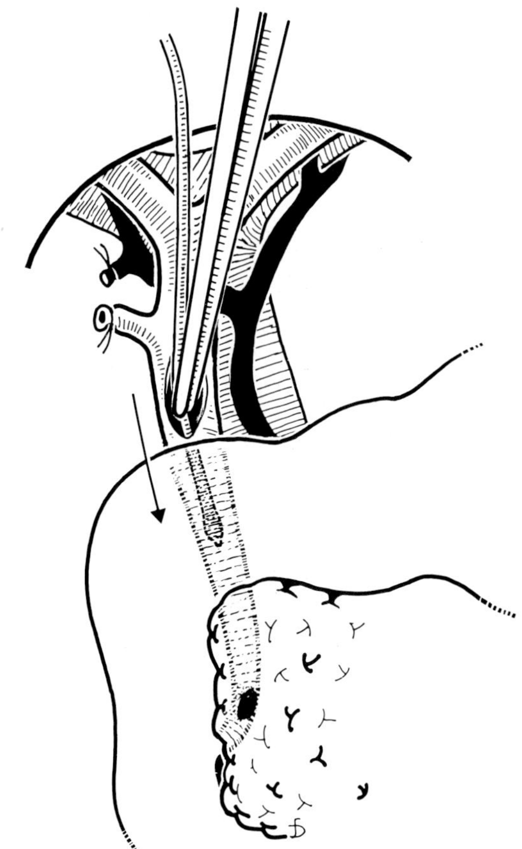

Fig. 52.7 a. The Fogarty catheter is fed into the duct with Desjardins forceps. b. The Fogarty catheter is fed into the duct with long forceps

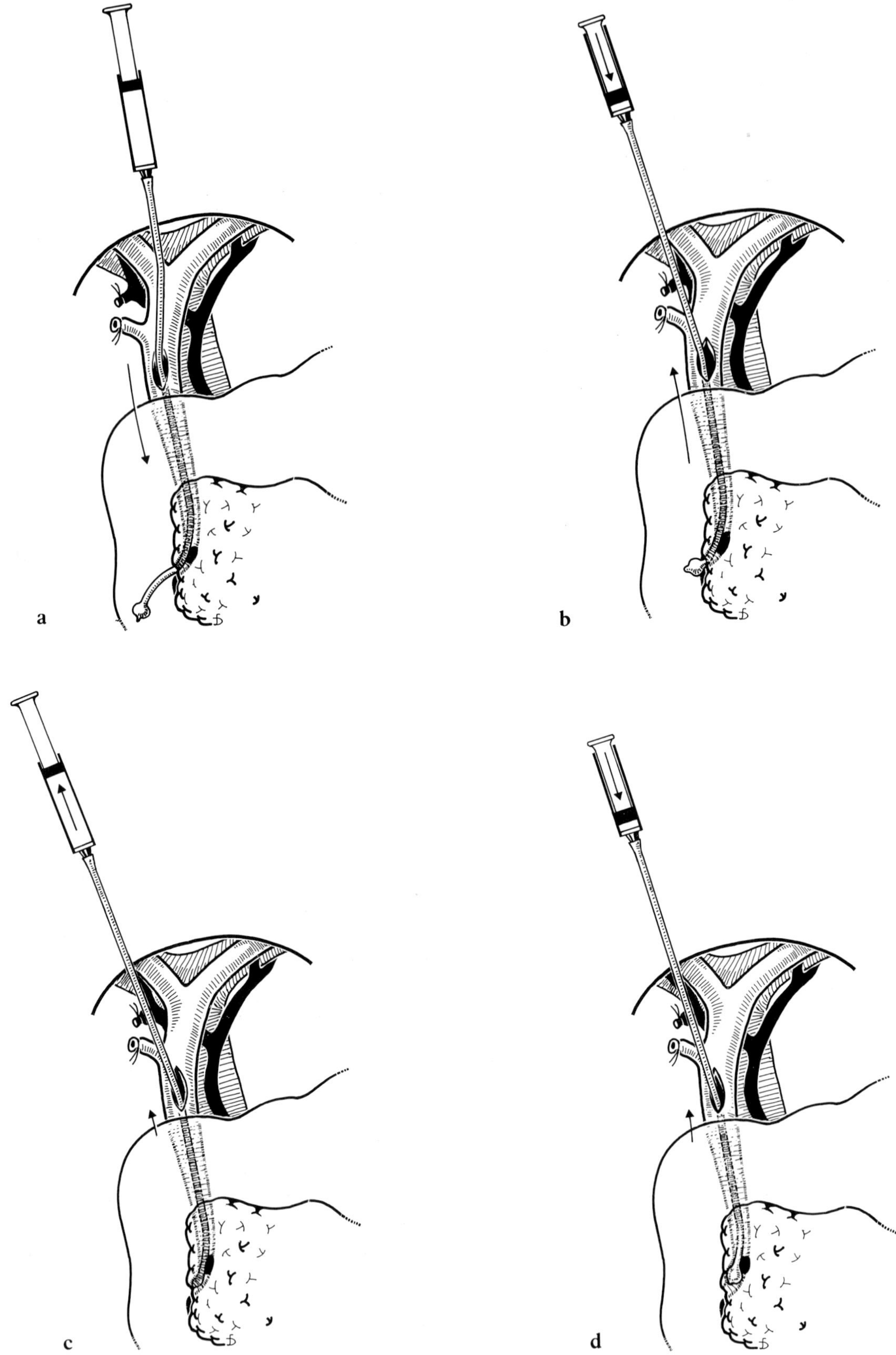

Fig. 52.8 a. The Fogarty catheter is attached to the syringe and the balloon inflated in the duodenum. b. The Fogarty catheter is retracted with the balloon against the papilla. c. The balloon is deflated gently until it slips through the papilla when the balloon is reinflated. d. The Fogarty catheter is gently withdrawn with the balloon inflated

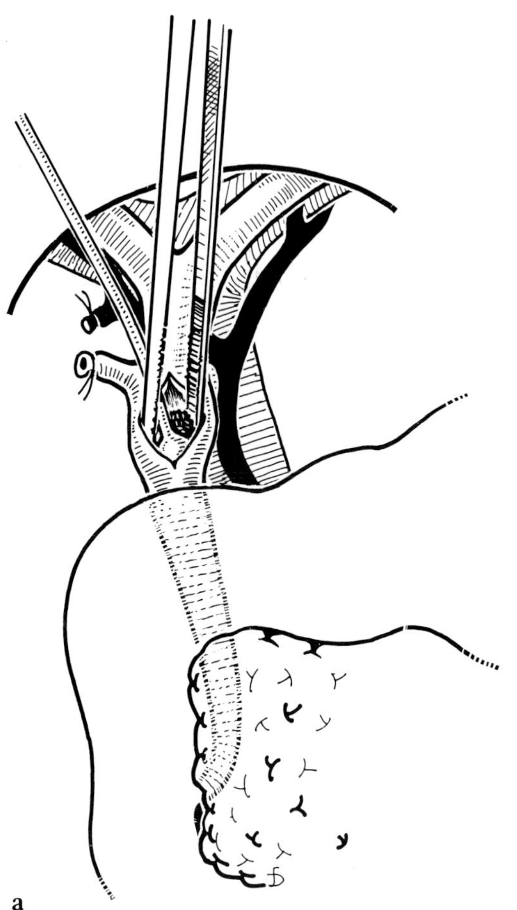

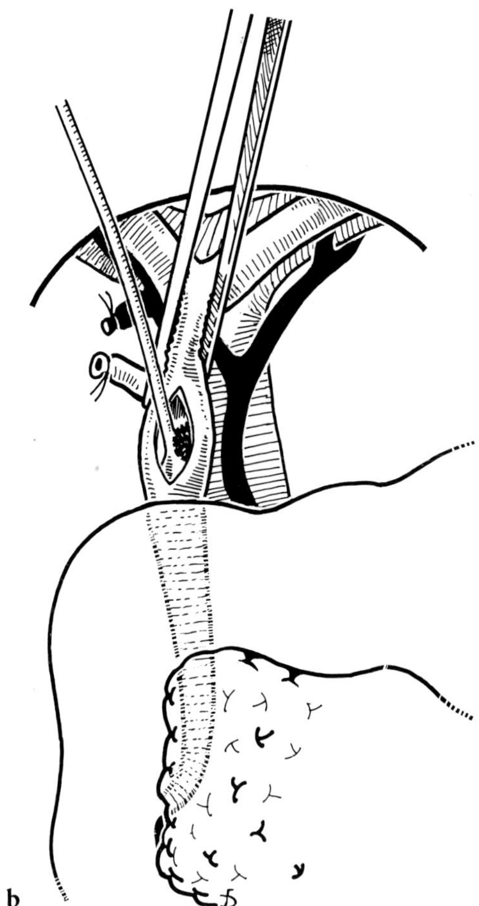

Fig. 52.9 a. The choledochotomy is widened with long forceps as the balloon is brought out revealing the stone. b. The long forceps can be used to obstruct the common hepatic duct preventing the stone slipping up

the papilla. This is detected by a sudden easing of the pull on the catheter (Fig. 52.8c). Immediately this happens the balloon is reinflated (Fig. 52.8d). The catheter is held by the syringe in the left hand and the degree of inflation controlled by the thumb on the plunger. With gentle traction superiorly the catheter is gradually pulled up to the dochotomy site (Fig. 52.9a), care being taken to prevent any stone slipping into the proximal biliary tree (Fig. 52.9b). If the traction is anteriorly rather than superiorly there is the risk of lacerating the opening into the duct (Fig. 52.10). The procedure is repeated until it is considered that the distal duct is clear.

The catheter is withdrawn and reinserted up each of the main hepatic ducts and the procedure repeated. It is important that the balloon inflation is correct; over inflation could damage the ducts and under inflation may miss any stone that is present. This can be achieved by inflating the balloon until the fingers feel the tension of the syringe plunger. This tension is maintained as the catheter is withdrawn into the gradually widening duct.

It is important to remove the stone when it appears at the choledochotomy opening and to avoid allowing it to fall into another part of the duct. Two techniques have proved helpful:

Firstly good visualization; fine dissecting forceps are placed in the choledochotomy opening and allowed to open transversely and the stone will be seen as it is brought up by the catheter. This also allows a sucker tip to be inserted into the duct (Fig. 52.9a).

Secondly, the common hepatic duct is obstructed by lightly grasping it with the flat atraumatic blades of long forceps while the stone is delivered from the common bile duct (Fig. 52.9b).

The last step in this technique is to repass the Fogarty catheter into the duodenum, inflate the balloon and retract it against the papilla. While the catheter is held in the right hand, the index and middle fingers of the left hand are placed posterior to the duodenum with the thumb anteriorly. This allows palpation of the duct against the wall of the catheter for any residual stones.

THE NORMALITY OF THE DUCTS

The surgeon must attempt to ensure that the duct system

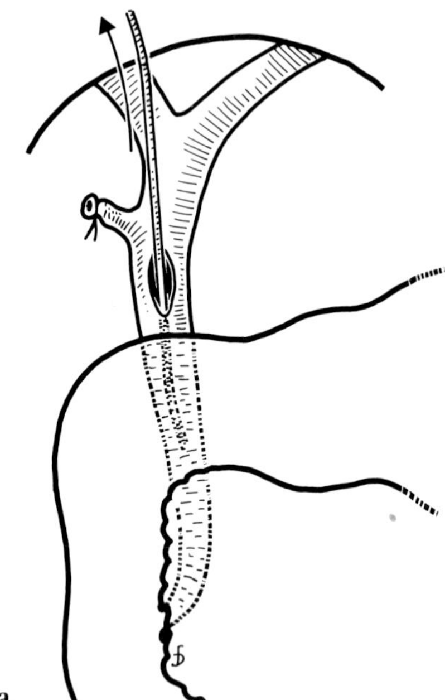

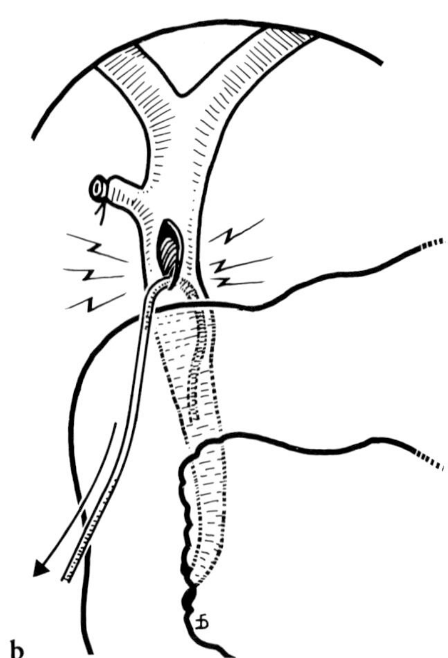

Fig. 52.10 a. Traction on the Fogarty catheter should always be in a superior direction. b. Angled traction on the Fogarty catheter results in tearing of the lower end of the choledochotomy

is normal even though nonoperative methods may be available for removing residual stones or dealing with residual strictures (Ch. 47, 48, 49). Choledochoscopy is one established method which has become more effective since the introduction of better instruments with improved optics (Ch. 29). Modern instruments are small enough to allow visualization of the major right and left hepatic ducts and intermediate hepatic ducts and to allow vision of the orifices of the smaller biliary radicals. However there are many hospitals where this facility is not currently available and one alternative is the Foley catheter technique of post-exploratory cholangiography first described by the author in 1970 (Lawson & Gunn 1970). The principle is to use the balloon of a Foley catheter to obstruct the lumen of the bile duct while allowing contrast medium to be injected beyond the catheter so as to demonstrate any residual pathology.

Foley catheter technique for post-exploratory cholangiography (Gunn 1982, Lawson & Gunn 1970, Leald & Peel 1985)

A 10 French gauge Foley catheter is modified by cutting off the end of the catheter beyond the balloon since the laterally placed orifice at this point can simulate a stone on radiographs. The balloon should be tested to see that it has not been damaged. The proximal end should be shortened so that its lumen will accept a syringe for a subsequent injection of contrast (Fig. 52.11).

The Foley catheter is introduced downwards into the common bile duct and inflated until it feels tight. Saline is injected to check that a watertight seal has been obtained.

The position of the X-ray head is checked and a syringe containing contrast attached to the Foley catheter ensuring that there are no air bubbles in the barrel of the syringe.

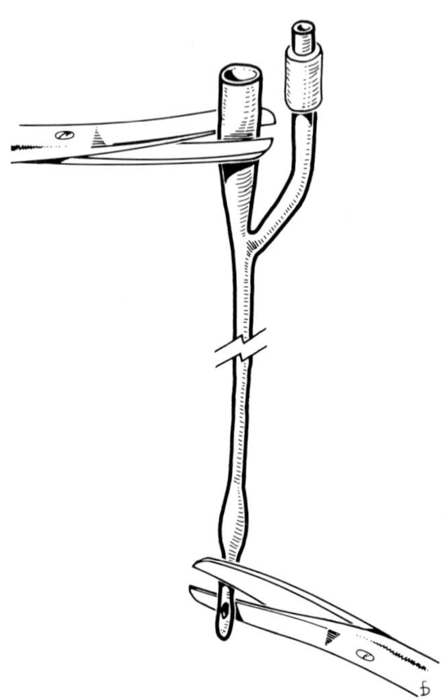

Fig. 52.11 The Foley catheter is modified at the proximal end to accommodate a syringe and distally to remove the tip that can look like a stone on cholangiography

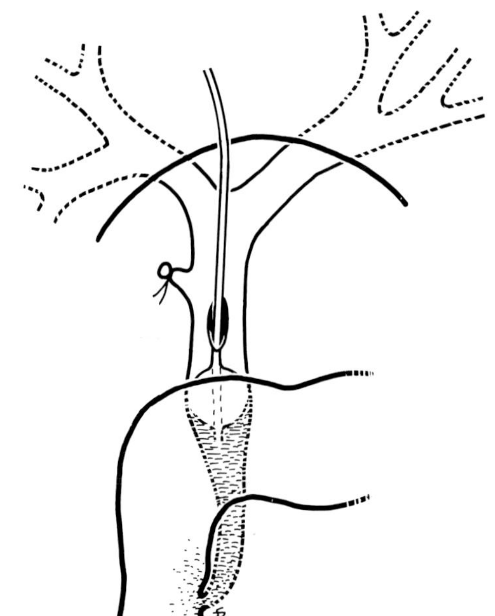

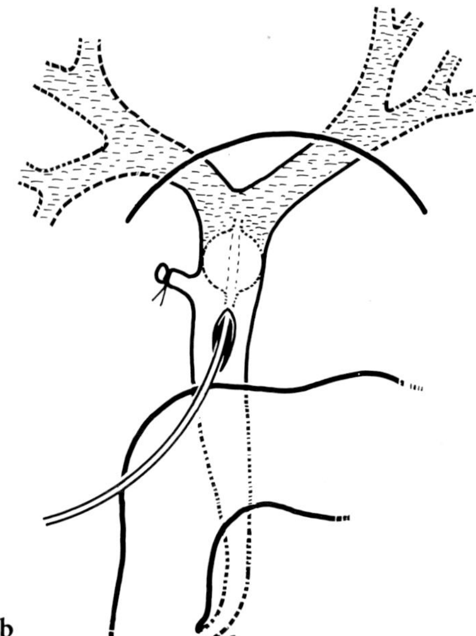

Fig. 52.12 The Foley catheter is inserted and the balloon inflated just below the choledochotomy and contrast medium injected. b. The Foley catheter is inserted into the common hepatic duct and the balloon inflated. Contrast medium is injected

The operative field is cleared of instruments and swabs and all scrub staff retreat while the surgeon injects contrast slowly down the common bile duct and one film is exposed (Fig. 52.12a).

The balloon is then deflated and the catheter placed in the common hepatic duct. The procedure is repeated with one exception, the contrast medium is injected until pressure is felt, indicating that the duct system is full (Fig. 52.12b). The catheter is clipped and the staff withdraw and a further film taken. This reduces the amount of radiation to the scrub staff.

Using this method only two films are taken since it has been found that additional views are unnecessary. Extension tubing allowing connection of the syringe to a Foley catheter has been tried but was associated with an increased risk of the introduction of air bubbles into the system which may masquerade as residual stones. This contributor wears a radiation badge which does not show excess radiation dosage provided the protocol outlined above is followed.

The results have been satisfactory, although there was some initial difficulty in interpreting the films. A review of the initial experience was carried out because some residual stones showed up on T-tube cholangiography despite a negative interpretation of the films at the time of operation. The majority of these stones could be seen, and therefore a policy was developed which ensured that the radiologists also saw the films to confirm or refute the surgeon's opinion before the duct was closed.

In a total series of 238 consecutive explorations of the common bile duct, the author found stones present at post-exploratory cholangiography in 36 cases, and unexpected strictures in a further 12. Residual stones were found in 15 of 196 patients (Table 52.4) submitted to postoperative T-tube cholangiography, 12 of these being in the first 100 patients; three have been seen subsequently in 91 patients. Assessment by T-tube cholangiography was not possible in the other patients because in the majority a choledochoduodenostomy was performed or a T-tube was not used. Recent reports from other authors have shown equally satisfactory results (Kelley & Blumgart 1985, Leald & Peel 1985).

Table 52.4 Exploration of the common bile duct
Intraoperative post-exploratory cholangiography
Foley catheter technique

Duct normal (no stones)	164
Residual stone	36
Unexpected stricture	12
?stone-repeated/normal no stones	10
Unsatisfactory	4
Not done	15
Total consecutive patients	238
Postoperative T-tube cholangiography	191
Retained stones	15

Problems with the Foley catheter

If the balloon is inflated too close to the choledochotomy it tends to prolapse. This is corrected by deflating the balloon and placing it a little further down the common duct and then reinflating the balloon until pressure is felt in the syringe.

Over-inflation of the balloon tends to make the balloon extrude and theoretically could damage the duct although this has not been seen in over 300 consecutive patients.

If the balloon is too low in the common duct it allows an adequate view of the ampulla and the flow through the papilla into the duodenum but will not show a stone in the proximal common duct which may have been bypassed by the catheter. This stone is occasionally lifted into the common hepatic duct when the catheter is withdrawn.

The balloon may be placed in the left or right hepatic duct rather than the common hepatic duct. This should be obvious on the films and the catheter is then replaced in the correct position.

THE USE OF A T-TUBE

The standard practice is to use a T-tube to allow spasm or oedema of the sphincter to settle following the trauma of the exploration. Failure to drain the duct might result in a build up of pressure in the system and leakage at or disruption of the closure of the duct with biliary peritonitis.

One other important reason for the use of a T-tube is the detection and subsequent treatment of residual stones. In the event of a stone being left behind, then the T-tube can be used for washouts, instillation of solvents and the later use of radiological techniques through the track created by the tube.

However, as has been indicated, the use of a T-tube creates a fistula between the skin and the lumen of the duct, both being potentially contaminated surfaces. The track of the fistula crosses the peritoneal surface. Theoretically, it would be better if the duct could be closed and not drained by a T-tube. This contributor uses a T-tube except where the stone extraction was simple and the post-exploratory X-rays showed no evidence of stone, stricture, papillary spasm, cholangitis or pancreatitis. The practice of primary duct closure without a tube is not recommended for inexperienced biliary surgeons and some might argue should never be used at all. Personal experience of primary closure of the duct using the principles already indicated has been satisfactory.

The choice of material

Latex-rubber is superior to the majority of plastic materials in that it stimulates a tissue reaction and the track is sealed quickly from the general peritoneal cavity. Initially when non- reactive tubes were introduced, surgeons experienced increased incidence of biliary leak, fistula, abscess or biliary peritonitis.

The size of the T-tube

A French gauge 16 is satisfactory and French gauge 14 the smallest that should be used if a satisfactory track is to be left for subsequent interventional radiology if necessary. This acknowledges the fact that a significant proportion of patients who have had choledochotomy for stone will have residual pathology (Ch. 46, 48). The use of post-exploratory choledochoscopy and cholangiography will greatly reduce the number of residual stones but the wise surgeon should accept that stones will be occasionally left.

Sometimes the duct is narrow and it is dangerous to attempt to use a tight-fitting T-tube as this can result in

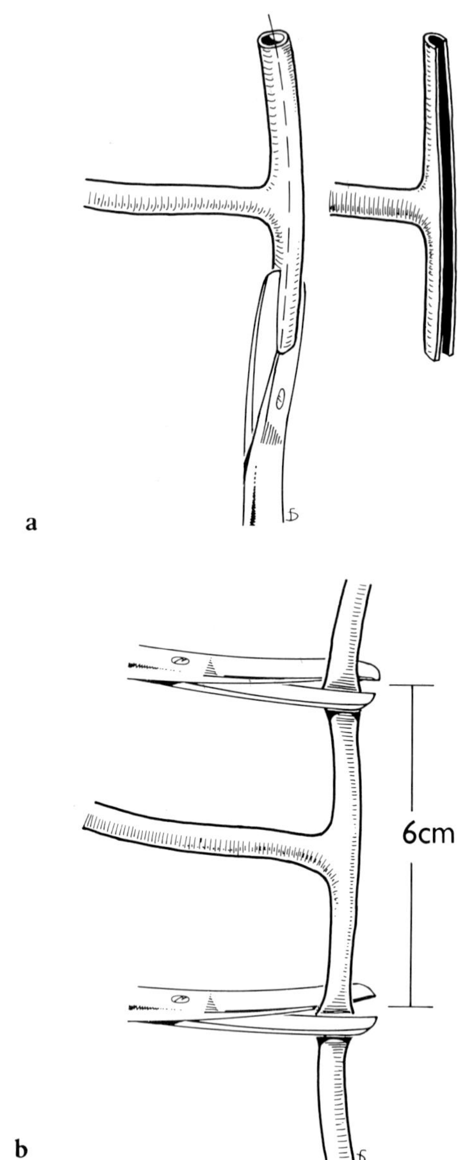

Fig. 52.13 a. The T-tube is modified by removing half the diameter to prevent obstruction and ease removal. b. The T-tube is modified by shortening the limbs to prevent proximal obstruction and distal entry into the duodenum

trauma to the duct or catching the tube with the suture used to close the choledochotomy. Some T-tubes are manufactured with a smaller diameter of cross piece than that of the long limb delivered at the surface.

The shape of the T-tube (Fig. 52.13a)

T-tubes can become obstructed particularly if they are tight fitting and can be difficult to extract. This can be avoided by cutting off a strip of the wall.

The length of the limbs of the T-tube (Fig. 52.13b)

If the proximal limb is long it may block one hepatic duct and a long distal limb may enter the duodenum creating a syphon of duodenal content. These difficulties can be avoided by shortening the limbs to 3 cm on either side of the T-junction.

Introduction of the T-tube (Fig. 52.14)

The modified T-tube is held in Desjardin's forceps which conveniently grasps the T-junction of the tube allowing it to be slipped into the choledochotomy (Fig. 52.14a). The long limb of the tube should be placed at the lower end of the opening and repair commenced just above the upper apex of the incision using continuous 3/0 or 4/0 chromic catgut. The final stitch should close the opening against the T-tube (Fig. 52.14b).

Avoiding problems in closure of the choledochotomy (Fig. 52.15)

Care must be ensure that the wall of the T-tube is not caught in one of the sutures and the end of the suture should not be tied around the tube (Fig.52.15a). Either of these faults may result in the tearing of the duct when the tube is withdrawn.

The proximal limb of the T-tube should not enter one of the hepatic ducts as this can produce obstruction (Fig. 52.15b). The distal end must not enter the duodenum as this can act as a syphon (Fig. 52.15c). In addition a tube through the papillary orifice may excite pancreatitis.

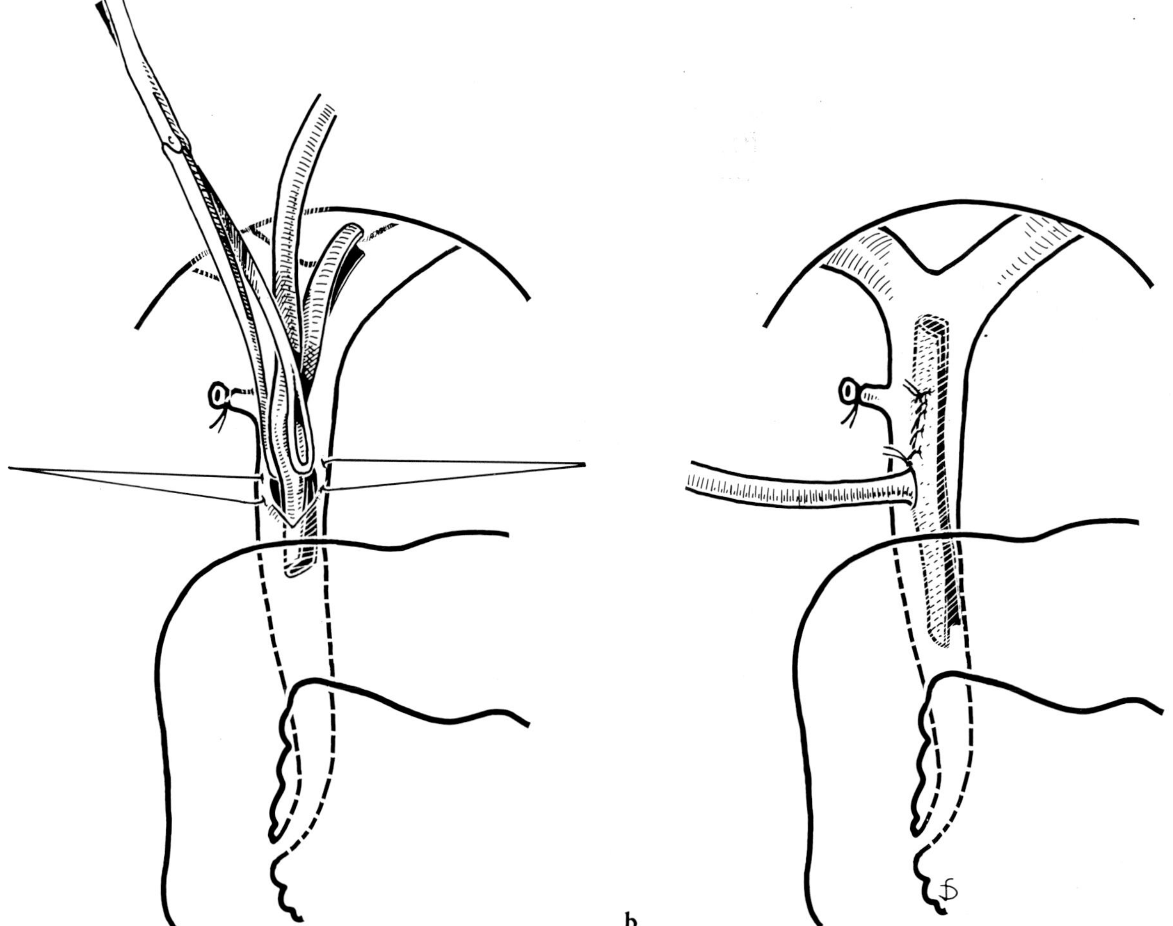

Fig. 51.14 a. The T-tube is introduced by Desjardins forceps. b. The choledochotomy closure is commenced above with the T-tube emerging at the lower end of the repair

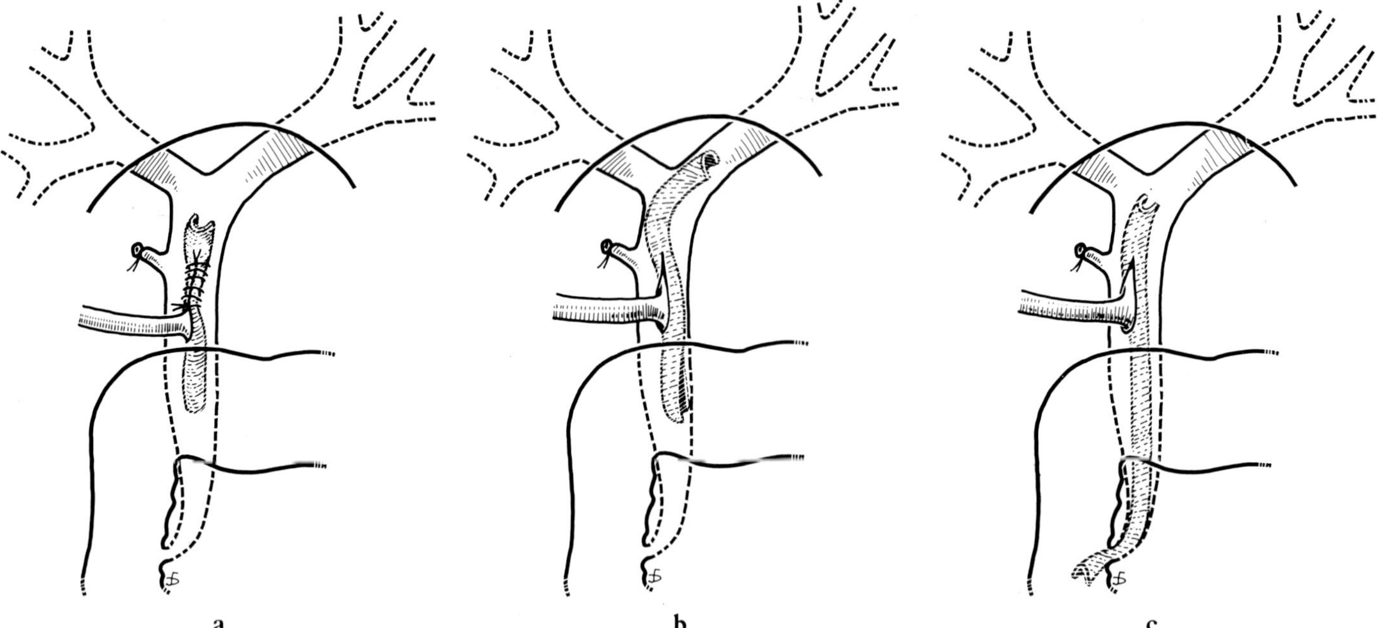

Fig. 52.15 a. The suture must not catch the T-tube as shown here. b. The T-tube limb should not enter the hepatic duct as here. c. The distal end of the T-tube should not enter the duodenum

The position of the T-tube in the abdominal wall (Fig. 52.16)

The correct position of the T-tube is with the long limb emerging under the costal margin laterally. For example, it should not come out below a Kocher's incision. This facilitates radiological techniques for later postoperative removal of stones should this be necessary. The contributor believes that two suction drains should be used, one emerging on the right, placed within the abdomen as high as possible in the hepatorenal pouch, and the other on the left, placed under the diaphgragm.

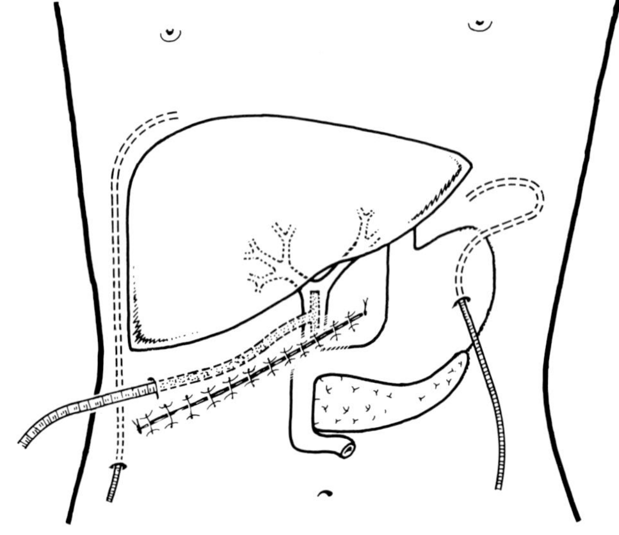

Fig. 52.16 The T-tube should be brought out superior and lateral to the wound. Suction drains should be placed under the left diaphragm and in the hepato-renal space under the right diaphragm

Postoperative management of the T-tube

Initially bile is allowed to drain freely into a bile bag to allow any spasm or oedema of the sphincter to settle before testing the suture line of the choledochotomy. The volume drained varies between 200 and 400 ml in 24 hours with decreasing amounts as flow increases through the sphincter. If the volume drained remains high or increases then the reason should be established. This may be due either to continuing distal obstruction or because the distal limb is lying within the duodenum.

Similarly, there is a problem if there is no drainage of the bile or bile drains around the T-tube. This suggests that the tube has either become blocked or has become dislodged from the duct.

The answer to all these problems is revealed by T-tube cholangiography.

Provided there have been no problems, the subsequent management is aimed at gradually directing the bile through the papilla into the duodenum. Some surgeons attain this by gradually lifting the bile bag until it is pinned to the patient's clothes above the level of the duodenum. Others, including this contributor, commence clipping the T-tube after meals on the fifth postoperative day for one hour. This is increased daily by one hour until the tube is completely clipped at nine days. Some surgeons do not aim to direct bile through the papilla at all but simply leave the bile draining freely into a bag. The use of a sealed drainage system (Ch. 37) probably reduces the incidence of ascending infection.

A T-tube cholangiogram is taken about 10 days after the operation; provided this is normal, the tube is removed by gentle traction but there may be a slight leakage over the first 24 hours and for that reason the patient should be kept in hospital for a further day after tube removal. The presence of a residual stone or stones seen at postoperative cholangiography demands decisions about subsequent management. Initially, the T-tube cholangiograph should be repeated after several days and should a stone still be demonstrated this may be managed either by lavage, gallstone dissolution (Ch. 49), endoscopic papillotomy (Ch. 47) or subsequently, after a period of some weeks, by means of interventional radiology (Ch. 48).

REFERENCES

Dawson J L 1965 Jaundice and anoxic renal damage. British Medical Journal 1: 82–86

Fogarty F J, Krippaeine W W, Dennis D L, Fletcher W S 1968 Evaluation of an improved operating technique in common duct surgery. American Journal of Surgery 116: 117–182

Fox J A, Gunn A A 1984 Common bile duct exploration by balloon catheter. Journal of the Royal College of Surgeons of Edinburgh 29: 81–84

Gunn A A 1982 Antimicrobial prophylaxis in biliary surgery. World Journal of Surgery 6: 301–305

Gunn A A 1983 Cholecystectomy, cholecystostomy and exploration of the common duct. In: Dudley H, Porries W, Carter D (eds) Rob and Smith, Operative surgery 2, 4th edn. Butterworth, London, p 616

Haw C S, Gunn A A 1973 The significance of infection in biliary surgery. Journal of the Royal College of Surgeons of Edinburgh 18: 209–212

Heimbalh D M, White T T Immediate and long term effects of instrumental dilatation of the sphincter of Oddi. Surgery, Gynecology and Obstetrics 148: 79–80

Keighley M R B 1982 Infection in the biliary tract. In: Blumgart L H (ed) The biliary tract. Churchill Livingstone, Edinburgh, p 219

Kelley C J, Blumgart L H 1985 Peroperative cholangiogram and post cholecystectomy biliary stricture. Annals of the Royal College of Surgeons of England 67: 93–96

Lawson R A M, Gunn A A 1970 The value of operative cholangiography. Journal of the Royal College of Surgeons of Edinburgh 15: 222–227

Leald A L, Peel A L G 1985 Choledochoscopy? Post-exploration fluorocholangiography? Or both? Annals of the Royal College of Surgeons of England 67: 99–100

Myat Thue Y A, Robinson D, Gunn A A 1973 Peroperative cholangiography. British Journal of Surgery 60: 711–712

Orloff M J 1978 Importance of surgical technique in prevention of retained and recurrent bile duct stones. World Journal of Surgery 2: 403–410

G. Ribotta, F. Procacciante

Transduodenal sphincteroplasty and exploration of the common bile duct

Sphincteroplasty consists of the incision of the common portion of the sphincter of Oddi with partial suture of the incision margin (Fig. 53.1). By this procedure the sphincters of the common bile duct (CBD) and the duct of Wirsung are not involved and therefore their function is not impaired. The procedure can also be defined as 'subtotal lower sphincteroplasty' (Fig. 53.2) (Stefanini et al 1977). The approach to the sphincter of Oddi is through a minimal duodenotomy in the second part of the duodenum. The following description is of the technique recommended by the authors.

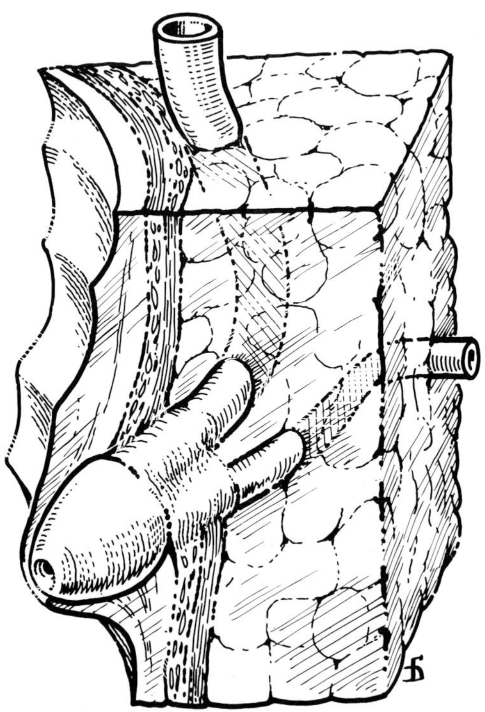

Fig. 53.1 A section of the sphincter of Oddi. Note the distinction between the papilla, the common portion of the sphincter and the sphincters of the common bile duct and duct of Wirsung

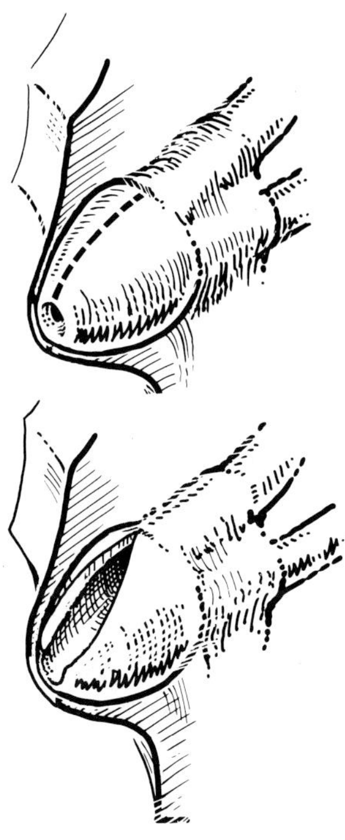

Fig. 53.2 Subtotal lower sphincteroplasty involves only the papilla while the sphincter of the common bile duct and that of the duct of Wirsung are preserved

TECHNIQUE

Preparation and positioning of the patient

Preoperative preparation is routine. A Levin tube is introduced preoperatively and maintained until the third or fourth postoperative day. The patient is placed in a supine position on a radiotransparent operating table.

Incision

The authors prefer a transverse incision below the right costal margin (Vogt & Hermann 1981). This allows

Table 53.1 Indications for sphincteroplasty

APPROACH TO THE CBD:
Bile duct stones
Hydatid cysts
NECESSITY OR THERAPEUTIC
Impacted stones
Fibrotic stenosis of the papilla
biliary mud and sludge
recurrent pancreatitis
CONTRAINDICATIONS
More than 2 cm dilation of the CBD
Long distal duct stricture
Peri-Vaterian diverticulum
Severe inflammatory changes in the area involving the duodenal wall and the head of the pancreas

(Arianoff 1980, Barraya et al 1974, Chigot et al 1978)

optimal light and excellent access. This approach is particularly suitable in obese patients and the incidence of postoperative incisional hernia is probably lower than with vertical and oblique incisions. A disadvantage is that self retaining retractors are not suitable and a third assistant is required.

The incision of the abdominal wall follows a transverse line, from the midaxillary to the median line at the level of the 11th/12th rib (Fig. 53.3).

Preparation of the operative field

The abdomen is opened and a large retractor is positioned at the upper margin of the wound. The right flexure of the colon is displaced inferiorly and the stomach to the left by means of two surgical pads. Viscera are maintained in this position with two large curved Deaver retractors.

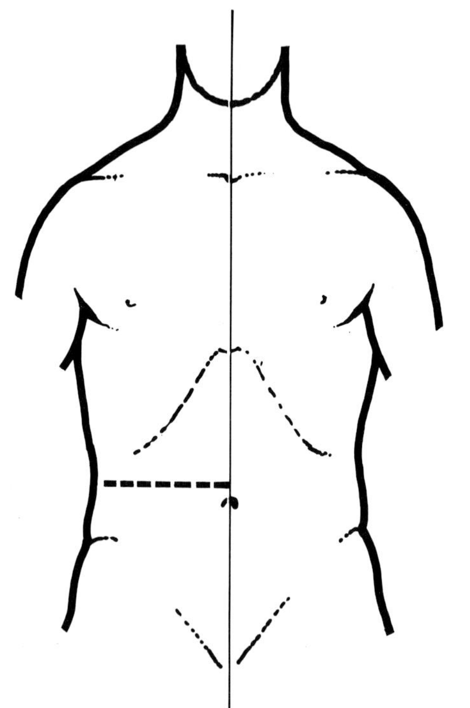

Fig. 53.3 Transverse subcostal incision. This offers excellent exposure with a low incidence of postoperative incisional hernia

Operative cholangiography

Operative cholangiography is carried out after cannulation of the cystic duct. In previously cholecystectomized patients, where a cystic duct remnant is present and a 5 to 6 mm stump can be isolated, this is employed. When this is not possible, contrast medium is injected by direct fine-needle puncture of the common bile duct. Image interpretation suggesting papillary stenosis is difficult and for this reason the authors favour radiological examination with biliary manometry and flow measurements (Jones 1978) (Ch. 28).

Exposure and mobilization of the duodenum

Kocher manoeuvre

For the performance of sphincteroplasty, extended mobilization of the duodenum and pancreas (Kocher manoeuvre) is mandatory (Moody et al 1983). The assistant surgeon displaces the second portion medially and forward. The peritoneum is incised posteriorly along the curved lateral margin of the duodenum (Fig. 53.4). The mesocolon of the right colic flexure is cleared inferiorly. At this point the assistant surgeon should also displace the duodenum superiorly (Fig. 53.5). Access is thus provided to the avascular space between the posterior aspect of the head of the pancreas anteriorly and the perinephric fat and inferior vena cava posteriorly; elevation of the structures should reach the left margin of the inferior vena cava. It is very important to expose and mobilize the third portion of the duodenum so as to allow easy access to the papilla and for closure of the duodenotomy without tension (Fig. 53.6).

Inframesocolic and extraperitoneal approaches

In some cases where the subhepatic space is obscured by adhesions as a result of previous surgery, access to the second portion of the duodenum using a different approach has been suggested. The authors are not familiar with these techniques since even in cases of extensive adhesions there has been little difficulty in access to the duodenum as described above.

In the inframesocolic approach (Villalba & Lucas 1978) the greater omentum and transverse colon are displaced superiorly and the small bowel inferiorly and to the left. Next, a transverse incision is made in the posterior peritoneum at the base of the transverse mesocolon from the superior mesenteric vessels extending laterally to expose the 2nd and 3rd duodenal portion.

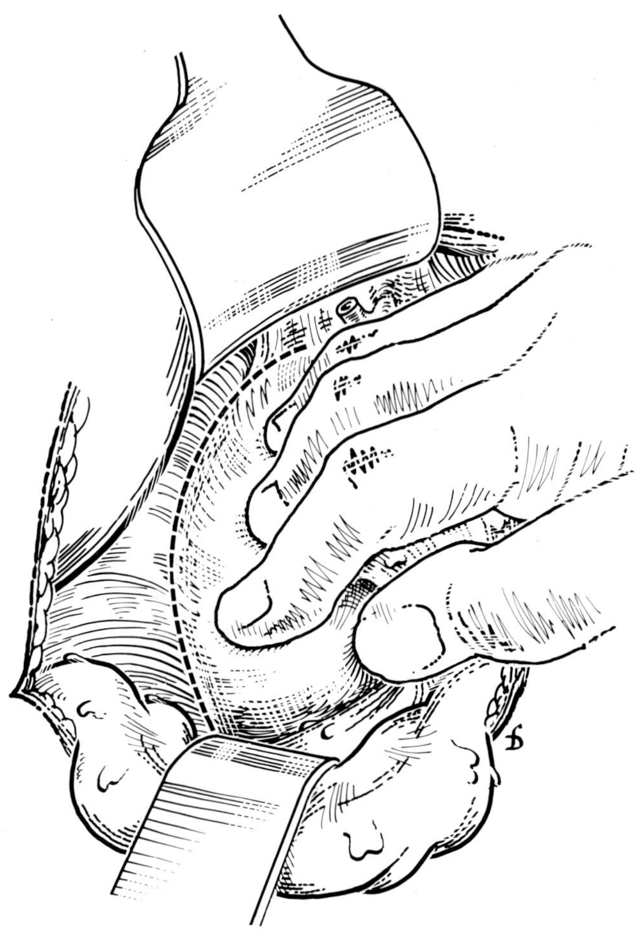

Fig. 53.4 Kocher maneouvre: this commences with an incision of the peritoneum laterally at the outer margin of the second portion of the duodenum (dotted line). Mesocolon related to the right colic flexure is stripped inferiorly

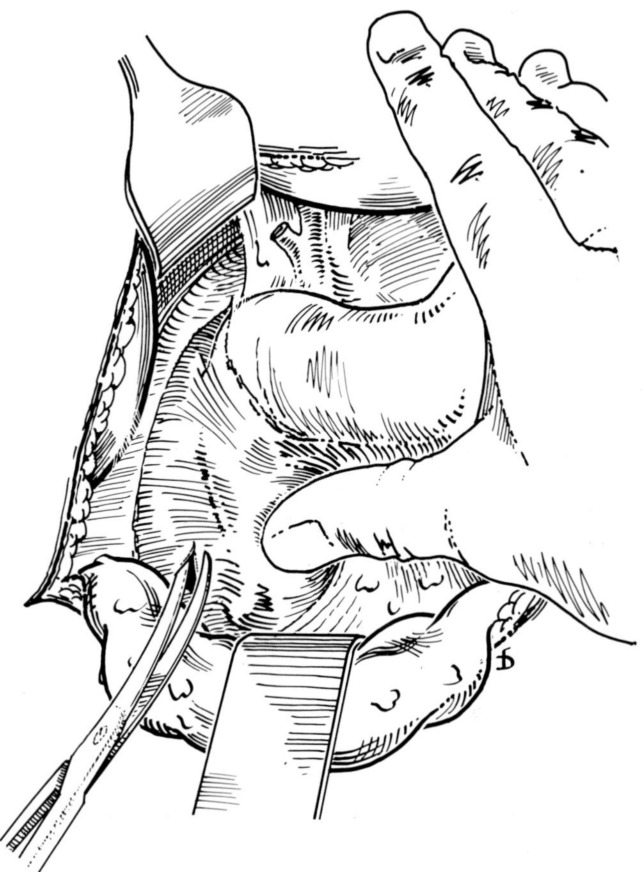

Fig. 53.5 To help mobilization of the duodenum the assistant surgeon displaces the second portion of the duodenum medially and superiorly

In the extraperitoneal approach (Choi et al 1982) (Ch. 77), an incision is made in the abdominal wall below the right costal margin from the midaxillary line to the lateral edge of the right rectus abdominis muscle. The peritoneum is displaced superiorly and medially. The right kidney and its perinephric fat are identified and the duodenum reached extraperitoneally.

Duodenotomy

Duodenotomy is performed in the lateral duodenal wall by surgical diathermy. The cut is 10 to 15 mm long, immediately above the inferior knee of the duodenum, the surgeon taking account of the fact that the papilla is usually located at the junction of the lower third with the upper two thirds of the second portion of the duodenum (Fig. 53.7).

The duodenal incision may be longitudinal or transverse, both types being suitable, provided that the suture of such incisions is always transverse. The authors prefer a longitudinal incision because if the retractor on the duodenum widens the duodenotomy, this occurs longitudinally; in the case of a transverse duodenotomy any inadvertent extension would cause a transverse enlargement of the wound.

Identification of the papilla

Following the duodenal incision the papilla is readily visualized on the medial duodenal wall in some 15 to 20% of cases; it appears as a roundish elevation with a central orifice. When the papilla is not readily visible it should be detected by displacement and flattening of the mucosal folds. This should be done with great care to avoid tearing of the mucosa which would hinder good visualization. Identification of the papilla, under direct vision, is possible in 80% of cases. If this is not the case, digital palpation can be used running the forefinger, introduced through the duodenotomy, across the medial duodenal wall; the papilla is then identified as a small elevation (Fig. 53.8).

Should digital palpation fail, a small (French gauge 5–6) Nelaton's catheter can be introduced via the cystic duct stump and advanced downwards to emerge at the papilla. This manoeuvre should never be performed with rigid catheters since they may result in the formation of false

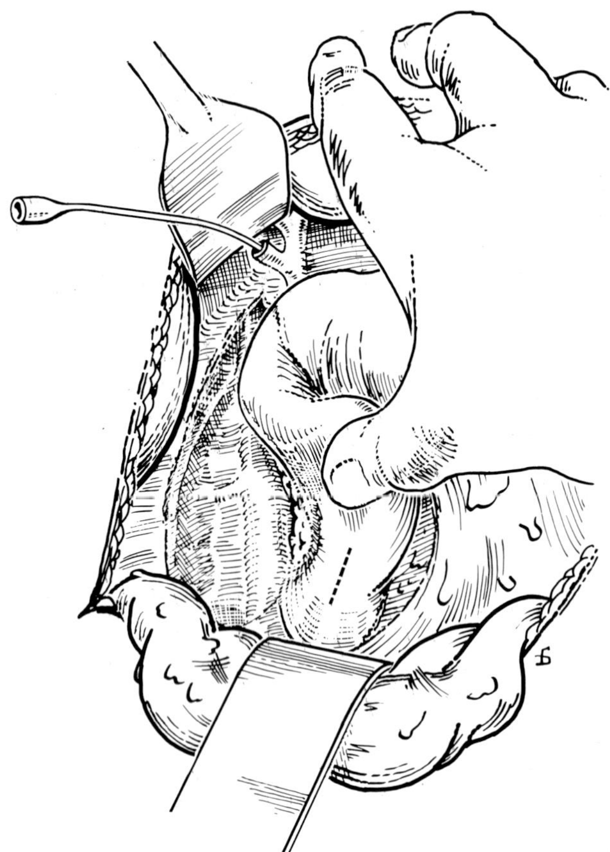

Fig. 53.6 It is important to expose and mobilize the third portion of the duodenum so as to make identification and operation on the papilla easy and to allow facile closure of the duodenotomy

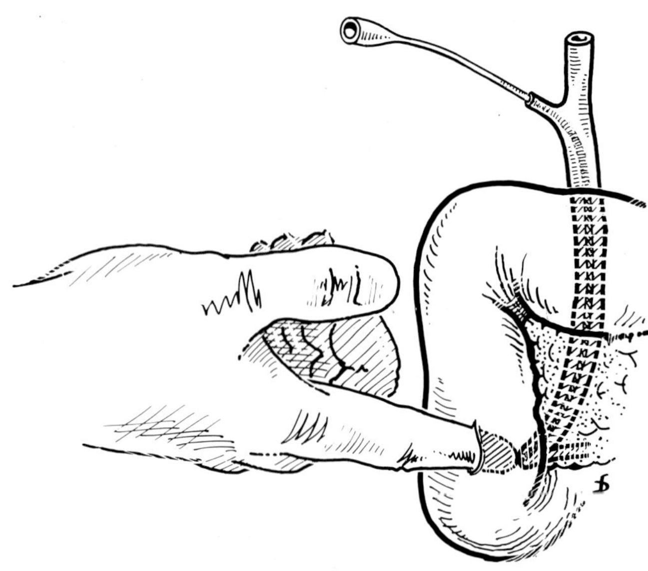

Fig. 53.8 If the papilla is not easily seen, a small Nelaton's catheter is introduced through the cystic duct stump until it is seen to protrude from the papillary orifice. The forefinger, introduced through the duodenotomy, detects the papilla as a small and thick elevation

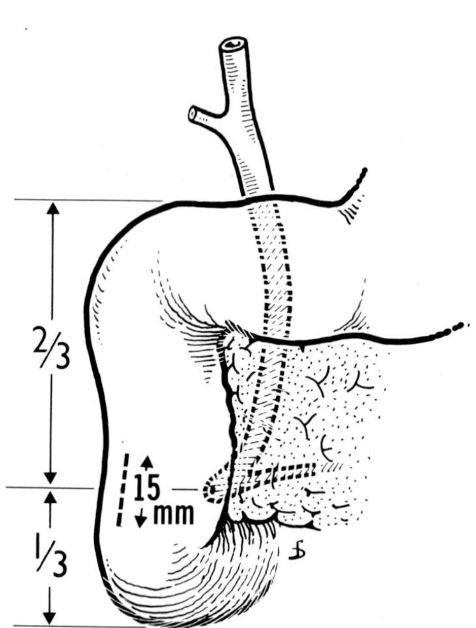

Fig. 53.7 The duodenotomy is performed above the junction of the second and third portions of the duodenum, the surgeon taking into account that the papilla is usually located at the junction of the upper two thirds and lower third of the second part of the duodenum

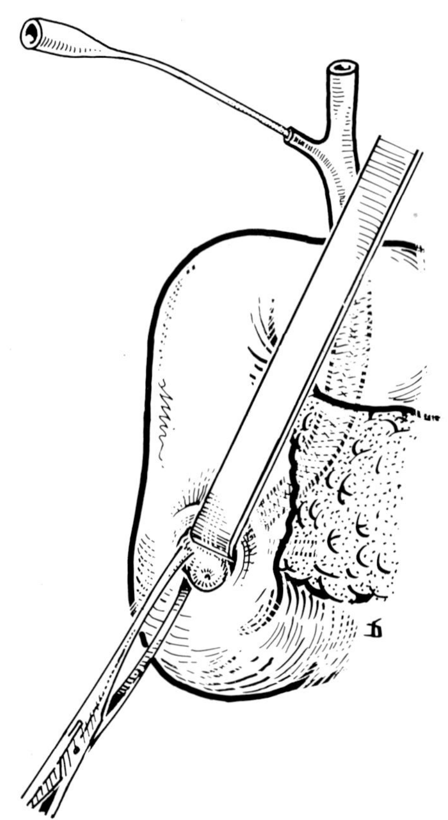

Fig. 53.9 The duodenotomy is kept open by a suitable retractor placed in the upper margin of the duodenal incision. The papilla is exposed by gentle traction with an Allis' clamp placed laterally (*never medially*) to avoid trauma to the duct of Wirsung

passages (Barraya et al 1974). A further recently introduced possibility consists of the passage of a 3 mm diameter fibreoptic light source introduced through the cystic duct which transilluminates the common bile duct as far as the papilla, making it identifiable even prior to duodenotomy, which can then be performed exactly at the level of the transillumination. The authors have no personal experience of this technique.

Sometimes a very small papilla is detected and its catheterization is difficult or impossible. In such cases the orifice is probably that of the duct of Santorini, while the major papilla should be searched for in a lower position.

Sphincteroplasty

Once the papilla has been identified it is exposed by gentle extraction with an Allis or similar clamp. This is applied laterally and never medially so as to avoid trauma to the duct of Wirsung (Partington 1977) (Fig. 53.9). A Nelaton's catheter (French guage 4–5) is introduced from the outside or via the cystic duct. Following the line of the catheter (and avoiding plastic catheters which melt when surgical diathermy is applied) make a cut using surgical diathermy. This is made superiorly (at '11.00 o'clock') for 4 to 5 mm (Fig. 53.10). The authors prefer surgical diathermy because good haemostasis is ensured by this instrument. When a sample for biopsy is required this should be done with a scalpel and taken only from the outer margin of the incision. Possible bleeding from the cut, usually modest, can be arrested with a stitch.

After sphincterotomy two or three stitches are placed between the duodenal mucosa and the wall of the common bile duct on the outer margin using an atraumatic needle and 3/0 silk. Traction is now applied to these sutures and incision of the sphincter is extended for a further 6 to 7 mm with sutures placed every 2 to 3 mm (all laterally) until the whole common tract of the sphincter of Oddi is incised (Fig. 53.11). The incision is complete when it is 10 to 12 mm long and an appropriate forcep can easily be introduced (Fig. 53.12). Its entry into the common bile duct allows an abundant flow of bile due to distension of its sphincter.

Sutures should be placed only on the outer margin of the sphincterotomy in order to prevent the risk of damage to the duct of Wirsung. The opening of the duct of Wirsung is usually identified as a small orifice from which clear, colourless pancreatic juice flows. (Fig. 53.11).

Instrumental exploration of the common bile duct

After sphincteroplasty, instrumental exploration of the common bile duct and extraction of stones is performed (Speranza et al 1983).

An angled Randall's forceps is introduced into the common bile duct and left and right hepatic ducts carefully

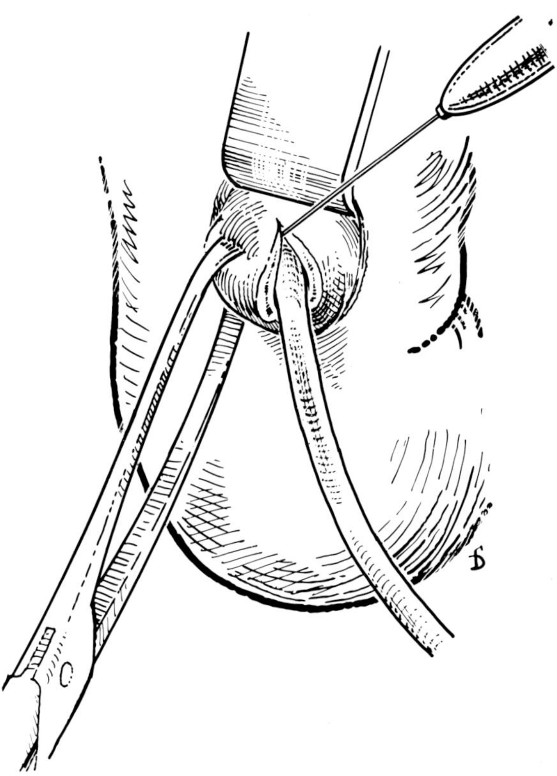

Fig. 53.10 With the Nelaton's catheter as a guide, a cut is made using surgical diathermy on the medial wall of the duodenum extending superiorly and slightly externally ('11 o'clock'). With diathermy good haemostasis is secured

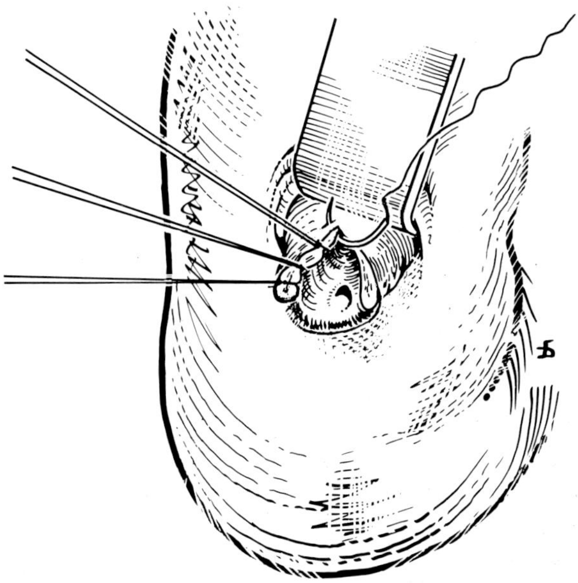

Fig. 53.11 After sphincterotomy is performed several stitches are placed between the duodenal mucosa and the wall of the common bile duct using an atraumatic needle and 3–0 silk. Sutures should be placed only on the outer margin of the sphincterotomy to avoid the risk of damaging the duct of Wirsung which in its distal portion runs inferiorly and medially along the length of the common bile duct

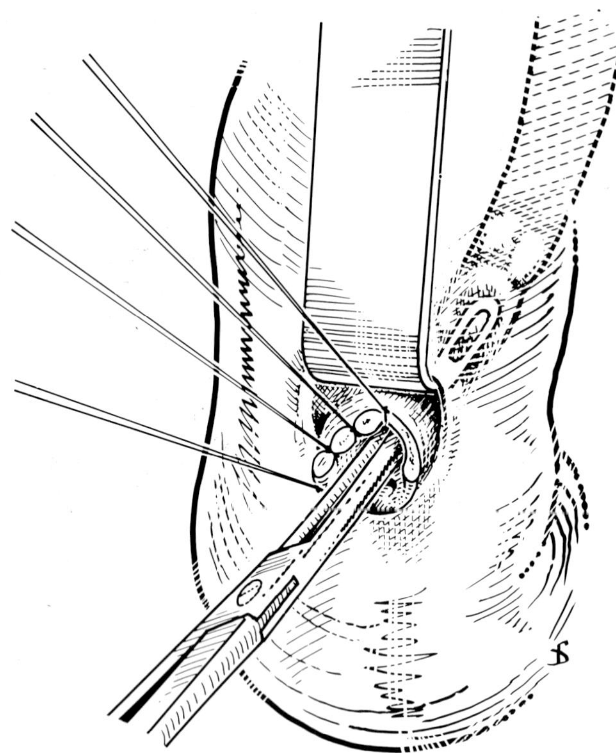

Fig. 53.12 Spincteroplasty is completed when a Randall's forceps can be easily introduced into the common bile duct extracting stones or other foreign bodies

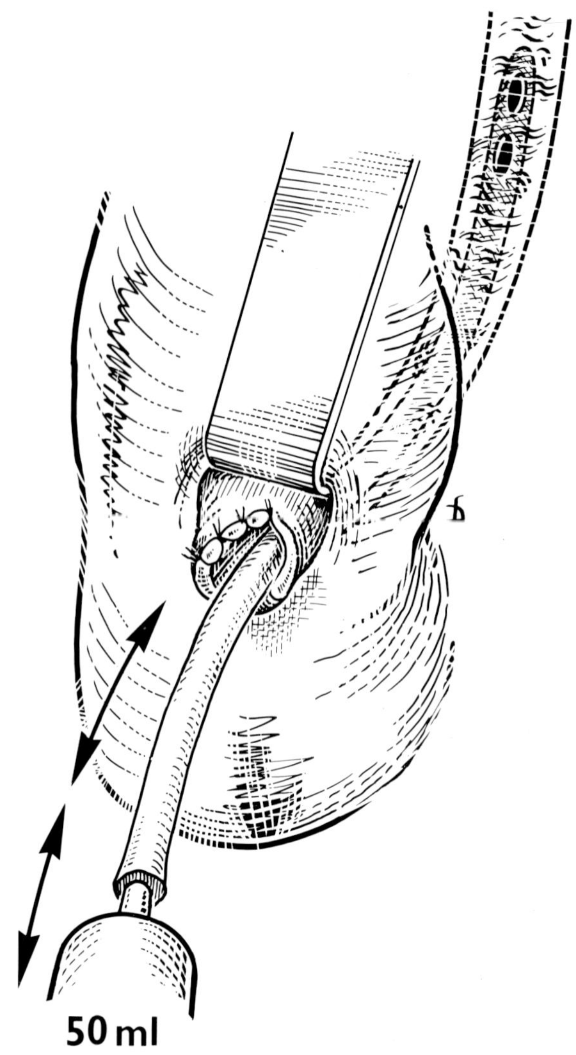

Fig. 53.13 After the extraction of stones the common bile duct is rinsed with saline solution introduced under slight pressure with a Nelaton's catheter and with subsequent siphoning so that small fragments can run downstream

explored. The manoeuvre should be repeated several times in order to extract all stones. The next step is to rinse with saline solution, introduced under slight pressure by a Nelaton's catheter (French gauge 8–9) and abruptly withdrawn so that, with the siphoning, small fragments flow downstream (Fig. 53.13).

Other means of extraction of stones from the common bile duct are the Fogarty catheter and Dormia basket. The authors have never used these instruments since Randall's forcep and rinsing and siphoning are effective.

The problem of residual stones exists and the best method of prevention is to use choledochoscopy introducing the endoscope via the sphincteroplasty.

Duodenal closure

As already emphasized, initial longitudinal duodenotomy should be always closed transversely. First, the superior and inferior margins of the incision are approximated and subsequently the resulting gaps are sutured with two extramucosal non-absorbable purse-string sutures. Three or four non-absorbable seromuscular sutures are then added (Fig. 53.14).

It is important that the suture should not be under tension and it is for this reason that preliminary extended mobilization of the duodenum and pancreas is mandatory. The authors have never experienced dehiscence of the duodenal suture using this procedure.

The operation is now complete and the wound is closed. The authors never use abdominal drains.

RESULTS

351 patients were operated upon between 1970 and 1984. 214 (61%) were females and 137 (39%) males, aged 18 to 92 (mean 54) years. 21.9% were in the sixth and 25.6% in the seventh decade of life.

Sphincteroplasty was most frequently performed to provide access to the common bile duct for the extraction of stones (Lechat et al 1976), although in 69 patients (19.6%) both stones and stenosing papillitis were thought to be present. In four cases hydatid cyst remnants and

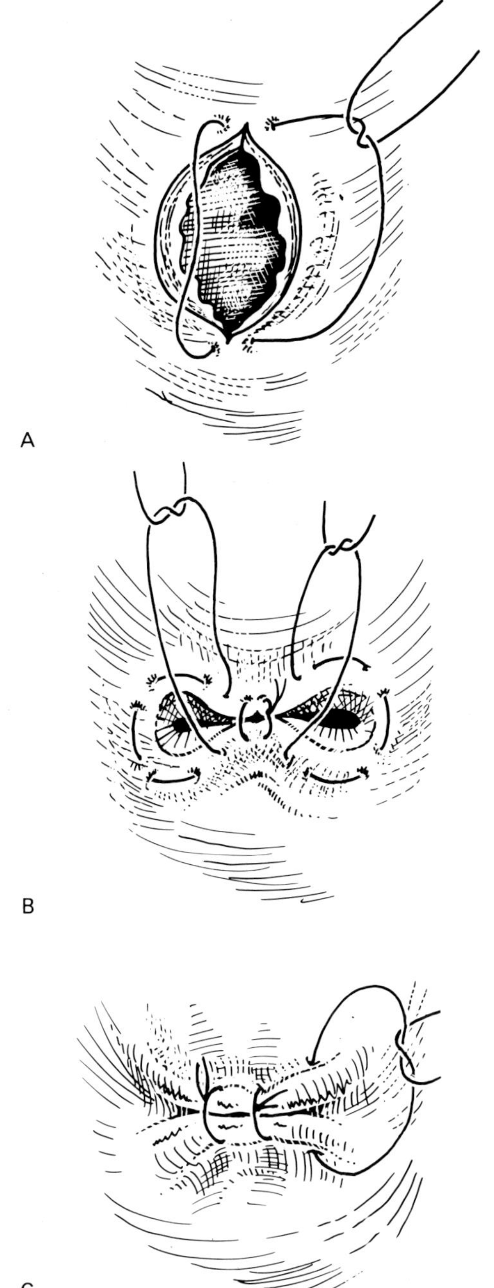

Fig. 53.14 The duodenotomy should always be closed transversely to avoid stenosis of the duodenum. (A) The superior and inferior angles are approximated; (B) The resulting lateral gaps are sutured with two extramucosal non-absorbable pursestring sutures; (C) 3–4 non-absorbable seromuscular stitches are added as a second layer. The sutures should not be under tension

membranes obstructing the biliary tree were the indication for operation.

Morbidity and mortality

In 18 cases (5.2%) postoperative complications occurred and four of these patients (1.1%) died. The most feared complication of this operation, acute pancreatitis, was

Table 53.2 Postoperative complications and mortality in 351 patients undergoing sphincteroplasty

Postoperative complication	Observed	%	Deaths	%
Acute pancreatitis	5	1.4	2	0.6
Bleeding from sphincteroplasty	4	1.4		
Bleeding from acute gastric ulcer	1			
Broncopneumonia	4	1.2	1	0.3
Retained stones	2	0.6	1	0.3
Wound infection	1	0.3		
Infection of haematoma	1	0.3		
Total	18	5.2	4	1.1

observed in five cases, two of which proved fatal. There were five cases of postoperative bleeding resulting from the sphincteroplasty in four and from an acute ulcer of the stomach in one. Re-operation was not necessary in these cases since bleeding arrested with simple conservative measures. Four bronchopulmonary complications were also observed, one of which was fatal. There was one case with an infected intra-abdominal haematoma and one case of wound infection. Residual stones in the common bile duct were found to be present in two cases, one of which presented with obstructive jaundice in the immediate postoperative period and required re-operation. The other patient presented with rapidly progressive and ultimately fatal suppurative cholangitis associated with the presence of a retained stone. In those patients without complication (94.9%) the mean hospital stay was 8.6 (range 7–10) days.

Long-term results

147 patients have been followed-up for periods of six months to 10 years (mean 5 years 7 months). At follow-up clinical data were recorded and when indicated laboratory investigations of liver function, ultrasonography, cholangiography, barium meal, gastroduodenoscopy and liver scanning with Tc-99m HIDA were carried out. Most recently, in selected cases, endoscopic manometry of residual sphincteric function was performed (Vassilakis, Manolas & Boundouris 1979).

The long-term results were classified (Choi et al 1981, Stefanini et al 1977) as *good* (134 cases) if there was a total absence of symptoms or only modest transient dyspepsia. Results were regarded as *fair* (10 cases) if dyspeptic symptoms were present; and were regarded as *poor* (three cases) in patients who complained of symptoms identical to those experienced preoperatively. One of these patients exhibited duodenal reflux to the common bile duct at barium meal, a second suffered recurrent attacks of cholangitis and a third presented with stenosis of a sphincteroplasty requiring hepaticojejunostomy three years after initial operation. In 23 of the 51 patients followed cholangiographically, a pharmacodynamic test was performed, consisting of the intravenous injection of cerulein, a synthetic analogue of cholecystokinin, following an intravenous injection of morphine hydrochloride. In 20 of these patients the administration of morphine caused the interruption of the flow of contrast into the duodenum. This was resumed with the administration of cerulein. This behaviour suggests the presence of residual sphincter activity likely to be due to that portion of the sphincter of Oddi pertaining to the common bile duct itself.

REFERENCES

Arianoff A A 1980 Analysis of 607 cases of choledochal sphincterotomy. World Journal of Surgery 3: 483–487

Barraya L, Pujol Soler R, Yvergneaux J P, Rozes J, Chauvin P 1974 Surgery of the sphincter of Oddi—Surgical techniques. In: Modern techniques in surgery—Digestive surgery. Editions Techniques, Paris, p 1–17

Chigot J P, Clot J P, Cassina I, Mercadier M 1978 La sphincterotomie oddienne, indications, complications, resultats. Annales de Chirurgie 32: 355–360

Choi T K, Wong J, Lam K H, Lim T K, Ong G B 1981 Late result of sphincteroplasty in the treatment of primary cholangitis. Archives of Surgery 116: 1173–1175

Choi T K, Lee N W, Wong J, Ong G B 1982 Extraperitoneal sphincteroplasty for residual stones. Annals of Surgery 196: 26–29

Jones S A 1978 The prevention and treatment of recurrent bile duct stones by transduodenal sphincteroplasty. World Journal of Surgery 2: 473–485

Lechat J R, Leborgne J, LeNeel J C, Visset J, Mousseau M 1976 La place actuelle de la sphincterotomie oddienne dans la chirurgie pour lesions benignes de la voie biliaire principale chez l'adulte. Annales de Chirurgie 30: 363–369

Moody F G, Becker J M, Potts J R 1983 Transduodenal sphincteroplasty and transampullary septectomy for postcholecystectomy pain. Annals of Surgery 197: 627–636

Partington P F 1977 Twenty-three years of experience with sphincterotomy and sphincteroplasty for stenosis of the sphincter of Oddi. Surgery, Gynecology & Obstetrics 145: 161–168

Speranza V, Lezoche E, Minervini S, Carlei F, Basso N, Simi M 1982 Transduodenal papillostomy as a routine procedure in managing choledocholithiasis. Archives of Surgery 117: 875–878

Stefanini P, Carboni M, Patrassi N, Be Bernardinis G, Negro P, Loriga P 1974 Transduodenal sphincteroplasty. Its use in the treatment of lithiasis and benign obstruction of the common duct. The American Journal of Surgery 128: 672–677

Stefanini P, Carboni M, De Bernardinis G, Negro P 1977 Long-term results of papillostomy. In: Delmont J (ed) The sphincter of Oddi. Karger S, Basel, p 206–212

Vassilakis J S, Manolas K, Boundouris J 1979 Transduodenal sphincteroplasty. Archives of Surgery 114: 181–184

Villalba M R, Lucas R J, 1978 Inframesocolic transduodenal approach to the distal biliary-pancreatic ductal system. Archives of Surgery 113: 496–499

Vogt D P, Hermann R E 1981 Choledochoduodenostomy, choledochojejunostomy or sphincteroplasty for biliary and pancreatic disease. Annals of Surgery 193: 161–168

M. L. Gliedman

Choledochoduodenostomy — technique

The following technique for choledochoduodenostomy has evolved over an 18-year period and some 400 choledochoduodenostomies. Two technical criteria are essential for a proper choledochoduodenostomy: a common duct of 1.4 cm in diameter at the minimum and a stoma size of 2.5 cm. As a corollary, a stoma size of 2.5 cm can not be accomplished with other than a single layer anastomosis.

The *indications* that have been utilized for a choledochoduodenostomy in benign diseases have been: multiple common bile duct calculi, papillary or ampullary stenosis, an impacted distal stone in the absence of pancreatitis,

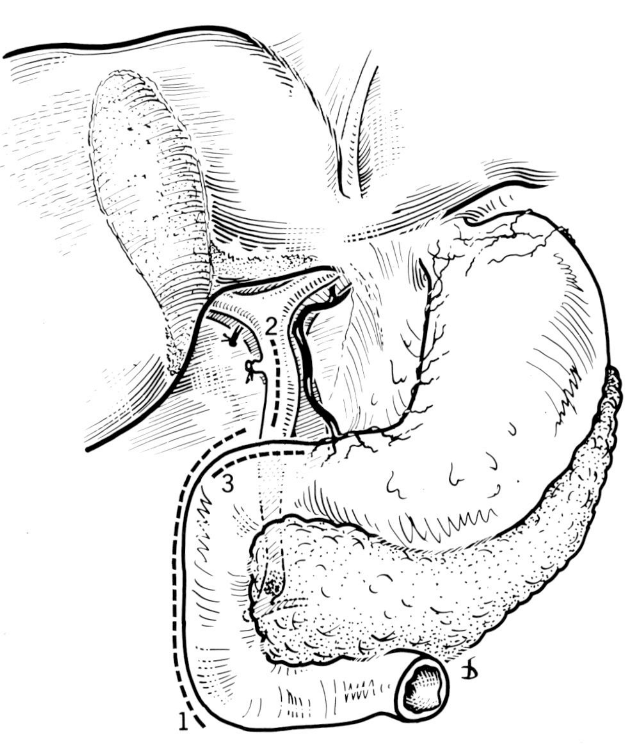

Fig. 54.1 After the gallbladder is removed, the common duct is opened through a conventional longitudinal incision following a Kocher incision (1) freeing the lateral duodenum around to the common duct. Routine common duct exploration is carried out. If the indications for a choledochoduodenostomy exist, the anastomosis is performed if the duct is 1.4 cm or wider. The incision in the common duct (2) is extended to 2.5 cm by direct measurement. In almost all instances, the incision in the duct will carry into the common hepatic duct. The incision in the post bulbar duodenum (3) is slightly smaller since the stoma in the duodenum stretches to approximate the choledochal incision.

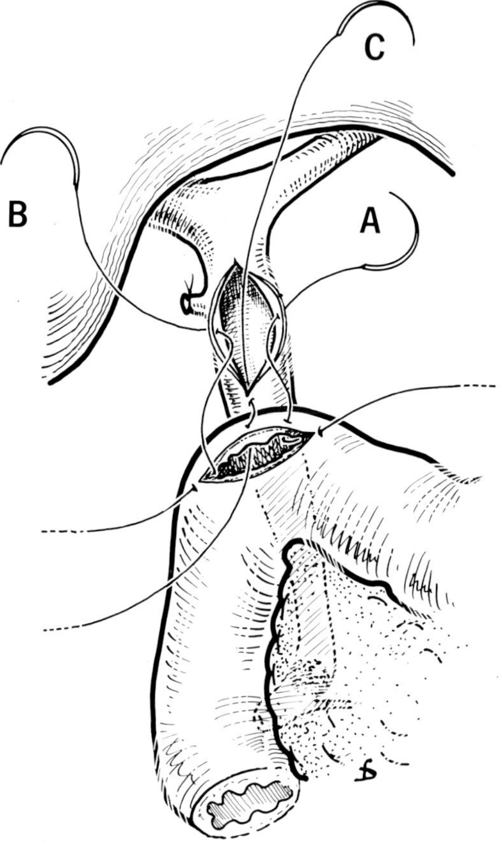

Fig. 54.2 Each side of the choledochoduodenostomy is bisected by a stitch (A & B) of absorbable material (chromic catgut or polyglycolic acid) that passes from the end of the duodenal incision through the mid-point of the choledochal incision. Likewise the duodenal incision is bisected by a stitch through the posterior wall of the duodenal incision and the lower apex of the choledochal incision (C). These stitches convert part of the longitudinal choledochotomy incision into a transverse ostium. A lax approximation of the duodenal and choledochal incision occurs, with the duodenum mobilized, by placing tension on a lateral stay suture (A or B) and the middle stay suture (C).

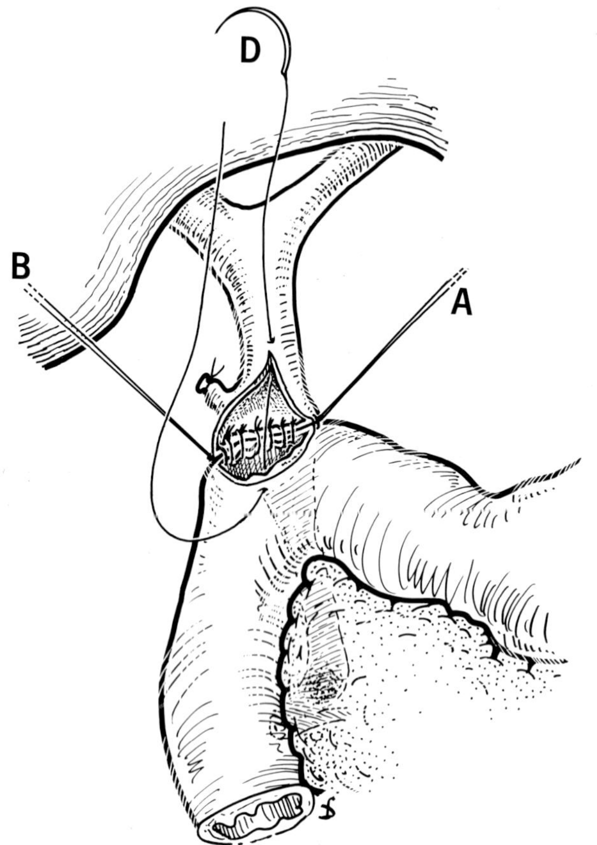

Fig. 54.3 Sutures may then be placed to complete the posterior suture line approximating the common bile duct to the posterior duodenal incision. Following placement of the sutures they are tied so that the knots are within the lumen. The anterior wall is similarly approximated utilizing a suture bisecting the anterior duodenal incision (D) and through the original apex of the bile duct incision.

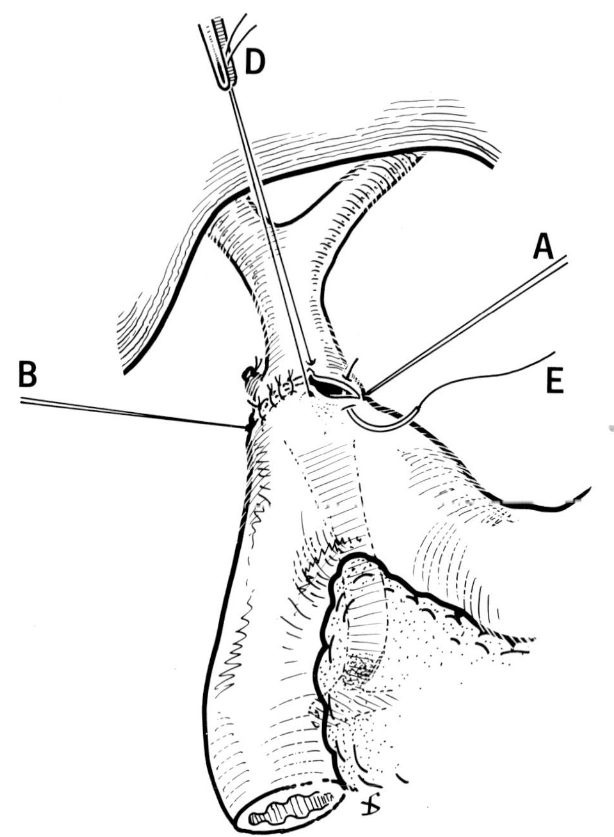

Fig. 54.4 With this bisecting suture (D) tented forwards, each of the segments, between the tied lateral stay suture and this anterior suture, is similary approximated using interrupted sutures with the knots tied on the outside. The anastomosis is completed by completing the third segment of this triangle by sutures placed between the remaining lateral stay suture and the suture 'D'. It is important in the placement of these last sutures that they do not catch the posterior suture line. The benefit of placing all the sutures in one line of the triangular closure and then tying them all following placement is that it allows an internal inspection before the lumen of the choledochoduodenostomy is obscured. A single row of sutures is all that is utilized. A second row does nothing but decrease the choledochoduodenostomy orifice size and is to be avoided. The sutures should be placed close enough so that there is a bile-tight approximation. Digital pressure on the duodenum or the common duct should give no evidence of leakage.

intrahepatic calculi, tubular narrowing of the distal common bile duct segment (usually secondary to pancreatitis), periampullary duodenal diverticula causing recurrent cholangitis, a massively dilated common bile duct without stones, residual stones, and a low iatrogenic stricture. The procedure is not indicated in a non-dilated common bile duct, in sclerosing cholangitis, in the decompression of the pancreatic duct for pancreatitis or where there is significant duodenal oedema or inflammation.

The degree of satisfaction with the procedure will be dependent upon the development of a standard technique for the rapid construction of a stoma that allows free entry and egress from the common bile duct. The described technique has been demonstrated to be most advantageous in fulfilling the patient's needs with surgical ease and with minimal postoperative difficulties.

While attempts are made to remove stones and particulate matter from the common bile duct. Impacted stones at the distal common bile duct that are not easily retrieved and stones in the hepatic duct are not too vigorously pursued prior to the anastomosis. Over 18 years we have not found these to represent a problem. Postoperative evaluation is carried out radiologically either by barium meal study or by HIDA scans which allow good anatomical visualization as well as assessment of the physiologic function of the anastomosis in emptying the biliary tree (Ch. 15). In our series we have not noted difficulties with post choledochoduodenostomy cholangitis or so-called 'sump syndrome'. We believe this is a result of a commitment to a measured anastomosis of 2.5 cm or greater in the duodenum and common bile duct.

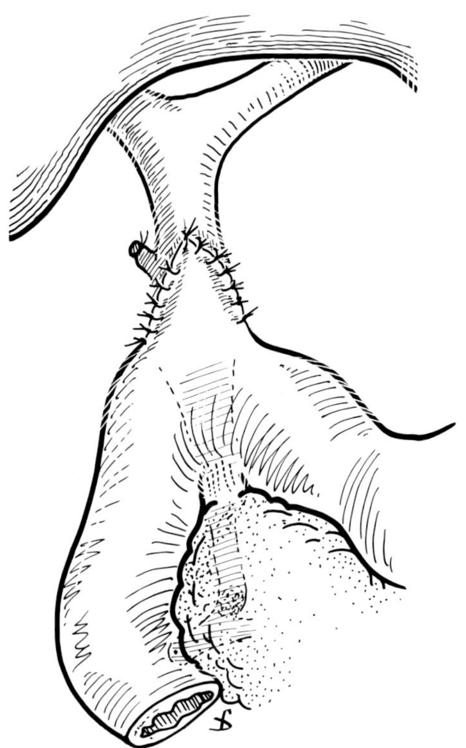

Fig. 54.5 The completed anastomosis allows a thumb-sized defect to be palpated through the duodenal tongue that has been brought on to the common bile duct and common hepatic duct. If the choledochoduodenostomy is done at the same time as a cholecystectomy, a closed suction drain is utilized. In general, if the choledochoduodenostomy is done as a second stage procedure, it is not accompanied by a drain.

ADDITIONAL READING

Degenshein G A 1974 Choledochoduodenostomy, An 18 year study of 175 consecutive cases. Surgery 76: 319–324

Gliedman M L, Gold M S 1985 Choledochoduodenostomy. In: Schwartz S I, Ellis H (eds) Maingot's Abdominal Operations, 8th edn. Appleton-Century-Crofts, Norwalk, Connecticut, ch 79 p 1909–1922

Gliedman M L, Schein C J 1980 The use and abuse of choledochoduodenostomy. In: Najarian J S, Delaney J P (eds) Hepatic, biliary and pancreatic surgery. Miami Symposia Specialists, p 91

Schein C J, Beneventano T C, Jacobson H S 1966 Choledochoduodenostomy — roentgen considerations. Surgery 60: 958–963

Schein C J, Gliedman M L 1981 Choledochoduodenostomy as an adjunct to choledocholithotomy. Surgery, Gynecology and Obstetrics 152: 797–804

Schein C J, Shapiro N L, Gliedman M L 1978 Choledochoduodenostomy as an adjunct to choledocholithotomy. Surgery, Gynecology and Obstetrics 146: 25–32

SECTION 7

Papillary stenosis and post-cholecystectomy problems

R. F. McCloy

Post-cholecystectomy symptoms

In most Western countries cholecystectomy remains the most common major abdominal operation yet not all patients are cured of their symptoms and some develop new complaints. These symptom complexes, irrespective of whether they have a causal relationship to cholecystectomy, present an important and often challenging clinical problem. Patients and their clinicians may attribute symptoms incorrectly to the cholecystectomy and if a positive line of investigation is to be pursued then biliary and non-biliary, organic and functional diagnoses must be entertained.

The diverse nature and temporal relations of these symptoms suggest that the use of the term 'post-cholecystectomy syndrome' is inappropriate (Burnett & Shields 1958) but unfortunately its usage still persists (Tondelli & Gyr 1983). In the past confusion has arisen over the terms used for the definition of post-cholecystectomy symptoms and only non-organic or functional causes have been designated as the 'post-cholecysectomy syndrome' (Schofield & Macleod 1966) whereas Bodvall (1973) uses the term 'biliary dyskinesia' for this group and defines post-cholecystectomy syndrome as biliary colic or dyspepsia which are similar to the symptoms prior to cholecystectomy. In this discussion biliary dyskinesia will be considered strictly in relationship to the dysfunction of the sphincter of Oddi (see below) and post-cholecystectomy symptoms include any symptom—old, new or recurrent — irrespective of aetiology (Tondelli et al 1979).

INCIDENCE

Post-cholecystectomy symptoms are common and can appear at any time after operation (Bodvall & Övergaard 1967). The incidence of significant symptoms after cholecystectomy has been reported as 12–68% and severe in 3–32% of cases (Table 55.1). Indeed many patients with symptoms never return to hospital and in a prospective series of 115 patients undergoing cholecystectomy (Bates et al 1984) 43% had symptoms 12 months after operation but only 19% consulted their family doctor and 8% were referred back to hospital.

The frequency of symptoms after cholecystectomy is related to the length of pre-operative history and occurs in 27% patients operated on for the initial attack of gall bladder disease and 50% of patients with a history longer than five years (Bodvall & Övergaard 1967). Stefanini et al (1974) reported this trend for mild but not severe symptoms. Women have the highest incidence of problems when the operation is performed between the ages of 40–49 (Bodvall & Övergaard 1967) but there is a lower incidence of post-cholecystectomy symptoms in men (sex ratio, men : women = 1 : 3.3) and with advancing age at operation. It is not surprising that problems are more frequent if a normal non-calculous gallbladder was removed (Bodvall 1973, Schofield & Macleod 1966) but this is not so if it was non-functioning on cholecystography (Nora et al 1984) or had a pathological diagnosis of adenomyomatosis (Meguid et al 1984).

Table 55.1 Incidence of symptoms after cholecystectomy

	Total no. patients	% post-cholecystectomy symptoms	
		all	severe
Burnett & Shields 1958	141	14	
Schofield & MacLeod 1966	407	18	
Bodvall 1964	1 930	40	5
Collected series 1920–1971 (Bodvall 1973)	20 000	12–68	3–32
Stefanini et al 1974	800	31	4
Hess 1977	919	26	
Bates et al 1984	115	43	

AETIOLOGY

It is arguable whether any of the symptoms that may occur after gallbladder surgery have ever been shown to be due to the absence of the gallbladder (Editorial, BMJ 1974).

Altered anatomy The bile ducts neither increase or decrease in size following cholecystectomy (Le Quesne et al 1959) but the diameter is increased in all the main bile ducts in patients who have had biliary tract disease and a cholecystectomy compared to normal patients (Hamilton et al 1982). Bodvall (1973) correlates increasing choledochal width with less severe post-cholecystectomy symptoms whereas Le Quesne and co-workers (1959) found no relationship between bile duct size and continuing symptoms after operation.

Altered physiology In recent years increasingly sophisticated manometric techniques in the bile ducts and sphincter of Oddi have been employed (Geenen 1983) (Ch. 9). Prior to cholecystectomy morphine-induced spasm of the sphincter fails to increase choledochal pressure, whilst after cholecystectomy morphine leads to a coarse and irregular rise in ductal pressure attributed to sphincter of Oddi spasm and possibly related to the loss of the gallbladder as a pressure reservoir (Tanaka et al 1984). The relationship between the bile duct pressure and post-cholecystectomy symptoms remains problematic. None of the nine patients in Tanaka's study developed abdominal symptoms. There is no evidence that intraductal biliary pressures relate to the diameter of the major bile ducts (Csendes et al 1979, Bar-Meir & Halpern 1984). Dysfunction of the sphincter of Oddi is considered in more detail below.

Altered metabolism Changes in metabolism are unlikely to lead to post-cholecystectomy symptoms (Tondelli & Gyr 1978). There is conflicting evidence concerning the effect of cholecystectomy on the bile salt pool (Editorial, BMJ 1974). After cholecystectomy bile is secreted at a constant concentration but in the gut the concentration remains above that necessary for emulsification and absorption of fat (Badley et al 1969) and the operation is not followed by steatorrhoea.

Complications of cholecystectomy Symptoms may develop in the immediate or early postoperative period, see Table 55.2 (Soehendra et al 1981). Symptoms ascribed to the cystic duct stump were amongst the first post-cholecystectomy problems to be diagnosed but have slipped from prominence in the last two decades almost certainly due to the widespread practice of peroperative cholangiography via the cystic duct. A cystic duct remnant of >10 mm has been reported in up to 84% of severe cases of post-cholecystectomy distress compared with an inci-

Table 55.2 Classification of causes of post-cholecystectomy symptoms

BILIARY	CBD stones*			
	Benign stricture*			
	Tumour*			
	Biliary-enteric fistula			
	'Sump' syndrome			
	Papillary disorders:	dysfunction		peri-ampullary problems
		primary stenosis*		
		secondary stenosis		
	Post-surgical*:	immediate,	trauma	
			bleed	
			biliary peritonitis	
		early,	haematoma	
			bile collection	
			abscess	
			fistula	
		late,	cystic duct stump problems,	neuroma
				stone
				inflammation
	Others			
EXTRA-BILIARY	Pancreatic disease:	post-surgical damage		
		concurrent disease		
	Liver disease			
	Flatulent dyspepsia syndrome			
	Peptic ulcer			
	Hiatus hernia			
	Irritable bowel syndrome			
	Diverticular disease			
	Renal disease			
	Post-surgical:	adhesions		
		others		
	Psychosomatic disorders			

* Considered in more detail in Chapters 46–50, 58, 65, 66.

dence of 40% in mild symptomatic or cured patients (Bodvall 1964, Bodvall & Övergaard 1966). The cystic duct remnant may act as the site of inflammation and retained or recurrent stones and up to 15% of patients with severe symptoms have some neuromatous tissue on pathological examination of the amputated duct stump (Bodvall 1964, Bodvall & Övergaard 1966) but only one patient had a typical neuroma and none of the patients with severe symptoms was improved by removal of the stump. In a review of the early literature on the clinical significance of the cystic duct or gallbladder remnant Bodvall (1973) concludes that the remnant per se does not seem to have any clinical significance.

Non-biliary disease Although symptoms can arise from abnormalities in the biliary tract they can also result from concurrent disease in other organs (Table 55.2) which may or may not relate to the cholecystectomy. Damage to the pancreas or liver can occur either from gallstone disease or from the performance of a cholecystectomy and these organs can also be the site for concurrent disease which leads to symptoms (Fig. 55.1). Flatulent dyspepsia is a frequent symptom in an ageing urban female population, independent of the presence of gallbladder disease (Price 1963), and Maingot (1956) stated that cholecystectomy has little or no effect in curing these symptoms. Yet cholecystectomy can be expected to improve or cure flatulent dyspepsia in 70–80% of patients (Johnson 1975, Kingston & Windsor 1975). Using tube techniques, Johnson (1972) found a close correlation between a history of flatulent dyspepsia and the detection of pyloric regurgitation and these findings have been confirmed more recently using a non-invasive isotopic method (Cheadle et al 1984). Flatulent dyspepsia after cholecystectomy may also be related to delayed gastric emptying (Watson & Love 1984) but the operation itself does not appear to alter gastric emptying (Kingston & Windsor 1975). Duodenal abnormalities including peptic ulceration have been reported in up to 32% of patients (Hunt & Blumgart 1982) and are more frequently recognized now that routine endoscopy is usual. Other associated Western diseases such as hiatus hernia and diverticular disease may contribute to the symptom complex. The possibility of diverse pathology should not be forgotten and cases of incisional hernia (McCloy et al 1984), adhesions (Burnett & Shields 1958) and renal calculi (Schofield & MacLeod 1966) have been reported in series of patients with post-cholecystectomy problems. Probably the most important non-organic disorder in patients with post-cholecystectomy symptoms is the irritable bowel syndrome (Tondelli & Gyr 1983), especially those with the 'hepatic flexure syndrome'. A psychosomatic origin for symptoms in young women has been proposed (Valberg et al 1971) and psychological stress may alter upper gastrointestinal function and lead to symptoms (Johnson 1975).

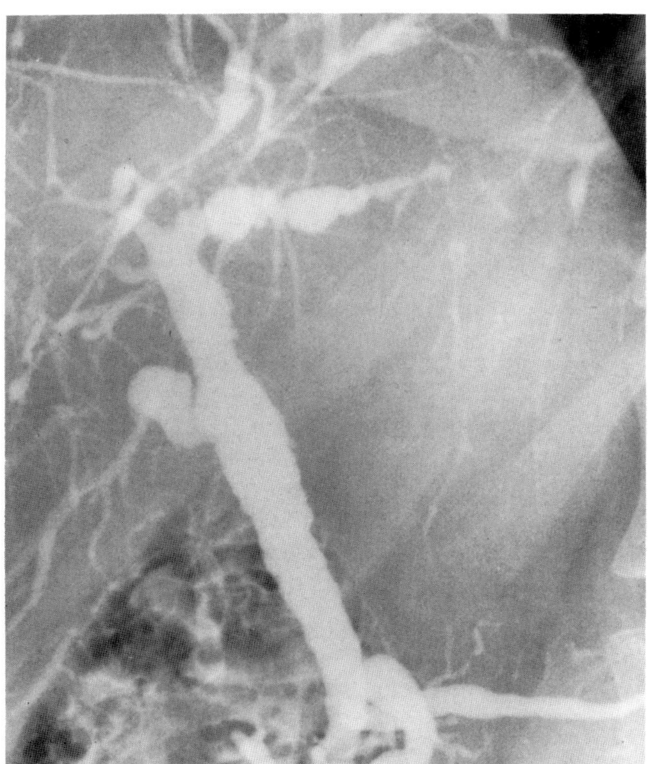

Fig. 55.1 Sclerosing cholangitis and moderate pancreatitic changes seen at ERCP in a 38-year-old woman presenting with cholangitis and pancreatitis two years after cholecystectomy

CLINICAL FEATURES

The symptom complex in the patient after cholecystectomy usually comprises dypepsia and upper abdominal pain, although a more clamant presentation with jaundice, cholangitis or pancreatitis is not uncommon. Post-cholecystectomy symptoms are often persistent and Bodvall & Övergaard (1967) found that 71% of patients with dyspepsia and approximately 50% of those with mild pain still had problems more than nine years after cholecystectomy.

Symptoms may appear immediately after operation. Pain and jaundice may herald bleeding into the biliary tree (Fig. 55.2) (Dos Reis & De Almeida 1981, Kelly et al 1983) and suggest that iatrogenic damage is likely (Soehendra et al 1981). In addition to jaundice, the early postoperative occurrence of bile peritonitis and persistent bile leak from a drain, or the drainage tract after removal, should alert surgeons to the possibility of iatrogenic biliary stricture (Ch. 58) (Collins & Gorey 1984), since in over 80% of cases damage to the biliary tree is not recognized at the time of cholecystectomy (Kelly & Blumgart 1985).

We have found that the pattern of symptoms at the time of presentation to our clinic is indicative of the final diagnostic outcome (McCloy et al 1984). In a series of 57 patients with post-cholecystectomy problems the diagnosis

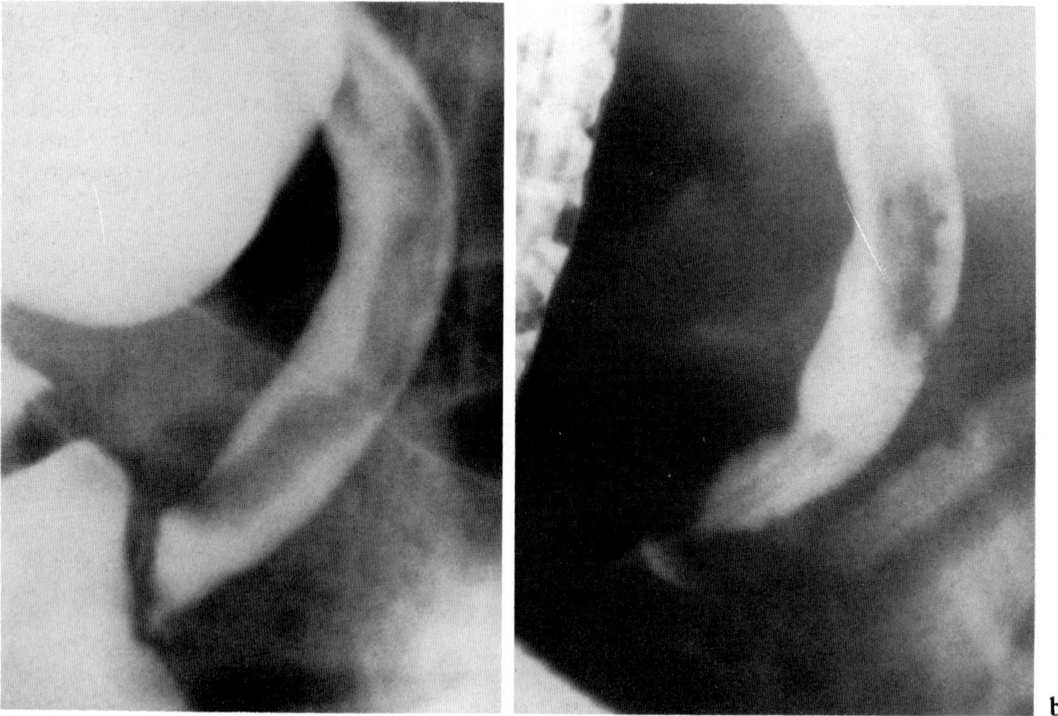

Fig. 55.2 Organized thrombus in the lower CBD of a man, aged 28, six months (a) and 18 months (b) after cholecystectomy and major hepatic resection for liver trauma. No symptoms could be directly attributed to this pathology identified at ERCP.

was not obvious in 16 cases yet in this sub-group definite organic pathology was established in 80% of patients with 'new' pain not present before cholecystectomy. If the pain was 'old', i.e., similar in nature to the pain prior to operation, organic pathology was identified in 60% of cases. This supported the findings of Schofield & MacLeod (1966) who reported that 68% of 74 patients with post-cholecystectomy symptoms had 'new' pain and 52% of this group had pathology, surprisingly all extra-biliary. In those with 'old' pain, 39% had pathology including 25% with stones in the common bile duct. In a study of 157 patients 36% presented with old and 64% with 'new' pain (Hunt & Blumgart 1982). The author has found that persistence of jaundice after cholecystectomy and exploration of the common bile duct is a particularly sinister predictor. In an experience of 215 patients with post-cholecystectomy problems eight cases (3.7%) of carcinoma of the ampulla of Vater, common bile duct, or pancreas were found and all presented with jaundice (Blumgart & McCloy 1986). However in a series of 102 patients undergoing ERCP for severe post-cholecystectomy symptoms 28% were jaundiced and 24% of these had a non-surgical cause (Ruddell et al 1980).

Patients with bile duct stasis distal to a choledochoduodenostomy or choledocho-jejunostomy—the 'sump' syndrome—often present with abdominal pain and pyrexia. Jaundice is frequently present, as are features of cholangitis and pancreatitis. A similar pattern of presentation is seen in cases of biliary-enteric fistulae.

Concurrent pancreatic disease is not uncommon (Ruddell et al 1980) but may be unsuspected at the time of cholecystectomy and pass unnoticed. However many of the cases of pancreatic disease which were recognized at operation do not have abdominal pain or signs of pancreatic malfunction and appear to remain silent (Schofield & MacLeod 1966).

INVESTIGATION AND DIAGNOSIS

Many clinicians have an ill-founded mistrust of the patient who returns with symptoms after cholecystectomy and seem reluctant to embark on a serious programme of investigations. Perhaps they feel it represents a criticism of their surgery? Yet, in all but one reported series, a significant majority of patients have definable organic disease which can reasonably account for the symptoms and most of these will benefit from appropriate treatment (see Table 55.3). Psychological disorders or psychiatric problems may be associated with post-cholecystectomy symptoms in 40–50% of cases (Christiansen & Schmidt 1971, Kakizaki et al 1976) but should only be regarded as causal after the exclusion of organic pathology.

Methods of investigation

The past two decades have witnessed a revolution in the diagnostic and imaging techniques which are now widely available for the investigation of biliary and pancreatic disorders (Ch. 25). At Manchester Royal Infirmary a modified programme of investigation (Fig. 55.3), initially developed for patients with jaundice in Glasgow and subsequently Hammersmith Hospital, London (Benjamin & Blumgart 1978), is used. Endoscopy and endoscopic retrograde cholangio-pancreatography (ERCP) play an early part in the investigative screen and a diagnostic laparotomy is not undertaken until all available information has been collated.

After a careful history and examination, routine blood tests include a coagulation screen and a full biochemical profile including liver function tests and serum amylase, which can be raised in up to 9% of cases (Hunt & Blumgart 1982). Many of the patients referred with post-cholecystectomy symptoms have already undergone many tests. However all existing records, operative notes and results of investigations are reviewed whenever possible. A surgeon's description of the cholecystectomy may give a clue to possible sites of damage to the biliary tree or other organs. Previous X-rays, including operative cholangiograms and T-tube cholangiograms are re-examined and may reveal a hitherto unsuspected diagnosis, such as common bile duct stones, strictures or tumour (Blumgart & McCloy 1985). Some patients are seen with a T-tube in site or an established fistula tract and in these cases further X-ray contrast studies are performed.

Ultrasonography

Ultrasound examination is particularly useful in the early postoperative period, when fluid collections and abscesses

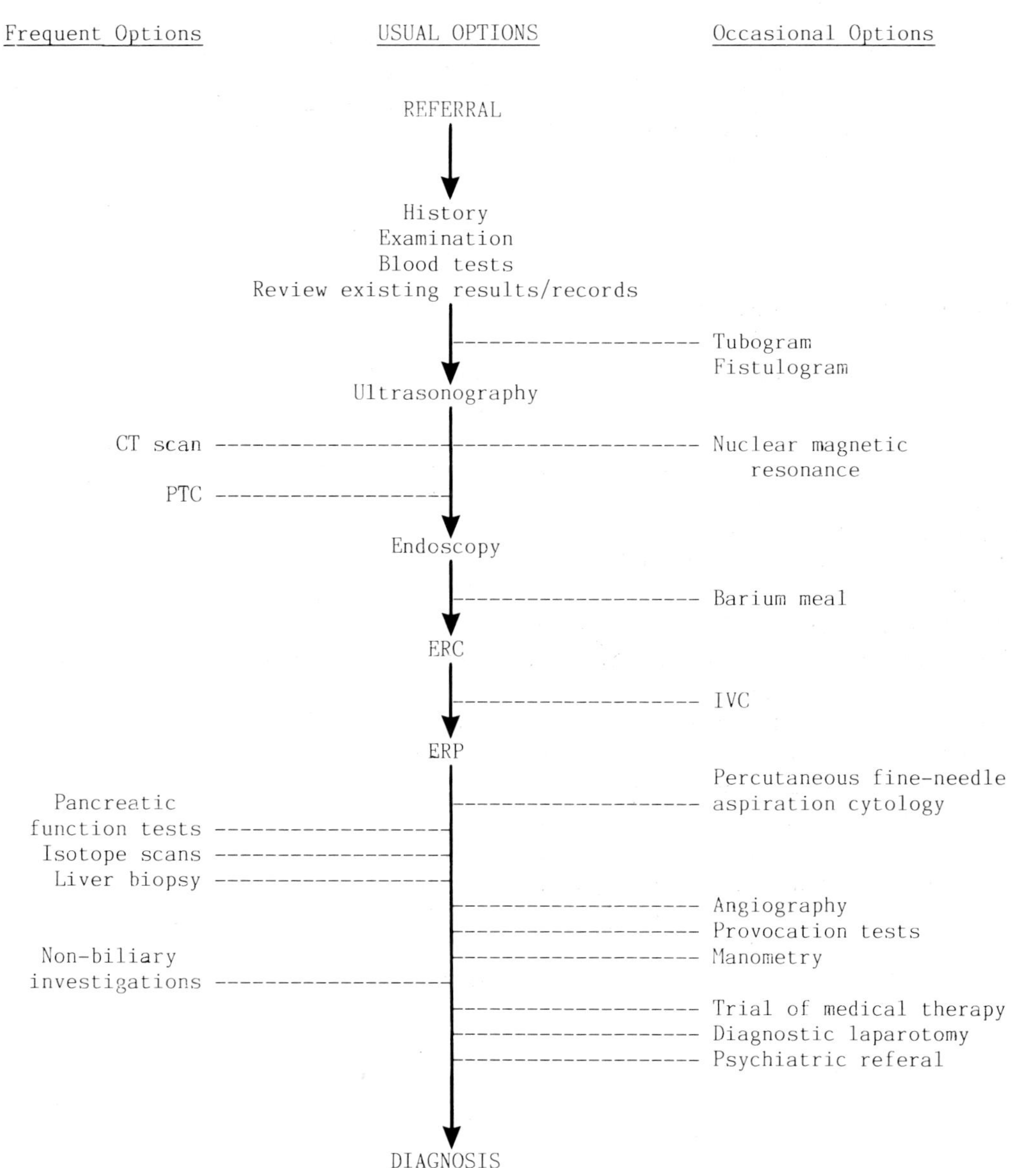

Fig. 55.3 Investigation plan for patients referred with postcholecystectomy symptoms

are reliably demonstrated and if jaundice is a presenting feature. However in patients with post-cholecystectomy problems the diameter of the extrahepatic biliary tree cannot be used as an indicator of biliary disease. After cholecystectomy the overlap in bile duct diameters between populations with and without further disease of the biliary tract makes this an unreliable discriminant for biliary lesions (Ruddell et al 1980, Hamilton et al 1982). Unfortunately ultrasound is less sensitive in identifying stones the lower they are in the biliary tree (Dewbury et al 1978) and this restricts its usefulness after cholecystectomy. However concurrent disease in the pancreas may be visualized. If abnormalities are seen on ultrasound examination then computerized tomography (CT scanning), and now nuclear magnetic resonance (NMR) in some centres, may be indicated to further define problems in the liver and pancreas. If dilated bile ducts are demonstrated by ultrasonography in jaundiced patients, then many would proceed to percutaneous transhepatic cholangiography (PTC) as the next investigational technique (Benjamin et al 1978) (Ch. 25). However in patients with post-cholecystectomy symptoms endoscopic retrograde cholangiopancreatography (ERCP) is preferred for its ability to diagnose both endoscopic abnormalities in the upper gastrointestinal tract and pancreatic disease (Hunt & Blumgart 1982, McCloy et al 1984) although both investigations may prove to be complimentary in delineating the extent and site of biliary pathology.

Endoscopy

A thorough examination of the upper gastrointestinal tract is possible with the standard side-viewing duodenoscope used for ERCP. It is even possible to view the lower end of the oesophagus with this instrument but if oesophageal varices are suspected then an end-viewing gastroscope should be passed first. A report of the endoscopic findings, including the nature of the ampulla and peri-ampullary diverticula are an important part of an ERCP in patients with post-cholecystectomy symptoms. A diagnosis on the basis of endoscopic findings alone may be made in up to 9% of cases (McCloy et al 1984) and duodenal abnormalities have been reported in 32% of patients (Hunt & Blumgart 1982). In two studies the combined experience (Hunt & Blumgart 1982, McCloy et al 1984) of 178 examinations of the ampulla in patients who have undergone cholecystectomy, have revealed that endoscopic abnormalities of the ampulla, which include redness, inflammation, oedema, and protuberance — collectively termed papillitis by many observers — correlate with abnormalities on ERCP in virtually every case. Carcinoma of the ampulla can be identified (see above) and surgical stomata inspected (see below). Upper gastrointestinal pathology is especially common in patients complaining of flatulent dyspepsia and duodenal ulceration is often found even when a previous barium meal has been reported normal. In this group of patients it is particularly useful if ERCP shows that the biliary tract and pancreas are normal and not involved.

ERCP (Ch. 20)

The majority of patients with symptoms after cholecystectomy are likely to have abnormalities within the biliary or pancreatic ductal system which can be identified by ERCP (Table 55.3) and a radiological diagnosis is obtained in the majority of cases. In all patients an attempt should be made to outline both the biliary and pancreatic duct systems. However if an abnormality has been demonstrated in either system and the diagnosis is clear cut, then prolonged attempts to cannulate the remaining duct are not always pursued. ERCP should be considered in the early postoperative period if there is obstructive jaundice without an obvious cause, a persistent biliary fistula and abscess formation or upper gastro-intestinal haemorrhage (Soehendra et al 1981). The techniques of ERCP are now standard and widely available (Ch. 20). In patients with a history which includes attacks of pancreatitis, ERCP should be preceded by an ultrasound examination to exclude pancreatic cyst or pseudocyst formation since sepsis following ERCP under these circumstances carries a high morbidity and mortality (Cotton 1977). It is our policy to use an appropriate antibiotic prophylactically as soon as pancreatic or biliary duct obstruction, irrespective of the presence of calculi, has been demonstrated (McCloy et al 1983). An update (Blumgart & McCloy 1986) of previously published figures (Hunt & Blumgart 1982) has allowed definition of the diagnosis in 93% of 75 patients undergoing ERCP for post-cholecystectomy symptoms, with only 4% failed cannulations and 3% complications. In common with other groups of workers in this field (Blumgart et al 1977, Hamilton et al 1982, Sugawa et al 1983) the author concludes that ERCP is the investigation of choice in diagnosis and management of patients with problems following cholecystectomy. It should be remembered that cholestasis may lead to changes in the pancreatogram (ERP) (Palmer et al 1984) and abnormal cholangiograms (ERC) may be observed in pancreatic disease (Warwick et al 1985) (see Fig. 55.1).

In the past intravenous cholangiography (IVC) has been a prime investigation in this group of patients. However it is valueless in the presence of jaundice and inaccurate and imprecise in many non-jaundiced patients (Blumgart et al 1975). The advantages of direct contrast examinations have been clearly established (Osnes et al 1978) and nowadays we employ IVC only on rare occasions when the biliary tree cannot be outlined by ERCP or PTC.

If a mass lesion is identified at the time of ERCP then percutaneous fine-needle aspiration cytology (Ch. 24) can be usefully employed whilst the bile or pancreatic ducts are opacified (Chia-Sing 1977) since this may improve the chances of making a positive tissue diagnosis.

Provocation tests and manometry

There are a sub-group of patients with attacks of biliary-type pain who have no demonstrable 'stenosis' (see below) of the papilla but who may have transiently abnormal liver function tests and some delay in emptying of injected contrast from the biliary tree and pancreas. This, probably heterogeneous, group of patients has been variously said to be suffering from 'biliary dyskinesia', 'biliary spasm', 'papillary dysfunction' or 'papillary stenosis' (Burnett 1984). Tests designed to raise intraductal pressure such as the morphine-prostigmine test (Nardi & Acosta 1966) and the morphine-choleretic test (Debray et al 1962) and so provoke symptoms and biochemical abnormalities have failed to become widely accepted. Results of trials with the morphine-prostigmine test have been disappointing and do not correlate with sphincter manometry and operative findings of paillary stenosis (LoGiudice et al 1979) and should not form the basis for clinical decisions (Steinberg et al 1980). The combination of the morphine-choleretic test with either dynamic hepatobiliary scintography or PTC has been claimed to identify hypertonic sphincter dysfunction as an independent clinical entity (Varro et al 1983). Pancreatic exocrine stimulation with secretin, combined with duct diameter measured by ultrasonography, has been shown to correlate with papillary stenosis at operation and may be more specific than morphine-prostigmine combined with ultrasound assessment (Warshaw et al 1985). The possibility of higher sphincter tone or phasic pressure waves rather than frank anatomical stenosis in these patients suggests that manometric techniques may be more successful in establishing not only a clinical diagnosis but the pathophysiology of this ill-defined condition (Bortolotti et al 1983). However techniques vary (Geenen 1983, Tanaka et al 1983a) and result in different relative values. Since any criterion for sphincter dysfunction available at the present time can be disputed the diagnosis must be based on the presence of more than one determinant and in practice it is difficult to meet more than one or two criteria (Sivak 1983).

Diagnostic laparotomy

When performed on the basis of symptoms alone a diagnostic laparotomy may result in an operative diagnosis but, this is frequently not the case. Indeed 46% of patients in the author's series (McCloy et al 1984) had another operation after cholecystectomy and some had up to five further surgical procedures prior to referral, resulting in frustration for the surgeon and continuing problems for the patient. Adhesions may hinder the exploration and peroperative cholangiography may be difficult to perform. Abnormalities at the site of existing surgical anastamoses cannot be readily assessed by external inspection at laparotomy. Precise information, obtained by a selected programme of investigations before operation, is essential both in the selection of the correct patients with post-cholecystectomy symptoms for operative treatment and as a guide to the surgeon during the operation (Blumgart et al 1977). A trial of medical therapy might be more appropriate, and carry less morbidity for the patient, than an ill-considered and hasty diagnostic laparotomy.

Other investigations

Isotope scans, liver biopsy and angiography all play a role in the investigational process but since the indications are similar to those in patients with biliary tract obstruction (Blumgart 1978) (Ch. 25) they will not be discussed further here. Although pancreatic function tests are negatively correlated with ERCP changes, the secretory overlap between disease groups renders the prediction of the pancreatogram appearance impractical in any individual case in whom an ERP was not obtained (Braganza et al 1982). Investigations of neighbouring organ systems, such as the colon, renal tract, heart, lungs and musculo-skeletal structures, may have to be entertained if the diagnosis proves elusive.

Diagnostic yield

Patients with post-cholecystectomy symptoms are worthy of careful investigation which will define a relevant diagnosis in 45–96% of cases (Table 55.3). Frequently, reported series represent highly selected groups of patients referred to major teaching centres (McCloy et al 1984) which might be expected to present with complex pathological problems but the incidence of pathology in patients with symptoms after cholecystectomy seen in a District General Hospital setting is also high (McCloy & Kirwan 1983). Since the advent of ERCP in the early 1970s, and the increasing accuracy of diagnostic ultrasound techniques, there has been a steady rise in the reported incidence of patients with biliary tract disease, from up to 14% in early series to 80% in recent years.

Not surprisingly, the most frequent cause of symptoms, in about one-third of cases with post-cholecystectomy symtoms, is recurrent or retained stones in the common bile duct (Ch. 46–50) and low and high bile duct strictures (Ch. 58) have a reported incidence of 0–35%.

Peri-ampullary problems

One of the recent advances in our recognition and understanding of patients with post-cholecystectomy symptoms has been the identification of peri-ampullary problems in 17–22% of cases (Table 55.3). These include papillitis,

Table 55.3 Incidence of pathology in symptomatic patients after cholecystectomy

	No. patients	% organic disease	% non-biliary disease	% pan-creatic disease	% biliary disease			% peri-ampullary problems*
					total	stone	stricture	
Burnett & Shields 1958	20	90	80	—	10	5	0	0
Schofield & MacLeod 1966	74	45	37	0	8	8	0	0
Bodvall & Övergaard 1967	764	—	—	—	9	8	—	—
Christiansen & Schmidt 1971	77	66	53	8	13	—	—	—
Stefanini et al 1974	249	—	—	0	14	9	0	6
Brandstätter et al 1976	47	66	23	—	43		—	—
Hess 1977	199	58	54	—	4	—	—	—
Ruddell et al 1980	102	51	24	21	27	23	4	0
Hamilton et al 1982	109	—	—	—	36	33	3	—
Hunt & Blumgart 1982	157	81	18	10	63	25	9	22
Sugawa et al 1983	164	73	22	17	34	28	5	17
McCloy & Kirwan 1983	21	76	5	0	71	67	0	19
McCloy et al 1984	70	96	16	4	80	35	35	19

* Peri-ampullary problems include papillitis, papillary stenosis, biliary-enteric fistulae, abnormalities of choledocho-duodenostomy (including 'sump' syndrome), ampullary tumours and low bile duct disease.

(secondary) papillary stenosis (Ch. 56), biliary-enteric fistulae and ampullary tumours. They all contribute to the incidence of low bile duct disease and concurrent pancreatic disease which is found in 0–21% of cases. Typically they are the result of surgical trauma or post-operative complications involving the biliary tree, ampulla of Vater and the pancreas (Fig. 55.4).

Biliary-enteric fistulae (Ch. 61) Spontaneous biliary-enteric fistulae due to calculous disease are most commonly cholecyst-duodenal (Glenn et al 1981) and represent a separate surgical problem (Stubbs et al 1983). After cholecystectomy, biliary-enteric fistulae are typically choledocho-duodenal, in the region of the ampulla and Vaterian segment of bile and pancreatic ducts, and may have multiple openings (Tanaka & Ikeda 1982). The most frequent cause is the spontaneous passage of stones (Tanaka & Ikeda 1982) but the relationship to iatrogenic damage to the common bile duct at the time of cholecystectomy and exploration of the biliary tree, either supra-duodenal or trans-sphincteric, as well as endoscopic sphincterotomy, is well described (Hunt & Blumgart 1980, Martin & Tweedle 1984, McCloy et al 1984, Van Linda & Rosson 1984). In the experience of Blumgart and McCloy at three centres (Glasgow, Hammersmith and Northampton) we have seen 14 cases of biliary-enteric fistulae out of 248 patients (5.7%) with post-cholecystectomy symptoms. ERCP proved a successful technique for defining this pathology and both the fistula tract and the papilla were successfully cannulated with opacification of bile and pancreatic ducts in all cases (Fig. 55.5). The typical radiological appearances may include the presence of a small 'rose-thorn' deformity at the lower end of the common bile duct (Fig. 55.6) but occasionally the fistulous tract can be gross (McCloy et al 1984). At the time of presentation of six cases of biliary-enteric fistulae all had pancreatitis, three had cholangitis and two a previous history of jaundice (McCloy et al 1984). Contrary to Martin & Tweedle (1984) who considered that in only one of their 13 patients could symptoms be directly attributed to the fistula, we considered this was the primary cause of symptomatology in all our cases.

Choledocho-duodenostomy (Ch. 54) It was first recognized in the early 1960s (Smith 1964, Stock & Fung 1964) that the blind part of the lower common bile duct below a side-

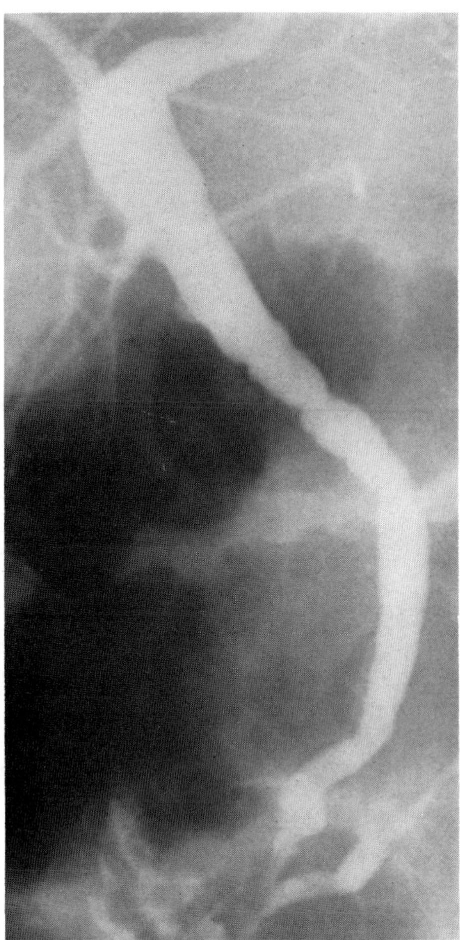

Fig. 55.4 Typical cholangitic changes in the CBD seen at ERC in a 59-year-old man following a cholecystectomy, exploration of CBD and a surgical sphincteroplasty. Deformity of the lower CBD is due to extrinsic compression by chronic pancreatitis (diagnosed on ERP)

to-side biliary-enteric anastomosis could become filled with vegetable debris and cause cholangitis and possible pancreatitis, the 'sump' syndrome. Choledocho-duodenostomy has its advocates (Degenshein 1974, Lygidakis 1981, de Almeida et al 1984) and opponents (Bodvall 1973, Jones 1973) and has recently been attracting further surgical interest (Fry 1984). The incidence of cholangitis following choledocho-duodenostomy has been reported as 0–4% (Johnson & Harding Rains 1978) and the 'sump' syndrome occurs in 5–25% of cases (Tondelli & Gyr 1978, Sugawa et al 1983). There seems little doubt that problems are unlikely if the initial stoma is more than 2.5 cm in length (Johnson & Harding Rains 1972, Degenshein 1974). However stenosis of the stoma can and does occur (Fig. 55.7) and ERCP is the investigation most suited for this problem (Reuben et al 1980). Similar 'sump' problems can occur after side-to-side choledocho-jejunostomy and other inadequate biliary-enteric anastamoses (Blumgart & Lygidakis 1983). Whether endoscopic and radiological abnormalities of the blind 'sump', including the persistence of stone, are a direct cause of the patients' pain and problems has not yet been resolved since the successes claimed for treatment (see below) remain anecdotal.

Papillary stenosis (Ch. 56) Since all the patients under consideration in this review have been submitted to previous biliary tract surgery the diagnosis of primary papillary stenosis should never be made. This distinction is often not present in reports from European centres and may account for some of the confusion over the incidence of this clinical entity. Secondary papillary stenosis has been reported in 11–17% of patients with post-cholecystectomy symptoms (Hunt & Blumgart 1982, Sugawa et al 1983). In the former series this was not an endoscopic diagnosis relying upon failure to cannulate the ampulla but based upon dilatation of the common bile duct with no other cause; additional criteria in the latter series included abnormal liver function tests and delay in drainage of contrast material from the common bile duct in excess of 45 minutes. Stenosis implies anatomical fibrosis and rigidity and it remains to be seen whether ampullary sphincter manometry (see above) can provide the objective assessment that has been lacking to date (Bodvall 1973, Tondelli & Gyr 1983).

TREATMENT, RESULTS AND OUTCOME

The successful management of residual stones in the biliary tree and benign bile duct strictures is likely to be of primary importance in the care of the majority of patients presenting with post-cholecystectomy symptoms. Detailed discussion of these important clinical problems is not entertained in this chapter, and reference should be made to Chapters 47–51. Similarly tumours of the bile ducts and ampulla, which are relatively infrequent in patients with problems after cholecystectomy, are considered further in Chapters 58 and 59. However, there are certain aspects of treating patients with peri-ampullary problems which require review since they are the subject of continuing debate and controversy.

Biliary-enteric fistulae

The treatment for biliary-enteric fistulae lies first in prevention. The morbidity of these fistulae could be avoided in many patients by the adoption of atraumatic techniques for exploring the common bile duct at the primary operation. Supraduodenal choledochotomy is the preferred approach (Blumgart & McCloy 1986) and there should be no attempts to dilate the ampulla of Vater with metal dilators or sounds from above. This is unnecessary if operative cholangiography demonstrates free-flow of contrast into the duodenum and, in the few instances where no flow is seen, a fine gum-elastic bougie or biliary balloon catheter is passed into the duodenum and the

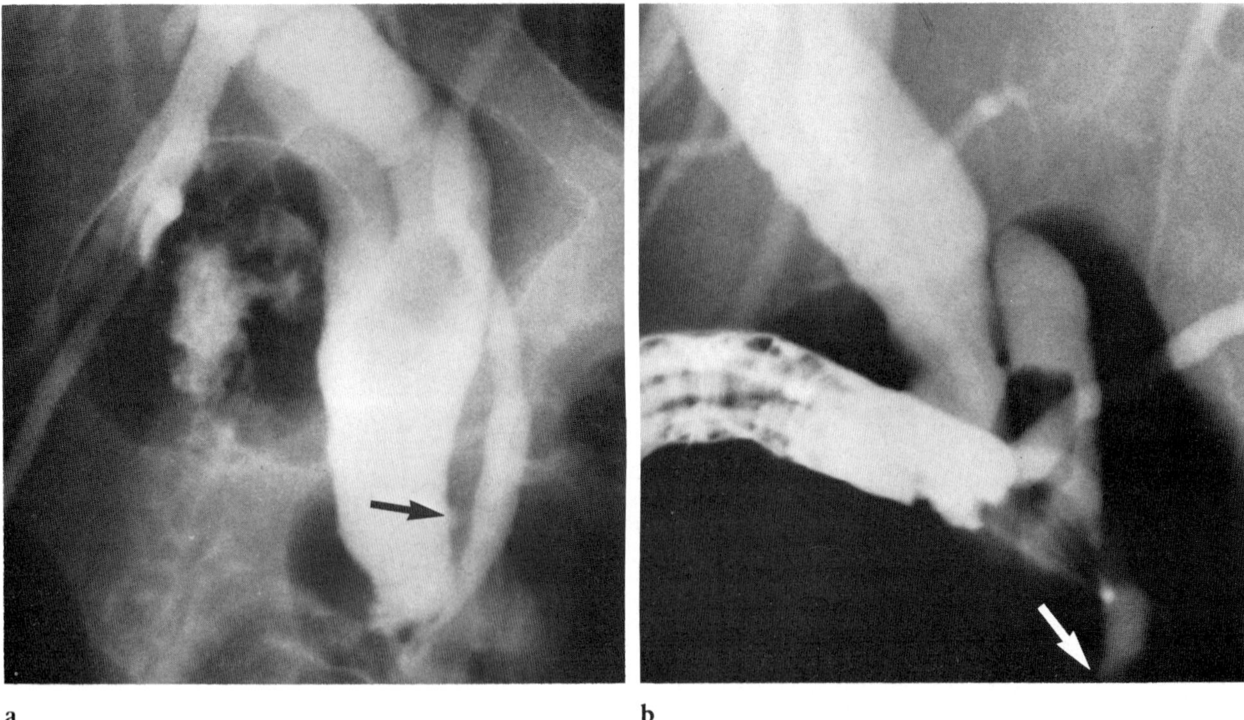

Fig. 55.5 ERCP demonstration of a biliary-enteric fistula in a woman aged 68 years, seven years post-cholecystectomy and exploration of the CBD. In (a) the site of the fistula is marked (arrow) and the ampulla has been cannulated whilst in (b) the fistula has been cannulated and the ampulla marked (arrow). A large recurrent stone, later shown to contain suture material, is seen at the origin of the low-entry cystic duct stump

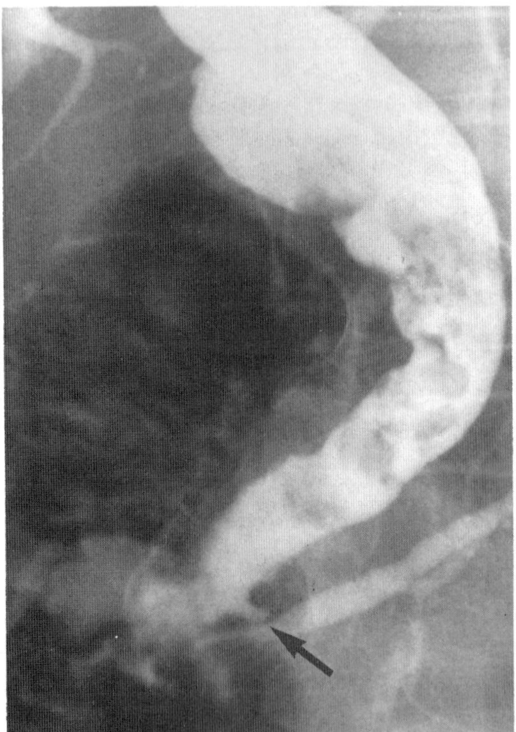

Fig. 55.6 A typical 'rose-thorn' appearance of a biliary-enteric fistula (arrowed) at the lower end of the CBD. The ERC also demonstrates multiple residual calculi, 16 years after cholecystectomy, some of which lie in a long cystic duct stump

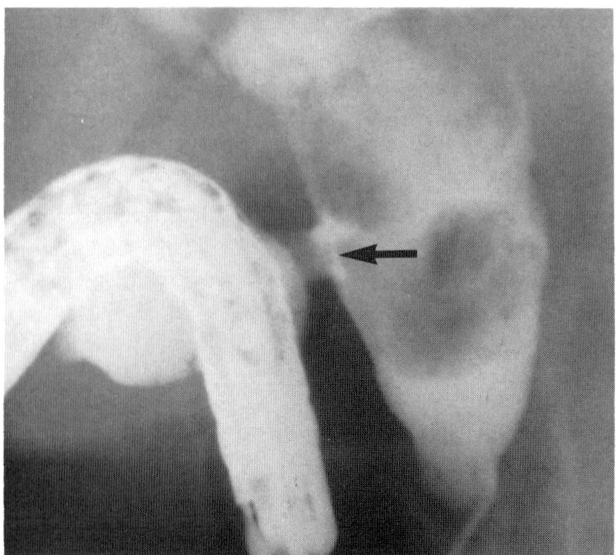

Fig. 55.7 Large stones and debris in a grossly dilated CBD diagnosed by ERCP in a 61-year-old woman, 12 years after cholecystectomy. A totally inadequate choledocho-duodenostomy stoma, performed nine years earlier for recurrent stones, is marked (arrow)

lower end of the common bile duct inspected by choledochoscopy to ensure that a peri-ampullary tumour is not missed. Any exploration of the bile ducts should be thorough, gentle, and ideally under direct vision using a choledochoscope. Rigid stone grasping forceps of the Desjardins type should be abandoned in favour of balloon and basket catheters since any rigid instrument can easily perforate the wall of the common bile duct proximal to the ampulla, produce a biliary-enteric fistula and persistent, late symptoms for the patient (Hunt & Blumgart 1980). The management of an established biliary-enteric fistula depends on its site and the problems it is causing. Martin & Tweedle (1984) described biliary-enteric fistulae opening within 1 cm of the main ampullary in 12 of their 13 cases. In six cases they joined the orifices of these fistulae to the main papillary opening by de-roofing the tract using the diathermy sphincterotome with clinical success, yet in none of these cases were symptoms directly related to the fistulae. Van Linda & Rosson (1984) report a similar success in five cases. Only one of Martin & Tweddle's cases was a more complex, symptomatic patient of the type we have previously reported (Hunt & Blumgart 1980, McCloy et al 1984). The presence of pancreatitis, cholangitis and jaundice in many of these patients presents a serious clinical picture requiring biliary bypass, either by end-to-side hepaticodocho- or choledocho-jejunostomy.

'Sump' syndrome

Madden et al (1970) challenged the traditional concept of ascending infection in the bile ducts and suggested that it was more likely that descending infection from the liver produces cholangitis if there is distal outlet obstruction. This is taken further by Jones (1973) who states that cholangitis does not occur as long as no obstruction of the common bile duct is present, and advocates surgical sphincteroplasty for patients suffering from the 'sump' syndrome following side-to-side choledocho-duodenostomy. However, even a widely-patent sphincteroplasty, in the absence of other anastomoses, has been reported as causing a form of 'sump' syndrome with the accumulation of considerable amounts of vegetable matter in the common bile duct (Blumgart 1978). Endoscopic sphincterotomy appears to be a logical treatment for the distal bile duct obstruction in this frequently high risk group of patients. As yet there is insufficient data, in a very small number of cases, to allow conclusions to be drawn as to the efficacy and safety of endoscopic sphincterotomy in patients with 'sump' problems, although the initial results are encouraging (Reuben et al 1980, Tanaka et al 1983b, Leese et al 1985). Siefert (1982) has attempted to enlarge stenotic choledocho-duodenal stomas using endoscopic techniques but severe bleeding was experienced and food debris continued to accumulate in the ducts. As with biliary enteric fistulae, a formal conversion to an end-to-side biliary bypass should be considered in selected cases.

Papillary stenosis (Ch. 56)

Sphincter of Oddi dysfunction has yet to be established as a pathophysiological entity and has been bedevilled by confused terminology (see above and Burnett 1984) and a lack of hard data. Any discussion of therapy must await more objective evidence and a better definition of this condition. Relaxation of the sphincter with nitrate therapy resulting in resolution of pain and decrease in sphincter activity was the subject of a single case-report (Bar-Meir et al 1983). Further studies are required to determine whether such a trial of therapy can distinguish between functional and organic pathology of the sphincter of Oddi. On the other hand secondary papillary stenosis, with fibrosis and scarring of the sphincter of Oddi, requires either a biliary-bypass procedure or a direct attack on the sphincter mechanism itself by endoscopic or open surgical methods. The author's preference is for the former approach and the formation of a Roux-en-Y choledocho-jejunostomy or a choledocho-duodenostomy in a high risk older patient. Biliary-bypass for papillary stenosis is not supported by Bodvall (1973) or Jones (1973). A far more radical transduodenal sphincteroplasty than that advocated by Jones is the Moody transampullary septectomy which has been used in a series of 92 patients with severe upper abdominal pain; 79 patients had a prior cholecystectomy (Moody et al 1983). The operation ablates the high pressure zone at the outlets of both the pancreatic and bile duct and one to 10 year follow-up revealed good or fair relief of pain in three-quarters of patients.

The use of endoscopic sphincterotomy (ES) has met with varying success in patients with papillary stenosis, independent of whether they had a prior cholecystectomy. The use of ERCP manometry (Bar-Meir et al 1979) and its combination with morphine provocation (Tanaka et al 1983) has improved the selection of cases. Geenen and co-workers (1984) have published the only randomized prospective study of ES for patients with presumptive sphincter dysfunction. All 45 patients in this study had unexplained biliary-type pain after cholecystectomy and one or more of the following features: a dilated CBD (> 12 mm); delayed contrast emptying at ERCP (> 45 minutes); abnormal liver function tests on two or more occasions. After ES significantly more patients were improved compared with a sham procedure (68% compared with 30%) and, if the sphincter pressure on ERCP manometry was elevated, the difference between the ES and sham groups was more marked (91% and 25% respectively). However it should be remembered that endoscopic sphincterotomy carries with it a significant morbidity and mortality which appears to be greater when the technique is used for papillary stenosis than for choledocholithiasis (Bodval 1973, Classen et al 1983). The most appropriate perspective on this controversial subject comes from Blumgart & Wood (1974) in a discussion on the use of endoscopic sphincterotomy: 'When commenting on papillary stenosis it seems reasonable to try and prevent the waves of endoscopic enthusiasm washing up on the same shore as the receding tide of surgical endeavour in the same ill-defined area'.

SUMMARY AND CONCLUSIONS

Selective investigation of patients with symptoms after cholecystectomy, especially by ultrasonograpy, endoscopy and ERCP, will provide a positive diagnosis of pathology which can account for the symptomatology in the vast majority of patients. However, in patients presenting with biliary colic or dyspepsia, particularly when these are similar in nature to the symptoms before cholecystectomy, there is often less identifiable pathology than in patients presenting with jaundice. In patients with cholangitis or pancreatitis there is likely to be a demonstrable abnormality in every case. The treatment of radiological abnormalities is usually straightforward and carries a high success rate but endoscopic abnormalities such as papillitis and papillary stenosis represent management problems. A proportion of patients with post-cholecystectomy symptoms are found to have a condition, such as pancreas divisum or peri-ampullary diverticulum (Fig. 55.8), whose precise clinical role has yet to be defined and in this group it is equally difficult to determine the most appropriate therapy. Coincidental upper gastrointestinal pathology is most frequently found in patients with persistent dyspepsia, and duodenal ulcer is not uncommon even when there has been a previously normal barium meal. In these patients ERCP plays a useful role in demonstrating that the biliary tract and pancreas are normal. In our own experience, one patient in five had peri-ampullary pathology, nearly all of which were a consequence of previous surgery or operative endoscopy, and determining a successful outcome in these patients is more problematic. Many post-cholecystectomy problems stem from misguided and inept approaches to exploration of the biliary tree at the time of primary operations for gallstones, together with failure to perform perioperative or post-exploratory cholangiography or choledochoscopy and a lack of understanding of the indications for drainage procedures of the bile ducts.

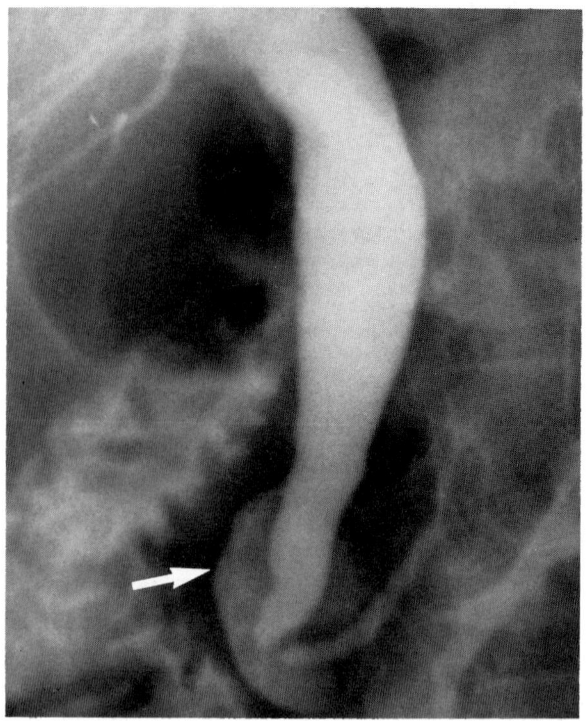

Fig. 55.8 A large peri-ampullary duodenal diverticulum (arrowed) and pancreas divisum in a woman, aged 63, presenting with acute relapsing pancreatitis after cholecystectomy

REFERENCES

Badley B W D, Murphy G M, Bouchier I A D 1969 Intraluminal bile-salt deficiency in the pathogenesis of steatorrhoea. Lancet ii: 400

Bar-Meir S, Geenen J E, Hogan W J, Dodds W J, Stewart E T, Arndorfer R C 1979 Biliary and pancreatic duct pressures measured by ERCP manometry in patients with suspected papillary stenosis. Digestive Diseases and Sciences 24: 209–213

Bar-Meir S, Halpern Z, Bardan E 1983 Nitrate therapy in a patient with papillary dysfunction. American Journal of Gastroenterology 78: 94–95

Bar-Meir S, Halpern Z 1984 The significance of the diameter of the common bile duct in cholecystectomized patients. American Journal of Gastroenterology 79: 59–60

Bates T, Mercer J C, Harrison M 1984 Symptomatic gall stone disease: before and after cholecystectomy. Gut 25: A579–60

Benjamin I S, Blumgart L H 1978 Biliary bypass and reconstructive surgery. In: Wright R, Alberti G, Karran S R, Sadler H M (eds) Liver and biliary disease: A pathophysiological approach. Saunders, London, Ch 54, p 1219–1246

Benjamin I S, Allison M E M, Moule B, Blumgart L H 1978 The early use of fine needle percutaneous transhepatic cholangiography in an approach to the diagnosis of jaundice in a surgical unit. British Journal of Surgery 65: 92–98

Blumgart L H 1978 Biliary tract obstruction: new approaches to old problems. American Journal of Surgery 135: 19–31

Blumgart L H, Sokji G S, Duncan J G 1975 Endoscopy and retrograde choledochopancreatography in the diagnosis of post cholecystectomy symptoms. Bulletin de la Societe International de Chirurgie 6: 587–591

Blumgart L H, Carachi R, Imrie C W, Benjamin I S, Duncan J G 1977 Diagnosis and management of post-cholecystectomy symptoms: the place of endoscopy and retrograde choledochopancreatography. British Journal of Surgery 64: 809–816

Blumgart L H, Wood C B 1979 Endoscopic treatment of biliary tract disease. Lancet i: 274

Blumgart L H, Lygidakis N J 1982 The post-cholecystectomy patient. In: Blumgart L H (ed) The biliary tract. Churchill Livingstone, London, ch 9, p 143–156

Blumgart L H, McCloy R F 1986 Endoscopic techniques after cholecystectomy. In: Way L W, Pellegrini C A (eds) Surgery of the gall bladder and bile ducts. Saunders, Philadelphia

Bodvall B 1964 Late results following cholecystectomy in 1930 cases and special studies on postoperative biliary distress. Acta Chirurgica Scandinavica Supplement 329: 1–155

Bodvall B 1973 The postcholecystectomy syndromes. Clinics in Gastroenterology 2(1): 103–126

Bodvall B, Övergaard B 1966 Cystic duct remnant after cholecystectomy. Annals of Surgery 163: 382–390

Bodvall B, Övergaard B 1967 Computer analysis of postcholecystectomy biliary tract symptoms. Surgery, Gynecology, and Obstetrics 124: 723–732

Bortolotti M, Caletti G C, Brocchi E et al 1983 Endoscopic manometry in the diagnosis of the postcholecystectomy pain syndrome. Digestion 28: 153–157

Braganza J M, Hunt L P, Warwick F 1982 Relationship between pancreatic exocrine function and ductal morphology in chronic pancreatitis. Gastroenterology 82: 1341–1347

Brandstätter G, Kratochvil P, Weidner F 1976 Die diagnostische bedeutung der endoskopisch retrograden cholangio-pankreatikographie beim sogenannten postcholezystektomiesyndrom. Wiener Klinische Wochenschrift 88: 806–810

Burnett D A 1984 Taking the pressure off the sphincter of Oddi. Gastroenterology 87: 971–976

Burnett W, Shields R 1958 Symptoms after cholecystectomy. Lancet i: 923–925

Cheadle W G, Pathi V, Mackie C R, Cuschieri A 1984 Effect of gall bladder function on duodenogastric reflux. Gut 25: A1138

Chia-Sing H O 1977 Percutaneous fine needle aspiration biopsy of the pancreas following endoscopic retrograde cholangiography. Radiology 125: 351

Christiansen J, Schmidt A 1971 The postcholecystectomy syndrome. Acta Chirurgica Scandinavica 137: 789–793

Classen M, Leuschner V, Schrieber H W 1983 Stenosis of the papilla Vateri and common bile duct calculi. Clinics in Gastroenterology 12(1): 203–229

Collins P G, Gorey T F 1984 Iatrogenic biliary stricture: presentation and management. British Journal of Surgery 71: 980–982

Cotton P B 1977 Progress report: ERCP. Gut 18: 316–341

Csendes A, Kruse A, Funch-Jensen P et al 1979 Pressure measurements in the biliary and pancreatic duct system in controls and in patients with gallstones, previous cholecystectomy, or common bile duct stones. Gastroenterology 77: 1203–1210

De Almeida A M, Cruz A G, Aldeia F J 1984 Side-to-side choledochoduodenostomy in the management of choledocholithiasis and associated disease. American Journal of Surgery 147: 253–258

Debray C H, Hardouin J P, Fablet J 1962 Le Test 'cholérétique — morphine'. Gastroenterology 97: 137–146

Degenshein G A 1974 Choledochoduodenostomy: an 18 year study of 175 consecutive cases. Surgery 76: 319–324

Dewbury K C, Meire H B, Husband J E 1983 Ultrasound imaging and computed tomography. In: Wright R, Alberti G, Karran S R, Sadler H M (eds) Liver and biliary disease: A pathophysiological approach. Sanders, London, ch 21, p 474–495

Dos Reis L, De Almeida C C 1981 Post-cholecystectomy jaundice due to intracholedochal blood clot. British Journal of Surgery 68: 885

Editorial 1974 Effects of cholecystectomy. British Medical Journal 1: 72–73

Fry D E 1984 Choledochoduodenostomy revisited. American Journal of Surgery 147: 304

Geenen J 1983 Direct choledochography and related diagnostic methods. Part 2: sphincter of Oddi manometry. Clinics in Gastroentrology 12(1): 108–114

Geenen J, Hogan W, Toouli J, Dodds W, Venu R 1984 A prospective randomized study of the efficacy of endoscopic sphincterotomy for patients with presumptive sphincter of Oddi dysfunction. Gastroenterology 86: 1086

Glenn F, Reed C, Grafe W R 1981 Biliary enteric fistula. Surgery, Gynecology and Obstetrics 153: 527–531

Hamilton I, Ruddell W S J, Mitchell C J, Lintott D J, Axon A T R 1982 Endoscopic retrograde cholangiograms of the normal and post-cholecystectomy biliary tree. British Journal of Surgery 69: 343–345

Hess W 1977 Nachoperationen an dem gallenwegen. Im: Praktische Chirurgie. Enke F, Stuttgart, Heft 91

Hunt D R, Blumgart L H 1980 Iatrogenic choledochoduodenal fistula: an unsuspected cause of post-cholecystectomy symptoms. British Journal of Surgery 67: 10–13

Hunt D R, Blumgart L H 1982 Endoscopic abnormalities in patients with postcholecystectomy symptoms. Surgical Gastroenterology 1: 155–158

Johnson A G 1972 Pyloric function and gall-stone dyspepsia. British Journal of Surgery 59: 449–454

Johnson A G 1975 Cholecystectomy and gallstone dyspepsia. Clinical and physiological study of a symptom complex. Annals of the Royal College of Surgeons of England 56: 69–80

Johnson A G, Harding Rains A J 1972 Choledochoduodenostomy. A reappraisal of its indications based on a study of 64 patients. British Journal of Surgery 59: 277–280

Johnson A G, Harding Rains A J 1978 Prevention and treatment of recurrent bile duct stones by choledochoduodenostomy. World Journal of Surgery 2: 487–496

Jones S A 1973 Sphincteroplasty (not sphincterotomy) in the treatment of biliary tract disease. Surgical Clinics of North America 53: 1123–1137

Kakizaki G, Kato E, Fujiwana Y, Hasegawa N 1976 Post-biliary surgery complaints. Psychosomatic aspects. American Journal of Gastroenterology 66: 62–68

Kelly C J, Blumgart L H 1985 Per-operative cholangiography and post-cholecystectomy biliary strictures. Annals of the Royal College of Surgeons of England 67: 93–95

Kelly C J, Hemingway A P, McPherson G A D, Allison D J, Blumgart L H 1983 Non-surgical management of post-cholecystectomy haemobilia. British Journal of Surgery 70: 502–504

Kingston R D, Windsor C W O 1975 Flatulent dyspepsia in patients with gallstones undergoing cholecystectomy. British Journal of Surgery 62: 231–223

Leese T, Neoptolemos J P, Carr-Locke D L 1985 Successes, failures, early complications and their management following endoscopic sphincterotomy: results in 394 consecutive patients from a single centre. British Journal of Surgery 72: 215–219

Le Quesne L P, Whiteside C G, Hand B H 1959 The common bile duct after cholecystectomy. British Medical Journal 1: 329–332

LoGiudice J A, Geenen J E, Hogan W J, Dodds W J 1979 Efficacy of the morphine-Prostigmin test for evaluating patients with suspected papillary stenosis. Digestive Diseases and Sciences 24: 455–458

Lygidakis N J 1981 Choledochoduodenostomy in calculous biliary tract disease. British Journal of Surgery 68: 762–765

McCloy R F, Kirwan M 1983 unpublished data

McCloy R F, Jaffe V, Blumgart L H 1984 Endoscopy and postcholecystectomy problems. In: Salmon P R (ed) Gastrointestinal endoscopy, Advances in diagnosis and therapy, vol 1. Chapman & Hall, London, ch 18, p 199–206

McCloy R F, Wood C B, Blumgart L H 1983 Surgical endoscopy. In: Goldsmith H S (ed) Practice of surgery. Harper & Row, Philadelphia, ch 26

Madden J L, Chun J Y, Kandalaft S, Parekh M 1970 Choledochoduodenostomy: an unjustly maligned surgical procedure? American Journal of Surgery 119: 45

Maingot R 1956. In: Rob C, Smith R (eds) Operative surgery, vol 2. Butterworths, London, p 390

Martin D F, Tweedle D E F 1984 The aetiology and significance of distal choledochoduodenal fistula. British Journal of Surgery 71: 632–634

Meguid M M, Aun F, Bradford M L 1984 Adenomyomatosis of the gallbladder. American Journal of Surgery 147: 260–262

Moody F G, Becker J M, Potts J R 1983 Transduodenal sphincteroplasty and transampullary septectomy for postcholecystectomy pain. Annals of Surgery 197: 627

Nardi G L, Acosta J M 1966 Papillitis as a cause of pancreatitis and abdominal pain. Annals of Surgery 164: 611–618

Nora P F, Davis R P, Fernandez M J 1984 Chronic acalculous gallbladder disease: a clinical enigma. World Journal of Surgery 8: 106–112

Osnes M, Larsen S, Lowe P et al 1978 Comparison of endoscopic retrograde and intravenous cholangiography in diagnosis of biliary calculi. Lancet ii: 230

Palmer K R, Cotton P B, Chapman M 1984 Pancreatogram in cholestasis. Gut 25: 424–427

Price W H 1963 Gall-bladder dyspepsia. British Medical Journal 2: 138–141

Reuben A, Jourdan M H, Isaacs P E T, McColl I 1980 Spontaneous closure of choledochoduodenostomy: diagnosis by endoscopy and ERCP. British Journal of Surgery 67: 283–286

Ruddell W S J, Ashton M G, Lintott D J, Axon A T R 1980 Endoscopic retrograde cholangiography and pancreatography in investigation of post-cholecystectomy patients. Lancet i: 444–447

Schofield G E, MacLeod R G 1966 Sequelae of cholecystectomy. British Journal of Surgery 53: 1042–1045

Siefert E 1983 Endoscopy and biliary disease. In: Blumgart L H (ed) The biliary tract. Churchill Livingstone, London, ch 4, p 61–81

Sivak M W 1983 How good is the manometric evidence for postcholecystectomy dyskinesia? Gastrointestinal Endoscopy 2: 134–136

Smith R 1964. In: Smith R, Sherlock S (eds) Surgery of the gall-bladder and bile ducts. Butterworths, London, p 297

Soehendra N, Kempeneers I, Eichfuss H P, Reynders-Frederix V 1981 Early post-operative endoscopy after biliary tract surgery. Endoscopy 13: 113–117

Stefanini P, Carboni M, Patrassi N, Loriga P, De Bernardinis G, Negro P 1974 Factors influencing the long term results of cholecystectomy. Surgery, Gynecology and Obstetrics 139: 734–738

Steinberg W M, Salvato R F, Toskes P P 1980 The morphine-Prostigmin provocative test — is it useful for making clinical decisions? Gastroenterology 78: 728–731

Stock F E, Fung J H Y 1964. In: Smith R, Sherlock S (eds) Surgery of the gall-bladder and bile duct. Butterworths, London, p 318

Stubbs R S, McCloy R F, Blumgart L H 1983 Cholelithiasis and cholecystitis: surgical treatment. Clinics in Gastroenterology 12(1): 179–201

Sugawa C, Clift D, Walt A J 1983 Endoscopic retrograde cholangiopancreatography after cholecystectomy. Surgery, Gynecology and Obstetrics 157: 247–251

Tanaka M, Ikeda S 1982 Multiple choledochoduodenal fistulas in the periampullary region. Endoscopy 14: 200–202

Tanaka M, Ikeda S 1983 Parapapillary choledochoduodenal fistula: an analysis of 83 consecutive patients diagnosed at ERCP. Gastrointestinal Endoscopy 29: 89–93

Tanaka M, Ikeda S, Nakayama F 1983a Continuous measurement of common bile duct pressure with an indwelling microtransducer catheter introduced by duodenoscopy: new diagnostic aid for postcholecystectomy dyskinesia — a preliminary report. Gastrointestinal Endoscopy 29: 83–88

Tanaka M, Ikeda S, Nakayama F 1984 Change in bile duct pressure responses after cholecystectomy: loss of gallbladder as a pressure reservoir. Gastroenterology 87: 1154–1159

Tanaka M, Ikeda S, Yoshimoto H 1983b Endoscopic sphincterotomy for the treatment of biliary sump syndrome. Surgery 93: 264

Tondelli P, Gyr K, Stalder G A, Allgower M 1979 The biliary tract. Clinics in Gastroenterology 8(2): 487–505

Tondelli P, Gyr K 1983 Postsurgical syndromes. Clinics in Gastroenterology 12(1): 231–254

Valberg L S, Jabbari M, Kerr J W et al 1971 Biliary pain in young women in the absence of gall stones. Gastroenterology 60: 1020–1026

Van Linda B M, Rosson R S 1984 Choledochoduodenal fistula and choledocholithiasis: treatment by endoscopic enlargement of the choledochoduodenal fistula. Journal of Clinical Gastroenterology 6: 321–324

Varro V, Dobronte Z, Hajnal F et al 1983 The diagnosis of hypertonic Oddi's sphincter dyskinesia. American Journal of Gastroenterology 78: 736

Warshaw A L, Simeone J, Schapiro R H, Hedberg S E, Mueller P E, Ferrucci J T 1985 Objective evaluation of ampullary stenosis with ultrasonography and pancreatic stimulation. American Journal of Surgery 149: 65–70

Warwick F, Anderson R J L, Braganza J M 1985 Sclerosing-cholangitis-like changes in pancreatic disease. Clinical Radiology 36: 51–56

Watson P, Love H G 1984 Gastric emptying in patients with flatulent dyspepsia, with and without gall bladder disease. Gut 25: A1137

56

P. Tondelli, J. P. Schuppisser

Papillary stenosis

INTRODUCTION

The nature of benign papillary stenosis, which Del Valle and Donovan in their original description in 1926 called 'papillitis stenosans', has remained controversial. While surgeons on the European continent appeared somewhat over enthusiastic in diagnosing and treating papillary stenosis the condition was declared non-existent and papillotomy considered an unnecessary if not criminal procedure by most of their Anglo-Saxon colleagues. The authors agree that the incidence of papillary stenosis might be a topic for discussion but that there is no doubt as to its existence.

The problem is well demonstrated by the case history of a 50-year-old lady whose history began in 1964. At that time she underwent cholecystectomy for stones without cholangiography or common duct exploration. The initial postoperative course was uneventful but after 1970 she suffered from repeated bouts of upper abdominal pain and jaundice due to cholangitis. In 1980 these attacks became more frequent and in 1981 she was admitted with acute pancreatitis. Evaluation at this time included intravenous cholangiogram which revealed a distended common bile duct without stones. Endoscopic retrograde cholangiography (ERC) and endoscopic papillotomy (EP) was then planned, papillary stenosis being suspected. It was however not possible to cannulate the common bile duct for which reason the patient was referred for surgery.

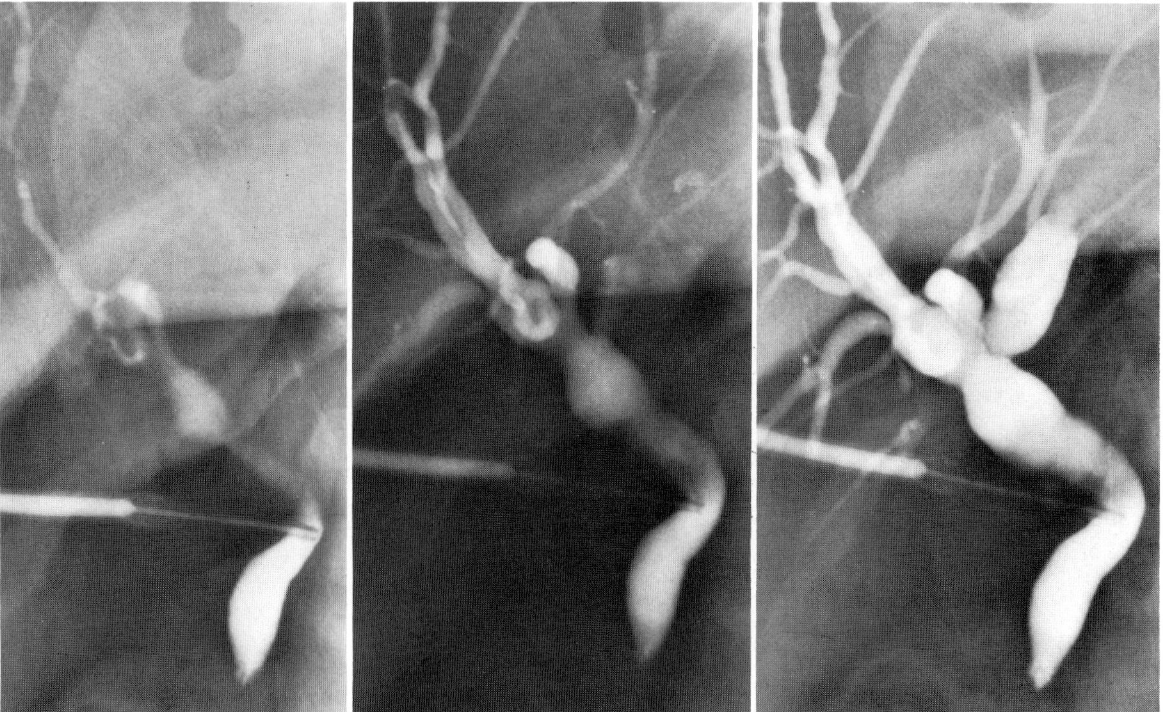

Fig. 56.1 Intraoperative pressure controlled cholangiogram. Papillary stenosis: no flow of contrast medium to the duodenum on the radiographs taken at a pressure of 14, 20 and 30 cm of water

Operative findings included a wide common bile duct without stones and in the pressure controlled cholangiogram no flow of dye into the duodenum at pressures of 14, 20 and 30 cm of contrast medium (Fig. 56.1). Transpapillary flow at a pressure of 30 cm of dye was zero and after application of CCK 6 ml/min which is clearly less than the minimally expected 14 ml/min. In addition it was not possible to pass a rubber catheter which measured 3 mm in diameter through the papilla. Transduodenal papilloplasty was then performed excising a specimen for histological examination. Microscopic examination revealed marked chronic inflammation with sclerosis of the papilla. The patient has been asymptomatic since the operation. This case clearly demonstrates the existence of papillary stenosis. The existence of this condition is especially obvious in those patients with postcholecystectomy symptoms who do not have common duct stones or pancreatic pathology and who are cured by papillotomy. Before endoscopic papillotomy was possible these patients had to be re-operated on but recent publications document the efficacy of endoscopic papillotomy (Safrany 1977, Seifert et al 1982, Viceconte etal 1981). One must admit however that in the endoscopically treated group an unknown number of patients with functional motility disorders of the papilla and no organic obstruction is included. In addition there is no representative specimen for histological examination obtained in this group, and final proof of papillary stenosis is therefore lacking.

DEFINITION

Papillary stenosis may be defined as follows:

An *obstructing* disease of the papilla
1. which is organic (excluding functional motility disorders);
2. which is benign and histologically consists of severe inflammation, fibrosis and sclerosis or hyperplasia, i.e. adenomyomatosis (excluding stones and tumours);
3. which causes symptoms (dyspepsia and mild pain, or severe pain, possibly with jaundice, cholangitis and pancreatitis) by impeding the passage of bile and pancreatic juice.

The problem with this definition is the lack of generally accepted criteria. The criteria for the diagnosis of an obstruction at the papilla vary widely and so do the frequencies of diagnosis of this disease in the literature.

FREQUENCY

The reported frequency of stenosis of the papilla varies from nil to 40% of all cholecystectomies (Arianoff 1968, Fernandez-Cruz et al 1977, Larrieu & Benoit 1978, Tondelli & Allgöwer 1980). In the authors' series from 1968 to 1975, papillary stenosis was diagnosed in 4.6%; today using CCK to differentiate between functional and organic obstruction, the frequency of diagnosis has dropped to 2.3% (Table 56.1, 56.7). Similarly, the frequency with which papillary stenosis is reported to cause postoperative syndromes also varies. Before endoscopic papillotomy was possible these patients were re-operated. In a series of 131 biliary re-operations in 10 years the authors found papillary stenosis as sole pathology in 15 patients (11%) (Bordley & White 1979, Gregg et al 1980, Stefanini et al 1974, Tondelli et al 1982). The reported frequency varies from 10% to 39%. As mentioned the lack of a clear and generally accepted quantitative definition and standardized diagnostic approach may account for this discrepancy as well as regional differences in patients and referral practices in different areas and hospitals.

The influence of the intraoperative diagnostic procedure on the frequency of the diagnosis of papillary stenosis is well demonstrated in a study recently performed in Switzerland (Tondelli 1983). In two years (1980/1981) papillary stenosis was diagnosed intraoperatively in 231 of 6912 (3.3%) consecutive biliary tract operations performed in the 21 major surgical departments (A-Kliniken) of Switzerland. This rate varied according to the intraoperative diagnostic procedure from 0.9% to 6.9% (Table 56.2).

Table 56.1 Papillary stenosis: frequency and diagnosis

3365 operations between 1968–1982 (cholecystectomy, re-operation) at the Department of Surgery, University Hospital, Basel/Switzerland	
1968–1975 (8 years) pressure controlled cholangiography	97 2106 = 4.6%
1976–1982 (7 years) flow measurement, CCK test	29 1259 = 2.3%
total 1968–1982 (15 years)	126* 3365 = 3.7%

* a histological examination was performed in 39/126 cases		
inflammation, fibrosis	9/39	23%
sclerosis	22/39	56%
adenomyomatosis	8/39	21%

AETIOLOGY

Primary papillary stenosis, which is an entity of its own, has to be differentiated from secondary papillary stenosis. This latter is a result of several primary pathological conditions (see also Fig. 56.2).

Primary papillary stenosis

Primary papillary stenosis is a rare condition. It is only diagnosed if the biliary tree, the pancreas and the

Table 56.2 Frequency of papillary stenosis in correlation with intraoperative diagnostic procedure
Survey in Switzerland 1980/1981

Intraoperative test	Frequency of papillary stenosis in all biliary tract operations (cholecystectomy, re-operation)
Syringe cholangiography	
without pharmacological test	16/1733 = 0.9%
with pharmacological test	13/1490 = 0.9%
Pressure controlled cholangiography	
without pharmacological test	56/ 919 = 6.1%
with pharmacological test	70/1010 = 6.9%
Pressure controlled cholangiography and flow	
without pharmacological test	57/ 899 = 6.3%
with pharmacological test	19/ 807 = 2.4%
Total	231/6912 = 3.3%

duodenum are free of disease. It can nevertheless not reliably be differentiated from secondary papillary stenosis: despite the presence of gallstones papillary stenosis could have pre-existed and caused biliary lithiasis as a result of stasis. Presumably primary papillary stenosis on the other hand could have been caused by passage of a small solitary stone.

The pathogenesis of primary papillary stenosis is largely unknown. One explanation is the occurrence of hyperplastic changes as is seen in adenomyomatosis.

Secondary papillary stenosis

Secondary papillary stenosis is more often the result of disease of the biliary tree than of a pancreatic or duodenal pathology. As mentioned before it is not always possible to separate cause and effect in relation to biliary calculi.

Papillary stenosis and cholelithiasis This represents by far the most frequent combination. Biliary calculi may be found in the gallbladder only or may coexist in the common bile duct. Papillary stenosis is most likely the result of direct mechanical trauma from passing stones. Subsequent scarring of the papilla eventually causes obstruction.

Papillary stenosis and pancreatic or duodenal pathology Pancreatitis and duodenal ulcer may involve the papillary region and result in stenosis.

Papillary stenosis secondary to surgical exploration Probing of the papilla with rigid instruments may injure the tissue and cause stenosis by scarring.

Relative incidence of the various types of papillary stenosis

The authors' experience supports the general opinion that primary papillary stenosis is a rare disease (Arianoff 1968). Secondary papillary stenosis is most often (86%) caused by biliary calculi and occurs with stones in the gallbladder only or when stones are present in the common bile duct with similar frequency (Table 56.3). In the experience of other authors the most frequent aetiology of secondary papillary stenosis is iatrogenic and due to previous surgical probing of the papilla (Blumgart 1978, Hunt & Blumgart 1980, McCloy et al 1982).

PATHOLOGY

In the original description of Del Valle inflammatory

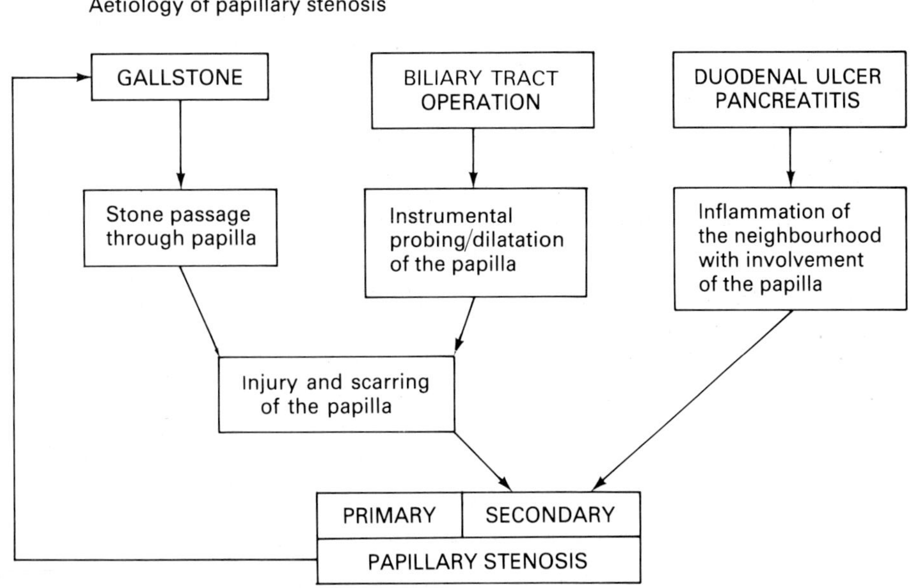

Fig. 56.2 Aetiology of papillary stenosis

Table 56.3 Underlying pathology in papillary stenosis
126 cases 1968–1982 Department of Surgery, University Hospital, Basel/Switzerland

Gallstones present			86%
in gallbladder	59/126	47%	
in gallbladder and common duct	49/126	39%	
No gallstones			14%
chronic pancreatitis	10/126	8%	
other pathology	7*/126	5.5%	
no pathology (primary papillary stenosis?)	1/126	0.5%	
total	126/126		100%

* 7 cases with *other pathology*:
re-operation after cholecystectomy and common duct exploration (instrumental probing, dilatation of the papilla): 4
history of typical colic in the upper abdomen (migration of a solitary small stone?): 3

changes were most prominent, for which reason it was named 'papillitis stenosans'. Numerous subsequent investigations of peroperative biopsies and post mortem specimens have also revealed hyperplastic changes (Acosta & Nardi 1966, Födisch 1972, Roux et al 1959, Stolte 1979):

Inflammation Various stages of acute (oedema, infiltration with leucocytes) and chronic (fibrosis, sclerosis (Fig. 56.3)) inflammation.

Hyperplasia Mucosal hyperplasia exclusively, a combination of mucosal and muscular hyperplasia: adenomyomatosis.

Mixed types

Problems with the definition of papillary stenosis exist also from a pathological point of view.

Normal histology of the papilla

It is difficult to define what the normal papilla looks like. If normality corresponds with the morphological findings of specimens from people less than 20 years of age then the papillae of people more than 20 years old will reveal pathological findings in 50% of the cases (Födisch 1972). The diagnosis of papillary stenosis cannot therefore be based exclusively on histological appearance.

Relation between histology and aetiology of papillary stenosis

The microscopic appearance of papillary stenosis will not permit its allocation to any one particular aetiology. Although a connection of primary papillary stenosis and adenomyomatosis is very likely other hyperplastic and inflammatory changes are found in primary as well as the different types of secondary papillary stenosis.

Relation between histology and degree of stenosis

There is no correlation between the histological appearance and the degree of stenosis. But histological changes are always found in specimens obtained from patients who fulfilled the peroperative criteria for papillary stenosis.

Reversibility of histological changes

This is a very important question with regard to secondary papillary stenosis. Does treatment of the biliary pathology alone result in disappearance of the papillary obstruction? To date a firm answer cannot be given. Although acute

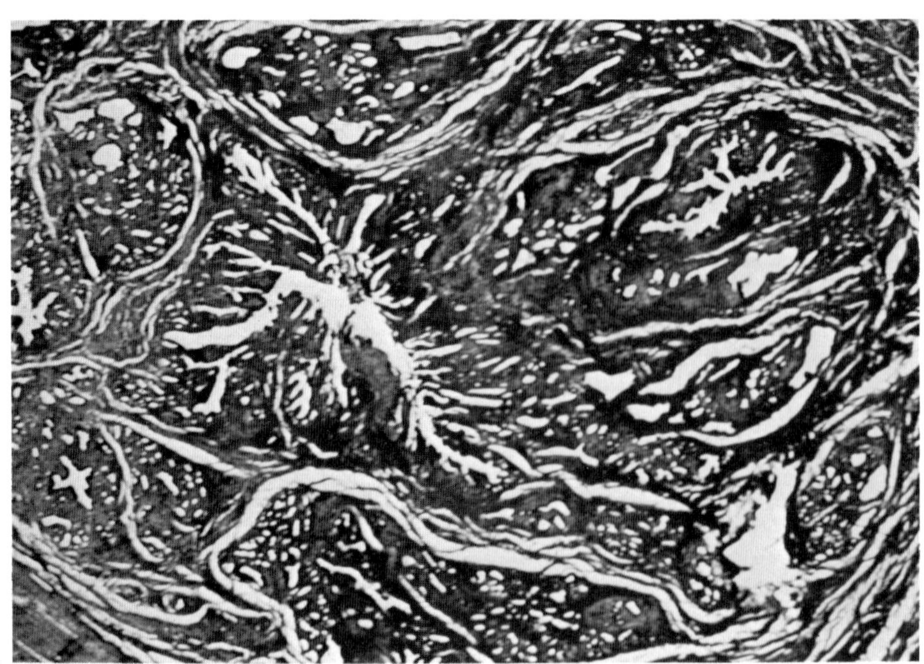

Fig. 56.3 Papillary stenosis: histology of sclerosis

inflammatory changes are likely to be reversible, this is not true for fibrosis, sclerosis and hyperplasia. Only a randomized prospective study using a properly defined diagnosis and long-term follow-up could establish criteria allowing the peroperative judgement of reversibility.

DIAGNOSIS

Preoperative examinations

If symptoms occur in a patient who has already had his gallbladder removed the indication for another operative procedure will depend on the findings of the ERCP. Inability to cannulate the papilla, an enlarged common duct (>12 mm) and delayed emptying of contrast from the common duct may be indicative of papillary stenosis as well as an elevated alkaline phosphatase. These criteria are quite subjective and tend to be interpreted on an individual basis. Recently developed methods allow objective data to be obtained by endoscopic manometry of the sphincter of Oddi but as yet this is not a routine procedure (Toouli 1984). However it has not been possible to establish values of sphincteric pressure consistent with the diagnosis of papillary stenosis. Intravenous cholangiogram is only performed when ERCP fails and is not conclusive for papillary stenosis. The same is probably true for the function test described by Nardi. For this provocation test morphine (10 mg i.v.) is administered leading to an additional papillary spasm and evoking the typical symptoms, possibly with an associated rise of hepatic enzymes (Anderson et al 1985, Gregg et al 1977, Nardi 1973, Steinberg et al 1980).

Whether the test described by Warshaw (Warshaw et al 1985) which assesses a dilatation of the pancreatic duct by ultrasonography after administration of Secretin (1 μg/kg i.v.) will improve preoperative diagnosis of papillary stenosis still needs further evaluation.

Intraoperative examination before opening the common duct (Fig. 56.10)

If on the other hand papillary stenosis exists in a patient with cholelithiasis and an intact gallbladder, the symptoms are usually attributed to gallstones. For this reason papillary stenosis has to be sought intraoperatively. This is especially true for patients referred for operation with sonography as the only preoperative examination. The intraoperative examinations consist of:
cholangiography
flow measurement
pharmacological test of papillary function.

Cholangiography

If cholangiography is performed *manually* through a catheter in the cystic duct connected to a syringe, judgement of papillary patency relies on the radiographic diameter. Such evaluation is unreliable because, with an anatomically measured diameter of 1–2 mm, the papilla is normally very narrow (Fig. 56.4). Due to peristaltic changes it may even appear occluded (Fig. 56.5). The diameter of a normal papilla may therefore easily simulate papillary stenosis on the cholangiogram. Indeed the authors reviewed the operative notes of patients who underwent common duct exploration. In 148 records the surgeon noted a narrow, stenotic papilla on the intraoperative cholangiogram. This diagnosis was later, after opening the common duct and probing the papilla, shown to be wrong in 62 out of 148 cases, i.e. 42%. Probes with a diameter greater than 2 mm easily passed the papilla.

For many years *pressure controlled cholangiography* (Tondelli & Allgöwer 1980) has been used in the Department of Surgery, Basle, in order to obtain objective infor-

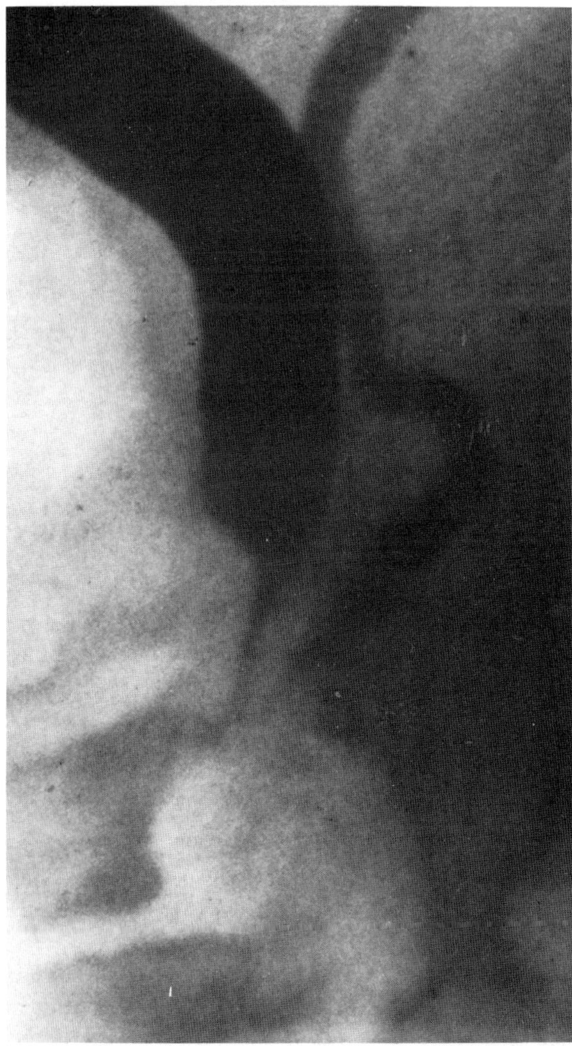

Fig. 56.4 Anatomy of the papilla. Large and narrow (sphincter) segment of the common duct

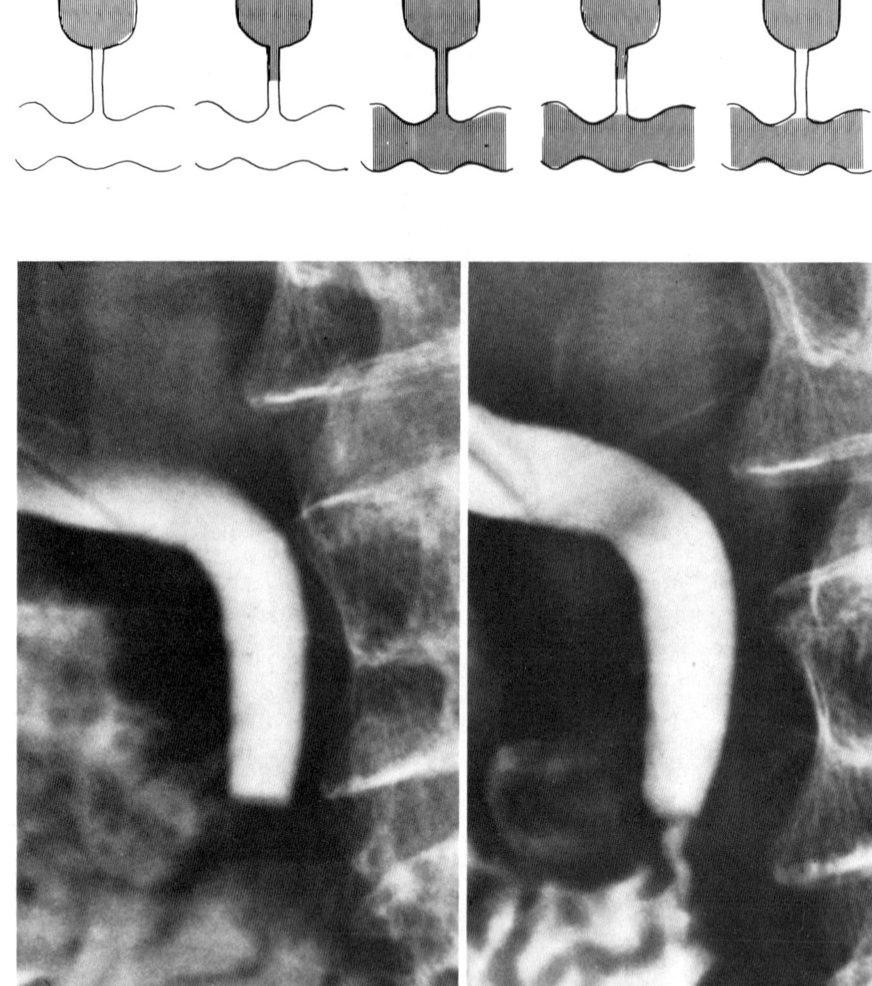

Fig. 56.5 Papillary peristalsis. a. Opening of the narrow (sphincter) segment of the common duct from proximal to distal, closing in the opposite direction. b. Cholangiography demonstrates opening

mation about the papilla. Pictures are taken at pressures of 14, 20 and 30 cm of contrast medium. For this purpose we have designed an apparatus which is a modification of the original described by Caroli (Fig. 56.6). The main component is a vertically mobile syringe. It is constructed so that a constant pressure can be maintained despite a falling fluid level. Passage of contrast into the duodenum is expected to occur at a pressure of 20 cm of contrast medium at the most and accordingly papillary stenosis is diagnosed if this is not observed (Fig. 56.7, 56.8). Between 1968 and 1975 the authors diagnosed papillary stenosis in this manner in 97 out of 2106 biliary tract operations (4.6%) (Table 56.1, 56.7). Pressure controlled cholangiography includes pressure measurement. The only well defined pressure value is the residual pressure (Tondelli & Allgöwer 1980), i.e. the pressure in the common duct when the flow of dye through the papilla falls to zero. X-ray shows that the residual pressure is just below the pressure at which the first evidence of dye is seen in the duodenum.

If an *image intensifer* is used, observation of papillary peristalsis can be another criterion in addition to the above-mentioned criteria on the X-ray film. Evident peristalsis excludes papillary stenosis. The absence of papillary peristalsis on the other hand is of relative value only; peristalsis is not always visible in the normal papilla.

Flow measurement

More recently the authors have relied more heavily on observations of flow (Tondelli & Allgöwer 1980) as a diagnostic aid in papillary disorders. With the same apparatus the quantity of contrast flowing into the duodenum within one minute at a constant pressure of 30 cm of contrast

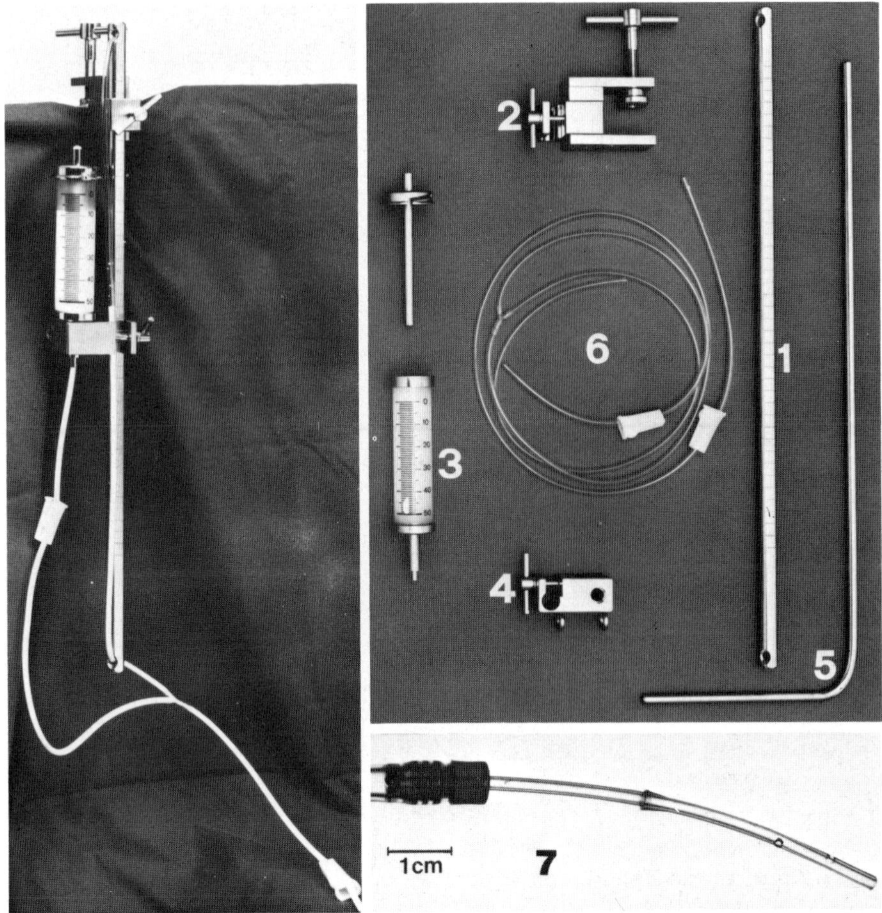

Fig. 56.6 Debitomanometer: apparatus for intraoperative pressure controlled cholangiography and flow measurement. The parts are easy to dismantle and to clean. The whole tubing system including the catheter for cannulation of the cystic duct are of plastic and disposable

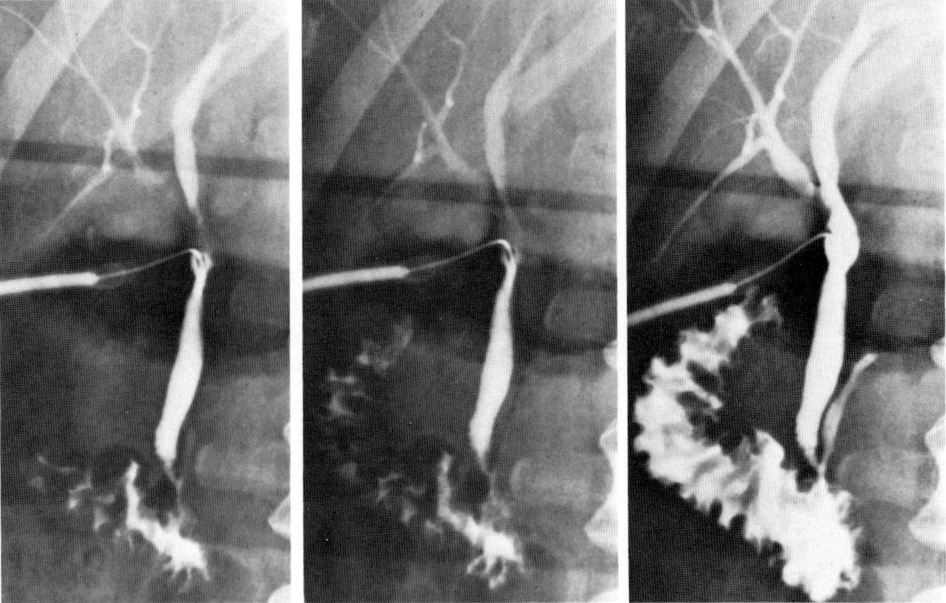

Fig. 56.7 Intraoperative pressure controlled cholangiogram: normal papilla. Flow of contrast medium to the duodenum on the radiographs taken at a pressure of 14, 20 and 30 cm of water

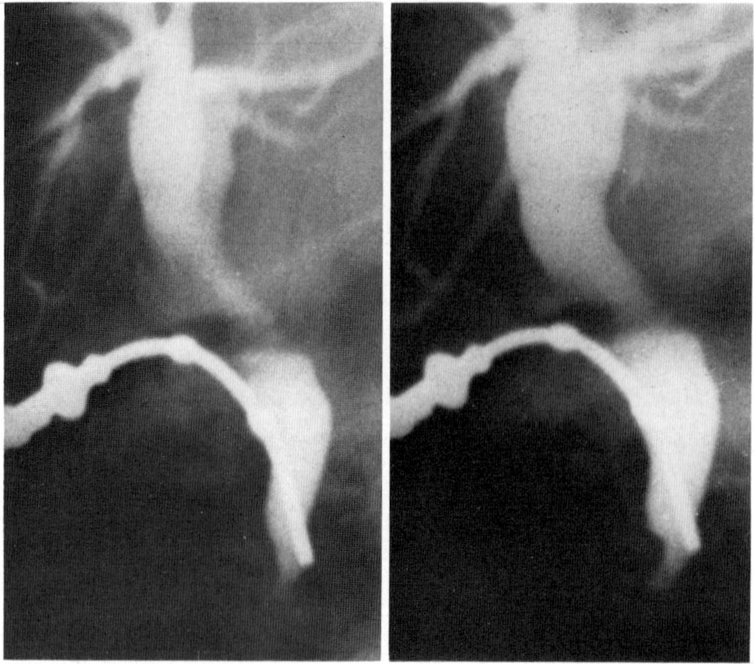

Fig. 56.8 Intraoperative pressure controlled cholangiogram: papillary stenosis. No flow of contrast medium to the duodenum on the radiographs taken at a pressure of 20 and 30 cm of water

medium is measured. This quantity is defined as standard flow. The papillary diameter is proportional to the flow value and inversely proportional to the square root of the pressure used. In an experimental model with glass capillaries of different diameters it was determined that a diameter of 0.5 cm corresponds with a flow of 14 ml/min. In a series of 152 cholecystectomies the mean standard flow was 26 ± 9 ml/min corresponding with a functional papillary diameter of 0.6–0.7 mm. The normal value for standard flow was then defined as greater than 14 ml/min corresponding with a normal value of the functional papillary diameter as greater than 0.5 mm (Table 56.4).

Using these two measurements, i.e. *pressure controlled cholangiography and standard flow*, the authors have tested their accuracy in diagnosing papillary obstruction in a combined retrospective and prospective analysis of 193 cases with papillary stones and stenosis (Table 56.5). Papillary stenosis was proved by the inability to pass a catheter with a diameter of 3 mm through the papilla. Histological confirmation was obtained in most of these cases. The accuracy of pressure controlled cholangiography alone was felt to be unsatisfactory with 80% and 85% in the prospective and retrospective parts of the study respectively and accordingly some small papillary stones and some papillary stenoses were missed. The addition of standard flow improved the diagnostic accuracy to 96%. In the prospective series, seven additional papillary obstructions were found: four stones and three histologically confirmed stenoses.

Table 56.4 Flow before and after pharmacological test with CCK
Department of Surgery, University Hospital, Basel/Switzerland

Papilla	Number of patients	Flow in ml/min	
		before CCK	after CCK
Normal	152 (73%)	26 ± 9	30 ± 9
Functional obstruction (spasm)	40 (19%)	9 ± 3	24 ± 6
Organic obstruction (stone, stenosis)	17 (8%)	3 ± 3	4 ± 6
total	209 (100%)		

Table 56.5 Accuracy of pressure controlled cholangiography and flow measurement in the intraoperative diagnosis of papillary obstruction (stone, stenosis)
Department of Surgery, University Hospital, Basle/Switzerland

	Retrospective study $n = 147$		Prospective study $n = 46$	
	False negative	Accuracy rate	False negative	Accuracy rate
Pressure controlled cholangiogram	22/147	85%	9/46	80%
Additional flow measurement	—	—	2/46	96%

Pharmacological papillary function test

One other important aspect of performing flow measurements concerns the possibility of differentiating between merely *functional spasm* and organic obstruction by the administration of CCK (Schuppisser et al 1981). In a prospective study of 209 procedures on the biliary tree this pharmacological test was performed with the following results (Table 56.5): In 152 cases (73%) standard flow was normal, i.e. more than 14 ml/min at the initial examination. Application of CCK resulted in an insignificant increase from 26 to 30 ml/min. In 57 cases (27%) standard flow was initially subnormal but increased markedly in 40 cases after application of CCK, i.e. from 9 to 24 ml/min (Fig. 56.9). In the other 17 cases CCK did not influence standard flow, i.e. 3 ml/min before and 4 ml/min after application. Accordingly these 17 cases underwent papillotomy and an organic obstruction was found in every single case: ten stones and seven stenoses. This type of functional evaluation has resulted in a decreased rate of papillotomy for papillary stenosis from 4.6% of all biliary procedures between 1968 and 1975 to 2.3% in the years 1976 to 1982 (Table 56.1, 56.7).

Two problems of intraoperative examinations before opening the common duct must be considered:

1. In about 40% of cases papillary stenosis and common duct stones coexist. If the common duct is obstructed by the stones the above criteria with regard to papillary patency are of course not applicable.

2. Reversible and irreversible papillary pathology cannot reliably be differentiated although clinical circumstances may serve as a clue: acute inflammatory conditions, e.g. acute cholecystitis, may result in coexistent oedema and thus reversible papillary stenosis which does not require surgical treatment.

Intraoperative examinations after opening the common duct and the duodenum respectively (Fig. 56.10)

If during cholecystectomy papillary obstruction is diagnosed by cholangiography, flow measurement and pharmacological testing of papillary function, the common duct has to be explored. Papillary stenosis is then confirmed by

1. probing of the papilla
2. histology of the papilla.

Probing of the papilla

Probing of the papilla is a relatively crude manoeuvre which easily injures this delicate structure. In addition a false passage may be created. It is, on the other hand, the only available diagnostic tool with regard to papillary stenosis, if obstructing common duct calculi are present, because pressure controlled cholangiography and flow measurement are not reliable after removal of the stones. Surgical manipulation of the common duct results in spasm and oedema of the sphincter which cannot be modulated pharmacologically. This situation corresponds with the one encountered at peroperative T-tube cholangiography which, after common duct exploration, will only rarely show passage of contrast into the duodenum. If it is necessary to probe the papilla, the authors prefer to use a rubber catheter. Compared with the metallic probe, it carries less risk of injury and its passage into the duodenum is assured by irrigation. If the irrigation fluid does not reappear at the choledochotomy site, passage of the catheter tip into the duodenum is proven (Fig. 56.11).

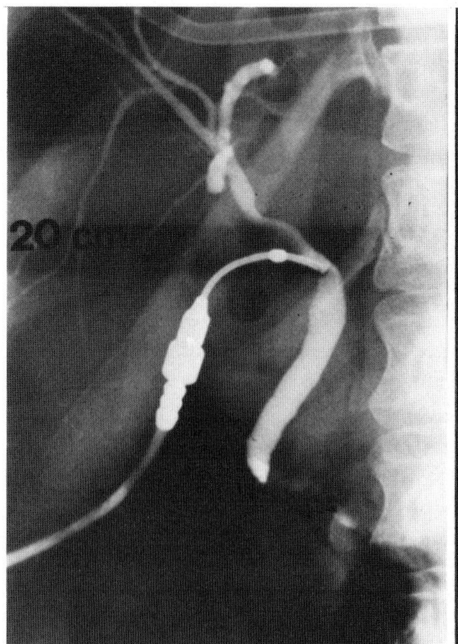

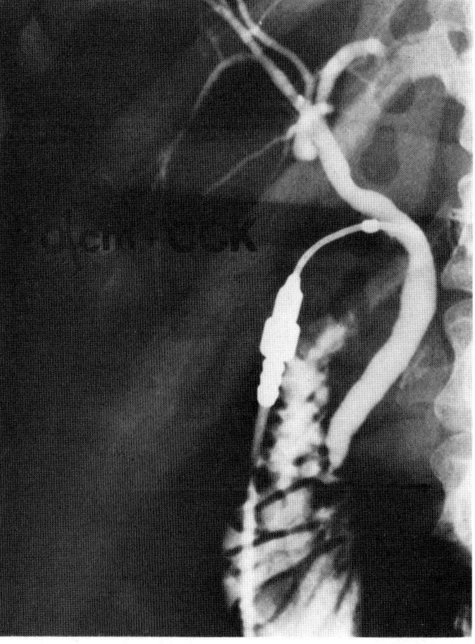

Fig. 56.9 Intraoperative pressure controlled cholangiograms: papillary spasm. No flow of contrast medium to the duodenum on the radiographs taken at a pressure of 20 cm of water. Good flow after application of CCK 100 Units intravenously

Intraoperatively during cholecystectomy

BEFORE OPENING COMMON DUCT

1. pressure controlled cholangiography: no flow into duodenum at pressure 20 cm contrast medium
2. flow measurement: < 14 ml/min. at pressure 30 cm contrast medium
3. CCK-test: no normalization of above results

AFTER OPENING OF COMMON DUCT

1. calibration of the papilla: catheter with diameter ≦ 3 mm does not pass

AFTER THERAPY (PAPILLOTOMY, PAPILLOPLASTY)

1. histological examination: fibrosis, sclerosis, adenomyomatosis

Postoperatively after cholecystectomy

ERCP

1. enlarged common duct > 12 mm?
2. delayed emptying of contrast medium into duodenum?
3. cannulation of papilla not possible

MANOMETRY

?

Fig. 56.10 Diagnosis of papillary stenosis

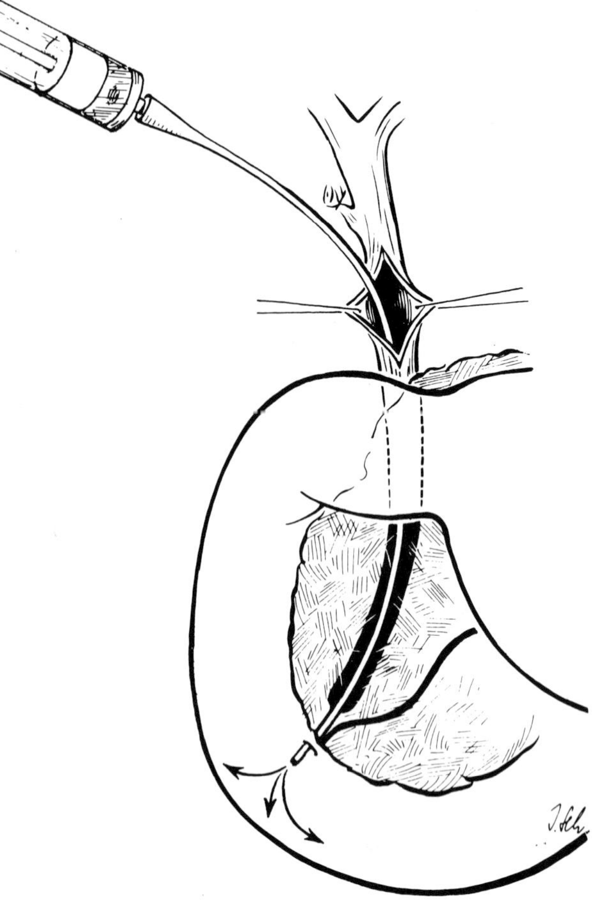

Fig. 56.11 Probing the papilla. The passage of the rubber catheter into the duodenum is assured by irrigation

The minimal outer diameter of a catheter which should be able to pass the papilla is considered to be 3 mm by various authors (Acosta & Nardi 1966, Anderson et al 1985, Arianoff 1968, Braasch & McCann 1967). If, due to insufficient catheter stiffness, cannulation of the papilla from above is not successful, then the last resort consists of opening the duodenum and passing a stiff calibrated probe under visual control in order to either confirm or rule out papillary stenosis.

Histology

The value of peroperative biopsy is diminished by the fact that often only the very tip of the papilla or even the duodenal mucosa are biopsied. In addition, microscopic morphology cannot be used to draw conclusions about the degree of narrowing of the papilla. Histology is therefore not considered helpful in deciding for or against papillotomy. Frozen section of a specimen obtained by choledochoscopy may represent a rare exception. All other attempts at biopsy require incision of the papilla.

THERAPY

Treatment of papillary stenosis during cholecystectomy (Fig. 56.12)

If papillary stenosis is diagnosed intraoperatively transduodenal papillotomy or papilloplasty respectively are the procedures of choice. Papillotomy consists of simple division of the sphincter. Papilloplasty adds suturing of duodenal to choledochal mucosa to this division. The length of the stenotic sphincter dictates the length of the incision. Partial division of the sphincter without severing the proximal parts is the rule. Complete division of the sphincter necessarily involves the posterior duodenal wall. We do not recommend dilatation of the papilla and choledochoduodenostomy as alternative procedures. Papillotomy is ineffective in the treatment of a long papillary and choledochal stricture due to pancreatitis or if the common duct is dilated more than 15 mm. Due to technical

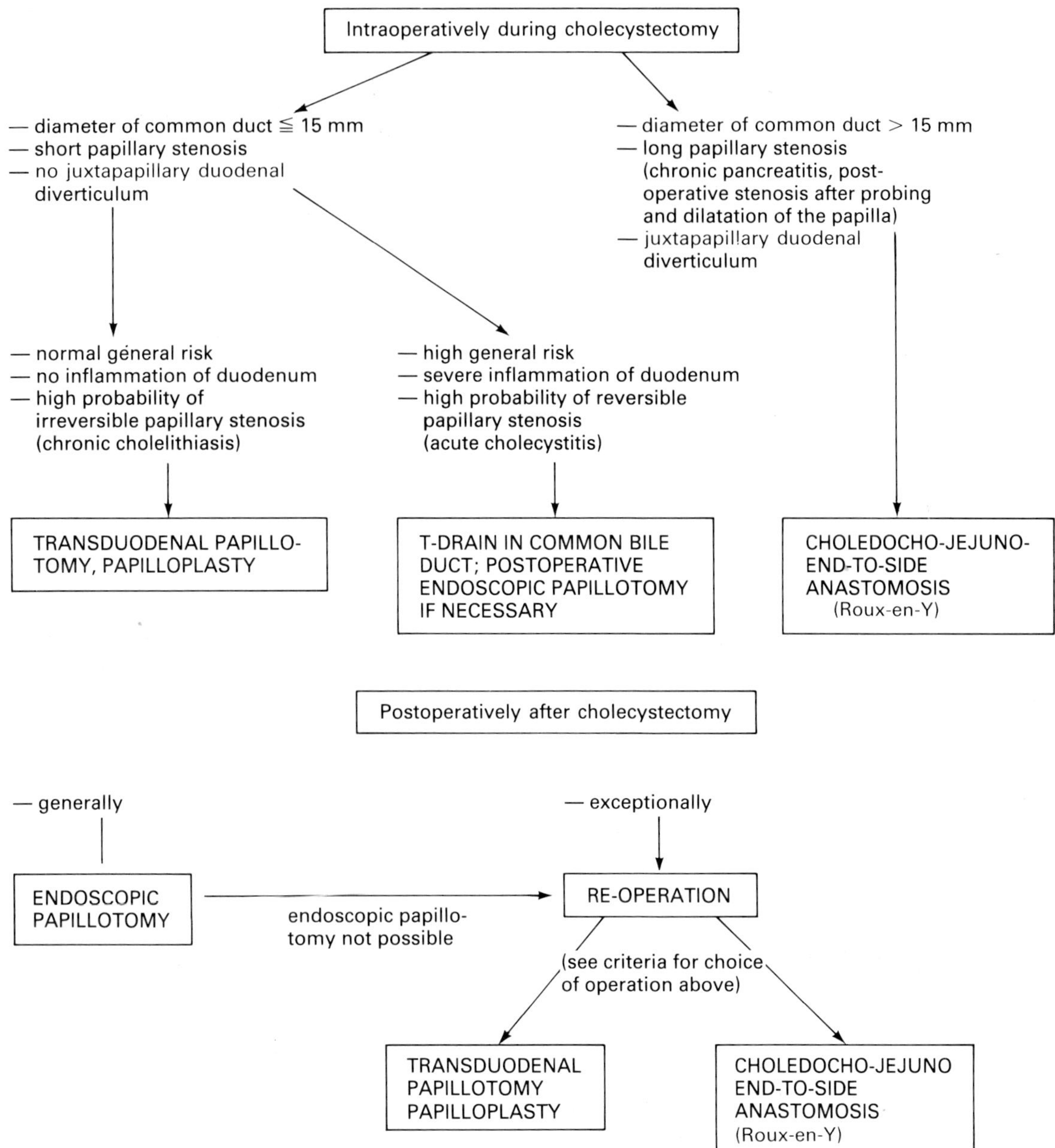

Fig. 56.12 Therapy of papillary stenosis

difficulties papillotomy is dangerous to perform in the presence of a duodenal diverticulum in the immediate vicinity of the papilla. In these cases end-to-side choledochojejunostomy using a Roux-en-Y jejunal loop is the most suitable procedure. Some surgeons advocate T-tube drainage of the common duct only if the papilla is found to be stenotic intraoperatively. They argue that they cannot discriminate reversible from irreversible papillary obstruction. If a stenosis of the papilla is confirmed at postoperative T-tube cholangiography, endoscopic papillotomy is recommended. The authors disagree with this procedure for the following reasons: By using the diagnostic criteria outlined above the rate of papillotomy/papilloplasty has dropped to 2–3% of all cholecystectomies. It is thus unlikely that patients are unnecessarily exposed to the additional risk of an extended operation on the biliary tree. In addition, if papillary stenosis is present, endoscopic papillotomy is technically successful in only 60 to 80% and its mortality exceeds 1% (Seifert et al 1982) under these circumstances. The authors therefore accept endoscopic alternatives only if surgical papillotomy is fraught with prohibitive local or systemic risk and if the likelihood of reversibility of the stenosis is overwhelming (e.g. in acute cholecystitis).

Treatment of papillary stenosis after cholecystectomy (Fig. 56.12)

If papillary stenosis is recognized as the cause of post-cholecystectomy symptom, we consider endoscopic papillotomy as the first therapeutic choice (Pitt 1984, Safrany 1977, Seifert et al 1982, Viceconte et al 1981). The only reason to prefer operation is a lengthy stricture mainly encountered after previous common duct surgery and not suitable for endoscopic papillotomy. The choice of the operative procedure then depends on previously discussed criteria.

Alternative procedures

Dilatation of the papilla

Dilatation is performed by passing metallic probes of gradually increasing diameter through the papilla until a desired diameter is reached. Although some authors employ this manoeuvre routinely or at least as an alternative procedure in the treatment of papillary stenosis, we regard this forceful rupture as dangerous. It not only carries the risk of creating a false passage but restricture due to scarring is likely to occur. For this reason we prefer deliberate surgical section of the papilla (Blumgart 1978, Hunt & Blumgart 1980, McCloy et al 1982) and have reserved transpapillary probing for diagnostic purposes only.

Side-to-side choledocho-duodenostomy

The main arguments for side-to-side choledocho-duodenostomy instead of papillotomy have traditionally been the technical ease with which it can be performed and its low morbidity/mortality. Mainly as a result of a low incidence of postoperative pancreatitis and decreasing mortality after papillotomy, this reasoning is no longer valid. Side-to-side choledocho-duodenostomy has been called into question by some authors in recent years because of its long-term complication. The so-called sump syndrome is reported to occur in 5–25% of cases (Classen et al 1979, Hoerr & Hermann 1973, Siegel 1981, White 1973) although others report good results. The procedure only bypasses the obstacle, leaves the pancreatic duct obstructed and gives rise to a choledochal 'blind sac' between the anastomosis and papilla where refluxed food is retained or recurrent stones formed. This may lead to pain. In addition the sludge may obstruct the anastomosis intermittently and may lead to jaundice and cholangitis. In the authors' view the indication for this procedure should be restricted to palliation of jaundice in tumour patients with a limited life expectancy and when the gallbladder cannot be used for biliary digestive anastomosis.

End-to-side choledocho-duodenostomy

Although this procedure does not create a blind pouch it nevertheless leaves the pancreatic duct obstructed. In addition reflux is the rule. Although the long-term significance of this is uncertain, the authors regard it as an argument against end-to-side choledocho-duodenostomy and do not employ this procedure in the treatment of papillary stenosis.

Techniques of transduodenal papillotomy and papilloplasty

Exploration of the common bile duct

Localization of the papilla of Vater (Fig. 56.13)

A Fogarty biliary catheter with an outer diameter of 2 mm is advanced into the duodenum. The balloon is inflated with 1 ml of air and the catheter withdrawn up to the point of firm resistance. The balloon is now situated at the papilla and can be felt through the duodenal wall. Compared with the use of metallic probes this procedure has no risk of perforation and localizes the papilla reliably.

Opening the duodenum

The duodenal wall is incised transversely for a length of 2 cm at the location where the balloon is palpable.

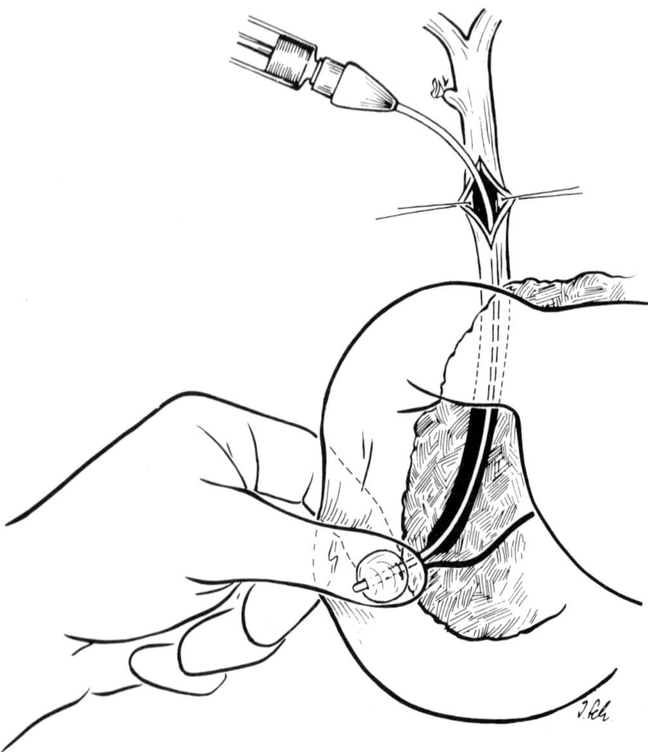

Fig. 56.13 Transduodenal papillotomy. Localization of the papilla with a Fogarty biliary catheter

Presentation of the papilla

As a rule we advance a probe with a stepwise, increasing diameter (step-probe) (Fig. 56.14) through the papilla as with the Fogarty catheter (Fig. 56.15). If the papilla is too narrow to allow passage of the smallest diameter probe, the probe is withdrawn and the manoeuvre repeated with the Fogarty catheter. A thread is attached to its tip and then

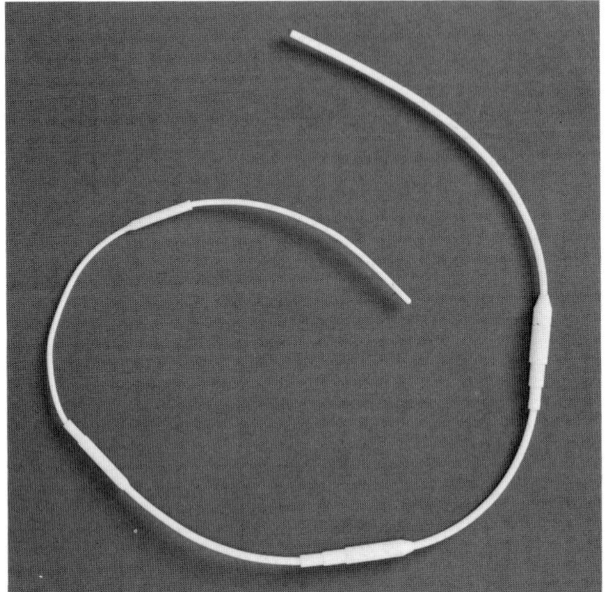

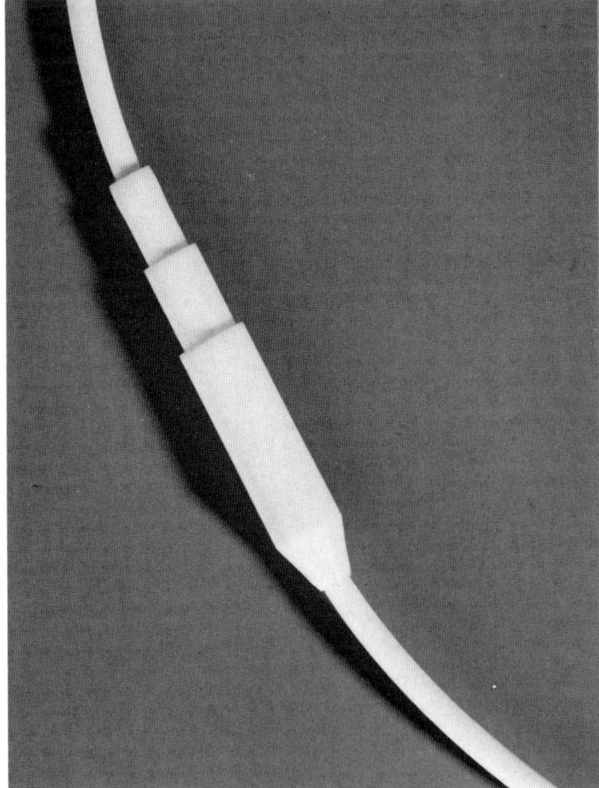

Fig. 56.14 Transduodenal papillotomy. Probe with stepwise increasing diameter (step probe) for presentation and incision of the papilla

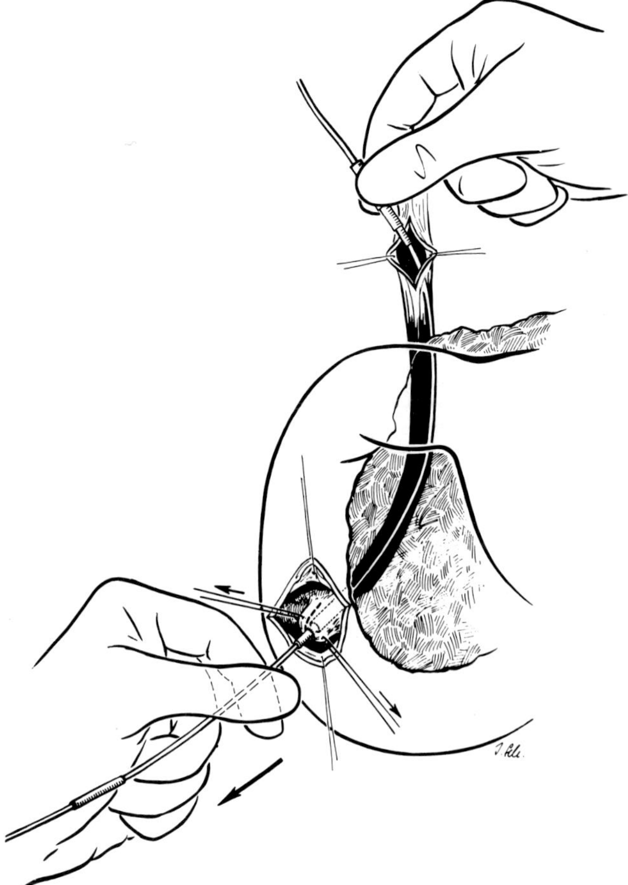

Fig. 56.15 Transduodenal papillotomy. With the help of a transpapillary probe (step probe) the papilla is exposed

it is pulled back until the thread is retrievable at the site of choledochotomy. The thread is sutured to the tip of the probe which is then gently pulled through the papilla. The papilla will resist the passage of the next step of the probe. By slight traction on the tip of the probe, the papilla can easily be delivered into full vision and accessibility. If of course the papilla is too narrow for even the Fogarty catheter, the papilla will have to be identified from the duodenal side exclusively.

Papillotomy, papilloplasty

Stay sutures are placed laterally to the tip of the papilla and held with fine clamps. The papilla is incised towards the right of the midline in a 45° angle between cephâlad and strictly lateral (Fig. 56.16). This direction is recommended because it carries least risk of injury to the duct of Wirsung. Stepwise incision of the papilla and placement of atraumatic 4–0 absorbable sutures through mucosa of duodenum and common duct is carried out. These sutures are not tied but held with fine clamps. The incision proceeds until the largest diameter of the probe which

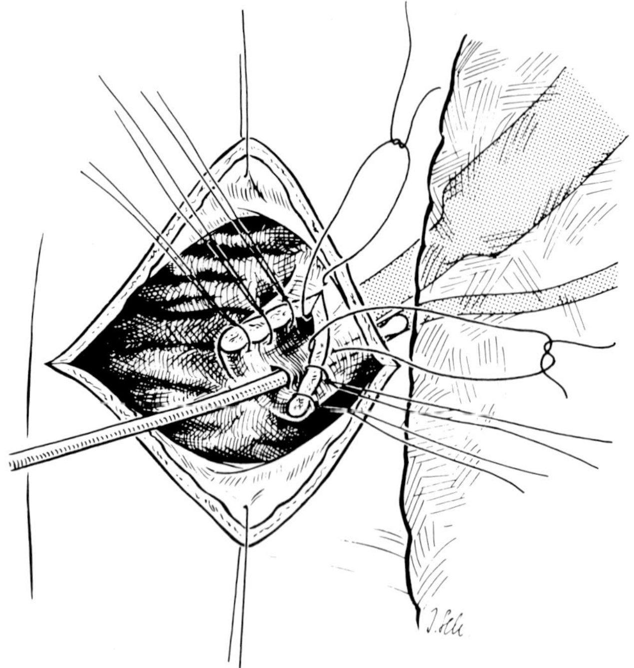

Fig. 56.16 Transduodenal papillotomy and papilloplasty. With the help of a transpapillary probe (step probe) the papilla is incised (papillotomy). Choledochal and duodenal mucosa are approximated with fine sutures once the opening of the pancreatic duct is identified (papilloplasty)

Table 56.6 Results of papillotomy/papilloplasty
Department of Surgery, University Hospital, Basle/Switzerland

Early results: 318 cases 1968–1982		mortality	
Specific complications		5/318	1.6%
acute pancreatitis	2 (0.6%)		
bleeding of incised papilla	1		
leak of duodenal suture	2		
General complications		8/318	2.5%
total		13/318	4.1%

Long-term results
223 cases 1968–1975, 131 re-evaluated 1 to 9 years after operation by clinical examination, laboratory investigation and ERCP

excellent	103/131	78.5%
good	22/131	17.0%
bad*	6/131	4.5%

* six cases with bad long-term results	
common duct stone	4
common duct stricture by chronic pancreatitis	1
no biliary pancreatic pathology	1

measures 5 mm passes through the papilla. The probe is then removed and the orifice of the pancreatic duct identified. Visualization can be helped by injecting 100 μg Secretin intravenously which results in a relatively copious secretion of clear pancreatic juice. The previously placed sutures may only be tied if identification of the pancreatic duct orifice is successful and the duct is therefore not at risk of being incorporated into one of the sutures. If the orifice cannot be identified the sutures are removed and the procedure terminated as a simple papillotomy.

Completing the operation

The duodenotomy is closed with single seromuscular sutures and the common duct is always drained with a T-tube. A T-tube cholangiogram is obtained before closing the abdomen.

Results of transduodenal papillotomy and papilloplasty

Early results

Operative mortality, which in the recent literature is given as 0–10%, depends mainly on the selection of patients (Anderson et al 1985, Lygidakis 1982, Moody et al 1983, Pitt et al 1981). Mortality in the authors' series was 4.1% (Table 56.6); 2.5% were due to nonspecific complications which occur after upper abdominal procedures of any kind and 1.6% were thought to be directly related to papillotomy. The indication for papillotomy and papilloplasty in these patients is shown in Table 56.7. Acute pancreatitis, haemorrhage and dehiscence of the duodenotomy closure are the most frequent local complications of papillotomy. Retroduodenal abscess and duodenal stenosis are seen less often. Severe acute pancreatitis after papillotomy is not a specific complication of this procedure but also occurs after common duct exploration alone. It has to be differentiated from an asymptomatic rise in serum amylase and lipase which are observed in up to 20% of cases. Frequency of severe pancreatitis with high mortality occurs in 1–2%. In our series the incidence was only 0.6% (Table 56.6). Atraumatic operative technique, identification of the pancreatic duct orifice and omission of transpapillary drainage will help to avoid this feared complication.

Late results

Long-term results after papillotomy are good: postoperative symptoms occur in only 1.5% to 5% of patients (Anderson et al 1985, Kozloff & Joseph 1975, Moody et al 1983, Stefanini et al, 1974). Residual papillary stenosis due to incomplete incision or recurrent papillary stenosis due to secondary accretion are the main causes of post-surgical symptoms. In our experience recurrent stenosis may be prevented by papilloplasty. In contrast to papillotomy (simple incision of the papilla) secondary accretion of the incised duodenal mucosa occurs rarely after papilloplasty (incision of the papilla plus suture of the choledochal and duodenal mucosae). Duodeno-biliary reflux may be a sequela of papillotomy. It occurs when a sphincter muscle is split over its whole length. Aerobilia

Table 56.7 Frequency and indications for papillotomy, papilloplasty Department of Surgery, University Hospital, Basle/Switzerland

3365 cases 1968–1982 (cholecystectomy, re-operation)

	incarcerated papillary stone	papillary stenosis	other indication	total
1968–1975 (8 years)	87/2106 = 4.1%	97/2106 = 4.6%	39/2106 = 1.9%	223/2106 = 11%
1976–1982 (7 years)	39/1259 = 3.1%	29/1259 = 2.3%	27/1259 = 2.1%	95/1259 = 7.5%
1968–1982 (15 years)	126/3365 = 3.7%	126/3365 = 3.7%	66*/3365 = 2%	318/3365 = 9.5%

* 66 cases with other indication:

suspicion of papillary stone	21
suspicion of papillary stenosis	33
suspicion of papillary tumour	12

is then found on the plain abdominal X-ray film and the duodeno-biliary pressure gradient determined by endoscopic manometry is abolished. This reflux however has no clinical significance as long as it is not combined with bile stasis (see choledocho-duodenostomy side-to-side). On the other hand splitting of the whole muscle is rarely indicated. Incision of the papilla over the length necessary to extract an incarcerated stone or to split the stenotic part is sufficient. In this case postoperative pressure and flow measurement show nearly normal function of the papilla. In the patients we studied good long-term results were found in 95.5% of the patients from one to nine years after the operation (Table 56.6) (Tondelli et al 1978).

REFERENCES

Acosta J M, Nardi G L 1966 Papillitis. Archives of Surgery 92: 354–361

Anderson T M, Pitt H A, Longmire W P 1985 Experience with sphincteroplasty and sphincterotomy in pancreatobiliary surgery. Annals of Surgery 201: 399–406

Arianoff A 1968 La Sphincterotomie de l'Oddi en Chirurgie Biliaire. Arscia, Brussels

Blumgart L H 1978 Biliary tract obstruction — new approaches to old problems. American Journal of Surgery 135: 19–31

Bordley J, White T T 1979 Causes of 340 reoperations on the extrahepatic bile ducts. Annals of Surgery 189: 442–446

Braasch J W, McCann J C 1967 Normal luminal size of choledocho-duodenal junction as determined by probe at choledochostomy. Surgery 62: 258–259

Classen M, Ossenberg F W, Schreiber H W 1979 The biliary tract II. Papillotomy and bilio-digestive anastomosis. Clinics in Gastroenterology 8: 506–524

Del Valle D, Donovan R 1962 Coledoco-Odditis retractil cronica concepto clinico y quirurgico. Arch. Argent. em Farm. Apar. Digest. 1: 605

Fernandez-Cruz L, Palacin A, Pera C 1977 Benign strictures of the terminal common bile duct In: Delmont J (ed) The sphincter of Oddi. S. Karger, Basel, 137–144

Födisch H J 1972 Normale und pathologische Anatomie. Heft 24: Feingewebliche Studien zur Orthologie und Pathologie der Papilla Vateri. Thieme, Stuttgart

Gregg J A, Taddeo A E, Milano A et al 1977 Duodenoscopy and endoscopic pancreatography in patients with positive morphine prostigmine tests. American Journal of Surgery 134: 318–321

Gregg J A, Clark G, Barr C, McCartney A, Milano A, Volcjak C 1980 Postcholecystectomy syndrome and its association with ampullary stenosis. American Journal of Surgery 139: 374–378

Hoerr S O, Hermann R E 1973 Side-to-side choledochoduodenostomy. Surgical Clinics of North America 53: 1115–1122

Hunt D R, Blumgart L H 1980 Iatrogenic choledochoduodenal fistula: an unsuspected cause of post-cholecystectomy symptoms. British Journal of Surgery 67: 10–13

Kozloff L, Joseph W L 1975 Transduodenal sphincteroplasty for biliary tract disease. American Journal of Surgery 41: 125–130

Larrieu H, Benoit G 1978 Kinésimétrie et oddite. A propos de 500 observations. Chirurgie 104: 178–183

Lygidakis N J 1982 A prospective randomized study of recurrent choledocholithiasis. Surgery, Gynecology and Obstetrics 155: 679–684

McCloy R F, Jaffe V, Blumgart L H 1982 Endoscopy and post-cholecystectomy problems. In: Salmon P (ed) Proceedings of growing points in endoscopy. Associate Book Publishers, Andover

Moody F G, Becker J M, Potts J R 1983 Transduodenal sphincteroplasty and transampullary septectomy for postcholecystectomy pain. Annals of Surgery 197: 627–636

Nardi G L 1973 Papillitis and stenosis of the sphincter of Oddi. Surgical Clinics of North America 53: 1149–1160

Pitt H A 1984 Is endoscopic sphincterotomy a safe and effective method for the management of stones in the distal common bile duct? In: Gitnick G (ed) Controversies in gastroenterology. Churchill Livingstone, New York, 97–109

Pitt H A, Cameron J L, Postier R G, Gadacz T R 1981 Factors affecting mortality in biliary tract surgery. American Journal of Surgery 141: 66–72

Roux M, Rettori R, Debray Ch, Le Canuet R, Laumonier R 1958 Roentgen and pathologic appearance of chronic odditis. Journal of International College of Surgeons 32: 599–612

Safrany L 1977 Duodenoscopic sphincterotomy and gallstone removal. Gastroenterology 72: 338–343

Schuppisser J P, Tondelli P, Allgöwer M 1981 Cholezystokinin in der intraoperativen Prüfung der Papillendurchgängigkeit. z. Gastroenterolog 19: 504–505

Seifert E, Gali K, Weismüller J 1982 Langzeitresultate nach endoskopischer Sphinkterotomie. Deutsche Med Wschrift 107: 610–614

Siegel J H 1981 Duodenoscopic sphincterotomy in the treatment of the 'sump syndrome'. Digestive Diseases and Sciences 26: 922–928

Stefanini P, Carboni M, Patrassi N, De Bernardinis G, Negro P, Loriga P 1974 Transduodenal sphincteroplasty: its use in the treatment of lithiasis and benign obstruction of the common duct. American Journal of Surgery 128: 672–677

Steinberg W M, Salvato R F, Toskes P O 1980 The morphine prostigmine test: is it useful for making clinical decisions? Gastroenterology 78: 728–731

Stolte M 1979 Some aspects of the anatomy and pathology of the papilla of Vater. In: Classen M, Geenen J, Kawai K The papilla Vateri and its diseases. Verlag Gerhard Witzstrock, Baden-Baden, Köln, New York

Tondelli P, 1983 Benigne Papillenstenose — Bericht aus der Schweiz. Langenbecks Archiv fur Chirurgie 361 (Kongressbericht)

Tondelli P, Gyr K, Lüscher N, Schuppisser J P, Stalder G A, Allgöwer M 1978 Papillotomie und Papillenplastik? Klinische und endoskopische Spätuntersuchungen nach chirurgischer Papillenspaltung. Helvetica Chirurgica Acta 45: 687–692

Tondelli P, Allgöwer M 1980 Gallenwegschirurgie. Springer-Verlag, Berlin

Tondelli P, Gygli Th, Harder F, Allgöwer M 1982 Reoperationen an den Gallenwegen: Indikationen und Resultate. Helvetica Chirurgica Acta 49: 145–150

Toouli J, 1984 Spincter of Oddi motility. British Journal of Surgery 71: 251–256

Viceconte G, Viceconte G W, Pietropaolo V, Montori A 1981 Endoscopic sphincterotomy: indications and results. British Journal of Surgery 68: 376–380

Warshaw A L, Simeone J, Schapiro R H, Hedberg S E, Mueller P E, Ferrucci J T 1985 Objective evaluation of ampullary stenosis with ultrasonography and pancreatic stimulation. American Journal of Surgery 149: 65–72

White T T 1973 Indications for sphincteroplasty as opposed to choledochoduodenostomy. American Journal of Surgery 126: 165–170

SECTION 8

Biliary stricture and fistula

57

E. R. Howard

Biliary atresia

DEFINITION

Biliary atresia may be defined as the end result of a destructive inflammatory process of unknown aetiology which may affect bile ducts of newborn infants. The incidence throughout the world is constant with a frequency of approximately one case per 12 000 live births.

Affected infants present with jaundice (conjugated hyperbilirubinaemia) which is usually noted within the first few weeks of life. Spontaneous bleeding secondary to vitamin K malabsorption may occur but the infants are usually well nourished and have no stigmata of chronic liver disease at the time of presentation. Examination of the stools shows a complete absence of bile pigment.

The best description of the inflammatory process in the bile ducts likens it to a form of sclerosing cholangitis which starts as an extrahepatic lesion of variable distribution (Hays & Kimura 1981). The inflammatory process eventually destroys the whole of the bile duct system and death from cirrhotic liver disease occurs in a majority of untreated cases before two years of age (Hays & Snyder 1963).

HISTORICAL

Early single case reports of infants with biliary atresia were published by Home (1813) and Cursham (1840). Thomson (1982), in the first major review of the condition, described the clinical history and gross pathology of the biliary system in 49 cases collected from published reports, and added a further personal case. He described clearly the progressive nature of the inflammatory lesion.

In 1916 Holmes analysed more than 100 reported cases and stated that the condition was not as rare as was supposed at that time. The important observation was that on gross macroscopic examination at least 16% were suitable for operation with a bile duct to bowel anastomosis. He also discussed diagnosis and suggested that laparotomy was justified as soon as the diagnosis could be established with reasonable certainty — which is in complete agreement with the modern approach to treatment. From the time of Holmes report, cases of biliary atresia were classified into 'correctable' or 'non-correctable' depending on the presence or absence of a residual segment of bile duct suitable for a conventional type of biliary-enteric anastomosis.

Ladd (1928) gave the first reports of successful surgery in six out of 11 cases submitted to laparotomy. However it now seems that the early reports often confused biliary atresia with choledochal cyst, neonatal hepatitis and inspissated bile syndrome and the overall results of surgical treatment remained extremely poor. Bill (1978), for example, found only 52 reported successes from operation on patients with biliary atresia between 1927 and 1970. A variety of techniques were attempted to try and improve these dismal results including resection and anastomosis of the left lobe of the liver (Longmire & Sandford 1948), the implantation of intrahepatic tubes (Sterling & Lowenburg 1963) and the anastomosis of hepatic lymphatics to the bowel (Fonkalsrud et al 1966). Kasai & Suzuki (1959) developed the present treatment of biliary atresia from their observation that bile drainage could be established after resection of all remnants of the obliterated extrahepatic ducts in a number of cases of 'non-correctable' atresia. Microscopic studies of residual tissue in the porta hepatis showed channels up to 300 μm in diameter which frequently communicated with intrahepatic ducts. Anastomosis of a Roux-en-Y loop of jejunum to the cut surface of the tissue in the porta hepatis is now known as the portoenterostomy procedure, and effective bile drainage has been described in large numbers of patients during the last 20 years. The oldest survivors are now in their third decade.

AETIOLOGY

Experimental

Many attempts have been made to produce an experimental model of biliary atresia. Bile duct lesions have been produced but usually without the progressive hepatic disease typical of the condition.

Okamoto et al (1980) devascularized the whole length of the extrahepatic bile ducts of newborn puppies. Atretic changes with cord-like segments of bile ducts were produced with destruction of epithelium and fibrous thickening of the muscle in the duct wall, but only one animal showed intrahepatic effects. Animals operated on after 14 days of age did not develop atretic lesions, and it was suggested that they were protected by larger intramural vascular channels.

Other experiments have given conflicting results and have been reviewed in detail by Hashimoto et al (1983). Ligation and devascularization of the common bile duct in foetal rabbits, pigs and lambs may cause lesions resembling biliary atresia, but a theory of vascular catastrophe is not really borne out by the clinical observation of normal hepatic arteries and the excellent blood supply to tissue of the porta hepatis in most patients. The production of sclerosing inflammation of the biliary tract in animals is possible after the administration of toxic substances such as Sporidesmin (Ito et al 1980) and the direct injection of sodium morrhuate (Holder & Ashcraft 1967), but these experiments shed little light on aetiology. No link has been demonstrated with either ionizing radiation (Brent 1962) or teratogenic drugs (Gourevitch 1971), and simple ligation of the common bile duct in foetal lambs caused choledochal cysts rather than atresia (Spitz 1977).

Development

Miyano et al (1979) have described an abnormally long common channel at the junction of bile and pancreatic ducts in infants with atresia, similar to the abnormality found in some cases of choledochal cyst; but whether this is aetiological or coincidental remains unclear. Biliary atresia has also been reported in association with the trisomy syndromes 17–18. (Alpert et al 1969) and 21 (Danks 1965).

Metabolic

Vacanti & Folkman (1979) investigated the effect of the amino acid L-proline on the development of the biliary tract of the mouse. Intraperitoneal infusion was associated with epithelial proliferation and enlargement of proximal bile ducts although there was no effect on intrahepatic structures. Investigation of four infants with biliary atresia, three with bile duct hypoplasia and one each with choledochal cyst and neonatal hepatitis revealed low levels of L-proline and high levels of the precursor L-glutamic acid. The authors postulated that reduced hepatic synthesis of the amino acid L-proline during postnatal growth of the biliary tree may result in anatomical abnormality of the bile ducts. A toxic effect of monohydroxy bile acids on the hepatobiliary system has also been proposed (Jenner & Howard 1975) and injection of lithocholic acid into pregnant rabbits was associated with obstructive lesions in the biliary tract in two of the offspring.

Viral studies

An aetiological relationship between biliary atresia, choledochal cyst and neonatal hepatitis syndrome was proposed by Landing (1974), and he suggested that all of these conditions could be included in the term 'obstructive infantile cholangiopathy'. A viral origin had previously been suggested (Strauss & Bernstein 1968) but attempts to isolate viruses from the liver and biliary tracts of patients with 'obstructive cholangiopathy' were unsuccessful. However Morecki et al (1983) have now reported studies of the Reo 3 virus. Antibodies to this virus are detectable in 50% of adults. Phillips et al (1969) reported that 21-day-old weanling mice developed chronic liver disease and obstructive jaundice after exposure and Morecki et al (1983) studied the development of the pathological changes in the porta hepatis which have a remarkable similarity to those found in the biliary tract of infants with biliary atresia. Epithelial necrosis, chronic inflammation and fibrosis were observed but the virus could be recovered from the tissues for only eight days after infection and had disappeared before the onset of jaundice. Reo 3 virus was not identified in a study of infants with biliary atresia, but 68% of patients possessed antibodies compared with 8% of age-matched controls. The authors suggested a causal relationship between Reo 3 virus and human biliary atresia.

PATHOLOGY

The intrahepatic histology in infants with biliary atresia is typical of any bile duct obstruction in this age group, showing widening of all the portal tracts with oedema and fibrosis and proliferation of bile ductules. Bile stasis is present within canaliculi and hepatocytes. In contrast with hepatitis the liver architecture is preserved in the first few weeks of life but unrelieved cholestasis leads eventually to hepatocellular damage associated with the formation of multinucleate giant hepatocytes. Hepatocelluar necrosis, giant cell formation and inflammatory cell infiltrate in the hepatic parenchyma are classic features of hepatitis but all may be seen occasionally in biliary atresia and this reduces the accuracy of liver biopsy in the two conditions to approximately 82% (Manolaki et al 1983). Intrahepatic changes similar to those of biliary atresia are seen in alpha-1-antitrypsin deficiency which accounts for between 10 and 20% of infants presenting with the hepatitis syndrome and PAS-positive inclusions, which are characteristic of this disease in later life, may be absent. Alpha-1-antitrypsin phenotyping is therefore essential in the investigation of infants with conjugated hyperbilirubinaemia. Histological confusion may also occur with intrahepatic biliary hypoplasia which also presents as persistent jaundice in infancy and which may be associated with failure to thrive. Liver biopsy shows inflammatory changes within the parenchyma as well as the portal tracts but in contrast with biliary atresia the bile ductules are absent or sparse. A syndromic form of hypoplasia includes a characteristic facial appearance, pulmonary stenosis, vertebral anomalies, hypogonadism and other abnormalities (Alagille et al 1975).

The morphology of the extrahepatic ducts is very variable and the original description of 'correctable' or 'non-correctable' atresia which depended on the presence or absence of a residual segment of patent bile duct has now been replaced by the classification of the Japanese Society of Pediatric Surgeons (Hays & Kimura 1980) which describes three principal types (Fig. 57.1): atresia of the common bile duct which may be associated with a cyst in the porta hepatis (1); atresia of the common hepatic duct (2); and atresia of the right and left hepatic ducts (3) (Hays & Kimura 1980). The classification is extended into subtypes to indicate patency or occlusion of the distal common bile duct and gallbladder as well as the morphological features of the tissue at the porta hepatis but these subdivisions have doubtful prognostic significance on the outcome of surgery. Non-communicating cystic dilatations may occur in any segment of the extrahepatic bile ducts and may suggest an erroneous diagnosis of type 1 atresia or even choledochal cyst. Unless the lumen of any cystic dilatation contains bile it must be regarded as non-

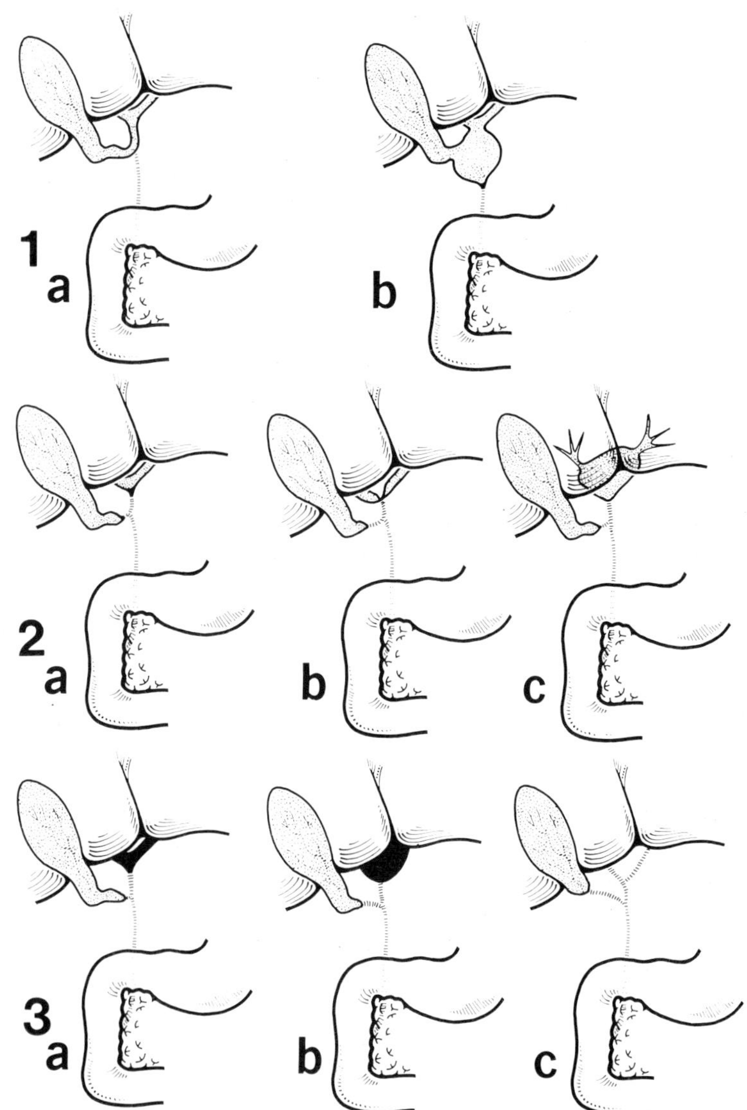

Fig. 57.1 Diagrams of the main types of extrahepatic bile duct lesions in biliary atresia. Types 1 and 2 include the 'correctable' atresias of previous classifications

communicating and must be resected during surgery.

Kasai et al (1980) have shown that during the first few weeks of life atresia patients possess patent intrahepatic bile ducts which reach the porta hepatis. Three-dimensional studies of the porta hepatis have revealed that, in type 3 disease, the major intrahepatic ducts divide into many small branches which terminate in the fibrous tissue which replaces the extrahepatic ducts. The number of major intrahepatic ducts progressively decreases with increasing age and this process is accompanied by a proliferation of ductules in the portal tracts which is maximal between six and 10 months of age, after which time it starts to decline. These studies suggest that attempts to establish bile drainage might be most successful if performed before six or eight weeks of age.

Microscopic examination of extrahepatic duct remnants has shown a variety of features which include duct-like structures, inflammatory cell infiltrates and fibrosis. The duct-like structures may be biliary glands, collecting ductules, or residual lumina of true bile ducts and the latter generally show at least partial loss of the epithelial lining (Ohi et al 1984). Gautier & Eliot (1980) classified the histological appearances into three main types. Type 1 cases show a complete absence of ducts and few inflammatory cells in the surrounding connective tissue. Type 2 tissue contains small lumina, usually less than 50 μm in diameter, lined by cuboidal epithelium and thought to be biliary glands. Type 3 tissue is identified by the presence of true bile ducts, lined at least in part by epithelium of the columnar type (Fig. 57.2). Bile may be identified within macrophages in more than two-thirds of the type 3 cases.

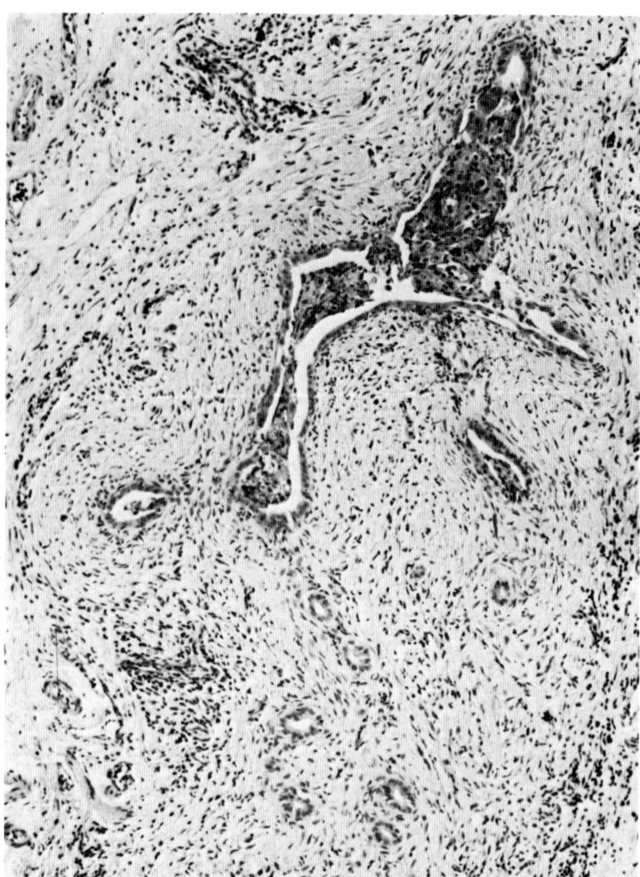

Fig. 57.2 Histological appearances of tissue excised from the porta hepatis of a 10-week-old infant with non-correctable atresia. A large bile duct with partial destruction of its epithelium and smaller biliary ductules are surrounded by fibrous tissue (H + E)

Several authors have compared the success of biliary drainage after surgical resection of tissue from the porta hepatis with the histological appearances of the bile duct remnants. It appears that bile flow may be anticipated when the maximum size of residual bile ducts exceeds 150 μm (Altman et al 1975, Ohi et al 1984). However bile flow has been noted in some cases with much smaller duct remnants and even in patients in whom duct structures were not identified at surgery (Lawrence et al 1981).

The response of the hepatobiliary system to surgery must be at least partly dependent on the severity of intrahepatic inflammation and fibrosis (or cirrhosis) as well as the morphological features of the extrahepatic bile duct tissue. Hass (1978) has suggested that the rapid onset of cirrhosis is due both to the bile duct obstruction and to a 'cholangiopathic' process akin to that seen in neonatal hepatitis.

ASSOCIATED ANATOMICAL ANOMALIES

Associated congenital anomalies have been reported in 12 to 27% of cases (Miyamoto & Kajimoto 1983). Cardiovascular, splenic (polysplenia and asplenia), gastrointestinal (malrotation and situs inversus) and genitourinary abnormalities are found most frequently and a preduodenal portal vein is not uncommon. All of these have been recorded in the author's personal series of 160 cases together with one example of an absent inferior vena cava.

INVESTIGATIONS

Obstructive jaundice in older children and adults can the readily separated from 'medical' jaundice in approximately 80% of cases by history, clinical examination and biochemical test of liver function. In early infancy, however, hepatocellular disease, intrahepatic bile duct disorders (hypoplasia) and obstructive lesions of the extrahepatic bile ducts (biliary atresia, choledochal cyst, etc), all have similar clinical and laboratory features. Jaundice, dark urine and pale stools, the signs of conjugated hyperbilirubinaemia, are found in all three groups. Hepatomegaly is common and all groups are prone to bleeding (e.g. intracranial haemorrhage) from malabsorption of the

Table 57.1 Investigation of infantile cholestasis

haematology
liver function tests
screening tests (for infective, metabolic, endocrine and genetic disorders)
ultrasonography
radioisotope excretion (^{131}I rose bengal faecal excretion or radionuclide hepatobiliary imaging)
duodenal aspiration
percutaneous liver biopsy
laparoscopy
operative cholangiography

fat soluble vitamin K. Liver function tests are usually unhelpful in infantile cholestasis as there is an element of hepatocellular injury in all types which is reflected in elevated serum transaminases, gammaglutamyl transpeptidase, alkaline phosphatase and alphafetoprotein levels. Further problems in diagnosis are caused by a lack of intrahepatic bile duct dilatation which limits the usefulness of ultrasonography except in the rare case of choledochal cyst. Radioisotope excretion studies have also proved disappointing in their lack of discrimination between extrahepatic bile duct obstruction and severe hepatocellular disease in the neonatal period.

A firm diagnosis of biliary atresia requires a battery of tests (Table 57.1) for the exclusion of infective, metabolic, genetic and endocrine causes of jaundice and a percutaneous liver biopsy which is often of crucial importance. Duodenal aspiration and analysis of the aspirate for bilirubin pigment is commonly used in Japan but, whilst the presence of bilirubin excludes a diagnosis of atresia, false negative results may be obtained in severe hepatitis syndromes. Laparoscopy and guided percutaneous cholangiography have also been used in infants (Sunaryo & Watkins 1983).

The difficulties in separating the causes of infantile obstructive jaundice were illustrated in an analysis of diagnostic tests in 85 jaundiced infants (Manolaki et al 1983). Serum bilirubin and liver enzyme values were unhelpful. Radioisotope excretion was reported absent in 97% of infants with biliary atresia but was also absent in 67% of the children with hepatitis syndromes. Percutaneous liver biopsy was the most reliable investigation with an accuracy greater than 82%.

An accurate preoperative diagnosis of bile duct obstruction is extremely important in the jaundiced infant as the patent extrahepatic bile ducts in hepatitis syndrome and bile duct hypoplasia are minute. Their patency may not be recognized even with the most careful intraoperative cholangiography and this may lead to a false diagnosis of biliary atresia and unnecessary surgery on the bile ducts (Kahn & Daum 1983).

SURGICAL TREATMENT

Before the advent of sophisticated investigations it was usual to confirm a diagnosis of biliary atresia by limited laparotomy. This was performed through a short transverse incision in the right hypochondrium when the diagnosis might be obvious from the atretic appearances of the gallbladder. Operative cholangiography through the gallbladder was performed whenever the gallbladder and cystic ducts were patent (approximately 25% of cases) and the procedure was terminated by taking a generous wedge biopsy of the liver. A more extensive laparotomy was undertaken a few days later if macroscopic appearances, cholangiography and histology suggested atresia rather than hepatitis.

Most cases of biliary atresia are now diagnosed preoperatively and the surgeon must be prepared to perform either hepaticojejunostomy for the type I cystic disease found in approximately 15% of cases, or the more radical portoenterostomy procedure for the remainder. Anomalies such as polysplenia, situs inversus and preduodenal portal vein, must also be expected in a significant number.

Preoperative preparation

The prothrombin time can generally be corrected to normal by the intramuscular injection of vitamin K (1.0 mg/day for four days). The bowel is prepared by the oral administration of neomycin (50 mg/kg/day in six divided doses for 24 hours) and one unit of blood is cross-matched. Oral fluids are withheld for four hours before operation. The child is placed supine on a heated operating table which is thermostatically controlled and which contains facilities for intraoperative cholangiography. An adequate intravenous line is set up, a rectal temperature probe inserted and the first intravenous dose of a broad-spectrum antibiotic (a cephalosporin) is given at the induction of anaesthesia.

Hepaticojejunostomy for cystic type 1 atresia (Fig. 57.3)

The abdomen is opened through a transverse upper abdominal incision which extends across both rectus muscles and divides the falciform ligament. A record is made of the size of the spleen, the size and texture of the liver and any ascites, portal hypertension or anatomical anomalies outside of the biliary tract. The gallbladder, which may be hidden within a cleft between segment V and the quadrate lobe, is examined for patency. A shrunken, fibrotic gallbladder suggests a diagnosis of atresia and precludes operative cholangiography. A patent gallbladder should be aspirated and intubated for X-ray studies. A clear mucoid fluid is generally present in the gallbladder but when bile is obtained in the aspirate the

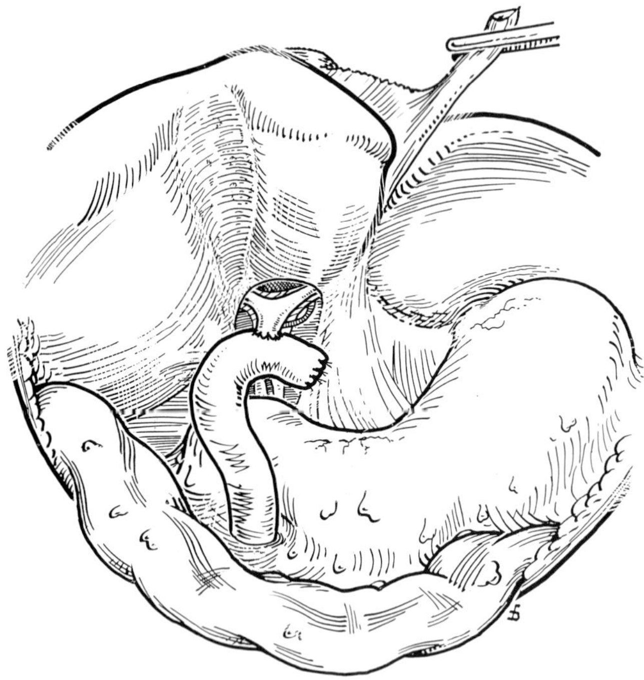

Fig. 57.3 Hepaticojejunostomy for type I-cystic atresia

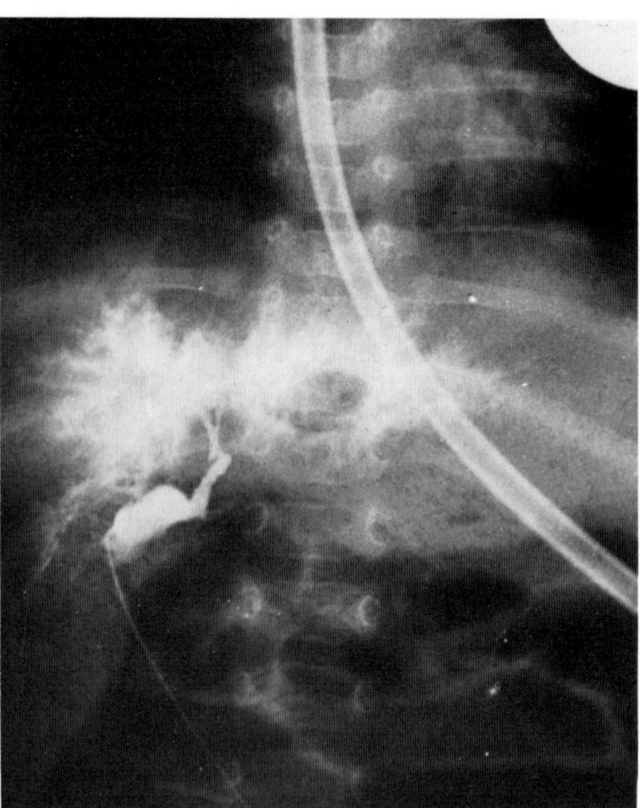

Fig. 57.4 Intraoperative cholangiogram in a 3-month-old infant with type 1 atresia. The hepatic ducts and gallbladder are patent but the common bile duct is occluded

diagnosis is either a cystic type-1 lesion or a hepatitis-syndrome with a patent extrahepatic biliary system and cholangiography is mandatory.

Cystic dilatation of the proximal hepatic ducts is usually visible during the examination of the gallbladder. An operative cholangiogram (Fig. 57.4) may show a communication via the cystic duct or bile may be aspirated from the cyst by direct puncture.

The confirmation of a cystic type-1 lesion is followed by the operation of hepaticojejunostomy. The gallbladder is dissected from its bed after division of the cystic artery between ligatures. Traction on the gallbladder allows identification of the atretic segment of distal common bile duct which is divided. The cystic segment is mobilized from the adjacent hepatic artery and portal vein and transected between stay sutures at its widest diameter. A Roux-en-Y loop of proximal jejunum, 40 cm in length, is prepared and passed in a retrocolic position to the porta hepatis. The open end of the Roux loop is closed in two layers and an end–to–side anastomosis constructed between the cyst and the bowel using interrupted sutures of 4/0 catgut, in a single layer (Ch. 70). Transanastomotic tubes are not used. A drain is placed in the subhepatic space and the abdominal wound closed in layers.

Portoenterostomy

A conventional biliary-enteric anastomosis is not possible in a majority of cases of biliary atresia, when the proximal hepatic ducts are either very narrow (type 2) or completely occluded (type 3). The demonstration of bile drainage from microscopic channels after transection of these abnormal hepatic ducts led Kasai to the development of the portoenterostomy procedure in which a Roux-en-Y loop of jejunum is anastomosed to the edge of the area left in the porta hepatis after excision of all remnants of extrahepatic bile ducts.

The initial stages of the portoenterostomy procedure are identical to those performed for hepaticojejunostomy. In a proportion of cases the cystic and distal common bile ducts are patent and contrast medium will flow from the gallbladder into the duodenum (Fig. 57.5). However the proximal atretic ducts will not be visualized even after occlusion of the supraduodenal portion of the common bile duct with a small vascular clamp. The operation commences with complete mobilization of the gallbladder which is used as a guide to the fibrous remnant of the common hepatic duct (Fig. 57.6b and 57.6c) which may be obscured by thickened peritoneum and enlarged lymph nodes. The bile duct remnants are dissected free of the hepatic artery and portal vein which are exposed throughout their course in the porta hepatis (Fig. 57.6d).

The distal portion of the common bile duct is divided between ligatures at the upper border of the duodenum and the gallbladder and attached ducts are dissected

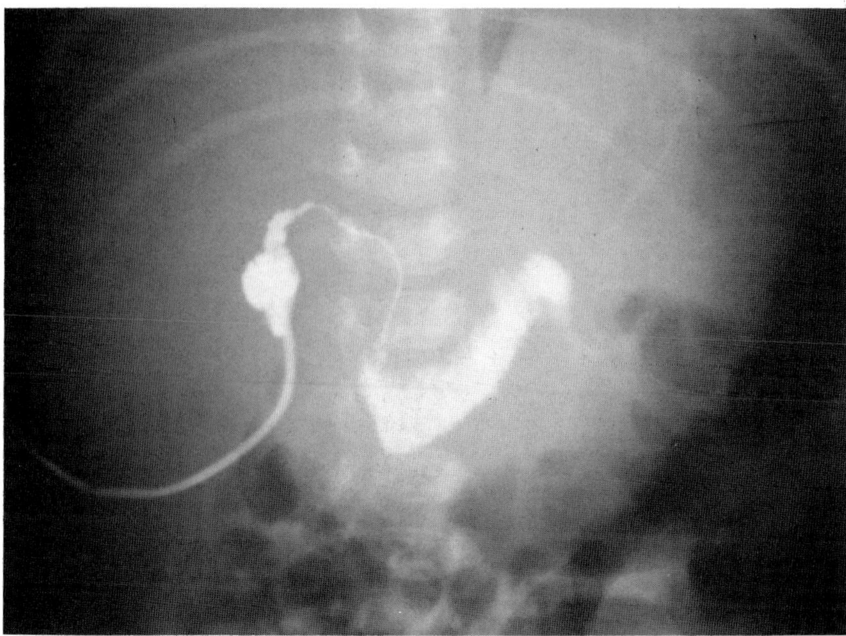

Fig. 57.5 Operative cholangiogram in a 10-week-old infant with type 3 atresia. The gallbladder and common bile duct are patent

towards the porta hepatis. Small vessels and lymphatics are ligated meticulously to prevent postoperative ascites from a leak of lymph. The dissection continues to the bifurcation of the portal vein (Fig. 57.6e) and both left and right veins are exposed. It is necessary to divide two or three short tributaries of the portal vein which run directly from the bile duct remnants. (Fig. 57.6f). The bile duct tissue is removed by a transection which is parallel to the liver capsule and which extends behind the posterior surface of the portal vein. The transection is made as wide as possible within the area bounded by the right and left portal veins. (Fig. 57.6g). Bleeding points in the porta hepatis are controlled by direct pressure.

Finally a 40 cm Roux loop of jejunum is prepared, the distal cut end oversewn, and passed in a retrocolic position to the hilum of the liver (Fig. 57.6h). An anastomosis is constructed between the edge of the transected area at the hilum and the side of the Roux loop with interrupted sutures of 4/0 catgut. All of the sutures of the posterior row are placed in position before the loop is 'rail-roaded' into position. The sutures are tied and the anterior row completed.

The operation is completed by placing a drain in the subhepatic space.

Cutaneous enterostomy

Episodes of ascending bacterial cholangitis occur in approximately 40% of patients after operation. Surgical attempts to reduce this complication have involved the cutaneous diversion of bile to prevent high intraluminal bowel pressure from reaching the portoenterostomy anastomosis. Many ingenious stomas have been described (Howard 1984) but their beneficial effect on the incidence of cholangitis has not been proven (Altman 1983). There was no reduction in the incidence of cholangitis in a personal series of cases in which the author added a cutaneous enterostomy and he has now returned to the original Kasai operation. Furthermore, complications of dehydration, hyponatraemia, intussusception and bleeding from the stoma edge were all encountered in the patients with cutaneous bile drainage. The enterostomy designed by Kasai is illustrated (Fig. 57.7), and it is recommended that closure of the stoma is delayed for one or two years after the portoenterostomy procedure.

Portocholecystostomy (Fig. 57.8)

An anastomosis between the gallbladder and the transected area in the porta hepatis may be possible after patency of the gallbladder and distal common bile duct has been demonstrated with cholangiography. There does appear to be a reduced incidence of cholangitis after this operation although technical problems including bile leaks, gallbladder obstruction and kinking of the common bile duct have been reported (Lilly 1979).

Postoperative care

Intravenous fluids and nasogastric drainage are continued until bowel activity returns. Any unexplained pyrexia accompanied by deteriorating liver function tests suggests cholangio-hepatitis and the responsible organism must be identified from blood and liver cultures. *E coli, Proteus and*

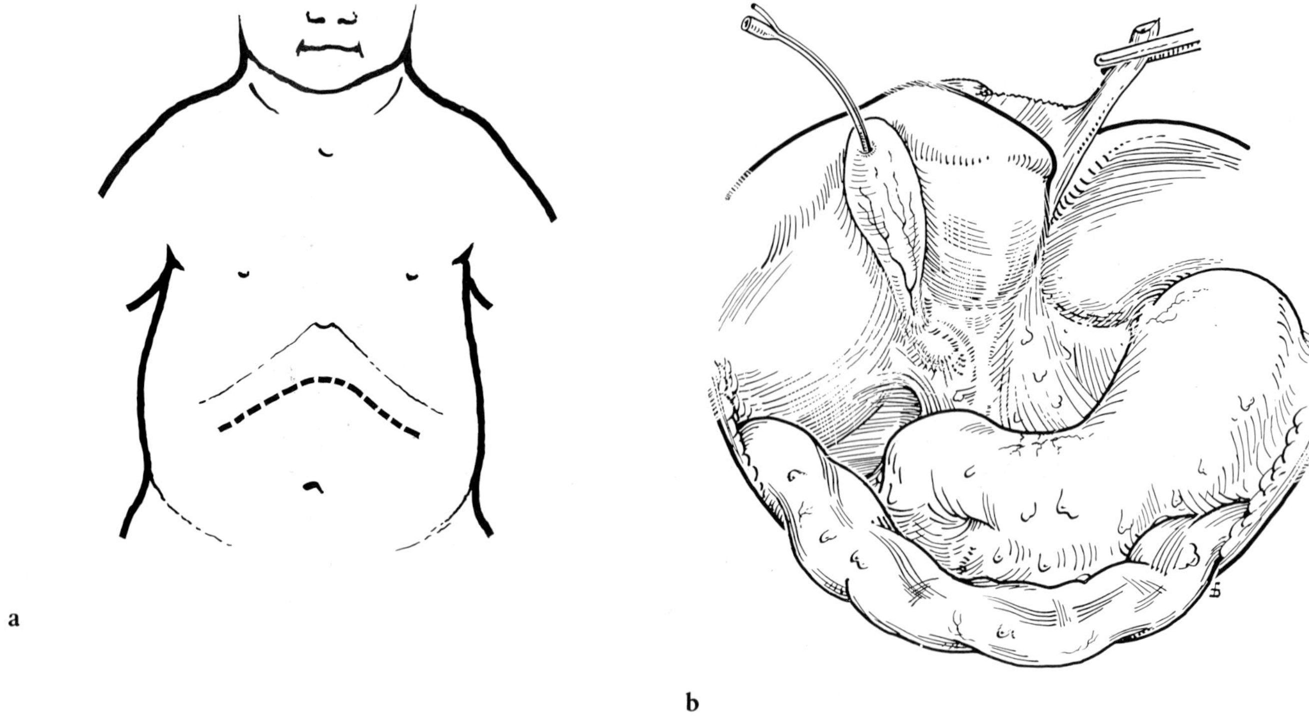

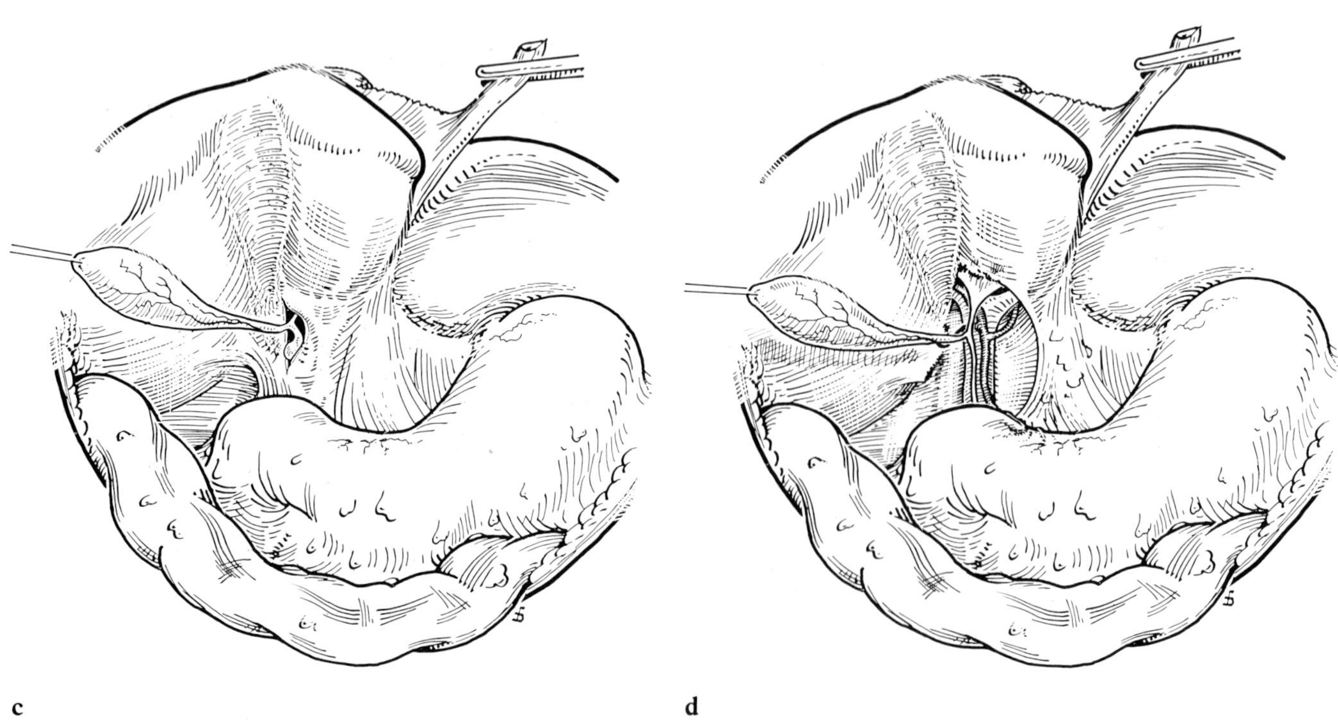

Fig. 57.6 a. Abdominal incision b. Exposure of gallbladder and cholangiogram c. Dissection of gallbladder from its bed d. Exposure of structures in the porta hepatitis e. Elevation of gallbladder and bile duct remnants after division of distal common bile duct f. Lateral view of proximal tissue showing site of residual bile duct tissue behind the bifurcation of the portal vein g. Transection of bile duct tissue flush with the liver capsule h. Construction of 40 cm Roux loop of jejunum; placement of posterior row of sutures in porta hepatis; application of Roux loop to transected tissue

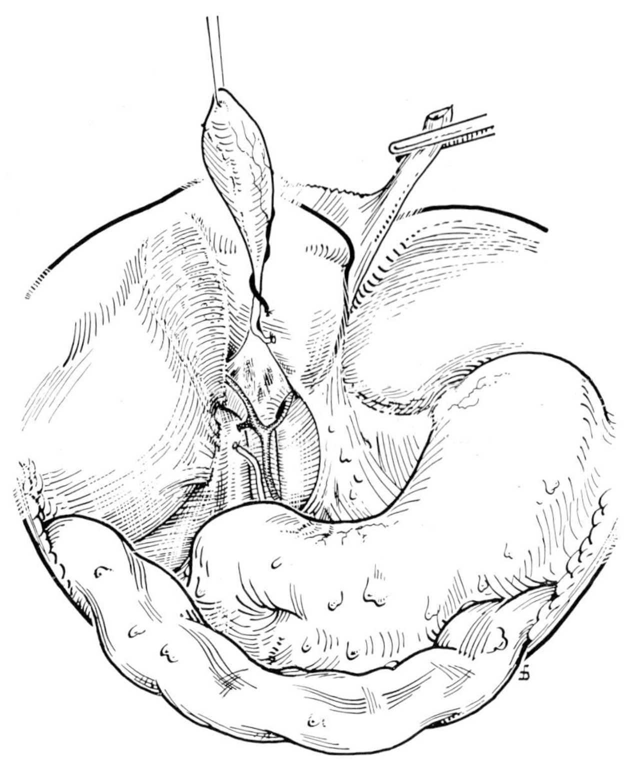

e

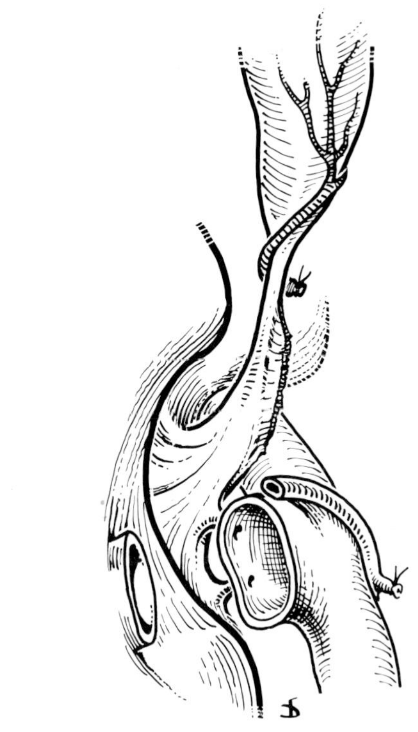

f

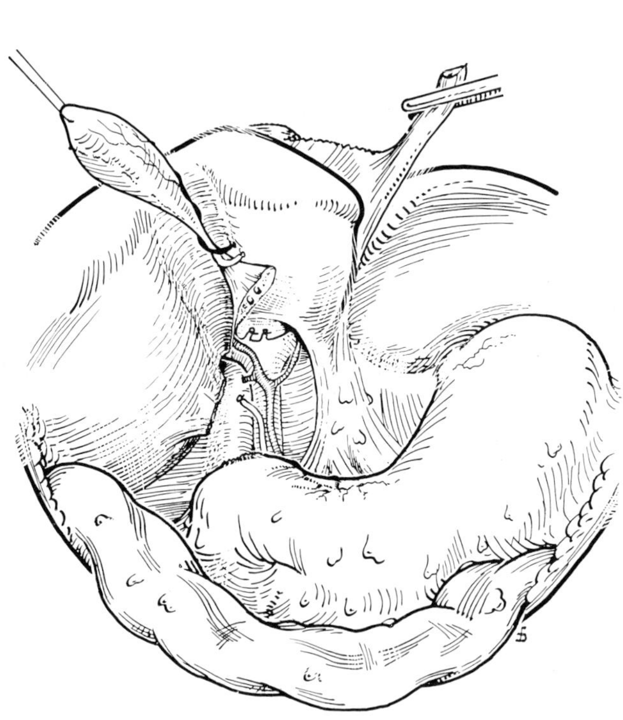

g

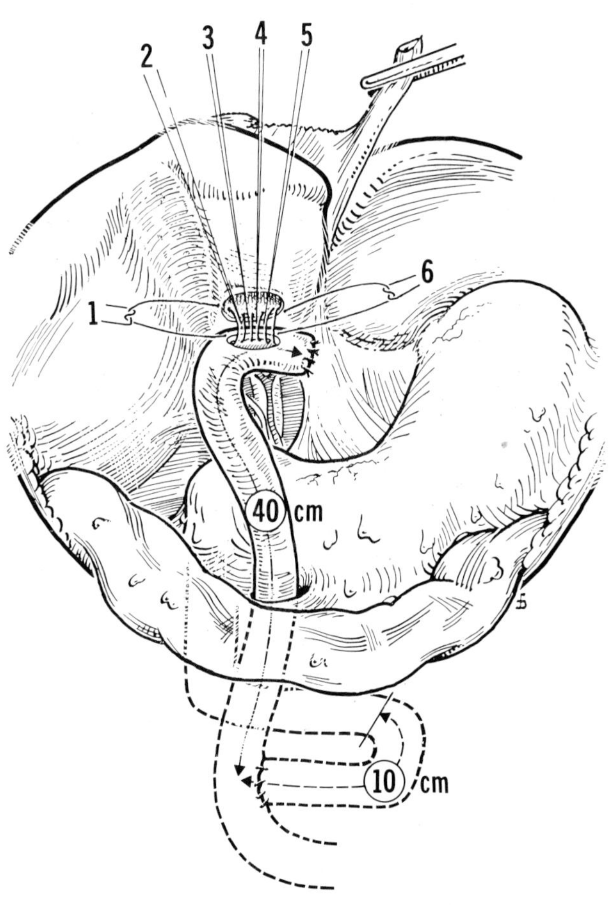

h

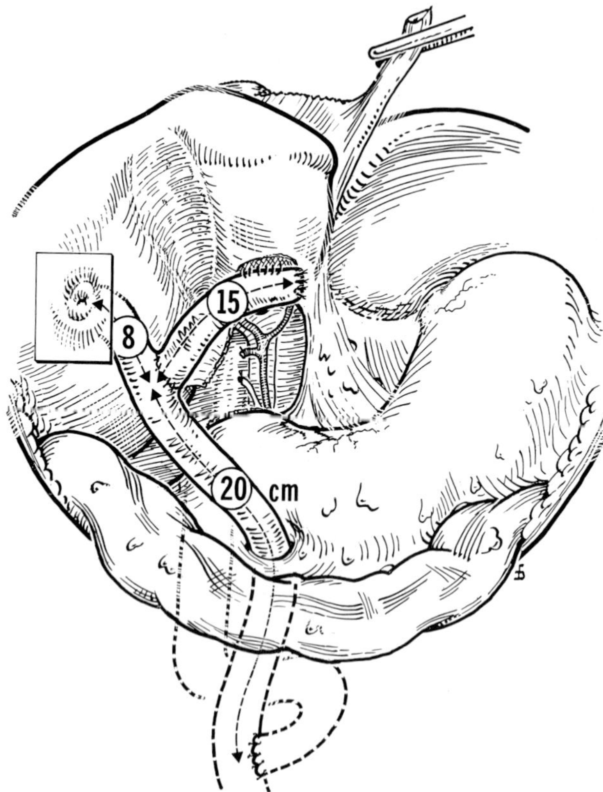

Fig. 57.7 The Kasai 2 cutaneous enterostomy in which a stoma is fashioned in the Roux loop. The recommended lengths of bowel are indicated in cm

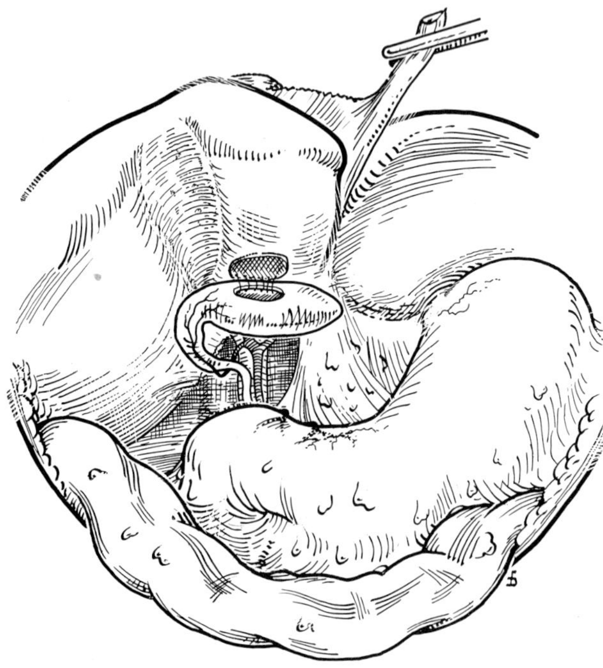

Fig. 57.8 Portocholecystostomy. A patent gallbladder may be anastomosed to the transected tissue in the porta hepatis in some cases of type 3 atresia

Klebsiella are commonly responsible for these infections. Systemic antibiotics are continued for five days after operation and are then replaced by oral prophylaxis for three weeks.

Phenobarbitone, cholestyramine and vitamins D and K are prescribed for at least one year after surgery in all cases. Bile drainage from cutaneous enterostomies is added to the infant's feeds and in these cases the serum electrolytes are checked regularly. When the child is discharged from hospital the parents and the referring hospitals are given full details of the operative procedure and information on the recognition, hazards and treatment of any attacks of cholangitis.

The establishment of satisfactory bile drainage and the loss of jaundice is difficult to predict after these operations. Serum bilirubin may fall to normal at any time between three weeks and six months later and histological analysis of the tissue from the porta hepatis is of prognostic significance only if ducts greater than 150 μm in diameter are identified.

Postoperative complications and treatment

Patients who fail to lose their jaundice after operation show a gradual deterioration in liver function and death commonly occurs between one and two years of age.

In contrast the prognosis for children who drain bile satisfactorily can be extremely good and there are now several survivors over 20 years of age. However, the postoperative progress of patients who lose their jaundice after either hepaticojejunostomy or portoenterostomy may be complicated by bacterial cholangitis, portal hypertension or a variety of metabolic disorders, and they probably need careful follow-up for the whole of their lives.

Bacterial cholangitis

Infection of the biliary tree may be confidently diagnosed from the triad of pyrexia, rising serum bilirubin and recurrence of acholic stools. These infections are most likely to occur during the first nine months after surgery, but are uncommon in older age groups. Experience with large numbers of patients in Japan suggests that cholangitis is rare after four years and that a late onset of infection should suggest a possible mechanical cause such as Roux loop obstruction (Fig. 57.9).

Ascending bacterial cholangitis is a serious complication as a permanent deterioration in liver function may follow each attack and, during the first few weeks after surgery, it may be severe enough to cause death.

It is generally believed that cholangitis arises by a direct infection from the bowel but other suggested portals of entry include the portal venous system (Danks et al 1974), the hilar hepatic lymphatics (Hirsig et al 1978) and the combination of an infected intestinal conduit with a partially obstructed biliary tree (Lilly 1978).

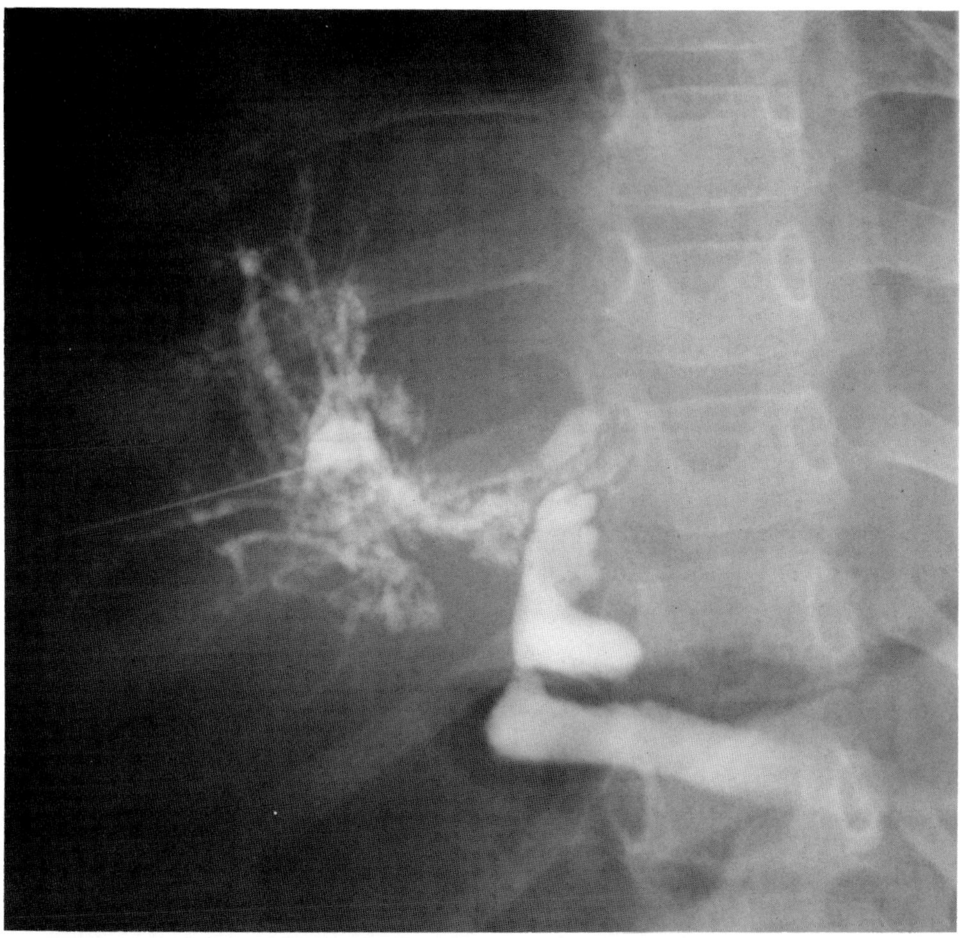

Fig. 57.9 Percutaneous cholangiogram six years after portoenterostomy in a child who developed recurrent attacks of cholangitis. The X-ray shows a stricture in the Roux loop of jejunum. Note the abnormal intrahepatic bile ducts which are typical of biliary atresia

A diagnosis of intrahepatic infection may be made from blood cultures or, if these are negative, from cultures of percutaneous liver biopsy material and a wide variety of gram negative organisms may be isolated. Treatment is empirical and usually consists of the systemic administration of a cephalosporin and gentamicin.

Prophylactic antibiotics have had little effect on the incidence of cholangitis and cutaneous diversion of bile has proved disappointing (Hays & Kimura 1980). It must be emphasized that investigations of patients who present with cholangitis after a long jaundice-free interval should include percutaneous cholangiography (Fig. 57.9) and radionucleide scanning to exclude a surgically correctable obstruction. Three patients in the author's series have benefited from reconstruction of the Roux loop three to six years after the original portoenterostomy.

Portal hypertension

Hepatic fibrosis is present at the time of diagnosis of biliary atresia and measurements of portal pressure at portoenterostomy have confirmed the presence of portal hypertension in a majority of cases. The fibrotic process often progresses even after successful surgery and follow-up measurements in 16 jaundice-free survivors showed portal pressures between 44 and 135 mm H_2O. Higher pressures (more than 200 mm H_2O) were recorded in eight out of 10 in children who had suffered attacks of cholangitis (Kasai et al 1981).

Endoscopy of jaundice-free survivors has revealed oesophageal varices in a large proportion of cases and variceal haemorrhage has been a major problem in 10 to 23% (Howard et al 1982, Lilly & Stellin 1984). Surprisingly the effects of portal hypertension may diminish with age (Odievre 1978) and for this reason injection sclerotherapy is currently regarded by the author as the treatment of choice for bleeding varices. Porto-systemic shunts and oesophageal transection have also been used for this difficult problem and Lilly & Stellin (1984) have reported the beneficial effects of splenic embolization in six cases.

Metabolic problems

Abnormalities in the metabolism of fat, protein, fat and

water soluble vitamins, iron, calcium, zinc and copper have all been described in children with chronic liver disease (Greene 1983). The effects are minimized by the regular administration of fat soluble vitamins, particularly D and K, and a multivitamin preparation which includes thiamine, riboflavine, pyridoxine, ascorbic acid and folic acid. Florid rickets may occur occasionally and seem to be the result of poor intestinal absorption rather than impaired metabolism of vitamin D. The condition is rapidly corrected by giving increased doses of vitamin D and ensuring that there is adequate calcium and phosphate in the diet.

Vitamin E deficiency is not uncommon in young children with cholestatic disease and has been associated with a progressive neurological disorder (Nelson et al 1983), which includes loss of tendon reflexes, a reduction in proprioception and sensation, abnormal eye movements and intellectual deterioration. Histological abnormalities have been described in large calibre sensory axons in the spinal cord and in peripheral nerves.

INTRAHEPATIC CYST FORMATION

Collections of bile (bile 'lakes') isolated from the biliary tree, are frequently found at autopsy within the central portion of the liver in patients who have never established satisfactory bile drainage. Large intrahepatic cysts, easily detected on ultrasound examination, may also occur occasionally in jaundice-free children and may be associated with attacks of ascending cholangitis. The author has seen one such case four and a half years after successful portoenterostomy. Percutaneous cholangiography and radionucleide scanning (Fig. 57.10) showed good drainage from the right intrahepatic ducts into the Roux loop but the left lobe was almost totally occupied by a cystic collection of bile. Cystogastrostomy was followed by rapid obliteration of the cyst. Saito et al (1984) reported a similar lesion in a 13-month-old child which also disappeared after surgical drainage through the abdominal wall. The origin of these cysts is not understood.

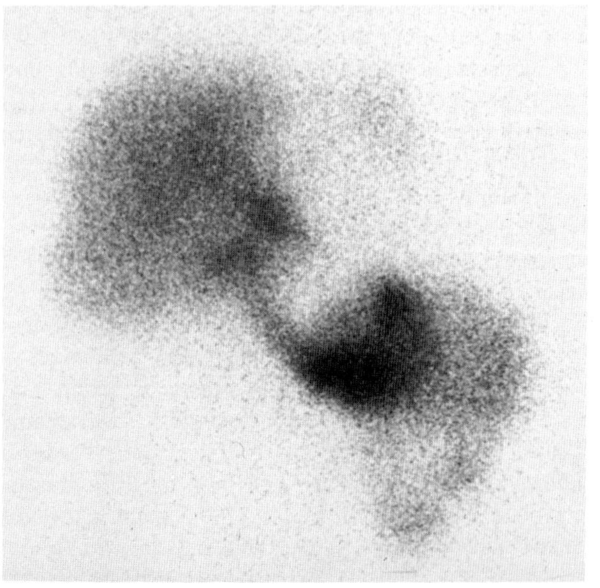

Fig. 57.10 Radionucleide scan (DISIDA) four and a half years after portoenterostomy, with good excretion from the right lobe of the liver 25 minutes after injection. A 'cold' area in the left lobe represents a cystic collection of bile

RE-OPERATION

The results of re-operation in a patient who has undergone a correct portoenterostomy procedure are not good unless there is a mechanical problem with the Roux loop of jejunum which can generally be excluded with ultrasound examination and percutaneous cholangiography. In a recent series of re-operations performed after failure of portoenterostomy only seven out of 33 achieved some increase in bile flow. Long-term results are not yet available (Suruga et al 1982). Only three out of 30 cases responded satisfactorily to re-operation in a series reported by Saito (1983).

RESULTS OF TREATMENT

Correctable (type 1) forms of biliary atresia treatable by conventional biliary-enteric anastomosis represent only eight to 15% of cases in most large series. Bile flow is usually seen immediately after surgery but the long-term results have often been disappointing. Kasai corrected 25 type 1 cases between 1953 and 1976 but only 49% achieved long-term jaundice-free survival (Hays & Kimura 1980) and Caccia et al (1983) reported long-term success in only two out of four type 1 cases in a series of 72 patients.

It is now clear that portoenterostomy can give long-term survival in cases previously thought to be uncorrectable. Hays & Kimura (1981), for example, have reported 85 patients alive and well for more than five years after operation and the oldest patient is now 25 years of age.

A survey by the surgical section of the American Academy of Pediatrics (1972–1982) collected 295 cases of 'non-correctable' atresia; 44% were alive at the time of the survey, 20% had normal serum bilirubin levels. 27 patients had lived longer than six years after surgery (Hays et al 1983). A further study of this series confirmed that most deaths (13.4%) occurred within the first year and that at six years after surgery the mortality rate was very low (0.3%).

The progressive inflammatory destruction of the biliary tract and the rapid onset of biliary cirrhosis suggests that surgery should be performed at the earliest possible age.

This has been confirmed in a personal series of 64 portoenterostomies. Jaundice cleared in 44.6% but a comparison of results with age at operation showed that success was greatest in the infants corrected before seven weeks of age (66%). Of those treated between eight and 11 weeks 52% were successful whereas only 27% of those over 12 weeks lost their jaundice. These results confirm the benefit of early operation which has been reported in many series.

Most long-term survivors show persistently abnormal liver function tests and severe changes in liver histology despite satisfactory bile drainage. Some examples of liver enzyme levels in 24 long-term survivors are given in Table 57.2.

Hadchouel et al (1983) examined liver biopsies from 20 patients who had survived at least five years after satisfactory surgery. Cirrhosis was present in all specimens but the degree of fibrosis and the size of regenerative nodules varied. Severe fibrosis was present in 15 and mild to moderate fibrosis in five patients. The portal tracts generally showed inflammatory infiltrate with mononuclear cells and a surprising observation was the absence of bile ductules within the portal tracts of four patients, all of whom were anicteric.

The long-term prognosis after operation for extrahepatic biliary atresia depends on many factors which include age at operation, histology of tissue resected from the porta hepatis, the incidence of ascending cholangitis, the severity of portal hypertension and the progress of intrahepatic inflammatory disease. The experience of the surgeon is also a factor and has been highlighted in a survey of surgical results in the United Kingdom (McClement et al 1984). Centres treating one case per year achieved jaundice-free survival in 11% compared with 29% in centres managing two to five per year. The success rate rose to 43% when more than five cases per year were seen.

Table 57.2 Liver enzyme values in 24 jaundice-free survivors after portoenterostomy

Enzyme (iu/l)	Range	Mean
alkaline phosphatase (n = 60–250)	125–1752	893
aspartate transaminase (n = 10–45)	45–302	131
gamma glutamyl transpeptidase (n = 0–45)	14–1880	481

Liver transplantation is now a recognized procedure for children in whom portoenterostomy is unsuccessful (Ch. 118, 119, 120, 121) and biliary atresia was the single most common indication for operation in a report of 48 paediatric transplants, 16 of whom survived for more than one year (Starzl et al 1979). Iwatsuki et al (1984) have reported the results in 17 children with either atresia or hypoplasia of the bile ducts and the one year survival figures have improved since the introduction of the immunosuppressive agent cyclosporin from 40 to 60%. In a further series of eight cases, five children were well from six weeks to nine months after transplantation. All had undergone a previous unsuccessful portoenterostomy and their ages at the time of transplant ranged from eight to 19 months (Ch. 119) (Ascher & Najarian 1984).

Advances in the treatment of biliary atresia over the last 25 years have increased the chances of four-year survival from 2% to approximately 40%. Ten-year survival after surgery is no longer unusual and liver transplantation may help to improve the overall results even more.

REFERENCES

Alagille D, Odievre M, Gautier M, Dommergues J P 1975 Hepatic ductular hypoplasia associated with characteristic facies, vertebral malformation, retarded physical, mental and sexual development and cardiac murmur. Journal of Pediatrics 86: 63–71

Alpert L I, Strauss L, Hirschhorn K 1969 Neonatal hepatitis and biliary atresia associated with trisomy 17–18 syndrome. New England Journal of Medicine 280: 16–20

Altman R P 1983 Longterm results after the Kasai procedure. In: Daum F (ed) Extrahepatic biliary atresia. Marcel Dekker, New York, ch 9, p 96

Altman R P, Chandra R, Lilly J R 1975 Ongoing cirrhosis after successful porticoenterostomy in infants with biliary atresia. Journal of Pediatric Surgery 10: 685–689

Ascher N L, Najarian J S 1984 Hepatic transplantation in biliary atresia: early experience in eight patients. World Journal of Surgery 8: 57–63

Bill A H 1978 Biliary atresia. World Journal of Surgery 2: 557–559

Brent R L 1962 Persistent jaundice in infancy. Journal of Pediatrics 61: 111–144

Caccia G, Dessanti A, Alberti D 1983 An 8 years experience on the treatment of extrahepatic biliary atresia: results in 72 cases. In: Kasai (ed) Biliary atresia and its related disorders. Excerpta Medica, Amsterdam, p 181–184

Cursham G 1840 Case of atrophy of the gallbladder with obliteration of the bile ducts. London Medical Gazette 26: 388–389

Danks D M 1965 Prolonged neonatal obstructive jaundice. A survey of modern concepts. Clinical Pediatrics 4: 499–510

Danks D M, Campbell P E, Clarke A M, Jones P G, Solomon J R 1974 Extrahepatic biliary atresia. American Journal of Diseases of Children 128: 684–686

Fonkalsrud E W, Kitagawa S, Longmire W P 1966 Hepatic lymphatic drainage to the jejunum for congenital biliary atresia. American Journal of Surgery 112: 188–194

Gautier M, Eliot N 1981 Extrahepatic biliary atresia: morphological study of 98 biliary remnants. Archives of Pathology and Laboratory Medicine 105: 397–402

Gourevitch A 1971 Duodenal atresia in the newborn. Annals of the Royal College of Surgeons of England 48: 141–158

Greene H L 1983 Nutritional aspects in the management of biliary atresia. In: Daum F (ed) Extrahepatic biliary atresia. Marcel Dekker, New York, ch 14, p 133–143

Haas J E 1978 Bile duct and liver pathology in biliary atresia. World Journal of Surgery 2: 561–569

Hadchouel M, Gautier M, Valayer J, Odievre M, Alagille D 1983 Histopathology of the liver five years after successful surgery for extrahepatic biliary atresia. In: Daum F (ed) Extrahepatic biliary atresia. Marcel Dekker, New York, ch 6, p 65–70

Hashimoto T, Yura J, Mahour G H, Warburton D, Landing B H, Stanley P et al 1983 Recent topics of experimental production of biliary atresia, and an experimental model using devascularization of

extrahepatic bile duct in fetal sheep. In: Kasai (ed) Biliary atresia and its related disorders. Excerpta Medica, Amsterdam, p 38–45
Hays D M, Snyder W H 1963 Life-span in untreated biliary atresia. Surgery 64: 373–375
Hays D M, Kimura K 1980 Biliary atresia: the Japanese experience. Harvard University Press, Cambridge, Mass.
Hays D M, Kimura K 1981 Biliary atresia: new concepts of management. Current Problems in Surgery 18:546
Hays D M, Altman R P, Hitch D C, Lilly J R, Smith E I, Uceda J E 1983 Biliary atresia in the United States: the survey of the surgical section, American Academy of Pediatrics. In: Kasai, M (ed) Biliary atresia and its related disorders. Excerpta Medica, Amsterdam, p 161–166
Hirsig J, Kara O, Rickham P P 1978 Experimental investigations into the etiology of cholangitis following operation for biliary atresia. Journal of Pediatric Surgery 13: 55–57
Holder T M, Ashcraft K W 1967 The effects of bile duct ligation and inflammation in the fetus. Journal of Pediatric Surgery 2: 35–40
Holmes J B 1916 Congenital obliteration of the bile duct: Diagnosis and suggestions for treatment. American Journal of Diseases of Children 11: 405–431
Home E 1813 On the formation of fat in the intestine of living animals. Philosophical Transactions of the Royal Society 103: 156–157
Howard E R 1984 Extrahepatic biliary atresia. In: Schwartz S I, Ellis H (eds) Maingot's Abdominal Operations, 8th edn. Appleton-Century-Crofts, Norwalk, Connecticut, ch 27, p 1775–1788
Howard E R, Driver M, McClement J, Mowat A P 1982 Results of surgery in 88 consecutive cases of extrahepatic biliary atresia. Journal of the Royal Society of Medicine 75: 408–413
Ito T, Sugito T, Shimoji H 1980 Obstructive jaundice produced by Sporidesmin, a product of Pithomyces Chartarum: experimental studies in the pathogenesis of biliary atresia in rabbits. In: Kasai M, Shiraki K (eds) Cholestasis in infancy. University Park Press, Baltimore, p 225–239
Iwatsuki S, Shaw B, Starzl T 1984 Liver transplantation for biliary atresia. World Journal of Surgery 8: 51–56
Jenner R E, Howard E R 1975 Unsaturated monohydroxy bile acids as a cause of idiopathic obstructive cholangiopathy. Lancet ii: 1073–1074
Kahn E I, Daum F 1983 Arterio hepatic dysplasia: evaluation of the extrahepatic biliary tract, porta hepatis and hepatic parenchyma. In: Daum F (ed) Extrahepatic biliary atresia, Marcel Dekker, New York p 194
Kasai M, Suzuki S 1959 A new operation for 'non-correctable' biliary atresia: hepatic portoenterostomy. Shujitsu 13: 733–739
Kasai M, Ohi R, Chiba T 1980 Intrahepatic bile ducts in biliary atresia. In: Kasai M, Shiraki K (eds) Cholestasis in infancy, University Park Press, Baltimore, p 181–188
Kasai M, Okamoto A, Ohi R, Yabe K, Matsumura Y 1981 Changes of portal vein pressure and intrahepatic blood vessels after surgery for biliary atresia. Journal of Pediatric Surgery 16: 152–159
Ladd W E 1928 Congenital atresia and stenosis of the bile duct. Journal of the American Medical Association 91: 1082–1084
Landing B H 1974 Considerations of the pathogenesis of neonatal hepatitis, biliary atresia and choledochal cyst: the concept of infantile obstructive cholangiopathy. Progress in Pediatric Surgery 6: 113–139
Lawrence D, Howard E R, Tzanatos C, Mowat A P 1981 Hepatic portoenterostomy for biliary atresia. Archives of Disease in Childhood 56: 460–463
Lilly J R 1978 Etiology of cholangitis following operation for biliary atresia. Journal of Pediatric Surgery 13: 559–560
Lilly J R 1979 Hepatic portocholecystostomy for biliary atresia. Journal of Pediatric Surgery 14: 301–304
Lilly J R, Stellin G 1984 Variceal hemorrhage in biliary atresia. Journal of Pediatric Surgery 19: 476–479
Longmire W P, Sandford M C 1948 Intrahepatic cholangiojejunostomy for biliary obstruction. Surgery 24: 264–276
Manolaki A G, Larcher V F, Mowat A P, Barrett J J, Portmann B, Howard E R 1983 The prelaparotomy diagnosis of extrahepatic biliary atresia. Archives of Disease in Childhood 58: 591–594
McClement J W, Howard E R, Mowat A P 1985 Results of surgical treatment for extrahepatic biliary atresia in the United Kingdom, 1980–1982. British Medical Journal 290: 345–347
Miyamoto M, Kajimoto T 1983 Associated anomalies in biliary atresia patients. In: Kasai (ed) Biliary atresia and its related disorders. Excerpta Medica, Amsterdam, p 13–19
Miyano T, Suruga K, Suda K 1979 Abnormal choledocho-pancreatico ductal junction related to the etiology of infantile obstructive jaundice diseases. Journal of Pediatric Surgery 14: 16–26
Morecki R, Glaser J H, Horwitz M S 1983 Etiology of biliary atresia: the role of reo 3 virus. In: Daum F (ed) Extrahepatic biliary atresia. Marcel Dekker, New York, ch 1, p 1–9
Nelson J S, Rosenblum J L, Keating J P, Prensky A L 1983 Neuropathological complications of childhood cholestatic liver disease. In: Daum F (ed) Extrahepatic biliary atresia. Marcel Dekker, New York, ch 16, p 153–157
Odievre H 1978 Long-term results of surgical treatment of biliary atresia, World Journal of Surgery 2: 589–594
Ohi R, Shikes R H, Stellin G P, Lilly J R 1984 In biliary atresia duct histology correlates with bile flow. Journal of Pediatric Surgery 19: 467–470
Okamoto E, Okasora T, Toyosaka A 1980 An experimental study on the etiology of congenital biliary atresia. In: Kasai M, Shiraki K (eds) Cholestasis in Infancy. University Park Press, Baltimore, p 217–224
Phillips P A, Keast D, Papadimitriou J M, Walters M N I, Stanley N F 1969 Chronic obstructive jaundice induced by reovirus type 3 in weanling mice. Pathology 1: 193–203
Saito S 1983 Reoperation for biliary atresia after hepatic portoenterostomy. In: Kasai M (ed) Biliary atresia and its related disorders. Excerpta Medica, Amsterdam, p 224–227
Saito S, Nishina T, Tsuchida Y 1984 Intrahepatic cysts in biliary atresia after successful hepatoportoenterostomy. Archives of Disease in Childhood 59: 274–275
Spitz L 1977 Experimental production of cystic dilatation of the common bile duct in lambs. Journal of Pediatric Surgery 12: 39–42
Starzl T E, Koep L J, Halgrimson C G, Hood J, Schroter G P J, Porter K A et al 1979 Fifteen years of clinical liver transplantation. Gastroenterology 77: 375–388
Sterling J A, Lowenburg K 1963 Increased longevity in congenital biliary atresia. Annals of the New York Academy of Sciences 111: 483–503
Strauss L, Bernstein J 1968 Neonatal hepatitis in congenital rubella; a histopathological study. Archives of Pathology 86: 317–327
Sunaryo F P, Watkins J B 1983 Evaluation of diagnostic techniques for extrahepatic biliary atresia. In: Daum F (ed) Extrahepatic biliary atresia. Marcel Dekker, New York, ch 2, p 17
Suruga K, Miyano T, Kimura A, Arai, Kojima Y 1982 Reoperation in the treatment of biliary atresia. Journal of Pediatric Surgery 17: 1–6
Thomson J 1892 Congenital obliteration of the bile ducts. Oliver and Boyd, Edinburgh
Vacanti J P, Folkman J 1979 Bile duct enlargement by infusion of L-Proline: potential significance in biliary atresia. Journal of Pediatric Surgery 14: 814–818

58

L. H. Blumgart

Benign biliary strictures

There is no aspect of biliary surgery in which imprecise treatment is associated with such disastrous results as in the management of benign bile duct stricture. On the other hand, early recognition and correct management at the first attempt at repair can lead to a successful outcome with good prognosis.

Benign stenosis and strictures of the bile ducts occur in a number of conditions and may affect the intrahepatic or extrahepatic biliary tree. They may be single or multiple. The following table details the causes of benign bile duct strictures:

1. Congenital strictures. Biliary atresia* (Ch. 57).
2. Bile duct injuries.
   a. Postoperative bile duct strictures following:
      (i) injuries at cholecystectomy and exploration of the common bile duct;
      (ii) injury after other operative procedures:
      biliary enteric anastomosis of previously normal bile ducts,
      operations upon the liver or portal vein,
      pancreatic operations,
      gastrectomy,
      following a variety of other operations (rarely).
   b. Stricture after blunt or penetrating injury.
3. Post-inflammatory strictures associated with:
   a. gallstones,
   b. chronic pancreatitis,
   c. chronic duodenal ulcer,
   d. abscess or inflammation in the subhepatic region or in the liver,
   e. parasitic infection* (Ch. 74, 75),
   f. recurrent pyogenic cholangitis* (Ch. 77).
4. Primary sclerosing cholangitis* (Ch. 59).
5. Following radiotherapy.
6. Papillary stenosis* (Ch. 28, 53, 56).

* Not discussed in this chapter.

BILE DUCT INJURIES

Injury to the bile ducts may follow damage inflicted during upper abdominal operations, usually during cholecystectomy, or may be due to blunt or penetrating abdominal injury. Injuries occurring during surgical operations are of importance firstly because they are preventable and secondly because they produce considerable mortality and morbidity far in excess of that recognized for the initial surgical procedure. The results may be particularly tragic since many of the patients so afflicted are young and in the most productive years of life.

Repair must be carried out in a precise and expert manner *at the first attempt* since repeated operative intervention is associated with less good results.

POSTOPERATIVE BILE DUCT STRICTURES

> 'Injuries to the main ducts are nearly always the result of misadventures during operation and are therefore a serious reproach to the surgical profession. They cannot be regarded as just an ordinary risk ... though I know only too well that even with all the care which may reasonably be expected of us, accidents will occasionally happen' (Grey-Turner 1944).

It is impossible to be accurate regarding the incidence of operative injury to the biliary tract. The risk of injury varies with the operation being performed and, with the exception of injury at cholecystectomy, there are no studies which reflect the frequency of such damage. Many injuries are not reported at all or are not detected, the patient's ultimate illness being ascribed to some other cause such as cholangiocarcinoma or sclerosing cholangitis.

While the great majority of injuries to the bile duct occur during cholecystectomy, with or without exploration of the common bile duct, a number also occur in association with other operations either on the stomach, the pancreas, the liver, or during surgery for portal hypertension. Stricture of biliary enteric anastomoses following reconstructive or bypass surgery in association with other operations, e.g. pancreaticoduodenectomy, also occur (Chadwick & Dudley 1984). It is important that such strictures are not misinterpreted as recurrent carcinoma. In addition to injury to a normal biliary tree damage may also follow operations performed on the diseased biliary tract, as e.g. after excision of choledochus cyst and following operations for the management of sclerosing cholangitis.

POST-CHOLECYSTECTOMY INJURIES

'Injuries to the bile ducts are unfortunately not rare and often turn out to be tragedies' (Grey-Turner 1944).

Cholecystectomy is probably the most commonly performed abdominal operation and has a high degree of safety. The surgical mortality is less than 0.5% in patients under the age of 65 although considerably higher in elderly patients submitted to emergency operation, in patients with coincident disease and where exploration of the common bile duct is required (Ch. 46, 50). Nevertheless, it is important to remember that *cholecystectomy is a major operation* and should never be lightly undertaken. While results are good, they are not uniformly so, and some reports suggest that 20–25% of patients will have some continuing symptoms (Bodvall 1973). Of those with continuing problems only 5% will have severe symptoms such as jaundice, pancreatitis or cholangitis (Blumgart et al, 1977, Blumgart & Lygidakis 1982). A minority of patients will suffer damage to the biliary tree. Figures are available from surveys carried out in Sweden, Finland, Germany, and France (Bismuth & Lazorthes 1981, Gutgemann et al 1965, Rosenquist & Myrin 1960, Viikari 1960) and all suggest the incidence of biliary injury is roughly 2 per 1000 operations for gallstones (Bismuth 1982). Kune & Sali (1981) suggest that the incidence is approximately 1 in 300–500 gallstone operations.

Causative factors and prevention

There are a number of factors which relate to bile duct injury during cholecystectomy.

Anatomical variations

There are a wide number of anatomical variations in the extrahepatic biliary tree and in the adjacent hepatic arteries and portal vein. These are so frequent that the surgeon must be aquainted with their range and should always expect the unusual.

The most common anomaly is an abnormal junction between the cystic duct and the main biliary channel. The cystic duct may join the common hepatic duct very high and almost at the hilus of the liver (Fig. 58.1A). In

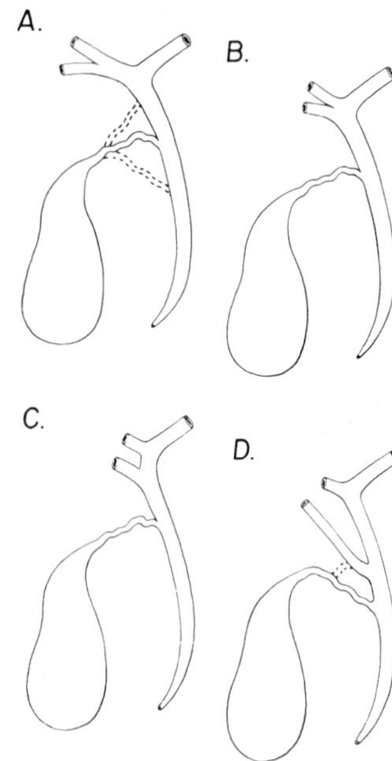

Fig. 58.1 Schematic representation of the manner of junction of the cystic duct with the main extrahepatic biliary channel. A. The cystic duct may join the main bile duct either very high and almost at the confluence of the hepatic ducts or at a much lower level. Indeed it may not join the common hepatic duct until almost at the ampulla. Note that in this figure the right hepatic sectoral ducts join to form a main right hepatic duct. B. The anterior and posterior sectoral ducts of the right liver join the left hepatic duct at a common confluence. C. The right anterior and posterior sectoral ducts join the left hepatic duct independently. D. The anterior (or posterior) right sectoral duct joins the common hepatic duct at a much lower level. The cystic duct may in fact drain into such a sectoral duct (previously published in: Blumgart L H 1984 Bile duct strictures. In: Fromm D (ed), Gastrointestinal surgery Vol. 2. Churchill Livingstone, London, p 755–811)

approximately 25% of patients the right hepatic duct as such is absent, and major ducts draining the anterior and posterior sectors of the right liver join the left hepatic duct directly (Fig. 58.1B, 58.1C). In some such cases a right sectoral duct may run a prolonged extrahepatic course to join the common hepatic duct. The cystic duct may drain directly into such a duct (Fig. 58.1D, 58.2) (Ch. 2).

Similarly bile duct injury may occur when the cystic duct is closely adherent to the common hepatic duct, running together with it in a common sheath before joining it low down. Injury may also occur if the cystic duct is short. In such cases misinterpretation of the anatomy and indeed of operative cholangiography can easily occur especially if a cannula has been advanced so far that it passes into the common bile duct. In this instance, if there is no distal obstruction, the contrast medium passes rapidly down the duct and into the duodenum, there being no display of the proximal ducts (Fig. 58.3a). The surgeon can then easily mistake the common bile duct for a long cystic duct, ligate it and remove it along with the attached gallbladder (Kelley & Blumgart 1985). This situation should not be confused with the almost obliterated cystic

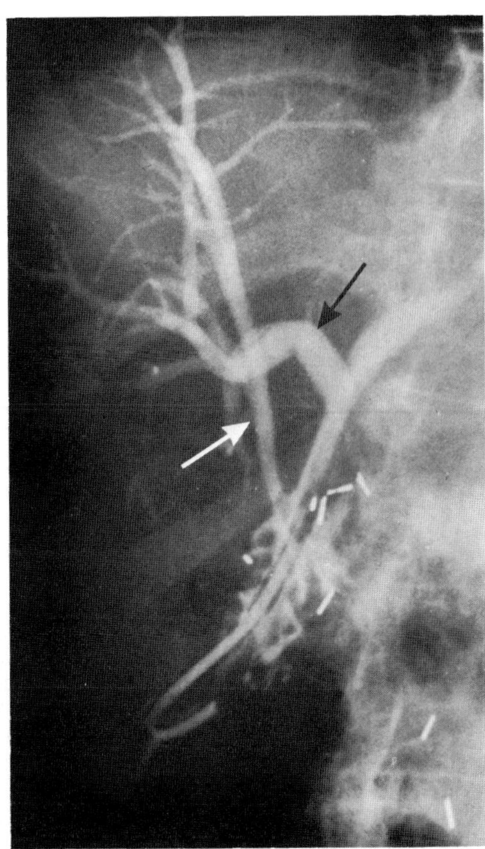

Fig. 58.2 The right anterior sectoral duct (white arrow) drains into the common hepatic duct and the right posterior sectoral duct (black arrow) joins a main left hepatic duct. The situation is as illustrated in Fig. 58.1D. Note that in this patient cholecystectomy was accompanied by a biliary injury at the point of confluence of the common hepatic duct and the right anterior sectoral duct (Bismuth Type 5). Repair has been carried out by hepaticojejunostomy Roux-en-Y

duct found in long standing chronic cholelithiasis and chronic cholecystitis (see below) (Kune 1970).

Anomalies of the vessels, in particular of the hepatic artery, are very frequent and occur in over 20% of patients (Ch. 3). The most common abnormality is for the right hepatic artery to arise in whole or in part from the superior mesenteric trunk. The anomalous vessel usually runs up to the right of the portal vein and just postero-lateral to the bile duct running close to the cystic duct at the neck of the gallbladder where it is prone to injury during cholecystectomy. During attempts to control bleeding there may be coincident damage to the bile ducts if clamps are blindly applied (Cattell & Braasch 1959a). The bleeding usually arises from the cystic artery or from the right hepatic arterial trunk, although injury to the common hepatic artery also occurs. In a recent series of 78 post-cholecystectomy biliary strictures studied at Hammersmith Hospital selective coeliac angiography was performed in 25 patients because of a history of vascular damage at operation prior to referral, haematemesis or melaena, oesophagogastric varices seen at endoscopy or a palpable spleen. Evidence of arterial damage or abnormality was noted in 14 (Fig. 58.4) and damage to the portal vein or one of its branches in five cases. In three patients portal venous obstruction was accompanied by segmental or lobar atrophy (Ch. 6) (Fig. 58.5). Oesophagogastric varices were demonstrated in five patients and splenomegaly in nine (Blumgart et al 1984). On occasion not only is there a bile duct stricture or stenosis but an hepatic artery aneurysm may form and erode into the biliary tree producing haemobilia (Ch. 85) (Kelley et al 1983).

In recent years the microcirculation of the extrahepatic biliary tree has been beautifully investigated by Northover & Terblanche (1979, 1982). The blood supply of the bile duct runs in three columns, one posterior and two lateral (Ch. 2) and it is suggested that damage to these vessels may result in ischaemia to the bile duct with consequent necrosis and stricture. The likelihood of such an event would be increased by dissection of the common bile duct during cholecystectomy or undue mobilization prior to choledochotomy. While there is no firm evidence for this proposition the anatomical studies are elegant and convincing. It would seem reasonable not to pursue extensive dissection of the common bile duct during cholecystectomy as is taught in some centres (Northover & Terblanche 1982). In addition, transection of the bile duct disturbs the blood supply and in particular arterial flow arising from its lower end. Ischaemia occurs in the upper transected duct and is undoubtedly responsible for the remarkable scarring and retraction of the stricture towards and into the hilus which is so frequently seen.

Pathological factors

Acute cholecystitis may be accompanied by extensive oedema in the region of the porta hepatis and Calot's triangle and there may be considerable friability during dissection. Under these circumstances, and in the presence of acute inflammation, damage might more easily occur and, if dissection appears hazardous, cholecystostomy may be a safer option than cholecystectomy (Dawson 1981).

Of undoubtedly greater significance is the small contracted fibrotic gallbladder with considerable surrounding inflammatory reaction, sometimes partly embedded in the liver tissue and obliterating Calot's triangle so as to lie close against the common hepatic duct. In such instances dissection of Calot's triangle is impossible. Cholecyst-choledochus fistula is not uncommon in long-standing disease, and there may already be pre-existing benign stenosis consequent upon the inflammation (Mirizzi 1948) (Fig. 58.6A). Any patient presenting with gallstones, jaundice and attacks of cholangitis who at operation has such a gallbladder present should be suspected of harbouring a cholecyst-choledochal fistula. In these circumstances it is wiser to remove the greater part of th gallbladder wall which is easily visible and to remove the stones. Such a

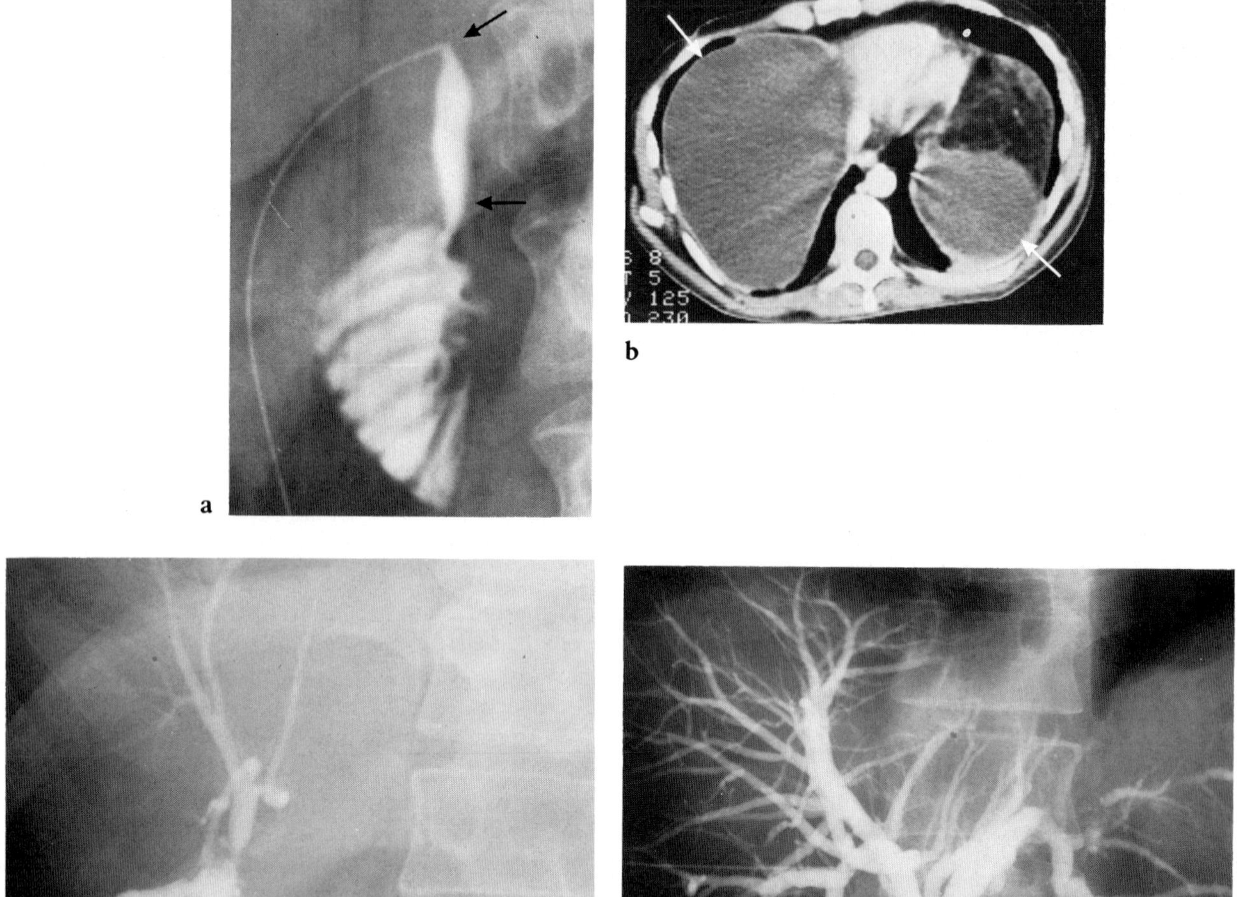

Fig. 58.3 a. Operative cholangiogram obtained after cannulation of the cystic duct. Note that the cannula has entered the common bile duct (upper arrow) and that only the common bile duct (lower arrow) has been outlined. The common hepatic duct has not been displayed at all. The surgeon proceeded with the cholecystectomy in the belief that he had cannulated the cystic duct. b. The patient became extremely ill following operation and was referred, jaundiced and with fever and incipient renal failure. CAT scan obtained on admission to Hammersmith Hospital revealed enormous intraperitoneal biliary collections (arrows). Operative drainage was instituted. c. Tubogram obtained after operative drainage revealed the presence of a fistulous tract with connections to both the right and left abdomen (arrow). A portion (the right anterior sectoral duct) of the biliary tree is outlined. The patient was treated expectedly and the fistula closed, but several weeks later the patient presented with recurrent cholangitis and jaundice. d. Percutaneous transhepatic cholangiogram obtained on re-admission reveals a high stricture at the confluence of the hepatic ducts (Bismuth Type 3). Repair was effected by hepaticojejunostomy Roux-en-Y using an approach to the left hepatic ductal system and extending the dissection to the right

'partial cholecystectomy' is a safe option and allows direct inspection of the depths of the gallbladder. If a fistula exists then it is almost always associated with some narrowing of the bile duct just distal to the fistula and is best managed by mobilizing the duodenum and carrying out a cholecyst-choledochoduodenostomy (Fig. 58.6B).

Technical factors

While it is true that some bile duct injuries occur following cholecystectomy performed by surgeons who have been inadequately trained or are inexperienced (Andren-Sandberg et al 1985), many occur after cholecystectomy done by well trained and often experienced surgeons who find that they have damaged the bile duct during an 'easy'

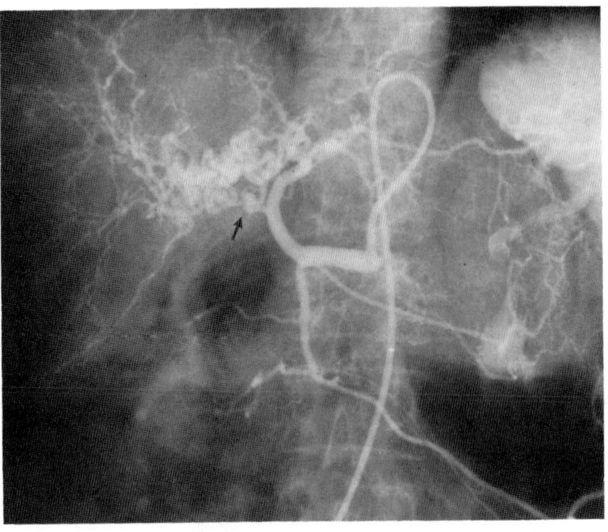

Fig. 58.4 Selective hepatic arteriogram in a patient with a high bile duct stricture. The investigation was carried out because of a history of severe haemobilia prior to referral. Note that there has been a complete occlusion of the right hepatic artery (arrow) and the development of an extensive collateral circulation (same case as in Fig. 58.22)

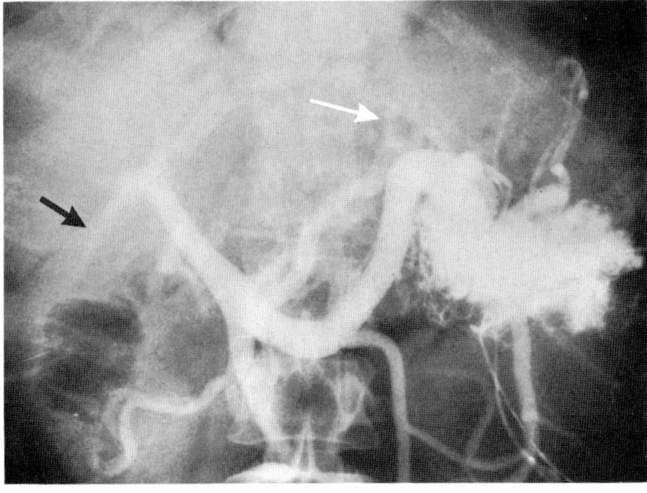

Fig. 58.5 Splenoportography in a patient with benign bile duct stricture and a history of vascular damage at the time of initial operation. Patient presented with portal hypertension and bleeding oesophageal varices. Note that only a portion of the right portal venous vasculature is outlined (black arrow). Note varices in the area of the gastric fundus (white arrow). Percutaneous transhepatic cholangiography revealed a severe stenosis (but no complete stricture) close to the hilar area. Liver biopsy revealed severe hepatic fibrosis. The patient was managed by a splenorenal shunt but no repair of the bile duct stricture since jaundice and cholangitis were not a problem. She remains well, seven years after porto-systemic shunt. Repair of the stricture has never been necessary

cholecystectomy. Indeed injury might occur even in the hands of the highly skilled and experienced (Grey-Turner 1944).

Cholecystectomy is a very common operation and it is easy for familiarity with the procedure to breed contempt.

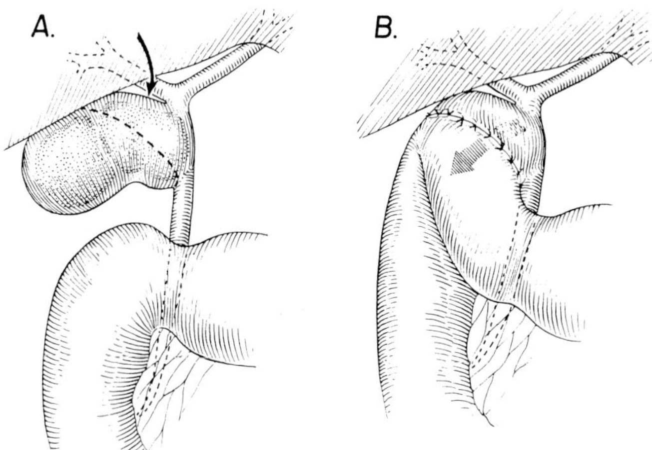

Fig. 58.6 A. Illustrates obliteration of Calot's triangle (curved arrow) by the inflammatory process accompanying severe chronic cholecystitis. There are two large gallstones in the gallbladder, one of which has eroded into the common hepatic duct producing a cholecysto-choledochal fistula. In such cases (which usually present with cholangitis and obstructive jaundice) there should be no attempt at cholecystectomy since this will be accompanied by inevitable biliary injury. B. Partial cholecystectomy (dotted line) can be performed with extraction of the calculi. Cholecyst-choledochoduodenostomy can be carried out with safety and adequate drainage of bile (Blumgart 1984) (previously published in: Blumgart L H 1984 Bile duct strictures. In: Fromm D (ed), Gastrointestinal Surgery, Vol. 2. Churchill Livingstone, London, p. 755–811)

Injury is much more likely to occur if the surgeon is attempting to operate single handed and without adequate assistance. In general one good assistant and preferably two should be employed so as to allow deliberate operation with good visualization. In this manner hurried or careless procedures will be minimized.

The reason for error is often difficult to determine in a particular case and frequently the surgeon has no memory of what might have occurred. It has been assumed that the common error is that the hepatic duct or common bile duct is mistaken for the cystic duct and is partially excised, or a portion of the common biliary channel is ligated along with the cystic duct. Of 78 cases seen at the Royal Postgraduate Medical School (Blumgart et al 1984) it was possible to incriminate this error in six and certainly the high nature of the injury in most cases suggests direct damage or ligation of the common hepatic duct (Smith 1979).

Abdominal incisions must be adequate in length and appropriately sited. Early demonstration of the cystic artery and cystic duct is desirable and the cystic artery should then be ligated close to the gallbladder wall so as to avoid any possible damage to the common hepatic artery or the right hepatic artery (Ch. 44). A cystic duct cannula can then be introduced and operative cholangiography performed which in addition to its advantage of indicating the necessity for bile duct exploration will on occasion reveal anatomical abnormalities (Morgenstern & Berci 1982) (Ch. 27). Peroperative cholangiography is important in this respect, but acceptance of poor cholangiographic pictures may mislead the surgeon, especially if there is not full demonstration of the biliary tree (Fig. 58.3) (Kelley & Blumgart 1985). However, knowledge gained at cholangiography is in general valuable. It is interesting that of 72 patients with post-cholecystectomy biliary strictures studied at Hammersmith Hospital and in whom adequate information was available, 71% did not have perioperative cholangiography at the time of initial cholecystectomy. Care must be taken to perform the examination early during the operation, to ensure suitable positioning of the cannula and to obtain adequate filling of both proximal and distal bile ducts. Although it is unlikely to prevent biliary ductal damage in all cases the information obtained may help reduce the incidence of biliary ductal injuries at cholecystectomy.

In jaundiced patients preoperative cholangiography is advisable and may be obtained by means of percutaneous transhepatic cholangiography or endoscopic retrograde choledochopancreatography (Benjamin & Blumgart 1979).

Dense fibrosis in the area of Calot's triangle should lead to a change in policy with either a partial cholecystectomy being performed as described above (Grey-Turner 1944) or alternatively a dissection of the gallbladder from the fundus carried out slowly and cautiously, proceeding and keeping close to the gallbladder wall. In this manner most cases can be safely dissected. If difficulty is encountered as the neck of the gallbladder is approached, then the attempted total cholecystectomy should be abandoned in favour of a partial procedure. In such densely fibrosed cases the cystic duct is always obliterated and postoperative biliary leakage does not occur. Excessive traction on the gallbladder during cholecystectomy should be avoided. If this is done, tenting of the common bile duct/common hepatic duct junction occurs and creates a situation likely to result in excision of a segment of common duct. Some authors argue that the precise point of junction of the cystic duct with the common hepatic duct should be clearly demonstrated and regard it as important to separate the cystic duct when adherent to the common hepatic duct and trace it to its termination (Kune & Sali 1981). Indeed Kune recommends deliberate choledochotomy in the supraduodenal part of the common bile duct and insertion of a probe or dilator in a proximal direction in order to allow satisfactory delineation of the common and right hepatic duct. This is totally unnecessary nor is there need to go to excessive lengths to display the cystic duct because such dissection might well lead to injury.

Should bleeding occur during operation then its control must be precise. Blood is removed by suction. Arterial haemorrhage can be controlled by pressure with the finger and thumb on the hepatic artery at the free edge of the lesser omentum or by the application of a soft gastrointestinal clamp across this region. The offending vessels are then dissected and deliberately controlled. An anomalous right hepatic artery arising from the superior mesenteric artery usually runs close to the common biliary channel behind the cystic duct and may be damaged during cholecystectomy (see above). This is common and careful dissection will avoid damage with subsequent bleeding.

Should operative cholangiography reveal a very small common bile duct with a filling defect indicating a *possible small stone* or stones within it, and in the presence of multiple small stones within the gallbladder, some surgeons, including the author, advocate simple cholecystectomy without exploration of the common duct. Virtually all such stones will pass asymptomatically. Furthermore, operative exploration of such a small duct in pursuit of a tiny stone is difficult, often unrewarding, and more likely to result in damage to the biliary system than exploration easily carried out within a normal size duct. The likelihood of further symptoms for the patient and of complications is almost certainly less when such a stone is left in situ than in an attempt at common bile duct exploration.

Exploration of the common bile duct should involve careful exposure of a sufficient length of duct to allow choledochotomy but no extensive dissection or stripping of the bile duct of its surrounding connective tissue. Exploration should be carried out gently utilizing soft gum elastic bougies, Fogarty type balloon catheters and choledochoscopy. If forceps are employed they should not be forced through the papilla of Vater.

There is a danger that should metal bougies, such as Bakes dilators, be passed downwards through the papilla into the duodenum, subsequent secondary post-inflammatory stenosis of the papilla of Vater might occur and that in addition false passages may be created. The dilator may pass either into the pancreatic tissue or through the bile duct wall proximal to the papilla and into the duodenum creating a choledochoduodenal fistula. Choledochoduodenal fistulae either due to passage of an instrument as described above or following an erroneously placed sphincteroplasty may result in symptoms of jaundice, cholangitis and pancreatitis (Hunt & Blumgart 1980). Passage of a dilator into the pancreas may result in postoperative pancreatitis (Schein 1978) and secondary bile duct stricture may result. Stenosis or stricture of the peripapillary common bile duct may also follow surgical or endoscopic sphincteroplasty.

Exploration of the common bile duct at the time of cholecystectomy should usually be carried out in a supraduodenal fashion. Sphincteroplasty is reserved by most surgeons only for patients with a stone impacted at the papilla of Vater (Benjamin & Blumgart 1979, Stubbs et al 1983) although some employ the approach for almost all bile duct exploration (Ch. 53).

In patients with multiple stones or primary stasis stones or where there is distal obstruction such as might occur with stenosis of the papilla of Vater. The surgeon might

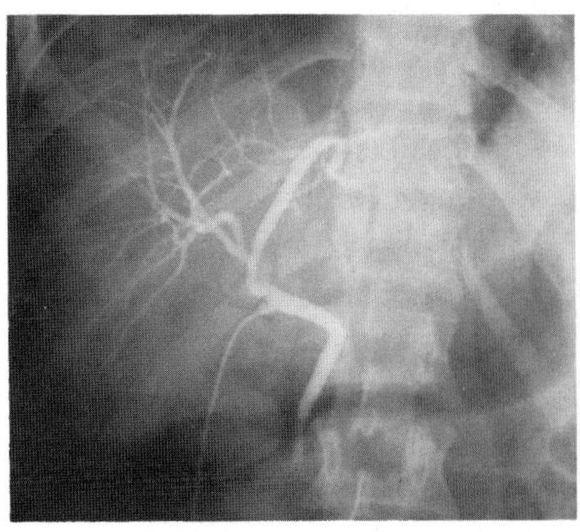
a

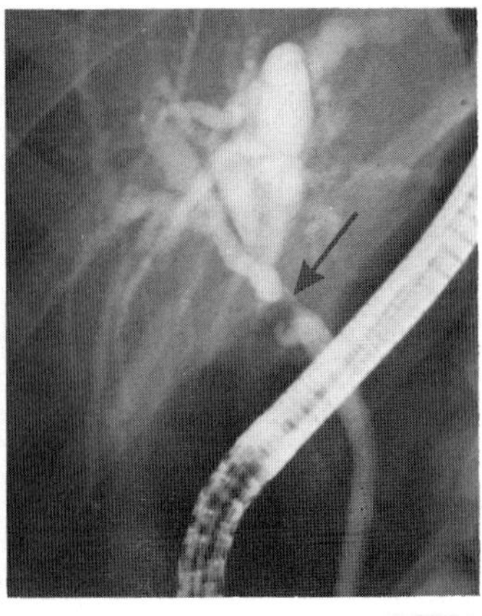
b

Fig. 58.7 a. T-tube cholangiogram obtained at the time of cholecystectomy during which a stone was suspected to be present in a small calibre common bile duct. Exploration was carried out and no stone was found despite repeated exploration. b. The patient developed recurrent attacks of cholangitis. Endoscopic retrograde cholangiography reveals a bile duct stricture at the point of choledochotomy (arrow)

elect to carry out choledochoduodenostomy (Ch. 54). Choledochoduodenostomy should generally not be performed if the common bile duct is less than 15 mm/diameter and if a stoma of at least 2 cm cannot be created. If an adequate stoma is created the results are good and late stenosis or cholangitis are rare (Lygidakis 1981, Madden 1973, Schein & Gliedman 1981). On the other hand should choledochoduodenostomy be performed to a narrow common bile duct, then stenosis perhaps associated with bile duct stricture is more likely.

After exploration of the common bile duct, post-exploratory cholangiography or choledochoscopy should be performed. Care must be taken in performing post-exploratory cholangiography and in immediate re-exploration of the common bile duct not to damage the duct by repeated suture about a T-tube (Fig. 58.7). The author prefers the method of post-exploratory cholangiography described by Gunn and his colleagues (Myat et al 1973) (Ch. 52). With this approach a small Foley catheter (with the tip amputated) is used to occlude the ducts, allowing proximal and distal cholangiography after exploration without the necessity to close the choledochotomy at the time of X-ray. In addition good radiographs of the proximal and distal duct are obtainable.

Pathological effects

Fibrosis

Biliary obstruction is associated with the formation of high local concentrations of bile salts at the canalicular membrane and these initiate pathological changes in the biliary system (Schaffner et al 1971). Bile thrombi form within dilated centrilobular bile canaliculi and secondary changes are seen in adjacent hepatocytes. An inflammatory exudate forms leading to collagen deposition and eventually fibrosis and scarring around bile ducts and ductules. As these progress they may lead to mechanical interference with bile flow and continuing cholestasis.

The fibrosis is accompanied by liver cell hyperplasia (Weinbren et al 1985). This is not a true secondary biliary cirrhosis since the lobular structure of the liver is usually well preserved (Fig. 58.8) and the marked fibrosis which occurs in long-standing cases only rarely proceeds to a true cirrhotic pattern (Ch. 100). This knowledge is of importance in planning therapy since many of the changes are potentially reversible and there may be a return to near normality of such a liver following relief of biliary obstruction (Blumgart 1978).

Changes also occur in the extrahepatic ducts which are subject to fibrosis and upward retraction especially in the presence of infection and perhaps ischaemia. This is accompanied by a sequence of mucosal atrophy, squamous metaplasia, inflammatory infiltration and fibrosis in the subepithelial layers of the ducts seen especially in long-standing obstruction.

Patients with biliary obstruction and secondary biliary fibrosis are at high risk (see below). Evidence of liver fibrosis associated with portal hypertension usually takes four or five years to become evident although it may present as early as two years after the onset of stricture.

Major stigmata of hepatocellular dysfunction such as spider naevia, asterixis, and portal-systemic encephalopathy may develop although these are not common in benign biliary obstruction and should make the clinician suspicious that there may be associated parenchymal disease. If liver biopsy reveals a major component of primary hepatocellular disease (e.g. alcoholic cirrhosis) in association with benign stricture then the prognosis is especially poor.

Atrophy

Distribution of liver mass is regulated by a complex balance in which bile flow, portal venous flow and hepatic venous flow are the main regulators. Quality and quantity of portal venous inflow are important in maintenance of liver cell size and mass (Ch. 6, 7). Segmental or lobar

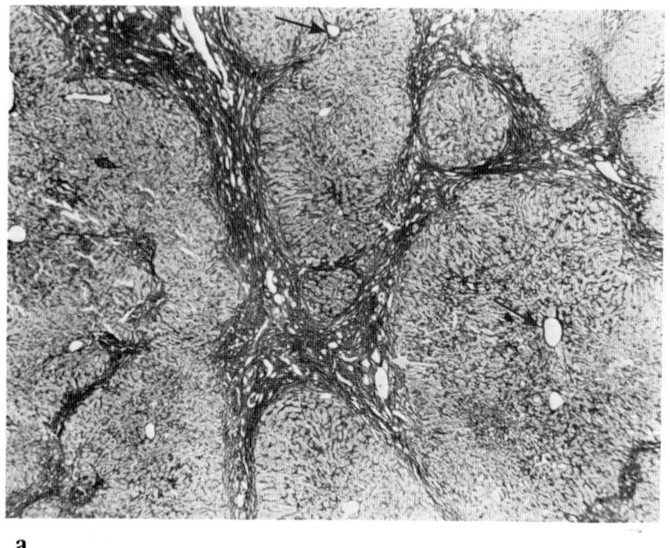

a

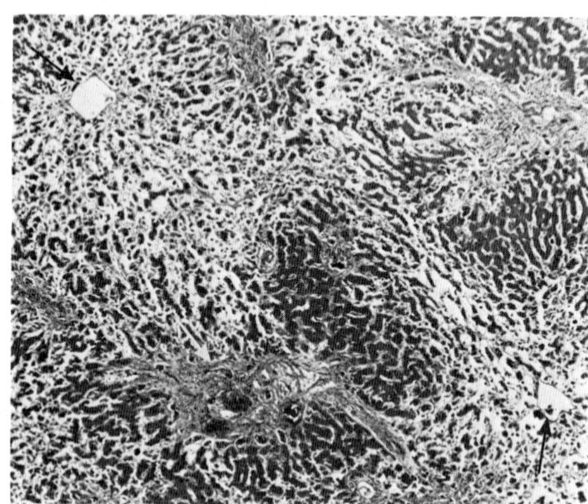

b

Fig. 58.8 a. Photomicrograph reveals the effect of long standing biliary obstruction due to benign biliary stricture. There is hepatic fibrosis present but preservation of the basic hepatic architecture, portal tract (white arrow) and hepatic venous radicles (black arrows) being normally related. The fibrosis extends between the lobules. Note that the pattern is not one of true cirrhosis in which there is destruction of the basic hepatic architecture. b. Extensive fibrosis with substantially normal relation of hepatic venous radicles (black arrows) to portal tracts (white arrow) in a patient with portal hypertension (Weinbren et al 1985)

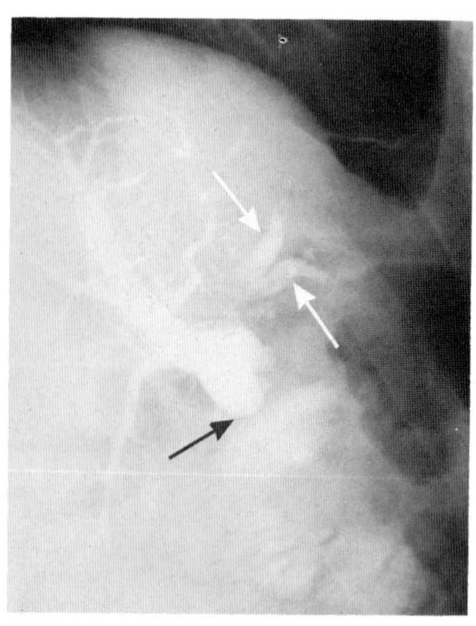

a

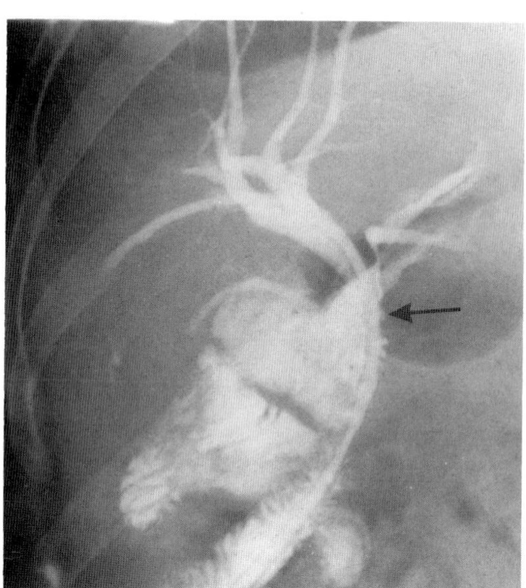

b

Fig. 58.9 a. Percutaneous transhepatic cholangiogram in a patient with recurrent post-cholecystectomy stricture following two previous attempts at hepaticojejunostomy Roux-en-Y. The right hepatic ductal system is dilated and there is a recurrent stricture (black arrow) of the common hepatic duct. The previous Roux-en-Y loop is faintly outlined. Note particularly (white arrows) the atrophic left hepatic ducts within a small left lobe. There are intrahepatic calculi. HIDA scan in this patient failed to reveal any evidence of left lobe function at all. b. Cholangiogram obtained via a transjejunal transanastomotic tube following refashioning of hepaticojejunostomy Roux-en-Y. There is a wide anastomosis (arrow). The stones have been removed from the left hepatic ductal system and they are draining freely. The tube was removed two months after surgery and the patient remains well and symptom free four years later

atrophy results from a degree of portal venous occlusion or bile duct occlusion to that area of liver tissue. Unilobar atrophy is associated with hypertrophy of the contralateral lobe and may present diagnostic and operative difficulty. Changes of this nature are frequently found in benign stricture (Fig. 58.9) and may be associated with asymetrical involvement of lobar or sectoral hepatic ducts, interference with the blood supply particularly the portal venous supply, or with decreased portal perfusion consequent on secondary fibrotic changes. In benign bile duct stricture, even though drainage of grossly dilated ducts within an atrophic segment may not be effective in relieving obstruction, the dilated ducts within the atrophic remnant are nearly always filled with infected bile and continued cholangitis is inevitable unless drainage is obtained not only of ducts within the hypertrophic area of liver tissue, but also in the atrophic portion.

Diagnosis

The diagnosis of benign bile duct stricture requires confirmation of suspicion that damage to the biliary tree has occurred together with a precise demonstration of the level and extent of the stricture particularly in its proximal portion. Any associated damage to adjacent blood vessels should also be shown.

Of course the fact that damage to the biliary tree has occurred may be recognized at operation, but this is often not so. It becomes evident early in the postoperative period or sometimes months later that a biliary fistula or stricture is present.

Excessive biliary drainage from the wound or drain sites in the early postoperative period may indicate a major injury to the bile ducts. In others localized or generalized peritoneal signs become evident and an intra-abdominal collection of bile is drained at a second operation, it then being clear that bile duct injury has occurred (Fig. 58.3b,c,d)

In some cases there is a history of postoperative biliary drainage and fever and perhaps even of a subphrenic or subhepatic abscess, the patient then being free of symptoms for some months before developing recurring bouts of pyrexia, rigors and jaundice. In other patients a steadily progressive obstructive jaundice may be the first sign of ductal injury and this, although usually evident immediately after operation, may come on weeks to months after initial operation.

On physical examination jaundice is usually present although it may be intermittent in nature or even absent, depending on whether bile duct obstruction is complete or partial (Fig. 58.10) and whether or not a biliary fistula is present. Sometimes a bile duct injury associated with fever may present without jaundice and in such cases an internal or external biliary fistula may have been established or the stricture involve only one sectoral duct (Fig. 58.10). In the presence of recurring bouts of cholangitis or an established biliary fistula, weight loss and debility are invariable. The patient may complain of itching and scratch marks may be evident upon the limbs.

Hepatomegaly is frequently present and indicates usually long-standing obstruction. Splenomegaly may be the result of secondary liver fibrosis with associated portal hypertension, but the possibility of direct damage or thrombosis of the portal vein must be considered and indeed is present in a number of patients. Splenomegaly, oesophageal varices or the presence of frank signs of liver failure such as spider naevi or a liver flap or of ascitis should alert the clinician to the possibility of associated hepatocellular disease. Exclusion of this as a factor in the illness is of importance not only in planning management but also in a medico-legal context.

Laboratory investigation

The majority of patients are jaundiced at presentation and the liver function tests reveal a cholestatic pattern. The serum bilirubin is elevated and the serum alkaline phosphatase raised. With incomplete or sectoral obstruction the serum alkaline phosphatase is usually elevated even though

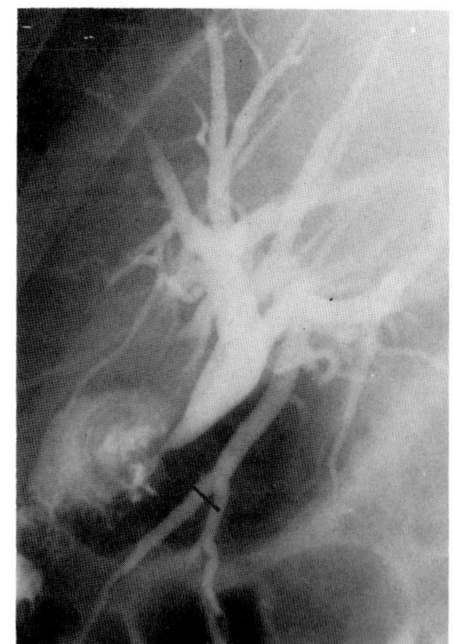

a

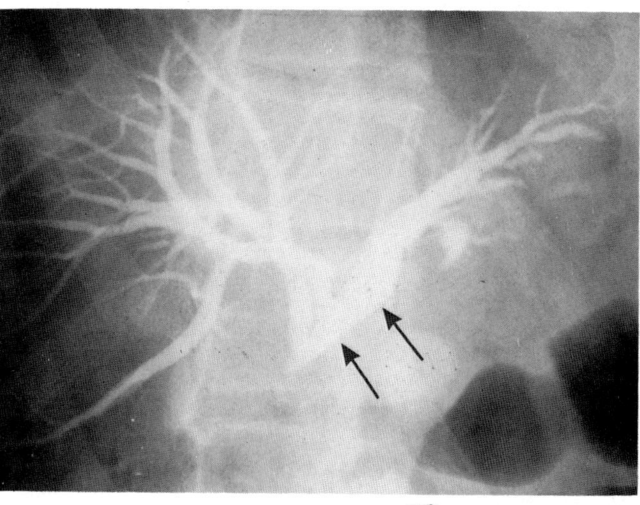

b

Fig. 58.10 a. Percutaneous transhepatic cholangiogram reveals a recurrent post-cholecystectomy bile duct stricture. Roux-en-Y hepaticojejunostomy had been created. There is a very fine stricture (arrow) present which just allows flow of bile. The ductal system is only very modestly dilated. The patient presented with recurrent attacks of fever and malaise but not jaundice. The serum bilirubin was normal but the alkaline phosphatase grossly raised. b. Anteroposterior view of the same case reveals a good length of left hepatic duct available (arrows). Repair was effected by hepaticojejunostomy Roux-en-Y utilizing the left duct approach (see text). The patient remains well, symptom free and with normal liver function tests two years after surgery

the serum bilirubin level may be normal. Serum transaminase levels may be within normal limits or may be elevated, especially if there is cholangitis. In cases of prolonged obstruction the serum albumin may be depressed. Nutritional status and especially the total body potassium may be related to surgical outcome in jaundiced patients (Ch. 32).

In patients with advanced secondary biliary fibrosis or associated hepatocellular disease or cirrhosis it may be very difficult to distinguish the effects of stricture from those consequent on hepatocellular dysfunction and in this instance, particularly where the patient is anicteric and the serum alkaline phosphatase raised, HIDA scanning may be of value (Ch. 15) (see below).

Blood urea should be measured and it is advisable to record the serum creatinine as an index of renal function.

Radiological investigations

On occasion an external fistula or a tube is in situ and contrast medium can be injected so as to outline the biliary ductal system (Fig. 58.11). Since biliary infection in such cases is inevitable it is wise to protect the patient with antibiotic prophylaxis against bacteraemia which may follow fistulography.

Ultrasonography is an excellent means of demonstrating dilatation of the intrahepatic ducts but is of little value in a precise demonstration the extent of stricture and of no value if the ducts are not dilated. Percutaneous transhepatic cholangiography (PTC) is the key investigation. Some investigators are wary of its use preoperatively because of the risk of cholangitis and bile leakage (Bismuth 1982), but the procedure has become much safer with the introduction of the fine needle (Okuda et al 1974) and, provided antibiotic cover is used and the ducts not overfilled, cholangitis and leakage are uncommon. The biliary ductal system is entered in almost 100% of cases and a successful cholangiogram will demonstrate the level and extent of the stricture (Fig. 58.3d, 58.10). Great care must be taken to outline all branches of the intrahepatic biliary tree, particularly in high bile duct stricture and in the diagnosis of a recurrent stricture after previous reconstruction. Modern surgical technique allows an ordered approach to the selection of a reconstructive operation (Ch. 70) so that full demonstration is necessary and in particular a display of the confluence of the bile ducts (if intact) and of the left ductal system and its branches.

Endoscopic retrograde cholangiopancreatography (ERCP) is seldom of value in the precise diagnosis of complete high bile duct stricture since there is usually discontinuity of the common bile duct preventing display of the intrahepatic structures. However, the procedure is of value in demonstrating incomplete stricture (stenosis). In addition it is important to carry out ERCP in any patient in whom there is a history of sphincteric damage at the time of initial exploration of the common bile duct and particularly if there is associated unexplained upper abdominal pain, since papillary stenosis and perhaps associated pancreatitis may be demonstrated. Furthermore, cholangitis may occur in association with stenosis of the high bile duct, continuing infection being related to the presence of sphincteric incontinence consequent on surgical or endoscopic sphincterotomy or an associated choledochoduodenal fistula (Fig. 58.12) (Hunt & Blumgart 1980, Blumgart & Lygidakis 1982). This combination of high stenosis and low incontinence is easily misinterpreted (Kracht et al 1986). Oesophagogastroduodenoscopy is also important if there is any suspicion of oesophageal varices.

If there has been excessive bleeding at the time of cholecystectomy or if there is any suspicion either from a history, access to previous notes, the presence of a palpable spleen or endoscopic evidence of varices that the patient has portal hypertension then arteriography and portography are necessary (Fig. 58.4, 58.5). The latter is usually obtainable by examination of late phase films after splenic arterial injection, but occasionally direct percutaneous splenoportography is necessary.

It is of some importance to recognize that unilateral bile duct and/or portal venous obstruction can lead to segmental liver atrophy (see above) (Ham 1979). Despite widely dilated ducts in such atrophic segments, the liver

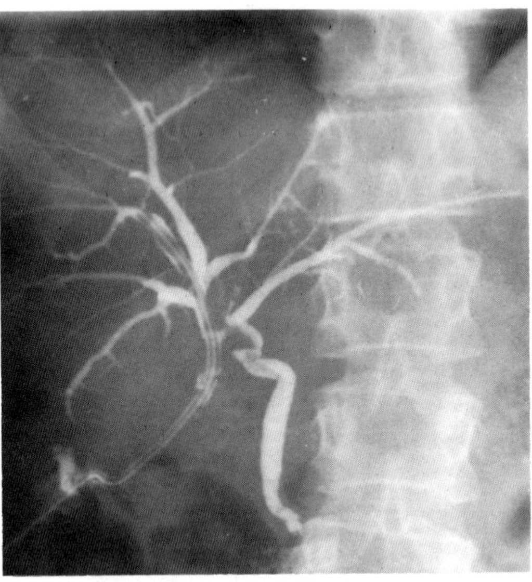

Fig. 58.11 Tubogram obtained after injection of a tube which had been placed into the ductal system following a hilar ductal injury recognized at the time of operation. The patient was referred draining aproximately 200 ml of bile per day but with normal liver function tests and no fever. Note that the tube has been passed into the right hepatic ductal system, but there is filling of the entire intrahepatic bile duct. There appears to be a complete division of the common hepatic ducts. A fistulous connection has established between the left hepatic ductal system and the common hepatic duct. The tube was withdrawn and no repair carried out. There was subsequent atrophy of the right liver but the patient remains well and symptom free and with normal liver function tests over a four-year follow-up period

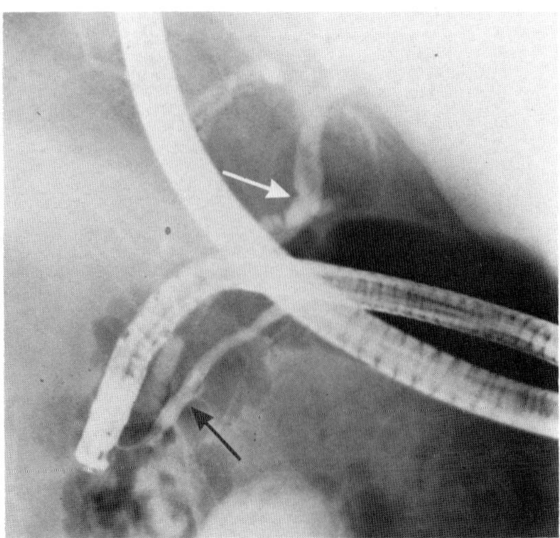

a

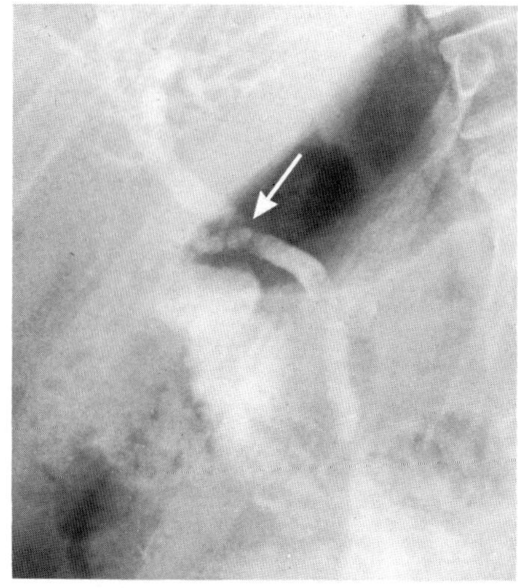

b

Fig. 58.12 a. Endoscopic retrograde choledochopancreatogram in a patient with recurrent cholangitis following a previous cholecystectomy and transduodenal sphincteroplasty. Endoscopic inspection of the papillary region revealed choledochoduodenal fistula 0.5 cm proximal to the papillary orifice, which was intact. Cannulation of the papilla showed the catheter lying within the pancreatic duct (black arrow) which was quite normal. Separate cannulation of the fistulous tract outlined the biliary tree (white arrow). b. Cholangiogram after withdrawal of the instrument. There is a significant stricture in the region of the cystic duct/common hepatic duct junction (arrow). Repair was effected by hepaticojejunostomy Roux-en-Y

tissue draining into these ducts is not healthy. The radiological signs of atrophy include crowding and irregularity of the smaller biliary radicles (Fig. 58.9) and arteries within the affected area. In addition isotope scanning may show what appears to be a filling defect in the related area and CAT scanning may reveal segmental liver atrophy (Czerniak et al 1986).

Isotopic scanning techniques may be of value in the assessment of bile duct strictures and in particular of the functional assessment of incomplete strictures and of anastomoses carried out at previous reconstructive attempts. HIDA scanning methods allow a dynamic and quantitative assessment of liver function and of the clearance of bile across anastomoses and strictures (Fig. 58.13a). Studies at the Royal Postgraduate Medical School, London (McPherson et al 1984) suggest that HIDA scanning may be of particular value in those cases where there is incomplete stricturing or re-stenosis and where ultrasonographic examination shows a non-dilated ductal system. Similarly in patients with hepatocellular disease HIDA scanning may be of value in distinguishing the contribution of restricture to the biochemical and symptomatic problem as distinct from that of liver disease. In such cases the bilirubin level may be normal but the alkaline phosphatase raised. PTC is invasive and may be difficult, especially if the liver is fibrous and tough and endoscopic retrograde cholangiography of no value since the previous construction of a Roux loop makes the investigation impossible. HIDA scanning is also valuable during follow-up of patients after surgical repair since it can be repeated and is non-invasive. It is of a special value in demonstrating anastomotic patency and function in patients in whom no tube has been left across the anastomosis at the time of repair (Fig. 58.13b).

Clinical interpretation

It should be emphasized that discovery at cholangiography of an area of stenosis or incomplete stricture is not necessarily an index for immediate operation. It is important not

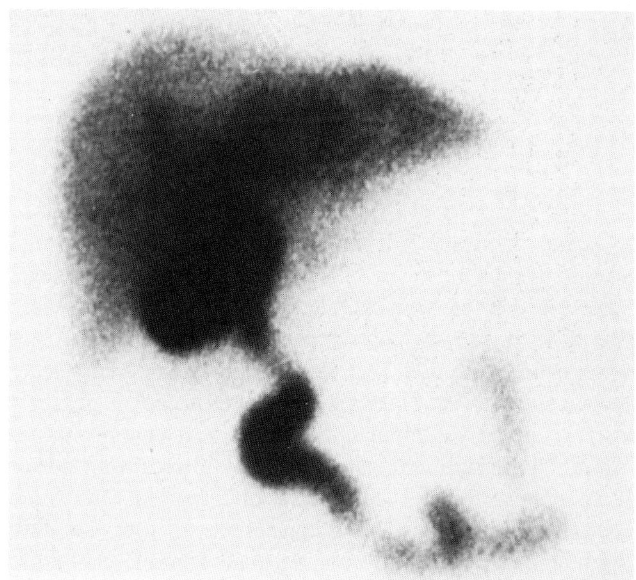

a

Fig. 58.13 a. Anterior view of liver at 2 minutes after the intravenous injection of 120 MBq (3 mC)$^{HIDA\ 99mTC}$ (Dimethyl imino diacetic acid) in a patient with a hepatojejunostomy for benign stricture. This shows tracer in the liver, major bile ducts and also in upper small bowel.

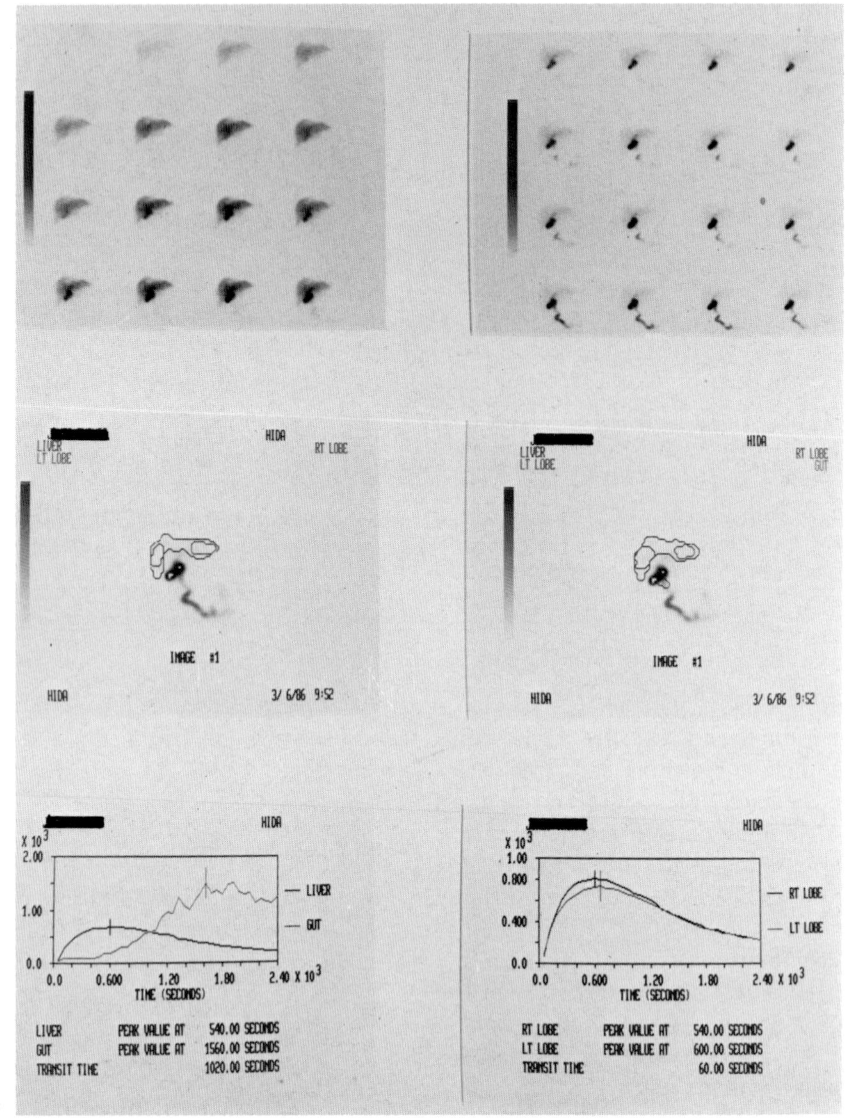

Fig. 58.13 b. Upper images show 32 $6\frac{1}{4}$ second sequential frames on the same patient as in a. Regions of interest have been selected over right and left lobes of the liver, and also the gut (shown on central images). Time activity curves, (lower left and right) show prompt uptake of tracer and rapid clearance with a rising curve over the bowel. These are normal findings

'to treat X-rays'. An established internal fistula may provide good long-term biliary drainage and quite severe degrees of stenosis on cholangiography may be associated with little in the way of symptoms and near normal liver function tests. Similarly it may be permissible in selected cases, especially in elderly patients, to accept a degree of obstruction or segmental obstruction if symptoms are minimal and easily controlled (e.g. by intermittent administration of antibiotics). In a series of 78 patients the author has chosen conservative management in four on these grounds and successfully managed all for periods of nine months to five years without resort to operation and without evidence of progressive illness. Balloon dilatation of benign strictures has recently been carried out (Toufanian et al 1978, Molnar & Stockum, 1978, Teplick et al 1980, Schwarz et al 1981, Vogel et al 1985) and may be successful but long-term results are not yet available. The results must be judged against no treatment at all. In addition balloon dilatation resulting in incomplete relief of obstruction may prove to be associated with relief of symptoms yet progressive liver damage (see below). Indeed it is particularly important in all cases in whom operative treatment is not selected or in whom dilatation has been carried out to observe the patients regularly, since progressive liver damage may be insidious and a persistently elevated alkaline phosphatase the only index of incomplete obstruction.

Finally it is important to emphasize that endoscopic examination of the papilla of Vater and of the peripapillary area is advisable in patients with pain as well as cholangitis since abnormalities in this region may be contributory to or causative of symptoms despite the presence of a severe degree of stenosis higher in the biliary tree (Kracht et al 1986).

Classification and severity

The ease of management, operative risk and ultimate prognosis of benign bile duct stricture varies very considerably. In a recent review of 34 series published since 1900, 7643 procedures were performed in 5586 patients with an overall operative mortality of 8.3% (Warren et al 1982). The factors influencing the outcome have been discussed by many. It is considered that younger patients have in general a better prognosis than older subjects and that patients with coincident disease, such as cardio-respiratory disease, have a worse outlook. The presence of hepatocellular disease or established secondary liver fibrosis and of portal hypertension are important adverse features (Sedgwick et al 1966). It has also long been recognized that strictures involving the common bile duct or low common hepatic duct are easier to repair than higher strictures, which may compromise the confluence of the bile ducts. In recognition of these factors Bismuth (1982) has proposed an anatomical classification of bile ducts strictures into five types (Fig. 58.14):

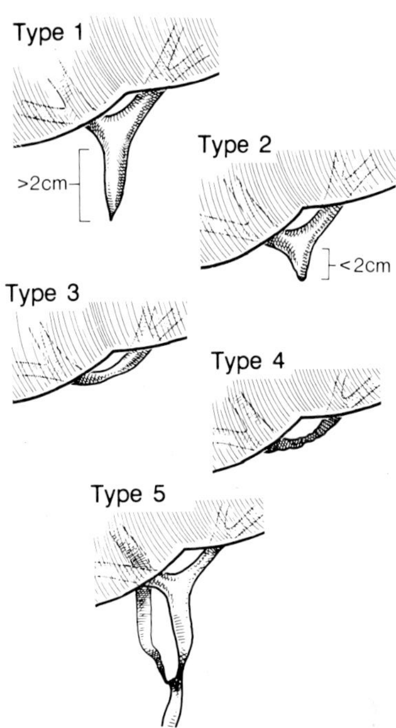

Fig. 58.14 Classification of bile duct strictures based on the level of the stricture related to the confluence of the hepatic ducts (after Bismuth 1982)

Type 1 Low common hepatic duct stricture. Hepatic duct stump > 2 cm (Fig. 58.12).

Type 2 Mid common hepatic duct stricture. Stump > 2 cm (Fig. 58.9).

Type 3 High stricture (hilar) no hepatic duct. Confluence intact (Fig. 58.3d, 58.10).

Type 4 Destruction of hilar confluence. Right and left hepatic ducts separated (Fig. 58.15).

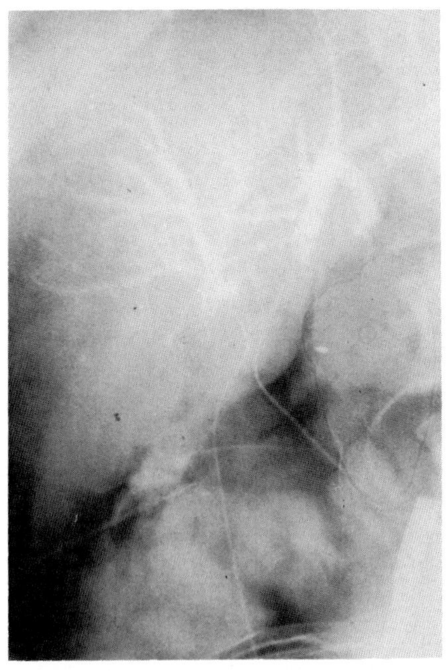

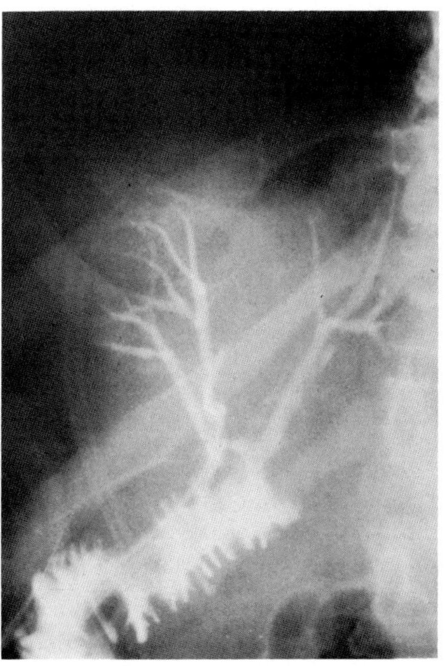

Fig. 58.15 a. Type 4 bile duct stricture outlined at operative cholangiography. Note that catheters have been introduced into the right and left hepatic ductal systems which are completely separated. Removal of the anterior part of the quadrate lobe was necessary to obtain access. b. Roux-en-Y hepaticojejunostomy carried out by separate anastomosis to the right and left hepatic ducts. The patient remains well, symptom free and with normal liver function tests 5.5 years after surgery

Type 5 Involvement of sectoral right branch alone or with the common duct (Fig. 58.2).

In addition the presence of infection and importantly re-operation has a bearing on outcome. Many have commented that the best chance of repair of bile duct injuries is the first attempt and that morbidity and mortality will probably rise at each subsequent effort (Warren et al 1982). While many would argue that injury to the bile duct could occur at primary cholecystectomy in the hands of any surgeon and that the error is excusable, it is hard to justify inadequate attempts at repair by the uninitiated. Once an injury is established then, unless recognized and repaired immediately, the first repair should be carried out by a surgeon well versed in the problems and with the experience likely to allow the highest chance of a successful outcome.

The factors influencing outcome are tabulated below:

General — age
coincident disease
Local — level of stricture
liver fibrosis/cirrhosis
portal hypertension
infection
previous surgery
technical experience of the surgeon

In a study at Hammersmith Hospital a number of preoperative indices of outcome, based on the history and biochemical assessment of the patient obtained in 78 cases of post-cholecystectomy stricture, were defined. It was found that portal hypertension occurred more often in patients with prolonged duration of obstruction and with frequent episodes of cholangitis. Major infection was significantly more common in patients who had had more than one operation before referral. There was also a highly significant relationship between the presence of liver fibrosis and a history of major infection and between depressed serum albumin and postoperative mortality. Similarly, patients with high strictures (Bismuth Type 3 and 4) fared worse than patients in whom some part of the common hepatic duct was still intact (Blumgart et al 1984). In essence, patients with multiple previous operations, with high strictures and particularly with liver disease and portal hypertension fared badly and infection was a major determinant in the progress of disease. Such prognostic indices are of importance in planning therapy and should be taken into account in the assessment of the new interventional radiological approaches to bile duct stricture.

Preoperative management

Except in the case of strictures recognized at the time of primary cholecystectomy or in patients in whom emergency operation is dictated by virtue of peritonitis, there is no hurry in proceeding to surgical reconstruction for bile duct stricture. The patient should be afforded full investigation and allowed time to be brought to optimal condition for operation.

In the presence of recurrent cholangitis administration of antibiotics is important as a preliminary to surgical treatment and the correct antibiotic can be selected on the basis of cultures obtained from aspiration of bile at percutaneous transhepatic cholangiography. While adequate surgical decompression is the only certain way of treating established cholangitis preoperative antibiotics are important in managing recurrent attacks and in the prevention of infective complications. Antibiotic regimens should take into account the not infrequent presence of anaerobic organisms in the presence of bile duct stricture (Blenkharn & Blumgart 1985). The most frequently used antibiotic regime at Hammersmith Hospital is piperacillin and tobramycin commenced immediately preoperatively and maintained for five days in the postoperative period.

Anaemia should be corrected, if necessary, by blood transfusion and coagulation defects, usually a prolongation of the prothrombin time, by the administration of vitamin K. The nutritional status of patients with bile duct stricture is important. Some patients are anorexic and grossly malnourished. We have found that, while feeding through a fine bore trans-nasal catheter may be successful in some cases, enterally administered nutrients are often not tolerated and that parenteral nutrition is frequently necessary. Despite all these measures, however, weight gain is sometimes difficult to achieve in a patient with biliary tract obstruction. If there is a significant external biliary fistula the patient will lose electrolytes and hyponatraemia in particular is a risk (McPherson et al 1982). Fluid replacement and electrolyte repletion are important (Cass et al 1955) (Ch. 60).

Treatment

The treatment of patients with benign bile duct stricture involves reconstruction of biliary enteric continuity. This holds out the only real possibility of cure. However, the management of complications such as biliary peritonitis, subphrenic and subhepatic abscess, haematemesis either due to erosive gastritis or varices, and of liver failure consequent on liver fibrosis are also important and often require treatment preliminary to biliary repair.

In general, drainage of abscess formation and control of erosive gastritis takes precedence and is carried out before definitive attempts to repair strictures. On the other hand, if sepsis arising from the obstructed biliary tree is a feature, especially in the causation of erosive gastritis, then immediate biliary drainage is essential and this also applies to patients with bacteraemia and renal failure (Ch. 72). Drainage may be obtained at operation but in such desperately ill patients it may be preferable to attempt percutaneous transhepatic biliary drainage as a temporary measure to allow resuscitation. The question of the management of portal hypertension occurring in association with stricture is discussed below. If a biliary fistula is present this should in general be managed conservatively in the first instance (see below).

The operative management of biliary stricture depends upon whether the injury is recognized at the time of original operation, presents in the postoperative period or occurs as a late event.

Injury recognised at the time of operation

If injury to the extrahepatic biliary tree is recognized at the time of initial cholecystectomy, then the surgeon should immediately consider his experience and competence to deal with the situation. Certainly, if a more experienced operator is available within the hospital or nearby, then advice should be sought. The situation is not an immediately desperate one and there is always time to insert a pack, cover the wound and wait a short while for another opinion.

The damaged area and the bile ducts on either side require careful dissection to define the extent of the injury. Operative cholangiography may be helpful at this time. In general the injury may be high, close to the hilus of the liver or lower in the supra-duodenal area, involving the common bile duct/cystic duct confluence. The injury may be partial with maintenance of mucosal continuity along one wall of the bile duct, or there may be complete transection or even excision of a length of common bile duct/common hepatic duct with loss of continuity.

Whether the lesion be high and close to the hilus of the liver or low, initial repair of injury *recognized at the time of cholecystectomy* should have two basic aims:

1. To maintain ductal length below the hilus and not to sacrifice tissue;
2. To affect a repair which does not result in postoperative biliary leakage.

It is important to recognize that initial repair may not be the final definitive reconstruction. This is particularly true of injury to very small ducts where repair may be difficult and the prime aims of preventing fistulation and maintaining length should guide the surgeon rather than elaborate attempts at initial reconstruction under difficult circumstances. It is probably preferable to provide external biliary drainage by means of a tube inserted proximally and refer the patient for specialist treatment than to complicate the situation by an attempted repair which causes further damage to the proximal ducts.

Unfortunately the injury is almost always total and *involves transection or excision* of a length of bile duct. Occasionally only a right sectoral duct is transected or ligated (Type 5, Bismuth) (Fig. 58.2) and there may or may not be involvement of the common hepatic duct or common bile duct as well. Injury is particularly likely to occur if the common biliary channels are small, thus allowing easy error by the surgeon. For this reason repair is likely to be difficult.

Several options are open to the surgeon. Firstly, if the bile duct has been transected and the ends can be apposed without tension, then an end-to-end anastomosis may be feasible. The duodenum and head of the pancreas should be completely mobilized so as to minimize tension and an end-to-end anastomosis is then done with a single layer of interrupted fine chromic catgut sutures or other absorbable sutures (e.g. Vicryl*). While some authors recommend silk as an alternative (Kune & Sali 1981), silk sutures may come to lie within the bile duct lumen and act as a foreign body or a nidus for stone formation. The anastomosis is made over a T-tube brought out of the bile duct away from the anastomotic line. Since 50–60% of such anastomoses may re-stricture (see below) and be accompanied by some loss of length, it is preferable to avoid direct repair for high injuries where initial hepaticojejunostomy Roux-en-Y is more likely to give good long-term results (Bismuth et al 1978).

Lateral injuries without loss of length are unusual but important to recognize since it may be possible to affect repair by direct suture of the defect over a T-tube. Longer lateral injuries which are not circumferential are much more difficult or impossible to suture transversely. Some authors have suggested, on the basis of experimental and clinical evidence, that a venous patch may be performed to cover such a defect and indeed vein grafts have been used to bridge gaps in the bile ducts (Belzer et al 1965, Ellis & Hoile 1980, Michie and Gunn 1964). Others have used flaps of the cystic duct stump or pedicled flaps of jejunum to close such defects (Okamura et al 1985). The author has no experience of these techniques and indeed in two cases has found the edges of the defect to be ragged and direct patching difficult. In this situation a Roux-en-Y loop of jejunum can be prepared and used as a serosal patch (Fig. 58.16). A T-tube is placed across the defect and its long limb led out across the Roux loop and developed as a transjejunal tube to the skin. Such a repair has three advantages. Firstly, length is maintained. Secondly, the serosa of the jejunum is used to bridge the defect and suture can be carried out with fine interrupted catgut sutures to the bile duct wall or adjacent connective tissue, without attempting direct approaches to the ragged wall of a damaged bile duct. Finally, the T-tube decompresses the biliary system across the jejunum, so that when it is removed, a fistula to the adjacent jejunum remains. Two cases managed in this manner have remained well with normal liver functions, four and six years after operation. This method is occasionally most useful and a help to the inexperienced surgeon caught in a difficult situation.

(*Ethicon, Edinburgh)

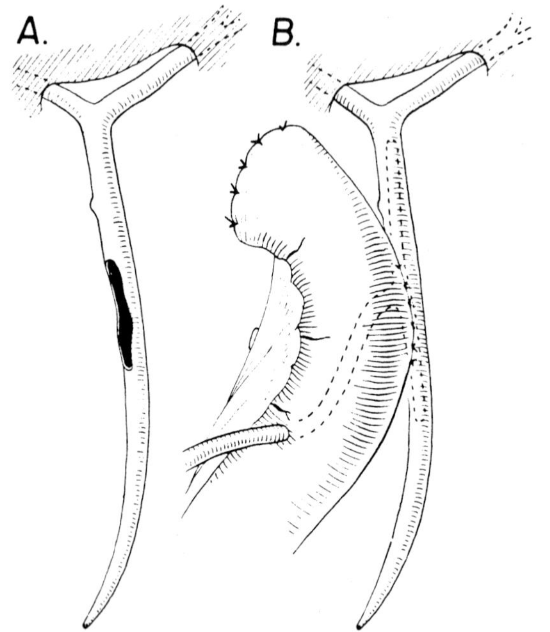

Fig. 58.16 Method of repair of a lateral biliary ductal injury. A. There is a lateral injury with loss of the ductal wall over some considerable length. B. A Roux-en-Y loop of jejunum is prepared and brought up. A T-tube is placed within the injured bile duct and the long limb led out across the jejunal loop which is then attached as a serosal patch across the defect (Blumgart 1984) (previously published in: Blumgart L H 1984 Bile duct strictures. In: Fromm D (ed), Gastrointestinal Surgery, Vol. 2. Churchill Livingstone, London, p. 755–811).

The frequency with which immediate repair of the common bile duct is effective and long lasting is difficult to ascertain. While many injuries presenting in the post-operative period (or later) are treated by specialists, injuries recognized at the time of operation may never come to the attention of referral centres and may not be documented. Some have suggested that the restricture rate is as high as 50% (Kune & Sali 1981), but the evidence for this is not strong and there is almost certainly a considerable underestimate of the number of bile duct injuries and of immediate repair done in district hospitals.

It is perhaps worth emphasizing again, that while the ultimate aim of the surgeon is to produce mucosa-to-mucosa suture with a long lasting repair, the primary aim in the acute situation is to preserve length and prevent biliary leakage and infection with resultant fibrosis, loss of length and re-stenosis.

Injuries recognized in the immediate postoperative period

Injuries not recognized at the time of operation present in the postoperative period in three ways.

Firstly, there may be postoperative drainage of bile from the wound or from a drain site with the formation of a biliary fistula. The essential in management in this situation is *not to re-operate rapidly*. It is wiser to take stock of the situation, to carry out fistulography, treat infection, nourish the patient and wait (Ch. 60). If fistulography reveals any continuity between the biliary system and the gastrointestinal tract, then a prolonged period of drainage, if well managed, may result in spontaneous closure of the fistula. Re-operation in such cases need never be hurried and the injury should be precisely documented. Eventual repair may be difficult because the bile ducts may be small, but the patient is not jaundiced and the adverse pathophysiological features associated with cholestasis are not present. It is a mistake to think that immediate repair of such a fistula is a simple matter, since definitive exposure of healthy bile duct mucosa within a sufficiently dilated duct to permit good anastomosis can be very demanding and indeed may be impossible. A cautious approach is preferable since even ultimate closure of the fistula with the development of jaundice is usually associated with proximal ductal dilatation and easier subsequent repair. Should fluid loss from the biliary fistula prove too heavy and too prolonged, then the external fistula can, after some weeks or months, be converted to an internal fistula-jejunostomy (Smith et al 1982). Definitive repair, if necessary, can then be carried out at a later date.

Secondly, presentation in the postoperative period may be as biliary peritonitis. This is a serious situation and the patient is often desperately ill, especially if the bile is infected. However, in some patients with sterile bile huge volumes may accumulate within the peritoneal cavity without overt signs of shock (Fig. 58.3b). The management of these cases demands closure of the biliary peritoneal fistula in order to save life. Definitive repair is seldom possible, the bile ducts having collapsed and the tissues being deeply stained with bile and friable. External drainage is the best initial approach and this may be carried out through a mobilized Roux-en-Y loop of jejunum, the external drainage tube simply being lead across in a transjejunal fashion to the exterior. Such a procedure allows initial control and the almost certain necessity for re-operation for stenosis at a later date should be accepted (Fig. 58.3c,d) (Ch. 60).

Finally the patient may become progressively jaundiced. In this case the injury should be managed as outlined below.

Injuries presenting at an interval after initial operation

The principles of management of late biliary stenosis and strictures are as follows:

1. Exposure of healthy proximal bile ducts draining *all* areas of the liver;
2. Preparation of a suitable segment of distal mucosa for anastomosis (usually a Roux-en-Y loop of jejunum);
3. Mucosa-to-mucosa suture anastomosis of the bile ducts to the intestinal mucosa (Ch. 70).

While excision of the stricture and end-to-end anastomosis or repair of the damaged bile duct may be carried out in some cases, this is not so in most series and almost invariably there is loss of length as a result of fibrosis of the common hepatic duct and common bile duct.

A staged procedure may be necessary because of the presence of abscesses, haematemesis consequent on erosive gastritis, oesophageal varices or other cause, or because of the poor general condition of the patient (see above). Certainly it is unwise to attempt definitive repair of a stricture in the presence of severe local sepsis or if significant bleeding is in progress. Initial drainage procedures to evacuate pus or biliary collections and establish external biliary flow are usually all that is advisable in such cases. Establishment of an external biliary fistula with drainage of pus allows the clinical condition to be improved and the metabolic state to be brought under control before definitive management (Cattell & Braasch 1959b). Percutaneous transhepatic drainage techniques may be of value in such a staged approach but there is scant published experience in this field. Similarly in portal hypertension initial porta-systemic shunting may be required to control variceal bleeding. Indeed biliary repair is substantially more difficult in the presence of portal hypertension. In particular the presence of dilated venous collateral channels lying within adhesions in the area of dissection are easily damaged and intraoperative haemorrhage may be difficult to control. In such patients radiological interventional procedures may be used for the management of some benign strictures with the introduction of transhepatic percutaneously placed tubes draining the biliary tree and simultaneous biliary dilatation of strictures (Molnar & Stockum 1978, Teplick et al 1980, Schwarz et al 1981, Vogel et al 1985). Indeed, although these methods may lead to immediate complications, are difficult to use in the presence of a fibrotic liver with minimally dilated ducts, and may be entirely inappropriate if the obstruction is of multiple ducts or segmental, some authors prefer this approach in patients with portal hypertension (Pellegrini et al 1984). Initial portal-systemic shunting may be carried out followed by later stricture repair and this may be an appropriate course in some cases. The author's experience is that such an approach is associated with less bleeding at subsequent operation.

End-to-end anastomosis

Excision of the stricture and end-to-end anastomosis may be carried out as reported by Cattell (Cattell & Braasch 1959b). This establishes repair with a normal anatomical status and drainage through an intact sphincter of Oddi. Cattell had reported such anastomosis even for high strictures after mobilizing the duodenum and lower common bile duct, if necessary splitting the pancreatic substance in an attempt at a tension-free anastomosis to the proximal hepatic duct. However, the procedure is now only used when the ends of the bile duct are close enough for anastomosis to be performed without any undue tension and where there is no appreciable discrepancy in the diameter of the proximal and distal ducts. The quality of the distal duct must also be satisfactory. These conditions are but rarely met in strictures at or near the hepatic hilus. In some series there is reported a high incidence of primary repair but this is not commonly possible in the author's experience (Blumgart et al 1984). A single row of interrupted fine chromic catgut or Vicryl® sutures is used, the anastomosis being created over a T-tube inserted at a separate point (Fig. 58.17).

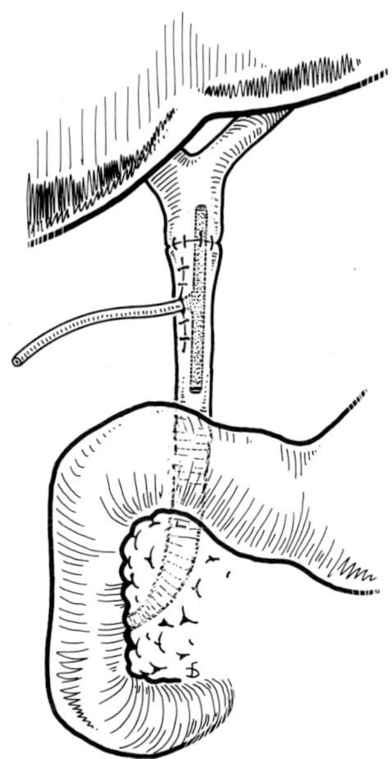

Fig. 58.17 Method of repair of a biliary ductal injury by end-to-end anastomosis over a T-tube

Biliary enteric repair procedures

In the vast majority of cases a biliary enteric repair procedure must be carried out in order to establish biliary drainage. There is abundant evidence that biliary intestinal anastomosis is superior to end-to-end anastomosis and there should be little hesitation in abandoning attempts at the latter if there is any difficulty.

For strictures of the retropancreatic portion of the common bile duct or of the common bile duct in its immediate supra duodenal portion, a choledochoduodenostomy is an ideal procedure, either performed side-to-side or end-to-side (Ch. 54). The procedure yields better results if the common bile duct is dilated. However, low injuries suitable for treatment in this manner are unusual after cholecystectomy but more often encountered after gastric operations (see below).

Strictures involving the common hepatic duct are more difficult, especially close to the hilus of the liver and are best dealt with by hepaticojejunostomy. When the stricture is of the Bismuth Type 1 or 2 then an approach to the common hepatic duct stump is usually not unduly difficult. When, however, the stricture involves the confluence of the right and left hepatic ducts (Type 3) or extends so as to separate these ducts (Type 4), the problem becomes much more complex and good results more difficult to obtain.

A variety of approaches to the proximal hepatic duct/s in order to expose ductal mucosa are described depending on the height and extent of the lesion (Ch. 70). The descriptions below are related to the classification as described by Bismuth (1982) (see above) and should be read in conjunction with Chapters 2 and 70.

An important feature is early division of the falciform ligament right back to the diaphragm thus freeing the liver from any adhesions. Dissection of the stricture should commence in the right subhepatic area and it may be necessary to completely mobilize the hepatic flexure of the colon, starting from below and working upwards and medially. The duodenum is exposed and very frequently is adherent, as a result of previous surgery, to the posterior hilar structures and almost always in its upper part to the area of the stricture. Indeed there is sometimes a fistula into the duodenum or a hole is made in the duodenum during dissection and must be repaired.

Some authors recommend that a search be made for the bile duct distal to the stricture (Kune & Sali 1981), but this is often difficult, tedious, may be dangerous and in any event is unnecessary, since it will be found that the distal duct is not suitable for anastomosis. *The essential and most important point* is identification of the bile duct proximal to the stricture. This can be difficult and a systematic, careful and patient approach is necessary.

While it is recommended that the area in the neighbourhood of the hilus be explored and the bile duct found lateral to the pulsation of the hepatic artery, and this is usually perfectly adequate for Type 1 lesions it is not, in the author's experience, the best approach; exposure is more reliable after incision at the base of the quadrate lobe and lowering of the hilar plate (Ch. 2, 70). This manoeuvre delivers the bile ducts and the confluence from the undersurface of the liver making identification of the strictured area much easier. Adhesions posterior to a damaged duct are often dense and it is not always necessary to dissect too extensively although it is usually possible to elevate sufficient posterior rim of common bile duct to hold sutures.

Once the duct is prepared for anastomosis this is carried out usually to a Roux-en-Y loop of jejunum (Fig. 58.9, 58.22) although some, in an attempt to obviate subsequent duodenal ulceration which occasionally occurs, have suggested anastomosis to an interposed loop of jejunum between the exposed bile duct (ducts) and the duodenum (McArthur & Longmire 1971, Sato et al 1982, 1983, Pappalorado et al 1982) (Ch. 70). The suture technique employed is that described by Voyles & Blumgart (1983) and Blumgart & Kelley (1984) (Ch. 70). If elevation of the posterior wall of the proximal bile duct from the underlying connective tissue is difficult because of adhesions, this may be only minimally elevated, suture then being carried out posteriorly without undue difficulty.

High strictures (Types 2,3,4) are much more demanding and a variety of approaches may be used for their repair. In addition to the height and extent of the stricture other complicating factors are the presence of secondary liver fibrosis, and of small ducts consequent upon incomplete obstruction or indistensability. In the vast majority of Type 2, Type 3 and Type 4 cases an adequate exposure of the bile ducts may be made by *dissecting the left hepatic ductal system.* The approach based on the studies of Couinaud (1953, 1955) has been well described (Hepp & Couinaud 1956) and extensively practised particularly in France by Hepp and later by Bismuth (Bismuth 1982, Bismuth et al 1978) and more recently by the author (Blumgart & Kelley 1984). Occasionally mobilization or even excision of the quadrate lobe may prove necessary in some Type 4 cases (Fig. 58.14, 58.15).

Once exposed the ducts are opened and anastomosis is performed as outlined in Chapter 70.

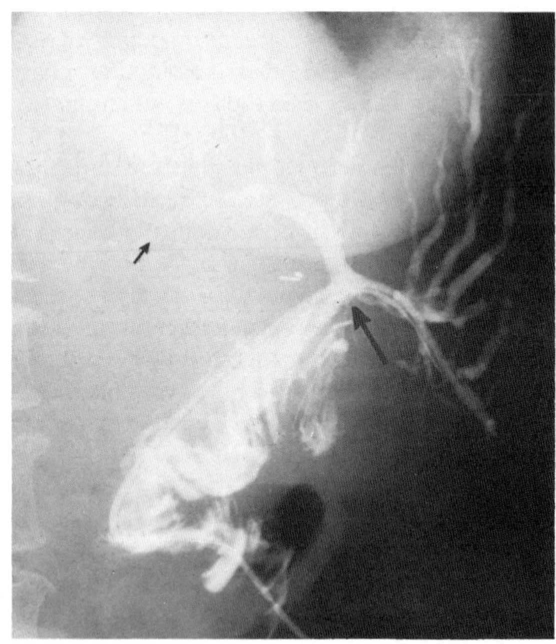

Fig. 58.18 Hepaticojejunostomy Roux-en-Y to the segment III duct following post-cholecystectomy stricture initially treated by hepaticojejunostomy using the mucosal graft technique with a transhepatic tube issuing through the right lobe of the liver. At referral the patient had a grossly atrophic right lobe and a high bile duct stricture (small arrow). At operation the left hepatic duct was exposed using the ligamentum teres approach and anastomosis carried out (large arrow). Subsequent re-stricture occurred one year later and was treated by refashioning of the anastomosis and subsequent transtubal balloon dilatation with a satisfactory outcome. The patient has remained well and symptom free for a period of two years

While the vast majority of high strictures can be approached and dealt with as described above it is occasionally very difficult to expose the left hepatic duct. This may be due to dense adhesions. Bleeding may be encountered or the quadrate lobe may be large and overhanging the area of the left duct. Sometimes the extrahepatic length of the left duct may be so short as to make the approach difficult. In such instances repair can be effected by dissection of the left hepatic duct within the umbilical fissure (*ligamentum teres approach*) (Fig. 58.18) (Soupault & Couinaud 1957) (Ch. 2, 70). This approach should not be used unless there is continuity at the hilus so that the whole biliary tree will be decompressed.

Smith (1969, 1979) described a method for treating the high stricture in which dissection at the area of the hilus is thought to be impossible and the ducts cannot be developed to reveal an adequate mucosa for anastomosis. This mucosal graft procedure (Ch. 70) has been hailed by some as an important advance in surgical technique (Kune & Sali 1981). The object of the procedure is to utilize a transhepatic tube to draw the jejunal mucosa high up into the hepatic ducts and thus allow apposition for subsequent healing without fibrosis. The procedure is claimed to be an easier operation than a formal anastomosis and is certainly quicker since no sutures are inserted. The transhepatic tube is allowed to drain and a cholangiogram is subsequently performed. The tube is left in place for a period, usually two to six months, but may be left longer for very difficult cases.

It must be emphasized that the mucosal graft procedure was originally advocated for those cases in which suture anastomosis was thought to be impracticable (Kune & Sali 1981; Smith 1979, 1981). On the other hand the procedure is by no means easy in the densely fibrous liver or if there is secondary biliary cirrhosis since, when the ducts are small, passage of a transhepatic tube may not be possible and it is easy to produce false passages. Indeed, of a series of bile duct strictures treated by Smith (1981) 8.4% were considered unsuitable for mucosal graft procedures as a result of liver fibrosis, secondary sclerosing cholangitis, sepsis, stones or various combinations. Furthermore, the method is a blind one without direct visualization (Bismuth 1982) and it is clear that the dome of mucosa pulled up into the hepatic ducts may block significant branches of the intrahepatic ductal system, thus occluding and isolating areas of liver tissue (Fig. 58.19) (Blumgart 1978, Blumgart et al 1984). Indeed, it is possible for the surgeon to erroneously 'graft' only one sectoral duct leaving the main stricture untouched. In addition the mucosa may 'pull away' postoperatively (Fig. 58.20) and

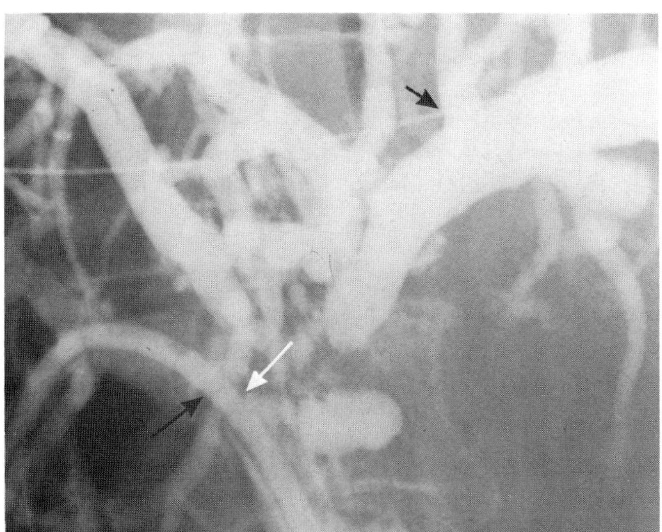

Fig. 58.19 Combined tubogram and percutaneous transhepatic cholangiogram in a complex case of high biliary stricture following two previous attempts at hepaticojejunostomy Roux-en-Y using the mucosal graft technique and during which it was considered that an approach by direct anastomosis was impossible. Injection of the indwelling tube (black arrow) reveals the area of a previous mucosal graft (white arrow). There is complete separation from the main left hepatic ductal system which was filled by percutaneous transhepatic cholangiography (small arrow). There is right lobe atrophy and left lobe hypertrophy

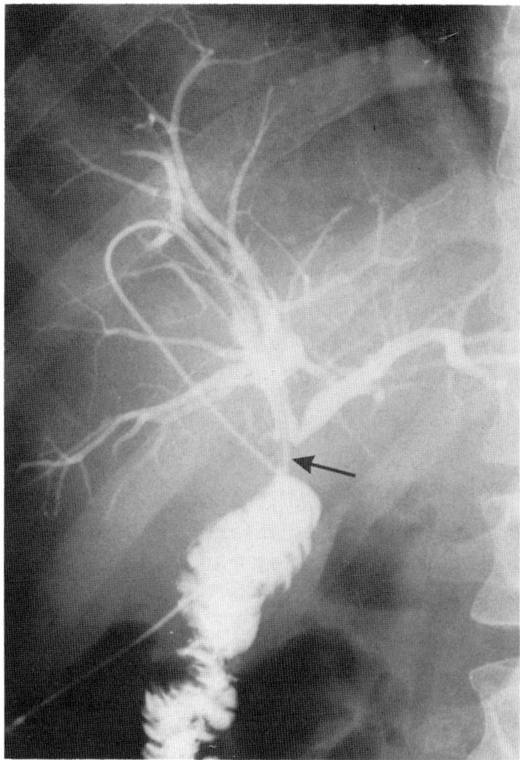

Fig. 58.20 Cholangiogram obtained by injection of a U-tube used to develop a mucosal graft repair of a high bile duct stricture carried out two weeks before this X-ray was obtained. It was considered that there were no ducts visible at the hilus of the liver which would allow formal anastomosis. Note that the mucosal graft is already widely separated from the biliary confluence (arrow). Repair was carried out by an approach to the left hepatic duct. A wide anastomosis was easily obtained. The patient remains well, symptom free and with normal liver function tests three and a half years after operation

the whole jejunal loop may become detached and lie at a distance from the hilus. Thus in an analysis of 22 cases with restricture after mucosal graft procedure the author found stricture at the site of the biliary enteric mucosal approximation in 15 cases. In two the right hepatic duct had been selectively occluded by the graft and the left hepatic duct in two further patients. Intrahepatic stones around and above the stent tube causing obstruction and cholangitis occurred in one and the Roux loop had pulled away from the hepatic duct in two patients.

Finally, doubts must be expressed as to those cases in whom it has been reported that dissection of bile duct mucosa for anastomosis is impossible. This statement is based on a misconception perpetuated by anatomical texts, by diagrams in the literature reporting the mucosal graft procedure (Smith 1969, 1981) and by the experience of surgeons who approach the scarred fibrotic hilum directly. However, as emphasized by Kelley and & Blumgart (1985) short segments of right hepatic duct and up to 4 cm of left hepatic duct are extrahepatic structures and can be approached by lowering the hilar plate (Ch. 2, 70). Thus in a series of 78 patients, many with complex high bile duct strictures (Blumgart et al 1984) of whom 67 came to operation, mucosa-to-mucosa anastomosis was carried out in all but two despite the fact that 20 had already been operated on previously by the mucosal graft technique. Similarly Bismuth (1982) has reported 180 consecutive cases, many of them of a serious nature, in whom mucosal suture has been possible and mucosal graft procedures never necessary.

As pointed out by Bismuth (1982) the performance of the mucosal graft leads to an imperfect mucosa-to-mucosa approximation due to the haphazard positioning of the graft in the absence of visual control and with the potential risk of intrahepatic duct obstruction. Unless carried out bilaterally the procedure of mucosal graft is unsuited for Type 4 cases where the stricture itself has separated the intrahepatic ducts, often quite widely.

The procedure should be considered only in patients in whom the biliary mucosa is really inaccessible despite a deep and adequate dissection. Currently available evidence indicates the approach is rarely indicated and is unlikely to stand the test of time.

Finally, some authors (Barker & Winkler 1985, Chen et al 1984) recommend that in difficult strictures hepaticojejunostomy is carried out over a transjejunal tube which is then brought to the exterior across the blind end of jejunum which is left long and brought up subcutaneously (Fig. 58.21). This allows easy subsequent interventional radiological or choledochoscopic procedures. The author has used this technique with success on five occasions.

Liver split procedures

Sometimes it is necessary to open the liver tissue as an hepatotomy in order to adequately expose bile ducts for repair (Blumgart 1980). The most frequent situation in which this is required is to more widely expose the umbilical fissure for approach to the segment III duct or in order to expose the origin of the right hepatic duct. This latter approach usually is an extension of the subhepatic approach to the left duct described above and involves opening of the liver tissue in the line of the scar of the gallbladder fossa. Liver split in this situation and opening of the umbilical fissure allows upward mobilization of the entire quadrate lobe (Ch. 70) (Bismuth 1982). These methods are usually only necessary for some Type IV lesions and especially where there is difficulty in access to the right hepatic ducts.

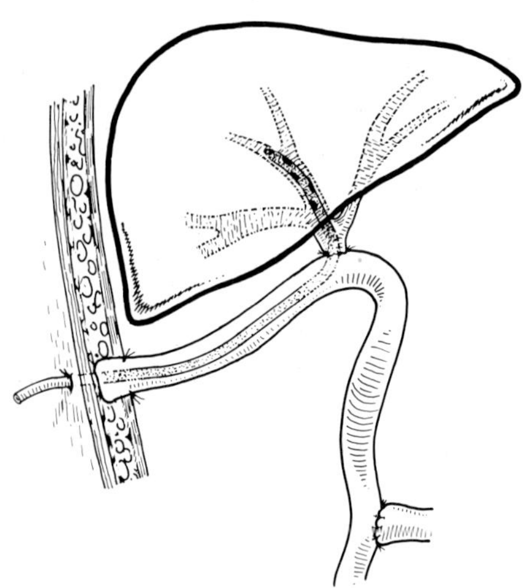

Fig. 58.21 Method of hepaticojejunostomy where it is desired to bring the jejunal loop to the abdominal wall so as to allow access for future instrumentation (see text)

The liver tissue must be patiently divided and this may be accompanied by a degree of haemorrhage. The technique should not be employed if approaches to the left hepatic duct are possible.

Liver resection in benign stricture

Resection of liver tissue may be necessary for exposure of the bile ducts. In general the form of liver resection necessary is of two varieties. Firstly, excision of a part of the quadrate lobe may be carried out, if exposure of the umbilical fissure and incision of the fibrous bed of the gallbladder is not sufficient to allow adequate exposure of the hepatic ducts or indeed to allow approaches to the ducts in Type 4 lesions (Fig. 58.15).

Secondly and very rarely, benign strictures of the bile ducts may be approached by means of intrahepatic hepatojejunostomy, as described by Longmire & Sandford (1949). In general, this procedure is difficult and can be dangerous in benign bile duct stricture since, if it is deemed necessary, the liver is always fibrous and resection of tissue is accompanied by haemorrhage. Furthermore, the bleeding vessels are in close proximity to the ducts required for anastomosis. However, the procedure can be valuable in exposing ducts for anastomosis where there is unilateral left sided liver hypertrophy (Johnson et al 1979, Czerniak et al 1986). Blumgart et al (1979) refer to the use of liver resection for benign stricture, but this is seldom necessary for post-cholecystectomy strictures which are usually approachable by exposure of the left hepatic ducts as described above. When necessary, liver resection usually involves removal of the anterior portion of the quadrate lobe (segment IV).

Liver atrophy/hypertrophy–influence on approach to repair

Segmental or lobar liver atrophy (Ch. 6) accompanied by compensatory hypertrophy and hyperplasia elsewhere in the liver may be encountered in segmental ductal obstruction, especially if there is also portal venous obstruction. If an entire half of the liver is affected then the combination of atrophy and hypertrophy leads to distortion and difficulties in dissection and anastomosis. The most common situation is gross hypertrophy of the left lobe accompanied by right lobe atrophy (Czerniak et al 1986).

The presence of liver atrophy should be suspected if, on cholangiography, one area of liver tissue is small and the ducts, although possibly dilated, are crowded together, the contralateral liver being larger and hypertrophied. Confirmation of the presence of the atrophy is obtainable often at CT scanning or by using HIDA scanning which will show an area of tissue with poor uptake and delayed excretion of the isotope. Similarly angiography may be carried out and where there is gross atrophy benign stricture may be accompanied by unilateral portal venous compromise.

The approach to such lesions demands drainage of the entire liver substance. If, as is frequently the case, there is discontinuity of the right and left hepatic ducts at the hilus, then drainage of the left ductal system via the ligamentum teres approach (Fig. 58.18) or by the Longmire-Sandford (Longmire & Sandford 1949) operation will only drain the left liver. This is usually unsatisfactory, the remaining obstructed area continuing to provide a focus of infection and a source of continued fever in the post-operative period. Anastomosis in the region of the hilus is still desirable but is always difficult. Bismuth suggests a thoraco-abdominal approach to such strictures in an effort to allow direct appreciation of the anatomy and access for suture repair (Bismuth & Lazorthes 1981). This approach through the right thorax and after division of the diaphragm allows rotation of the liver to the left and facilitates dissection.

Portal hypertension and biliary stricture

Patients with biliary stricture may develop portal hypertension and this may be associated either with the development of secondary liver fibrosis or with direct damage to the portal vein. Sometimes there is coincident hepatocellular disease.

Few reports specifically stress this problem. Sedgwick et al (1966) found portal hypertension to be present in about 20% of patients treated at the Lahey Clinic, Boston. Similarly Blumgart et al (1984) in a series of 78 patients treated at the Hepatobiliary Surgical Unit, Hammersmith Hospital, found 11 (14%) with portal hypertension at the time of referral. Patients with bile duct stricture who are found during investigation to have a palpable spleen or oesophageal varices or who have a history of gastro-intestinal bleeding, should be subjected to upper gastro-intestinal endoscopy and angiography including splenoportography. Bleeding oesophageal varices occur quite commonly and this complication, especially if accompanied by hypersplenism or ascites, renders the prognosis much worse (Sedgwick et al 1966, Way & Dunphy 1972). Furthermore, collateral venous channels in the subhepatic region and within vascular adhesions make dissection difficult and bloody. Finally the patient who develops portal hypertension is also frequently the patient with a high stricture who has had multiple previous attempts at repair.

While the difficulties encountered in the management of these cases have been detailed by some (Adson & Wychulis 1968, Blumgart et al 1984, Ekman & Sandblom 1962, Sedgwick et al 1966, Way & Dunphy 1972, Pellegrini et al 1984) there remain problems in the assessment of therapy. The developments of techniques for balloon dilatation of strictures by percutaneous means offers new possibilities but will seldom be a complete solution.

In seriously ill patients with jaundice, portal hypertension, and with a history of variceal bleeding it may be advisable to pass an initial percutaneous transhepatic drain or treat the stricture at least in the first instance by means of percutaneous balloon dilatation (Fig. 58.22b) (Toufanian et al 1978, Pellegrini et al 1984, Molnar & Stockum 1978, Teplick et al 1980, Schwarz et al 1981) and then to assess the possibilities of late definitive repair.

If haemorrhage is encountered during the course of a stricture repair then hepaticostomy drainage may be performed initially and a spleno-renal shunt undertaken at a later date. Biliary repair carried out at the time of shunting procedures can be extremely difficult and in any event is best not performed at a time of severely compromised liver function. Thus some authors (Kune & Sali 1981) recommend that, if profuse haemorrhage is encountered during attempted repair, a three-stage procedure be carried out. Hepaticostomy in the first instance followed by a shunt some three weeks later and then by re-construction of the bile duct at a third operation when liver function is at an optimum level. This approach is, however, now seldom necessary if percutaneous drainage is used judiciously as a first stage before attempted operation.

If a patient should present with *severe bleeding, oesophageal varices and with established biliary obstruction*, conservative measures should be tried in the first instance to control bleeding. The use of pitressin infusions, the Sengstaken tube and of peroesophageal injection of sclerosants into the varices (Ch. 105) are all reasonable first measures, but if the bleeding does not stop then a two-stage operation is recommended: an immediate spleno-renal shunt being performed in the first instance and bile duct reconstruction at a later date. Again, percutaneous transhepatic drainage or balloon dilatation may be used in association with the above measures.

Occasionally patients present *without jaundice and with bleeding oesophageal varices*, the stricture having been adequately repaired at an earlier date. In these instances a portal-systemic shunt is indicated (Fig. 58.5) occasionally as an emergency measure but preferably after initial conservative management of the bleed. Experience of injection sclerotherapy in the management of this group of cases is very small, but should be considered. However, there should be no hesitation in proceeding to shunting if acceptable criteria are present. In general the best and most convenient form of portal-systemic shunt in these patients is a spleno-renal shunt. Portacaval shunting is technically difficult or impossible because of previous surgery in the hilar area. It is possible, although not proven that adequate biliary repair in such cases is followed by slow improvement with resolution of fibrosis and an eventual fall in portal pressure and there is some evidence for this belief (Blumgart 1978).

Finally it should be emphasized that it is important to obtain a liver biopsy in patients with portal hypertension and benign bile duct strictures. Parenchymal liver disease, and in particular alcoholic cirrhosis, may exist in association with iatrogenic bile duct stricture and can be a cause of confusion. Thus in a series reported by Blumgart et al (1984) two of 11 patients with portal hypertension were found to have hepatocellular disease not consequent on obstruction. It is important to emphasize that many of these patients are the subject of medico-legal proceedings and precise documentation, in order to afford accurate assessment of the causation of symptoms and of prognosis, is essential.

The prognosis of this group of patients is much worse than for patients without portal hypertension and a hospital mortality approaching 40–80% is to be anticipated (Blumgart et al 1984, Sedgwick et al 1966). In a series of 78 patients reported by Blumgart et al (1984) preoperative indices of prognosis were investigated. It was found that portal hypertension was associated with a high mortality, three of 11 patients dying in the hospital and one of these of uncontrolled variceal haemorrhage before any operation was undertaken. Portal hypertension was found more frequently with prolonged obstruction and recurrent episodes of cholangitis and these in turn were more frequent in patients who had more than one operation before referral. There was a highly significant relationship between the presence of liver fibrosis and major infection.

Results

'We are still in considerable doubt about the best method of repairing the common duct and we want someone to analyse carefully the records of all the available cases to see if we can get guidance from the end-results' (Grey-Turner 1944).

There are a variety of factors which influence the prognosis and outcome of patients admitted to hospital with bile duct strictures. *Factors influencing a satisfactory stricture repair* are the number of previous operations, the site of the stricture and the type of repair; while *those which influence mortality* are the number of previous operations, a history of major infection, the site of the stricture, preoperative serum albumin concentration and particularly the presence of liver fibrosis and portal hypertension (Cattell & Braasch 1960a, Kune 1979, Blumgart et al 1984).

The adequacy of surgical repair is of great importance in determining ultimate long-term prognosis. While untreated cases have a fatal outcome, surgical treatment which offers only partial relief of the biliary obstruction results in progressive liver damage and ultimate death. Failure to drain all segments of the liver results in segmental liver atrophy. While some (Kune & Sali 1981) express the opinion that the mucosal graft technique is a recent advance which allows adequate drainage of all parts of the biliary tree, this is not the author's experience and published results (Smith 1981) reflect a significant proportion of patients with sustained elevations in the serum alkaline phosphatase suggesting incomplete drainage.

Operative morbidity and mortality

The postoperative *morbidity* of reconstructive surgery of bile duct stricture is high. Some estimate that at least one patient in 10 is likely to have one or more major non-fatal complications (Kune & Sali 1981). However, some report higher figures and more complications are to be expected from series including a high proportion of re-operated cases (Blumgart et al 1984). The common complications encountered are subphrenic, subhepatic, or pelvic infections, wound infections, cholangitis, bacteraemic shock, secondary haemorrhage, biliary fistula and pulmonary complications.

Mortality is very difficult to assess. Firstly, some reports do not define operative mortality and whether this includes hospital mortality. Furthermore, some patients die before operation can be embarked upon and others die of infection, renal failure or haematemesis consequent upon variceal bleeding. Other features which make assessment of mortality difficult are failure in some series to differentiate high strictures as distinct from low, to allow for the effects of multiple operations or to clearly differentiate mortality for one operative procedure as against another.

The operative mortality is reported as being between 5 and 8% (Cattell & Braasch 1959a, Kune 1979, Way & Dunphy 1972, Warren et al 1982). The most common causes of death in these series is uncontrolled haemorrhage, hepatic or renal failure, or a combination of these features. Biliary fistula, bacteraemia and pulmonary complications were responsible for the remaining operative deaths. In the recent Hammersmith series of 78 patients, the *overall* 30-day hospital mortality was 11.5%, this including one death due to bleeding oesophageal varices before operation could be undertaken. The operative mortality for *all procedures*, including surgery for drainage of abscesses, shunt procedures for control of bleeding and biliary repair was 8.3% (Table 58.1). There were no deaths in 58 patients treated by hepaticojejunostomy nor in three treated by choledochoduodenostomy. Two patients with complex high strictures were treated by mucosal apposition early in the series and both died. Thus of the 63 patients treated by stricture repair alone there was an operative mortality of 3.2%. A total of 84 patients have to date been subjected to stricture repair alone with a 30-day mortality of 2.4% (2 patients) there being no deaths in 82 consecutive cases treated by mucosa-to-mucosa suture.

There are in fact very few reports on series of patients operated upon for biliary repair by hepaticojejunostomy to the left hepatic duct system. The zero mortality for 82 cases in the author's series is comparable to that of Bismuth (1982), who reports 186 patients operated on by this approach since the introduction of the technique in 1956. 70% of these cases had one or more operations before referral and associated lesions which complicated operation and compounded the difficulty of the biliary repair. The associated lesions were mainly intrahepatic stones above the stricture, biliary fistula, hepatic atrophy and biliary fibrosis. Despite these complications all patients were operated on by a mucosa-to-mucosa suture and the left duct approach was possible in all but four, one of whom was subjected to intrahepatic cholangiojejunostomy. The operative mortality defined as intraoperative and immediate postoperative mortality was 0.6%.

Smith (1979, 1981) reports a review of 451 patients, 413 operated upon by the mucosal graft technique. There were 17 deaths postoperatively in the entire series (3.75%) but none for those patients submitted to the mucosal graft procedure.

It is important that the safety of repair in experienced hands and particularly in the uncomplicated case is appreciated and taken into account in assessing the newer techniques of transhepatic or transendoscopic biliary dilatation.

Late results

The late results of repair of bile duct injury are difficult to evaluate and there is a considerable variation in the criteria chosen to assess long-term results. Morbidity and mortality not associated with stricture repair must be taken into account and the results of stricture repair in an uncomplicated case should be distinguished from those with liver disease, portal hypertension or lobar atrophy. Similarly there is scant information on relative mortality and morbidity rates according to the level of stricture and only one author has proposed a formal classification of severity (Bismuth 1982). There is also variation in what is accepted as a satisfactory result. Thus Braasch (Braasch et al 1981) accepts as a good result patients without symptoms or with occasional attacks of cholangitis and jaundice three years after repair. Others define a satisfactory repair as the absence of symptoms two years after operation (Smith 1981). Bismuth (1982) suggests a follow-up of at least five years and preferably ten years symptom free with normal liver function tests and no stenosis as constituting a good result.

In a study reported by Blumgart et al (1984) the Bismuth classification was employed. It was found that Type 3 and 4 strictures were associated with less good results. Warren (Warren & Jefferson 1973) has reported 958 patients reviewed at the Lahey Clinic of which 77 were at or proximal to the common hepatic duct. While not differentiating Bismuth Type 3 and 4 strictures from Bismuth Type 2 this study emphasized the difficulties in the higher strictures. Indeed in a recent literature survey Warren (Warren et al 1982) has reported satisfactory results obtained in only approximately 47% of patients (72% of those patients followed for a suitable length of time) with an overall operative mortality of 8.3%. Pitt et al (1982) examined the factors influencing outcome of repair of benign strictures following cholecystectomy and showed that better results are achieved in patients less than 30 years old, with no previous attempt at stricture repair, by the use of a Roux-en-Y jejunal loop, and with the employment of transhepatic silastic tubal splinting for longer than one month, extended to nine months or more with changeable silastic splints in patients with difficult hilar strictures. Way and his colleagues (Pellegrini et al 1984) analysed the course of 50 consecutive patients with recurrent biliary stricture, all of whom had at least one previous repair, in order to determine the pattern of recurrence and the outcome of *reoperative* treatment. Presenting features included cholangitis in 40% of patients, jaundice in 30% and pain in 17%. Operative mortality was 4% and 76% of patients had no further recurrence of symptoms. However, in 11 patients (22%) recurrence developed although six did well after yet another operation. In 4 patients, a third recurrence developed and was successfully treated at a fourth operation in three of these.

It was concluded that two-thirds of recurrent strictures were evident by two years and 90% by seven years. The authors calculate that the chance of recurrence was about 25% after re-treatment of a first recurrent stricture. The authors do not outline the methods of repair employed but emphasize the necessity for hepaticojejunostomy by direct suture. They concluded that prolonged stenting did not contribute to a good result.

The study reported by Blumgart et al (1984) revealed that, in a series of 78 patients, a satisfactory result was achieved in 90% of cases treated by stricture repair only, over a mean follow-up period of 3.3 years. There were two late deaths within a year of surgery, one of liver failure and the other in a patient who developed a coincidental cholangiocarcinoma.

Bismuth in a series of 186 patients (1982) chose a 10-year follow-up period. Of 186 patients operated on by means of *hepaticojejunostomy to the left duct*, 141 were operated on between 1956 and 1972 and were recently studied for assessment of late results. Fourteen patients (11%) were lost to follow-up. Seven died from non-biliary causes thus leaving 120 patients for re-assessment at between 10 and 20 years. Of these 88% had an excellent result defined by the absence of any biliary troubles, 5% had transitory trouble shortly after operation, probably related to the procedure itself, but did not require re-operation and 7% had unsatisfactory results. Three developed recurrent stenosis and required re-operation and all three had a subsequently good outcome. Five, all with secondary biliary fibrosis, died. These result are essentially similar to those reported by Blumgart et al (1984) and to the estimate of Kune & Sali (1981) that 85% of patients who have sustained an operative injury to the bile ducts will be restored to normal health if surgical reconstruction is undertaken by an experienced surgeon. Duodenal ulceration appears to develop in a small proportion of patients after Roux-en-Y biliary enteric repair (McArthur et al 1971, Sato et al 1982, 1983, Pappalorado et al 1982) (Ch. 70) and constitutes an additional cause of late mobidity. The majority of cases will respond to the administration of H_2 inhibitory agents.

Late results for the *mucosal graft procedure* have been reported by Smith (1979, 1981). Of 451 patients reviewed 413 had mucosal graft procedures. At two years 15% of those submitted to mucosal graft had continuing symptoms. In 4% these symptoms were directly attributable to restenosis and the remaining 11% were seriously compromised having either liver disease, secondary sclerosing cholangitis and/or severe sepsis with stones. Patients with liver fibrosis, sclerosing cholangitis, sepsis and stones were considered a high risk group unlikely to derive lasting benefit from stricture repair and unsuitable for mucosal graft although it is noteworthy that 11% of those patients submitted to mucosal graft did in fact develop precisely these features. Many patients (indeed half of the cases reported as having an excellent result) had a persisting elevation of the serum alkaline phosphatase. It is possible that this might be due to segmental obstruction associated with the graft operation and Blumgart (1978) has shown that such segmental obstruction can occur. The results reported (Smith 1981) appear to offer no advantage in the treatment of the complex case. The reason for the procedure — namely that high strictures cannot be sutured — is open to question since precise direct anastomosis can be carried out with a very low mortality and excellent long-term follow-up even in patients with complex strictures previously submitted to mucosal graft operation (Fig. 58.22) (Blumgart et al 1984).

Techniques of follow-up have varied from simple observation and measurement of liver function tests to the performance of transtubal cholangiography and HIDA scanning (McPherson et al 1984). It has been repeatedly noted that some patients will remain asymptomatic but yet have a persistently raised alkaline phosphatase (Smith 1979, Way & Dunphy 1972). Studies carried out at the Royal Postgraduate Medical School in which both HIDA scanning and alkaline phosphatase were measured suggest that persistence of elevation of alkaline phosphatase over a prolonged period of time is consequent either on associated hepatocellular disease or incomplete relief of obstruction (McPherson et al 1984). It is probably correct to suggest that a result should not be regarded as excellent unless the alkaline phosphatase returns to normal levels. This is important in assessing late results and should be recognized in studying the results of percutaneous transhepatic dilatational techniques.

The influence of long-term transanastomotic tubal splinting on long-term patency has been debated. Transanastomotic splinting has been used by many (Deaver 1904, Ellsworth 1936) and a transhepatic tube by Grindlay et al (1953), Goetz (1951), Praderi (1963, 1974) and subsequently by Smith (1969, 1979). The length of time that the tube should be left in situ is a subject of controversy. One study (Kune et al 1969) suggested that better long-term results were obtained in anastomoses splinted for longer than 12 months than those splinted for six months. Three to six months is now generally considered to be the minimum period of splintage with the tube left for 12 months in more difficult cases. The median duration of splintage in a study carried out at Hammersmith Hospital (Blumgart et al 1984) was only four months. It should be noted that some authors (Bismuth et al 1978, Bismuth 1982) rarely use transanastomotic stenting and have obtained good results. It may well be that transanastomotic tubes are unnecessary (Pellegrini et al 1984) in the average patient and indeed the author has recently omitted tubes altogether in a series of 19 patients without noticeable problems.

Percutaneous transhepatic catheterization and dilatation can be a useful manoeuvre in patients with *recurrent stric-*

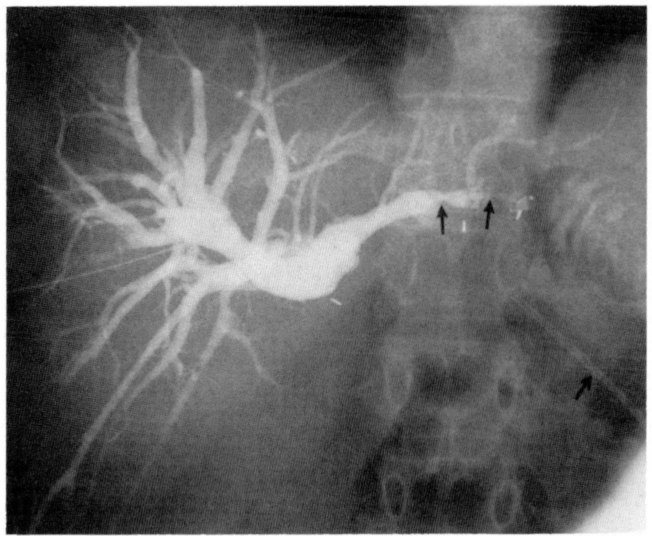

a

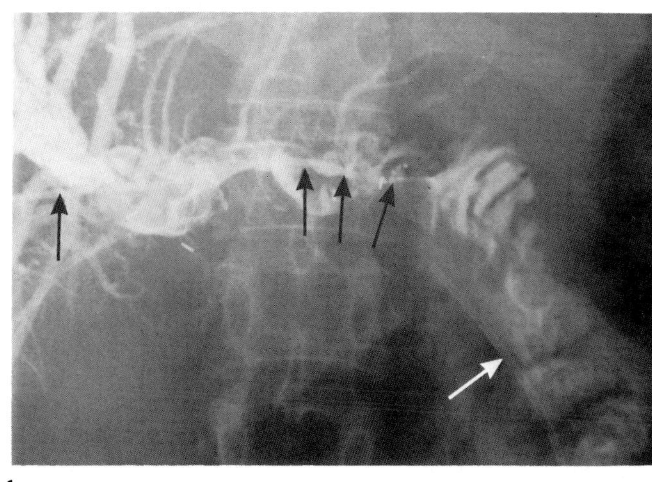

b

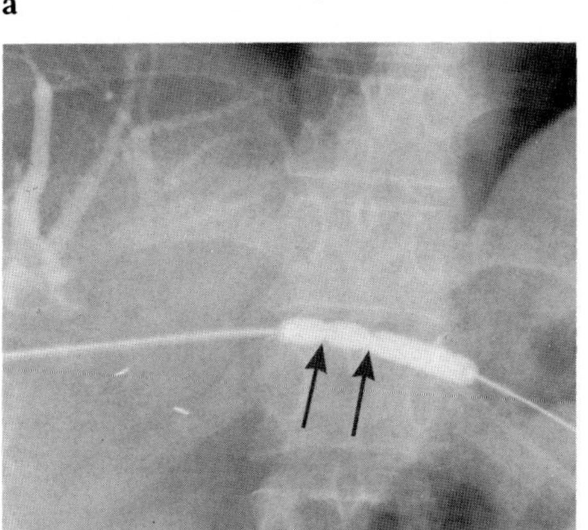

c

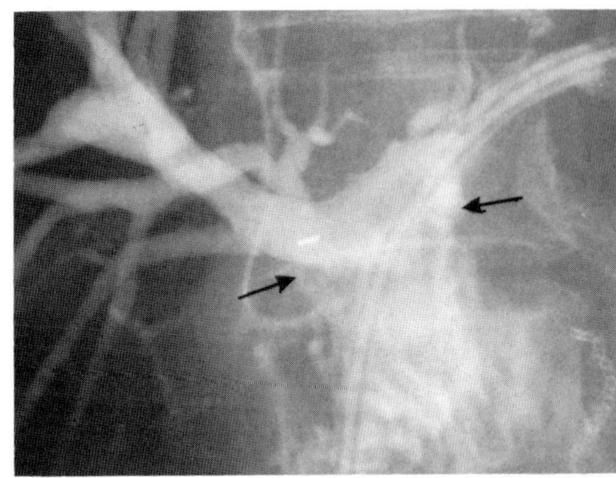

d

Fig. 58.22 a. Percutaneous transhepatic cholangiogram reveals a high (Type 3) post-cholecystectomy biliary stricture in a complex case following cholecystectomy in which there had been excision of the entire common hepatic duct. This was followed by two attempts at a mucosal graft procedure and then by a left sided hepaticojejunostomy by the Longmire-Sandford operation. On failure of this operation percutaneous intubation of the biliary ductal system was undertaken from the right side with attempted balloon dilatation of the hepaticojejunostomy on three consecutive occasions. The X-ray shows the area of the hilus (marked by surgical clip), two strictures in the left hepatic ductal system, one just proximal and the other at the hepaticojejunostomy Roux-en-Y (black arrows). A free endoprosthesis is seen (small black arrow) lying in the jejunum.

b. Cholangiogram obtained during attempted balloon dilatation of the stricture reveals the passage of the catheter (black arrows) and the biliary system full of blood clot. The guide wire crosses the stricture. A free endoprosthesis lies within the jejunal loop (white arrow). This procedure was followed by a severe episode of haemobilia requiring blood transfusion.

c. Radiograph obtained during balloon dilatation clearly illustrates the two strictures (arrows).

d. Hepaticojejunostomy Roux-en-Y was easily carried out using the left duct approach and a very wide anastomosis obtained (between the arrows). The previous hepaticojejunostomy to the left lobe was dismantled and the new anastomosis splinted by a tube passed through the left hepatic ductal system. The tube was removed two months later. The patient remains well and symptom free with normal liver function tests two years after operation

ture following hepaticojejunostomy and the author has used this approach with success. A planned *combined* surgical and interventional radiological approach is also useful especially if intrahepatic stones cannot be completely retrieved by the surgeon of if repair is difficult or unsatisfactory and recurrent stricture is anticipated. A tube is left across the anastomosis and delivered to the exterior, the tract subsequently being used by the radiologists. However, percutaneous approaches should not be used when anastomosis is easily possible and of course has its own risks (Fig. 58.22).

It should be emphasized that injury to the bile duct during cholecystectomy is a most serious problem. The mortality both initially and late is related largely to re-operative procedures, infection and the evolution of secondary biliary fibrosis and to the development of portal hypertension.

The following points summarize the problem:

1. Bile duct injury at cholecystectomy is inflicted as a result of imprecise dissection and poor visualization of anatomical structures.

2. Vascular damage to the hepatic artery and/or portal vein is not uncommon.

3. A prolonged history of high stricture involving the hepatic ducts, multiple attempts at repair, infection and the development of secondary liver fibrosis together with a low preoperative serum albumin are adverse prognostic features.

4. Precise diagnosis of the level of the stricture and demonstration of hepatic ducts prior to surgery is desirable.

5. Associated conditions such as abscess formation, gastrointestinal bleeding, fistula and portal hypertension are probably best treated *before* stricture repair.

6. There is a place for conservative management or transhepatic percutaneous dilatation in *selected high risk patients* especially in the presence of portal hypertension. However, non-operative approaches should be employed with care, since incomplete relief of a stricture may be dangerous in the long-term and associated with development of liver damage. In any event, most strictures can be safely repaired by biliary-enteric anastomosis.

7. Interventional radiological approaches may be used in an *adjunctive* manner with surgical repair in selected cases using either a percutaneous approach or the introduction of catheters along previously defined ductal tracts.

8. The majority of benign bile duct strictures can and should be managed by surgical restoration of biliary-enteric continuity by dissection of the left hepatic ductal system and confluence followed by direct mucosa-to-mucosa anastomosis of the bile duct usually to a Roux-en-Y loop of jejunum. For this approach and in the absence of liver disease the operative mortality is probably less than 1%.

9. Mucosal graft techniques, hepatotomy and left hepaticojejunostomy of the Longmire type have only a limited indication.

10. Future investigations of this subject should examine prognostic indices and classification of bile duct strictures so as to allow comparison of results and assessment of new methods of treatment.

11. *Repair of bile duct strictures is a specialist procedure and the best results are obtained by initial adequate repair.* Repeated attempts at anastomosis or intubation are associated with the development of high complex strictures and late liver disease both of which are associated with poor long-term results.

BILE DUCT INJURY AFTER OPERATIONS OTHER THAN CHOLECYSTECTOMY

Biliary operations

Operations which involve biliary enteric anastomosis may be complicated by postoperative stricture or fistula. Such procedures may be carried out for reconstructive purposes after primary pancreaticoduodenectomy (Chadwick & Dudley 1984), after deliberate excision of the bile duct for tumours in its middle third, after excision of choledochal cysts with subsequent hepatico-enteric anastomosis and after choledochoduodenostomy.

Late strictures are most likely to occur after such bypass procedures carried out with an enteric anastomosis to a normal calibre duct and particularly if the bile duct is itself diseased, as e.g. after excisional surgery or bypass for chronic pancreatitis, in which disease the duct is often involved in the inflammatory process (see below). Where biliary-enteric anastomosis has been carried out for long standing biliary obstruction, the duct is dilated and thickened, anastomosis is easy and late stenosis rare. Indeed if such stenosis occurs as, e.g. following pancreaticoduodenectomy for pancreatic or ampullary cancer, then recurrence of disease should be suspected rather than a stenotic process.

Post-gastrectomy biliary stricture

Injury to the bile duct can occur during performance of gastrectomy (Florence et al 1981) and particularly, if during the procedure, the pyloric region and first part of the duodenum is found grossly distorted or inflamed. The most common situation is biliary injury during the course of Polya gastrectomy. Such cases may present in the postoperative period with jaundice or a biliary fistula and there may be difficulty in distinguishing the presentation from a leaking duodenal stump.

The author has experienced four bile duct strictures after gastrectomy (Table 58.1). Two were of the nature described but two followed Bilroth I gastrectomy. In these two cases the surgeon carried out what was claimed to be an easy straightforward Bilroth I gastrectomy. It was remarked that the duodenal loop was mobile and the procedure not difficult. In one case after completing the anastomosis the surgeon realized that he had removed the entire first and second part of the duodenum from the pancreatic head, thus disconnecting the bile duct and pancreatic duct. In the second case a precisely similar injury occurred but the surgeon did not recognize the problem and closed the abdomen. The patient presented in the postoperative period with a biliary-pancreatic fistula. Surgical re-exploration revealed the denuded pancreatic head. A similar case has been treated at the University of Leiden, Holland, by Dr. H. Gooszen (Fig. 58.23) and communicated to the author.

Repair of the damaged bile duct following Polya gastrectomy is usually not difficult. The stricture usually lies in close proximity to the duodenal stump and it is a simple matter to identify the biliary tree and carry out a direct anastomosis at, or close to, the blind end of the duodenum. Where the entire duodenal head is denuded, as described above, a Roux-en-Y loop of jejunum may be

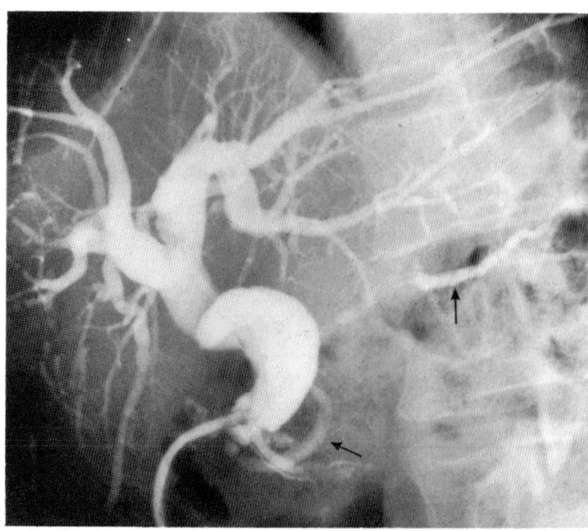

Fig. 58.23 A patient with ampullary disconnection which occurred during Bilroth I gastrectomy. The duodenal loop was completely detached from the peripapillary area. Fistulogram obtained through a T-tube which had been left in situ demonstrates both the biliary tree and the pancreatic duct (arrows) (case of Dr. H. Gooszen, University of Leiden, Holland)

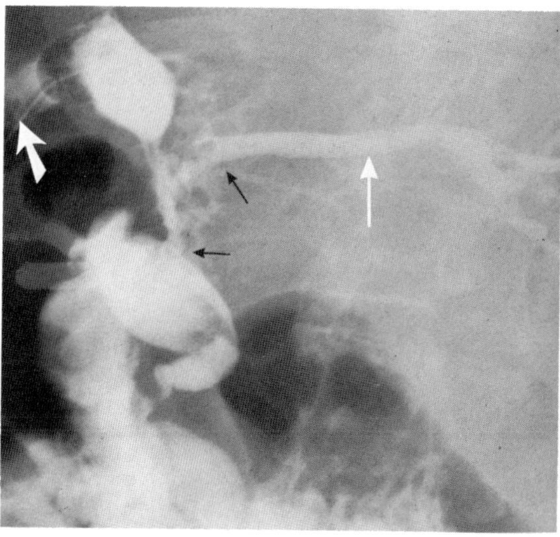

Fig. 58.24 Complex biliary stricture and fistula following right hepatic lobectomy performed for hydatid cyst. There was a biliary fistula through the right chest wall (thick white arrow). X-ray was obtained by injection of a tube within the fistulous tract. A cavity in the right chest and below the diaphragm were both outlined and there was an associated right empyema. There is complete disruption of the biliary ductal system (black arrows). The left hepatic duct in the liver remnant is shown (white arrow) and a fistula then filling the low common bile duct and the duodenum independently. The patient was managed by drainage of the right empyema, antibiotics and parenteral nutrition. Subsequently repair of the duodenal fistula and hepaticojejunostomy Roux-en-Y to the exposed bile duct were successfully carried out. The patient now remains well, symptom free and with normal liver function tests three years after operation

developed and brought up in a retrocolic fashion, the open end being used to envelop the pancreatic head. The two patients described have been followed up for periods of 10 and six years respectively. Both remain alive and well with normal liver function and normal pancreatic function. However, one patient developed a late biliary stenosis in the area of damage and secondary choledochojejunostomy had to be performed at the apex of the previously placed Roux-en-Y loop.

Other procedures

In a total series of 137 cases of benign bile duct stricture, the author has experience of a patient with late biliary stenosis following *portacaval shunt*, and a further case in whom bile duct stricture occurred following *irradiation* of para-aortic glands for testicular malignancy (Table 58.1).

Table 58.1 Benign biliary stricture*

Post-cholecystecomy	101
Associated with choledocholithiasis	3
Penetrating injury	5
Blunt injury (5 with liver injury)	6
Pancreatitis	9
Post-gastrectomy	4
Operation for choledochus cyst	4
Periportal inflammation (including 1 after DXR)	4
Portal shunt	1
Total	137

*Excludes peripapillary stricture, primary localized stricture (sclerosing cholangitis) and stricture secondary to cholelithiasis or associated with the Mirizzi syndrome

Liver resection may also be complicated by biliary damage. In cases of *liver injury*, biliary injury may be associated with the original trauma (see below) or be inflicted during the subsequent operative treatment. It may be difficult or impossible to precisely define the cause of a subsequent evident biliary fistula or stricture. Biliary damage may also occur during liver resection for tumour or cyst and is more likely for lesions involving the hilus where dissection renders the biliary tree more liable to injury (Fig. 58.24).

In general it is not necessary to insert a T-tube into the common bile duct after partial hepatectomy. However, should there be a ductal injury inflicted during operation, or if there is doubt as to the anatomy of the biliary tree at the time of surgery, then operative cholangiography can be valuable in displaying the anatomy; opening of the common bile duct with a passage of fine bougies into the right and left ducts may assist identification. If this has been carried out, then a T-tube should be inserted.

The management of injuries following partial hepatectomy can be extremely difficult (Johnson et al 1979, Smith et al 1982), the problems being similar to those encountered in the atrophy/hypertrophy complex (see above). It should be emphasized, however, that a biliary fistula occurring after partial hepatectomy should be treated expectantly for long periods and operation should only be proceeded with if the fistula fails to close after observation or if jaundice and cholangitis supervene (Ch. 60).

BILE DUCT INJURY DUE TO BLUNT OR PENETRATING ABDOMINAL TRAUMA

This problem is only briefly referred to here since it is discussed fully in Chapter 82. The gallbladder or biliary tree may be damaged following closed abdominal injury or by penetrating stab or gun shot wounds. The latter, while common in some parts of the world, are uncommon in the United Kingdom. In a total series of 137 bile duct strictures at the Royal Postgraduate Medical School, Hammersmith Hospital, six occurred in association with blunt injury (Fig. 58.25), five with associated liver injury and five following stab wounds (Table 58.1).

Occasionally late problems arise where prolonged fistulation occurs from a segment of the liver isolated by the injury so that discharge of the biliary product of a large portion of the liver occurs through the fistulous tract. Management of such cases is difficult and even prolonged observation may fail to see closure of the fistula, especially if this is associated with a distal stricture. Where such fistulation occurs management may be by one of three methods. Firstly *resection* of the isolated segment of liver tissue may be carried out. Such an approach can be difficult and is seldom warranted. In rare instances the fistula may be identified at operation and simply *oversewn*.

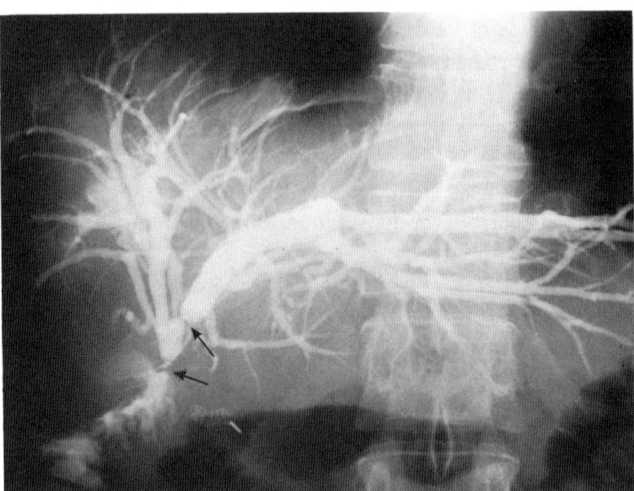

Fig. 58.25 Percutaneous transhepatic cholangiography obtained in a young man with recurrent attacks of cholangitis one year after repair of a hilar biliary stricture occurring at the site of damage to the common hepatic duct associated with a severe liver injury which had necessitated right hepatectomy. Note that there are two strictures present — one at the site of previous hepaticojejunostomy and the other in the main left hepatic duct. Rotation of the liver had made an approach to the left hepatic duct difficult. Hepaticojejunostomy was refashioned in the area of the confluence and the stricture within the left hepatic duct was treated by subsequent balloon dilatation with a good result

Alternatively, a well developed fibrous fistulous *tract can be anastomosed* either to a prepared loop of jejunum or to the gallbladder if this is near by. Such an operation may produce a permanent cure but late stenosis or stricture may still be a problem for which secondary repair must be carried out (Smith et al. 1982).

POST-INFLAMMATORY BILIARY STRICTURES

Bile duct stenosis and stricture may occur in association with any process which causes fibrosis of the common biliary channels or which causes a diffuse sclerotic process within the biliary tree. Such strictures may result from choledocholithiasis, granulomatous, lymphadenitis, chronic pancreatitis or recurrent pyogenic cholangitis.

Long-standing cholelithiasis

This results in repeated attacks of cholecystitis, the gallbladder being progressively fibrosed, shrunken and surrounded by inflammatory tissue. As this process proceeds and the gallbladder shrinks it may come to obliterate the triangle of Calot so that the gallbladder wall abuts against the common hepatic duct. In such instances the inflammatory process may spread to involve the common hepatic duct, causing inflammatory stenosis, stricturing and usually a presentation with jaundice and recurrent attacks of cholangitis (Mirizzi 1948). The presentation may be in association with a history of acute or chronic cholecystitis and a stricture may be present at the time of cholecystectomy. The surgeon who has proceeded to operation on the jaundiced patient without prior imaging of the biliary tree may find operative cholangiography difficult to obtain and may discover that he has created a bile duct injury inadvertently during attempts to remove the gallbladder. Furthermore, as outlined above, a large stone in the region of Hartman's pouch may erode into the common hepatic duct, causing a cholecyst-choledochal fistula (Fig. 58.6). In such instances removal of the gallbladder results in an opening into the common hepatic duct or inadvertent removal of a portion of the common hepatic duct. This situation should be suspected in any patient with a long history of gallstones who presents with jaundice and cholangitis. Operation should never be performed in such cases without preliminary percutaneous transhepatic or endoscopic retrograde cholangiography.

Finally, inflammatory strictures of the common hepatic duct in association with chronic cholelithiasis may present with radiological features indistinguishable from those produced by cholangiocarcinoma. This possibility must be borne in mind in any patient suspected of having hilar cholangiocarcinoma in whom there is coincident cholelithiasis. While such stricturing in association with choledocholithiasis is rare, four such cases have been recorded in Hammersmith Hospital.

The key to management in these situations is preoperative recognition of the possibility of stricture in association with cholelithiasis and appropriate management at the time of surgery.

Chronic duodenal ulcer

Chronic peripapillary duodenal ulcer can erode the entire papillary area (Colovic 1986) resulting in stricture or a choledochoduodenal fistula. Presentation is with jaundice and cholangitis and is usually on a background of a prolonged history of duodenal ulcer.

Granulomatous lymphadenitis

This may also be responsible for stricture of the adjacent common hepatic or common bile duct. It may occur in association with tuberculosis and occasionally this can be proven, although the history is usually a prolonged one and positive proof may be difficult to obtain. In such cases there has almost always been long standing obstruction to the bile ducts and there is usually associated secondary biliary fibrosis and a degree of liver damage, occasionally unilateral with liver atrophy. Treatment can be difficult since not only is there compromised liver function but biliary drainage can be difficult to establish.

Recurrent pyogenic cholangitis

As seen in South East Asia, this condition is complicated by intrahepatic gallstones consisting of calcium bilirubinate. Intrahepatic bile duct strictures also occur (Choi et al 1982, Chen et al 1984, Maki et al 1972, Ong 1962). The best management of such intrahepatic strictures, particularly if unilateral, is a combination of Roux-en-Y hepaticojejunostomy and partial hepatectomy including the affected ducts (Ch. 77).

Chronic pancreatitis

Chronic pancreatitis may also result in bile duct stenosis and stricture. Jaundice occurs in up to one-third of patients with chronic pancreatitis (Sarles & Sahel 1978). This may be due be biliary stenosis or stricture. The characteristic lesion is long and narrow and occupies the retropancreatic portion of the common bile duct (Sarles et al 1976) (Fig. 58.26) but other variants of stricture may occur and have been described in detail (Sarles & Sahel 1978). Although this is more common in association with chronic alcoholic-related pancreatitis, it occasionally occurs in chronic pancreatitis with no relationship to alcohol. In addition to jaundice there may be associated pain which is usually intermittent in character. Cholangitis and fever is unusual but can occur (Warshaw et al 1976).

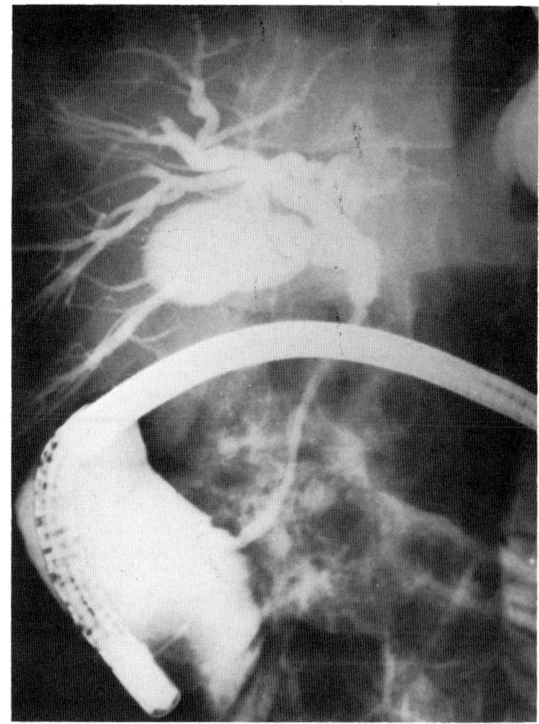

Fig. 58.26 Retrograde choledochography. Note the long stricture within the common bile duct as it passes through the head of a calcified pancreas. The stricture is a result of pancreatitis consequent to alcohol ingestion and the patient's symptoms were of intermittent attacks of jaundice and pain. The pancreatic duct could not be be outlined. Management included laparotomy and choledochojejunostomy (Blumgart 1975) (previously published in Blumgart L H 1975 Endoscopy of the upper gastrointestinal tract. In: Longmire W P (ed) Advances in Surgery Vol. 9, Year Book Medical Publishers Inc., Chicago.)

Diagnosis is made either at endoscopic retrograde cholangiography or by means of transhepatic percutaneous cholangiography and sometimes at the time of operation. The radiological appearance is of a long standing stenosis in the retropancreatic portion of the common bile duct but because the fibrotic process may affect the proximal duct, and because the process is gradual, there may be very little dilatation of the proximal bile duct. Stenosis, however, may be shorter or may only involve the immediate papillary area. Contrast medium usually traverses the stricture and passes into the duodenum but this is not always the case and *differentiation from carcinomatous obstruction may be very difficult*. While the long tapering narrow stricture of the bile duct is usually characteristic of chronic pancreatitis and especially when associated with demonstrable pancreatic ductal abnormality at ERCP, carcinoma may still very occasionally be present and caution is necessary in these cases since erroneous diagnosis may occur.

Discovery of a bile duct stenosis or stricture in association with chronic pancreatitis is not an indication for therapy and quite severe stenosis may be found in patients in whom there are absolutely normal liver function tests and in whom there has never been jaundice. If, however, cholestasis or cholangitis occur then biliary bypass is necessary. In addition, if operation is to be carried out for the management of chronic pancreatitis itself, and it is known that severe biliary stenosis is present, the surgeon may elect to perform a biliary bypass at the same time. Thus in a series of 240 patients with chronic pancreatitis, 39 of whom came to surgery, nine had symptomatic biliary tract obstruction and a total of 13 were subjected to some form of biliary enteric anastomosis either alone or in association with excisional surgery for pancreatic disease (Blumgart et al 1982).

While side-to-side choledechoduodenostomy may be employed in some cases, this is usually not the best procedure since the surrounding inflammatory reaction may render the duodenum rigid and less mobile and freqeuntly the common bile duct is not grossly dilated. Choledochojejunostomy Roux-en-Y is a preferable procedure in obstruction secondary to chronic pancreatitis and may be carried out side-to-side or end-to-side after division of the common bile duct. Cholecystjejunostomy should not be used in these circumstances nor is transduodenal sphincteroplasty suitable since the stricture is usually too long to allow this approach to the problem.

In patients with chronic pancreatitis in whom the primary presentation has been with cholestasis and in whom the pancreatic disease remains quiescent, biliary enteric anastomosis is an excellent operation with good long-term relief of symptoms (Blumgart et al 1982, Kune & McKenzie 1978).

CONCLUSION

Biliary stricture usually presents a complex problem in diagnosis and management. As such it is a specialized subject demanding an experienced surgical team working in close collaboration with others and, in particular, excellent diagnostic and interventional radiological backup and facilities for endoscopic diagnosis and operative endoscopy when indicated. Treatment decisions should be taken in consultation. Bile duct strictures, and in particular high strictures and stenoses extending to the confluence of the bile ducts, should not be treated by the occasional operator.

REFERENCES

Adson M A, Wychulis A R 1968 Portal hypertension in secondary biliary cirrhosis. Archives of Surgery 96: 604–612

Andren-Sandberg A, Alinder G, Bengmark S 1985 Accidental lesions of the common bile duct at cholecystectomy. Annals of Surgery 201: 328–332

Barker E M, Winkler M 1985 Permanent-access hepaticojejunostomy. British Journal of Surgery 71: 181–191

Belzer F O, Watts J McKay, Ross H B, Dunphy J E 1965 Autoreconstruction of the common bile duct after venous patch graft. Annals of Surgery 162: 346–355

Benjamin I S, Blumgart L H 1979 Biliary bypass and reconstruction. In: Wright R, Alberti K G M M Karran S, Millward-Sadler G D T (eds) Liver and biliary disease: Pathophysiology, diagnosis, management. Ch. 54, Saunders, London

Bismuth H 1982 Postoperative strictures of the bile duct. In: Blumgart L H (ed) The biliary tract. Clinical Surgery International Vol. 5. Churchill Livingstone, Edinburgh, p 209–218

Bismuth H, Franco D, Corlette M B 1978 Long term results of Roux-en-Y hepaticojejunostomy. Surgery, Gynecology and Obstetrics 146: 161–167

Bismuth H, Lazorthes F 1981 Les traumatismes operatoires de la voie biliaire principale Vol. 1. Masson, Paris

Blenkharn J I, Blumgart L H 1985 Streptococcal bacteraemia in hepatobiliary operations. Surgery, Gynecology and Obstetrics 160: 139–141

Blumgart L H 1978 Biliary tract obstruction — New approaches to old problems. American Journal of Surgery 135: 19–31

Blumgart L H 1980 Hepatic resection. In: Taylor S (ed) Recent advances in surgery 10. Churchill Livingstone, Edinburgh, p 1–26

Blumgart L H, Carachi R, Imrie C W, Benjamin I S, Duncan J G 1977 Diagnosis and management of post-cholecystectomy symptoms: the place of endoscopy and retrograde choledochopancreatography. British Journal of Surgery 64: 809–816

Blumgart L H, Drury J K, Wood C B 1979 Hepatic resection for trauma, tumour and biliary obstruction. British Journal of Surgery 66: 762–769

Blumgart L H, Lygidakis N J 1982 The post cholecystectomy patient. In: Blumgart L H (ed): The biliary tract. Clinical Surgery International Vol. 5. Churchill Livingstone, Edinburgh, p 143

Blumgart L H, Imrie C W, McKay A J 1982 Surgical management of chronic pancreatitis. Journal of Clinical Surgery 1: 229–235

Blumgart L H, Kelley C J 1984 Hepaticojejunostomy in benign and malignant biliary stricture: approaches to the left hepatic ducts. British Journal of Surgery 71: 257–261

Blumgart L H, Kelley C J, Benjamin I S 1984 Benign bile duct stricture following cholecystectomy — critical factors in management. British Journal of Surgery 71: 836–843

Bodval B 1973 The post-cholecystectomy syndrome. Clinical Gastroenterology 2: 103–126

Braasch J W, Bolten J S, Rossi R L 1981 A technique of biliary tract reconstruction with complete follow-up in 44 consecutive cases. Annals of Surgery 194: 635–638

Cass M H, Robson B, Rundle F F 1955 Electrolyte losses with biliary fistula: post-cholecystectomy acidotic syndrome. Medical Journal of Australia 1: 165–169

Cattell R B, Braasch J W 1959a General considerations in the management of benign stricture of the bile duct. New England Journal of Medicine 261: 929–933

Cattell R B, Braasch J W 1959b Two-stage repairs of benign strictures of the bile duct. Surgery, Gynecology and Obstetrics 109: 691–696

Cattell R B, Braasch J W 1960 Repair of benign strictures of the bile duct involving both or single hepatic ducts. Surgery, Gynecology and Obstetrics 110: 55–60

Chadwick S J K, Dudley H A F 1984 Stenosis at the choledochojejunostomy anastomosis following pancreaticoduodenectomy when the common bile duct is of normal calibre. Annals of the Royal College of Surgeons of England 66: 319–320

Chen H H, Zhang W H, Wang S S 1984 Twenty-two year experience with the diagnosis and treatment of intrahepatic calculi. Surgery, Gynecology and Obstetrics 159: 519–524

Choi T K, Wong J, Ong G B 1982 The surgical management of primary intrahepatic stones. British Journal of Surgery 69: 86–90

Colovic R 1986 Cholangitis caused by chronic duodenal ulcer. Digestive Surgery (in press)

Couinaud C 1953 Les hepato-cholangiostomies digestives. La Presse Medicale 61: 468–470

Couinaud C 1955 Recherches sur la chirurgie du confluent biliaire

superieur et des canaux hepatiques. La Presse Medicale 63: 669–674
Czerniak A, Søreide O, Gibson R N, Hadjis N, Kelley C J, Benjamin I S, Blumgart L H 1986 Liver atrophy complicating benign bile duct strictures in surgical and interventional radiological approaches. American Journal of Surgery (in press)
Dawson J L 1981 Cholecystectomy. In: Lord Smith of Marlow, Dame Sheila Sherlock (eds): Surgery of the gallbladder and bile ducts 2nd Edn. Butterworths, London, p 329
Deaver J B 1904 Hepatic drainage. British Medical Journal 2: 821–825
Ekman C A, Sandblom P 1962 Bilio-intestinal anastomosis as a cause of liver cirrhosis with portal hypertension. Acta Chirurgica Scandinavica 123: 383–388
Ellis H, Hoile R W 1980 Vein patch repair of the common bile duct. Journal of the Royal Society of Medicine 73: 635–637
Ellsworth E 1936 Benign scicatricial strictures of the bile duct. Annals of Surgery 104: 668–699
Florence M G, Hart M J, White T T 1981 Ampullary disconnection during the course of biliary and duodenal surgery. American Journal of Surgery 142: 100–105
Goetz O 1951 Die transhepatische Bile Drainage bei der hohen Gallengangstenose. Archiv für Klinische Chirurgie 270: 97–99
Grey-Turner R G 1944 Injuries to the main bile duct. Lancet i: 621–622
Grindlay J H, Eberle J, Walters W 1953 Technique for external drainage of the biliary tract which leaves the duct intact — Experimental study. Archives of Surgery 67: 289–296
Gutgemann A, Schriefers K H, Phillipp R, Wulfing D 1965 Zur rekonstruktiven Chirurgie des verletzten und strikturierten grossen Gallenganges. Beiträge zur klinischen Chirurgie 210: 129–150
Ham J 1979 Partial and complete atrophy affecting hepatic segments and lobes. British Journal of Surgery 66: 333–337
Hepp J, Couinaud C 1956 L'abord et l'utilisation du canal hepatique gauche dans les reparations de la voie biliaire principale. La Presse Medicale 64: 947–948
Hunt D R, Blumgart L H 1980 Iatrogenic choledochoduodenal fistula: an unsuspected cause of post-cholecystectomy symptoms. British Journal of Surgery 67: 10–13
Johnson A G, Murray-Lyon I M, Blumgart L H 1979 Stricture of common hepatic duct after right hepatic lobectomy treated by Longmire's operation. Journal of the Royal Society of Medicine 72: 136–139
Kelley C J, Hemingway A P, McPherson G A D, Allison D J, Blumgart L H 1983 Non-surgical management of post-cholecystectomy haemobilia. British Journal of Surgery 70: 502–504
Kelley C J, Blumgart L H 1985 Peroperative cholangiography and post-cholecystectomy biliary strictures. Annals of the Royal College of Surgeons of England 67: 93–95
Kracht M, Thompson J N, Bernhoft R A, Tsang V, Gibson R N, Blumgart L H 1986 Cholangitis following endoscopic sphincterotomy in patients with high biliary stricture. Surgery, Gynecology and Obstetrics (in press)
Kune G A 1970 The influence of structure and function in the surgery of the biliary tract. Annals of the Royal College of Surgeons of England 47: 78–91
Kune G A 1979 Bile duct injury during cholecystectomy. Causes, prevention and surgical repair in 1979. Australian and New Zealand Journal of Surgery 49: 35–40
Kune G A, Hardy J H, Brown G, McKenzie G 1969 Operative injuries of the common bile duct. Medical Journal of Australia 2: 233–236
Kune G A, McKenzie G G C 1978 The surgeon's role in chronic pancreatitis. Proceedings, First Australian Pancreas Congress, University of Melbourne
Kune G A, Sali A 1981 Benign biliary sttrictures. In: The practice of biliary surgery 2nd Edn. Blackwell Scientific Publications, Oxford
Longmire W P Jr, Sandford M C 1949 Intrahepatic cholangiojejunostomy for biliary obstruction — further studies: Report of 4 cases. Annals of Surgery 130: 455–460
Lygidakis N J 1981 Choledochoduodenostomy in biliary calculous disease. British Journal of Surgery 68: 762–765
Madden J L 1973 Common duct stones: Their origin and surgical management. Surgical Clinics of North America 53: 1095–1113
Maki T, Sato T, Matsushiro T 1972 A reappraisal of surgical treatment for intrahepatic gallstones. Annals of Surgery 175: 155–165
McArthur M S, Longmire W P Jr 1971 Peptic ulcer disease after choledochojejunostomy. American Journal of Surgery 122: 155–158
McPherson G A D, Benjamin I S, Habib N, Bowley N B, Blumgart L H 1982 Percutaneous transhepatic biliary drainage. Advantages and problems. British Journal of Surgery 69: 261–264
McPherson G A D, et al L H 1984 HIDA scanning and assessment of bile duct stricture.
Michie G, Gunn A 1964 Bile duct injuries. A new suggestion for their repair. British Journal Surgery 51: 96–100
Mirizzi P L 1948 Sindrome del conducto hepatico (Sindrome Hepaticiano). Journal International Chirurgie 8: 731–734
Molnar W, Stockum E 1978 Transhepatic dilatation of choledochoenterostomy strictures. Diagnostic Radiology 129: 59–64
Morgenstern L, Berci G 1982 Intraoperative diagnostic procedures. In: Blumgart L H (ed): The biliary tract. Clinical Surgery International Vol. 5. Churchill Livingstone, Edinburgh, p 99
Myat Thu Ya, Robinson D, Gunn A A 1973 Per-operative cholangiography. British Journal of Surgery 60: 711–712
Northover J M A, Terblanche I 1979 A new look at the arterial blood supply of the bile duct in man and its surgical implications. British Journal of Surgery 66: 379–384
Northover J M A, Terblanche I 1982 Applied surgical anatomy of the biliary tree. In: Blumgart L H (ed): The biliary tract. Clinical Surgery International Vol. 5. Churchill Livingstone, Edinburgh, p 1–16
Okamura T, Orii K, Ono A, Ozaki A, Iwasaki Y 1985 Surgical technique for repair of benign stricture of the bile ducts, preserving the papilla of Vater. World Journal of Surgery 9: 619–625
Okuda K, Tanikawa K, Emura T et al 1974 Non-surgical percutaneous transhepatic cholangiography — diagnostic significance in the medical problems of the liver. American Journal of Digestive Diseases 19: 21–36
Ong G B 1962 A study of recurrent pyogenic cholangitis. Archives of Surgery 84: 199–225
Pappalardo G, Correnti S, Mobarhan S, Frattoroli F, Castrini G 1982 Long term results of hepaticojejunostomy and hepaticoduodenotomy. Annals of Surgery 196: 149–152
Pellegrini C A, Thomas M J, Way L W 1984 Recurrent biliary stricture. Patterns of recurrence and outcome of surgical therapy. American Journal of Surgery 147: 175–180
Pitt H A, Miyamato T, Parapatis S K, Thompkins R K, Longmire W P 1982 Factors influencing outcome in patients with post-operative biliary strictures. American Journal of Surgery 144: 14–20
Praderi R 1963 E1 drenaje biliar externo o interno per el hepatico izquierdo. Revista Da Associacao Medica Brasileira 9: 401–403
Praderi R C 1974 Twelve years experience with transhepatic intubation. Annals of Surgery 179: 937–940
Rosenquist H, Myrin S O 1960 Operative injury to the bile ducts. Acta Chirurgica Scandinavica 119: 92–107
Sarles H, Payan N, Tasso F, Sahel J 1976 Chronic pancreatitis, relapsing pancreatitis, calcifications of pancreas. In: Bochus H L (ed): Gastroenterology. Saunders, Philadelphia, p 1040
Sarles H, Sahel J 1978 Cholestasis and lesion of the biliary tract in chronic pancreatitis. Gut 19: 851–857
Sato T, Imamura M, Sasaki I, Kameyama J 1982 Biliary reconstruction and gastric acid secretion. American Journal of Surgery 144: 599–553
Sato T, Mikio I, Sasaki I, Kameyama J 1983 Gastric acid secretion after biliary reconstruction. American Journal of Surgery 146: 245–249
Schaffner F, Bacchin P G, Hutterer F et al 1971 Mechanisms of cholestasis. 4. Structural and biochemical changes in the liver and serum in rats after bile duct ligation. Gastroenterology 60: 888–897
Schein C J 1978 Post cholecystectomy syndromes. Harper and Row, Hagerstown, Maryland
Schein C J, Gliedman M L 1981 Choledochoduodenostomy as an adjunct to choledocholithotomy. Surgery, Gynecology and Obstetrics 152: 797–804
Schwarz W, Roxen R J, Fitts W Jr et al 1981 Percutaneous transhepatic drainage pre-operative for benign biliary strictures. Surgery, Gynecology and Obstetrics 152: 466–468
Sedgwick C E, Poulantzas J K, Kune G A 1966 Management of portal hypertension secondary to bile duct stenosis: review of 18 cases with splenorenal shunt. Annals of Surgery 163: 949–953
Smith R 1969 Strictures of the bile ducts. Proceedings of the Royal Society of Medicine 62: 131–137

Smith R 1979 Obstructions of the bile duct. British Journal of Surgery 66: 69–79
Smith R 1981 Injuries of the bile ducts. In: Lord Smith of Marlow, Dame Sheila Sherlock (eds): Surgery of the gallbladder and bile ducts 2nd Edn. Butterworths, London, p 361
Smith E E J, Bowley N, Allison D J, Blumgart L H 1982 The management of post-traumatic intrahepatic cutaneous biliary fistulae. British Journal of Surgery 69: 317–318
Soupault R, Couinaud C L 1957 Sur un procede nouveau de derivation biliaire intra-hepatique. Les cholangio-jejunostomies gauches sans sacrifice hepatique. La Presse Medicale 65: 1157–1159
Stubbs R S, McCloy R F, Blumgart L H 1983 Cholelithiasis and cholecystitis: surgical treatment. In: Classen R, Schreiber H W (eds) Clinics in gastroenterology Vol. 12. Biliary Tract Disorders. W B Saunders, London, p 179–201
Teplick S K, Goldstein R C, Richardson P A et al 1980 Percutaneous transhepatic choledochoplasty and dilatation of choledochoenterostomy strictures. Journal of the American Medical Association 244: 1240–1242
Toufanian A, Carey L C, Martin E T Jr 1978 Transhepatic biliary dilatation: an alternative to surgical reconstruction. Current Surgery 35: 70–73
Viikari S J 1960 Operative injuries to the bile ducts. Acta Chirurgica Scandinavica 119: 83–92
Vogel S B, Howard R J, Caridi J, Hawkins I F 1985 Evaluation of percutaneous transhepatic balloon dilatation of benign biliary strictures in high risk patients. American Journal of Surgery 149: 73–74
Voyles C R, Blumgart L H 1983 A technique for the construction of high biliary-enteric anastomoses. Surgery, Gynecology and Obstetrics 154: 885–887
Warren K W, Jefferson M P 1973 Prevention and repair of strictures of the extrahepatic bile ducts. Surgical Clinics of North America 53: 423–433
Warren K W, Christophi C, Armendari Z R 1982 Surgical Gastroenterology 1: 141–154
Warshaw A L, Schapiro R H, Ferrucci J T Jr, Galdabini J J 1976 Persistent obstructive jaundice, cholangitis and biliary cirrhosis due to common bile duct stenosis in chronic pancreatitis. Gastroenterology 70: 562–567
Way L W, Dunphy J E 1972 Biliary stricture. American Journal of Surgery 124: 287–295
Weinbren H K, Hadjis N S, Blumgart L H 1985 Structural aspects of the liver in patients with biliary disease and portal hypertension. Journal of Clinical Pathology 38: 1013–1020

S. I. Schwartz

Sclerosing cholangitis

INTRODUCTION

Sclerosing cholangitis, also referred to as primary sclerosing cholangitis, is a disease of unknown aetiology. It is a progressive cholestatic disorder characterized by a fibrosing inflammatory process which affects the intrahepatic and/or extrahepatic ducts. The first case was reported by Delbet in 1924, and the second case appeared in the same French journal a year later (Lafourcade 1925). Miller recorded the first case in the English literature in 1927. A review in 1958 by Schwartz & Dale included only 13 previously recorded cases to which the authors added six cases of their own.

Sclerosing cholangitis occurs alone or in association with inflammatory bowel disease, and it is now the consensus that the presence of inflammatory disease does not negate the term 'primary sclerosing cholangitis' since no cause/effect relationship has been defined. Newly introduced radiological techniques suggest that the disorder is more common than previously appreciated. A distinction between this lesion and carcinoma of the bile duct may be extremely difficult (Ch. 65). Although the course is usually progressive, there may be a long quiescent asymptomatic period. No therapeutic approach has achieved complete success, but there has been recent enthusiasm for a more aggressive surgical approach.

INCIDENCE

Sclerosing cholangitis had been regarded as a very rare disorder when the diagnosis was based solely on the findings at laparotomy. At one institution the diagnosis increased more than twofold after the introduction of percutaneous transhepatic cholangiography (PTC) and endoscopic retrograde cholangiopancreatography (ERCP) (Wiesner & LaRusso 1980). Approximately 70% of patients with sclerosing cholangitis are men, most of whom are in the fifth decade. The youngest reported patient was four years old (Spivak et al 1982). The overwhelming majority of patients have been Caucasian, but the disease has been reported in blacks and orientals. Two large series (Schrumpf et al 1982, Dew et al 1979) of patients with ulcerative colitis have shown a 1% incidence of sclerosing cholangitis. The reported incidence of inflammatory bowel disease in patients with sclerosing cholangitis ranges between 25 and 74% (Meyers et al 1970, Thorpe et al 1976, Danzi et al 1978, Wiesner & LaRusso 1980).

AETIOLOGY

The aetiology of sclerosing cholangitis has not been defined. The two categories of causes which have received the greatest attention are infection and immunological factors. Warren et al (1966) have reported that *E. coli* has grown out of the bile in many of their patients. These authors also pointed to the association with ulcerative colitis in which the mucosal barrier is interrupted, facilitating the entrance of bacteria into the portal circulation and the evolution of an inflammatory sclerosing process in the ducts. Evidence for an autoimmune response is also indirect. Elevation of the serum immunoglobulin levels, as well as a reduction in the serum bilirubin and alkaline phosphatase levels following steroid therapy are offered as evidence of an immune aetiology. Two reported cases in which there was associated fibrosis and inflammation of the retroperitoneum (Bartholomew et al 1963) as well as the association with Riedel's thyroiditis, also suggest such a factor. Roberts (1958) has shown that in certain animals an induced immune reaction could result in chronic inflammation of the common bile duct.

The most cogent evidence of an immunological factor is the recent report of Chapman et al (1983) that defined a 60% incidence in the frequency of HLA-B8 in patients with sclerosing cholangitis compared with a 25% incidence in controls. Low titres of serum autoantibodies were frequently found in the primary sclerosing cholangitis group but did not correspond to the presence of HLA-B8. Raised concentrations of IgM and IgG also were not related to HLA-B8. The finding is suggestive of immunological dysfunction in patients with primary sclerosing cholangitis because the presence of HLA-B8 has been shown to be associated with disease involving immunological dysfunction and HLA-B8 appears to promote an immune response to many different antigens. The reports of the complex of sclerosing cholangitis, chronic pancreatitis and Sjogren's syndrome, in which there is an increase in the HLA-B8 antigen is also suggestive of an immune aetiology (Montefusco et al 1984).

An increased frequency of HLA-B8 has not been observed in patients with primary biliary cirrhosis, providing evidence that primary biliary cirrhosis and primary sclerosing cholangitis are not related diseases. A number of studies have shown that HLA-B8 is not increased in ulcerative colitis. The increased frequency of HLA-B8 was similar in sclerosing cholangitis patients whether or not ulcerative colitis was co-existent. Thus, the Chapman (1981) study has demonstrated that in patients with primary sclerosing cholangitis there exists in many individuals a disease susceptibility gene that may be modified by other factors such as ulcerative colitis.

PATHOLOGY

Diffuse thickening of the walls of the extrahepatic biliary ducts with concomitant encroachment upon the lumen result in marked luminal narrowing, which may be diffuse or segmental in distribution. The walls of the ducts may be up to eight times their normal thickness, while the lumen is generally between 3–5 mm in diameter. The bile in the ducts varies from a thin fluid to sludge. Histologically the areas of inflammation and fibrosis are in the submucosal portions of the ducts. The duct wall contains a diffuse infiltration of chronic inflammatory cells. Periluminal glands may be entrapped in the inflammatory and fibrous tissue, and mimic cholangiocarcinoma. The gallbladder is not usually involved, but if it is, the process is similar to that described for the remainder of the extrahepatic bile duct system. Papillary hyperplasia of the gallbladder mucosa may be present.

A review of cholangiograms of 36 patients (Cameron et al 1984) with sclerosing cholangitis demonstrated an involvement of the extrahepatic bile ducts in 33 patients, involvement of the hepatic duct bifurcation in 33 patients and of the intrahepatic bile duct in 35 patients. When the cholangiograms were graded for the area of most severe obstructive disease, the hepatic bifurcation was designated as the region in 32 patients.

There are no hepatic lesions that are diagnostic of sclerosing cholangitis. Changes in the portal tracts are suggestive. An infiltrate of plasma cells, neutrophils, and occasionally eosinophils are characteristic. As a consequence of bile secretion, bile salts are retained in the periportal hepatocytes. Copper, which is excreted in the bile, is accumulated in the periportal tissue. As the disease progresses, periductal fibrosis, diminished numbers of interlobular bile ducts, and piecemeal necrosis become more apparent. The spectrum of liver pathological changes is shown in Figure 59.1 (Lefkowitch 1982). Primary sclerosing cholangitis may be staged histologically according to the system proposed by Ludwig et al (1981):

Stage 1 Periductal fibrosis and inflammation confined to the portal tracts
Stage 2 Portal and periportal fibrosis and inflammation
Stage 3 Fibrosis and inflammation bridging portal tracts
Stage 4 Cirrhosis.

In the Royal Free Hospital series (Chapman et al 1980) the histological diagnosis of sclerosing cholangitis was made in only 40% of hepatic biopsy specimens of patients proven to have the disease. The hepatic histology of sclerosing cholangitis is most frequently confused with that of primary biliary cirrhosis.

CLINICAL MANIFESTATIONS

Some patients are asymptomatic at the time of diagnosis and may remain so for up to 15 years (Chapman et al 1981). These are patients in whom an elevated alkaline phosphatase led to a radiological study which established the diagnosis. In patients with clinically apparent disease there are no pathognomonic symptoms or signs. The symptoms include jaundice, pruritus, right upper quadrant abdominal pain and intermittent temperature elevations at times accompanied by shaking chills. Fevers, chills and abdominal pains are actually unusual in patients who have not had a previous bile duct operation. On physical examination, jaundice, hepatomegaly and splenomegaly are the most common findings, occurring in about one half of the patients. 80% of patients have noted symptoms for an average of two years before diagnosis. The incidence of symptoms at the time of presentation is shown in Table 59.1 (Chapman et al 1983).

Primary sclerosing cholangitis is characterized by relapses and remissions. In some patients, the disease remains quiescent for prolonged periods of time. In most cases the disorder is progressive, with the development of secondary biliary cirrhosis. At this time xanthomas may become apparent, and the manifestations of liver failure appear. Some patients with sclerosing cholangitis present with the signs of portal hypertension, hepatosplenomegaly, bleeding oesophagogastric varices and/or ascites.

In patients with inflammatory bowel disease, the symptoms and signs of ulcerative colitis or Crohn's disease are frequently dominant. In these patients sclerosing cholangitis is usually diagnosed in the course of investigating an elevated alkaline phosphatase. The findings of keratocon-

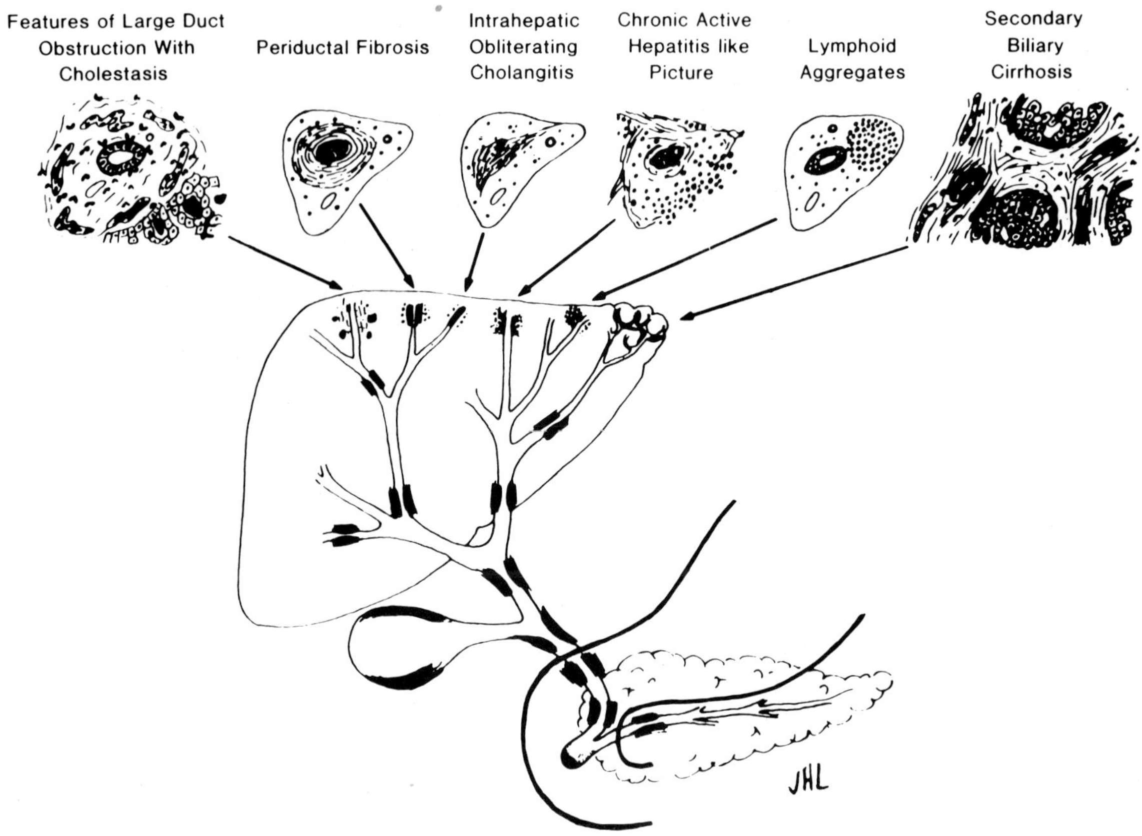

Fig. 59.1 Schematic representation of spectrum of liver histopathological changes in primary sclerosing cholangitis. Areas of black hatching indicate possible sites of biliary tree involvement. Various hepatic changes reflect both duration of disease and level of biliary tree involvement. From Lefkowitch 1982, with permission

junctivitis sicca, xerostomia, and swelling of the salivary glands are diagnostic of associated Sjogren's syndrome.

Other associated diseases are retroperitoneal fibrosis, mediastinal fibrosis, retractile mesenteritis, Peyronie's disease, pancreatitis, Riedel's thyroiditis, pseudotumour of the orbit and Weber-Christian disease.

Diagnostic studies

The results of laboratory tests are indicative of a cholestatic process and are not specific for sclerosing cholangitis. The alkaline phosphatase is almost always elevated, frequently out of proportion to the serum bilirubin which is normal in half the patients. The transaminase level may be normal or moderately elevated, particularly in icteric patients. Levels of serum IgM may be raised; elevations of IgA and IgG are less common; antinuclear or antismooth muscle antibodies may be present. Antimitochondrial antibodies, characteristic of primary biliary cirrhosis, are absent, providing additional evidence of a lack of association between primary sclerosing cholangitis and primary biliary cirrhosis. Eosinophilia is occasionally noted. The bile is frequently heavily infected with coliform bacilli, bacteroides, klebsiella or candida (Wood & Cuschieri 1980). Copper metabolism is almost always abnormal; urinary copper levels and serum caeruloplasmin values are elevated in 75% of the patients, often to the degree seen in primary biliary cirrhosis and Wilson's disease (LaRusso et al 1984). These tests of copper metabolism are of prognostic significance (Gross et al 1983).

Currently the diagnosis of sclerosing cholangitis is based on radiological findings in the majority of cases. Cholangiography provides the most relevant information and it is the 'gold standard', but scintigraphy, sonography and computed tomography are important addenda to the diagnostic armamentarium. None of these radiological studies can completely differentiate between sclerosing cholangitis and carcinoma of the bile ducts.

Cholangiography

Diagnostic cholangiograms are performed by endoscopic retrograde cholangiopancreatography (ERCP) or by percutaneous transhepatic cholangiography (PTC). ERCP usually is the preferred approach when a T-tube is not in place, because there is a greater likelihood of success in the absence of intrahepatic ductal dilatation and because the pancreatic ducts are better visualized. PTC, which is

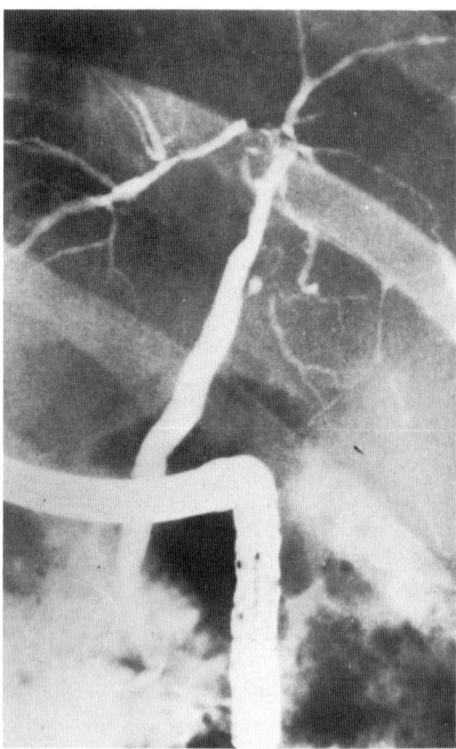

Fig. 59.2 Endoscopic retrograde cholangiogram in a 40-year-old male with sclerosing cholangitis not associated with inflammatory bowel disease. The disorder affects predominantly the intrahepatic duct system with multiple strictures. Although diseased, the common bile duct is not markedly involved. (Cuschieri 1985, with permission)

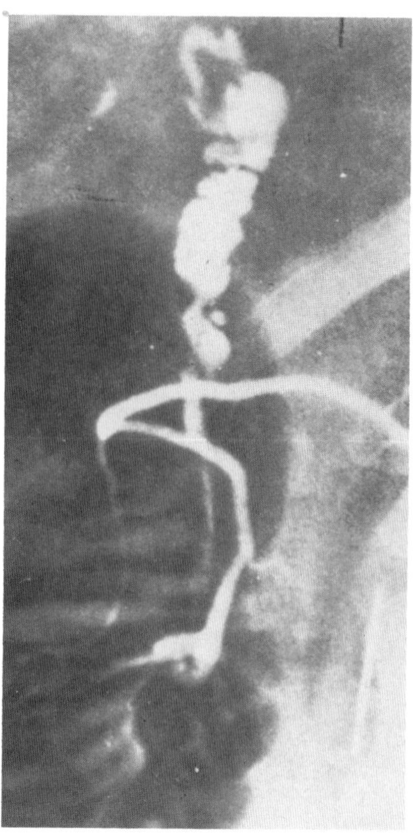

Fig. 59.3 Multiple short, band-like strictures involving the common hepatic duct can be seen, alternating with protruding, diverticulum-like pouchings. Portions of the main and accessory pancreatic ducts are superimposed on a long stricture of the lower common bile duct. From MacCarty et al 1983, with permission

successful in about half the cases, represents an excellent alternative and should be used if the ERCP has failed, or in a patient with a choledochojejunostomy. Intraoperative cholangiograms, which historically preceded ERCP and PTC as a method of making the diagnosis, continue to be used with success. Intravenous cholangiography rarely results in radiographs that are diagnostic of sclerosing cholangitis.

The characteristic cholangiographic finding is that of multifocal strictures of the intra- and extrahepatic ducts. In the experience of MacCarty et al (1983) the intrahepatic ducts were involved in all patients in whom they were visualized (Fig. 59.2). The extrahepatic ducts (Fig. 59.3) were involved in all but one patient. In 20% of the cases, only the intrahepatic and proximal extrahepatic ducts were involved. The strictures are typically short and annular, alternating with normal or minimally dilated segments, accounting for the 'beaded' appearance. In more advanced disease, the strictures become confluent and 'diverticula' of the ducts may be formed (Fig. 59.4). In the same series, focal dilatation of ductal segments occurred in 42% of the cases, but diffuse dilatation was uncommon. The cystic duct was considered abnormal in 18% of the cases in which it was visualized; the pancreatic duct was abnormal in 8% of the cases (Fig. 59.5). Gluskin & Payne (1983) suggest that the presence of marked cystic dilatation on cholangiography is highly suggestive of an associated cholangiocarcinoma (Fig. 59.6).

Sonography

Few reports regarding the sonographic manifestations of sclerosing cholangitis are available; ultrasound examination of these patients is often normal or inconclusive. Carroll & Oppenheimer (1982) presented a patient with biliary obstruction in whom the sonogram defined marked concentric thickening of the intra- and extrahepatic biliary tree (Fig. 59.7). The duct wall thickening is non-specific and may be indistinguishable from other inflammatory processes, such as suppurative cholangitis; it is also indistinguishable from primary or metastatic tumours.

Scintigraphy (Ch. 15)

An hepatobiliary agent, such as Tc-99m labelled DISIDA (diisopropylphenylcarbamoyl iminodiacetic acid) or one of its analogues, is injected intravenously and the patient is scanned with a gamma camera. Bilirubin levels up to 20 mg/100 ml do not compromise this study. Scintigraphic

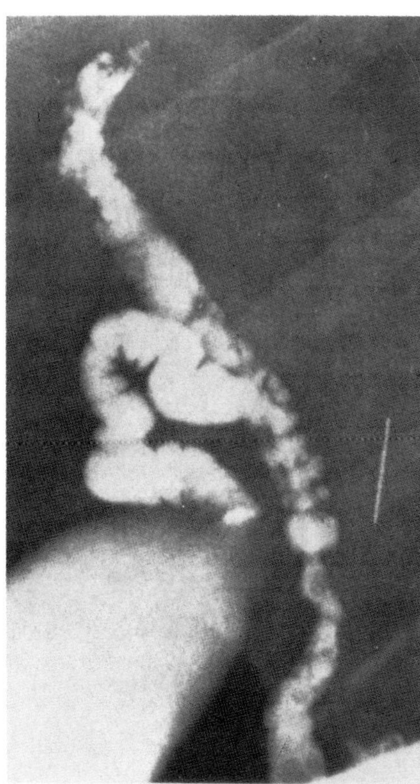

Fig. 59.4 Extensive, complex band strictures with diverticula involving the common hepatic and bile ducts. Note the normal valves of Heister in the cystic duct. From MacCarty et al 1983, with permission

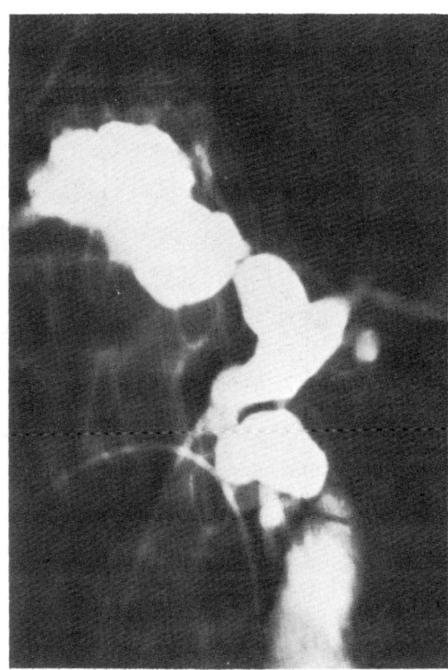

Fig. 59.6 Nasobiliary cholangiogram demonstrating dilated ducts and cystic dilatation of the biliary tree. From Gluskin and Payne 1983, with permission

findings are noted in both the biliary tract and the hepatic parenchyma. The most specific findings, reported by Ament et al (1984), consisted of multiple focal areas of increased radiotracer accumulations that were apparent as early as 15 minutes after injection and persisted for 60 minutes or longer (Fig. 59.8). These focal 'hotspots' corresponded to dilated ducts demonstrated on the cholangiogram. Another finding was delayed isotope clearance of various segments of the liver, corresponding to areas drained by stenosed ducts.

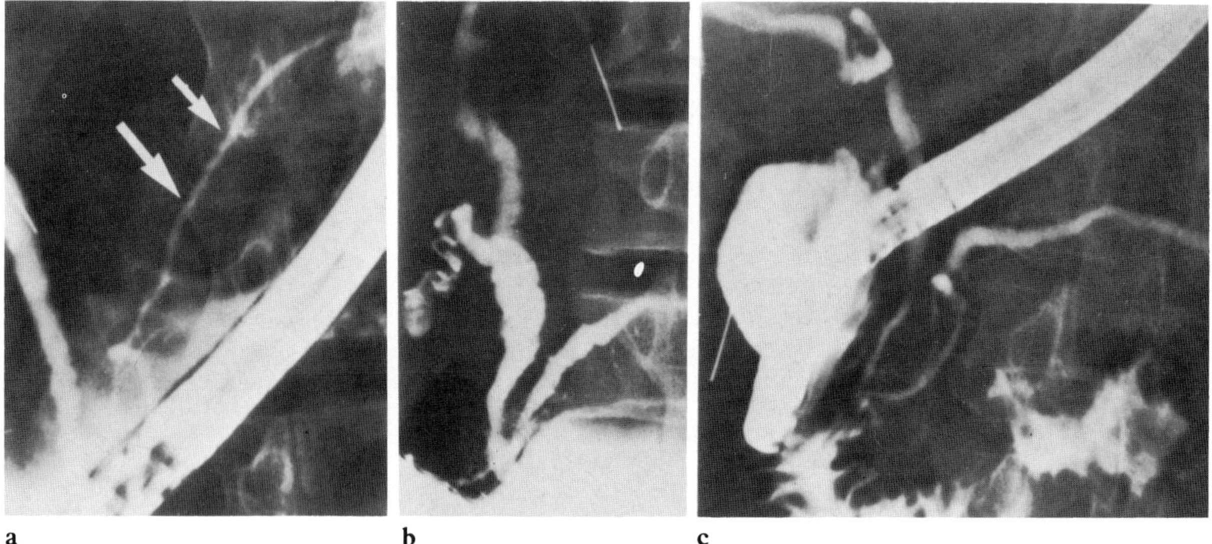

Fig. 59.5 a. Diffuse narrowing of the main pancreatic duct with multiple short strictures (arrows) in a patient with PSC. b. Slightly dilated main pancreatic duct proximal to a tapered stricture in the head of the pancreas. The margins of the pancreatic duct are irregularly serrated. Note the involvement of the common bile duct by PSC, producing fine mural irregularities. c. Undulating, smooth strictures of the main pancreatic duct, expecially in the head of the pancreas; the secondary branches are also involved. The intervening ductal segments are mildly ectatic. The common duct is involved by PSC, producing a smooth stricture at its lower end. From MacCarty et al 1983, with permission

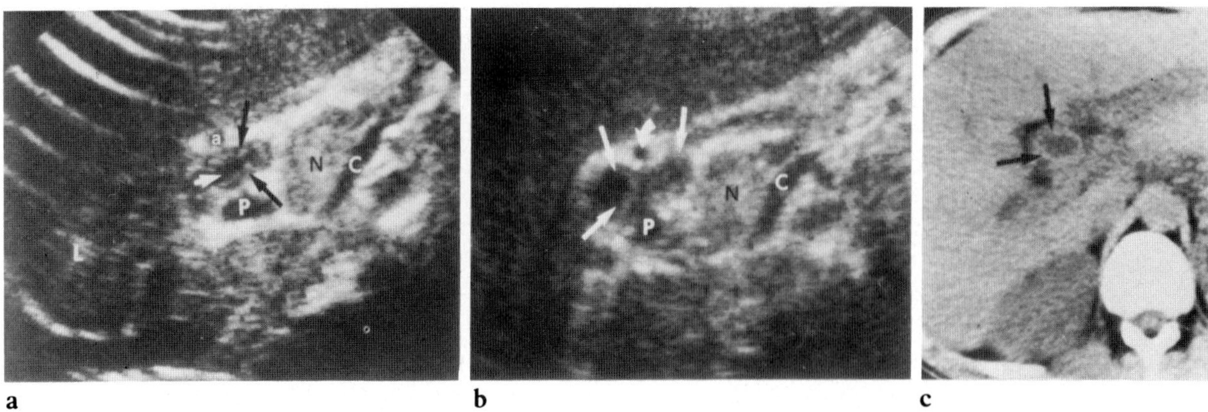

Fig. 59.7 a. Sagital left decubitus sonogram through porta hepatis. Concentric thickening of walls of common hepatic and common bile duct to 1.5 cm (arrows). Lumen of common duct (white arrow) less than 5 mm in diameter. L = liver, P = portal vein, N = portal adenopathy, C = inferior vena cava, a = hepatic artery. b. Oblique sonogram through porta hepatis. Concentric thickening of walls of right and left hepatic ducts (straight arrows). Hepatic artery (curved arrows). c. CT scan at level of porta hepatis. Concentric thickening of dilated common bile duct (arrows). From Carrol & Oppenheimer 1982, with permission

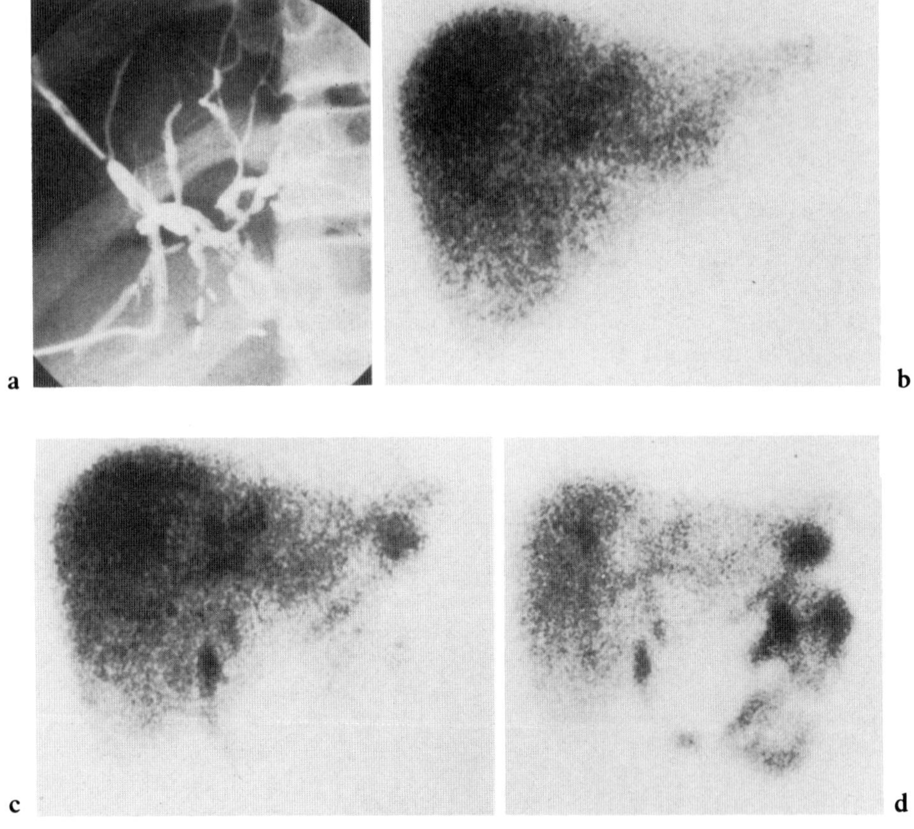

Fig. 59.8 a. Straight-tube cholangiogram demonstrates numerous strictures of the common duct and major intrahepatic ducts, characteristic of PSC. b. A 5-min DISIDA scan shows patchy hepatocellular isotope distribution. c. A 15-min DISIDA image demonstrates multiple areas of focal activity corresponding to the biliary tree. Note delayed clearance in the right lobe. Early bowel activity is present. d. DISIDA scan at 60 min shows more marked localized variation in hepatic clearance of activity, and persistence of intense activity in common bile duct. From Ament et al 1984, with permission

Computerized tomography

The findings in patients with sclerosing cholangitis were relatively consistent in a series of 10 patients evaluated by Rahn et al (1983). The intrahepatic biliary system showed focal areas of mild dilatation, usually located peripherally in the liver parenchyma; at times this produced a 'beaded' appearance (Fig. 59.9). The segments of the dilated biliary tree did not continue centrally to the hilus, distinguishing the lesion from biliary obstruction due to tumour or

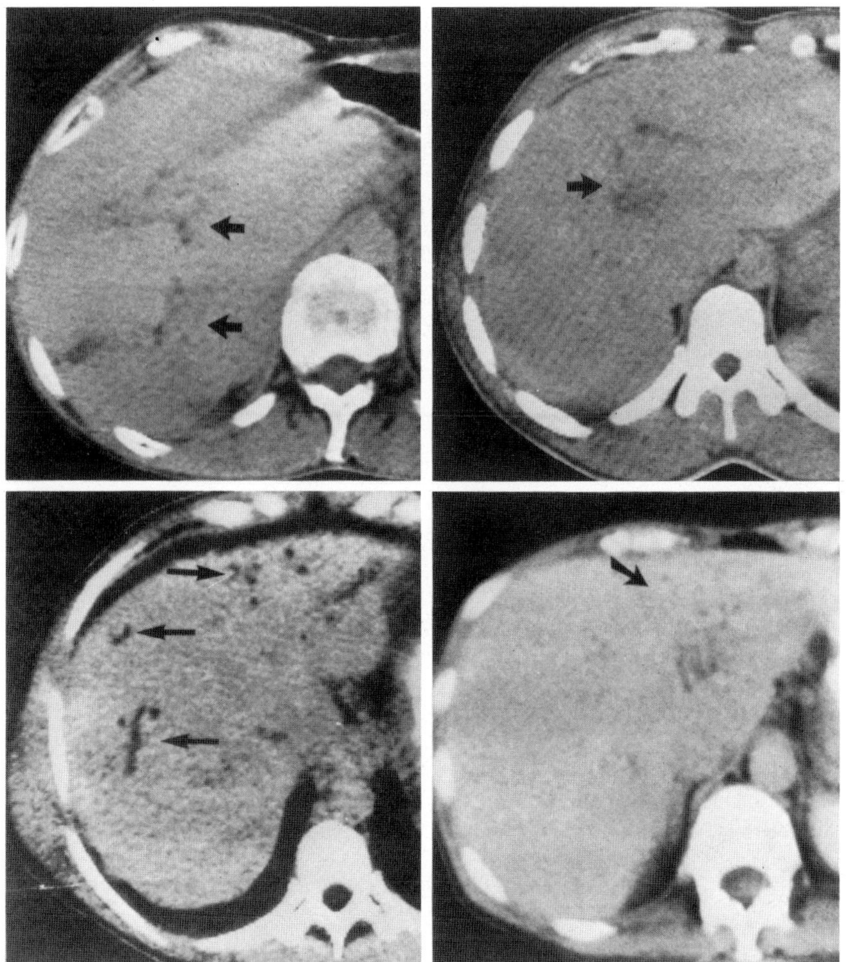

Fig. 59.9 CT appearance in proven sclerosing cholangitis. CT scans at comparable levels in four patients with biopsy-proven sclerosing cholangitis. There is focal, irregular dilatation of intrahepatic bile ducts (arrows) in each case. Similar appearance was seen in all 10 patients. From Rahn et al 1983, with permission

calculi. Gross dilatation of the extrahepatic bile ducts was never noted. The CT scan showed evidence of cirrhosis and venous collaterals of portal hypertension in three patients with advanced disease.

Exploratory laparotomy

Even with the radiological refinements that usually provide the diagnosis of sclerosing cholangitis, laparotomy may be required as the definitive diagnostic procedure. The presence of a dense, inflammatory reaction in the region of the gallbladder and extrahepatic bile ducts in patients who have not undergone a previous operative procedure in that area is suggestive of the disease. Palpation of the extrahepatic bile ducts gives the sensation of a cord-like structure of normal diameter because the luminal compromise is compensated for by the thickening of the wall. A cystic duct cholangiogram should be performed, and generally demonstrates areas of stenosis and, at times, of dilatation; characteristically there is free passage of the contrast medium into the duodenum, indicating absence of obstruction at the ampulla of Vater. Incision of the common hepatic duct or the common bile duct in the thickened area may be difficult and the edges of the incision usually pout, revealing a thick wall and a narrow lumen without mucosal abnormality. Generally only a fine probe can be passed either proximally or distally. Nothing about the appearance of the bile duct distinguishes sclerosing cholangitis from a sclerosing carcinoma of the ducts; the greatest confusion occurs in the region of the hilus of the liver (Ch. 65). The ducts may be biopsied, aspiration cytology may be performed, and the mucosa may be scraped in involved areas. Despite all these manoeuvres, the ultimate differentiation between sclerosing cholangitis and a sclerosing adenocarcinoma of the bile duct may depend upon the patient's course or autopsy findings (Altemeier et al 1966).

TREATMENT

The appropriate management of sclerosing cholangitis

remains unclear. No drug therapy has achieved consistent, or even usual, success. Operative intervention is no longer required for diagnostic purposes in most patients except to distinguish between sclerosing cholangitis and carcinoma of the bile ducts in some patients. Both the medical regimens and the operative procedures are palliative in nature. These facts, coupled with the variations in the clinical course of the patients, and the lack of any controlled trials, precludes any sense of assurance in prescribing a particular therapeutic approach.

Asymptomatic patients

Since it is now appreciated that sclerosing cholangitis may follow a less severe course than previously recognized, no drug treatment or surgical procedure is indicated for the asymptomatic, anicteric patient in whom the diagnosis has been made as a consequence of cholangiographic investigation of a persistently elevated alkaline phosphatase.

Symptomatic patients

Medical therapy

Anecdotal reports have recorded symptomatic improvement and reduction of jaundice with a wide variety of drugs, including corticosteroids, choleretics, bile-acid binding agents, immunosuppressants and D-penicillamine.

Our own experience (Schwartz & Dale 1958), and that of Meyers, Cooper & Padis (1970), present evidence for a favourable response to corticosteroids, while the most significant evidence against the use of this drug was the report of Wiesner & LaRusso (1980), which indicated that steroid use was significantly associated with the death of their patients. The decrease in bilirubin levels resulting from the use of steroids may be attributed to a direct choleretic action of the drug, but prednisone (40–50 mg daily) is preferred for long-term use because its anti-inflammatory effect is marked, and there is less salt retention. This drug is generally continued for several months after the patient becomes asymptomatic, when improvement is shown on liver function tests and when there is cholangiographic evidence of improvement of the disease. The recurrence of symptoms or jaundice is an indication for the reinstitution of steroid therapy; this has resulted in the relief of symptoms in three of our patients followed for prolonged periods.

Choleretics such as dehydrocholic acid (Decholin®, 250 mg three times daily) have been administered to increase the fluidity of bile. Cholestyramine has been effective in managing pruritus and in one case appeared to have prevented symptoms and normalized liver function tests (Polter et al 1980). Attacks of acute cholangitis are treated with appropriate antibiotics, and some reports have advised the prophylactic administration of antibiotics which achieve high biliary concentrations.

Javett (1971) reported a favourable response when steroids and azathioprine were administered as combined treatment. Immunosuppressive therapy, however, has not achieved consistent success, and death from liver abscesses has been reported when steroids were used in combination with immunosuppressive agents to treat sclerosing cholangitis (Wagner 1971). The cupruretic, antifibrogenic, and immunosuppressive actions of penicillamine, as well as the reported beneficial effect in primary biliary cirrhosis, has led to a controlled trial of this drug (LaRusso et al 1984).

Invasive radiological procedures

Martin et al (1981) reported using percutaneous radiologically controlled catheter dilatation of critical common bile duct stenoses in two patients with sclerosing cholangitis. The patients were free of jaundice at five and seven months respectively.

Surgical procedures

Management of hepatobiliary lesions

In my own reported experience (Schwartz 1973) nine of eleven patients treated with T-tube drainage and steroids improved and survived for as long as 20 years. Reduction in hyperbilirubinaemia and the alkaline phosphatase and ductal dilatation on sequential T-tube cholangiograms were noted (Fig. 59.10). Three of six patients treated since 1973 have shown similar improvement. By contrast, the combination of T-tube drainage and steroids was associated with death due to progressive disease in six of nine patients reported by Thompson and co-workers (1972). Pitt et al (1982) reported that this approach resulted in excellent or good results in only 40% of their patients. Wood & Cuschieri (1980) are advocates of T-tube drainage and lavage, and they suggest that this may actually reverse the disease process, but the experience has not been shared by Wiesner & La Russo (1980).

As a consequence of disappointment with T-tube drainage since 1974, Pitt and associates (1982) adopted a policy of performing an hepato- or choledochoenteric anastomosis in all patients with sclerosing cholangitis who had either a major hepatic blockage or primary involvement of the extrahepatic bile ducts. This approach was applied to 70% of the patients they managed surgically. Although more patients (77%) achieved an excellent or a good result, the length of follow-up was significantly longer among patients managed with T-tube drainage alone, and no significant differences in survival resulted. Similar favourable results have been reported by Warren et al (1966) and by Chapman et al (1980) respectively. Recently, Collier et al (1985) performed biliary-enteric anastomoses for sclerosing cholangitis in 12 patients with either localized stricture at the confluence of the hepatic ducts, isolated segmental dilatation of the left hepatic duct or predomi-

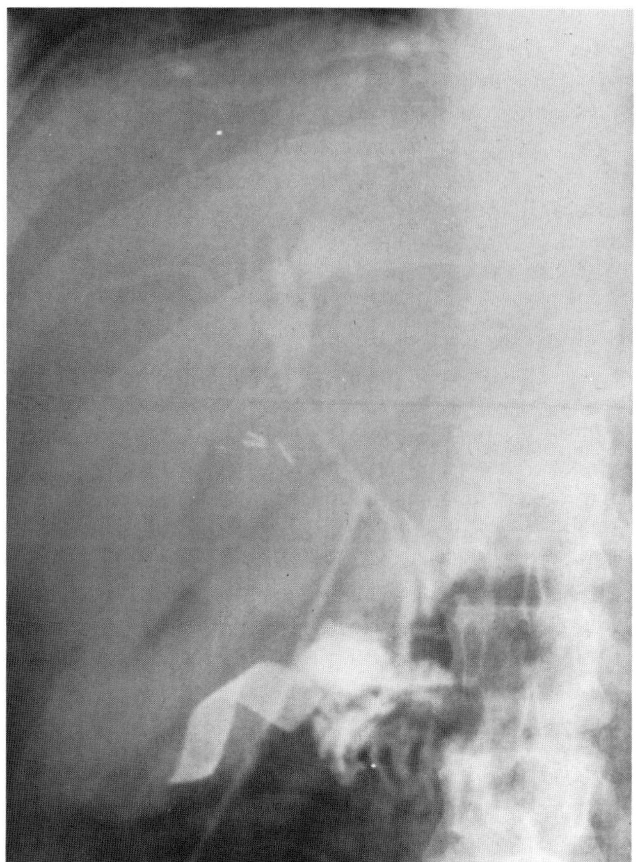

a

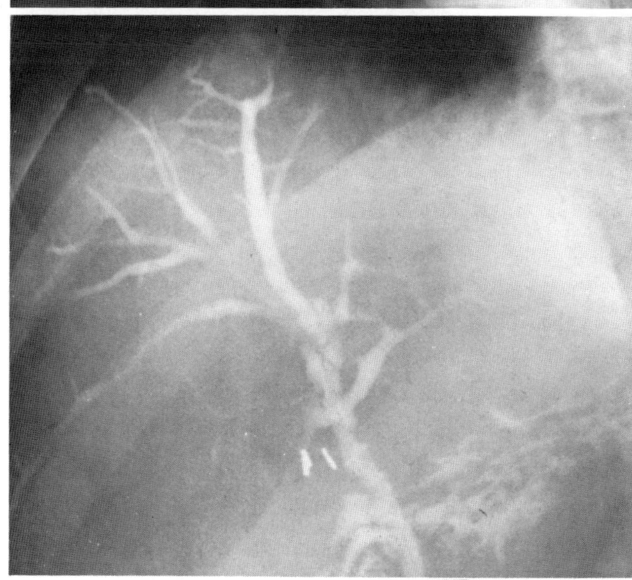

b

Fig. 59.10 Treatment with T-tube and steroids. a. Operative film b. Three weeks postoperative film showing improved filling of the ducts

nantly extrahepatic ductal disease. Nine remained symptom-free for a median of 13 months.

Cameron et al (1983) extended biliary-enteric anastomosis by combining resection of the extrahepatic biliary tree, including the bifurcation, with dilatation of the right and left hepatic ducts and their intrahepatic extensions,

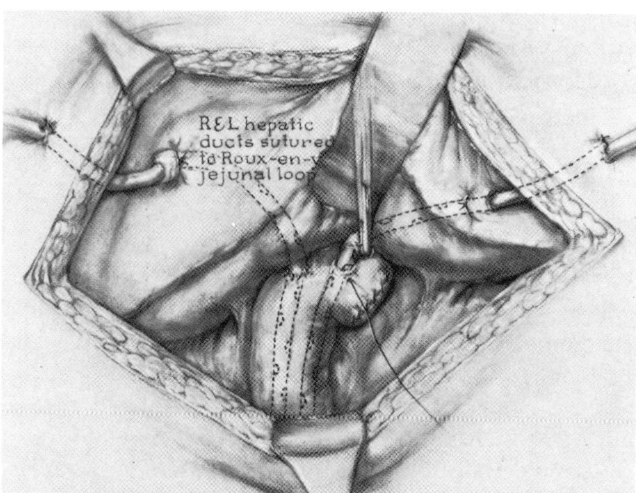

Fig. 59.11 Bilateral hepaticojejunostomy is performed over the Silastic stents. From Cameron et al 1984, with permission (See also Ch. 71).

and transhepatic insertion of laterally vented silicone rubber stents followed by bilateral hepaticojejunostomy (Fig. 59.11). Nine of ten patients discharged from the hospital were markedly improved over a mean follow-up of 18 months, during which time the stents were left in position, generally requiring change as an outpatient procedure every three to four months. Although these results are excellent, it is difficult to comprehend dilatation of the intrahepatic stenotic segments and improved drainage from a diffusely involved liver.

Extensive intrahepatic involvement represents an indication for orthotopic liver transplantation. Special problems pertain to patients with sclerosing cholangitis. A primary duct-to-duct anastomosis is often impossible because of a diseased distal common duct, and the homograft duct must be anastomosed to a Roux limb of jejunum. Also, the fact that most patients with sclerosing cholangitis have undergone previous procedures in the right upper quadrant, including portal decompressive operations, compromise the transplantation procedure (Starzl et al 1983). To date approximately 35 patients have received a transplant; 70% have survived for one year.

Author's current approach

The asymptomatic anicteric patient is not treated and is not studied with repeated cholangiograms if jaundice or cholangitis does not develop. The pruritic and icteric patient is treated for four to six weeks with prednisone; if there is no improvement, or if cholangitis is present or develops, an operation is performed with a preoperative cholangiogram as a guide. If there is minimal intrahepatic involvement and dilatation of a segment of the common bile duct or common hepatic duct proximal to marked stenosis, the stenotic segment is excised as a biopsy to rule out cholangiocarcinoma and a direct mucosa-to-mucosa anastomosis is effected between the dilated segment of duct and a Roux limb of jejunum, preferably without a stent. Stricture of the confluence of the hepatic ducts is managed by excision of the distal ducts for histological evaluation and anastomosis of the hepatic ducts to the Roux limb of jejunum by the mucosa-to-mucosa technique (Ch. 70). If the hepatic ducts are sufficiently dilated, no stent is used. If these ducts are small, transhepatic stents are used, but no attempt is made to dilate intrahepatic ducts. If the entire extra- and intrahepatic systems are dominated by areas of marked stenosis and narrowing, with minimal dilatation, a small T-tube is inserted and steroid therapy is used, and the patient is followed by sequential T-tube cholangiograms which will define improvement. If the disease has progressed to the stage of marked hyperbilirubinaemia and liver failure or cirrhosis, transplantation is advised, avoiding a shunt to decompress portal hypertension even if there has been variceal bleeding.

Management of associated disorders

There is little to offer surgically in the management of associated pancreatitis. The role of colectomy in patients with sclerosing cholangitis combined with ulcerative colitis has been debated. Although Wood & Cuschieri (1980) suggest that colectomy may be beneficial, the uncontrolled experience at the Mayo Clinic demonstrated no predictable benefit for patients with sclerosing cholangitis. Proctocolectomy and ileostomy in these patients resulted in peristomal varices in about one-quarter of the patients, often causing life threatening bleeding (Wiesner, Beaver & LaRusso 1982). I have personally performed mesocaval shunts on two such patients to control bleeding from an ileostomy stoma.

PROGNOSIS

The prognosis is difficult to define; there are no clinical, laboratory or histological factors of statistically significant prognostic value. Asymptomatic patients with the disease diagnosed by cholangiogram may experience a benign course for life expectancy. In symptomatic patients remissions and relapses are common, extending over many years. Although sclerosing cholangitis is not always associated with progression leading to death, many patients do have an unrelenting downhill course progressing to cirrhosis and liver failure despite early palliation. There is an increased risk of bile duct cancer, due either to erroneous initial diagnosis or to actual transformation of the disease process.

REFERENCES

Altemeier W A, Gall E A, Culbertson W R, Inge W W 1966 Sclerosing carcinoma of the intrahepatic (hilar) bile ducts. Surgery 60: 191–200

Ament A E, Bick R J, Miraldi F D, Haaga J R, Wiedenmann S D 1984 Sclerosing cholangitis: Cholescintigraphy with Tc-99m-labeled DISIDA. Radiology 151: 197–201

Bartholomew L G, Cain J C, Woolner L B, Utz D C, Ferris D O 1963 Sclerosing cholangitis: Its possible association with Riedel's struma and fibrous retroperitonitis: Report of two cases. New England Journal of Medicine 269: 8–12

Cameron J L, Gayler B W, Sanfey H, Milligan F, Kaufman S, Maddrey W C et al 1984 Sclerosing cholangitis: Anatomical distribution of obstructive lesions. Annals of Surgery 200: 54–60

Carroll B A, Oppenheimer D A 1982 Sclerosing cholangitis: Sonographic demonstration of bile duct wall thickening. American Journal of Radiology 139: 1016–1018

Chapman R W, Marborgh B A, Rhodes J M, Summerfield J A, Dick R, Scheuer P J et al 1980 Primary sclerosing cholangitis: a review of its clinical features, cholangiography and hepatic histology. Gut 21: 870–877

Chapman R W, Burroughs A K, Vass N M, Sherlock S 1981 Long standing asymptomatic primary sclerosing cholangitis: Report of three cases. Digestive Diseases and Sciences 26: 778–782

Chapman R W, Varghese Z, Gaul R, Patel G, Kokinon N, Sherlock S 1983 Association of primary sclerosing cholangitis with HLA-B8. Gut 24: 38–41

Collier N A, Armitage N C M, Hadjis N S, Blumgart L H (1985) Surgical approaches in primary sclerosing cholangitis. Australian and New Zealand Journal of Surgery 55: 437–442

Danzi J T, Makipour H, Farmer R G 1978 Primary sclerosing cholangitis. A report of nine cases and clinical review. American Journal of Gastroenterology 65: 109–116

Delbet P 1924 Retrecissement du choledoque: Cholecystoduodenostomie. Bulletin et Memoires de la Societe Nationale de Chirurgie 50: 1144–1146

Dew J M, Thompson H, Allan R N 1979 The spectrum of hepatic dysfunction in inflammatory bowel disease. Quarterly Journal of Medicine 48: 113–135

Gluskin L E, Payne J A 1983 Cystic dilatation as a radiographic sign of cholangiocarcinoma complicating sclerosing cholangitis. The American Journal of Gastroenterology 78: 661–664

Gross J B Jr, Beaver S J, McCall J T, Ludwig J, LaRusso N F 1983 Abnormalities in tests of copper metabolism in primary sclerosing cholangitis: prognostic and diagnostic significance. Gastroenterology 84:1176 (abstract)

Javett S L 1971 Azathioprine in primary sclerosing cholangitis. Lancet i:810

Lafourcade J 1925 Deux observations d'obliteration cicatricielle du choledoque. Anastomose laterale entre le choledoque et le duodenum dans le premier cas. Reconstitution par prothese avec tube de caoutchouc dans le second. Bulletin et Memoires de la Societé Nationale de Chirurgie 51: 828–831

LaRusso N F, Wiesner R H, Ludwig J, MacCarty R L 1984 Primary sclerosing cholangitis. New England Journal of Medicine 310: 889–903

Miller R T Jr 1927 Benign stricture of bile ducts. Annals of Surgery 86: 296–303

Lefkowitch J H 1982 Primary sclerosing cholangitis. Archives of Internal Medicine 142: 1157–1160

Ludwig L, Barham S S, LaRusso N F, Eleveback L R, Wiesner R H, McCall J T 1981 Morphologic features of chronic hepatitis associated with primary sclerosing cholangitis and chronic ulcerative colitis. Hepatology 1: 632–640

MacCarty R L, LaRusso N F, Wiesner R J, Ludwig J 1983 Primary sclerosing cholangitis: findings on cholangiography and pancreatography. Radiology 149: 39–44

Martin E, Fankuchen E I, Schultz R W, Casarella W J 1981 Percutaneous dilatation in primary sclerosing cholangitis: two experiences. American Journal of Radiology 137: 603–605

Meyers R N, Cooper J H, Padis N 1970 Primary sclerosing cholangitis. American Journal of Gastroenterology 53: 527–538

Miller R T Jr 1927 Benign stricture of bile ducts. Annals of Surgery 86: 296–303

Montefusco P P, Geiss A C, Bronzo R J, Randall S, Kahn E, McKinley M J 1984 Sclerosing cholangitis, chronic pancreatitis, and Sjogren's syndrome: A syndrome complex. The American Journal of Surgery 147: 822–826

Pitt H A, Thompson H H, Tompkins R K, Longmire W P 1982 Primary sclerosing cholangitis: Results of an aggressive surgical approach. Annals of Surgery 196: 259–268

Polter D E, Gruhl V, Eigenbrodt E H, Combes B 1980 Beneficial effect of cholestyramine in sclerosing cholangitis. Gastroenterology 79: 326–333

Rahn N H III, Koehler R E, Weyman P J, Truss C D, Sagel S S, Stanely R J 1983 CT appearance of sclerosing cholangitis. American Journal of Radiology 141: 549–552

Roberts S 1958 cited in the discussion by Warren H Cole of Schwartz S I and Dale W A Primary sclerosing cholangitis: Review and report of six cases. Archives of Surgery 77: 439–451

Schrumpf E, Fausa O, Kolmannskog F, Elgjio K, Ritland S, Gjone E 1982 Sclerosing cholangitis in ulcerative colitis: a follow-up study. Scandinavian Journal of Gastroenterology 17: 33–39

Schwartz S I, Dale W A 1958 Primary sclerosing cholangitis: Review and report of six cases. Archives of Surgery 77: 439–451

Schwartz S I 1973 Primary sclerosing cholangitis. Surgical Clinics of North America 53: 1161–1168

Spivak W, Grand R J, Eraklis A 1982 A case of primary sclerosing cholangitis in childhood. Gastroenterology 82: 129–132

Starzl T E, Iwatsuki S, van Thiel D H, Garter J C, Zitelli B J, Malatack J J et al 1982 Evolution of liver transplantation. Hepatology 2: 614–636

Summerfield J A 1983 Primary sclerosing cholangitis. Postgraduate Medical Journal 59 (Suppl 4): 99–105

Thompson B W, Read R C, White H J 1972 Sclerosing cholangitis. Archives of Surgery 104: 460–464

Thorpe M E, Scheur P J, Sherlock S 1976 Primary sclerosing cholangitis of the biliary tree and ulcerative colitis. Gut 18: 435–438

Wagner A 1971 Azathioprine treatment in primary sclerosing cholangitis. Lancet ii: 663–664

Warren K W, Athanassiades S, Monge J I 1966 Primary sclerosing cholangitis: A study of forty-two cases. American Journal of Surgery 111: 23–38

Wiesner R H, LaRusso N F 1980 Clinicopathologic features of the syndrome of primary sclerosing cholangitis. Gastroenterology 79: 200–206

Wiesner R H, Beaver S J, LaRusso N F 1982 Bleeding peristomal varices: a serious complication of proctocolectomy for chronic ulcerative colitis in patients with primary sclerosing cholangitis. Hepatology 2:699 (abstract)

Wood R A B, Cuschieri A 1980 Is sclerosing cholangitis complicating ulcerative colitis a reversible condition? Lancet ii: 716–718

60

G. A. Kune, L. H. Blumgart

External biliary fistula

An external biliary fistula is an abnormal, persistent discharge of bile or bile containing fluid usually through the abdominal wall. Excluded from the discussion in this chapter will be primarily internal biliary fistulae, as in broncho-biliary fistula which only secondarily discharge to the surface.

Biliary fistulae may be intentionally created by the surgeon, e.g. in the creation of a cholecystostomy or choledochostomy, but may also occur postoperatively following hepatobiliary or less commonly pancreatic or gastric surgery, in which instance they are usually due to surgical error. Finally biliary fistula may be pathological such as the rare fistulation which may occur in a grossly neglected empyema of the gallbladder or in association with malignancy involving the biliary tract and ulcerating at the skin surface.

From a practical point of view, purely pathological external biliary fistulae are extremely rare, while intentional surgically created fistulous tracts are of significance only if they continue to discharge bile unexpectedly. Almost all clinically significant external biliary fistulae follow some type of surgical procedure on or in the neighbourhood of the biliary ductal system. The persistent biliary discharge is the result of some unrecognized pathology in the bile ducts, of surgical error or of an unexpected complication of the operative procedure.

AETIOLOGY AND PREVENTION

When grouping the causes of external biliary fistula it is useful to classify them according to the type of previous intervention performed.

The following procedures are the more commonly associated surgical antecedents of fistula.

Postcholecystostomy fistula

Cholecystostomy is now infrequently performed. A persistent biliary or mucous fistula from the biliary system after cholecystostomy is usually due to an unrecognized retained gallstone lodged within Hartmann's pouch (Fig. 60.1) Less commonly it may be due to an unrecognized distal bile duct obstruction either as a result of retained bile duct stones or of malignant obstruction of the biliary tree.

Postcholecystectomy fistula

External biliary fistula continuing through the drainage tube track after elective cholecystectomy almost always indicates surgical error. Similarly, a bile duct injury should be suspected if a second operation has been done following cholecystectomy in which a large bile collection was drained externally, the patient subsequently being left with

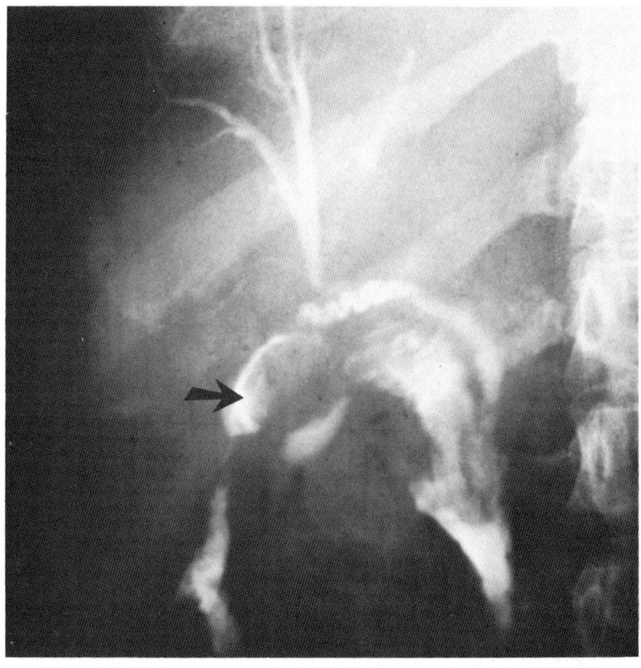

Fig. 60.1 Postcholecystostomy external mucous fistula caused by a large retained gallstone in Hartmann's pouch (arrow) as demonstrated by a fistulogram

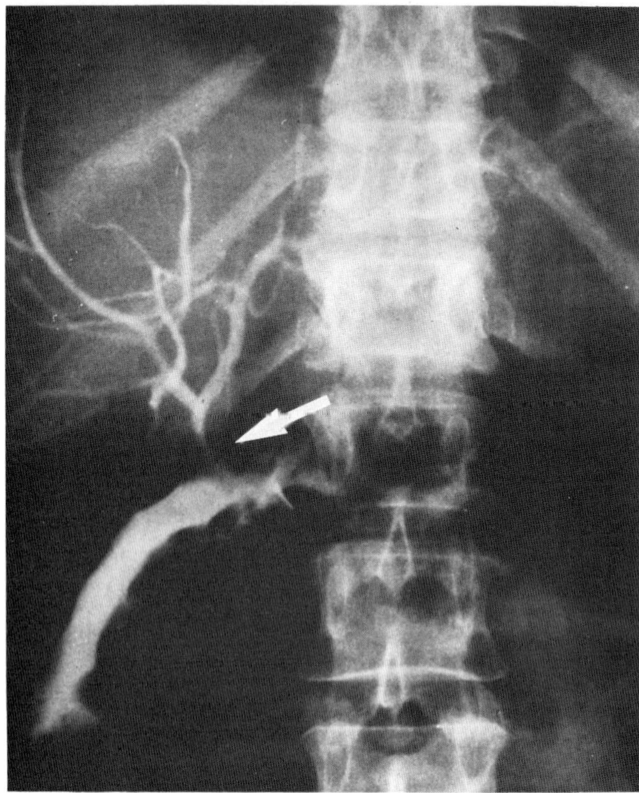

Fig. 60.2 Postcholecystectomy fistulogram. Biliary fistula caused by accidental transection of the common hepatic duct (arrow), the commonest cause of a persistent external biliary fistula

an external biliary discharge (Fig. 60.2). (Ch. 58). Such fistulation may arise from damage to an anomalous sectoral duct of the right hepatic duct (Ch. 2). Much less commonly a fistula may occur in the absence of any major bile duct injury and then it is usually associated with inadvertent damage to the subvesical duct (Ch. 2). This small duct has been variously reported to be present in normal subjects in between 20% and 50% of cases (Kune & Sali 1980). The recognition of biliary ductal anomalies and prevention of biliary injury at cholecystectomy is detailed in Chapter 58.

Slipped or sloughed ligatures on the cystic duct are responsible for postcholecystectomy external biliary fistulae in rare instances. For this reason the authors recommend ligation of the cystic duct with a transfixion suture. Finally, cholecystectomy may be required in difficult circumstances, e.g. in the presence of a gangrenous gallbladder in association with a pericholecystic abscess. In such cases it is often not possible to identify or ligate the cystic duct. Temporary external biliary fistula may follow and has been seen on five occasions by the authors (Fig. 60.3).

Postcholedochotomy fistula

Biliary fistula persisting after exploration of the common bile duct and after removal of a T-tube is almost always due to residual bile duct gallstones (Fig. 60.4) but much less frequently to overlooked malignant obstruction of the distal bile ducts (Fig. 60.5). Clearly post-exploratory cholangiography and/or choledochoscopy will be of value in preventing subsequent fistulous complications (Ch. 27, 29). T-tube cholangiography before removal of the tube is an essential routine in order to recognize retained gallstones. Preoperative definition of the cause of biliary obstruction in jaundiced patients (Ch. 25) avoids error in diagnosis, e.g. a malignant stricture co-existing with choledocholithiasis, which might result in subsequent fistulation.

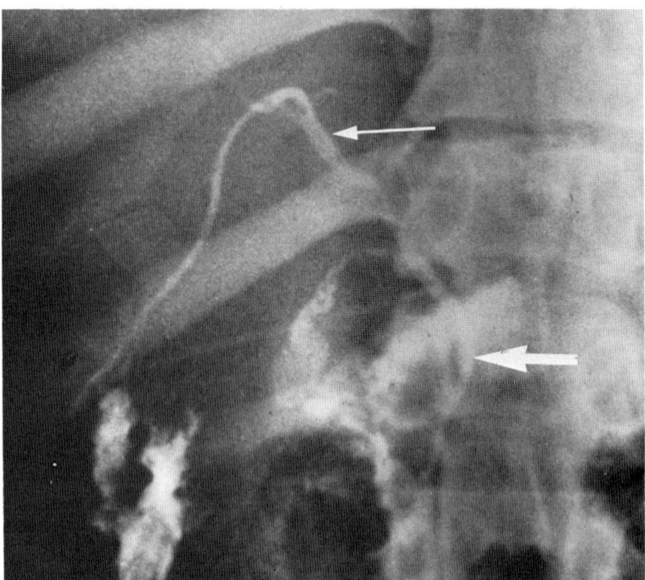

Fig. 60.3 Postcholecystectomy fistulogram outlining large irregular cavity (bottom arrow) and connecting with a faintly outlined, but apparently normal, biliary ductal system (top arrow)

Fistula following biliary-intestinal anastomoses

External biliary fistula following biliary intestinal anastomosis, while relatively uncommon, does occur and is due either to disruption of part of the suture line or to failure of the surgeon to appreciate ductal anatomy, so leaving one or more ducts outside the anastomotic line. This is particularly likely to occur in the hilar region where the mode of confluence of the major right and left ducts is extremely variable. (Ch. 2). Suture line disruption may be caused either by technical error, in which case the fistula becomes evident immediately after surgery, or due to some complicating factor such as local abscess formation, postoperative pancreatitis or ischaemic necrosis. Such fistulae only become evident some days after surgery. It is of some importance to ascertain whether the fistula is purely biliary or whether it is complicated in that it also contains duodenal and/or pancreatic juice. Meticulous technique with mucosa to mucosa anastomosis obviates most of such leakage (Ch. 70).

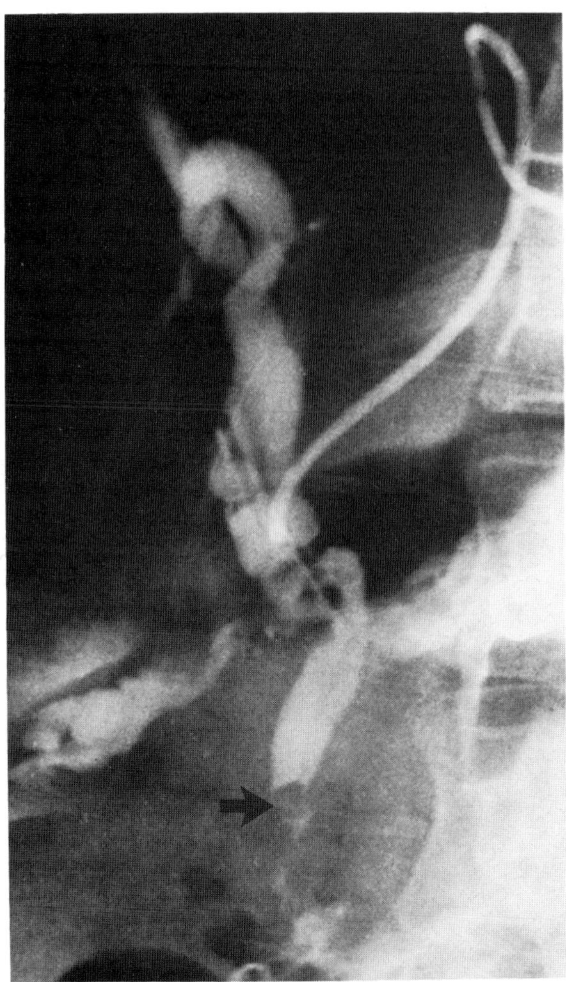

Fig. 60.4 Postcholedochotomy T-tube cholangiogram showing a retained stone obstructing the distal bile duct (arrow). The stone was removed six weeks after surgery by instrumental basket extraction through the T-tube track, preventing a persistent external biliary fistula

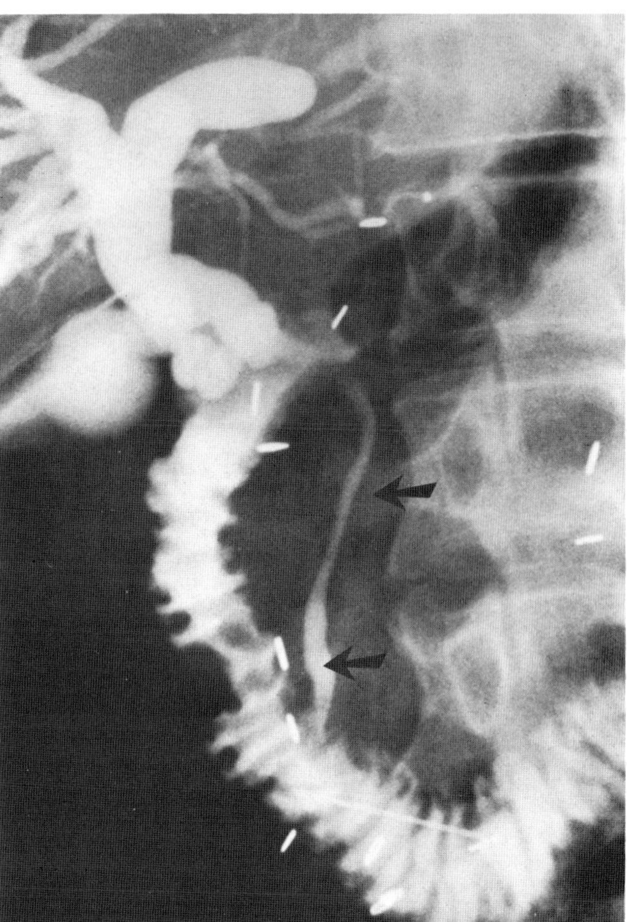

Fig. 60.5 Postcholedochotomy fistulogram showing that the external biliary fistula was caused by an extrinsic compression of the pancreatic portion of the bile duct (arrows). At reoperation, choledochal compression was shown to be due to cancer of the head of the pancreas

Biliary fistula after drainage of intra-abdominal collections

Drainage of intra-abdominal collections of pus, bile, duodenal or pancreatic juice may be followed by the establishment of an external biliary fistula (Fig. 60.6, Fig. 60.7). Such collections may be a complication of previous surgery (see above) or may be a complication of a spontaneously occurring pathological process, such as acute haemorrhagic pancreatitis, pancreatic abscess, drainage of sub-phrenic abscess after liver resection and, rarely, spontaneous perforation of a bile cyst of the liver. Again it is important to know whether the biliary fistula contains bile only or whether it also contains gastric, duodenal or pancreatic juice.

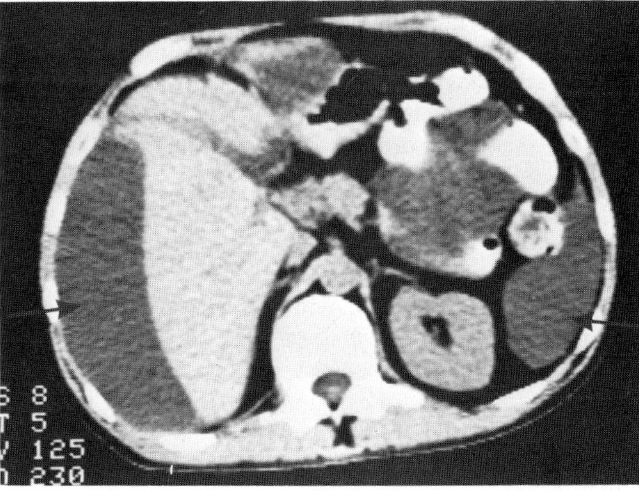

Fig. 60.6 CAT scan performed in the postoperative period following cholecystectomy. There are large collections of fluid within the peritoneal cavity (arrows). Subsequent open drainage revealed multiple encysted collections of bile with a total volume of 4 litres. A controlled external fistula was eventually obtained which was associated with transection of the common bile duct at initial cholecystectomy. Biliary repair with closure of the fistula was performed at a later date

Biliary fistula after interventional radiology

The passage of a percutaneous transhepatic biliary drainage catheter in obstructive jaundice may be a tempor-

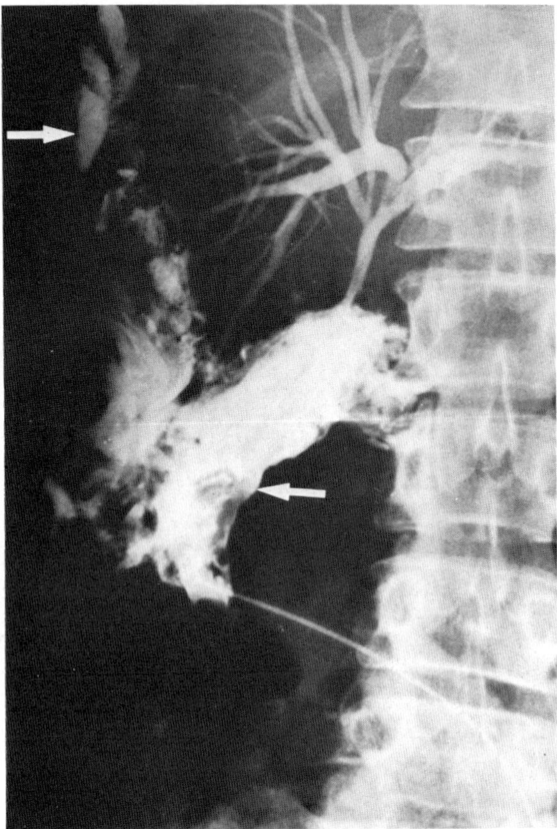

Fig. 60.7 Fistulogram in a neglected postcholecystectomy biliary fistula due to accidental transection of the common hepatic duct with associated subphrenic (top arrow) and subhepatic (bottom arrow) collections of infected bile

ary, initial procedure with deliberate external drainage prior to subsequent surgical intervention. Alternatively it may be carried out with a view to subsequent percutaneous transhepatic insertion of an endoprosthesis traversing the obstructing lesion (Ch. 36). In some instances, however, initial percutaneous drainage and successful puncture of an intrahepatic duct is followed by failure to bypass the obstruction within that segment of the liver. The patient is then left with an external biliary fistula. For this reason cholangiograms should be very carefully assessed before the institution of percutaneous transhepatic drainage and the possibility of successful subsequent surgical or percutaneous endoprosthetic drainage evaluated. Certainly in high malignant obstruction surgical access for drainage of the right intrahepatic ductal system is limited (Ch. 2) and the potential for biliary-enteric bypass utilizing the round ligament (segment III) approach should be fully considered before selecting percutaneous drainage of the right intrahepatic ducts as an initial procedure (Ch. 64, 65, 70).

Biliary fistula following liver injury and liver surgery

Liver injury may be followed by the formation of an external biliary fistula. Such fistulation may occur in association with damage to the bile ducts as well as the liver, may follow sequestration and infection of areas of liver necrosis or may be associated with the late consequences of major liver injury especially if liver resection has been carried out. Details of injuries likely to result in biliary fistulation are to be found in Chapter 82.

Liver resection carried out for tumour may also be followed by biliary fistula (Czerniak et al 1986). Operative injury to the biliary tract likely to result in fistulation is more common following resection of lesions involving or close to the hilar structures (Fig. 60.8). It is also more likely to occur after right liver resection or after resection of lesions involving the caudate lobe ducts since the anatomy of the right sectoral hepatic ducts and caudate ducts is variable in the hilar region (Ch. 2). For this reason, some consider it better to secure the bile ducts during transection of the

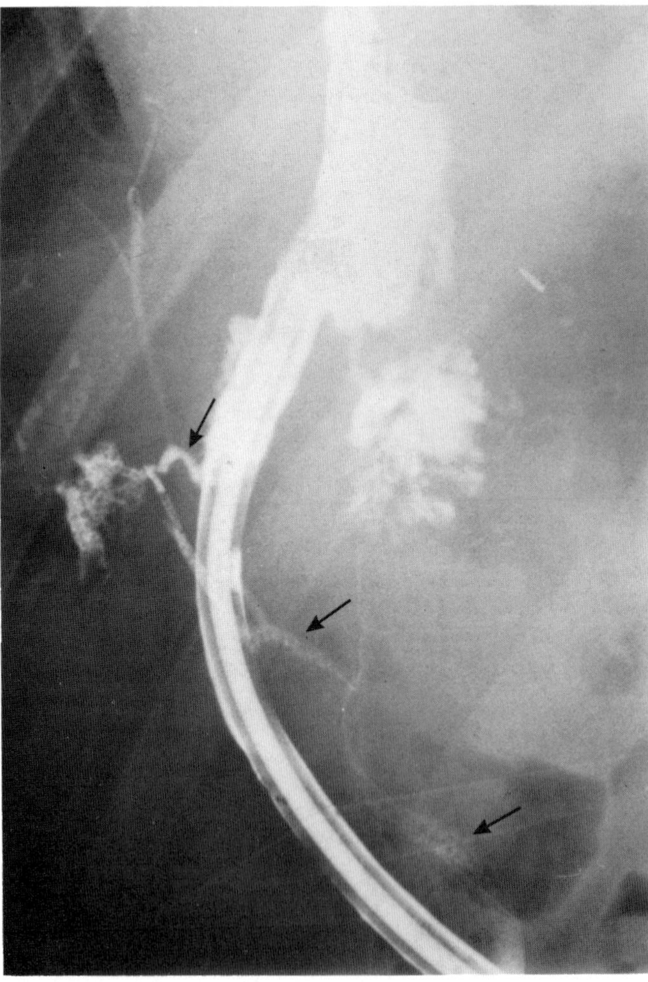

Fig. 60.8 Fistulography carried out via a tube drain demonstrates a biliary fistula following extended left hepatic lobectomy for primary hepatocellular cancer. The tumour was large and involved the hilar ducts in that tumour extension was demonstrated within the left hepatic duct. The fistula was managed conservatively and closed within four weeks. Arrows indicate the fistula and course of the right hepatic duct and common bile duct

liver parenchyma rather than to secure them at the hilus as described in Chapter 97.

Hydatid disease of the liver is associated with compression and stretching of adjacent tissues including the bile channels by the enlarging cysts. Indeed, the expanding cysts may erode the stretched ducts with the establishment of continuity between the cyst cavity and the biliary tree. Hydatid material may enter the biliary ductal system or bile may leak into the liver cyst.

External biliary fistula develops after surgery for liver hydatid disease in three situations. Firstly, a communication between the biliary duct and the residual cavity in the liver may not be recognized and is not directly sutured. This complication is particularly likely to develop if a hydatid cyst cavity is drained externally (Kune, Jones & Sali 1983) (Fig. 60.9). Secondly and rarely, biliary fistulation develops because hydatid material within the biliary tract produces biliary ductal obstruction (Fig. 60.10). After removal of the cyst a persistent fistula develops which is only relieved once the hydatid material passes or is surgically or endoscopically removed. Indeed, if there has been a history of jaundice or if cholangitis is a presenting feature in a patient with hydatid disease, it is probably wise to perform endoscopic cholangiography prior to surgery in order to assess the state of the biliary tree or, if not, to carry out intraoperative cholangiography. Finally, although liver resection is not the preferred method of treatment for liver hydatid disease (Ch. 75), it is occasionally performed and such patients are prone to all the complications of liver resection carried out for other reasons.

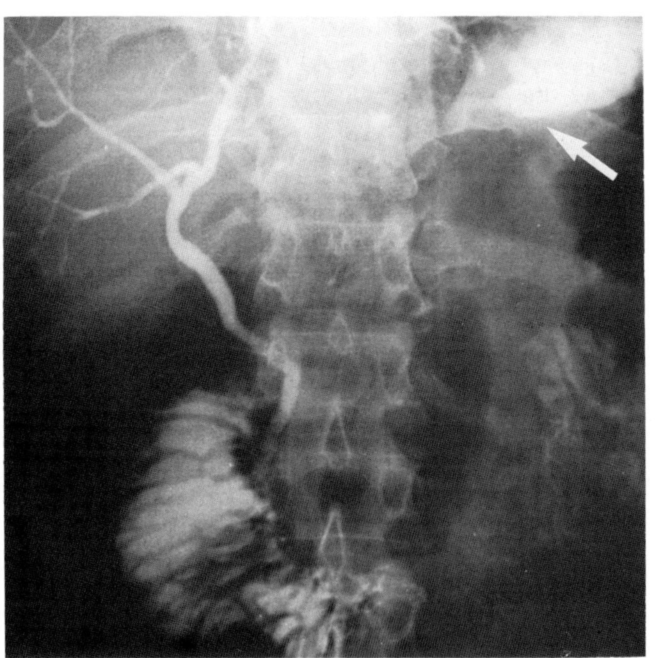

Fig. 60.9 Persistent external biliary fistula following external drainage of a hydatid cyst cavity (arrow) in the left lobe of the liver. The fistulogram shows clear communication between the cyst cavity and the left hepatic duct

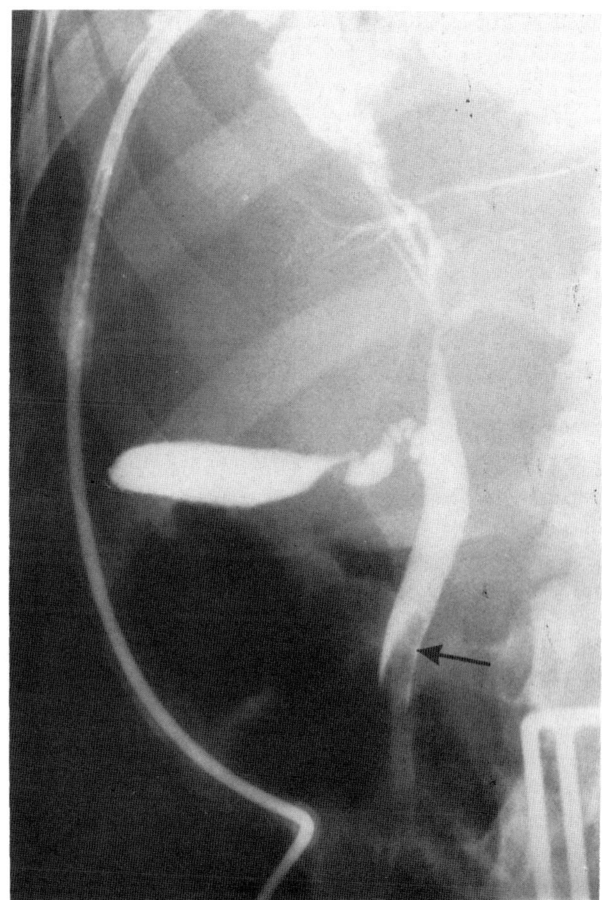

Fig. 60.10 Fistulogram obtained after excision of a right hepatic hydatid cyst. Note the persistent fistula consequent upon retained hydatid material in the common bile duct (arrow). Treatment was by exploration of the common bile duct and surgical removal of the retained hydatid material. The fistula rapidly closed

PATHOPHYSIOLOGICAL CONSEQUENCES OF EXTERNAL BILIARY FISTULA

The important pathophysiological effects of an external biliary fistula depend on the length of time the fistula has been present and the degree to which bile is diverted externally from the gastrointestinal tract. The consequences are due to depletion of electrolyte and fluid, to the absence of bile from the gut and occasionally to skin digestion caused by extra-biliary components present in the draining fluid. Ascending exogenously acquired infection is common.

Depletion of electrolyte and fluid

Bile secretion and composition is discussed in Chapter 8 and the reader is referred for details. For present consideration it is important to remember that the volume of bile secreted daily is of the order of 1000 ml per day, containing the ions of sodium, potassium chloride and calcium in concentrations equal to those found in blood.

Sometimes bile is secreted in volumes much greater than one litre per day and in particular this may occur in patients with chronic liver disease or in those who have had a long period of biliary tract obstruction (McPherson et al 1982). With the above exceptions, if fluid loss is much greater that one litre daily, it is likely that bile as well as some other associated internal secretion (pancreatic fluid, duodenal juice) is also present.

Short periods of total biliary diversion of up to three weeks may not cause serious depletion of electrolytes and the body is able to compensate for this loss. However, long term total external biliary fistula results in fluid and electrolyte disturbance if replacement is not meticulous. There is a decrease in the serum, potassium, and chloride. The sodium loss is usually in excess of the chloride loss, leading to an acidosis which Cass, Robson & Rundell (1955) called the choledochostomy acidotic syndrome. In such cases the serum potassium level is lowered initially but, if the plasma volume decreases due to dehydration, low output renal failure occurs followed by hyperkalaemia (Knochel, Cooper & Barry 1962).

Clinically, patients with an external biliary fistula, even in the short–term, feel unwell, weak and without energy. In advanced cases the electrolyte changes may result in stupor and vasomotor collapse.

Absence of bile in the gastrointestinal tract

In total biliary fistula, bile is absent from the gastrointestinal tract. The patient will have clay coloured stools and be unable to absorb fat adeuqately. There is interference in the absorption of the fat soluble vitamins A, D & K. In the usual instance, biliary fistulation is not present long enough for there to be significant clinical effects with the exception of Vitamin K deficiency which manifests early.

Calorie and protein malnutrition may also accompany external biliary fistula of long-standing and this is accompanied by gradual weight loss as a result of malnutrition.

Digestion of the skin

It is important to emphasize that bile alone never causes digestion or excoriation of the skin. If excoriation is present then it can be assumed that pancreatic, duodenal or jejunal juice is present and that there is enzymatic activation with skin digestion.

Biliary tract infection

External biliary fistulae are not necessarily associated with biliary tract infection in the first instance. However, rapid infection follows especially if the fistula is not draining directly from a bile duct but involves pooling and stasis of bile within a cavity in the abdomen (Fig. 60.9).

DIAGNOSIS

Clinical examination will confirm the presence of an external biliary fistula. The presence or absence of skin excoriation should be noted and the volume of drainage recorded.

Precise diagnosis of the site and often of the cause of the fistula is however radiological.

All contrast radiological examinations when performed in patients with an external biliary fistula, should be covered with appropriate antibiotic prophylaxis in order to minimize the risk of a bacteraemic episode.

Tube cholangiography

When cholecystostomy, choledochostomy, or tubal drainage across biliary-enteric anastomosis has been carried out and drained externally, tube cholangiography should be performed routinely before removal. This is of particular importance since there are now available a number of non-surgical means for dealing with retained bile duct stones utilizing the tube or tube track for instillation of solvent fluids or the passage of instruments (Ch. 48, 49).

Fistulography

Fistulography is a simple and effective means of demonstrating the site and cause of external biliary fistula (Fig. 60.1–60.3, 60.7–60.10). A fistulogram will frequently delineate the bile ducts, demonstrate whether distal obstruction is present or absent and in addition give information as to the underlying cause of the problem.

Percutaneous transhepatic cholangiography

If fistulography is not useful, or the findings are equivocal, or if further information is required, particularly in the jaundiced patient, then percutaneous transhepatic cholangiography is a useful means of confirming the diagnosis of the cause and level of external biliary fistula. (Fig. 60.11).

Endoscopic retrograde cholangiography

This modality is usually only of value in the patient with an external biliary fistula when additional information over and above fistulography is required and when percutaneous cholangiography is contraindicated. ERCP is of very little value in high fistulation arising as a result of iatrogenic bile duct injury (Ch. 58).

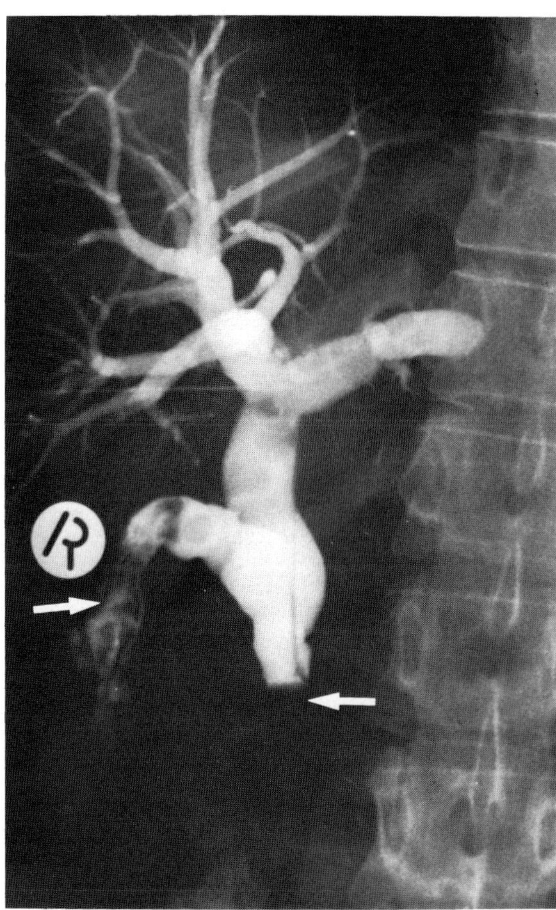

Fig. 60.11 Percutaneous transhepatic cholangiogram in a case of external biliary fistula (top arrow) and obstructive jaundice in which the fistulogram was not useful. The external fistula followed cholecystectomy with leakage through the cystic duct stump as a result of high intraductal pressure caused by multiple overlooked choledochal stones, including one in the distal choledochus (bottom arrow)

Isotope scanning

Scanning of the liver and biliary tract after injection of HIDA (Ch. 15) gives not only an index of liver function and biliary secretion but may be very useful in a demonstration of the origin of fistulous tracks not clearly demonstrated by other means (Fig. 60.12) (McPherson, Collier & Blumgart 1984). This modality is particularly useful in fistula arising from the liver surface.

In summary, if a tube is already present within the biliary tree in a patient with external biliary fistula, then tube cholangiography should be performed before removal of the tube. If no tube is present, then fistulography should be performed first. Percutaneous transhepatic cholangiography or endoscopic retrograde cholangiography are used as required. HIDA scanning may be useful in difficult situations.

TREATMENT

Treatment of external biliary fistula consists firstly of the correction of electrolyte and fluid imbalance and of malnutrition. Secondly skin excoriation and intra-abdominal infection are controlled. Finally the treatment of the fistula itself depends on clear knowledge of the cause of the problem with particular respect to the likelihood of spontaneous closure and the possibility of serious sequelae.

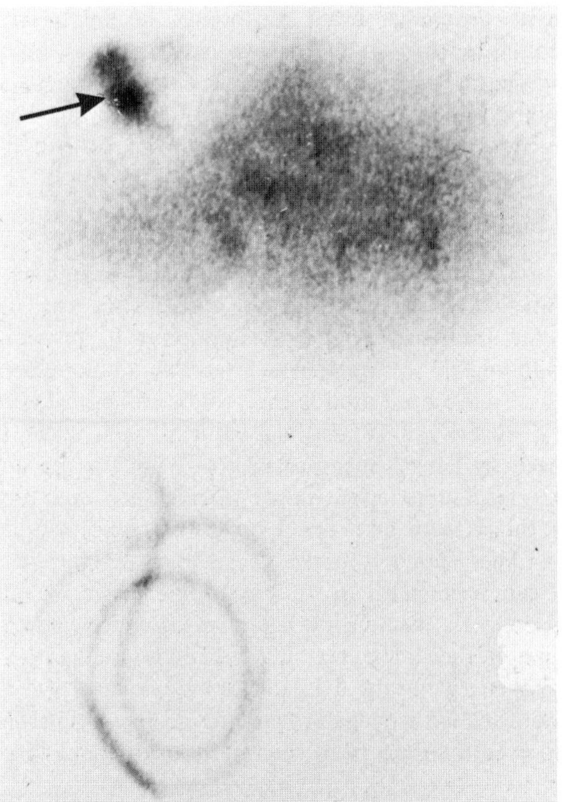

Fig. 60.12 HIDA scan demonstrating a fistula issuing from the liver surface (arrow). Same case as Fig. 60.10. Note drainage tube is also demonstrated (McPherson et al 1984). Reproduced with permission of Surgical Gastroenterology

Electrolyte and fluid replacement

The prevention of fluid and electrolyte depletion follows conventional lines. Estimation of the volume and composition of the loss and replacement either orally or, if volume cannot be replaced, by venous administration is performed.

In the presence of an established fistula and particularly if there is also loss of duodenal or pancreatic juice, total parenteral nutrition is valuable and often mandatory if further surgery is contemplated. Total parenteral nutrition is thought to be of value in both the healing of external fistulae and also in minimizing the rate of post surgical complications. Apart from the major components of total parenteral nutrition, namely calorie, protein, carbohydrate and fat requirements, there is increasing evidence that the addition of micronutrients such as vitamins and trace elements are valuable in promoting healing (Ch. 32). Parenteral nutrition is an essential element in the management of duodenal and pancreatic fistulae, where total prohibition of oral intake is important in allowing healing to occur.

Skin digestion

The presence of skin excoriation and digestion implies that activated digestive enzymes are present in the fistula effluent. In these cases it is important to protect the surrounding skin. Creams which have an aluminium paste as a basis have been used in the past but often make handling of overlying stoma bags difficult and have been replaced by flanges made of Karaya gum with an appropriately measured and tailored opening for each fistula. Over this Karaya gum flange an ostomy-type bag can be fitted. The Karaya gum flange protects the surrounding skin from excoriation. In the management of high volume fistulae or of a fistula shown to have an underlying collection within the abdomen acting as a reservoir, the insertion of a catheter along the fistula track and connected to a low pressure suction is valuable, not only in promoting healing but preventing fluid from reaching the surrounding skin.

Treatment of the underlying cause

With most external biliary fistulae, conservative management is the first line of approach. Biliary drainage is ideally carried out using a sealed drainage bag system (Blenkarn et al 1981) in order to limit ascending infection. During this period special radiological investigations are undertaken to define the site and cause of the fistula (see above). In general, conservative treatment is continued if closure can be anticipated and this is the case if there is no distal bile duct obstruction, abdominal collection or septic or necrotic focus. Surgical closure is required if there is evidence of major bile duct injury, particularly if there is ductal obstruction or for the drainage of abscesses and removal of necrotic tissue. These general principles are modified slightly according to the various types of external biliary fistula.

Postcholecystostomy biliary fistula

A persistent biliary fistula is almost always caused by some form of distal obstruction to the gallbladder outlet or to the common bile duct. Further surgery is usually required. This may mean removal of gallstones in the gallbladder, the bile duct or both (Fig. 60.1) or surgical excision or bypass of malignant obstruction unrecognized at the time of initial operation.

Postcholecystectomy biliary fistula

Small amounts of bile may drain for a few days in the immediate postoperative period following cholecystectomy. In such cases the general condition of the patient remains excellent, the drainage decreases and usually stops within a day or two and there are almost always no sequelae. While of some concern to the surgeon the cause is usually not evident. These transient biliary fistulae draining small amounts of bile may be caused by injury to tiny bile ducts in the liver around the gallbladder fossa. This is particularly likely to occur after removal of a gallbladder which is in part intrahepatic or when cholecystectomy involved some damage to the surrounding liver substance.

Occasionally, external fistulation is accompanied by overt signs of peritoneal irritation and biliary peritonitis. In this situation the patient is usually very ill, especially if the bile is infected. The management of such cases demands drainage of bile in order to save life. Definitive biliary repair is seldom possible, the bile ducts being collapsed and the tissues friable. Operation is directed at draining the peritoneal cavity and establishing external drainage which is then managed on the lines outlined above. It is sometimes possible to carry out drainage through a mobilized and approximated Roux-en-Y loop of jejunum, the drainage tube being led from the transected bile duct across the jejunum to the exterior (Fig. 60.13). This procedure allows initial control and the almost certain necessity of re-operation for re-stenosis at a later date should be accepted (Ch. 58).

If large quantities of bile, of the order of 100 ml per day or more, drain in the postoperative period then there is usually a serious cause and indeed operative injury of a major bile duct should be suspected. Such patients may become generally ill and superimposed sepsis is common. The essential in management in this situation is not to re-operate rapidly. It is wiser to take stock of the situation, treat infection, nourish the patient and wait (Ch. 58). If fistulography or cholangiography reveals any continuity between the biliary system and the gastrointestinal tract, then a prolonged period of drainage may result in spontaneous closure of the fistula. Re-operation for definitive repair of a bile duct stricture should be delayed. It is a mistake to think that immediate repair is a simple matter since exposure of healthy bile duct mucosa without a sufficiently dilated duct can be very demanding and indeed may be impossible. A cautious approach is preferable since even ultimate closure of the fistula with the development of jaundice is usually associated with proximal ductal dilatation and easier subsequent repair. Should fluid loss from the biliary fistula prove too heavy and prolonged, then the external fistula can, after some weeks, be converted to an internal fistulo-jejunostomy (Smith et al 1982) and subsequent definitive stricture repair performed if and when necessary.

Occasionally percutaneous transhepatic or endoscopic cholangiography will reveal a normal biliary ductal system. This unusual situation probably means that the external

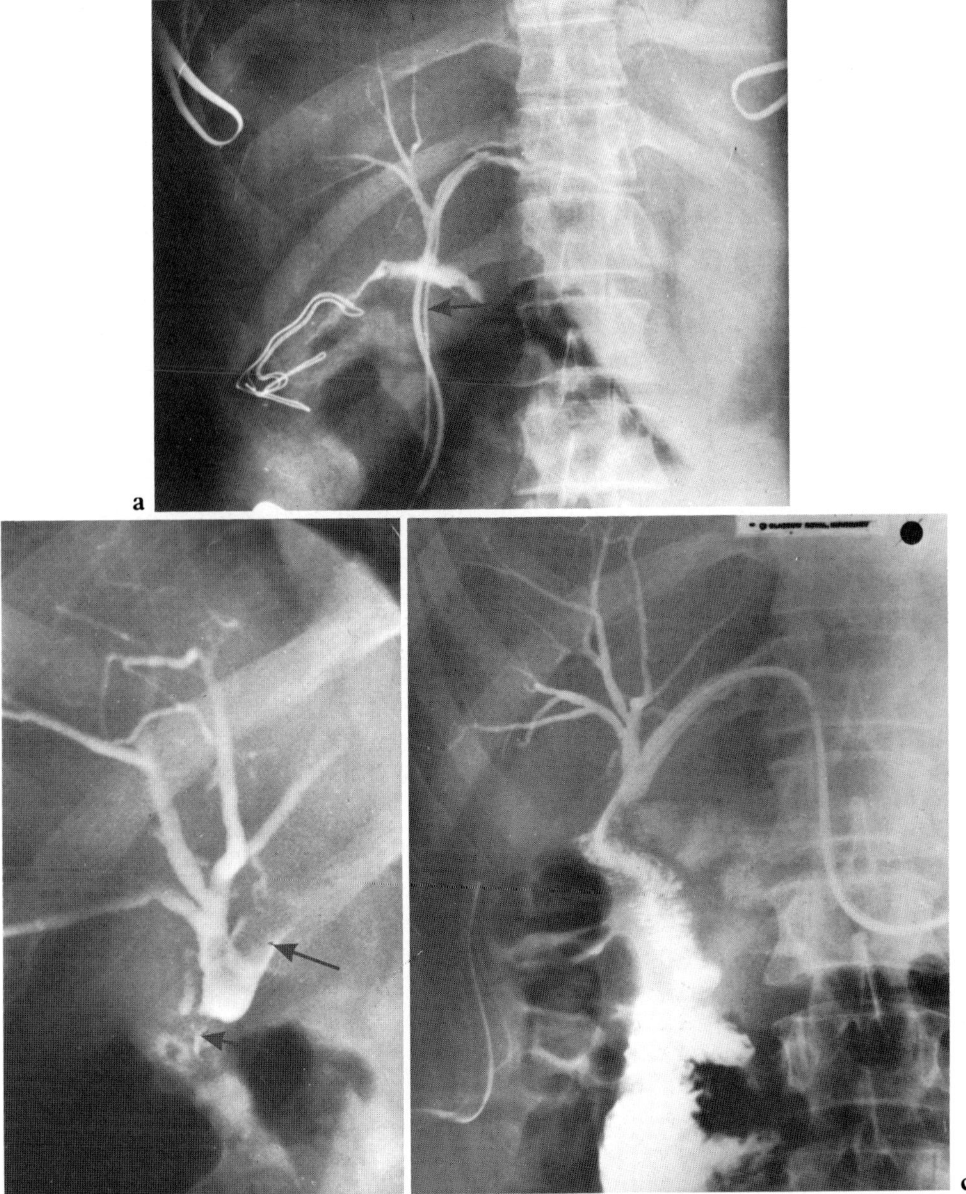

Fig. 60.13 Complete transection of the common bile duct at cholecystectomy occurred in this patient. Following cholecystectomy and closure of the abdomen without external drainage the patient became very ill and was found to have an intra-abdominal collection of bile. At laparotomy the common hepatic duct was found completely transected and was small, lying within grossly inflamed tissue in the hilus of the liver. Definitive repair was impossible

Two small catheters (arrow) were introduced into the biliary ductal system and led across a Roux-en-Y jejunal loop to the exterior creating a controlled external fistula. The patient recovered and the tubes were removed. b. One year later the patient presented with recurrent attacks of cholangitis and jaundice, a biliary stricture (small arrow) and intra-hepatic stones (large arrow). c. Treatment was carried out by means of hepaticojejunostomy Roux-en-Y over a transhepatic tube passed through the left hepatic ductal system. The tube was removed two months later. Patient remains perfectly well with normal liver function tests 12 years later

biliary fistula is due to injury to the subvesical duct in the gallbladder fossa (see above) (Ch. 2). In this situation it is safe to treat the patient expectantly since the biliary drainage will cease in due course without further sequelae.

Biliary fistula after choledochotomy

The usual cause of potential or actual postcholedochotomy fistula is a retained stone in the bile duct distal to the T-tube although it rarely may be due to undetected malignant obstruction in the low common bile duct or to surgical injury to the duct. The management of retained stones within the bile duct is covered in detail elsewhere in this book and it is important to recognize the very effective non-operative approaches now available. Previously unrecognized malignant obstruction or other forms of distal bile duct stenosis resulting in postcholedochotomy external biliary fistula, usually require re-operation and surgical excision of malignancy or appropriate biliary-enteric bypass.

Biliary fistula after drainage of intra-abdominal collections

Biliary fistula may occur following the drainage of sub-hepatic, perihepatic or periductal collections of pus and bile or may be associated with the complications of severe acute necrotizing pancreatitis.

Irrespective of the cause, initial management is drainage of the related cavity, removal of slough, fluid replacement and nutrition. The use of appropriate antibiotics is an important element. The majority of such fistulae close spontaneously within a month to six weeks without the need for further surgery. However, if the residual cavity remains inadequately drained or if there is still pancreatic or peripancreatic slough present, the fistula will not close spontaneously and further operative drainage is required.

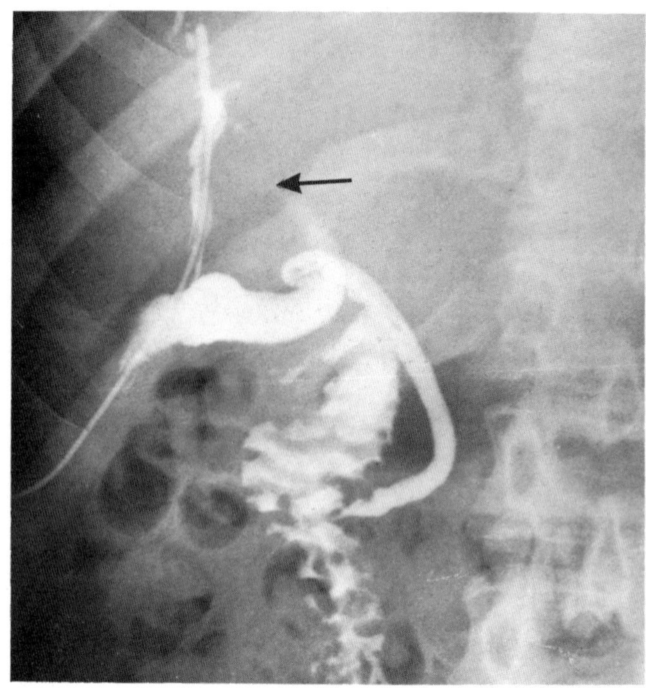

Fig. 60.14 External biliary fistula following blunt injury to the right lobe of the liver and subsequent drainage of a large right intrahepatic haematoma. The injury was associated with damage to the right hepatic duct and subsequent intrahepatic stricture (arrow). Following external drainage a high output biliary fistula developed. The tubogram illustrated was obtained after anastomosis of the fistulous track issuing from the liver to the adjacent mobilized gallbladder. Note that the cavity within the liver has collapsed and that the gallbladder fills and subsequently outlines the common biliary ductal cyst. The tube was removed and postoperative recovery was uneventful. The patient remains symptom free and with normal liver function tests five years after surgery (Smith et al 1982)

Biliary fistula after hepatic surgery or liver injury

Liver injury might involve intrahepatic biliary structures or be associated with transection of major biliary radicles. Initial management is that of the liver injury (Ch. 82) but complete transection of the bile duct requires immediate hepaticojejunostomy and lacerations of the main biliary channel may be sutured after placement of a T-tube. Occasionally problems arise where prolonged fistulation occurs from a segment of the liver isolated by the injury. Management of such cases is difficult and often even prolonged observation fails to see closure of the fistula especially if associated with distal stricture. Where such fistulation occurs, operation may be by one of three approaches. Firstly, resection of the isolated segment of liver tissue may be carried out. This can be difficult and is seldom warranted. In rare instances the fistula may be identified at operation and simply oversewn (Smith et al 1982). Alternatively a well developed fibrous fistulous tract can be anastomosed either to a prepared loop of jejunum or to the gallbladder (Fig. 60.13) if this is nearby. Such an operation may produce a permanent cure but late stenosis of the stricture may still be a problem for which secondary repair must be carried out (Smith et al 1982).

Biliary fistulation after partial hepatectomy for tumour may occur from the liver surface. If biliary reconstruction, e.g. following liver resection for hilar cholangiocarcinoma, has been performed leakage from the anastomosis or from bile ducts not identified and anastomosed at the time of surgery may occur. Such leakage is particularly prone to arise from caudate lobe ducts (Ch. 2). Management is conservative and most such fistulae will close in due course.

Biliary fistula after removal of a hydatid cyst is a difficult problem. As emphasized above the complication is usually avoidable (Kune, Jones & Sali 1983) (Ch. 75). Initial treatment should be conservative, but if the fistula fails to close then it is important to carry out fistulography and/or endoscopic retrograde cholangiography (Fig. 60.14) to determine that there is no biliary ductal obstruction. Re-operation is usually necessary, either to relieve biliary obstruction or to attempt to close biliary communications under vision. Such approaches can be combined with omentoplasty (Ch. 75). The cavity is not drained but the operative area adjacent to it is drained postoperatively.

REFERENCES

Blenkarn J I, McPherson G A D, Blumgart L H 1981 An improved system for external biliary drainage. Lancet ii: 781–782

Cass M H, Robson R, Rundle F F 1955 Electrolyte losses in biliary fistula: postcholedochotomy acidotic syndrome. Medical Journal of Australia 1: 165–168

Czerniak A, Benjamin I S, Thompson J W, Soreide O, Blumgart L H 1986 Biliary fistula complicating hepatic resection (in preparation)

Knochel J P, Cooper E B, Barry K G 1962 External biliary fistula: a study of electrolyte derangements and secondary cardiovascular and renal abnormalities. Surgery 51: 746–754

Kune G A, 1981 Surgical intervention in acute pancreatitis. Journal of Japanese Gastrointestinal Surgical Society 14: 1256–1261

Kune G A, Sali A 1980 The practice of biliary surgery, 2nd edn. Blackwell Scientific Publications, Oxford, Ch 1, p 9

Kune G A, Jones T, Sali A 1983 Hydatid disease in Australia. Prevention, clinical presentation and treatment. Medical Journal of Australia 2: 385–388

McPherson G A D, Benjamin I S, Habib N A, Bowley N B & Blumgart L H 1982 Percutaneous transhepatic drainage in obstructive jaundice: advantages and problems. British Journal of Surgery 69: 261–264

McPherson G A D, Collier N C, Blumgart L H 1984 The role of HIDA scanning in the assessment of external biliary fistula. Surgical Gastroenterology 3: 77–80

Smith E E J, Bowley N, Allison D J, & Blumgart L H 1982 The management of post-traumatic intrahepatic cutaneous biliary fistulas. British Journal of Surgery 69: 317–318

61

K. P. Morrissey, C. K. McSherry

Internal biliary fistula and gallstone ileus

As a consequence of several acquired or congenital pathological processes, an abnormal communication may develop between distinct parts of the biliary tract itself, or between it and other parts of the alimentary or respiratory passages. For the purposes of this chapter, such abnormal communications will be considered internal biliary fistulae. External biliary fistulae (Ch. 60) as well as some of the more rare and bizarre fistulous communications between the biliary tract and other internal structures, e.g. pericardium, major blood vessels, urinary bladder, uterus and vagina, will not be considered.

INCIDENCE AND AETIOLOGY

Whether occurring as a consequence of calculous biliary tract disease, trauma, neoplasm or congenital anomalies, biliary fistulae are uncommon. Estimates of their incidence are crude and may be learned only from many small series, usually of less than 50 patients. If all types of biliary fistulae are included, calculous biliary tract disease accounts for 90%, peptic ulcer disease for 6%, and neoplasm, trauma, parasitic infestation and congenital anomalies together comprise the remaining 4% (Piedad & Wells 1972).

Overall, from 1–3% of patients with cholesterol cholelithiasis in Western countries develop biliary-enteric fistula, with a female : male ratio of 3 : 1. At The New York Hospital — Cornell Medical Center, in 11 808 cases of non-malignant biliary tract disease encountered from 1932–1978, the incidence of biliary-enteric fistulae was 0.9% with a male : female ratio of 2.3 : 1 (Glenn et al 1981). Large series from Greece (Lygidakis 1981) report an incidence of 2%, while in American Indians it is 3.2% (Zwemer et al 1979). In Japan, where bilirubin and primary intraductal stone disease is dominant, the incidence of fistula is 13–18% and males slightly outnumber females (Urakami & Kishi 1978). The type of fistula noted in this group of patients usually involves the ductal system rather than the gallbladder.

The pathogenic sequence of events for calculous biliary tract disease has been well described by Glenn & Mannix (1958). It consists of pressure necrosis and erosion of part of the biliary tract wall into an adjacent structure to which it has become adherent in the course of repeated bouts of inflammation, often with distal biliary tract obstruction. The liability of the components of the hepato-biliary tree to become inflamed, as well as their anatomical proximity to several adjacent hollow viscera, largely determine the relative incidence of the different types of spontaneous biliary-enteric fistula due to calculous disease. Table 61.1 summarizes the distribution of biliary-enteric fistulae at The New York Hospital — Cornell Medical Center. The various types of biliary-enteric fistula can best be subclassified from an aetiological, as well as an anatomical point of view, by the names of the principal organs involved. The names for a particular fistula between two structures are variable in the literature, e.g. bronchobiliary vs. biliobronchial, and do not connote differences in aetiology or pathogenesis.

Fistulae involving the gallbladder

In Western countries where cholesterol cholelithiasis abounds, the gallbladder is most often the site of severe inflammation and obstruction. Thus cholecyst-enteric fistulae comprise from 70–85% of all biliary fistulae reported in the world literature up to 1982 (LeBlanc et al

Table 61.1 Distribution of 109 biliary-enteric fistulae
The New York Hospital-Cornell Medical Center (1932–1983)

	No. cases	per cent
Cholecystoduodenal	83	76.1
Cholecystocolic	17	15.5
Cholecystogastric	2	1.8
Cholecystocholedochal	3	2.7
Choledochoduodenal	1	0.9
Multiple	3	2.7
(cholecysto-duodeno-colic 1)		
(cholecysto-jejuno-colic 1)		
(cholecysto-choledocho-duodenal 1)		

1983, Rau et al 1980, Safaie-Shirazi et al 1973). Of these, 55–75% are *cholecystoduodenal*, 15–30% are *cholecystocolic*, and 2–5% are *cholecystogastric*. Multiple fistulae, e.g. *cholecystoduodenocolic*, are very rare (Shocket et al 1970). Of the 23 cases reported up to 1978, 21 were secondary to gallstone disease, and one each due to duodenal ulcer and a primary carcinoma of the gallbladder (Morris et al 1978).

Gallstone ileus, a dramatic clinical presentation of a cholecyst-enteric fistula, is reported in 8–20% of large series of patients with biliary-enteric fistulae (LeBlanc et al 1983, Rau et al 1980, Safaie-Shirazi et al 1973, VanLandingham and Broders 1982, Kasahara et al 1980, Heuman et al 1980). Indeed, in the cumulative experience at The New York Hospital-Cornell Medical Center, from 1932 to 1980, 23 of the 109 cases of biliary-enteric fistulae presented as intestinal obstruction. However, as a cause of intestinal obstruction alone, gallstone ileus accounts for 1–2% of cases, although in patients over 70, gallstone ileus may account for up to 20% of cases of small bowel obstruction.

Whereas most fistulae between the gallbladder and intestinal tract become obvious either pre- or intraoperatively, *cholecyst-choledochal* fistulae are insidious and may not be appreciated even at surgery. These 'bilio-biliary' fistulae develop between the ampulla of the gallbladder or cystic duct and the proximal common bile duct. In either instance, the mechanism of formation is the same — pressure necrosis into the common duct by a large solitary calculous impacted in either the ampulla of the gallbladder or in the intra-mural portion of the cystic duct. Cholecyst-choledochal fistula has been estimated to occur in 1–6% of biliary operations for calculous disease (Corlette & Bismuth 1975). Although this estimate appears high and is uncorroborated by other reports, an awareness of the possibility of cholecyst-choledochal fistula is important, and may help avoid damage to the common duct at operation (Ch. 58).

Fistulae involving the common bile duct

Proximal *choledochoduodenal* fistula is the principal form of abnormal communication between the common bile duct and adjacent structures. It represents 4–20% of all biliary-enteric fistulae and, of its type, 80% are caused by peptic ulcer erosion from the first portion of the duodenum into the proximal common bile duct. The sex distribution is representative of the peptic ulcer population, i.e., men outnumber women by 3 : 1; and the age of onset is in the 5th or 6th decade, slightly earlier than that for fistulae due to cholelithiasis. In fact, there is usually no associated cholelithiasis, or if so, it plays no role in the formation of the fistula. Other less common causes of choledochoduodenal fistula, cited by Saar et al (1981) and Feller et al (1980), include cholelithiasis, operative trauma, duodenal diverticula, echinococcosus, Crohn's disease and neoplasms of the stomach, distal bile duct, ampullary region and duodenum.

The incidence of distal choledochoduodenal fistula due to cholelithiasis or operative trauma may be higher than previously estimated. With the development of PTC and ERCP studies of pathological anatomy, it is becoming apparent that many patients with minor or major biliary-digestive complaints and gallstone disease may in fact have a distal choledochoduodenal or '*parapapillary choledochoduodenal fistula*'. In Japan, where there is a high incidence of primary intrahepatic calculous biliary tract disease, Tanaka & Ikeda (1983) have reported a 5.3% incidence of parapapillary fistula in ERCP studies of 1500 patients. The male:female ratio is about equal, in keeping with the Japanese sex distribution of gallstone disease. Ikeda & Okada (1975) have classified these as: Type I fistula, characterized by a small fistula opening on the longitudinal fold of the duodenum just proximal to the papilla, probably caused by penetration of a small calculous through the intramural portion of the common duct into the duodenum; and Type II fistula, a larger opening of the duodenal wall adjacent to the longitudinal fold, probably caused by a relatively large stone eroding from the extramural portion of a greatly dilated common duct into the duodenum. The incidence of parapapillary choledochoduodenal fistula is probably less in Western Europe, the United Kingdom and the United States; and perhaps a greater proportion of these are not due to spontaneous gallstone disease itself but rather to iatrogenic surgical injury (Ch. 55) or other instrumental damage to the distal common duct in operations directed against choledocholithiasis (Fig. 61.5). Hunt and Blumgart (1980) and Tytgat et al (1979) have recently published their experience with these fistulous complications of biliary tract surgery.

Unusual choledochal fistulae can only be mentioned briefly in this context. Spontaneous fistula formation between the common duct and the colon has been recorded only once in the English literature, by Bose & Sastry (1983), a rare case of agenesis of the gallbladder with erosion of a common duct stone into the hepatic flexure of the colon. We are aware of only two adult cases of fistulous communication of a pancreatic pseudocyst to the common bile duct (Ellenbogen et al 1981). Recently, DeVanna, et al (1983) have reported a similar case in a two-year-old baby. Chandar & Hookman (1980) reported one case of GI haemorrhage resulting from a choledochocolonic fistula, which developed from a cystic duct remnant 28 years post cholecystectomy and associated with a benign stricture in the ampullary segment of the common bile duct.

Fistulae involving the intrahepatic ducts, liver and lung

Bronchobiliary fistula are quite rare. There are three major categories of bronchobiliary fistula: 1. acquired and due to infection, especially parasitic, or iatrogenic injury during biliary tract surgery; 2. trauma; 3. congenital.

The many diverse causes of acquired bronchobiliary fistula have been well referenced by Sane et al (1971). The principal cause of bronchobiliary fistula in adults is either echinococcal or amoebic abscess (Ch. 75, 76) of the liver; however, even in large series of surgically treated cases of hepatic echinococcal disease in Greece and Turkey, only 2% were complicated by rupture into the lung or bronchi (Alestig et al 1972). On the other hand, amoebic abscess of the liver has been reported in association with broncho-biliary fistula in 8% of cases (Razemon et al 1963–64). These rare complications of parasitic disease are more likely to be suspected in patients from Mediterranean countries, as well as North Africa, Mexico and some of the southern border states of the USA.

The incidence of bronchobiliary fistula as a consequence of surgically treated calculous or neoplastic disease of the hepato-biliary tract or pancreas has declined over the past two decades as patients are operated upon earlier in the course of their disease and by better trained surgeons (Warren et al 1983).

Thoraco-abdominal injuries rarely lead to bronchobiliary fistulae. Although penetrating or blunt trauma to the abdomen and chest is a common enough civilian and wartime occurrence, the number of fistulae resulting has remained small, often because their initial surgical treatment has been excellent and because no obstruction to proper flow of bile existed (Oparah & Mandal 1978).

Of the 10 cases reported since congenital bronchobiliary fistula was first described in 1952, four were associated with biliary tree malformations, e.g. biliary atresia, hypoplasia of the common duct (Chan et al 1984), and one with oesophageal atresia and tracheo-oesophageal fistula (Dyon et al 1978). The fistula appears to be composed of an accessory bronchus arising at or near the tracheal bifurcation and passing down the posterior mediastinum through the oesophageal hiatus to communicate with the left hepatic duct. Theories of embryogenesis are conjectural (Sane et al 1971, Dyon et al 1978).

ROLE OF DIAGNOSTIC TESTS

There are no specific serological tests for biliary-enteric fistulae. Nevertheless, in the evaluation and management of elderly, high risk or critically ill patient with a symptomatic biliary fistula, tests of liver function, electrolytes and blood count are very useful.

Plain and barium contrast radiographs

Pneumobilia, the presence of air in the biliary tree, may be noted on the plain film of 30–50% of patients with gallstone ileus. Other less common causes of pneumobilia include: an incompetent sphincter of Oddi (Fig. 61.1), emphysematous cholecystitis or suppurative cholangitis and prior biliary-enteric bypass surgery. Hricak & Molen (1978) suggest that the low incidence of pneumobilia in gallstone ileus is due to the cystic duct obstruction which led to the acute cholecystitis and perforation into an adjacent viscus. It also prevents retrograde passage of air into the extrahepatic and intrahepatic bile ducts.

As well as pneumobilia with intestinal obstruction, other classic radiographical signs of gallstone ileus are: visualization of a calcified gallstone in the peritoneal cavity at a distance away from the gallbladder region; change on repeat films in the position of a previously observed calcification; and a change in the level of mechanical intestinal obstruction, the so-called 'tumbling obstruction' (VanLandingham & Broders 1982, Day & Marks 1975). However, only 30% of gallstones are sufficiently calcified to be radio-opaque.

A barium meal or upper gastrointestinal series demonstrates reflux of contrast material into the fistula in up to 40% of cholecystoduodenal communications, and up to 75% of choledochoduodenal fistulae of peptic ulcer origin (Balthazar & Gurkin 1976, Kourias & Chouliaras 1964). If both the plain film and barium swallow are employed in concert, more than 60% of biliary enteric fistulae will be correctly diagnosed preoperatively (Fig. 61.3) (Balthazar & Schecter 1975). A negative upper gastrointestinal series in the presence of pneumobilia is an indication for a barium enema which will disclose greater than 95% of cholecysto-colic fistulae (Fig. 61.4).

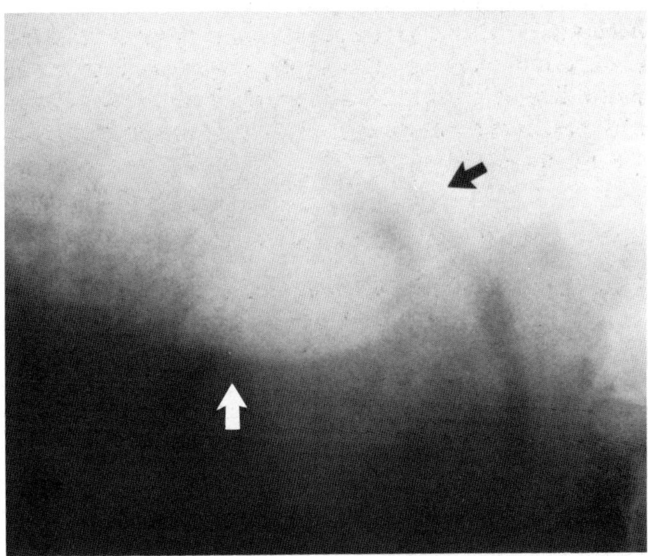

Fig. 61.1 Pneumobilia without biliary-enteric fistula (plain film). A 74-year-old man with multiple radio-opaque calculi (lower arrow) presented with epigastric pain and the signs and symptoms of common duct obstruction. He expired shortly after admission, and autopsy revealed a small calculus in the second duodenum adjacent to a patulous sphincter of Oddi as well as a myocardial infarct

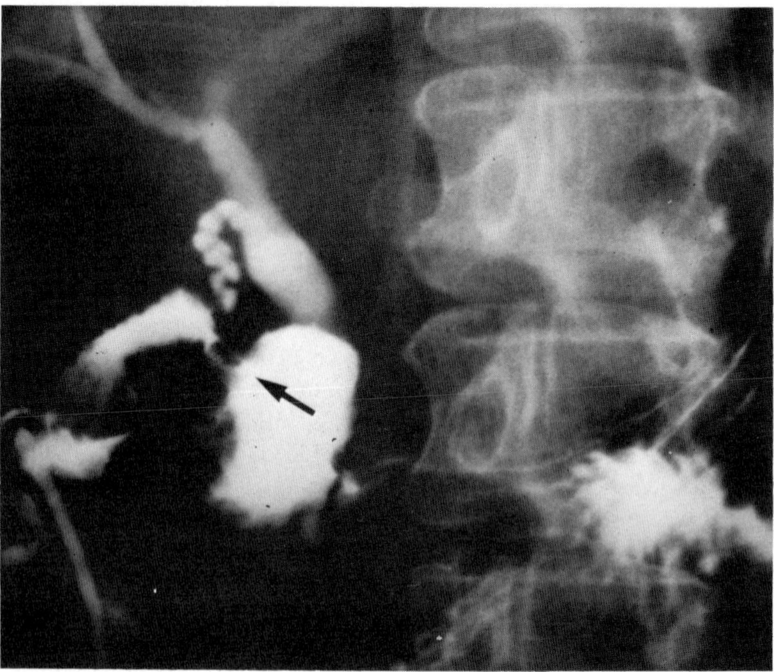

Fig. 61.2 Cholecystoduodenal fistula (arrow) demonstrated by cholecystostomy tube cholangiogram, one month following operation for acute cholecystitis

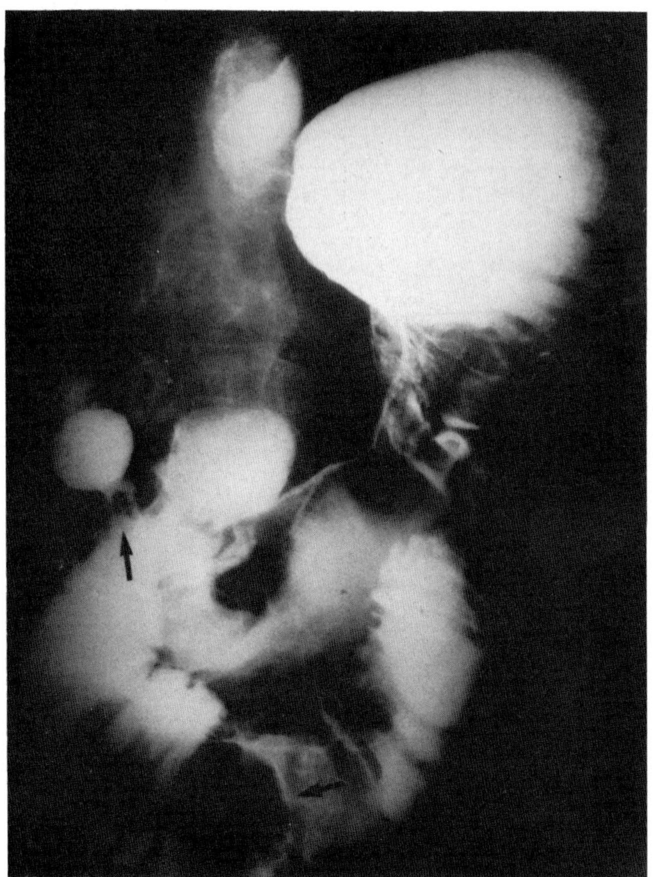

Fig. 61.3 Gallstone ileus with duodenal obstruction. Upper GI series demonstrates a cholecystoduodenal fistula (upper arrow) and the leading edge of a large, non-opaque calculus (lower arrow) in a dilated transverse segment of duodenum

Iodinated dye studies and endoscopy

Indirect imaging techniques, with the exception of CAT scanning, are not helpful. The oral cholecystogram is misleading and non-diagnostic in the case of biliary-enteric fistulae because orally administered dye, and often intravenously given contrast agents, flow through the fistula and usually cannot be sufficiently concentrated within the biliary tract to show the pathological anatomy let alone the presence of gallstones. Whereas the CAT scan may disclose fusion of the biliary tract to an adjacent viscus, it may not precisely demonstrate a fistula, but should be used to demonstrate other important pathological changes which may be helpful in case evaluation, e.g. distal common duct stones or other obstructive processes, the presence of a subphrenic abscess, pleural effusion or parasitic disease of the liver (Porta et al 1981).

Direct injection of iodinated contrast material is the best way to outline the normal and the pathological anatomy of the biliary tract. Preoperatively, this is accomplished either by endoscopic retrograde cholangiopancreatography (ERCP) or percutaneous transhepatic cholangiography (PTC), and, in situations where an external bile fistula exists, a fistulagram should be performed (Ch. 60). Intraoperative or postoperative cholangiograms are often invaluable. (Fig. 61.2).

Since 1970, numerous reports have appeared in the literature supporting the efficacy of ERCP in documenting surgical or spontaneous biliary fistulae (VanLinda & Rosson 1984, Tanaka & Ikeda 1983, Nakib et al 1982, Tytgat 1979, Fruhmorgan et al 1971). Endoscopically, one

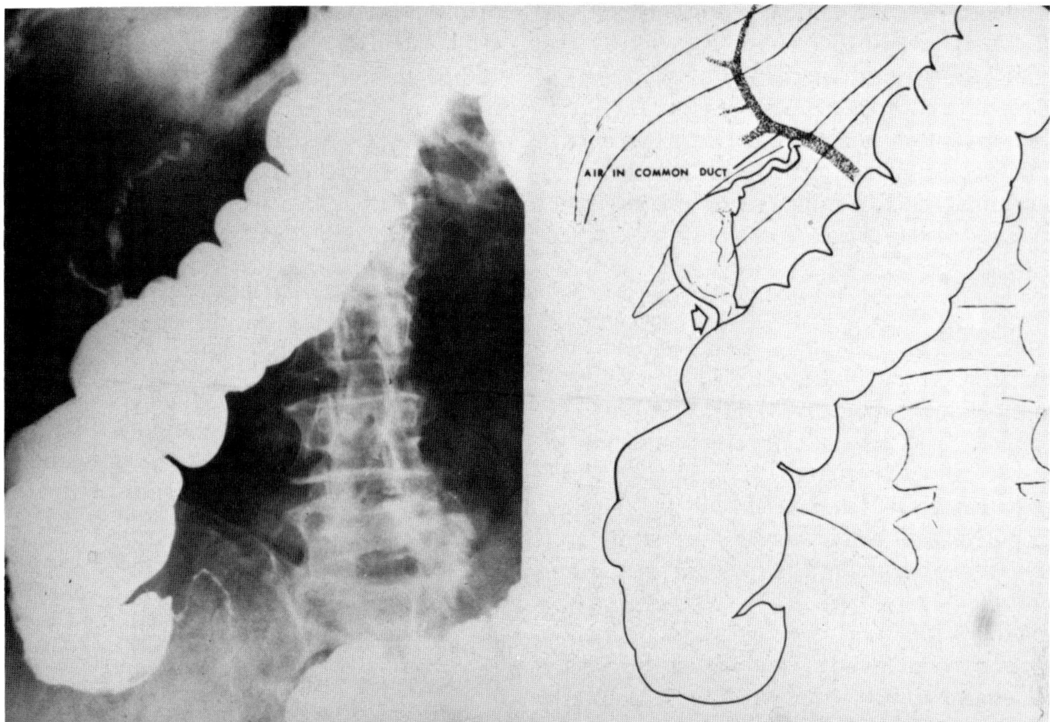

Fig. 61.4 Cholecystocolic fistula demonstrated by barium enema

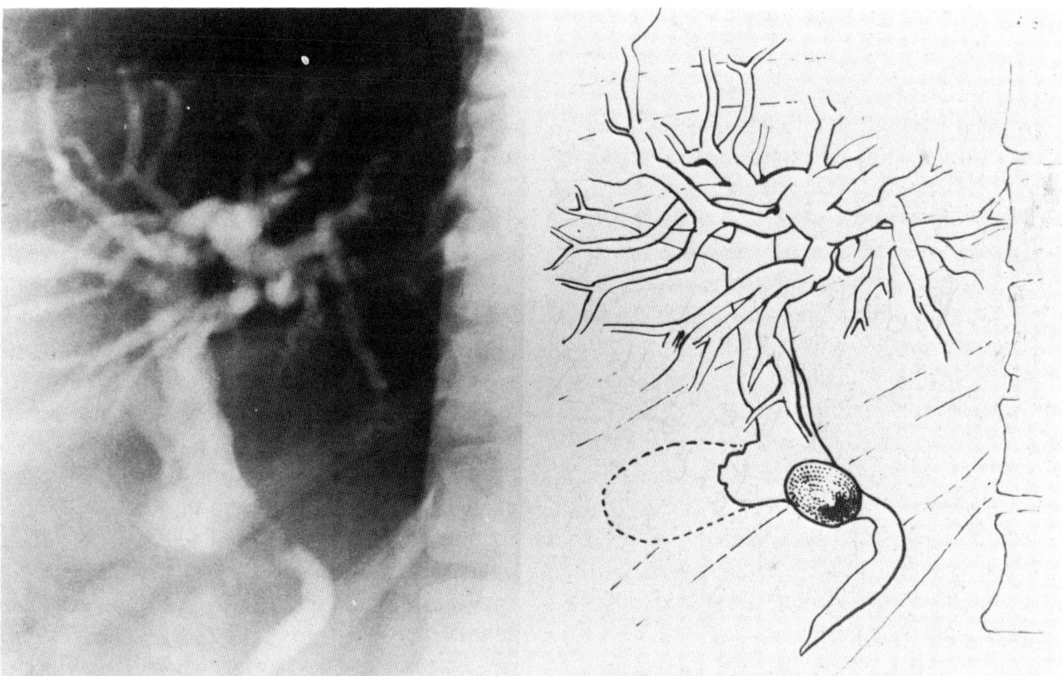

Fig. 61.5 Mirizzi Syndrome — Type I (without cholecyst-choledochal fistula). PTC demonstrates an impacted cystic duct stone with extrinsic compression of the proximal hepatic ducts

can not only directly visualize the alimentary side of a given fistula, be it gastric (Stempfle & Diamantopoulos 1976), duodenal or colic, but also cannulate either the fistula itself or the ampulla of Vater to obtain a high quality roentgenogram of the communicating biliary anatomy. In this way, the heretofore elusive anatomy of bronchobiliary fistulae has been repeatedly clarified (Watkins et al 1975, Moreira et al 1984). Similarly, the largely unappreciated and frequently asymptomatic parapapillary choledochoduodenal fistulae have been demonstrated and found to be quite common (Tanaka & Ikeda 1983, Hunt & Blumgart 1980).

There have been far fewer reports of the role of PTC in demonstrating biliary fistulae. It has been helpful in the diagnosis and treatment of bronchobiliary fistula in association with echinoccocal disease of the liver and in icteric patients with common duct obstruction and dilated intrahepatic ducts, e.g. cholecyst-choledochal fistula (Cornud et al 1980).

Radionuclide imaging

With the introduction of the imidoacetic acid agents bound to technetium (99T-Pipida and 99T-Hida), radionuclide scans have rapidly become the preferred method of outlining the normal and pathological anatomy of the extrahepatic bile passages. These relatively non-invasive procedures do not rely on hepatocellular concentration of bile or on short critical time flow periods for satisfactory visualization of the biliary tree. In fact, prolonged (24 hour) accumulation of radioactivity, measured either by patient scanning or by quantitative isotopic counts of body secretions, e.g. sputum, have been used to demonstrate very small or intermittent fistulae from the biliary tract to the respiratory passages and the colon (Bretland 1983, Taillefer et al 1983, Henderson et al 1980, Edell et al 1981).

Sonography

Sonography is a most useful non-invasive diagnostic aid in the preoperative evaluation of a patient with a suspected biliary fistula (Porta et al 1981, Renner et al 1982). Whereas the radionuclide scan may readily demonstrate a fistula, the sonogram will indicate the presence of calculi in the gallbladder, common duct dilatation or echogenic foci suggestive of common duct stones, as well as the presence of inflammatory, cystic or infiltrative disease of the liver and pancreas (Griffin et al 1983). This information is important in the decision making process, e.g. the need or advisability of cholecystectomy and dismantling of a fistula at the time of operation for gallstone ileus in an elderly or high risk patient. Paradoxically, this information may be obtained more rapidly, safely and probably with equivalent accuracy by a preoperative sonogram rather than by intraoperative manipulations about a mass of inflamed tissue in the right upper quadrant.

SPECIFIC CLINICAL PRESENTATIONS AND TREATMENT

Gallstone ileus

Gallstone ileus is the blockage of the intestinal tract by a gallstone large enough to partially or completely occlude its lumen. This dramatic presentation of intestinal obstruction is too indelibly fixed in the medical imagination to permit amendment of the inappropriate term 'ileus'; perhaps it is derived from the frequent initial clinical impression of an unexplained ileus, in that many patients with gallstone obstruction present without a clinical history or physical signs to suggest mechanical intestinal obstruction. As with other patients in Western European and English speaking countries in which cholesterol cholelithiasis predominates, those presenting with this manifestation of advanced biliary tract disease are usually elderly, more often than not female, and beset by multiple other medical conditions which may cloud or complicate their prompt diagnosis and appropriate treatment.

When an elderly person presents with typical signs and symptoms of intestinal obstruction, or perhaps less dramatically an unexplained ileus, but without obvious incarcerated abdominal wall hernia, scar of a previous laparotomy and little suspicion of an occult malignancy, then calculous obstruction by a gallstone must be considered. Approximately half of the patients so presenting with gallstone ileus will indeed, on close questioning, give a history suggestive of prior calculous biliary tract disease. However, at the time of clinical presentation with gallstone obstruction, there may be no signs of active gallstone disease such as pain, tenderness in the upper abdomen, cholangitis or jaundice. Laboratory data will be consistent with fluid and electrolyte disturbances appropriate to the degree and duration of intestinal obstruction; and some abnormalities of liver function tests may suggest chronic disease of the liver and biliary tract in up to one quarter of the patients.

The plain abdominal film, in addition to characterizing the patient's condition as one of mechanical obstruction, will demonstrate air in the biliary tree and so be diagnostic for gallstone ileus in about 20%–50% of patients. However, pneumobilia is often not appreciated even in restrospect, but if biliary-enteric fistula is suspected and a barium meal administered as well, reflux of barium into the biliary tree will yield a correct preoperative diagnosis in up to 60% of patients. Calculi large enough to obstruct the intestine usually do so in the last 50 cm of ileum but occasionally also in the jejunum or duodenum (Fig. 61.3) and rarely in the sigmoid colon. Such calculi are usually larger than 2.5 cm and, if partially calcified, will be readily apparent on the plain film. Additional stones still in the gallbladder, or more importantly in the common duct, may be demonstrated preoperatively by abdominal sonography.

The clinical presentation of gallstone ileus has not changed over the past 40 years. However heightened awareness of the possibility and use of the barium meal in patients presenting with mechanical intestinal obstruction, have led to an improvement in preoperative diagnostic accuracy in our clinic, from 30–40% for the period from 1932–56 to 75% for the years 1956–1978 (Glenn et al 1981). The reported experience in other clinics in the preoperative diagnosis of gallstone ileus is about 50–60%. This improved preoperative diagnostic accuracy, as well as other advances in our understanding and treatment of these critically ill patients, have contributed to an improved outcome of therapy, to be discussed next.

The overriding consideration in patients presenting with gallstone obstruction of the intestine should be relief of the life-threatening cause of obstruction, i.e. enterolithotomy. This surgical emergency should be approached expeditiously, and without a period of waiting in hope that a suspected stone will pass; it will not. The only reason for delay should be to provide adequate preoperative fluid and electrolyte resuscitation of these critically ill patients and, if possible, to assess the presence of other gallstones in the gallbladder and common duct by means of sonography or CAT scan. Nasogastric decompression and peroperative antibiotics are strongly urged to minimize the risks of aspiration and postoperative wound infection.

The terminal ileum is the site of obstruction in 70% of cases. Unless the obstructed segment is ischaemic, or has perforated requiring a small bowel resection, the obstructing calculous can be manipulated proximally to a healthy dilated jejunum where a safe enterotomy and stone removal may be executed. Jejunal impaction, often by stones larger than 4 cm, occurs approximately 15% of the time and enterotomy may be made at that site or just proximal to it. Duodenal obstruction, usually in the bulb, is known as Bouvret's Syndrome (Argyropoulos et al 1979, Cooper & Kucharski 1978, Thomas et al 1976). It occurs in 10% of cases and may be handled by duodenotomy and primary closure or by tube duodenostomy or pyloroplasty. Occasionally it may be possible to manipulate the stone back into the stomach and remove it via a gastrotomy. Rarely will a gastroenterostomy and vagotomy be necessary to protect a duodenotomy or severely traumatized duodenum at the site of impaction. In rare instances, the sigmoid colon is the site of obstruction of a calculus that has managed to get through the terminal ileum via a cholecystoduodenal fistula. In either instance, a colostomy will be necessary to decompress the proximal bowel. If the impacted stone cannot be manipulated proximally to a transverse colostomy, consideration should be given to exteriorization of the impacted segment.

Almost as important as removing the obstructing stone is to determine, by careful palpation of the entire bowel and the gallbladder region, whether other gallstones are in transit more proximally or still reside in the diseased gallbladder. These calculi may be poised for passage through the fistula, possibly to induce a recurrent episode of gallstone ileus. This phenomenon is estimated to occur in 5% of cases and by these simple manoeuvres can be avoided (Haq et al 1981, Levin & Shapiro 1980).

There is still considerable debate in the surgical literature whether cholecystectomy and/or common duct exploration, with dismantling and closure of the cholecystenteric fistula, should accompany enterotomy and relief of the obstruction or await a second operation. Our own experience (Table 61.2), as well as recent reports of others (VanLandingham et al 1982, Heuman et al 1980, Kasahara et al 1980) indicates that operative mortality is lower in these critically ill, elderly patients when only the gallstone obstruction is relieved. Moreover, careful follow-up of a number of these patients indicates that between one-third and one-half will become minimally or completely asymptomatic following relief of the gallstone ileus and nothing more need have been done either at the emergency procedure or at a later time. Of course, if the patient has both jaundice and intestinal obstruction at the outset, then common duct exploration or at least tube decompression of the common duct may also be necessary as a life saving procedure. For those patients who continue to be symptomatic following relief of gallstone ileus, careful preoperative evaluation and bowel preparation can precede a later operation adding to its safety. Since common duct stones are found in up to 40% of patients with biliary-enteric fistula, it is likely that those patients who continue to be symptomatic will require common duct exploration in addition to cholecystectomy and repair of the fistula.

When Courvoisier first discussed 44 cases of surgically treated gallstone ileus in 1890, he reported an operative mortality of 44%. This figure had slowly declined to 15–25% in large reported series up to the early 1970s. Now, our clinic (Glenn et al 1981) and others (VanLandingham & Broders 1982, Heuman et al 1980, Kasahara et al 1980) are able to report a further reduction in mortality figures to 4–10%. It should be stressed, however, that this improvement includes some patients treated by enterotomy and stone removal alone, with no further surgical therapy indicated or performed.

Cholecystoduodenal fistula

Most cholecystoduodenal fistulae do not result in gallstone

Table 61.2 Operative experience in 98 patients with biliary enteric fistulae
The New York Hospital-Cornell Medical Center (1932–1983)

	No. of operations
Cholecystectomy, repair of fistula	39
Cholecystectomy, repair of fistula, CDE	39
Choledochotomy, repair of fistula	3
Choledochotomy, repair of fistula, repair of stricture	1
Cholecystostomy	5
Choledochostomy	1
Ileotomy, second stage repair	9
Ileotomy	5
Ileotomy, cholecystectomy	2
Ileotomy, cholecystectomy, repair of fistula, CDE	1
Gastrotomy, cholecystectomy, repair of fistula, CDE	1
Duodenotomy, second stage repair	1
Sigmoid colotomy	2
Total	109

ileus. Rather, they are asymptomatic or occur in association with the usual digestive complaints consistent with gastric or biliary tract disease. They may be found during an upper gastrointestinal barium study or, under less welcome circumstances, at the time of abdominal surgery for an unrelated problem.

Should an asymptomatic or mildly symptomatic cholecystoenteric fistula be diagnosed preoperatively, many of the management decisions regarding gallstone ileus discussed above may apply. Elective surgery may never be necessary in a completely asymptomatic individual or may present an unfavourable risk–benefit ratio in an elderly, minimally symptomatic patient. Other alternatives to cholecystectomy with dismantling of the fistula and probable common duct exploration must be considered; e.g. a period of expectant management with careful observation, endoscopic papillotomy and stone extraction with the gallbladder left in situ, or interval cholecystectomy if symptoms of pain or cholangitis persist after endoscopic biliary surgery. However, in a relatively healthy person under 70 years, we feel that surgical extirpation of the gallbladder and closure of the fistula, as well as treatment of any common duct pathology, still promise the best long-term therapeutic result.

If an incidental cholecystoduodenal fistula is discovered at the time of surgery or is found unexpectedly in the course of a biliary tract procedure, the major intraoperative decision revolves around the patient's need for and ability to tolerate additional surgical manipulations at that time. In this regard, knowledge of the patient's intestinal complaints and general state of well-being are most valuable to the surgeon. If the patient is judged an unsound risk, and/or the biliary tract pathology not felt to be pertinent to the major indication for operation, then nothing need be done. Rarely, a cholecystostomy (Fig. 61.2) and extraction of large calculi can be accomplished with little additional risk. Usually, however, the gallbladder is shrunken and barely palpable as it is stuck to the duodenum. If the patient can tolerate additional surgery, and sufficient indication exists to proceed at the present operation rather than at a subsequent one, then an attempt should be made to demonstrate the biliary-enteric anatomy and state of the common duct by an operative cholangiogram before proceeding with a definitive procedure.

Cholecystocolic fistulae and choleric enteropathy

The acute development of a cholecystocolonic fistula may present in patients with long-standing mild or moderately symptomatic biliary tract disease and be heralded by a sudden change in bowel habit with multiple, loose stools and the development of fever, chills and other signs of cholangitis from colonic bacterial reflux into the biliary tract. Interestingly, many elderly patients either weather or ignore these symptoms without seeking medical attention, and some develop signs and symptoms which may incriminate the entire gastrointestinal tract. Thus increased stool frequency, particularly after ingestion of food, will persist while bouts of fever and malaise subside. Then other characteristic symptoms appear such as eructation, nausea, weight loss and increasing diarrhoea and steatorrhoea. These latter symptoms precede the onset of choleric enteropathy, a dramatic complication of cholecystocolonic fistula. This enteropathy is also seen in other major disturbances of bile acid metabolism, e.g. major ileal resection, or blind loop syndrome (Brandt 1984).

Choleric enteropathy consists of a wide spectrum of anatomical, physiological and biochemical changes produced by a significant alteration of the entero-hepatic circulation of bile acids. The malabsorption syndrome secondary to cholecystocolonic fistula was first clinically documented by Augur (1970) and has since been studied by others (Rau et al 1980). Ordinarily 95% of the bile acids are passed down the jejunum, aiding in fat and cholesterol absorption, before being largely reabsorbed in the terminal ileum and then resecreted into bile. Up to two or three cycles of the bile acid pool per meal occur with very little loss and further metabolism of bile acids in the colon. However, with a cholecysto-colonic fistula, a large part or all of the primary bile acid pool may be shunted immediately into the colon. Depending upon the amount of bile still passing via the common duct into the small bowel, fat absorption is affected and in time may result in fatty acid diarrhoea. More immediately, however, colonic secretion of water and electrolytes is maximally stimulated by the dihydroxy bile acids. Chenodeoxycholic acid gains access to the colon in large quantities and massively increased amounts of deoxycholic acid are formed by bacterial dehydroxylation of cholic acid. The primary bile acids as well as their metabolites are no longer actively absorbed and so are lost from the body, in time causing a chronically lowered bile salt pool beyond the liver's capacity to synthesize new bile acids to replete it. At this point, even with a partial shunt to the colon, the bile acid concentration still normally passing down the common duct and through the small intestine may be too small to affect micellar solubilization of dietary fat. Unlike a blind loop syndrome, where bacterial overgrowth contributes to the choleric enteropathy, and can be largely corrected, at least temporarily by antibiotics, cholecystocolonic fistula does not respond adequately to antibiotics. Until the fistula is dismantled, massive shunting of bile acids to the intestine persists and promotes continued watery diarrhoea, diminished bile salt pool and a variable degree of fat malabsorption.

Cholangitis appears to be a more prominent feature of cholecystocolonic fistula when the fistula is narrow and liable to intermittent obstruction of bile flow (Safaie-Shirazi et al 1973, Edell et al 1981) whereas diarrhoea with a lesser incidence of fever and chills is more common with a wide open fistula (Lygidakis 1981). In either instance, a fistula to the colon is more likely than other biliary-enteric fistulae to have associated cholangitis. If so, the serum levels of bilirubin, SGPT and γ-glutamyl transferase may be slightly elevated and direct attention to the biliary and upper digestive tract.

Because of the patients' unusual presenting complaints, full investigations for malabsorption, including upper GI studies and GB sonography and jejunal biopsy, may be undertaken but usually do not pinpoint the diagnosis. The plain abdominal film is reported to reveal air in the biliary tree in only 50% of cases. Only if a barium enema examination is done, preferably with air contrast, will the diagnosis become evident as both barium (Fig. 61.4) and air fill the gallbladder and extrahepatic bile ducts. Failure of even a barium enema to demonstrate a cholecystocolic fistula has been reported, but that is quite rare.

There is little controversy about the appropriate treatment for cholecystocolic fistulae. Except in the most extenuating circumstances, they all should be dismantled because of the ever present risk of sepsis. If the diagnosis can be made preoperatively, suitable mechanical and antibiotic bowel preparation will reduce the chance of infectious complications of surgery, and permit primary closure of the large bowel. Cholecystectomy and, if indicated, common duct exploration should be carried out at the same time.

Cholecyst-choledochal fistula, including the Mirizzi syndrome

In cases of bilio-biliary fistula between the ampulla of the gallbladder or cystic duct and common duct, the offending stone often remains impacted and only partially traverses the fistula it has produced. Thus it may cause common duct obstruction. The large size of the stone and the acute cholecystitis with marked pressure necrosis and inflammatory reaction at the site of stone intrusion into the common hepatic duct combine to produce a clinical picture of bile duct obstruction with variable components of both extrinsic compression and intrinsic calculous blockage of bile flow.

In the formative stages of this bilio-biliary fistula when a large gallstone is impacted in either the ampulla of the gallbladder or in the intra-mural portion of the cystic duct, it is not uncommon to have extrinsic compression of the common hepatic duct indistinguishable from choledocholithiasis. This 'functional hepatic syndrome' in patients was first described by Mirizzi in 1948. McSherry et al (1982) have suggested a further subclassification of the Mirizzi Syndrome: Type I category in which there is compression of the common hepatic duct by an impacted ampullary or cystic duct calculous (Fig. 61.5); Type II in which a fistula has formed and the offending calculus is in the common duct. The surgical approach to these impacted stones is influenced by the recognition either pre- or intraoperatively of the fistula.

The large and solitary nature of the ampullary or cystic duct stones may be a hint to the preoperative diagnosis. Conventional, non-invasive biliary imaging studies such as ultrasonography may incorrectly indicate the findings to be a common duct stone. An ERCP or PTC done preoperatively may delineate the condition and so markedly alter surgical strategy. Cornud et al (1981) have demonstrated the X-ray appearance of bilio-biliary fistulae by PTC, while Heil & Belohlavek (1978) have relied upon ERCP. In the six patients documented by McSherry et al (1982), PTC and ERCP were equally effective in elucidating the cause of common duct obstruction.

Bilio-biliary fistula have been referred to as a trap in the surgery of cholelithiasis. This is most appropriate because often the presence of such a fistula is not recognized until the time of surgery, and often not soon enough to prevent injury to the common duct in the attempt to dissect the ampulla of the gallbladder or the cystic duct (Ch. 58). Lygidakis (1981) emphasized the technical problems in operating on these patients. If a large adherent mass at the hilum of the gallbladder and common duct is encountered at surgery, an operative cholangiogram may delineate the presence of true choledocholithiasis or of either the impacted cystic duct stone, without fistula (Mirizzi — Type I) or the biliobiliary fistula itself (Mirizzi — Type II). For the Type I situation, the impacted stone may often be manipulated back into the gallbladder without having to open the common duct, or the gallbladder can be transected several centimeters from its junction with the common hepatic duct and the stone extracted from the dilated cystic duct stump. Often choledochotomy is unnecessary because multiple stones are infrequent in this entity. For the Type II situation, direct choledochotomy is carried out and the obstructing stone removed. The gallbladder is then dissected 1–2 cm proximal to the fistula between the ampulla and the common hepatic duct, at which point it is transected and sutured closed. T-tube drainage of the common duct is achieved through the longitudinal choledochotomy. Alternatively the opened gallbladder ampulla may be anastomosed to the duodenum as described in Ch. 58.

Choledochoduodenal fistula secondary to peptic ulcer disease

Patients with these fistulae may be asymptomatic or present with GI complaints suggestive of peptic ulcer. Biliary tract symptoms are usually absent and indeed these patients generally do not have associated cholelithiasis. In rare instances, cholangitis, jaundice or abnormal liver function tests are part of the clinical picture and indicate concomitant biliary tract infection and obstruction. The diagnosis may be suggested by pneumobilia in 15–60% of patients. More often, it is made as contrast material from a barium meal refluxes up the common duct to outline a normal-sized, functioning gallbladder. Endoscopy, with direct visualization of the ulcer and fistula, and ERCP is the best way to confirm the diagnosis and evaluate the extent of disease (Fig. 61.6).

Given the paucity of reported experience with choledochoduodenal fistula: only 149 cases in the world literature up to 1964 (Kourias & Chouliaras 1964), and long-standing differences of opinion about the correct approach to peptic ulcer disease, it is not surprising that until recently treatment recommendations have been controversial. Excellent discussions of the natural history, clinical presentation and management of these fistulae have been reported by Constant & Turcotte (1968), Feller et al (1980) and Sarr et al (1981). Most authors now agree that treatment should be directed at the ulcer diathesis and not at the biliary tract or the fistula itself. Current medical management is often sufficient to control the ulcer disease and even bring about closure of the fistula. As in other instances of severe disease, surgery is not indicated unless there is uncontrollable haemorrhage, free perforation, obstruction or intractability. Many types of ulcer operation have been used successfully; however, if technically possible, an exclusion type of gastric resection or duodenal bypass procedure such as a Bilroth II or gastroenterostomy should be performed in addition to a vagotomy. There is no need to close the fistula; in fact, doing so may injure the duodenum or bile duct. As a group, these patients are younger and healthier than those with biliary-enteric fistula due to calculous biliary tract disease, and the results of medical and surgical treatment are very good.

Parapapillary choledochoduodenal fistula

Whether caused by spontaneous gallstone erosion or by iatrogenic damage to the distal common duct, parapapillary fistula have a clinical presentation similar to that of other patients with advanced calculous biliary tract diseases. In the series of Tanaka & Ikeda (1983) the following observations were made: a history of biliary symptoms longer than 10 years duration in 46%; pain and jaundice 88% and 69% respectively; prior biliary surgery 54%; air or barium in the biliary tree 41%; cholelithiasis 71%; choledocholithiasis 38%. The anatomical diagnosis rests on meticulous endoscopic observation and expertise in the technique of ERCP (Fig. 61.7). In Japan the incidence of primary intrahepatic stone disease is reported to be as high as 17–30% (Tanaka & Ikeda 1983). Thus, particularly in Japanese patients with parapapillary fistula, careful and complete evaluation of the intrahepatic ductal system is important.

The management of these recently recognized biliary fistulae is still controversial. Various endoscopic techniques have been advocated by Osnes & Kahrs (1977), Urakami & Kishi (1978), and by VanLinda & Rosson (1984). Surgical procedures such as hepaticodochojejunostomy have been successfully used by Hunt & Blumgart (1980).

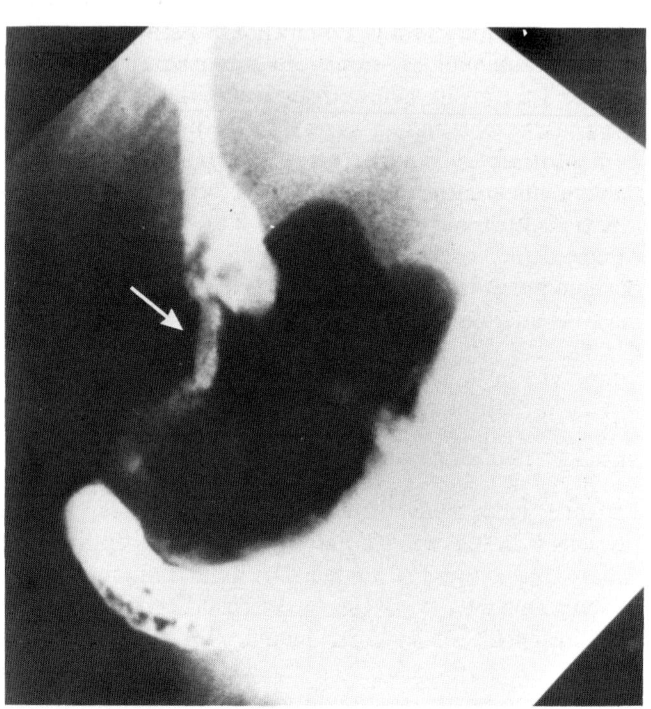

Fig. 61.6 Choledochoduodenal fistula secondary to gallstone disease, demonstrated radiographically by ERCP

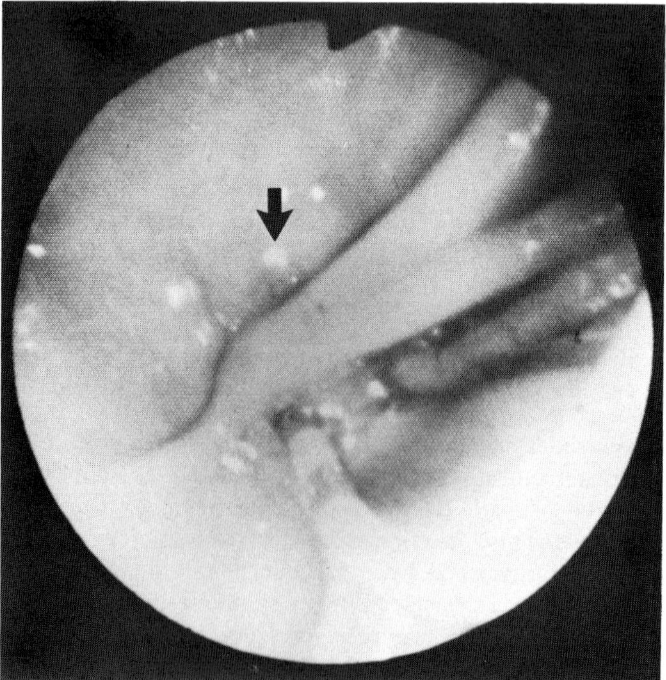

Fig. 61.7 Parapapillary choledochoduodenal fistula demonstrated endoscopically. The ERCP catheter is in the ampulla of Vater. The fistulous opening into the duodenum (arrow) is immediately superior to the horizontal fold of duodenal mucosa

Further experiences and a longer period of follow-up will be necessary before setting guidelines for an established treatment.

Bronchobiliary fistula

The aetiology of a bronchobiliary fistula largely determines its clinical presentation and treatment.

In acquired echinococcal or amoebic bronchobiliary fistula, the Mediterranean, Middle Eastern or North African origin of the patient, as well as a history of prior parasitic disease, is often evident. Hepatic calcification on abdominal roentgenograms, or a history of prior abdominal surgery with mention of hepatic cysts is often suggestive. The patient may have fever, malaise, right upper quadrant pain, fluctuating jaundice or other signs of an enlarging, possibly obstructing, hepatic inflammatory process. There may be a persistent, dry or productive cough, elevated right hemidiaphragm and basal pleural reaction or evidence of a chronic pneumonia. Then the patient will suddenly begin expectorating frothy, green, bitter-tasting sputum in large amounts. Depending on whether a biliopleural or a bilio-bronchial fistula has formed, chest films will demonstrate a large pleural effusion, empyema or air-fluid level in the lung parenchyma.

The rare adult presenting with a bronchobiliary fistula secondary to complicated calculous biliary tract disease almost invariably gives a history of multiple prior upper abdominal operations; usually a cholecystectomy and multiple common duct explorations, or less frequently, an hepatic or pancreatic resection or bypass procedure. A chronic cough complicated by acute dyspnoea and the production of copious infected sputum followed by frank biloptysis are the usual symptoms. As the bronchobiliary fistula forms for the first time, or re-opens and drains again, the level of jaundice suddenly subsides. If there are no adhesions matting the diaphragm to the lung periphery, a biliopleural effusion, with empyema, is more likely than fistula to the bronchial tree (Boyd 1977).

The treatment of parasitic infestation, and of external biliary fistulae, with which a bronchobiliary fistula is occasionally associated, is discussed elsewhere in this text. Echinococcal disease of the liver extending to the lung may require thoracotomy, resection of damaged lung tissue, possible decortication, closure of the diaphragmatic defect and prolonged drainage (Alestig 1972), in addition to appropriate surgical treatment of the hepatic disease. Pleuropulmonary complications of hepatic amoebic disease usually respond to medical treatment with emetine or chloroquine, although repeated aspiration of an empyema and, rarely, thoracotomy with surgical drainage may be necessary (Cleve 1958, Shaw 1949). Bronchobiliary or pleurobiliary fistulae secondary to complicated calculous biliary tract disease requires adequate drainage of all abscesses, as well as relief of distal bile duct obstruction. Warren et al (1983) and Boyd (1977) believe these fistulae can be largely treated via an abdominal approach; rarely is a thoracic procedure also indicated.

The clinical presentation of bronchobiliary or pleurobiliary fistula due to trauma is usually one of injury to the right chest wall, hemidiaphragm and liver as consequence of a fall or penetrating wound, with an interval of from two to three weeks from the time of injury to development of symptoms. These include fever, pleuritic chest pain and cough, often productive of bile. Jaundice occasionally develops. Chest X-ray reveals a pleural effusion and elevated right hemidiaphragm.

Once diagnosed, a well-developed thoracobiliary fistula should be operated upon without delay in order to minimize destruction of lung parenchyma or pleural scarring. Thoracotomy is usually necessary. The fistula tract should be interrupted, the diaphragmatic defect securely closed, and any subphrenic bile collection separately drained. Depending on the degree of intrathoracic damage, limited lung resection and/or decortication may also be indicated (Oparah & Mandel 1978, Ferguson & Buford 1967).

The clinical presentation of congenital bronchobiliary fistula has two general patterns: 1. immediate onset within the first days of life in the newborn whose fistula is the only or major outlet of bile, and 2. a later, more variable onset from age 3–33 months in other reported cases. The presenting signs and symptoms of cough and respiratory distress are similar; however in the newborn, biloptysis is often mistaken for vomiting, and the associated severe dyspnoea and intermittent cyanosis may not be correctly recognized as indicative of a bronchobiliary fistula until pulmonary function has severely deteriorated. Chest X-ray may reveal bilateral pulmonary markings, patchy pneumonia or pneumonitis. Abdominal films may show air in the gallbladder or in a proximally distended intrahepatic bile duct. The anatomical diagnosis is best made preoperatively by bronchoscopic examination and/or bronchography (Chan et al 1984).

Five of the 10 reported cases of congenital bronchobiliary fistula have been successfully treated, usually by right thoracotomy with resection and/or ligature of the intrathoracic segment of the fistula. If hypoplasia or atresia of the bile duct system is present, a biliary-digestive anastomosis is also indicated.

REFERENCES

Alestig K, Holm C, Nystrom G, Schersten T 1972 Biliobronchial fistula secondary to echinococcal abscess of the liver. Acta Chirurgica Scandinavica 138: 90–94

Argyropoulos G D, Velmachos G, Axenidis B 1979 Gallstone perforation and obstruction of the duodenal bulb. Archives of Surgery 114: 333–335

Augur N A, Gracie Jr W A 1970 Cholecystocolonic fistula associated with malabsorption. American Journal of Gastroenterology 53: 558–563

Balthazar E J, Schechter L S 1975 Gallstone ileus. The importance of contrast examinations in the roentgenographic diagnosis. American Journal of Roentgenology, Radium Therapy, Nuclear Medicine 125: 374–379

Balthazar E J, Gurkin S 1976 Cholecystoenteric fistulas: significance and radiographic diagnosis. American Journal of Gastroenterology 65: 168–173

Bose S M, Sastry R A 1983 Agenesis of gallbladder with choledochocolonic fistula. American Journal of Gastroenterology 78: 34–35

Boyd D P 1977 Bronchobiliary and bronchopleural fistulas. The Annals of Thoracic Surgery 24: 481–487

Brandt L J 1984 Gallbladder and biliary tree. In: Gastrointestinal disorders of the elderly. Raven Press, New York, Ch 11, p 578

Bretland P M 1983 Biliary-bronchial fistula due to old hydatid cyst demonstrated with Tc-HIDA. British Journal of Radiology 56: 757–759

Chan Y T, Ng W D, Mak W P, Kwong M L, Chow C B 1984 Congenital bronchobiliary fistula associated with biliary atresia. British Journal of Surgery 71: 240–241

Chandar V P, Hookman P 1980 Choledochocolonic fistula through a cystic duct remnant. A case report. American Journal of Gastroenterology 74: 179–181

Cleve E A, Correa Jr J L 1958 Bronchobiliary fistulas secondary to amoebic abscess of liver. Gastroenterology 34: 320–324

Constant E, Turcotte J G 1968 Choledochoduodenal fistula: the natural history and management of an unusual complication of peptic ulcer disease. Annals of Surgery 167: 220–228

Cooper R A, Kucharski P 1978 Ectopic gallstone as a cause of gastric outlet obstruction. American Journal of Gastroenterology 70: 175–178

Corlette M B, Bismuth H 1975 Biliobiliary fistula: a trap in the surgery of cholelithiasis. Archives of Surgery 110: 377–383

Cornud F, Grenier P, Belghiti J, Breil P, Nahum H 1981 Mirizzi syndrome and biliobiliary fistulas: roentgenologic appearance. Gastrointestinal Radiology 6: 265–268

Day E A, Marks C 1975 Gallstone ileus. Review of the literature and presentation of thirty-four new cases. American Journal of Surgery 129: 552–558

DeVanna T, Dunne M G, Haney P J 1983 Fistulous communication of pseudocyst to the common bile duct: a complication of pancreatitis. Pediatric Radiology 13: 344–345

Dyon J F, Sarrazin R, Baudain P, Lebranchu Y, Brambilla C 1978 Congenital tracheobiliary fistula. Report of a case with choledochal hypoplasia (author's transl.). Chirurgie Pediatrive 19: 189–195

Edell S L, Milunsky C, Garren L 1981 Cholescintigraphic diagnosis of cholecystocolic fistula. Clinical Nuclear Medicine 6: 303–304

Ellenbogen K A, Cameron J L, Cocco A E, Gayler B W, Hutcheon D F 1981 Fistulous communication of a pseudocyst with the common bile duct: demonstration by endoscopic retrograde cholangiopancreatography. Johns Hopkins Medical Journal 149: 110–111

Feller E R, Warshaw A L, Schapiro R H 1980 Observations on management of choledochoduodenal fistula due to penetrating peptic ulcer. Gastroenterology 78: 126–131

Fruhmorgan P, Classen M, Kozu T 1971 Endoskopisch-radiologische darstellung biliodigestiver fisteln. Zeitshrift fur Gastroenterologie 72: 415–420

Ferguson T B, Burford T H 1967 Pleurobiliary and bronchobiliary fistulas. Archives of Surgery 95: 380–386

Glenn F, Mannix H 1957 Biliary enteric fistula. Surgery, Gynecology and Obstetrics 105: 693–705

Glenn F, Reed C, Grafe W R 1981 Biliary enteric fistula. Surgery, Gynecology and Obstetrics 153: 527–531

Griffin J, Jennings C, Owens A 1983 Hepatic amoebic abscess communicating with the biliary tree. British Journal of Radiology 56: 887–890

Haq A U, Morris A H, Daintith H 1981 Recurrent gall-stone ileus. British Journal of Radiology 54: 1000–1001

Heil T, Belohlavek D 1978 Das Mirizzisyndrom als besonder form des verschlussikterus. Chirurg 49: 57–59

Henderson R W, Telfer N, Halls J M 1981 Gastrobiliary fistula: pre- and postoperative assessment with 99m Tc-PIPIDA. American Journal of Radiology 137: 163–165

Heuman R, Sjodahl R, Wetterfors J 1980 Gallstone ileus: an analysis of 20 patients. World Journal of Surgery 4: 595–598

Hricak H, Uander-Molen R L 1978 The radiology corner: duodenocolic fistula with gallstone ileus. American Journal of Gastroenterology 69: 711–715

Hunt D R, Blumgart L H 1980 Iatrogenic choledochoduodenal fistula: an unsuspected cause of post-cholecystectomy symptoms. British Journal of Surgery 67: 10–13

Ikeda S, Okada Y 1975 Classification of choledochoduodenal fistula diagnosed by duodenal fiberoscopy and its etiological significance. Gastroenterology 69: 130–137

Kasahara Y, Umemura H, Shiraha S, Kuyama T, Sakata K, Kubota H 1980 Gallstone ileus. Review of 112 patients in the Japanese literature. American Journal of Surgery 140: 437–440

Kourias B G, Chouliaras A 1964 Spontaneous gastrointestinal-biliary fistula complicating duodenal ulcer. Surgery, Gynecology and Obstetrics 119: 1013–1018

LeBlanc K A, Barr L H, Rush B M 1983 Spontaneous biliary enteric fistulas. Southern Medical Journal 76: 1249–1252

Levin B, Shapiro R A 1980 Recurrent enteric gallstone obstruction. Gastrointestinal Radiology 5: 151–153

Lygidakis N J 1981 Spontaneous internal biliary fistulae: early surgery for prevention, radical surgery for cure. A report of 75 cases. Med-Chir-Dig 10: 695–699

McSherry C K, Ferstenberg H, Virshup M 1982 The Mirizzi syndrome: suggested classification and surgical therapy. Surgical Gastroenterology 1: 219–225

Mirizzi P L 1948 Sindrome del conducto hepatico. Journal international de chirurgie 8: 731–732

Moreira V F, Garcia E M, Marco S 1984 Endoscopic retrograde cholangiography (E.R.C.P.) and complicated hepatic hydatid cyst in the biliary tree. Endoscopy 16: 124–126

Morris S J, Greenwald R A, Barkin J S, Tedesco F J, Snyder R 1978 Cholecystoduodenocolic fistula secondary to carcinoma of the gallbladder. American Journal of Digestive Diseases 23: 849–852

Nakib B A, Jacob G S, Liddawi A I, Commen J 1982 Choledochoduodenal fistula due to tuberculosis. Endoscopy 14: 64–65

Oparah S S, Mandal A K 1978 Traumatic thoracobiliary (pleurobiliary and bronchobiliary) fistulas: clinical and review study. The Journal of Trauma 18: 539–544

Osnes M, Kahrs T 1977 Endoscopic choledochoduodenostomy for choledocho-choledocholithiasis through choledochoduodenal fistula. Endoscopy 9: 162–165

Piedad O H, Wels P B 1972 Spontaneous internal biliary fistula; obstructive and non-obstructive types. 20 year review of 55 cases. Annals of Surgery 175: 75–80

Porta E, Borgstrom M S, Giampaglia F, Carrillo F, Angelillo M 1981 Contribution of CT and ultra sound to the preoperative diagnosis of biliobronchial fistula caused by echinococcosis of the liver. Computertomographie 5: 349–350

Rau W S, Matern S, Gerok W, Wenz W 1980 Spontaneous cholecystocolonic fistula: a model situation for bile acid diarrhea and fatty acid diarrhea as a consequence of a disturbed enterohepatic circulation of bile acids. Hepatogastroenterology 27: 231–237

Razemon P, Salembier Y, Ribet M, Gautier C, Laget J 1963 Abces amibiens du foie fistulises dans les bronches. Lille Chirurgie 18: 201–207

Renner W, Went J, McLean J, Plattner G 1982 Ultrasound demonstration of a non-calcified gallstone in the distal ileum causing small-bowel obstruction. Radiology 144:884

Saar M G, Shepard A J, Zuidema G D 1981 Choledochoduodenal fistula: an unusual complication of duodenal ulcer disease. American Journal of Surgery 141: 736–740

Safaie-Shirazi S, Zike W L, Printew K J 1983 Spontaneous biliary fistula. Surgery, Gynecology and Obstetrics 137: 769–772

Sane S M, Sieber W K, Girdany B R 1971 Congenital bronchobiliary fistula. Surgery 69: 599–608

Shaw R R 1949 Thoracic complications of amebiasis. Surgery, Gynecology and Obstetrics 88: 753–762

Shocket E, Evans J, Jonas S 1970 Cholecystoduodeno-colic fistula with gallstone ileus. Archives of Surgery 101: 523–526

Smith E E, Bowley B, Allison D J, Blumgart L H 1982 The management of post-traumatic intrahepatic biliary fistulas. British Journal of Surgery 69: 317–318

Stempfle B, Diamantopulos G 1976 Spontaneous cholecysto-gastric fistula with massive gastrointestinal bleeding. Endoscopic diagnosis and concrement extraction. Fortschritte der Medizin 94: 444–447

Taillefer R, Leveille J, Lefebvre B, Pomp A, Bourbeao D 1983 Demonstration of a bronchobiliary fistula by 99mTc HIDA cholescintigraphy. European Journal of Nuclear Medicine 8: 37–39

Tanaka M, Ikeda S 1983 Parapapillary choledochoduodenal fistula: an analysis of 83 consecutive patients diagnosed at ERCP. Gastrointestinal Endoscopy 29: 89–93

Thomas T L, Jaques P F, Weaver P C 1976 Gallstone obstruction and perforation of the duodenal bulb. British Journal of Surgery 63: 131–132

Tytgat G N, Bartelsman J, Huibregtse K, Agenant D 1979 Common duct complications of choledocholithiasis revealed by ERCP. Gastrointestinal Endoscopy 25: 63–66

Urakami Y, Kishi S 1978 Endoscopic fistulotomy (EFT) for parapapillary choledochoduodenal fistula. Endoscopy 10: 289–294

VanLandingham S B, Broders C W 1982 Gallstone ileus. Surgical Clinics of North America 62: 241–247

VanLinda B M, Rosson R S 1984 Choledochoduodenal fistula and choledocholithiasis: treatment by endoscopic enlargement of the choledochoduodenal fistula. Journal of Clinical Gastroenterology 6: 321–324

Warren K W, Christophi C, Armendariz R, Basu S 1983 Surgical treatment of bronchobiliary fistulas. Surgery, Gynecology and Obstetrics 157: 351–356

Watkins L, Laufer I, Evans G, Mullens J E 1975 Biliary-bronchial fistula demonstrated by endoscopic retrograde cholangiography. Canadian Medical Association Journal 113: 870–872

Zwemer F L, Coffin-Kwart V E, Conway M J 1979 Biliary enteric fistulas. Management of 47 cases in native Americans. American Journal of Surgery 138: 301–304

Index

Vol 1 pp 1–789   Vol 2 pp 791–1544

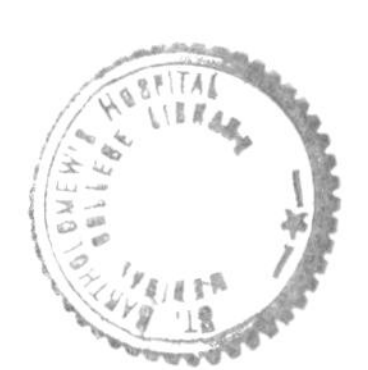